Small Animal Cytologic Diagnosis

This second edition of *Small Animal Cytologic Diagnosis* presents clinically applicable information about the use of cytology in small animals and indicates when advanced diagnostic testing can be beneficial to diagnose underlying disease processes. It includes more images, additional cases, and a new user-friendly chapter organization.

This book discusses the pathophysiology of inflammation, cancer biology, and comparisons to histology to help readers fully comprehend the cytologic changes that can occur with inflammation and neoplasia. Also covered are some of the limitations and advantages of cytology compared to histopathology, important gross findings (e.g. body cavity effusions), and parasites and the associated diagnostic methods required. Further information is provided on oncogenes, reference values for effusions and bone marrow aspirates, laboratory handling of samples, and how to carry out certain diagnostics. The book:

- Includes chapters written by experts from around the world
- Provides multiple cytological images for the same sample, providing different views of what may be seen
- Uses technical language where appropriate but without overcomplicating the information presented; it is very accessible and easy to understand

This book includes tissue-specific chapters focusing on diseases of a particular area, always in comparison to normal tissue. Each of these chapters concludes with various cases that include information on signalment, history, pertinent laboratory data, specimen images, final outcome, and the underlying pathology causing the cytologic lesions, when possible. With more than 1,500 superb illustrations, this comprehensive resource provides ample practical information for students as well as practicing veterinarians.

Small Animal Cytologic Diagnosis

Canine and Feline Disease

Second Edition

Edited by
Anne M. Barger DVM, MS, DACVP and
Amy L. MacNeill DVM, PhD, DACVP

CRC Press
Taylor & Francis Group
Boca Raton London New York

CRC Press is an imprint of the
Taylor & Francis Group, an **informa** business

Designed cover image: Editors

Second edition published 2025

by CRC Press
2385 NW Executive Center Drive, Suite 320, Boca Raton FL 33431

and by CRC Press
4 Park Square, Milton Park, Abingdon, Oxon, OX14 4RN

CRC Press is an imprint of Taylor & Francis Group, LLC

ISBN: 9781032192970 (hbk)
ISBN: 9781032192994 (pbk)
ISBN: 9781003258551 (ebk)

DOI: 10.1201/9781003258551

Typeset in Minion Pro
by Deanta Global Publishing Services, Chennai, India

For Product Safety Concerns and Information please contact our EU representative:
GPSR@taylorandfrancis.com
Taylor & Francis Verlag GmbH, Kaufingerstraße 24, 80331 München, Germany

CONTENTS

PREFACE

Small Animal Cytologic Diagnosis is the combined effort of veterinary clinical pathologists and other board-certified specialists working across the globe. The goal of this text is to provide small animal clinicians, veterinary students, clinical and anatomic pathology residents, and residents from other specialties with current, clinically applicable information about the diagnostic utility of cytology and provide guidance on the necessity of advanced testing.

The text uses images to illustrate the wide variety of cytologic lesions. Within each chapter, the underlying pathology is discussed, as it relates to the cytologic findings. Unique chapters reviewing general principles of oncology and inflammation that influence the appearance of cytologic lesions are included to aid veterinary students and residents with their study of pathology. Additionally, each chapter contains one or more cases, demonstrating the clinical practicality of cytology.

We hope readers find this text to be a valuable resource that is complete, easy to use, and adds to the excellent information already provided by other veterinary cytology texts.

ABOUT THE EDITORS

Dr. Anne M. Barger graduated from the University of Illinois in 1996 and, after graduation, went on to a clinical pathology residency program at North Carolina State University. After completion of her residency, she worked for Antech Diagnostics for two years, before accepting a faculty position at the University of Illinois in 2002. Her research interests include clinical cytology and immunocytochemistry as it pertains to the diagnosis of canine and feline neoplasia. Currently, she is the department head of Veterinary Clinical Medicine at the University of Illinois.

Dr. Amy L. MacNeill graduated from the University of Florida College of Veterinary Medicine in 1998. Following a year in private practice, she returned to the University of Florida to complete her clinical pathology residency and a PhD in virology and immunology. In 2005, she joined the faculty at the University of Illinois. In 2014, she accepted a clinical pathology faculty position at Colorado State University. Her research interests include the isolation and characterization of canine and feline tumor cells and the study of poxviruses as anticancer agents.

LIST OF CONTRIBUTORS

Linda Berent BS, DVM, PhD, DACVP
IDEXX
Columbia, Missouri, USA

Dorothee Bienzle, DVM, PhD, DACVP
Department of Pathobiology
Ontario Veterinary College
University of Guelph
Guelph, Ontario, Canada

Nathalie Bourges-Abella PhD
Unité d'Histologie et Anatomie Pathologique
Université de Toulouse,
Toulouse, France

Melinda S. Camus, DVM, DACVP
Department of Pathobiology
College of Veterinary Medicine
Auburn University
Auburn, Alabama, USA

Stefano Comazzi, DVM, PhD, DECVCP
Department of Veterinary Science and Public Health
University of Milan
Milan, Italy

Sara Connolly, DVM, MS, DACVP
Department of Veterinary Clinical Medicine
College of Veterinary Medicine
University of Illinois
Urbana, Illinois, USA

Chandler C. Carter, DVM
Department of Veterinary Clinical Medicine
College of Veterinary Medicine
University of Illinois
Urbana, Illinois, USA

Timothy M. Fan, DVM, PhD, DACVIM (oncology)
Department of Veterinary Clinical Medicine
College of Veterinary Medicine
University of Illinois
Urbana, Illinois, USA

Laura Garrett, DVM, DACVIM (oncology)
Department of Veterinary Clinical Medicine
College of Veterinary Medicine
University of Illinois
Urbana, Illinois, USA

Amelia Goddard, BVSc, BVSc(Hons), MMedVet, PhD
Department of Companion Animal Clinical Studies
Faculty of Veterinary Science
University of Pretoria
Pretoria, Gauteng, South Africa

Elena Gorman, DVM, MS, DACVP
Department of Biomedical Sciences
College of Veterinary Medicine
Oregon State University
Corvalis, Oregon, USA

Fanny Granat, DVM
Laboratoire Central de Biologie Médicale
Université de Toulouse
Toulouse, France

Catherine Layssol, DVM
Unité d'Imagerie
Université de Toulouse
Toulouse, France

Samantha Lee, DVM, MS, DACVP
Department of Veterinary Clinical Medicine
College of Veterinary Medicine
University of Illinois
Urbana, Illinois, USA

Marie-Noëlle Lucas, DVM, DECVP
Unité d'Histologie et Anatomie Pathologique
Université de Toulouse
Toulouse, France

Cheryl Moller, BSc BVMS, DACVP
Antech Diagnostics
Fountain Valley, California, USA

A Russell Moore, DVM, MS, DACVP
Department of Microbiology, Immunology and Pathology
Colorado State University
Fort Collins, Colorado, USA

K. Marcia Murphy, DVM, DACVD
Department of Companion Animals and Special Species
College of Veterinary Medicine
North Carolina State University
Raleigh, North Carolina, USA

Jennifer A. Neel, DVM, DACVP
Antech Diagnostics
Tucson, Arizona, USA

Ashleigh W. Newman, VMD, DACVP
Department of Population Medicine and Diagnostic Sciences
College of Veterinary Medicine
Cornell University
Ithaca, New York, USA

Indira Pargass, DVM, MVSc, DACVP
School of Veterinary Medicine
St. Augustine Campus
Trinidad & Tobago, West Indies

Yolandi Rautenbach, BVSc, BVSc(Hons), MMedVet, DECVCP
Department of Companion Animal Clinical Studies
Faculty of Veterinary Science
University of Pretoria
Pretoria, Gauteng, South Africa

Michael F. Rosser, DVM, MS, DACVP
Department of Veterinary Clinical Medicine
College of Veterinary Medicine
University of Illinois
Urbana, Illinois, USA

Samantha N. Schlemmer, DVM, MS, DACVP
Department of Pathology
College of Veterinary Medicine
University of Georgia
Athens, Georgia, USA

Amy N. Schnelle, DVM, MS, DACVP
Department of Veterinary Clinical Medicine
College of Veterinary Medicine
University of Illinois
Urbana, Illinois, USA

Ilse Schwendenwein, DVM, DECVCP
Clinical Pathology/Central Laboratory
University of Veterinary Medicine Vienna
Vienna, Austria

Emmeline Tan, DVM, DVSc, DACVP
Idexx Laboratories
Markham, Ontario, Canada

Catherine Trumel
Laboratoire Central de Biologie Médicale
Université de Toulouse
Toulouse, France

Julie L. Webb DVM, DACVP
Department of Population Medicine and Diagnostic Sciences
College of Veterinary Medicine
Cornell University
Ithaca, New York, USA

CHAPTER 1

SAMPLE ACQUISITION AND PREPARATION

Laura Garrett, Linda Berent, and Anne M. Barger

INTRODUCTION

The use of cytology – the examination of cells from the body – in small animals has gained recognition and clinical application at a rapid rate. It is a powerful tool that can be employed successfully in a wide variety of anatomic locations and disease processes. Cytology can provide a definitive diagnosis in many cases, including infections and some tumors. Even if a definitive diagnosis is not possible, sample evaluation often will rule out many differentials and point the clinician towards the next best diagnostic test to run. The first step, and a critical one, in the application of cytologic analysis on a patient's sample is obtaining and preparing a good sample. Items that can be sampled and evaluated include solid tissues and fluids.

SAMPLING AN ORGAN OR A MASS – FINE NEEDLE ASPIRATION

Equipment needed

Limited equipment is needed to obtain good cytology samples and includes a 22- or 20-gauge needle, a 6 ml syringe, and 5–8 glass microscope slides laid out individually (Figure 1.1). Needle gauge size is not a critical issue; for very small masses a 25-gauge needle may be used, and for bone lesions an 18 gauge is sometimes beneficial. Needle gauge size does not appear to affect cellularity but smaller gauge needles, like 25-gauge, can result in more cellular damage (Arai et al., 2019). For best results, all the needed materials should be set out and ready to use prior to getting the tissue sample. Once the sample is obtained, it can rapidly clot and lead to poor smear preparation. Also, once the sample is expelled onto a slide, it will begin to dry, which will also limit the ability to make good smears.

TECHNIQUES FOR SAMPLE ACQUISITION

There are two ways in which to use a needle to obtain a sample of a tissue from a patient for subsequent dispelling of the needle contents onto a slide for smearing and then cytologic assessment: fenestration and aspiration. 'Fine needle aspiration' (FNA) is typically the term used to describe either way of sampling, but the term 'aspiration' is often a misnomer, as fenestration, the easiest FNA technique and one that will provide a good sample the majority of the time, does not actually involve aspiration. With fenestration, the needle is rapidly inserted repeatedly into the tissue without drawing back on the plunger of an attached syringe to create negative pressure. The needle may be held and used on its own, or a syringe may be attached to the needle to act as an extension to allow for an improved grip. The syringe-attached fenestration technique is often used when sampling intrathoracic or intra-abdominal structures, as it not only creates an easier way to hold the needle but also maintains a closed system and prevents air from entering the body cavity. Preparation of the skin with clipping and scrubbing prior to FNA is almost never needed, the exception being if a culture is going to be obtained from the aspirate.

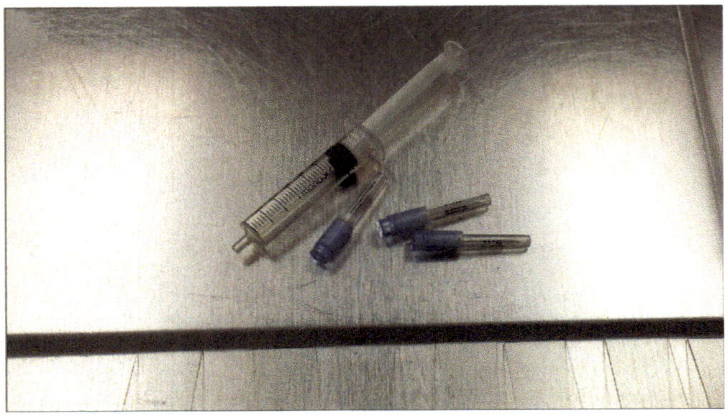

Figure 1.1 Glass slides, 22-gauge needles, and a 6 ml syringe filled with air set up prior to sampling the patient.

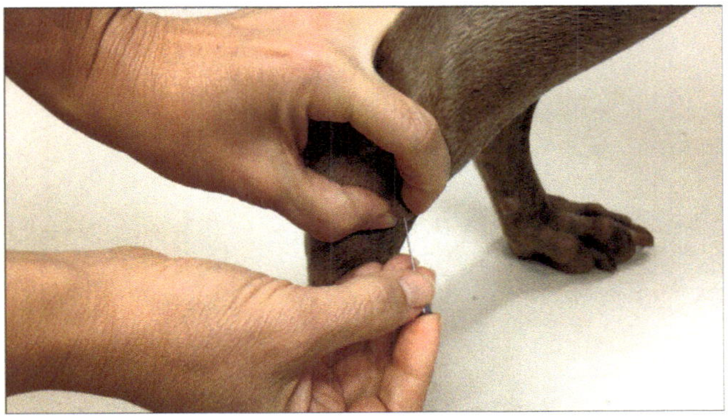

Figure 1.2 Holding only the needle for the fenestration technique. Note the finger over the hub of the needle; this keeps fluid from squirting out in the case of a fluid-filled mass.

DOI: 10.1201/9781003258551-1

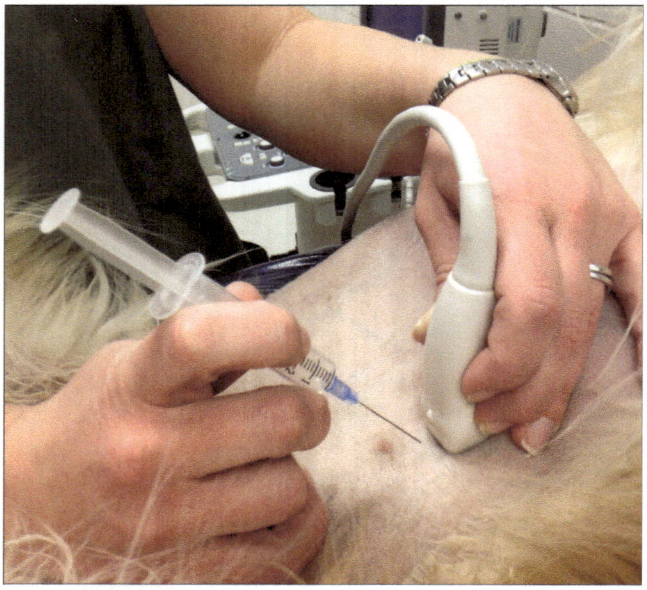

Figure 1.3 **Ultrasound-guided aspirate, fenestration technique. The syringe is used solely as a handle for the needle. The syringe has air in it for ease of expelling the sample once obtained.**

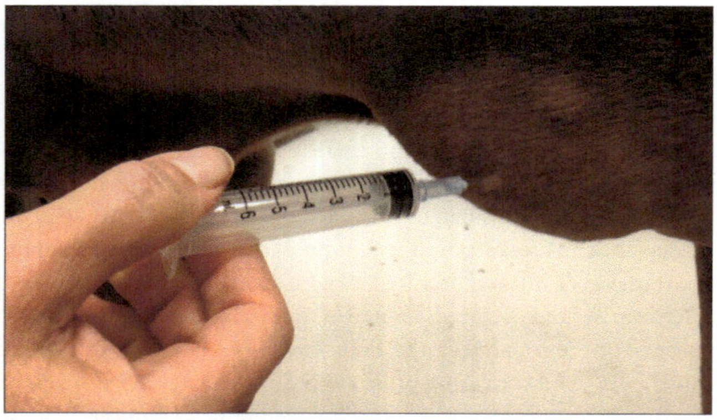

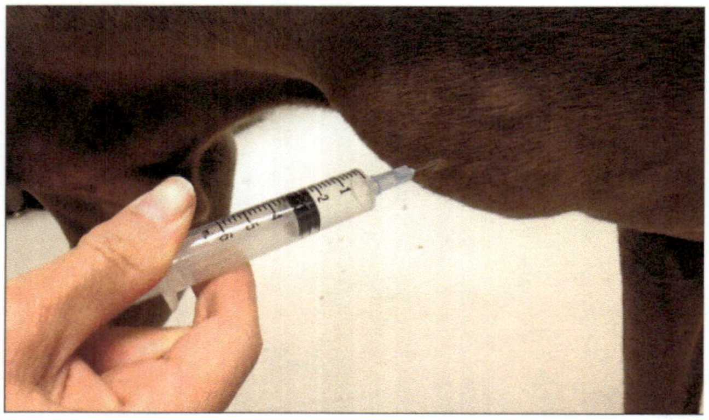

Figures 1.4, 1.5 **FNA performed with aspiration technique. (1.4) The needle is attached to the syringe prior to entering the mass. (1.5) Once the needle is inserted, the plunger is pulled back to obtain 2–3 mL of negative pressure.**

For the fenestration technique without the syringe attached, first prepare the syringe that is laid out near the slides by drawing back the plunger so that there is 4–6 ml of air in the syringe. Having the syringe ready to dispel the needle contents as soon as the sample is obtained will help in creating an efficient process, thus keeping the sample from clotting. Next, the tissue to be sampled is held firmly with the non-dominant hand (Figure 1.2). The needle is inserted, using the dominant hand, through the skin and into the tissue. Then, the needle is rapidly moved back and forth, 4–8 times, into the tissue, keeping the needle under the skin at all times. If the area to be sampled is large, the needle can be redirected in a fan shape during multiple fenestrations. Lastly, the needle is withdrawn, the syringe is attached, and the sample is expelled onto a slide (see Techniques for smearing samples onto slides). As mentioned earlier, if the tissue to be sampled is internal, a syringe with air in it may be attached to the needle and used simply as an extension without any negative pressure applied (Figure 1.3).

Alternatively, true aspiration can be used for sample attainment. In this situation, a 6 ml syringe, with the seal broken but all air expelled, is attached to the needle, and the needle is inserted into the tissue of interest with the syringe held in the dominant hand (Figure 1.4). Once the opening in the beveled part of the needle is completely inserted, so that negative pressure is obtained with aspiration, the plunger on the syringe is drawn back 1–3 ml and released rapidly 3–5 times (Figure 1.5). Be sure to release the suction on the syringe prior to withdrawing the needle from the tissue. Once the needle is withdrawn from the lesion, the needle is removed from the syringe, and 4–6 ml of air are aspirated into the syringe. It is critical to remove the needle prior to drawing air into the syringe, or the sample will be pulled into the syringe and the amount expelled will be poor. The sample is then expelled onto a slide (see Techniques for smearing samples onto slides).

For internal organs or lesions, if a mass can be felt, it can generally be aspirated blindly. However, for lesions that cannot be palpated, or for lesions near critical structures such as major blood vessels, ultrasound (Figure 1.6) or computed tomography (Figures 1.7, 1.8) can be useful for guiding FNAs.

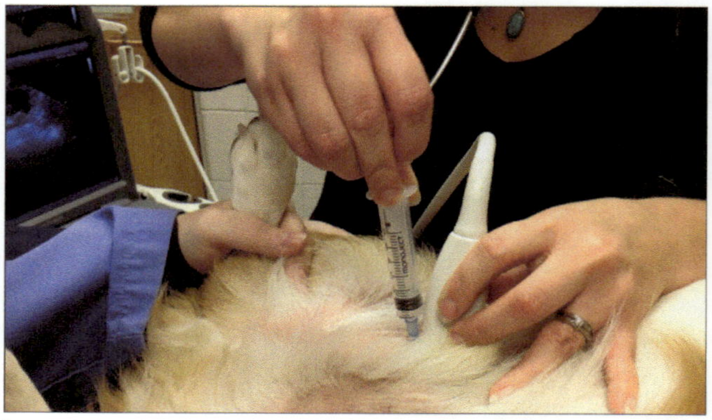

Figure 1.6 **Ultrasound can be used to guide the sampling of internal lesions. In this example the aspiration technique is shown.**

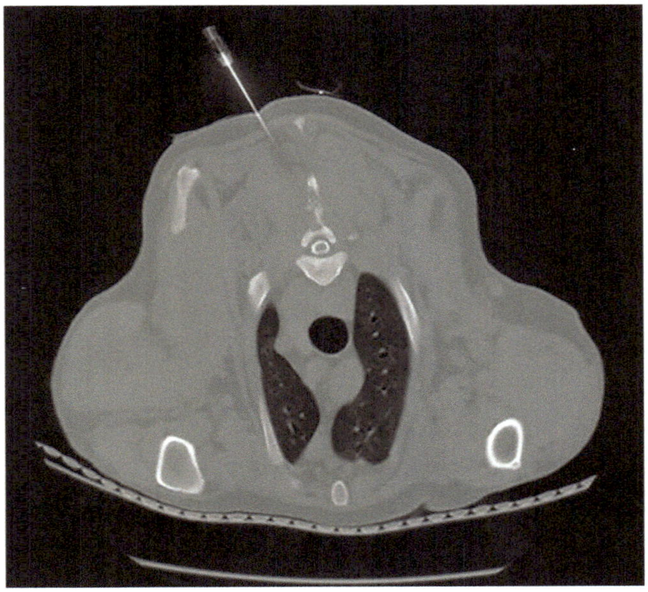

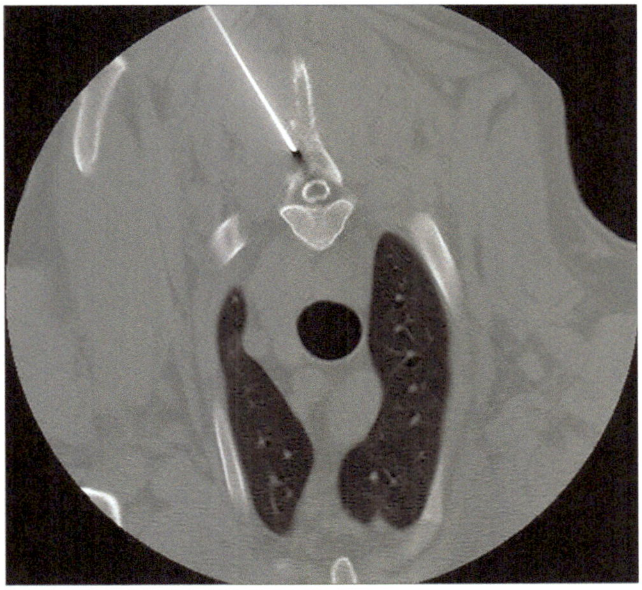

CT-guided FNA of a bone lesion.

Figures 1.7 The needle is just entering the patient.

Figures 1.8 The needle is entering the lesion.

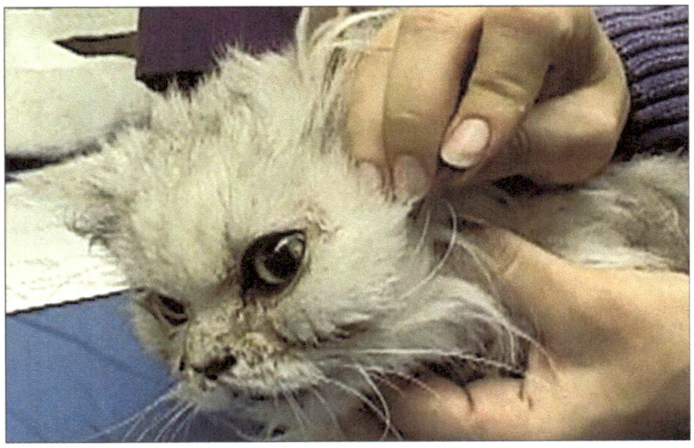

Figure 1.9 Fenestration technique used to sample the mandibular lymph node in a cat. The lack of bulky equipment makes sampling small targets easier.

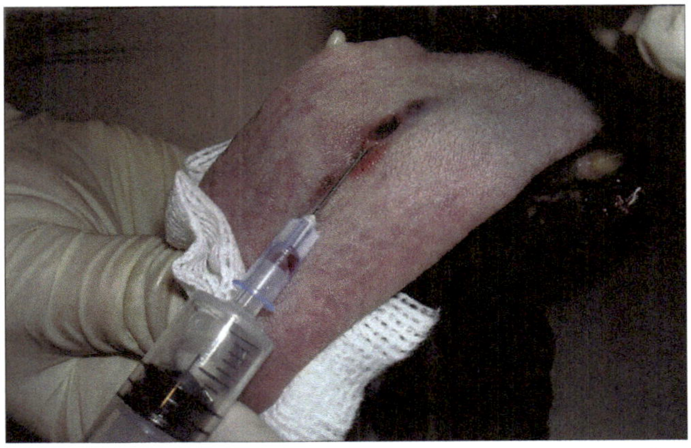

Figure 1.10 Lingual melanoma in a lightly sedated patient. This small, sensitive area can be better sampled with aspiration than with fenestration.

Fenestration versus aspiration

The greatest advantage of fenestration is the ease of sample collection. For most lesions, it is easier to handle only a needle as opposed to the more cumbersome syringe with a needle, and for all solid tissues, rapidly 'poking' the tissue several times is less difficult than holding a needle still and having to pull back and release the syringe plunger repeatedly. For very small areas of interest (e.g. feline lymph nodes [Figure 1.9], small masses), aim is improved with decreased volume of equipment and distance of the dominant hand from the sampling site with fenestration. Additionally, there may be higher cellularity and less blood contamination with the fenestration method (Leblanc et al., 2009).

The aspiration technique can be of advantageous in situations where the mass is extremely firm and does not release cells with the fenestration technique. In these cases, the added force of the negative pressure generated in the syringe may pull firmly attached cells into the needle. Note, however, that most firm masses will exfoliate very well with the fenestration method. Another situation in which aspiration is of benefit is in areas to be sampled that are extremely sensitive or painful, such as an inflamed digit or the tongue (Figure 1.10), or near a critical structure that should not be punctured, such as the eyelid margin (Figure 1.11). Entering the tissue with the needle only once and holding the needle still while aspirating with a syringe can be less uncomfortable than multiple fenestrations and is less likely to cause the needle to enter a tissue that is contraindicated. Two recent studies evaluated lymph node aspiration in dogs and cats. One study used ultrasound guidance and found that aspiration, rather than fenestration, resulted in more cellular samples (Whitlock et al., 2020). The

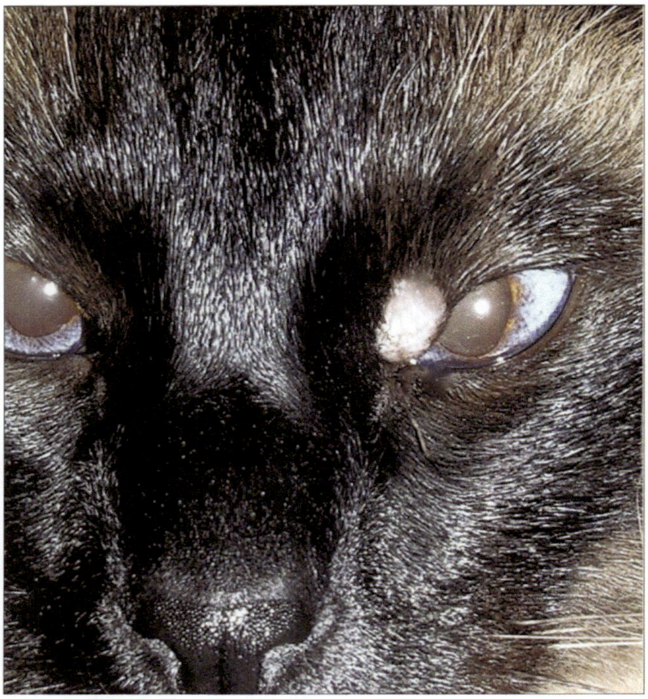

Figure 1.11 **A mast cell tumor at the medial canthus in a Siamese cat. Aspiration of a lesion in this location in an awake patient may be less irritating and safer than fenestration.**

second study evaluated canine lymph nodes and found no difference between the two techniques (Karakitsou et al., 2022).

For internal organs, fenestration is generally the preferred technique, but is usually performed with the needle attached to the syringe to prevent air from entering a body cavity through an open needle hub. Complications associated with FNA of internal organs are rare; hemorrhage from the liver or spleen or pneumothorax in cases with severe lung disease is very unlikely, but is a potential sequela to discuss with owners (Wood et al., 1998; Reichle & Wisner, 2000; Bonfanti et al., 2004; Zekas et al., 2005; Barrouin-Melo et al., 2006; Ballegeer et al., 2007; Watson et al., 2011; Bahr et al., 2013; Feeney et al., 2013; Glinska-Suchocka et al., 2013; Crain et al., 2014).

TECHNIQUES FOR SMEARING THE SAMPLE ONTO SLIDES

The main goal in creating slides for cytologic assessment is to make smears that are thin and evenly distributed without rupturing the cells. It is best to create multiple slides from one FNA, enabling the clinician to stain one with an in-house stain (Diff-Quik®) for sample assessment while allowing for unstained slides to be sent to the cytology laboratory for a Wright–Giemsa based stain and potentially other special stains. Additionally, making multiple slides from one sample creates the thin slides that are desired. The key to getting a thin, even sample is to start with a very small sample to smear. This small amount of tissue can be put on the slides in one of two ways. With either method, the sample is expelled onto the slide with the needle bevel pointing down towards the slide and the bevel over the slide near the frosted edge to give the most room for smearing (Figure 1.12). It is helpful to stabilize the syringe-holding non-dominant hand against the table or countertop while the dominant hand presses down on the plunger to expel the sample.

The first technique involves gently and carefully expelling a very small amount of the sample onto as many slides as possible (most FNAs will yield enough for 4–6 slides; Figure 1.13). Next, another empty, or 'smearing', slide is used to smear each small sample across each slide. The same smearing slide can be used to smear every slide from one sampling procedure. A new smearing slide must be used for every new sample to avoid contamination of the new sample with cells on the smearing slide from the first sample. To create a thin, even, and unruptured sample, the smearing slide is placed crosswise to the sample slide and gently pressed down to flatten the sample (Figure 1.14). Keeping the slides touching via the same gentle pressure, the smearing slide is pulled to the end of the sample slide (Figures 1.15, 1.16). If the slides stay flat against each other, the sample will be smooth and

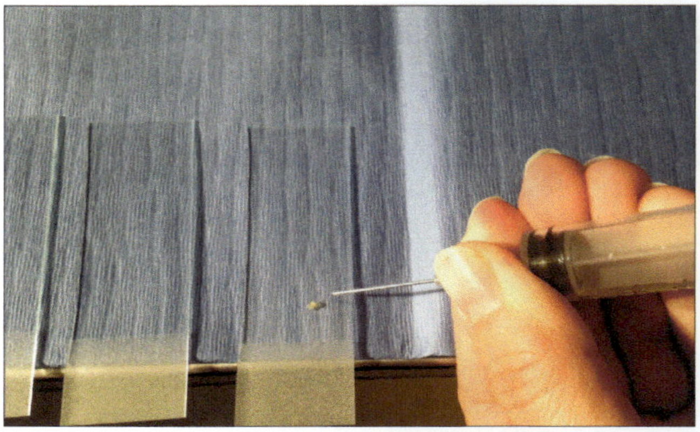

Figure 1.12 **Expelling the sample onto a slide. Expel the contents with the needle bevel down and near the frosted edge of the slide. Stabilizing the hand holding the syringe and needle against the table surface while depressing the plunger with the other hand can help to maintain good needle position.**

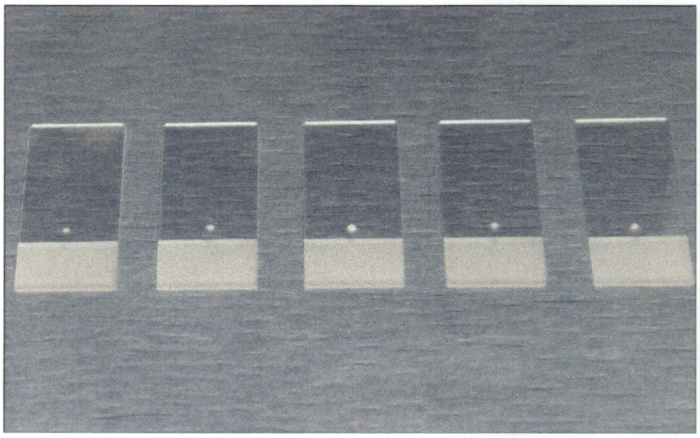

Figure 1.13 **Slides on which a small amount of material, from one aspirate, has been expelled.**

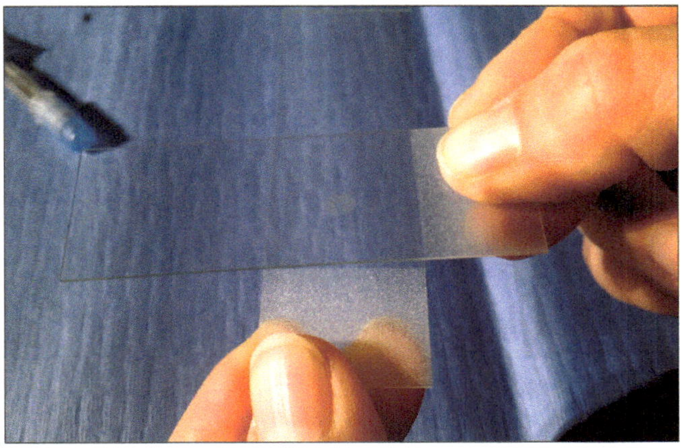

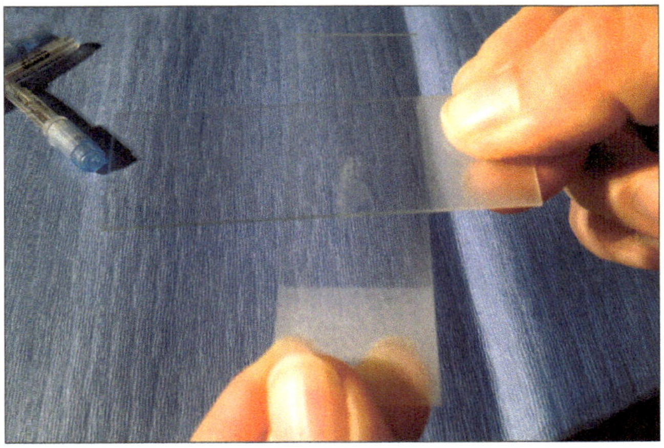

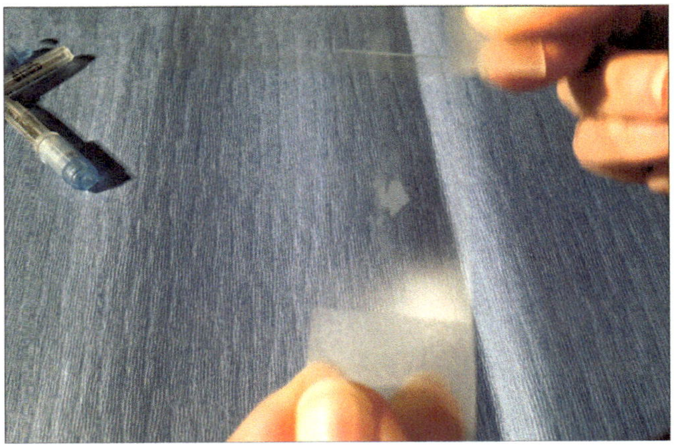

Figures 1.14–1.16 A clean 'smearing' slide is used to smear the material on each of the slides shown in Figure 1.13. (1.14) First, the smearing slide is used to press the sample flat. (1.15) Next, the smearing slide is pulled across the sample slide, while maintaining even pressure and contact, to create a smear. (1.16) The smearing slide is pulled all the way off of the sample slide, and the even smear that was created can be seen.

even. If one of the smearing slide edges touches the sample slide with disproportionate pressure, the sample will get dragged and will have ruptured areas and areas that are too thick (Figure 1.17).

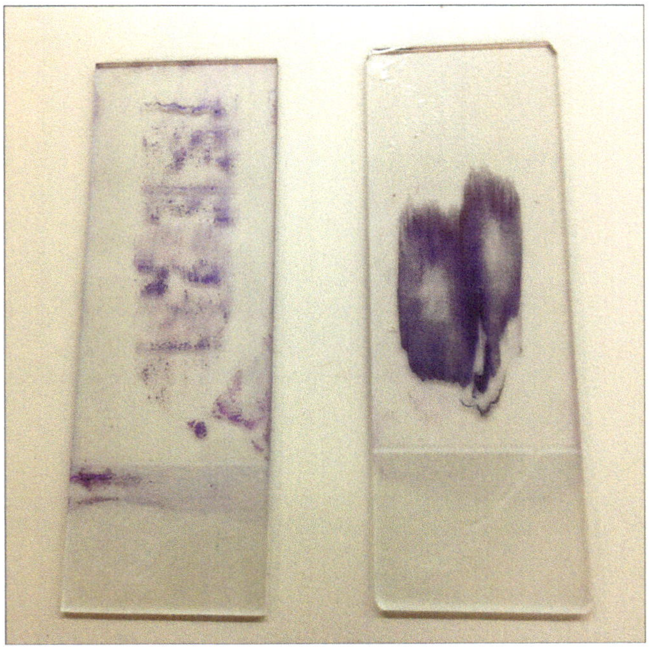

Figure 1.17 Sample slides stained with Diff-Quik®. The slide on the right is the goal of good sample creation. The slide on the left shows what unequal pressure from the smearing slide can result in. Note the irregular shape of the smear with very thin and thick areas.

The second, and authors' preferred, technique for making smears is to expel all of the sample onto one slide (Figure 1.18). From there, the smearing slide is used to lightly touch the top of the sample drop, pick up a small amount of sample, then smear that sample evenly across a new slide (Figures 1.19–1.25). The same smearing slide is then used to pick up another small bit of sample and smear it onto a new slide. This goes on until only a very small amount of sample is left on the first slide, which is then smeared itself. In this manner, at least 3–5 good slides are generally produced from one FNA (Figure 1.26).

Both of these techniques for sample distribution and smearing on slides will produce better slides than the traditional 'squash prep' technique, as squash preps create many areas in the sample that are too thick for microscopic evaluation (Figure 1.27).

IMPRESSION SMEARS

Cytologic assessment of tissues that have been biopsied can be a worthwhile diagnostic tool for several reasons. The turnaround time for results is much quicker for cytology versus histopathology, and such results may be critical to guide decisions in time-sensitive situations. Additionally, some diagnoses can be made more readily with cytology compared with histopathology, including the diagnosis of round cell tumors and mycobacterial infections. Preparing slides for possible cytologic evaluation is a quick and easy procedure to do after a tissue sample has been obtained. Even if the slides are not submitted immediately to save cost when a biopsy is going to be submitted, it is

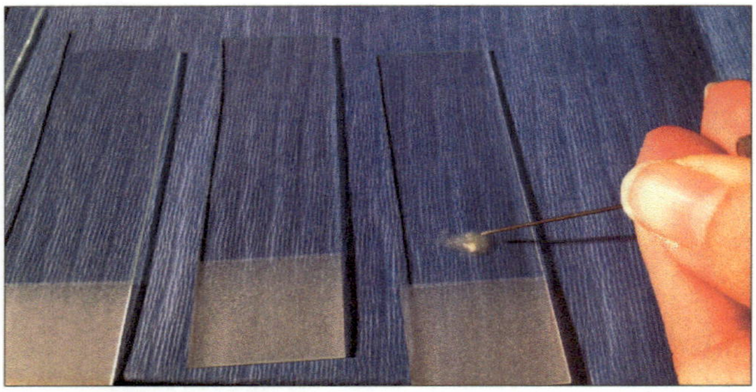

Figures 1.18 Demonstration of expelling all of the sample onto one slide.

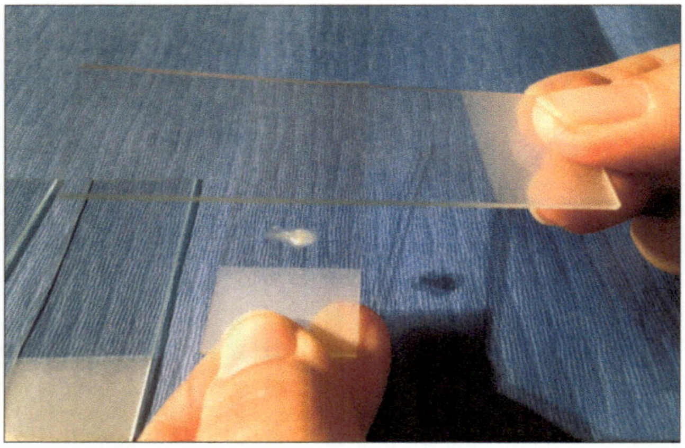

Figures 1.19 The smearing slide is used to barely touch the large sample and pick up a small amount on its underside.

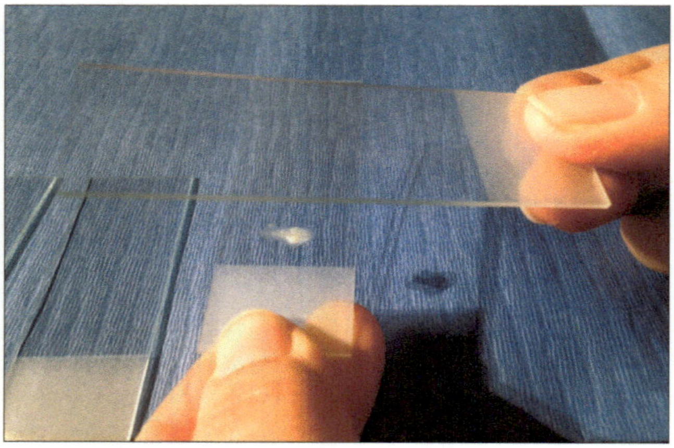

Figures 1.20 Here both slides can be seen, the original sample slide with sample remaining and the top smearing slide with a drop of sample on the underside.

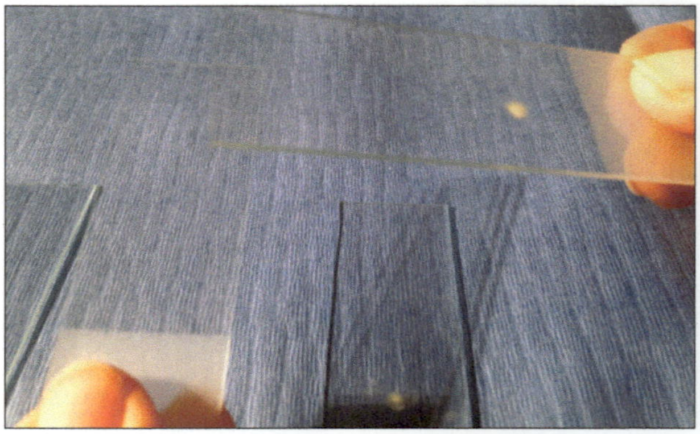

Figures 1.21 The sample slide has been set down and a clean slide is picked up in the left hand. The right hand still holds the smearing slide.

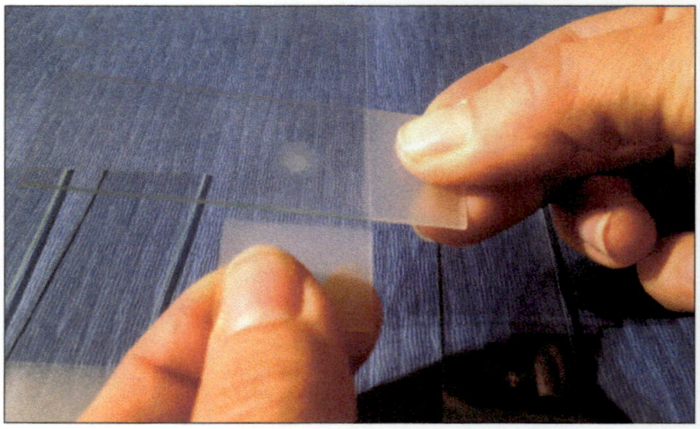

Figures 1.22 The smearing slide now presses down on the clean slide and flattens the sample, as in Figure 1.14.

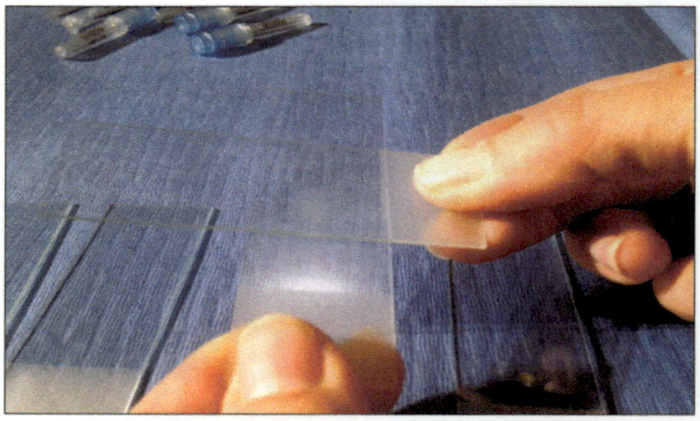

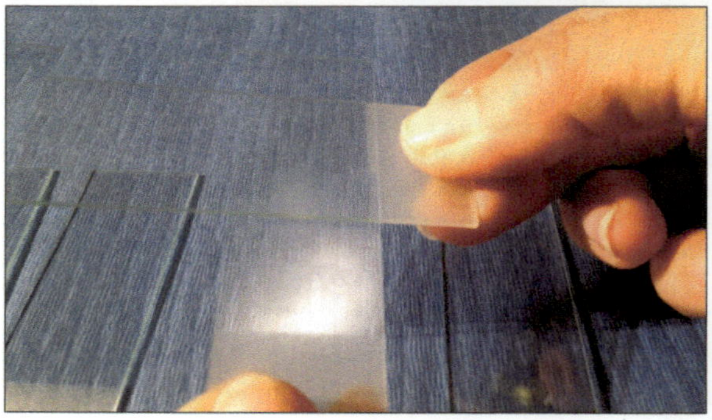

Figures 1.23, 1.24 The sample is smeared as in Figures 1.15 and 1.16.

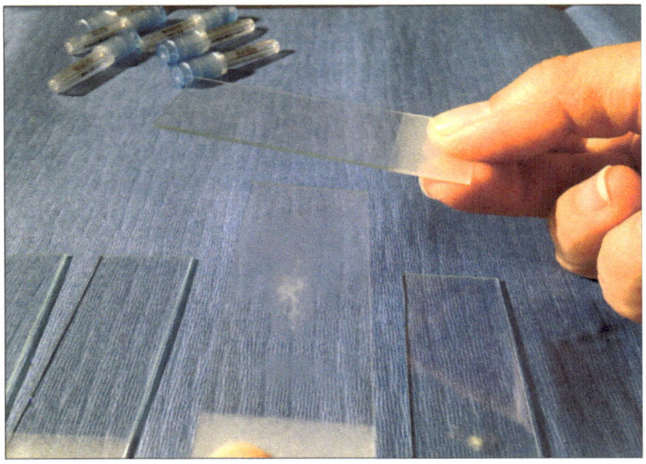

Figure 1.25 The first smear is complete, and will now be set down. The sample slide to the right in the photo will be picked up with the left hand, another drop of sample is picked up on the underside of the same smearing slide seen in the right hand, and this is smeared onto a new slide, repeating Figures 1.19–1.24. At the end, the sample on the original sample slide is smeared flat.

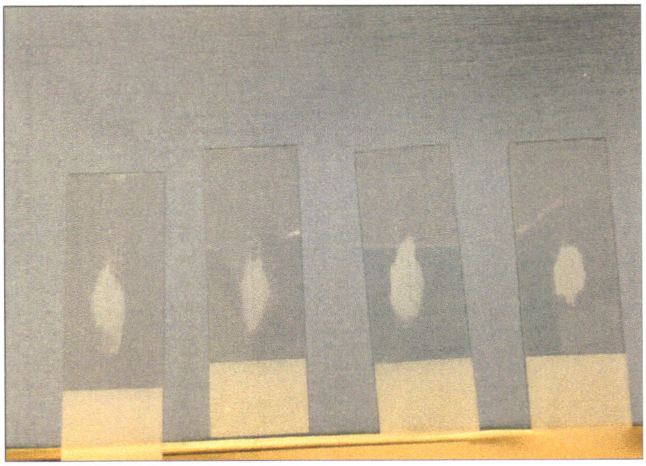

Figure 1.26 The line-up of evenly smeared slides that can be made from one fenestration procedure.

worthwhile saving the slides for later submission if the histopathology suggests that cytology could be of additional advantage.

To make an impression smear, the tissue of interest is blotted with gauze to remove surface blood (Figure 1.28). The cut surface of the tissue can then be pressed, quite firmly, to a slide (Figure 1.29). Multiple impressions are made along the length of the slide, and multiple slides are created in this way. For very firm masses, a scalpel blade can be used to scrape at the cut surface in an effort to increase exfoliation (Figure 1.30). Any material on the blade can be smeared onto a slide, and the surface of the tissue itself can again be pressed against slides. When stained, the impression smears will look similar to squash prep samples, with thick and thin areas (Figure 1.31).

It is important to remember that the presence of formalin near cytology slides will fix the slides and ruin them for evaluation. Be sure

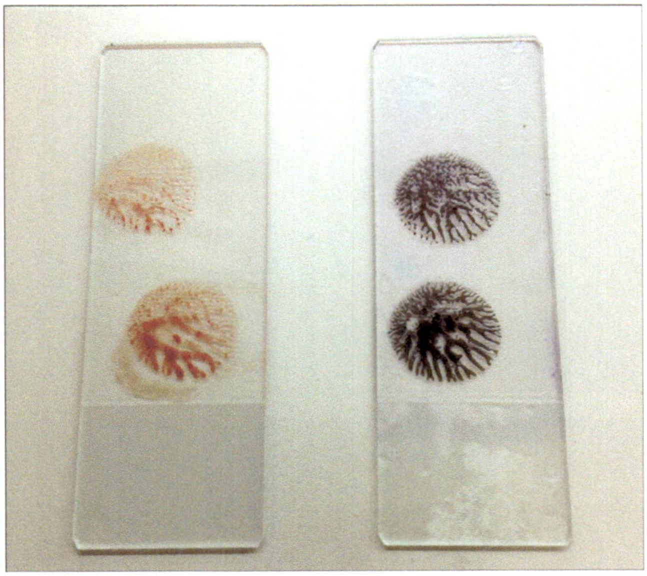

Figure 1.27 The slides, unstained and stained, that result from the squash prep technique. Note the thick and thin areas.

to keep the slides away from the formalin jar, even when it is closed. Histopathology and cytology samples should not be submitted in the same package. Also, if the biopsy samples are very small, care must be taken not to destroy the sample for histologic evaluation. Care and gentle pressure are needed when making impressions of small pieces of tissue, and if multiple biopsies of the same lesion are obtained, only use one or two for impressions.

SAMPLING OF INTRA-ABDOMINAL OR INTRATHORACIC FLUIDS

Fluid analysis with cytology can be extremely helpful in identifying processes leading to fluid development, including infectious and neoplastic causes. Thoracocentesis and abdominocentesis are fast procedures with a very low risk of complications. For either body cavity, if a moderate to large amount of fluid is present, it is easy to obtain a sample blindly. Equipment needed includes a 3/4 inch 22-gauge needle, a 3–6 ml syringe, and red and purple top tubes. Unlike when sampling tissues, the needle is always placed on the syringe for this procedure.

For abdominocentesis, similar to the standard procedure for cystocentesis, the skin is not usually clipped or scrubbed. To avoid the liver and spleen, the sampling site should be mid-abdomen and towards the right side of the midline. In an upright patient, the needle is inserted into the ventral abdomen, as fluid will sink (Figure 1.32). If the patient is recumbent, the needle is directed into the cavity from below the midline point. The plunger on the syringe is then withdrawn and the sample obtained (Figure 1.33). Several milliliters of fluid can be obtained rapidly. Pressure on the syringe is released before the needle is extracted. The sample is then divided between red and purple top tubes.

For thoracocentesis, the best place to sample is between the 6th and 8th ribs. The patient is placed in ventral recumbency or may be

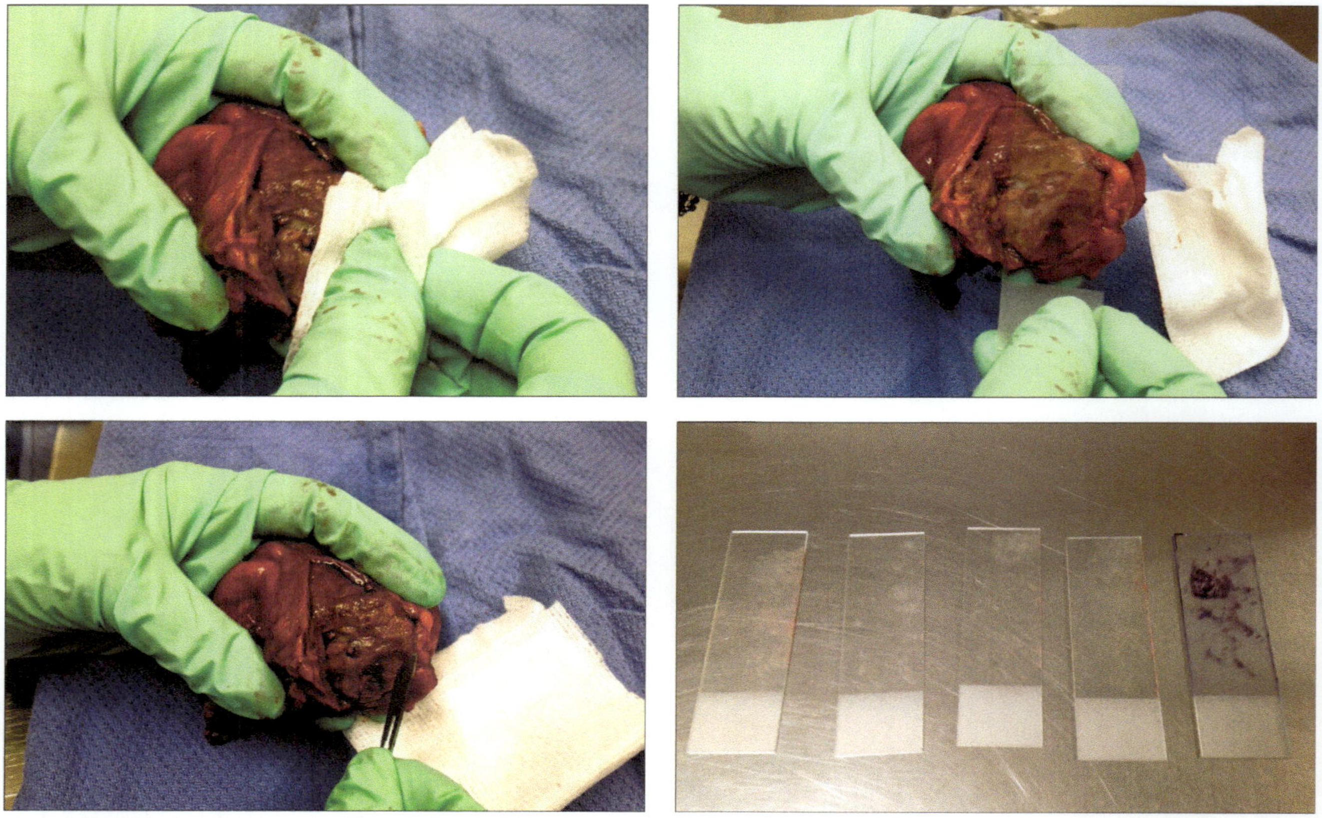

Figures 1.28–1.31 **Preparing a surgically excised mass to obtain an impression smear. (1.28) First, gauze is used to dry blood from the surface. (1.29) A slide is pressed firmly against the surface of the mass. (1.30) A scalpel blade is used to scrape cells from the mass; the material on the blade will then be smeared on a slide. (1.31) Impression smear slides, both unstained and stained, showing thick and thin regions.**

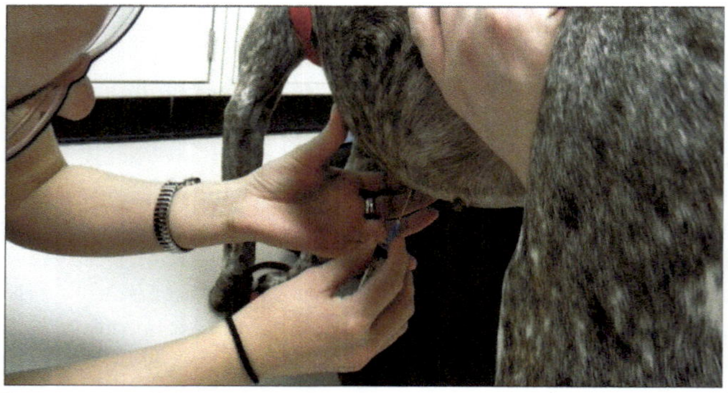

Figure 1.32 **Abdominocentesis using a 22-gauge 1½ inch needle and a 6 ml syringe.**

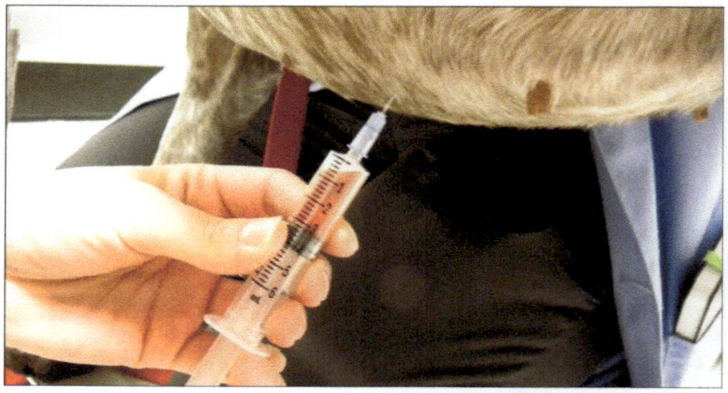

Figure 1.33 **The fluid easily obtained from the abdomen of a dog with marked effusion.**

left standing but restrained. The skin is usually clipped and scrubbed. The needle is inserted between the ribs and ventrally on the chest wall. Depending on the size of the animal, only half the length of the needle may be needed to reach the fluid. Alternatively, an intravascular or butterfly catheter can be used. As with abdominocentesis, the plunger is drawn back and fluid is obtained; pressure on the plunger is released and the needle is withdrawn. For situations where minimal fluid is present in either body cavity, ultrasound guidance can be used to help direct the needle into a pocket of fluid.

SLIDE SUBMISSION

Labeling of the slides is an invaluable component of slide submission whether the slides are being sent out to a clinical pathology laboratory

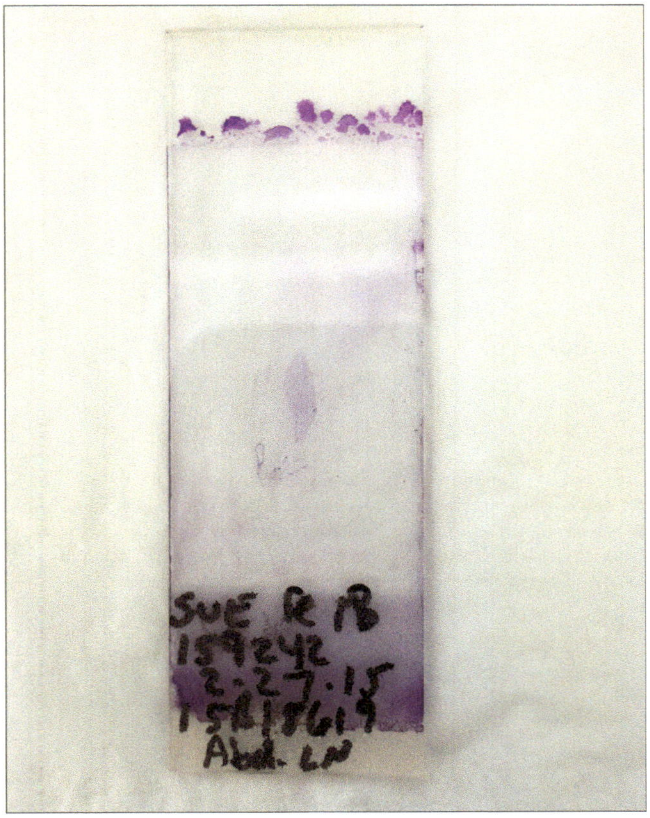

Figure 1.34 FNA from a cat. The slide is labeled with the patient's name, medical record number, date, and source of the aspirate.

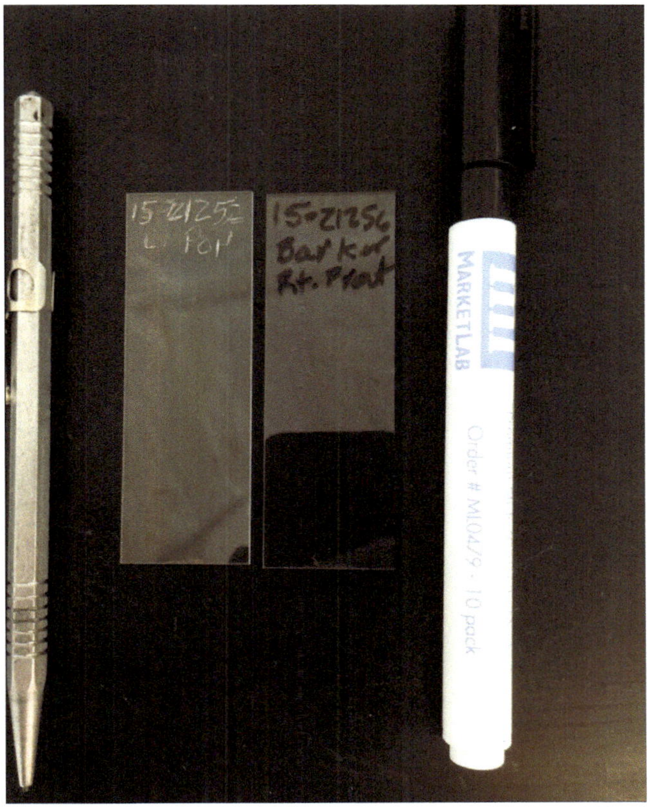

Figure 1.35 Diamond tipped pencil (left) and slide marker (right) used for permanent labeling of samples.

or being evaluated in-house. Pertinent information to write on the slides includes the patient's identification information (either name or medical record number) and the site sampled, particularly if multiple sites were sampled (Figure 1.34). Slides with a frosted edge are ideal because then the slides can be labeled with pencil. Special markers or diamond-etched pencils are necessary to label slides without frosted edges (Figure 1.35). Ink from other markers, such as Sharpie® markers, will wash off during the staining process.

If sending slides to a laboratory for evaluation, it is important to package the slides appropriately because they are quite fragile. Many types of slide boxes are available and include cardboard, polystyrene, and plastic (Figure 1.36). Cardboard carriers are the least expensive; however, they are also the least stable (Figure 1.37). The plastic containers are the most stable, but even these should be wrapped in additional padding or sent in a padded envelope. Accompanying the slides should be a form containing necessary patient information including signalment and pertinent historical data as well as the source(s) of the aspirates. This information is vital for the clinical pathologist to be able to provide the most complete cytologic diagnosis, as well as a thorough list of differential diagnoses and suggestions for appropriate additional diagnostic testing.

STAINING OF SLIDES

If sending slides to a laboratory, it is recommended that unstained slides be submitted. It is beneficial, however, to examine at least one slide to determine if an adequate sample was obtained and/or the appropriate tissue sampled (Figure 1.38).

Many types of stains are available for cytologic preparations, and some are available for easy in-house use. Common types used in veterinary medicine include Romanowsky stains, Pap stain, and new methylene blue. Each of these will be described in more detail.

Romanowsky stains

In veterinary medicine, Romanowsky stains are the most commonly used and readily available stains. These stains include May–Grünwald–Giemsa, Leishman–Giemsa, Wright–Giemsa, and Diff-Quik® and its variants. The Romanowsky stains include a combination of reagents that include azure B/polychromed methylene blue and the eosin family of stains (Horobin, 2011). The characteristic staining with this combination results in a classic purple staining of the nucleus (Figure 1.39). If the nucleus of the cell is not purple, concern for inappropriate staining, inadequately dried sample, overly thick preparation, or

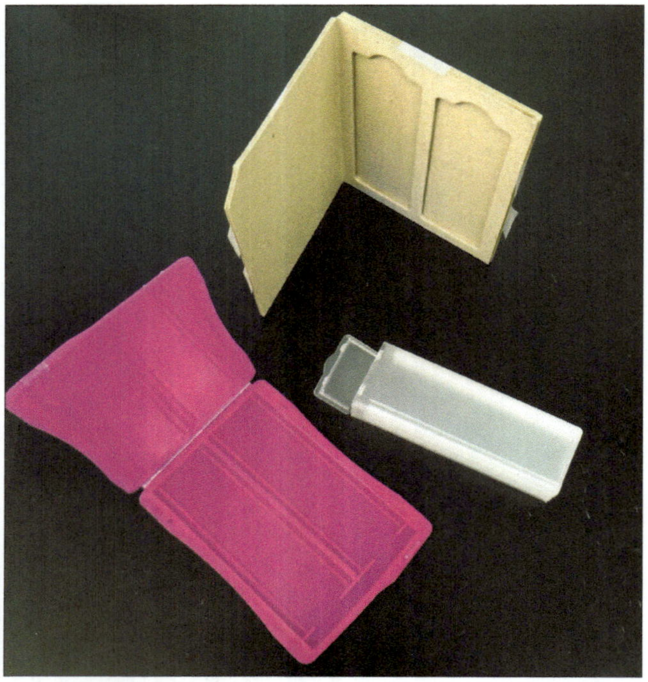

Figure 1.36 Options for containers for slide transport. Plastic slide boxes are more durable than cardboard.

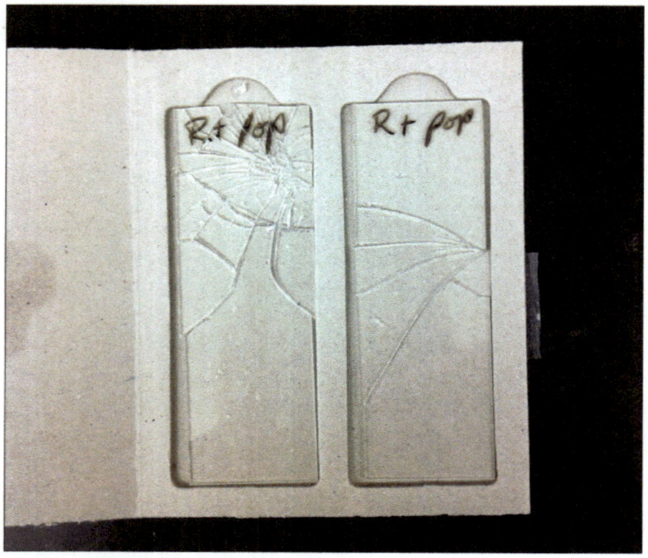

Figure 1.37 Slides sent in a cardboard container, inappropriately packaged. Both slides are severely damaged.

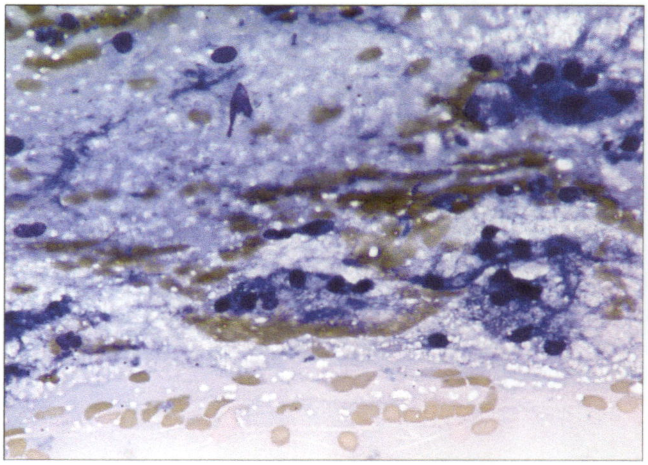

Figure 1.38 Mandibular lymph node aspirate from a dog reveals cytologically unremarkable salivary tissue. Clusters of vacuolated salivary epithelial cells and thick mucus are observed in the background. No lymphoid tissue is observed, so this is likely inadvertent aspiration of healthy salivary tissue (Wright–Giemsa, 1,000× magnification).

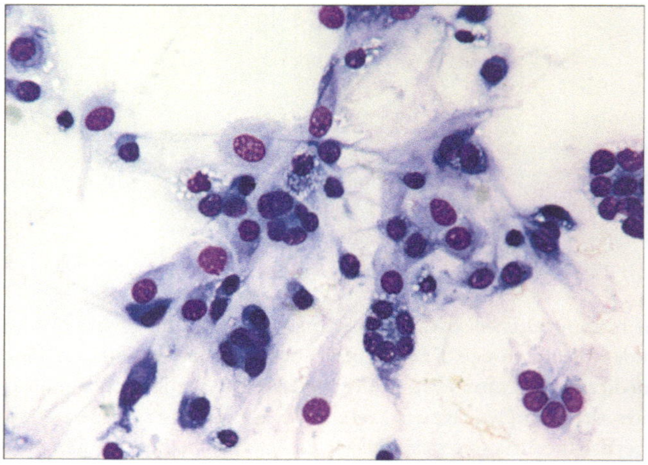

Figure 1.39 Subcutaneous mass on the carpus of a dog. The sample is highly cellular and consists of a population of neoplastic mesenchymal cells. The sample is adequately stained with basophilic cytoplasm, classic purple staining of the nucleus and basophilic nucleoli (Wright–Giemsa, 1,000× magnification).

exposure to aldehyde fixatives should be considered (Horobin, 2011; Kraft's, 2011).

One of the many advantages of Romanowsky stains is the ease of fixation. Air drying is all that is required. Even heat fixation is unnecessary for these types of stains. A recent study showed that even for ear swabs, heat fixation provided no benefit (Toma et al., 2006). Slide preparation, therefore, is so important because quick, even drying is essential for uniform staining. Prolongation of the drying time can result in cellular rupture and poor cell preservation (Jörundsson et al., 1999). Additionally, fixation will influence the uptake of the stain. The result of an inappropriately fixed slide is poorly stained cells with blue rather than purple nuclei (Horobin, 2011). Incomplete staining or understaining of samples is a common problem. As mentioned earlier, the nuclei of cells stained with Romanowsky stains should be purple. If the nuclei are blue, the sample may have not stained long enough, had prolonged drying time, be too thick, or been exposed to aldehyde fixatives (Figures

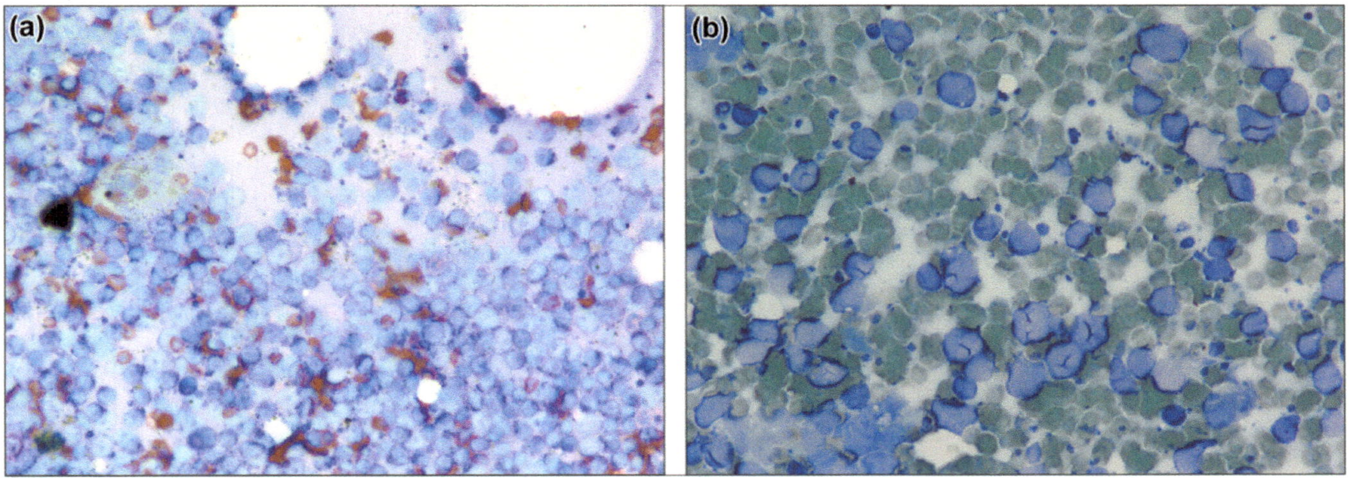

Figure 1.40a, b Lymph node aspirate from a dog with lymphoma. (a) Represents a sample that is poorly stained. The nuclei are staining blue rather than purple and individual cytologic features are difficult to discern. (b) Represents a sample exposed to formalin fumes. Note the green staining of the erythrocytes and the blue staining of the nuclei (Wright–Giemsa: a, 500× magnification; b, 1,000× magnification).

1.40a, b). A blue–green appearance to the erythrocytes indicates the sample has been exposed to aldehyde fixatives or the pH of the stain is too high (Horobin, 2011).

There are several different Romanowsky stains available. Many practices will use a manual stain like Diff-Quik®. The manual stains are presented as three solutions: methanol, solution 1 or eosin, and solution 2 consisting of azure A and B. The slides are dipped in each solution. This is an easy stain to use; however, there are some limitations. The solutions must be changed frequently to limit sedimentation and bacterial growth. Additionally, mast cell granules, basophils, and granules from granular lymphocytes do not stain as reliably with the aqueous Romanowsky stains (Allison & Velguth, 2010). For this reason, many clinical pathology laboratories use Wright–Giemsa or May-Grünwald–Giemsa because the Giemsa component stains mast cell granules vibrantly. If performing in-house cytology, it is important to leave some of the slides unstained so one of these stains can be used.

There are several advantages to the use of Romanowsky stains for cytology, including detailed staining of the cytoplasm, background material, and microorganisms (Kraft's, 2011). A more complete list is shown in Table 1.1.

Papanicolaou stain

The Papanicolaou (Pap) stain has a long history of use in cytology. It was developed by George Papanikolaou and is most commonly associated with the Pap smear used to diagnose cervical cancer. The classic stain involves a combination of five dyes including hematoxylin, orange G, and eosin 50, which is a combination of eosin, Bismark brown, and light green. The eosin gives a pink color to the cytoplasm of mature squamous epithelial cells, nucleoli, and cilia. Light green stains the cytoplasm of metabolically active cells blue, such as parabasal cells, squamous epithelial cells, and intermediate and columnar epithelial cells. Hematoxylin is used to stain nuclei (Pérez et al., 2005).

The original Pap stain is a little cumbersome for in-house cytology, requiring many reagents and steps. However, simplified Pap stains have been evaluated for easy cytologic use. Sawa et al. (2012) evaluated RADPap® and found the stain was easy to perform and only took 15 minutes; however, there were still 18 steps, which diminishes the clinical utility. The Ultrafast Papanicololaou staining protocol has 14 steps but only takes 5 minutes to perform (Pérez et al., 2005).

The Pap stain requires wet fixation such as 95% ethanol, 100% ethanol, or 80% isopropanol (Jörundson et al., 1999). To improve the clinical utility of wet fixation, techniques have also been developed for air-dried smears to be rehydrated with saline (Jörundson et al., 1999).

There are significant advantages of the Pap stain when compared with Romanowsky stains in exhibiting nuclear detail and for evaluating thick tissue samples (Table 1.1; Jörundson et al., 1999; Krafts, 2011).

Table 1.1 **Advantages and limitations of the common stains used for cytologic preparations**

	Romanowsky	Papanicolaou	New methylene blue
Advantages	Excellent cytoplasmic detail. Adequate staining of background material.	Excellent nuclear detail. Useful in staining cells in thick preparations.	Consistent staining of mast cell granules. Nuclear detail is adequate. Easy to use.
Limitations	Staining of cells challenging in thick samples. Nuclear detail is minimal.	Wet fixation or rehydration of samples required. Not useful for evaluation of microorganisms or background material.	Use of stain on air-dried smears for cytology is not permanent.

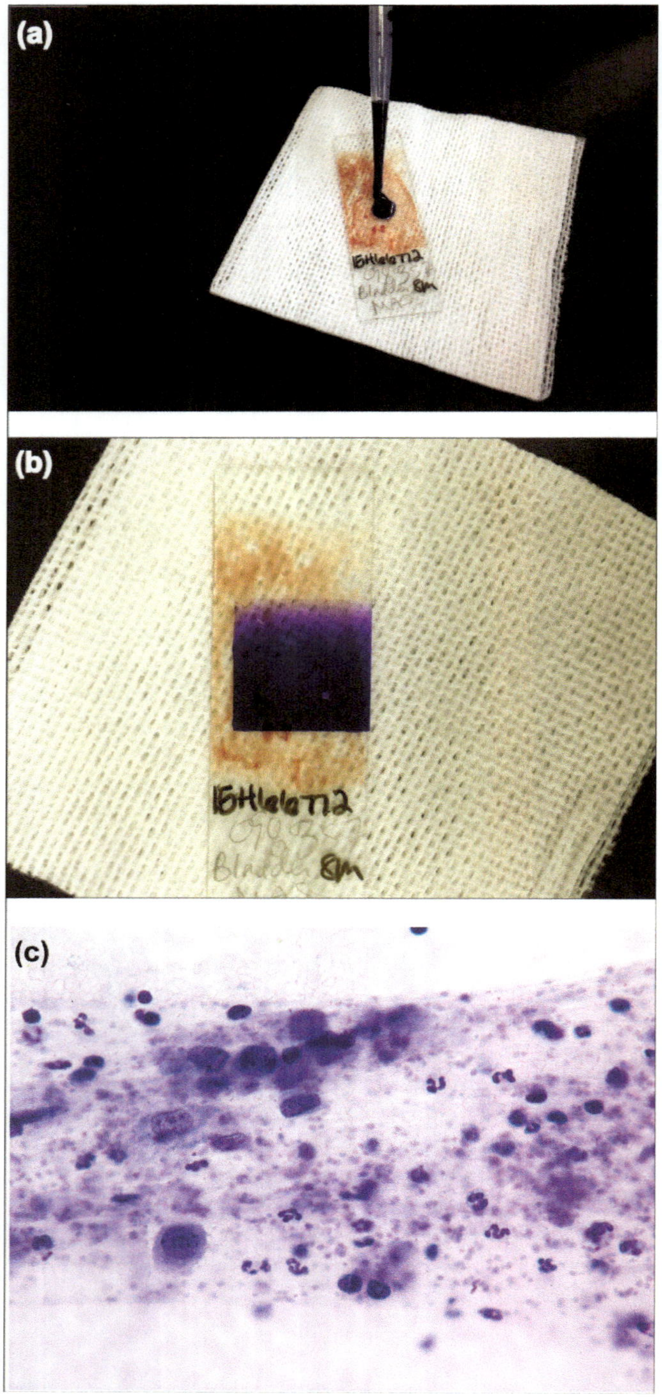

Figure 1.41 New methylene blue staining of cytology specimens. (a) The stain is applied to an unstained cytologic specimen. (b) A coverslip is placed on the slide. (c) Microscopic evaluation reveals reasonable nuclear staining; neutrophils and macrophages are identified in this sample (500× magnification).

New methylene blue

New methylene blue (NMB) is a supravital stain and is very easy to use. It is commonly used to quantify reticulocytes in the peripheral blood because it will stain organelles vibrantly. Its use in cytologic preparations is a little different. A drop of stain is placed on an air-dried smear and then a coverslip is placed on the droplet to evenly spread the stain on the smear (Figures 1.41a–c). This stain provides excellent nuclear and nucleolar detail and also stains mast cell granules (Table 1.1). The stain is a wet mount stain so it is not permanent. As the NMB stain dries, the cellular staining diminishes. Therefore, this may be a limitation for its use in laboratories required to save slides for an extended period of time.

Additional techniques for immunostaining

Immunocytochemical staining can be performed on regular unstained or destained cytology preparations. Formalin fixation and antigen retrieval are not required. A limitation of this is the variability in cellularity and cellular preservation. There are some interesting techniques available to improve the consistency of cellularity, but these require formalin fixation and antigen retrieval. Needle rinse cell blocks can be used to prepare cells obtained with cytology for paraffin embedding. These samples are fixed and undergo similar processing as histopathology samples (Marrinhas et al., 2021). The advantage of this technique is to get multiple uniform slides for evaluation, and multiple stains can be performed if needed. An additional technique of placing the aspirate directly in formalin and using a micromesh strainer to place the material in a cassette for processing and paraffin embedding has also been evaluated (Etzioni, 2022). This cyto-histo technique can be useful for immunostaining.

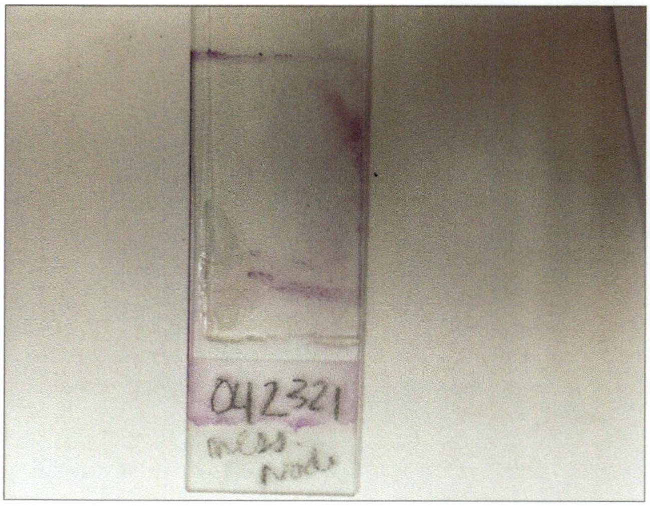

Figure 1.42 FNA from a mass on a dog. Macroscopic evaluation of the slide is beneficial to identify the best area to evaluate. Some aspirates provide a very small sample.

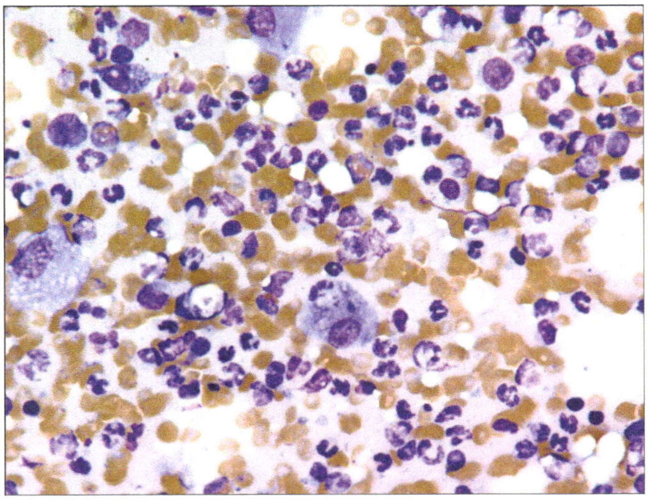

Figure 1.43 FNA from a dog reveals a mixed cellular population consistent with an inflammatory response (Wright–Giemsa, 500× magnification).

CYTOLOGIC EVALUATION

Once the slide is stained, it is ready to be evaluated cytologically. Low-power microscopic evaluation is critical. Many different patterns, processes, and background material can be very easily identified with low-power evaluation. Generally, for cytology, this is done at 10× magnification; however, visual evaluation of the stained slide itself is also beneficial to determine the position of the sample on the slide (Figure 1.42). Microscopic low-power evaluation will allow the evaluator to determine if the sample is cellular enough for diagnostic quality. Patterns of cellular association can be identified. Epithelial cells will commonly form clusters whereas round cells and mesenchymal cells are more likely to be arranged in a loose sheet or as individualized cells. Low-power evaluation can also allow for evaluation of the diversity of a population. Recognition of one cell population versus a pleocellular population can help determine the overall process. One cell type being present is more consistent with aspiration of a tumor or of a specific tissue (for example, aspiration of the liver may result in the identification of primarily hepatocytes), while a mixed or pleomorphic population of cells is more consistent with inflammation (Figure 1.43). Low-power evaluation should also be used to identify well-stained, diagnostic areas on the slide. Thick areas of the smear make full evaluation of cellular morphology difficult. Thinner areas, where cells have the opportunity to spread out, are more useful for evaluating individual cellular morphology (Figures 1.44a, b).

At higher magnification, individual cellular features, such as chromatin pattern, presence of nucleoli, and cytoplasmic features, can be identified as well as smaller microorganisms such as bacteria (Figure 1.45). It is important to clearly identify the presence of cytoplasm and a nucleus in the cells. Cells may rupture during the aspiration or slide preparation process, resulting in bare nuclei or streams of nucleoproteinaceous debris (Figure 1.46). Nuclei that have lost their cytoplasm will swell and become much larger, and it is important not to overinterpret their value. A diagnosis should always be made on intact cells.

Higher magnifications can include 40×, 50×, and 100× objective lenses. Often 100× is necessary to fully evaluate the sample for bacteria and smaller yeast. If using a 40× objective that is not oil immersion, remember to place a coverslip over the sample to improve the crispness of the objective. Features of individual cells will be described in each of the chapters.

Finally, the material present in the background should be examined. Blood contamination is possible with every aspirate, although some organs such as the spleen and liver are more vascular than others and are prone to lead to significant hemodilution when sampled. Accompanying white blood cells can be seen in samples with significant peripheral blood contamination; therefore care should be taken not to confuse inflammation with blood contamination. Proteinaceous material can also be observed, either as a pathologic process or potentially as a healthy cellular product, such as mucin

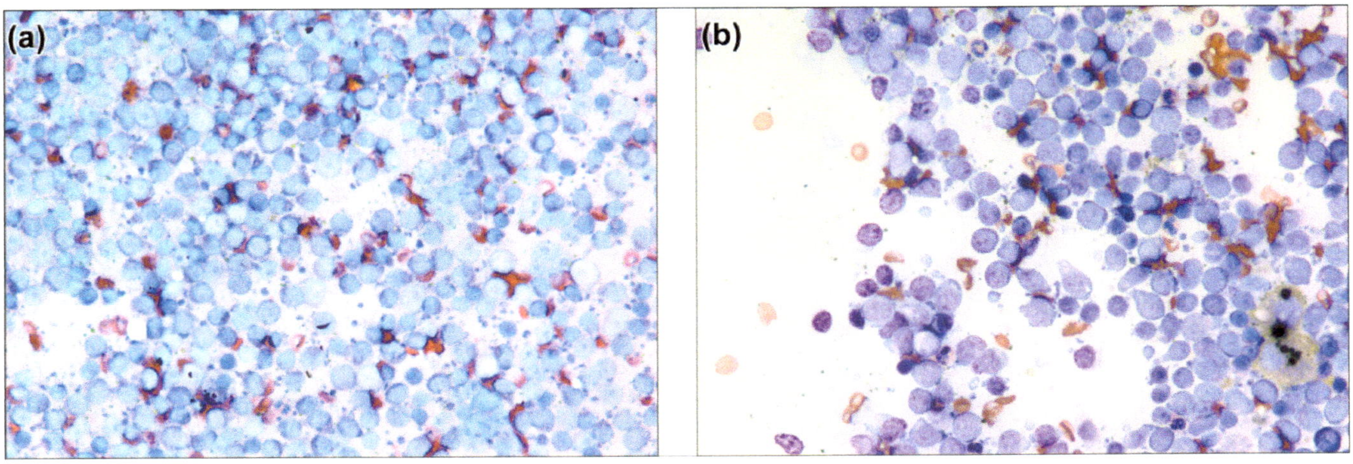

Figures 1.44 Lymph node aspirate from a dog. (a) Reveals a thick area of the smear. The cells are crowded and inappropriately stained. (b) Represents a thinner area of the smear. The cells are more spread out and appropriately stained (Wright–Giemsa, 500× magnification).

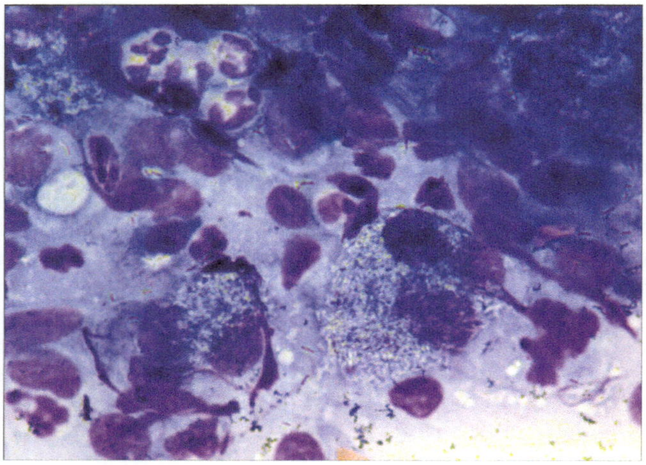

Figure 1.45 Lymph node aspirate from a dog. At higher magnification, macrophages containing negative staining rod-shaped bacteria (*Mycobacteria* sp.) can be more easily identified (Wright–Giemsa, 1,000× magnification).

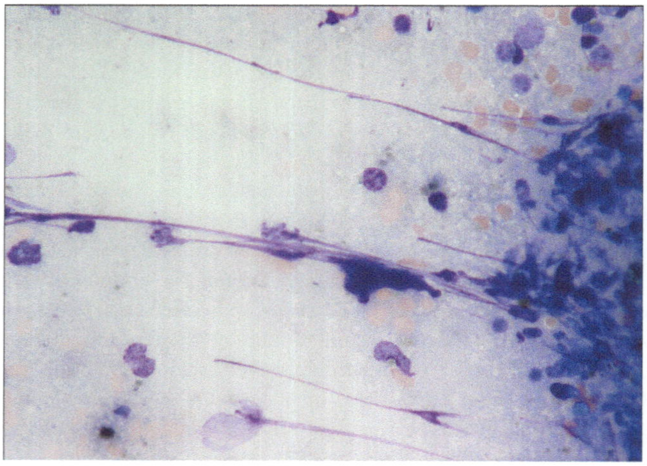

Figure 1.46 FNA from a mass on a dog. Streams of nucleoproteinaceous debris can be identified and are often caused during slide preparation. These structures should not be confused with fungal hyphae (Wright–Giemsa, 500× magnification).

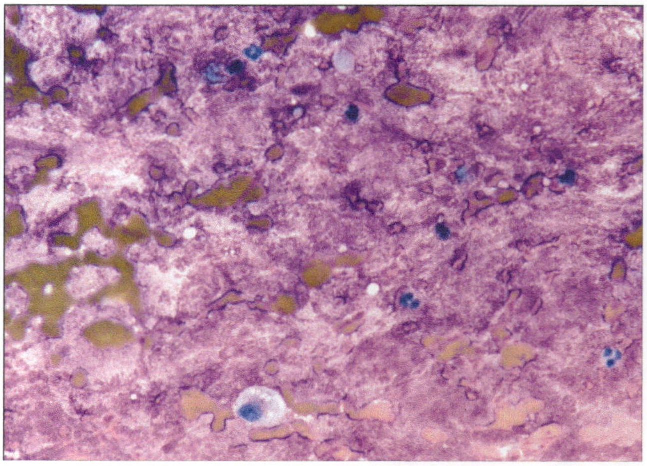

Figure 1.47 Aspirate from a lytic bone lesion in a dog. The deeply eosinophilic material in the background is consistent with chondroid. The material is so thick, it is difficult to fully evaluate the nucleated cells in the sample (Wright–Giemsa, 500× magnification).

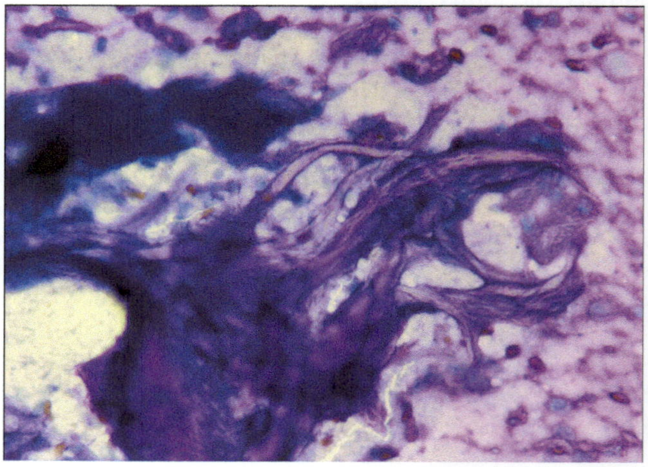

Figure 1.48 Aspirate from a mast cell tumor in a dog. Thick aggregates of collagen bundles are present (Wright–Giemsa, 500× magnification).

production in joint aspirates. If the sample is highly proteinaceous, the individual cellular features may be difficult to evaluate, so identification of a thin area in the smear is recommended (Figure 1.47). Thick eosinophilic-staining proteinaceous material may indicate the presence of osteoid, chondroid, fibrin, or collagen in a sample. Collagen may be seen accompanying mast cell tumors or epithelial neoplasms (Figure 1.48). Granules can also be seen in the background from ruptured melanocytes, mast cells, eosinophils, and, less likely, basophils. It is important not to confuse these structures with microorganisms. Again, it is important to try to identify the intact cells and compare the background material with any granules in the cytoplasm of the cell population (Figure 1.49).

In order to interpret the cytology appropriately, it is important to consider the histologic appearance of the tissue and the underlying architecture. The term exfoliate cytology refers to looking at individual cells been exfoliated from a tissue – literally the tissue has been 'stripped of leaves'. In order to accurately interpret the cytologic findings, it is essential to know the structure of the 'tree' from which the cells originate. There is a close relationship between cytologic findings and the histologic structure of common tissues and tumors. One frustration for the beginner cytologist is the question of identifying normal, particularly as normal structures are rarely intentionally aspirated. For those without a strong background in histology, a good reference text in the clinic can aid in the recollection of which types of cells are normally found in each tissue. This is particularly helpful in the identification of cell types in aspirates from unusual locations, such as the esophagus or reproductive organs. Also bear in mind that there are some species differences in what is normal in various locations (Bacha & Bacha, 2012).

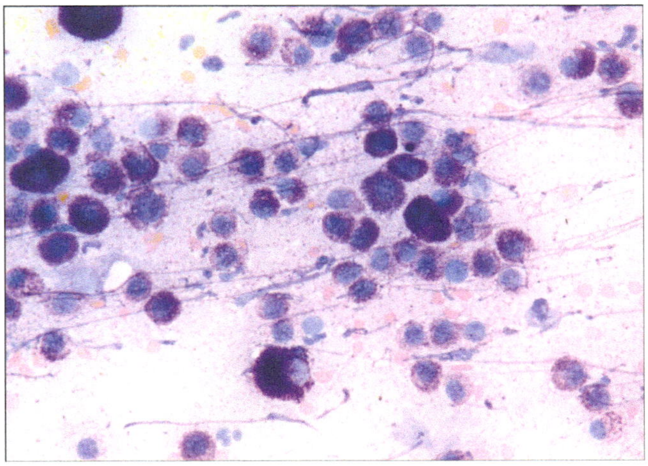

Figure 1.49 Aspirate from a mast cell tumor in a dog. Metachromatic granules are visible in the cytoplasm of the cells but also in the background (Wright-Giemsa, 500× magnification).

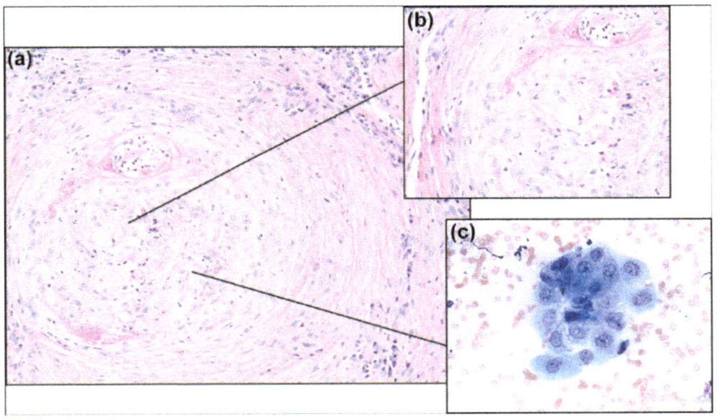

Figure 1.50 Histologic (a, 200× magnification; b, 400× magnification) and cytologic (c, 500× magnification) examples of a squamous cell carcinoma from a dog exhibiting a pavement pattern of loosely cohesive cells (H&E and Wright-Giemsa).

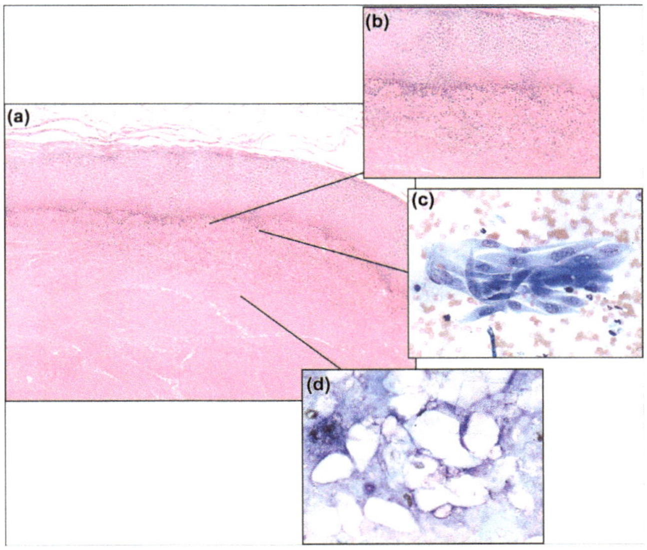

Figure 1.51 Histologic (a, 100× magnification; b, 400× magnification) and cytologic (c & d, 500× magnification) examples of a type of cystic skin tumor (pilomatricoma) from a cat. The epithelial cells (c) form a flattened pavement pattern on the perimeter while the center of the cyst (d) contains cholesterol crystals and poorly staining keratin debris (H&E and Wright-Giemsa).

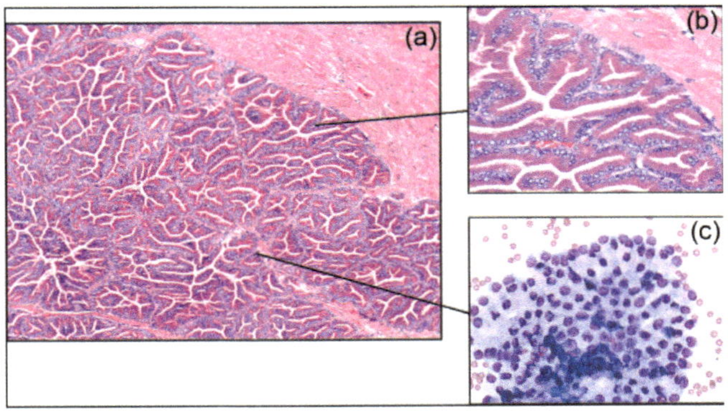

Figure 1.52 Histologic (a, 100× magnification; b, 400× magnification) and cytologic (c, 500× magnification) examples of benign prostatic hyperplasia in a dog. The cells exhibit a classic honeycomb pattern. They are columnar cells with basal nuclei and a moderate amount of cytoplasm, which stains eosinophilic on histology and basophilic on the cytology preparation (H&E and Wright-Giemsa).

A recent article highlighted common patterns in cytologic samples and stressed the importance of careful attention to collection and smear preparation (Masserodotti, 2006). Patterns are found more easily if the relationships among cells are maintained and cells are intact. These patterns correlate to the parent tissue architecture and can be explained by the normal function of the tissue.

Pavement pattern

Pavement patterns are found in squamous, conjunctival, and urogenital epithelium. These cells often exfoliate in loose cohesive sheets or individualized cells. They tend to be flat with somewhat angular margins. This pattern is often confused with individual spindle cells because of the angular cell margins and poor cohesion (Figure 1.50). Additionally, many of these tissues have multiple layers of cells with distinct morphology that may be aspirated in the same cytologic sample. The prime example of this is the presence of variable maturing cells in cystic skin tumors. The cells range from mature anuclear keratin flakes to squamous cells with nuclei in various stages of pyknosis (Figure 1.51). The architecture of the various benign skin tumors explains the variability of the cystic epidermal neoplasms seen on cytology (Gross, 2006).

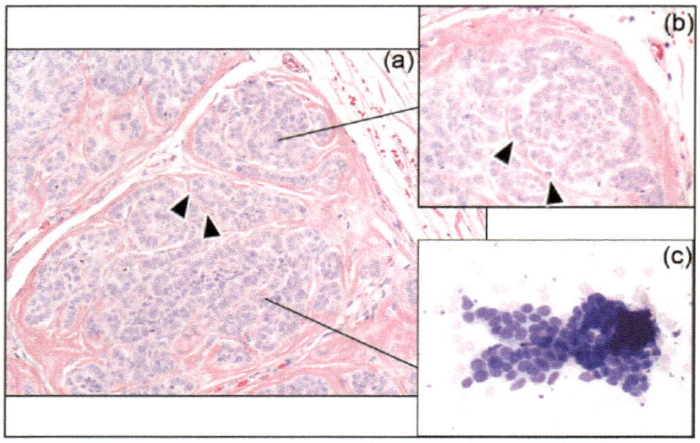

Figure 1.53 Histologic (a, 200× magnification; b, 400× magnification) and cytologic (c, 500× magnification) examples of trichoblastoma from a dog. This is one of several different skin tumors that are classified as basaloid epithelial tumors on cytology as they exfoliate palisading ribbons of cuboidal cells. Collagen and fibrocytes in surrounding matrix (arrowheads) can be seen on the histology slides but not on the cytology preparation (H&E and Wright–Giemsa).

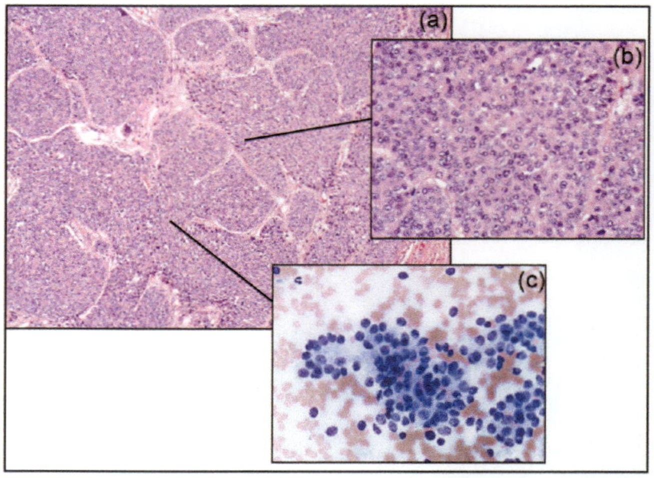

Figure 1.55 Histologic (a, 100× magnification; b, 400× magnification) and cytologic (c, 500× magnification) examples of an apocrine anal gland adenocarcinoma from a dog. The acinar arrangement can be seen on the edge of the sheets of loosely cohesive epithelial cells (H&E and Wright–Giemsa).

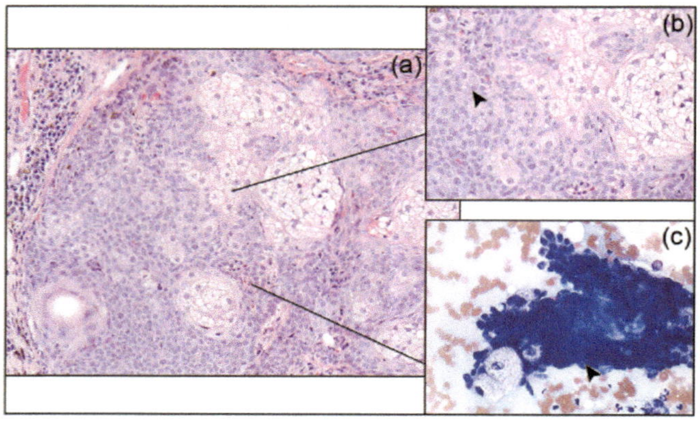

Figure 1.54 Histologic (a, 100× magnification; b, 400× magnification) and cytologic (c, 500× magnification) examples of a sebaceous epithelioma from a dog. Dense cuboidal cells and large foamy sebaceous cells can be seen on both preparations. Arrowheads (b, c) indicate the cells in a palisade pattern similar to those seen in Figure 1.53 (H&E and Wright–Giemsa).

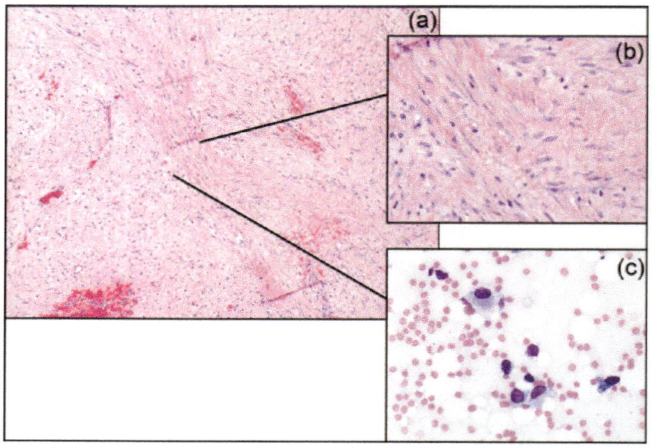

Figure 1.56 Histologic (a, 100× magnification; b, 400× magnification) and cytologic (c, 500× magnification) examples of granulation tissue from a healing surgical site in a dog. The individual spindle cells seen in the cytology panel are difficult to distinguish from a well-differentiated sarcoma (H&E and Wright–Giemsa).

Honeycomb and palisade patterns

The honeycomb and palisade patterns are related to the pavement pattern; however, they tend to maintain a more cohesive appearance. These are cuboidal or columnar cells that maintain distinct cell margins and cohesiveness. The most common site in which to observe the honeycomb pattern in veterinary cytologic samples is the normal prostate or benign prostatic hyperplasia (Figure 1.52). It can also be seen in the normal stomach and intestine; however, these tissues are less commonly sampled for cytology. The palisade pattern presents as ribbons and small aggregates of cuboidal to elongated cells and is common in benign skin tumors (Figures 1.53, 1.54).

Acinar pattern

The acinar pattern reflects the secretory nature of glandular epithelium. When the cells exfoliate intact, they are arranged around an empty or secretion-filled central area. Many of these tissues are prone

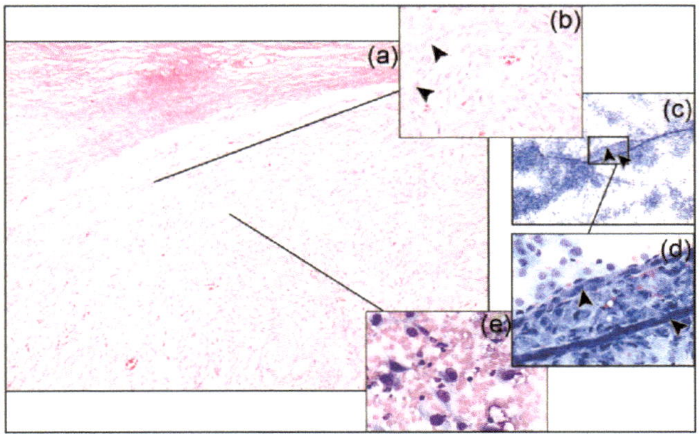

Figure 1.57 Histologic (a, 100× magnification; b, 400× magnification) and cytologic (c, 100× magnification; d & e, 500× magnification) examples of a soft tissue sarcoma from a dog. The spindle cells are seen both individually and in a storiform arrangement near capillaries. Arrowheads (b, c, d): capillaries (H&E and Wright–Giemsa).

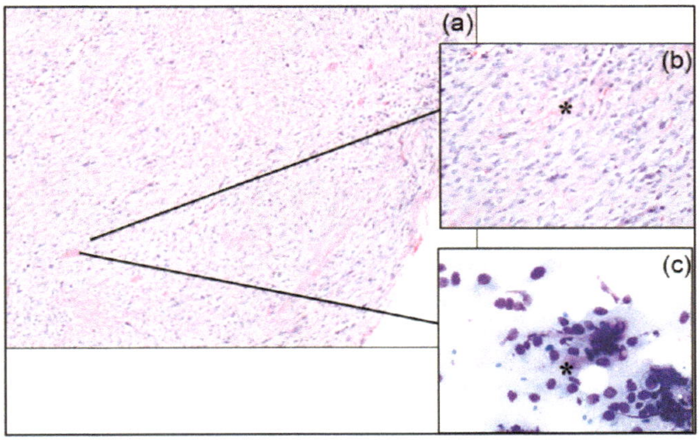

Figure 1.58 Histologic (a, 100× magnification; b, 400× magnification) and cytologic (c, 500× magnification) examples of an osteosarcoma from a dog. The asterisks (b, c) represent osteoid seen as a pink matrix material on both stains (H&E and Wright–Giemsa).

to mechanical disruption, resulting in loosely cohesive sheets or nuclei floating in a 'sea of cytoplasm'. Thyroid carcinomas and anal gland carcinomas are known for this type of presentation (Figure 1.55).

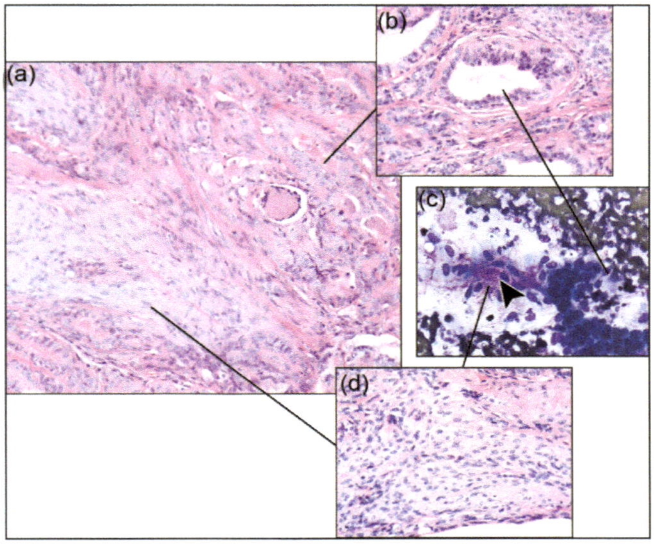

Figure 1.59 Histologic (a, 100× magnification; b & d, 400× magnification) and cytologic (c, 500× magnification) examples of a complex mammary tumor from a dog showing both epithelial and mesenchymal differentiation. The spindle cells are intermixed with extracellular matrix material consistent with osteoid (arrowhead, c) and are adjacent to cuboidal cells in a palisade pattern (H&E and Wright–Giemsa).

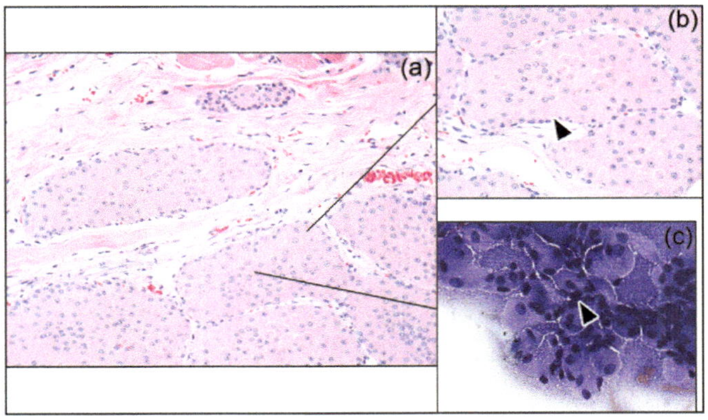

Figure 1.60 Histologic (a, 100× magnification; b, 400× magnification) and cytologic (c, 500× magnification) examples of a perianal adenoma from a dog. Arrowheads (b, c): cuboidal reserve cells (H&E and Wright–Giemsa).

Supporting stroma

Mesenchymal cells create the supportive framework of all tissues. They provide a tight interwoven matrix, which is more difficult to aspirate and thus typically yields fewer cellular samples. Normal fibrocytes can be seen as the pink bundles between the cellular islands of the trichoblastoma in the histopathology sample of Figure 1.53 but they were not present in the cytology sample from that tumor. Abnormal mesenchymal populations such as tumors or granulation tissue will exfoliate more readily than normal fibrous tissue, and the resulting slides have increased cellularity. They present as individual spindle cells in a storiform pattern (Figure 1.56). In some cases, the vascular elements of a tissue will be present on a cytology sample. These small capillaries are commonly seen in thicker preparations of some soft tissue sarcomas (Figure 1.57). In addition, the spindle cells may be associated with extracellular stromal elements such as chondroid or osteoid, which have an amorphous purple–pink appearance (Figure 1.58).

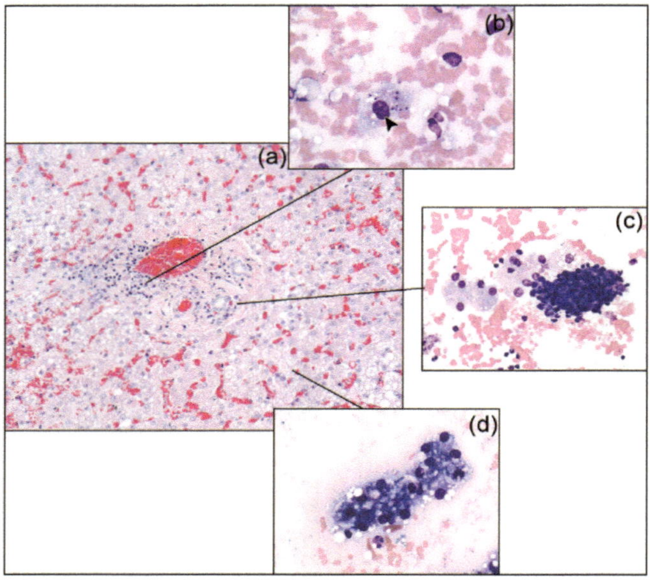

Figure 1.61 Histologic (a, 400× magnification) and cytologic (b, c & d, 500× magnification) examples of a liver. Arrowhead (b): macrophage containing *Histoplasma capsulatum* yeast. Macrophages and biliary epithelial cells (c) are mixed with vacuolated hepatocytes (d) (H&E and Wright–Giemsa).

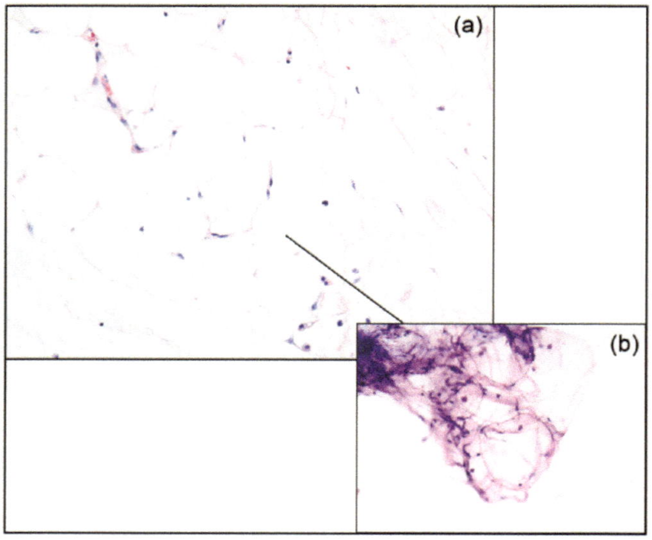

Figure 1.62 Histologic (a, 200× magnification) and cytologic (b, 200× magnification) examples of a lipoma. The fat-filled cells are similar in both preparations (H&E and Wright–Giemsa).

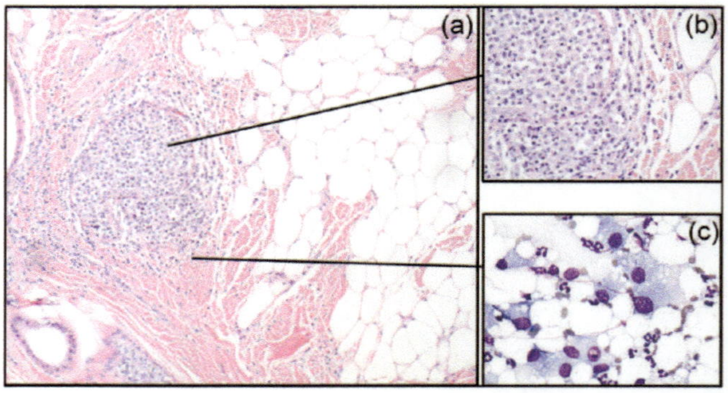

Figure 1.63 Histologic (a, 200× magnification; b, 400× magnification) and cytologic (c, 500× magnification) examples of an infiltrating lipoma with inflammation. The majority of cells in this cytology preparation are large activated macrophages and non-degenerate neutrophils. There is a background of fatty material but only rare intact adipocytes (H&E and Wright–Giemsa).

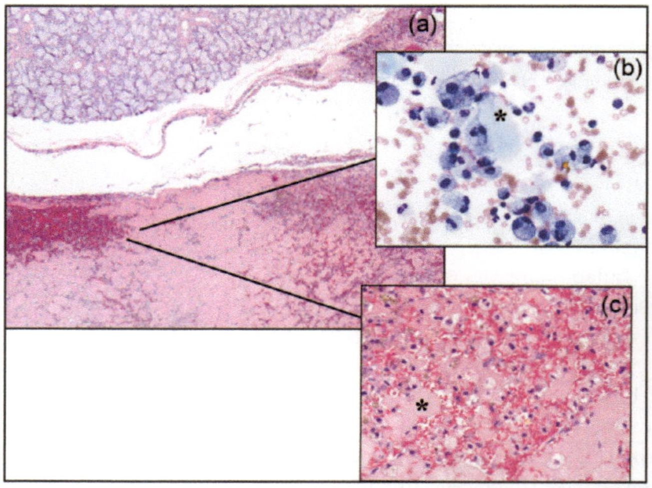

Figure 1.64 Histologic (a, 200× magnification; c, 400× magnification) and cytologic (b, 500× magnification) examples of a sialocele. The normal gland can be seen above the dilated sialocele. The aspirate (b) revealed abundant vacuolated macrophages, some of which contained hematoidin crystals. The blue inspissated saliva on the cytology (asterisk, b, c) stains pink in the histology section (H&E and Wright–Giemsa).

Complex tissues

Samples such as internal organs, inflammatory samples, and tumors with multiple tissue types can lead to confusing cytologic samples. The normal architecture and proportion of different cell types should correspond to what exfoliates on cytology. Mammary tumors are a prime example of tissues that yield multiple cell types on cytology. They often have a mixture of glandular epithelial cells and mesenchymal cells. These mesenchymal cells can range from spindeloid fibrocytes to chondrocytes and osteoblasts if the tumor contains complex features such as cartilage or bone (Figure 1.59). Some tumors, such as the perianal gland adenoma in dogs, have both large polygonal epithelial cells and smaller cuboidal reserve cells. Understanding the histology helps explain the presence of these two cell types (Figure 1.60).

The liver is another tissue in which multiple cell types are normal. The majority of the cells seen on cytology should be hepatocellular,

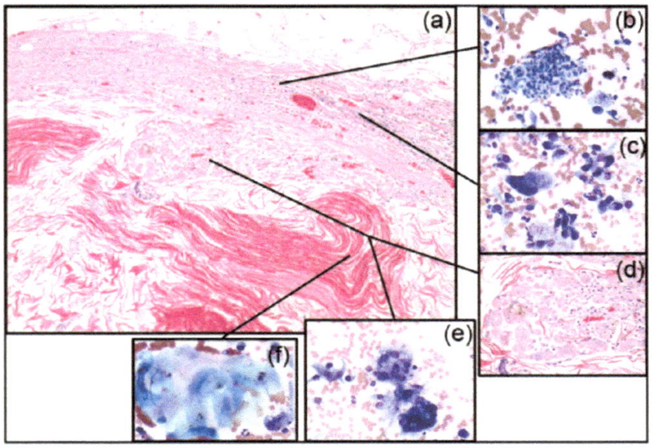

Figure 1.65 **Histologic (a, 100× magnification; d, 400× magnification) and cytologic (b, c, e & f, 500× magnification) samples from a cat skin tumor. The majority of the cells on this cytology were the spindle cells and multinucleate cells seen in c and e. The inflammatory cells in b and the keratin debris in f were rare on the cytology slide. Biopsy revealed a keratin-filled cyst with a border of multinucleate inflammatory cells, fibrosis, and inflammation (H&E and Wright–Giemsa).**

with a smaller proportion of biliary epithelial cells. Inflammatory cells can be diffuse but are often overrepresented in the periportal area. An example of a liver from a cat with histoplasmosis is shown (Figure 1.61).

Inflammatory lesions can have a myriad of cell types present. The cells seen may not reflect the underlying pathology in the case of a tumor with a devitalized center or when the inflammation is incidental to the final diagnosis. As seen in Figure 1.56, reactive spindle cells can mimic neoplastic processes and are often intermixed with inflammatory lesions. An example of the drastic difference inflammation can make in your ability to diagnose simple lesions on cytology is when there is granulomatous inflammation in a simple lipoma. Fat has a characteristic cytologic appearance (Figure 1.62), but when traumatized it produces an intense granulomatous steatitis. Aspiration of this inflammatory population can be misinterpreted as a primary inflammatory or even a neoplastic process such as a histiocytic sarcoma (Figure 1.63).

A normal salivary gland has a characteristic appearance of foamy epithelial cells in small sheets, but when there is inflammation and dilation of the salivary duct, a sialocele may form, producing a marked granulomatous inflammation (Figure 1.64).

A case that caused a diagnostic dilemma serves as the final example to instill caution in the overzealous cytologist (Figure 1.65). The spindle cells and multinucleate cells were the majority of the cells on the slide; there was relatively little keratin debris and inflammation, and a sarcoma was suspected. Histopathology revealed the lesion to be a benign cystic skin tumor with inflammation. This example highlights the need for caution in the interpretation of cytologic samples without the correlation of the tissue architecture.

ADDITIONAL DIAGNOSTIC TESTING

The use of cytology is growing. Additional testing is available to help obtain more specific diagnoses. The immunophenotyping of lymphoma is possible using several techniques including immunocytochemistry, flow cytometry, and polymerase chain reaction. The identification of certain microorganisms can be assisted via special stains such as acid-fast for *Mycobacteria* spp.; *Nocardia* spp., and *Actinomyces* spp., Gomori methenamine silver and periodic-acid Schiff stains are useful for the identification of fungal organisms. Special stains can also be useful for the identification of specific tumors. For example, staining for alkaline phosphatase activity is very useful in the diagnosis of osteosarcoma, and currently is used only in cytology and not formalin fixed tissues. Each of these techniques will be expanded on in the appropriate chapters.

REFERENCES

Allison R.W., Velguth K.E. (2010) Appearance of granulated cells in blood films stained by automated aqueous versus methanolic Romanowsky methods. *Vet Clin Path 39*:99–104.

Arai S., Rist P., Clancey N. et al. (2019) Fine-needle aspiration of cutaneous, subcutaneous, and intracavitary masses in dogs and cats using 22- vs 25-gauge needles. *Vet Clin Pathol 48*:287–292.

Bacha W., Bacha L. (2012) *Color Atlas of Veterinary Histology*, 3rd edn. Wiley-Blackwell, Ames.

Bahr K.L., Sharkey L.C., Murakami T. et al. (2013) Accuracy of US-guided FNA of focal liver lesions in dogs: 140 cases (2005–2008). *J Am Anim Hosp Assoc 49*:190–196.

Ballegeer E.A., Forrest L.J., Dickinson R.M. et al. (2007) Correlation of ultrasonographic appearance of lesions and cytologic and histologic diagnoses in splenic aspirates from dogs and cats: 32 cases (2002–2005). *J Am Vet Med Assoc 230*:690–696.

Barrouin-Melo S.M., Larangeira D.F., de Andrade Filho F.A. et al. (2006) Can spleen aspirations be safely used for the parasitological diagnosis of canine visceral leishmaniosis? A study on assymptomatic and polysymptomatic animals. *Vet J 171*:331–339.

Bonfanti U., Bussadori C., Zatelli A. et al. (2004) Percutaneous fine-needle biopsy of deep thoracic and abdominal masses in dogs and cats. *J Small Anim Pract 45*:191–198.

Crain S.K., Sharkey L.C., Cordner A.P. et al. (2014) Safety of ultrasound-guided fine-needle aspiration of the feline pancreas: A case-control study. *J Feline Med Surg 17*:858–863.

Etzioni A. (2022) Osteosarcoma diagnosed in a dog using a formalin-fixed fine-needle aspirate biopsy. *Vet Clin Pathol 51*:349–355.

Feeney D.A., Ober C.P., Snyder L.A. et al. (2013) Ultrasound criteria and guided fine-needle aspiration diagnostic yields in small animal peritoneal, mesenteric and omental disease. *Vet Radiol Ultrasound 54*:638–645.

Glinska-Suchocka K., Jankowski M., Kubiak K. et al. (2013) Fine needle biopsy of abdominal organs in dogs: Indications, contraindications and performance technique. *Pol J Vet Sci 16*:835–842.

Gross T. (2006) Section two: neoplasms and other tumors: Part one: Epithelial neoplasms. In: *Skin Diseases of the Dog and Cat*, 2nd edn. (eds. P.J. Ihrke, E.J. Walder) Wiley-Blackwell, Ames, pp. 561–703.

Horobin R.W. (2011) How Romanowsky stains work and why they remain valuable, including a proposed universal Romanowsky staining mechanism and a rational troubleshooting scheme. *Biotech Histochem 86(1)*:36–51.

Jörundsson E., Lumsden J.H., Jacobs R.M. (1999) Rapid staining techniques in cytopathology: A review and comparison of modified protocols for hematoxylin and eosin, Papanicolaou and Romanowsky stains. *Vet Clin Path 28(3)*: 100–108.

Karakitsou V., Christopher M.M., Meletis E. et al. (2022) A comparison of cytologic quality in fine-needle specimens obtained with and without aspiration from superficial lymph nodes in the dog. *J Small An Pract 63*:16–21.

Krafts K.P., Pambuccian S.E. (2011) Romanowsky staining in cytopathology: History, advantages and limitations. *Biotech Histochem 86(2)*:82–93.

Leblanc C.J., Head L.L., Fry M.M. (2009) Comparison of aspiration and non-aspiration techniques for obtaining cytologic samples from the canine and feline spleen. *Vet Clin Path 38*:242–246.

Marrinhas C., Oliveira L.F., Sampaio F. et al. (2022) Needle rinse cell blocks as an ancillary technique: Diagnostic and clinical utility in gastrointestinal neoplasia. *Vet Clin Pathol* (Suppl 1):47–54.

Masserodotti C. (2006) Architectural patterns in cytology: Correlation with histology. *Vet Clin Path 35(4)*:388–396.

Pérez C.C., Rodríguez I., Dorado J. (2005) Use of ultrafast Papanicolaou stain for exfoliative vaginal cytology in bitches. *Vet Rec 156*:648–650.

Reichle J.K., Wisner E.R. (2000) Non-cardiac thoracic ultrasound in 75 feline and canine patients. *Vet Radiol Ultrasound 41*:154–162.

Sawa M., Yabuki A., Miyoshi N. et al. (2012) Rapid-Air-Dry Papanicolaou stain in canine and feline tumor cytology: A quantitative comparison with the Giemsa stain. *J Vet Med Sci 74(9)*:1133–1138.

Toma S., Cornegliani L., Persico P. et al. (2006) Comparison of 4 fixation and staining methods for the cytologic evaluation of ear canals with clinical evidence of ceruminous otitis externa. *Vet Clin Path 35(2)*:194–198.

Watson A.T., Penninck D., Knoll J.S. et al. (2011) Safety and correlation of test results of combined ultrasound-guided fine-needle aspiration and needle core biopsy of the canine spleen. *Vet Radiol Ultrasound 52*:317–322.

Whitlock J., Taeymans O., Monti P. (2020) A comparison of cytological quality between fine-needle aspiration and non-aspiration techniques for obtaining ultrasound-guided samples from canine and feline lymph nodes. *Vet Record 188(6)*: 1–6.

Wood E.F., O'Brien R.T., Young K.M. (1998) Ultrasound-guided fine-needle aspiration of focal parenchymal lesions of the lung in dogs and cats. *J Vet Intern Med 12*:338–342.

Zekas L.J., Crawford J.T., O'Brien R.T. (2005) Computed tomography-guided fine-needle aspirate and tissue-core biopsy of intrathoracic lesions in thirty dogs and cats. *Vet Radiol Ultrasound 46*:200–204.

CHAPTER 2

GENERAL PRINCIPLES OF INFLAMMATION

Amy L. MacNeill

INTRODUCTION

Inflammation is a complex interaction between chemical mediators and cells that occurs when tissue is injured. Inflammatory reactions are designed to eliminate the cause of the injury and repair the damaged tissue. There are five classic signs of inflammation. Celsus, an ancient Roman philosopher, described four signs of inflammation: redness (*rubor*), swelling (*tumor*), heat (*calor*), and pain (*dolor*). Rudolf Virchow added loss of function (*functio laesa*) as a sequela of inflammation. Inflammatory cells (leukocytes) were first described by the Nobel laureate, Ilya Metchnikoff.

Inflammation is initiated when mechanical barriers (skin and mucous membranes) are damaged by trauma or infection. Initially, inflammation is a nonspecific reaction designed to destroy the inciting agent, limit the spread of the injury, and stimulate an acquired immune response. Acquired immunity is more specific and limits repeated injury by agents via recognition of foreign antigens. Inflammation relies on interaction between damaged tissue cells, cell mediators, inflammatory leukocytes, and the blood vascular system. Note that the inflammatory process is critically linked to the blood vascular system; vascular endothelial cells regulate the inflammatory response and blood transports inflammatory mediators and cells to the site of injury. The subsets of inflammatory leukocytes present at the site of injury provide valuable information about what caused the injury, when the injury occurred (acute or chronic), and which medical treatment is most appropriate. A simplified overview of the steps involved in inflammation will be discussed; they include: (1) recognition of injury, (2) acute vascular response, (3) acute cellular response, (4) chronic cellular response, and (5) resolution. The final section of this chapter reviews important diagnostic information that is provided by cytologic evaluation of inflammatory lesions.

RECOGNITION OF INJURY

Initiation of an inflammatory response requires that an inflammatory stimulus be recognized by the body. Endogenous proinflammatory molecules, including cytokines and danger-associated molecular patterns (DAMPs) that are released from dying cells, can stimulate inflammation. Proinflammatory mediators are also derived from extracellular components such as the extracellular matrix and plasma. Exogenous stimuli, including infectious organisms, are commonly recognized by the body by pattern recognition receptors (PRRs) on tissue cells and macrophages, which recognize specific pathogen-associated molecular patterns (PAMPs), and by receptors that recognize the constant region (Fc) of antibodies bound to pathogens. Signaling through these cellular receptors leads to the release of mediators by cells present at the site of injury.

Inflammatory mediators typically have more than one function and can have redundant functions. Mediators often synergize with one another and can have a cascade effect where the action of one mediator depends on previous actions of other mediators. Mediators may have autocrine, paracrine, and/or endocrine effects (Figure 2.1). Importantly, these effects are not antigen specific. Mediators generally exist in inactive forms in the plasma or in intracellular storage pools and are synthesized, released, or activated at the site of injury. They are responsible for hemodynamic and vascular permeability changes that occur during acute inflammation and attract inflammatory leukocytes to the site of injury.

Plasma-derived inflammatory mediators

Kinins

Kinins are potent, slow-acting vasodilators that increase capillary permeability. They mediate pain and produce sustained *rubor*, *calor*, and *dolor* associated with inflammation. They can stimulate the release of

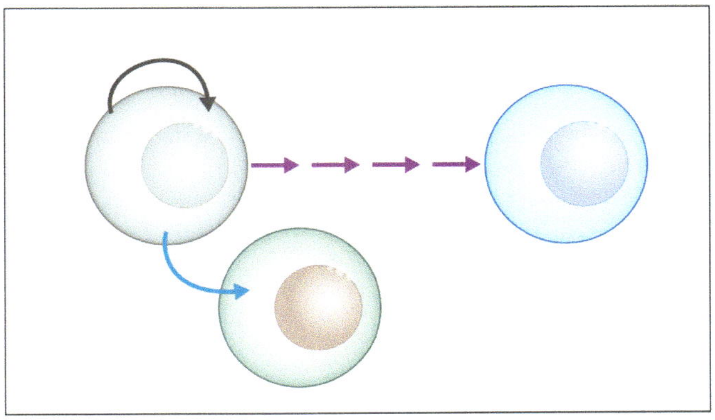

Figure 2.1 Autocrine, paracrine, and endocrine effects. Cell mediators with autocrine effects (gray arrow) signal changes in the same cell that the mediator was secreted from. Paracrine effects (blue arrow) signal nearby cells to alter their function. Endocrine effects (purple arrows) are observed when cell mediators signal changes in distant cells after being secreted into the plasma or extracellular fluids.

DOI: 10.1201/9781003258551-2

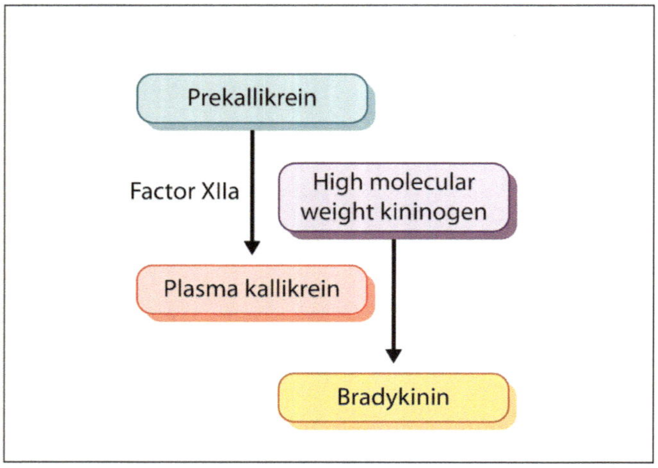

Figure 2.2 **Kinins. Inactive precursor kininogens are cleaved to form active kinins, including bradykinin.**

Table 2.1 Selected acute phase proteins (APPs) in the dog and cat

Positive APPs	Negative APPs
al acid glycoprotein	Albumin
C-reactive protein*	Antithrombin
Complement factors	Transferrin
Haptoglobin	
Hepsidin	
Ferritin	
Fibrinogen	
Fibronectins	
Mannose-binding lectin	
Serum amyloid A*†	

*Major APPs in dogs.
*Major APPs in dogs.
†Major APPs in cats.

histamine and activate the eicosanoid cascade to form leukotrienes and prostaglandins. Kinins are comprised of short peptides derived from plasma protein precursors. Inactive precursor kininogens are broken down by active kallikreins into the shorter, active kinins (Figure 2.2). Bradykinin is the prototype short chain peptide.

Components of the coagulation cascade, including activated Hageman factor (factor XII) and plasmin, can activate pre-kallikreins and initiate production of bradykinin (Del Rosso et al., 2008; Schmaier, 2008). Leukocytes also produce kinins that are similar to bradykinin. Additionally, there are tissue kallikreins, which are released when parenchymal cells are lysed, that bind high molecular weight kininogen and activate it to form bradykinin (Schulze-Topphoff et al., 2008). Kinins are rapidly inactivated by other enzymes in tissues and plasma, especially in the lung, to prevent excessive tissue damage.

Acute phase proteins

When acute injury has occurred in the body, the serum concentrations of acute phase proteins change by >25% during the first few days of an inflammatory response. There is an increase in the concentration of positive acute phase proteins and a decrease in negative acute phase proteins (Table 2.1). Most acute phase proteins are synthesized in the liver. Changes in acute phase protein concentrations reflect the presence and intensity of inflammation and are important diagnostic indicators of inflammation in some species (Figure 2.3). The major responding acute phase protein differs slightly in different species (Eckersall & Bell, 2010).

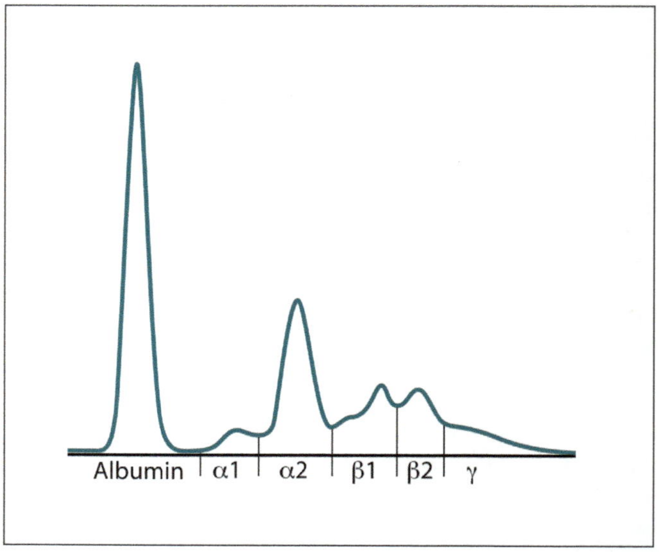

Figure 2.3 **Serum protein electrophoresis tracing. An acute phase protein reaction is occurring with increases in alpha- and beta-globulins.**

FIBRINOGEN

Fibrinogen is a positive acute phase protein. Most fibrinogen is utilized at the site of inflammation. The fibrin that results from cleavage of fibrinogen serves to wall off bacterial agents and form a scaffold for the healing process to begin. Fibrinogen increases erythrocyte aggregation, leading to an increased sedimentation rate, which can also be used as an indicator of inflammation (Késmárky et al., 2008).

Fibronectins

Fibronectins are important positive acute phase reactants. Tissue fibronectins bind fibrocytes and epithelial cells to the extracellular matrix, maintain cell shape, and promote fibroblast growth. Insoluble fibronectins bridge fibrin to cells and promote platelet adhesion (Stoffels et al., 2013). Soluble fibronectins opsonize bacteria to decrease bacterial adherence to tissues and stimulate phagocytosis by inflammatory leukocytes (Butler et al., 1987).

Transferrin and hepsidin

Transferrin and hepsidin are acute phase proteins involved in iron transport. Iron is an essential nutrient for most pathogenic bacteria, so protective mechanisms have developed to sequester iron away from bacteria (Johnson & Wessling-Resnick, 2012). During inflammation, transferrin is downregulated and neutrophils release lactoferrin, which removes iron from iron–transferrin complexes in tissues and produces oxidizing agents that can kill bacteria. Macrophages then take up iron–lactoferrin complexes and sequester iron within ferritin. Hepcidin is a positive acute phase protein that binds to the iron uptake protein of the intestine to prevent iron uptake from the gastrointestinal (GI) tract.

Complement

Complement components are small plasma glycoproteins, mostly synthesized in the liver, that become activated by a series of enzymatic cleavages (Figure 2.4). There are three pathways to complement formation: (1) the mannose-binding lectin pathway, (2) the alternative pathway, and (3) the classical pathway.

The mannose-binding lectin pathway is activated by unique sugars on the surfaces of bacterial and fungal pathogens that are not present on vertebrate cells. Mannose-binding lectins recognize foreign sugars and activate complement components C2 and C4. This leads to the activation of C3 and C5 and the formation of a membrane attack complex (MAC), made up of a complex of C5b, C6, C7, C8, and C9 molecules, which induces cell lysis.

The alternative pathway is microorganism dependent. This pathway protects the host during the early phases of microbial invasion when sufficient antibodies have not yet been produced. The alternative pathway is nonspecific and is activated when C3b binds to a pathogen, preventing plasma proteins from inactivating C3b. Factor B in the plasma binds to C3b. Factor D then cleaves factor B. The cleaved segment of factor B combined with C3b activates additional C3 molecules.

The classical pathway is immune complex dependent. Antibody–antigen (Ab–Ag) complexes bound to an infectious organism activate C1. Activation of C1 leads to the sequential activation of other C proteins in the cascade.

Complement fragments C3a, C4a, and C5a are anaphylatoxins; they mediate histamine release from mast cells, leading to increased vascular permeability. Fragment C5a also is a chemoattractant for neutrophils and increases neutrophil respiratory burst. Complement component C3b opsonizes bacteria to make them more prone to phagocytosis by neutrophils and macrophages. Other C3 fragments can mobilize cells from the bone marrow. Neutrophils and macrophages have receptors for C fragments and are resistant to MAC lysis (Sacks, 2010). Lymphocyte functions are also modified by complement components (Clark & Tenner, 2014).

Cell-derived inflammatory mediators

Vasoactive amines

Vasoactive amines (histamine and serotonin) are stored in mast cells, platelets, and basophils and are secreted extremely early following tissue injury. They initiate the first phase of vascular permeability in the inflammatory response. Vasoactive amines cause dilation of pre-capillary sphincters of arterioles and induce venule and capillary endothelium to round up and develop intercellular gaps that allow fluid to escape (Figure 2.5).

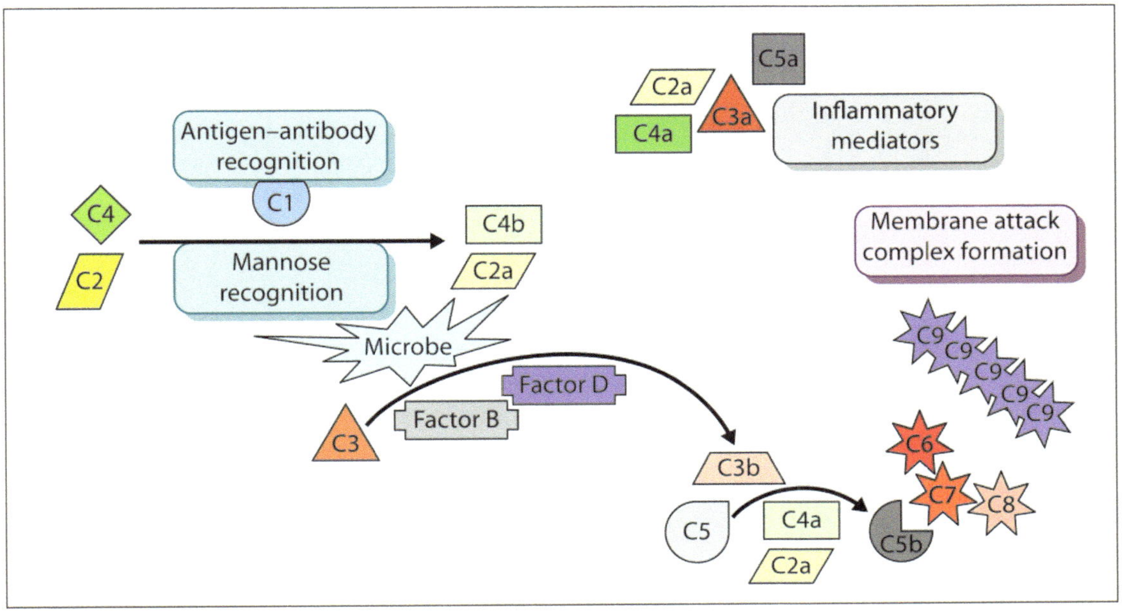

Figure 2.4 Complement cascade. Inactive complement proteins are cleaved by activated complement proteins to form inflammatory mediators and the membrane attack complex.

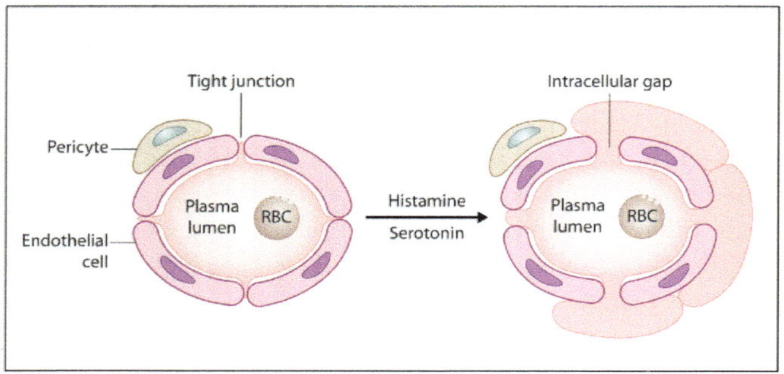

Figure 2.5 **Effect of vasoactive amines on capillaries. Histamine and serotonin induce endothelial cells to round up and develop intercellular gaps that allow fluid to escape.**

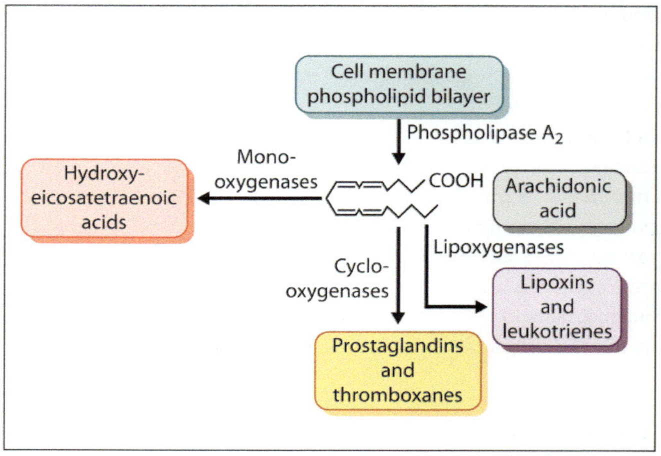

Figure 2.6 **Formation of eicosanoids. Membrane phospholipids are digested by phospholipase A_2 to form arachidonic acid and lysophosphatidylcholine. Mono-oxygenases in the cell process arachidonic acid into hydroxyleicosatetraenoic acids, whereas cyclo-oxygenases produce prostaglandins and thromboxanes and lipoxygenases stimulate the formation of lipoxins and leukotrienes.**

Histamine and serotonin

Histamine induces vasodilation and causes endothelial cells to express adhesion molecules for neutrophils and macrophages. The effects of histamine are short-lived (15–20 minutes) but immensely important for the initiation of inflammation. Serotonin has many of the same physiologic effects as histamine and acts very early during the inflammatory response to mediate smooth muscle contraction and pain. These vasoactive substances are rapidly inactivated (Rutkowski et al., 2012).

Eicosanoids

Eicosanoids are derivatives of arachidonic acid (AA), which is one of the fatty acids released from cell membranes during cell membrane metabolism, injury, or death. Membrane phospholipids are broken down by phospholipases to form free AA and lysophosphatidylcholine (Figure 2.6). AA-derived eicosanoids include prostaglandins, thromboxanes, leukotrienes, lipoxins, and hydroxyeicosatetraenoic acids. The type of eicosanoid produced is dependent on which enzymes mediate the AA breakdown. The enzymes present in a cell are dependent on the cell type.

Prostaglandins and thromboxanes

Prostaglandins are produced by the action of cyclo-oxygenase (COX). Prostaglandin Es (PGEs) are key mediators of inflammation and are produced by macrophages, platelets, and several other cell types. Most PGEs affect vasodilation, increase blood flow, and mediate pain. They also induce the release of neutrophils into the circulation from the bone marrow and peripheral storage pools. Thromboxanes are also produced by COX, mainly in platelets. Thromboxane A_2 acts as a vasoconstrictor and facilitates platelet aggregation.

Leukotrienes

Leukotrienes (LTs) induce leukocytes to move out of blood vessels towards an inflammatory stimulus and are extremely potent mediators of vascular responses. Some forms of LTs are more than 1,000× more potent than histamine (Dahlén et al., 1981). Lipoxygenase initiates the LT cascade and is activated when cytosolic Ca^{2+} levels are elevated. Endotoxin from Gram-negative bacteria can be a potent stimulator of LT production (Rossi et al., 2005). Neutrophils produce a large amount of the precursor form LTA_4 while other cells help to convert LTA_4 to more active forms of LTs. Myeloid cells (neutrophils, eosinophils, and basophils) can produce both LTBs as well as LTC_4, LTD_4, and LTE_4. Nonmyeloid cells (platelets, endothelial cells, Kupffer cells, and hepatocytes) can only synthesize LTC_4, LTD_4, and LTE_4.

Leukotriene B_4 is chemotactic for neutrophils and makes them more adherent to endothelium (Sadik & Luster, 2012). The respiratory burst and release of enzymes by neutrophils are enhanced by LTB_4. Also, immunoglobulin production by B lymphocytes is indirectly stimulated by LTB_4 (Terawaki et al., 2005). Leukotriene B_4, LTC_4, LTD_4, and LTE_4 synergize to increase capillary permeability. In addition, LTC_4, LTD_4, and LTE_4 induce airway smooth muscle contraction in asthma and anaphylaxis in certain species.

LIPOXINS

Lipoxins are produced later in the inflammatory response and tend to have anti-inflammatory properties (reducing granulocyte recruitment). Lipoxins are important in the induction of the resolution phase of inflammation and promotion of repair (Serhan et al., 2008a).

HYDROXYEICOSATETRAENOIC ACIDS

Hydroxyeicosatetraenoic acids (HETEs) regulate vasoconstriction in many tissues. Alterations in HETEs have been associated with vascular diseases including ischemia and hypertension, indicating that these eicosanoids are important in cardiovascular function (Miyata &

Roman, 2005). They may also play a role in cancer biology (Panigraphy et al., 2010).

Platelet activating factor

When phospholipase A_2 cleaves AA from phospholipids, platelet activating factor (PAF) is formed. PAF is produced by leukocytes, platelets, and vascular endothelium. It causes platelets and leukocytes to aggregate and adhere to vascular endothelium, inducing leukocytes to marginate and become pavemented to the endothelial surface. PAF causes leukocytes to release enzymes and free radicals. It also has a role in increasing vascular permeability (Uhlig et al., 2005).

Reactive oxygen species

Reactive oxygen species are by-products of oxidative metabolism and are produced by nearly all cells. Reactive oxygen intermediates (ROIs) include O_2^- and OH^- (free radicals), which cause harmful effects to cells through DNA damage, lipid peroxidation, the oxidation of proteins, the oxidation of enzymatic co-factors, and the release of inflammatory cytokines. Cells have several defenses against ROIs. Superoxide dismutases, catalase, glutathione peroxidase, lactoperoxidase, peroxiredoxins, and α_1-microglobulin enzymatically reduce ROIs and prevent oxidative damage to cells (Bartz & Piantadosi, 2010). Other antioxidants in the body include vitamins C and E, uric acid, glutathione, and polyphenol antioxidants, which neutralize harmful free radicals.

CYTOKINES

Cytokines are small proteins produced by all nucleated cells, particularly leukocytes. They provide an important way for cells to communicate, limit injury, and drive an appropriate immune response. These molecules have been subdivided based on molecular structure and biologic activities. Types of cytokines include interferons, interleukins, chemokines, mesenchymal growth factors, the tumor necrosis factor (TNF) family of proteins, and adipokines.

INTERFERONS

Type I interferons (IFNa and IFNβ) are produced by all cell types and are particularly important in cellular defense against viral infection. Expression of type I IFNs is triggered by virus infection, PAMPs, and proinflammatory cytokines. Type I IFNs are expressed by a virus-infected cell to inhibit intracellular viral protein synthesis by inhibiting the translation of viral proteins, degrading viral mRNAs, and inhibiting RNA synthesis (Gibbert et al., 2013). They are also secreted to stimulate type I IFN expression by adjacent cells. This protects neighboring cells from viral infection and inhibits virus spread.

Type II IFNs (e.g. IFNγ) are produced by T helper 1 (Th1)-type T cells and conventional innate lymphoid cells (ILCs, aka conventional natural killer [cNK] cells), which are components of a cell-mediated immune response. IFNγ induces inflammatory cells to express Fc and C3b receptors, which enhance phagocytosis of organisms opsonized by antibodies and C3b, respectively. IFNγ is the most important mediator for activating macrophages and stimulates nitric oxide (NO) synthetase so that macrophages can produce NO. IFNγ also induces the synthesis of antiprotozoal enzymes (Zhao et al., 2009). IFNγ stimulates ILC subsets to infiltrate into an area infected by a virus and kill the virus-infected cells. Additionally, IFNγ enhances major histocompatibility (MHC) class II Ag processing and recognition.

Type III IFNs (e.g. IFNλ) also have important antiviral functions, but receptors for these cytokines are predominantly found on epithelial cells. Type III IFNs may also play a role in the differentiation of hematopoietic cells (Rauch et al., 2013).

INTERLEUKINS

Interleukins (ILs) were classically defined as cytokines that are secreted by one leukocyte to affect other leukocytes; however, it is now known that many cell types produce these mediators. Some of the more well-known ILs are listed in Table 2.2. Over 30 ILs have been characterized.

Activated macrophages produce several key proinflammatory cytokines (Ferrante & Leibovich, 2012). For example, IL-1 stimulates the synthesis of acute phase proteins by the liver, causes the endothelium to express adhesion molecules and promote coagulation, stimulates neutrophil migration, affects the hypothalamus (producing fever), stimulates PG production and the respiratory burst of neutrophils, and acts synergistically with IFNγ and IL-2 to enhance inflammation and the immune response. IL-1 also stimulates the resorption of bone and cartilage by stimulating osteoclasts. This role of IL-1 may partially explain the hypercalcemia that is seen with some chronic granulomatous diseases. IL-1 is important for granuloma formation and enhances the size and persistence of these inflammatory lesions. Bacterial endotoxin is a very potent stimulator of IL-1. Like IL-1, IL-6 is a key mediator of acute phase protein synthesis by hepatocytes.

Table 2.2 **Selected interleukins and their primary functions**

Interleukin	Primary function
IL-1	Fever, T-cell, and macrophage (M1) activation
IL-6	Acute phase protein production
IL-12	IFNγ production, cell proliferation, innate lymphoid cell, and T-cell cytotoxicity
IL-2	T-cell proliferation
IL-15	T-cell proliferation
IL-10	Suppresses M1 functions
IL-13	Inhibits M1 cytokine production
TGFβ	Inhibits cell growth
IL-5	Eosinophil chemotaxis
IL-8 (CXCL8)	Neutrophil chemotaxis

It also triggers immunoglobulin synthesis by B lymphocytes. IL-12 is often released by macrophages with IL-1 and IL-6. This cytokine induces differentiation of naïve T lymphocytes into Th1 cells; stimulates the proliferation, maintenance, and activation of Th1 lymphocytes and cNK cells; stimulates the production of IFNγ, IL-2, and TNF; and inhibits the development of Th2 cells.

CHEMOKINES

Chemokines are promiscuous in that they can bind several G-protein-coupled receptors and function either as homeostatic or chemotactic proteins (Martins-Green et al., 2013). There are four classes of chemokines: CC chemokines, CXC chemokines, C chemokines, and CX_3C chemokines. The chemokine CXCL8 (IL-8) is particularly important for neutrophil chemotaxis. It is produced by many cell types (e.g. neutrophils, macrophages, keratinocytes, airway smooth muscle cells, endothelial cells). It induces chemotaxis and phagocytosis by neutrophils and is pro-angiogenic (Baggiolini & Clark-Lewis, 1992).

Mesenchymal growth factors

Mesenchymal growth factors are cytokines that are extremely important for hematopoiesis. Erythropoietin, thrombopoietin, and colony-stimulating factors are included in this category of cytokines.

Tumor necrosis factors

The most well-characterized member of the TNF family of cytokines is TNFα. This protein induces apoptosis in some cells it interacts with, while other cells are stimulated to proliferate and differentiate. TNFα is a potent stimulator of acute phase protein production by the liver. It is associated with fever via the stimulation of IL-1 secretion and cachexia associated with chronic inflammatory diseases. TNFs induce endothelial cell dysfunction, leading to thrombosis, inflammation, and increased vascular permeability (Zhang et al., 2009). They also stimulate leukocyte functions.

ADIPOKINES

Adipokines are released by adipocytes and several other cell types. Adipokines include leptin, adiponectin, and resistin, among others (Lee et al., 2013). Leptin is critical for food satiation and induces Th1 immune responses. Adiponectin increases insulin sensitivity and may have anti-inflammatory functions. Resistin is an important factor in the development of insulin resistance and also promotes Th1 responses.

LYSOSOMAL ENZYMES

Lysosomal enzymes contained within leukocyte granules are very important immune mediators and are critical for the removal of pathogens and cellular debris. Each leukocyte cell type contains slightly different lysosomal enzymes. Important enzymes in mast cells include chymase and tryptase. Neutrophils contain myeloperoxidase, defensins, elastase, lactoferrin, and many proteases. Eosinophils and basophils have major basic protein, which is important for antiparasitic defense mechanisms. Macrophages contain β-glucuronidase, β-galactosidase, acid hydrolases, and many other mediators.

DEFENSINS

Defensins are peptide mediators made by many cell types of both animals and plants. They are host defense peptides that have antibacterial, antifungal, and antiviral properties. They often function by forming pores in microbial cell membranes that lyse the organism.

Cells involved in the recognition of injury

Epithelial cells

Epithelial cells recognize inflammatory stimuli through the expression of several transmembrane receptors, including PRRs (Fukata & Arditi, 2013; Salazar & Ghaemmaghami, 2013). They initiate inflammatory responses by releasing soluble proteins including eicosanoids and ROIs. They also secrete several cytokines when they are injured or infected. Many of these mediators attract leukocytes to the area including IL-16, granulocyte colony-stimulating factor, granulocyte monocyte colony-stimulating factor (GM-CSF), and several chemokines (e.g. CCL2, CXCL8, CCL11).

Mast cells

Mast cells are one of the first cell types involved in the inflammatory response because they are already present in the tissue and are close to the site of injury. Mast cells are bone marrow derived, but differentiate within connective tissues. They are found in small numbers in the skin, respiratory tract, and GI tract as well as around vessels and peripheral nerves.

The morphologic characteristics of mast cells are very distinctive if the mast cell granules stain well. In cytology samples, mast cells have abundant, rounded cytoplasm that is filled with metachromatic (pinkish-violet) granules and a large, rounded nucleus (20–60 μm in diameter), which is often centrally located in the cell (Figures 2.7–2.9). The granules are metachromatic due to the heparin they contain. With toluidine blue or Giemsa stains, the granules will stain bright pinkish-violet, whereas with other Romanowski stains (e.g. Diff-Quik® stain), the granules may be nonstaining, which makes it difficult to distinguish mast cells from other round cells. Two cytologic details can help with the identification of mast cells that lack well-stained granules: (1) unlike some other round cells, the mast cell nucleus is typically in the center of the cell, and (2) mast cells commonly attract eosinophils, which can be seen in the background of the sample.

Mast cell granules contain preformed heparin, histamine, serotonin, eosinophil chemotactic factor, PAF, tryptase, and more (Pohlman, 2010). Granules are released in response to proinflammatory molecules including C fragments, cytokines, and foreign

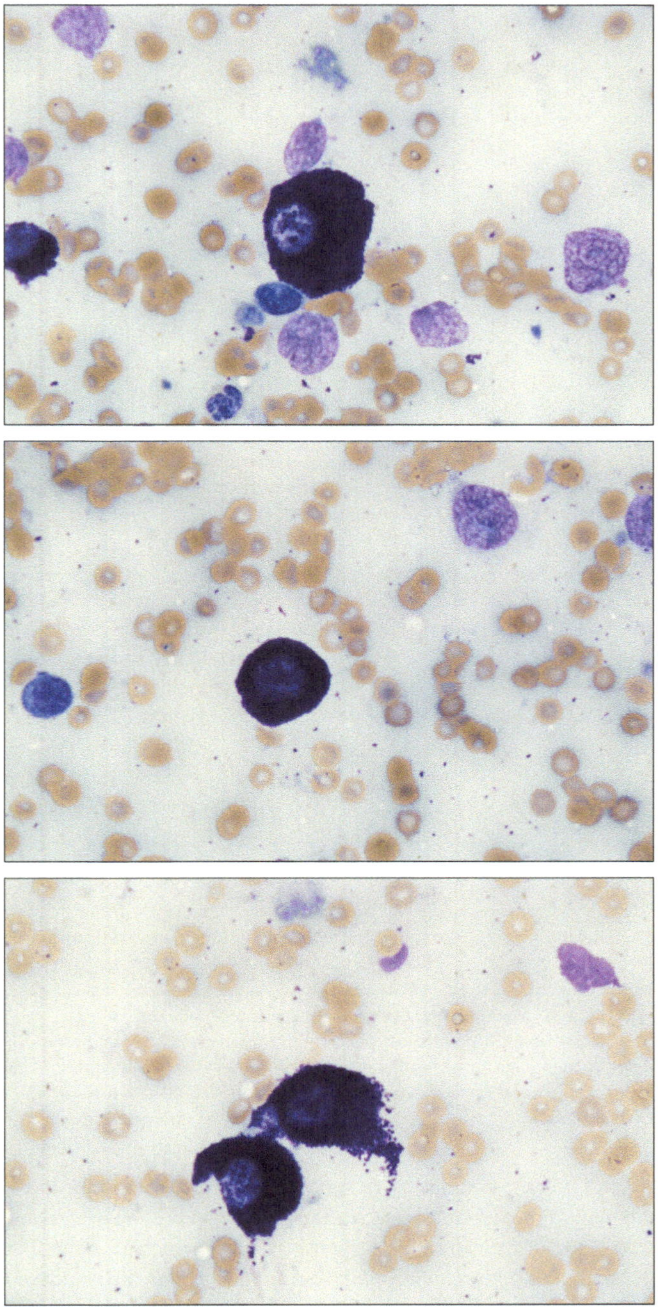

Figures 2.7–2.9 **Mast cells. Mast cells are individualized, round cells with abundant cytoplasm and a round nucleus. The cytoplasm is usually filled with small, metachromatic granules (Wright–Giemsa, 1,000× magnification).**

substances. Mast cell receptors for inflammatory stimuli include immunoglobulin E receptors (FceRI), PRRs, and complement receptors. Mast cells are not killed when they degranulate; instead, they are partially regulated by macrophages and endothelial cells, which ingest and degrade released granule contents (Kokkonen & Kovanen, 1989; Wang et al., 1996).

Additional mast cell functions include the production of PGs and LTs that attract leukocytes to the site of injury. Mast cells are associated with inflammatory reactions involving parasite infections and type I hypersensitivity reactions, including anaphylactic reactions. Mast cells have a regulatory role on eosinophils; they produce IL-5, which is the major cytokine that affects the differentiation, activation, and maintenance of eosinophils, and primes eosinophils for the effects of other cytokines.

PLATELETS

Platelets are a key component of coagulation and have an active role in inflammation. Platelets are fragments of cytoplasm that are smaller than erythrocytes (Figures 2.10, 2.11). They frequently aggregate and accumulate at sites of inflammation. Platelets have Fc and C3 receptors (Hamad et al., 2010; Berlacher et al., 2013). They are activated by collagen to release several inflammatory mediators including agents that increase vascular permeability (e.g. serotonin, histamine, and LTs), complement activators, PAF, and coagulation factors. Platelets interact extensively with neutrophils. For example, platelets convert the LTA_4 released from neutrophils to LTC_4, LTD_4, and LTE_4 (Tornhamre et al., 1998).

Resident histiocytes

Monocytes that enter the tissues when no inflammation is present will differentiate into histiocytic macrophages, which often localize near endothelial cells. These are termed Kupffer cells along the space of Disse in the liver, alveolar macrophages and pulmonary intravascular macrophages in the lung (Figure 2.12), and Langerhans cells in epithelial tissue. They can also localize to lymphoid organs (Figure 2.13). Resident macrophages have varying functions including the removal of dead cells and debris associated with tissue remodeling. These macrophage functions do not typically induce an inflammatory response, but histiocytes can become activated when stimulated by proinflammatory mediators.

Dendritic cells (DCs) are specialized histiocytes that reside in tissues. Conventional DCs are important antigen-presenting cells (APCs) and plasmacytoid DCs secrete large numbers of inflammatory mediators. Many subtypes of DCs have been isolated and described; these cells help direct the specific immune response to individual pathogens.

VASCULAR RESPONSE

The vascular response to an injury is essential to the development of inflammation. Trauma can cause transient vasoconstriction. Arteriolar dilation then occurs, which increases blood flow into the area. Pre-capillary sphincters open to allow capillary beds and venules to fill with blood resulting in hyperemia. At the same time, the permeability of the vasculature in the area of injury is altered and plasma proteins leak out of the vessels, causing edema. One reason for the edema is increased hydrostatic pressure from the increased blood flow. Endothelial changes also occur that permit large molecules and leukocytes to exit through gaps between endothelial cells. These changes are caused directly by injury to the endothelium and

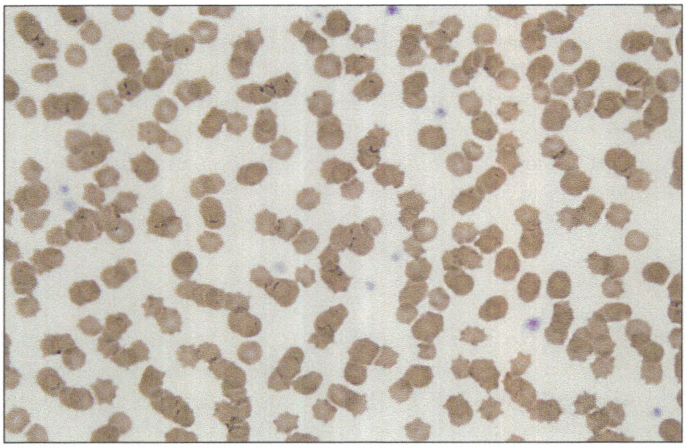
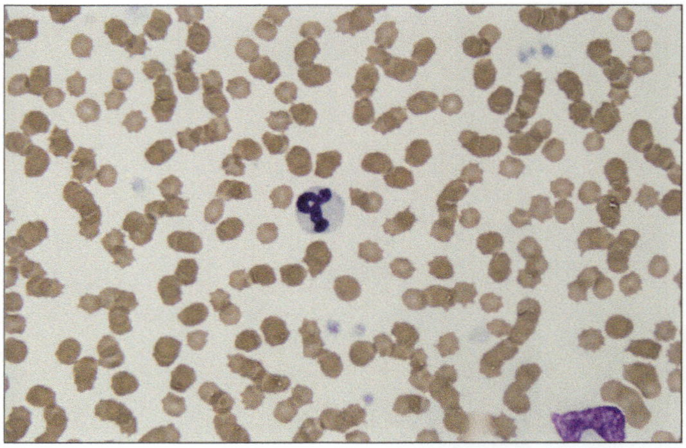

Figures 2.10, 2.11 Platelets. Peripheral blood smear from a 13-year-old, spayed female domestic shorthair cat. Mammalian platelets are lightly basophilic to eosinophilic, anucleated, cytoplasmic fragments. They are typically smaller than erythrocytes. Several erythrocytes are seen in these images for size comparison. A segmented neutrophil and a monocyte are also present in 2.11 (Wright–Giemsa, 1,000× magnification).

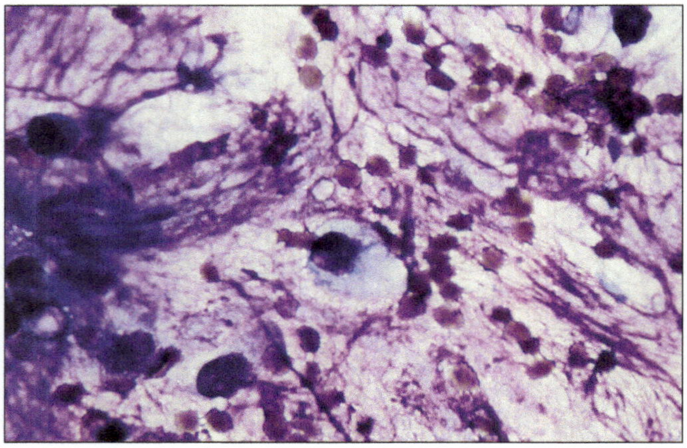

Figure 2.12 Alveolar macrophage. Transtracheal wash from a 9-year-old, spayed female Shih Tzu. An intact macrophage is shown (center) entrapped in a large amount of mucus. The macrophage has abundant, pale basophilic cytoplasm and an eccentrically located, rounded nucleus. There are several erythrocytes and a few ruptured nucleated cells present in the background (Wright–Giemsa, 1,000× magnification).

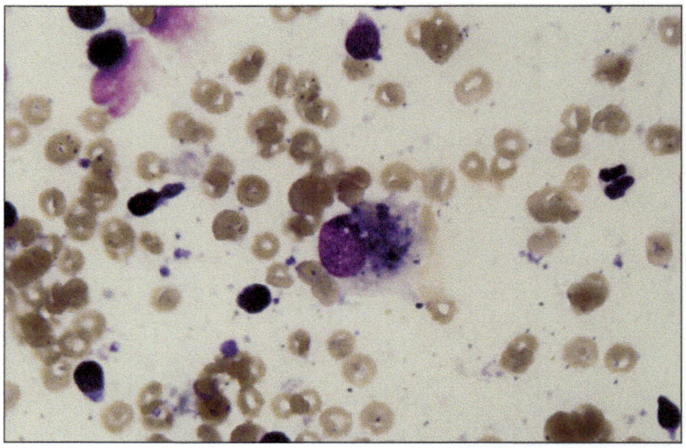

Figure 2.13 Macrophage. Lymph node aspirate from a dog. A macrophage containing phagocytized cellular material is present at the center of the image. Low numbers of small lymphocytes, a neutrophil (right), and several erythrocytes are also present (Wright–Giemsa, 1,000× magnification).

indirectly by mediators released by mast cells, by injured cells in the area, or by activated inflammatory leukocytes.

CELLULAR RESPONSE

Acute cellular response

Once vascular dilation occurs, an acute cellular response to an inflammatory stimulus can begin. An early leukocyte response to inflammation is the increased release of neutrophils from the marginating pool in blood vessels and the storage pool in the bone marrow into the circulating pool in the bloodstream. This can be transiently mediated by epinephrine and corticosteroids (Webb & Latimer, 2011a). Glucocorticoids also cause mild, transient lymphopenia and eosinopenia. After the initial response, inflammatory mediators (including ILs and colony-stimulating factors) promote the division and differentiation of progenitor cells in the marrow and drive a persistent leukocytosis. Typically, this response results in increased numbers of circulating mature neutrophils and monocytes. If the response is severe, band neutrophils may be released by the bone marrow, resulting in neutrophilia with a left shift (Figure 2.14). If the stimulus is overwhelming, a neutropenia may occur as the neutrophils are rapidly consumed at the site of inflammation and the marrow response to inflammatory mediators is unable to meet demand. An eosinophilia may be induced by parasitic or allergic inflammation, whereas a lymphocytosis can be seen with more chronic antigenic stimulation and viral infection. Leukocytes move from the bloodstream into inflamed tissues by adhering to endothelium then migrating by diapedesis between cell junctions in the capillary walls (Figure 2.15). They follow a gradient of chemical mediators to the site of an inflammatory

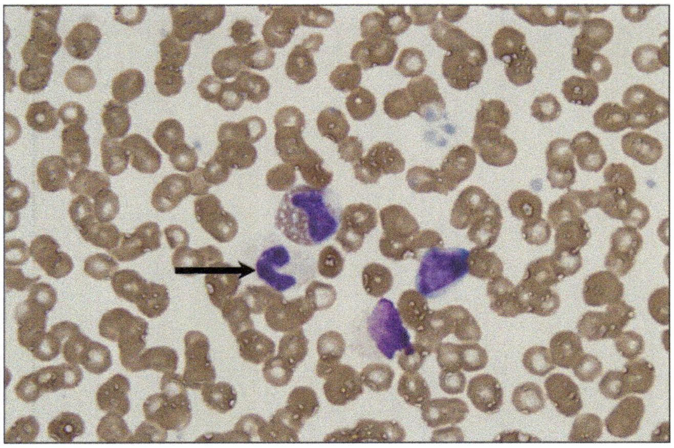

Figure 2.14 **Immature granulocytes in circulation. Peripheral blood from a 10-year-old, intact male mixed-breed dog. A band neutrophil (arrow) and a band eosinophil (upper center) are shown. A small lymphocyte (right), a lysed nucleated cell (lower center), platelets, and erythrocytes are also present (Wright–Giemsa, 1,000× magnification).**

stimulus. Adherence/adhesion of leukocytes to endothelial cells has a reversible and an irreversible phase.

Reversible adherence occurs as vascular changes and inflammatory mediators cause the cells to marginate toward vessel walls. Blood flow through affected tissue is slowed by vasodilation, allowing leukocytes to interact with the endothelium and adhere to it. This is mediated by endothelial cell expression of P-selectin in response to histamine, thrombin, PAF, and other mediators. P-selectin is pre-formed in endothelial granules called Weibel–Palade bodies. Within 2 or 4 hours, the endothelium expresses E-selectin in response to TNFα or IL-1, respectively (Wyble et al., 1997). Leukocytes express P-selectin glycoprotein ligand 1 (PSGL-1), which interacts with endothelial selectins. Binding of PSGL-1 to P-selectin initiates rolling. Binding to E-selectin slows down rolling (Choi et al., 2009). Leukocytes also express L-selectin, which recognizes mucosal addressin cell adhesion molecules on high endothelial venules in the intestine and other sites (Ogawa et al., 2005). Similarly, L-selectin recognizes glycosylation-dependent cell adhesion molecules in vessels of lymph nodes, mammary glands, the uterus, and lung (Hemmerich et al., 1994). If there is no further activation of the leukocytes or endothelium by mediators, then selectins are shed by the leukocytes and recycled by the endothelium, and the leukocytes return to circulation. If further stimulation occurs, an irreversible process called pavementing occurs. This is induced by continued IL-1 and TNFα stimulation and is mediated by β2-integrins (CD11/CD18) on leukocytes and intracellular adhesion molecule 1 on endothelial cells (Dimasi et al., 2013; Figure 2.16).

Diapedesis begins when platelet/endothelial-cell adhesion molecule (PECAM-1) and junctional adhesion molecules (JAMs) on leukocytes bind to PECAM-1 and JAMs expressed within endothelial junctions (Dimasi et al., 2013). This occurs at postcapillary venules and sometimes capillaries. Neutrophils are particularly good at extravasation and they are the first to get into a site of inflammation. Monocyte/macrophage migration through the endothelium is partially dependent on initial neutrophil migration (Soehnlein et al., 2009).

Chemotaxis enables leukocytes to migrate to the site of an inflammatory stimulus. A chemoattractant binds to its receptor on the leukocyte cell membrane. This is followed by changes in membrane fluidity that allow the leukocyte to send out long pseudopodia. The front end of the cell then moves toward the stimulus, and the rest of the cytoplasm is pulled along by contraction of actin and myosin (Weninger et al., 2014).

The first cell types recruited to an inflammatory lesion are often granulocytes, specifically neutrophils and/or eosinophils. Basophils are also granulocytes, but they are rarely observed in an inflammatory response; if they are present, they are typically associated with chronic inflammation. Granulocytes, or polymorphonuclear cells,

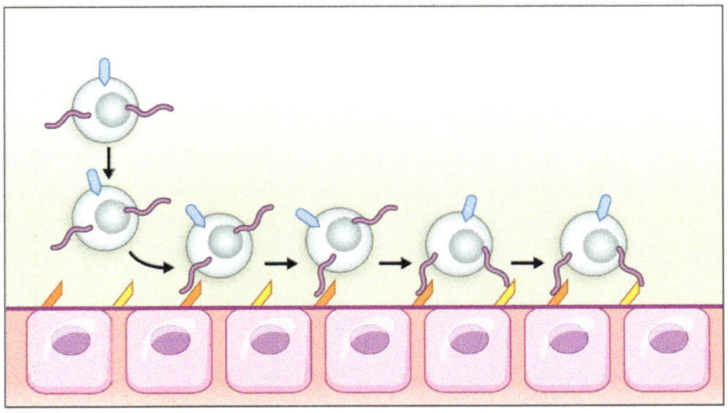

Figure 2.15 **Diapedesis. During an inflammatory event, leukocytes are triggered to alter the expression of cell surface proteins and follow a gradient of chemical mediators to the site of an inflammatory stimulus. During this process, leukocytes adhere to endothelial cells. Purple lines indicate P-selectin glycoprotein ligand 1 (PSGL-1), expressed by leukocytes. Orange structures are endothelial P-selectins, which allow for leukocyte rolling on binding PGSL-1. Yellow structures are endothelial E-selectin, which slows leukocyte rolling. Teal structures on the leukocytes are β2-integrins, utilized in pavementing and illustrated in Figure 2.16. (Courtesy Veronica Kinn.)**

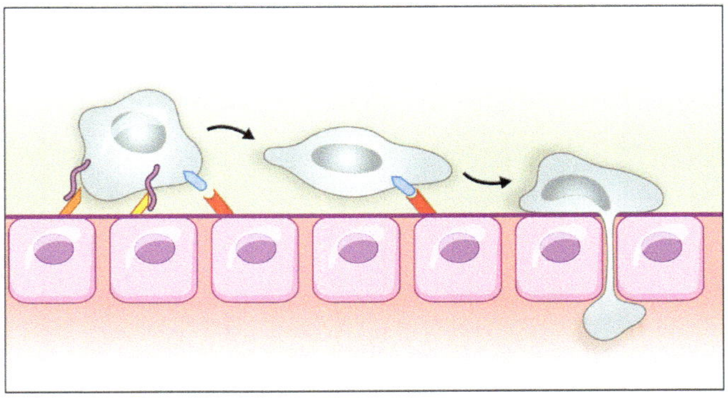

Figure 2.16 **Pavementing is an irreversible process of leukocyte adherence to endothelial cells that leads to the migration of leukocytes between cell junctions in the capillary walls and toward a site of inflammation. It is induced by continued IL-1 and TNFα stimulation and mediated by β2-integrins (CD11/CD18) on leukocytes (teal structures) and intracellular adhesion molecule 1 on endothelial cells (red structures). (Courtesy Veronica Kinn.)**

have a lobed or segmented nucleus and contain cytoplasmic granules with various characteristics, due to their contents. The staining characteristics of the granules are the basis for the names of the different granulocytes. Neutrophils contain three types of granules (azurophil granules, specific granules, and tertiary granules); all are neutral staining or nonstaining with Romanowski stains. Eosinophil granules take up eosins to stain bright red or orange. Basophil granules take up basophilic stains to stain dark blue. Granulocytes are terminally differentiated and have short half-lives. Granulocytes normally circulate in the blood with neutrophils being the most common, eosinophils less common, and basophils rare.

NEUTROPHILS

Most types of injury cause the release of mediators that are chemotactic for neutrophils. The primary chemokine that draws neutrophils to a site is CXCL8 (IL-8). Large numbers of neutrophils may accumulate in one area and form pus. Neutrophils are 10–12 μm in diameter and have a highly segmented nucleus (Figure 2.17). The number of nuclear segments can vary in segmented neutrophils. Neutrophils with fewer than two segments are considered immature, band neutrophils (Figure 2.18). Those with more than five segments are termed hypersegmented neutrophils, and are near the end of their life span (Figure 2.19). If not activated to migrate into tissues, neutrophils will die via apoptosis about 10 hours after release into the circulation. If activated to migrate into tissues, neutrophils will live for 1–2 days (Webb & Latimer, 2011b). When activated, neutrophils move rapidly by ameboid motion and are intensely phagocytic.

A key function of neutrophils is to phagocytize foreign material or injurious agents and neutralize them (van Kessel et al., 2014). Neutrophils send out processes that surround and enclose the offending particle in a vacuole. They utilize Fc and C receptors to detect Ab–Ag complexes and complement proteins on the surface of a particle,

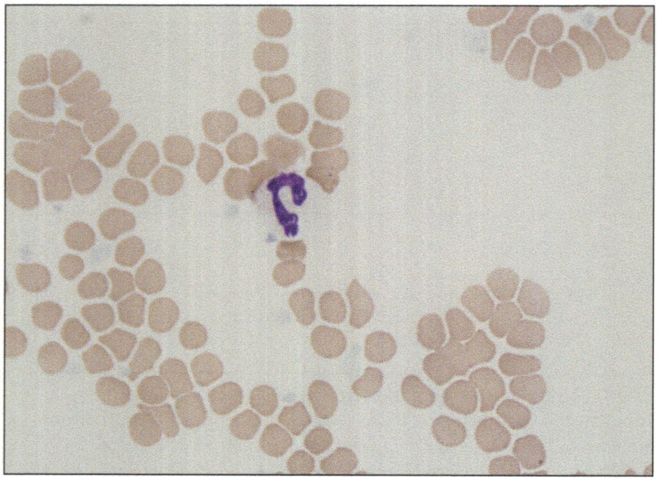

Figure 2.17 Segmented neutrophil. Peripheral blood from a 10-year-old, intact male mixed-breed dog. The neutrophil is mature with nonstaining cytoplasm and a segmented nucleus with dense chromatin (Wright–Giemsa, 1,000× magnification).

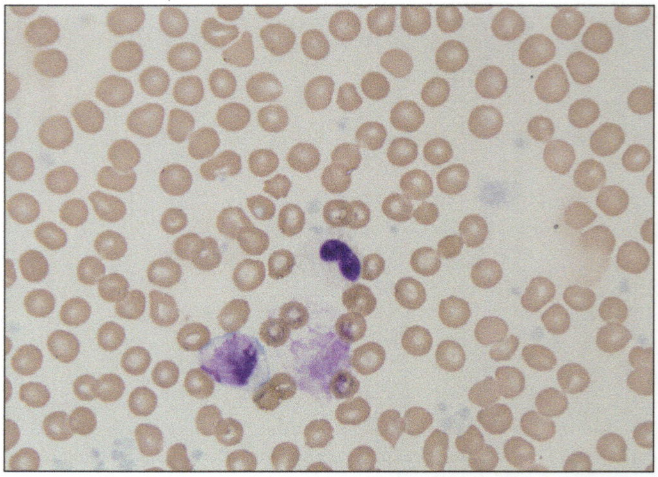

Figure 2.18 Band neutrophil. Peripheral blood from a 10-year-old, intact male mixed-breed dog. The neutrophil is immature with nonstaining cytoplasm that is speckled with small pink primary granules. The nucleus is horseshoe-shaped and has dense chromatin and a dark, round chromocenter (Wright–Giemsa, 1,000× magnification).

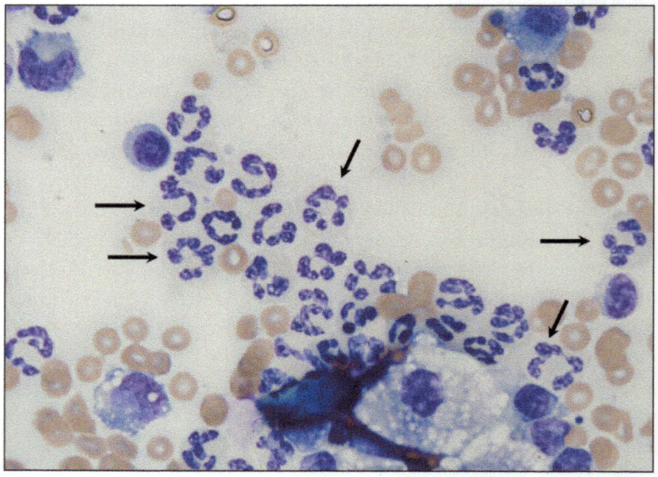

Figure 2.19 Hypersegmented neutrophils. Synovial fluid from an 8-year-old, neutered male Labrador Retriever. Several neutrophils and lower numbers of large mononuclear cells are present. Neutrophils have segmented nuclei with crisp edges and dense chromatin. Neutrophil nuclei with more than five segments are considered hypersegmented (examples indicated by arrows) (Wright–Giemsa, 1,000× magnification).

respectively. These receptors are upregulated by inflammatory mediators. The phagocytized material stimulates a respiratory burst by the neutrophil. During this process, the phagocytic vacuole fuses with a neutrophil lysosome to begin degrading the particle. If the neutrophil cannot ingest the particle, it will release its lysosomal enzymes out onto the surface of the particle, which can inadvertently digest and harm the surrounding tissues. Elastases, collagenases, and gelatinase released by neutrophils are especially damaging because they destroy the stromal framework of the tissue.

The respiratory burst is essential for killing bacterial and fungal agents by the neutrophil. First there is a dramatic increase in respiratory activity due to an increase in O_2 consumption. The enzyme NADPH oxidase in the membrane of the phagocytic vacuole converts O_2 to O_2^- (superoxide anion). This molecule is toxic and reacts with water to form H_2O_2. If iron is present, hydroxyl radicals are generated. Lactoferrin in the specific granules of neutrophils serves as a source of iron for this reaction. Azurophil and tertiary granules contain cytochrome b, which also generates free radicals. Additionally, myeloperoxidase (MPO) is present (mainly in azurophil granules) and converts Cl^- ions to oxidizing agents.

Another way neutrophils eliminate pathogens is through the formation of neutrophil extracellular traps (NETs, Nauseef & Borregaard, 2014). NETs are comprised of DNA, proteins, and granule constituents that are released from neutrophils following NETosis, a type of programmed cell death for neutrophils, which occurs in response to neutrophil receptors binding PAMPs and certain inflammatory mediators. Neutrophils can either actively release NETs from their cytoplasm or can depolarize and rupture, subsequently releasing NETs (Papayannopoulos, 2018). These form a fibrillar matrix, which entraps bacteria, yeast, and other pathogens. Neutrophil extracellular traps are effective at killing bacteria. They also limit the spread of released granule constituents to minimize tissue damage.

Neutrophils also stimulate the inflammatory response by generating kinins, PGs, LTs, PAF, chemotaxins, and many cytokines. They cleave complement as well as activating mast cells and platelets to release histamine. Neutrophil granule proteins promote synthesis of monocyte-attracting chemokines by endothelial cells and macrophages. Dying neutrophils also attract monocytes/macrophages.

EOSINOPHILS

Eosinophils are typically present in allergen- and parasite-mediated inflammatory reactions. Eosinophils are particularly good at activating mast cells. Another major function of the eosinophil is to regulate acute hypersensitivity reactions. Eosinophils are 12–15 µm in diameter and have a segmented nucleus and several large, brightly eosinophilic, cytoplasmic granules (Figure 2.20). A major component of eosinophil granules is eosinophil major basic protein (MBP). This protein kills parasites by creating pores in the cuticle of the organism. Tissue damage by MBP is prevented by ingestion of the protein by mast cells. Reciprocally, MBP neutralizes heparin secreted by mast cells. Eosinophils also contain per-oxidases, eosinophil cationic protein, and other degradative enzymes (Acharya & Ackerman, 2014).

Eosinophils are attracted to inflammatory sites where cells are secreting IL-5, which is the major mediator affecting eosinophil production and activation. It is produced by mast cells, Th2 lymphocytes, and eosinophils. Eosinophils are ameboid and phagocytic, like neutrophils, but they are more selective in their responses to chemotactic stimuli. Eosinophils are stimulated by antibody–antigen complexes and histamine. However, they are not as responsive to complement. Eosinophils can reside in tissues for several days to weeks.

Large mononuclear cells

Monocytes, macrophages, and DCs are histiocytic cells. Monocytes are present in the peripheral blood. Once they migrate through

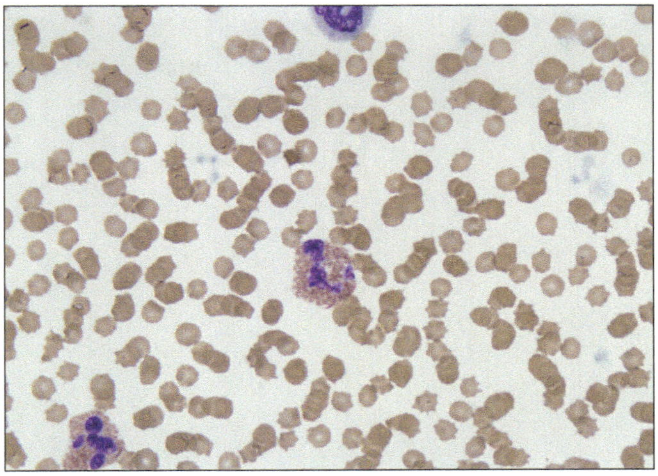

Figure 2.20 **Eosinophil. Peripheral blood smear from a 13-year-old, spayed female domestic shorthair cat. Two eosinophils are shown, in the bottom left and in the center of the image. The cell has abundant cytoplasm, filled with eosinophilic granules. The nucleus is segmented and has dense chromatin (Wright–Giemsa, 1,000× magnification).**

the endothelium, they begin to differentiate into macrophages. Macrophages migrate to the site of injury after neutrophils, partly because their migration is enhanced by the extravasation of neutrophils through the endothelium. Released neutrophil granule proteins anchor on endothelial proteoglycans and are adhered to by monocytes rolling along the endothelium (Soehnlein et al., 2009). Macrophages take about 24 hours to accumulate in the lesion. If the agent becomes persistent, then the macrophage will become a prominent cell type in the lesion. Unlike granulocytes, macrophages can enter a tissue site and divide there (Weiss & Souza, 2010). Macrophages regulate inflammatory responses and clean up damaged cellular and microbial debris, making them very important for preparing the site for healing and repair. DCs tend to reside in tissues and play a major role in directing the immune response to injury.

Monocytes have an oval to bean-shaped nucleus and gray–blue cytoplasm with small vacuoles and occasional granules (Figure 2.21). These cells are 15–20 µm in diameter. Tissue macrophages have a more pleiomorphic morphology. They tend to have a large round to oval nucleus, abundant blue–gray cytoplasm, and vacuoles (Figure 2.22). Macrophages can be up to 80 µm in diameter and can be swollen and filled with phagocytized debris (Figure 2.23). They can have an epithelioid morphology, making sheets of macrophages difficult to differentiate from epithelial cells (Figure 2.24). Additionally, macrophages can fuse together and become multinucleated giant cells (Figures 2.25, 2.26). Multinucleated giant cells tend to occur when large, hard-to-digest foreign bodies are encountered or when there is chronic infection.

If there is inflammation present when the monocyte leaves the vasculature, it differentiates into an active inflammatory macrophage (M1), which is microbicidal, proinflammatory, and phagocytic (Ferrante & Leibovich, 2012). IL-12 and IFNγ help to activate histiocytes to become the typical inflammatory macrophage. Recognition of PAMPs and DAMPs is also an important trigger for M1 activation. If other cytokines (IL-4 and IL-13 produced by Th2 lymphocytes) are

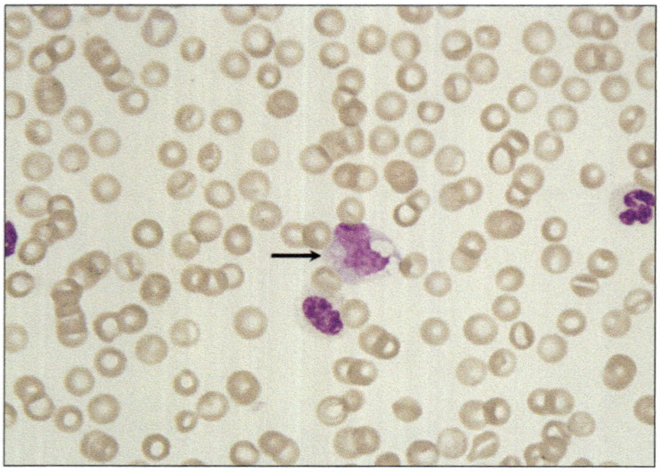

Figure 2.21 Monocyte. Peripheral blood smear from a dog. The monocyte has abundant basophilic cytoplasm that contains several distinct cytoplasmic vacuoles and has an irregularly shaped nucleus with slightly open chromatin (arrow) (Wright–Giemsa stain, 1,000× magnification).

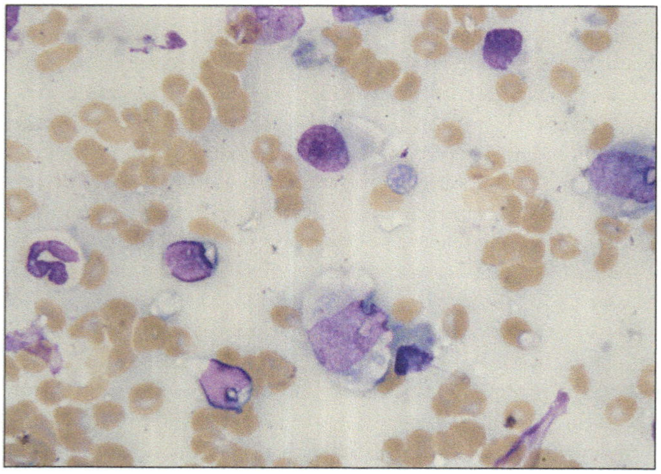

Figure 2.22 Tissue macrophage. FNA from a mass on the ear pinna of an 8-year-old, neutered male Boxer. A mixture of inflammatory cells was observed. A mildly degenerate neutrophil is shown at the left of the image. Three lymphocytes with scant cytoplasm and a smooth, round nucleus are present. The lymphocytes are smaller than the neutrophil. The three cells that are larger than the neutrophil are macrophages (two in the center and one to the far right in the image). Macrophages have abundant, lightly basophilic cytoplasm and a round to oval nucleus. The nuclei of macrophages typically have more stippled chromatin than lymphocyte nuclei. A small amount of eosinophilic material is observed within the cytoplasm of the largest macrophage. A few lysed nuclei and several erythrocytes are present in the background (Wright–Giemsa stain, 1,000× magnification).

present, the macrophages tend to differentiate into a classic APC that stimulates the adaptive immune response. The cytokines produced by M1 macrophages drive the inflammatory response. Important examples of cytokines released by M1 macrophages include IL-1, TNFα, IL-6, IL-12, and IL-23.

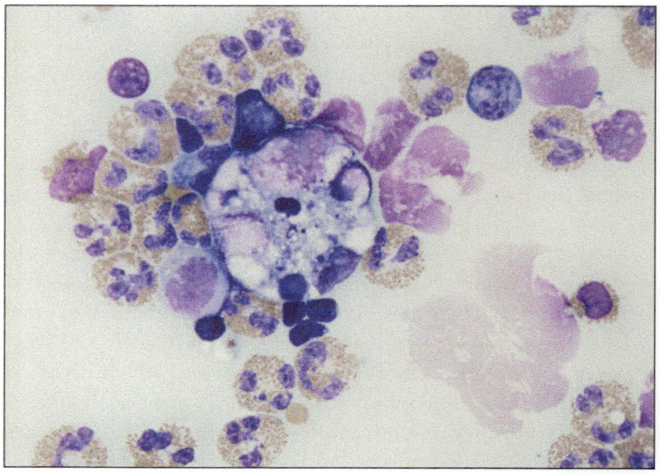

Figure 2.23 Tissue macrophage with phagocytized debris. Cytocentrifuged abdominal fluid from an 8-year-old, spayed female domestic shorthair cat with a history of vomiting and hypoalbuminemia. A thickened gastrointestinal wall and peritoneal effusion were detected ultrasonographically. This image contains several eosinophils and low numbers of macrophages and lymphocytes. The macrophage in the center is large with distended cytoplasm that contains phagocytized cellular debris (Wright–Giemsa, 1,000× magnification).

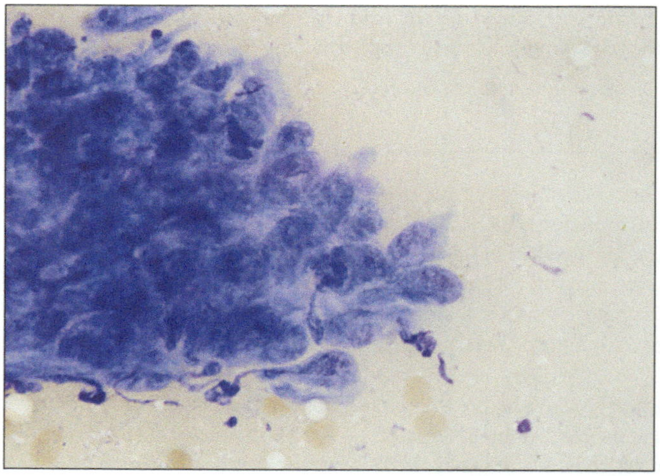

Figure 2.24 Epithelioid macrophages. FNA of a skin mass on a 13-year-old, spayed female Labrador Retriever. A large aggregate of macrophages is shown. Cells have wispy, basophilic cytoplasm and appear cohesive in some areas. Nuclei are rounded with stippled chromatin. Some of the cell nuclei have dark chromocenters (Wright–Giemsa, 1,000× magnification).

Like neutrophils, M1 macrophages contain lysosomes that store MPO. They also generate free radicals through a membrane oxidase that converts O_2 to O_2^- when an opsonized organism is ingested. Inducible nitric oxide synthase is synthesized, which takes O_2^- and arginine and forms NO. The NO then reacts with more O_2^- to produce additional free radicals, NO_2^- and OH^-. During the last phase of the process, lysosomal enzymes degrade what is left of the organism.

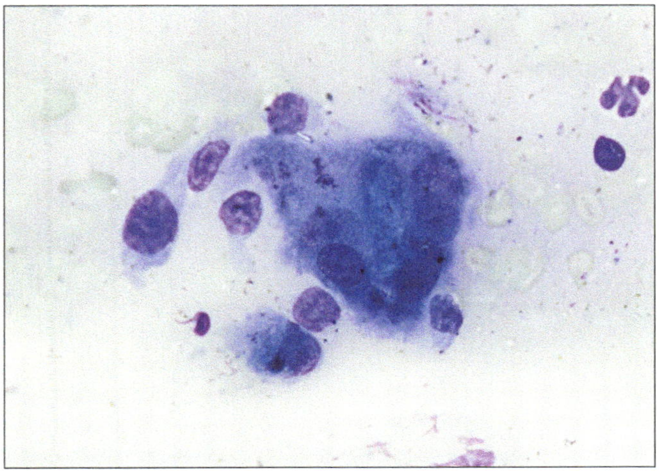

Figure 2.25 Multinucleated giant cell. FNA from an ulcerated dermal mass between the fourth and fifth digits of the left rear limb of a 13-year-old, spayed female Labrador Retriever. There is a large macrophage with several nuclei in the center of the image (the multinucleated giant cell). A few intact macrophages and a neutrophil are also seen (Wright–Giemsa, 1,000× magnification).

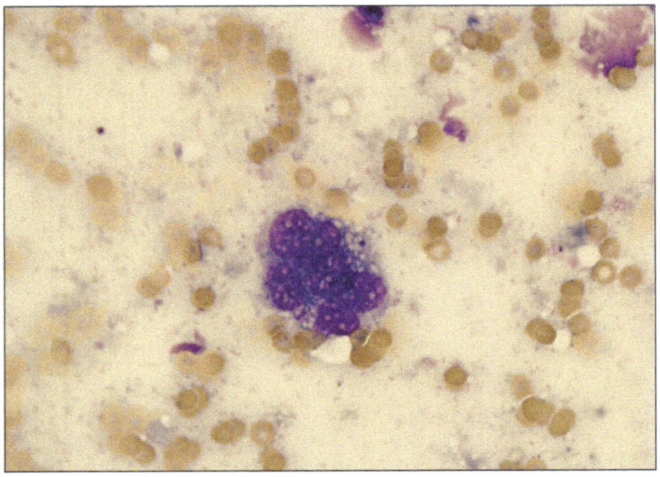

Figure 2.26 Multinucleated giant cell. FNA from a subcutaneous mass on the left hip of a 4-year-old, neutered male domestic shorthair cat. A large vacuolated cell containing several nuclei is shown. Moderate numbers of erythrocytes and a few fragments of lysed nuclei are present in the background (Wright–Giemsa stain, 1,000× magnification).

Macrophages are essential in cleaning up an area for healing and repair. Wound healing macrophages (M2 macrophages) have immunomodulatory functions but are poorly microbicidal (Ferrante & Leibovich, 2012).

Chronic cellular response

Lymphoid cells

Lymphocytes are mononuclear leukocytes that indicate an adaptive immunologic response is ongoing. They are often associated with a response to viral infections. Lymphocytes may be observed several days to weeks after injury occurs. Small lymphocytes are 7–10 µm in diameter and have very sparse basophilic cytoplasm and a small, round nucleus with a dense chromatin pattern (Figure 2.27). Plasma cells are derived from B lymphocytes and are approximately 15 µm in diameter with abundant basophilic cytoplasm and a small, dense, eccentrically located nucleus. These cells often have a pale halo near one side of the nucleus, which is the Golgi apparatus filled with antibody (Figure 2.28).

Lymphocytes are a major source of polarizing cytokines in inflammatory responses. Several subtypes of CD4+ T lymphocytes are recognized. Each cell subset has a slightly different immune function. Th1 cells secrete IL-2, IL-12, IFNγ, and other proinflammatory cytokines that stimulate cell-mediated responses. Th2 cells tend to produce IL-4, IL-5, IL-10, and other cytokines that promote immunoglobulin production and tend to induce allergic responses. Regulatory T cells predominantly produce IL-10 and are critical in downregulating immune responses. Other subsets of Th cells include Th9, Th17, and Th22 cells (Raphael et al., 2014). Similarly, CD8+ T cell subsets have different functions, driven in part by the cytokines they produce (Mosmann et al., 1997). Tc0 cells secrete IFNγ and IL-4, and Tc1 cells produce IFNγ and TNFα. These cells are cytotoxic through perforin and Fas/FasL pathways. Tc2 cells release IL-4, IL-5, IL-10, IL-13, and low levels of IFNγ. The cytotoxicity of Tc2 cells occurs primarily through perforin.

ILCs are morphologically identical to B and T lymphocytes. Conventional NK cells are a subtype of ILCs that produce large amounts of IFNγ, TNFα, and GM-CSF. These cells inhibit viral replication, induce MHC class I expression, activate macrophages, stimulate granulocytes, and cause apoptosis of certain cells. Several other ILC subsets have recently been identified. The functions of these ILCs are actively being studied (Diefenbach et al., 2014).

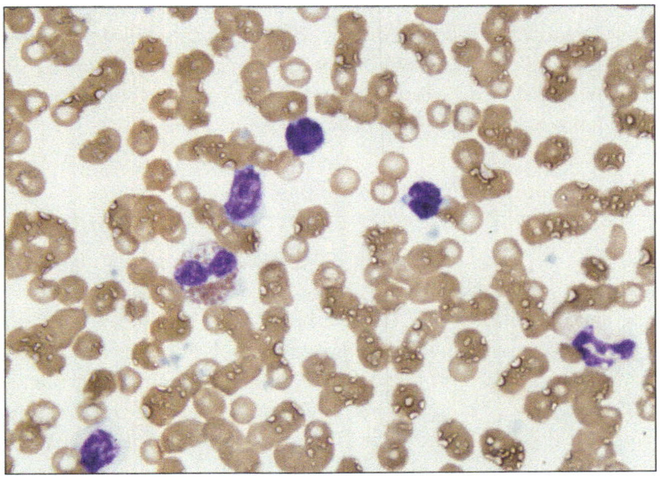

Figure 2.27 Lymphocyte. Peripheral blood from a 10-year-old, intact male mixed-breed dog. Three small lymphocytes (at the top of the image) and a partially lysed lymphocyte (lower left) are shown. Lymphocytes have scant, lightly basophilic cytoplasm and a round to cleaved nucleus. The nuclear chromatin is dense to clumped in mature, intact cells. An eosinophil, a neutrophil, and several erythrocytes are also present (Wright–Giemsa, 1,000× magnification).

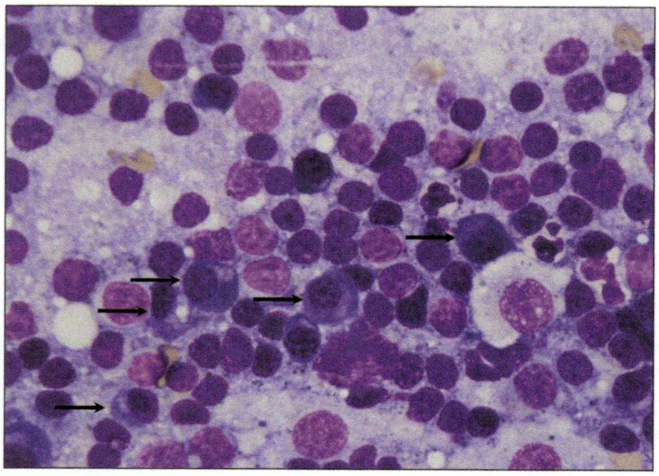

Figure 2.28 **Plasma cells. Reactive lymph node from a dog. The sample contains several lysed cells and small lymphocytes, fewer intermediate-sized lymphocytes, and increased numbers of plasma cells (arrows). A few neutrophils and macrophages are also present (Wright–Giemsa, 1,000× magnification).**

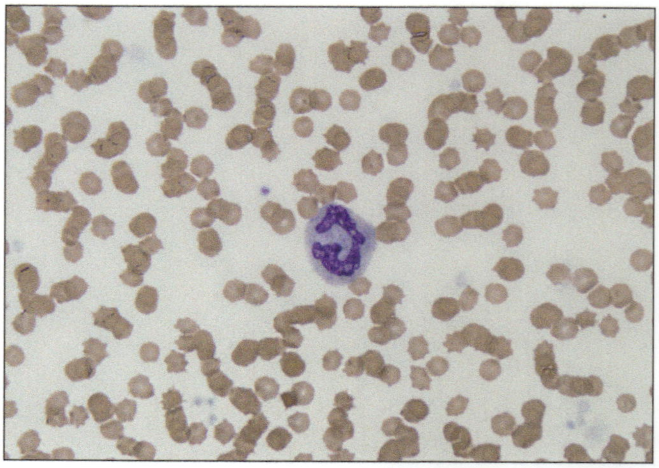

Figure 2.29 **Basophil. Peripheral blood smear from a 13-year-old, spayed female domestic shorthair cat. A basophil is shown in the center of the image. The cell has abundant cytoplasm, filled with pale, lavender granules. The nucleus is segmented and has dense chromatin. Several erythrocytes and platelets are also observed (Wright–Giemsa, 1,000× magnification).**

Most lymphocytes within inflammatory lesions originate from the regional lymph nodes that drain the site of injury (Halin et al., 2005). Lymph nodes are key sites for the formation of an adaptive immune response to eliminate the agent causing inflammation. Molecules from damaged cells and infectious organisms drain into lymphatics around the site of inflammation. The lymph nodes filter lymphatic fluid and begin processing the antigens present in the fluid to mount an appropriate immune response. In response to antigenic stimulation, T cells proliferate in paracortical regions of lymphoid tissues and begin to coordinate the immune response. This process stimulates B cells to proliferate in follicles. Many of these B cells will develop into plasma cells and migrate to the medulla of the node to form cords. The activated T cells and antibodies produced by this reaction limit the spread of pathogens and protect against reinfection.

BASOPHILS

Basophils are rarely observed in inflammatory lesions, but have been associated with chronic inflammation and delayed hypersensitivity reactions (Borriello et al., 2014). Basophils are 12–15 µm in diameter and have a segmented nucleus and purple cytoplasm that contains a few basophilic granules in dogs and several lavender granules in cats (Figure 2.29). As with mast cells, basophil granules contain heparin, histamine, serotonin, eosinophil chemotactic factor, and tryptase. Basophils release mediators of inflammation in response to certain C fragments, lymphokines, and foreign substances. Basophils can also synthesize PGs and LTs to induce infiltration of other inflammatory cells.

FIBROCYTES

Fibrocytes and fibroblasts are often observed in chronic inflammatory lesions. They arrive after macrophages have cleared the area of tissue debris and produce collagen to repair defects in the injured tissue. Fibrocytes are mesenchymal cells that typically have lightly basophilic, spindle-shaped cytoplasm and an oval nucleus (Figures 2.30, 2.31). Collagen production by fibroblasts is induced by cytokines (including tumor growth factor-β) released from macrophages and T cells during resolution of inflammation (Leask, 2013). Fibroblasts proliferate at sites of tissue injury and synthesize collagens, matrix metalloproteinases, and tissue inhibitors of metalloproteinases that construct and remodel extracellular matrix and can lead to fibrosis.

RESOLUTION

The restoration of tissue homeostasis is the desired outcome of an inflammatory process. Lipid mediators, such as lipoxins and resolvins, limit the influx of neutrophils (Serhan et al., 2008b; Lee & Surh, 2012). Lactoferrin from apoptotic neutrophils also reduces neutrophil infiltration, promotes the influx of M2 macrophages, and interacts with fibroblasts to promote wound healing (Takayama & Aoki, 2012).

If inflammation persists, negative systemic effects of unchecked inflammatory mediators can be seen. Cachexia is a serious side-effect of chronic inflammation that leads to an overall loss of fat and muscle. Cachexia is due to prolonged release of TNFα, IL-1, IL-6, and IFNγ (Argiles et al., 2012). TNFα (cachectin) prevents adipocyte differentiation and synthesis of enzymes needed to make triglycerides by inhibiting lipoprotein lipase in nonadipose tissues and preventing fat absorption from the gut. Skeletal muscle atrophy, which is observed in cachexic animals, is likely due to the inhibition and proteolysis of protein synthesis mediated by NO and/or TNF. Osteoporosis also occurs in longstanding inflammation as a result of osteoclast stimulation by cytokines.

Systemic inflammatory response syndrome (SIRS) is an excessive inflammatory response that can lead to organ failure. It is a possible

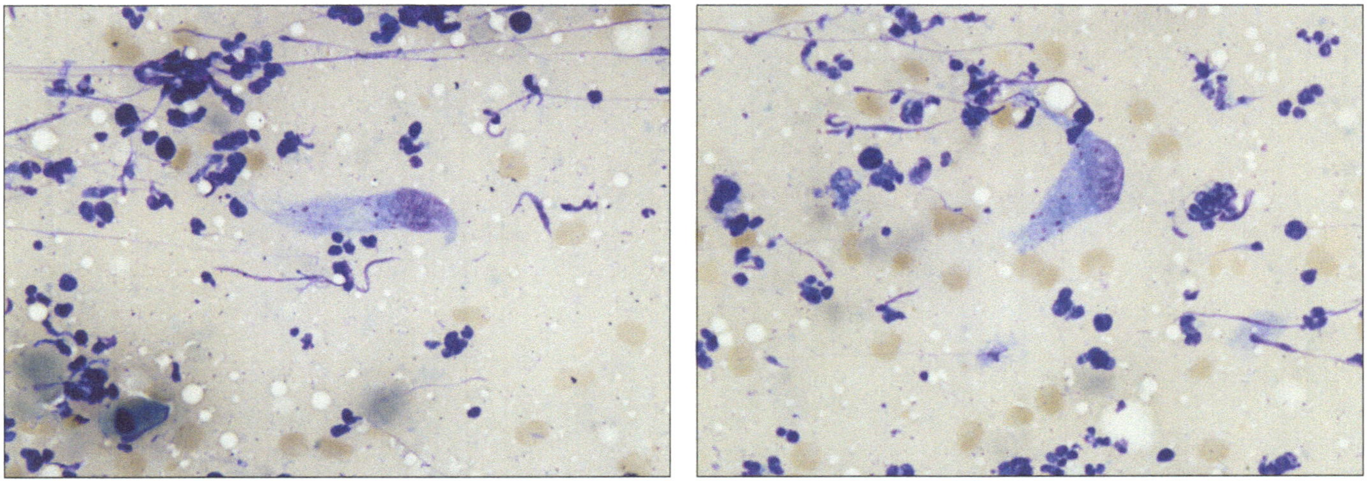

Figures 2.30, 2.31 **Fibroblasts. FNA of a skin mass on a 13-year-old, spayed female Labrador Retriever. The sample contains several lysed neutrophils. A single spindle-shaped fibroblast is shown in each image. The fibroblasts have wispy, lightly basophilic cytoplasm, and an oval nucleus (the fibroblast in 2.30 is binucleate). The nuclei have a stippled chromatin pattern with an indistinct nucleolus. Small eosinophilic cytoplasmic product is present in some of the fibroblasts in this sample (Wright–Giemsa, 1,000× magnification).**

complication of bacterial sepsis and some viral infections. It can also be caused by massive tissue injury (e.g. trauma, tumor lysis syndrome). Clinical signs associated with SIRS include tachycardia, tachypnea, and generalized peripheral vasodilation, which may progress to septic shock and multiple organ dysfunction syndrome. The diagnostic criteria used to diagnose SIRS in dogs and cats are indicated in Table 2.3; two of the listed abnormalities must be present (Hauptman et al., 1997; Brady et al., 2000).

CLASSIFICATION OF INFLAMMATION

Often, diagnosis of the cause of inflammation is sought several days after the initial injury has occurred. Cytologically, inflammatory processes are classified by the cell types present in the lesion. The differential diagnoses typically associated with each category of inflammation are summarized in Table 2.4.

Suppurative inflammation

Suppurative (purulent, neutrophilic) inflammation is predominated by neutrophils. Degenerate neutrophils with karyolytic chromatin are associated with bacterial or fungal infection (Figures 2.32, 2.33). Nondegenerate neutrophils are suggestive of a sterile inflammatory process, but infection may still be occurring (Figures 2.34, 2.35). Causes of sterile inflammation include immune-mediated disease, caustic injury, and trauma. Karyorrhectic and pyknotic neutrophils are observed in chronic inflammatory processes (Figures 2.36, 2.37).

EOSINOPHILIC INFLAMMATION

Lesions with eosinophilic inflammation contain >10% eosinophils (Figures 2.38, 2.39). Differential diagnoses for these lesions include parasitic, allergic, and immune-mediated diseases as well as paraneoplastic conditions and type I hypersensitivity reactions. Also, eosinophilic granuloma is a differential in cats that have a raised, erythematous mass with alopecia.

Granulomatous inflammation

There are large numbers of macrophages in lesions with granulomatous inflammation. Multinucleated giant cells are often seen (Figures 2.40, 2.41). Foreign body reaction, fungal infection, atypical bacterial

Table 2.3 **Criteria for diagnosis of systemic inflammatory response syndrome (SIRS). At least two of the indicated abnormalities must be observed to diagnose SIRS**

Factor	Dogs	Cats
Temperature (°F [°C])	>102.6 [39.2] or <100.6 [38.1]	>103.5 [39.7] or <100.0 [37.7]
Heart rate (beats per minute)	>120	>225 or <140
Respiratory rate (breaths per minute)	>20	>40
Leukocyte count (cells/µl)	>16,000 or <6,000	>19,500 or <5,000
Band neutrophils (%) if other leukocyte counts are within reference intervals	>3	>5

Table 2.4 **Category of inflammation and selected associated differential diagnoses**

Type of inflammation	Duration of injury	Differential diagnoses	
Infectious	**Noninfectious**		
Suppurative	Acute	Bacterial	Traumatic; immune-mediated
Eosinophilic	Acute	Parasitic	Allergic; paraneoplastic
Granulomatous	Chronic	Fungal; bacterial (often atypical forms)	Foreign body
Pyogranulomatous	Chronic	Fungal; bacterial (chronic or atypical)	Foreign body; chronic suppurative processes
Lymphocytic/plasmacytic	Chronic	Viral	Vaccination; insect bite

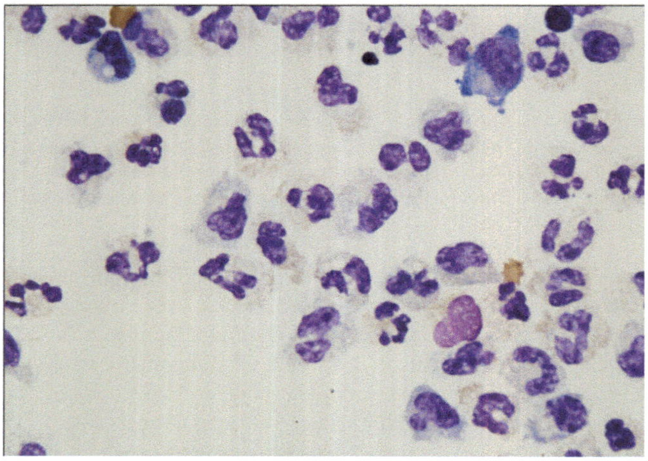

Figure 2.32 **Suppurative inflammation with degenerate neutrophils. Direct smear of abdominal fluid from a 16-year-old, spayed female Bulldog. Neutrophils are the predominant cell type. Most neutrophils have a pale, swollen nucleus with more open chromatin than neutrophils in a peripheral blood smear, which indicates that they are degenerate (Wright–Giemsa stain, 1,000× magnification).**

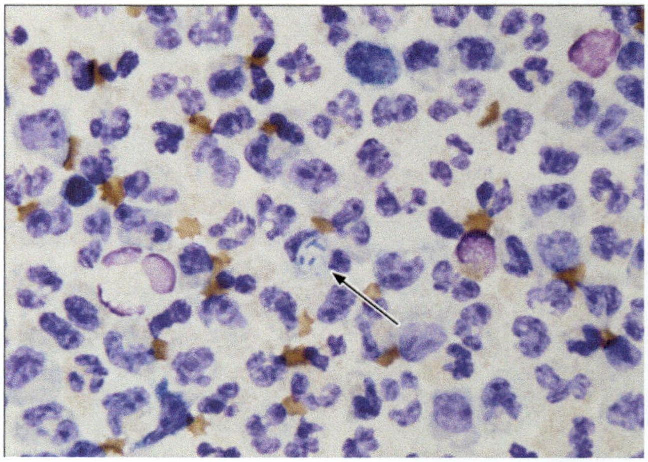

Figure 2.33 **Suppurative inflammation with degenerate neutrophils and bacterial sepsis. Cytocentrifuged abdominal fluid from a 16-year-old, spayed female Bulldog. Neutrophils are the predominant cell type. Most neutrophils are degenerate; they have a pale, swollen nucleus with more open chromatin than neutrophils in a peripheral blood smear. Bacterial rods are contained within a cytoplasmic vacuole of a neutrophil (arrow) (Wright–Giemsa, 1,000× magnification).**

infection, and chronic irritation should be considered if granulomatous inflammation is diagnosed.

Pyogranulomatous inflammation

When a mixed population of macrophages and neutrophils is present, the lesion is described as pyogranulomatous (Figures 2.42, 2.43). As with granulomatous inflammation, the differential diagnoses include foreign body reaction, fungal infection, atypical bacterial infection, and chronic irritation. Close evaluation of the sample for fungal organisms and filamentous bacteria is highly recommended in these lesions. Special staining (e.g. silver stains and periodic acid–Schiff stain) can aid in the identification of infectious organisms.

Lymphocytic/plasmacytic inflammation

Lymphocytic inflammation is diagnosed when large numbers of small, well-differentiated lymphocytes predominate (Figure 2.44). If moderate numbers of plasma cells are also seen, the inflammation can be diagnosed as lymphoplasmacytic (Figure 2.45). Antigenic stimulation and type IV (delayed) hypersensitivity reactions are differentials for this type of inflammation. Sources of antigen are varied and include vaccines, insect bites, and viral infection.

Mixed inflammation

Chronic inflammatory lesions can involve all inflammatory cell types (Figures 2.46, 2.47). The predominant cell type should be identified, if possible, so that a more targeted list of differential diagnoses can be made.

SUMMARY

Cytology is a powerful diagnostic tool that provides clinicians with immediate information about the cause of lesion formation. Although inflammation is a complex process (involving interactions of several cell types, cell surface receptors, and chemical mediators), the cell types present in a cytologic sample indicate the duration of the

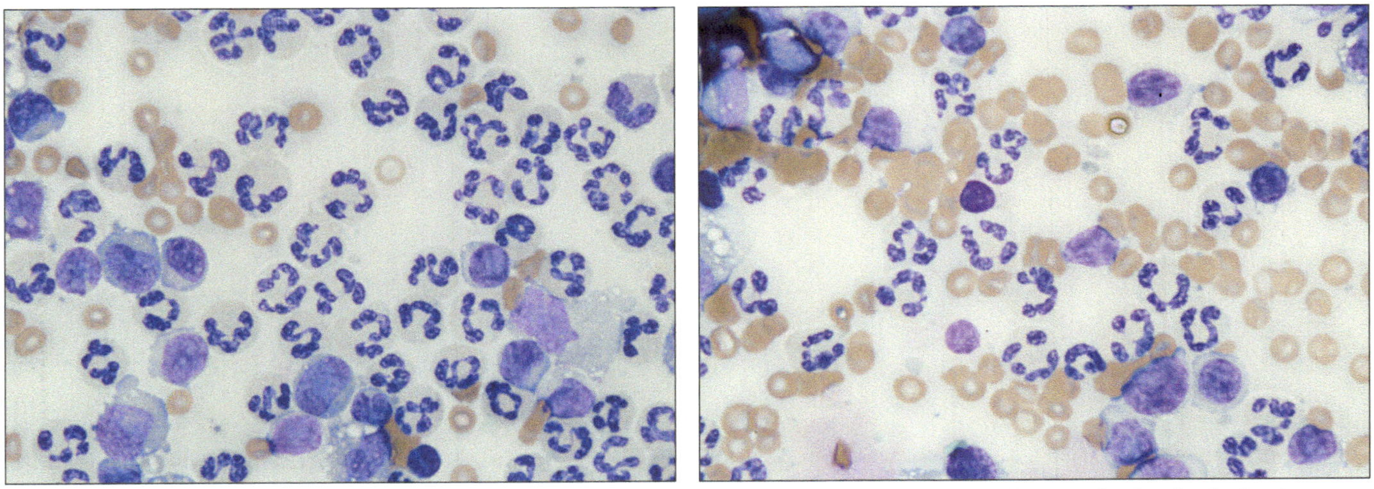

Figures 2.34, 2.35 Suppurative inflammation with nondegenerate neutrophils. Synovial fluid from an 8-year-old, neutered male Labrador Retriever. Several neutrophils and lower numbers of large mononuclear cells are present. Neutrophils are nondegenerate; they have segmented nuclei with crisp edges and dense chromatin, similar to neutrophils in a peripheral blood smear. Moderate numbers of erythrocytes are present in the background (Wright–Giemsa stain, 1,000× magnification).

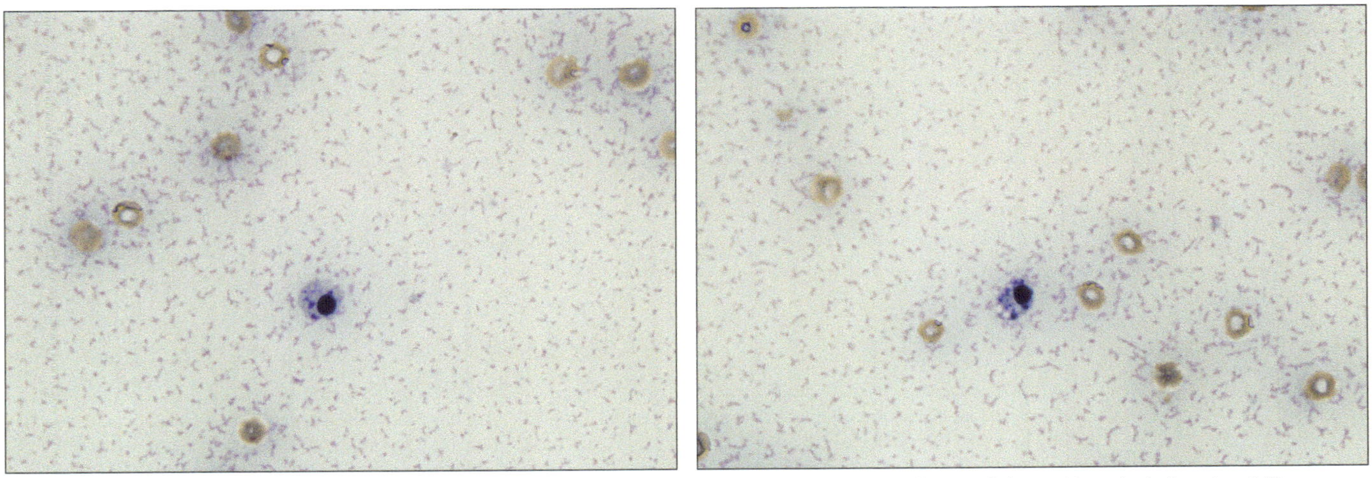

Figures 2.36, 2.37 Pyknotic cells. Synovial fluid from a 3-year-old, spayed female mixed-breed dog. The sample has a thin, stippled, eosinophilic background consistent with joint fluid of decreased viscosity. Each image has a cell with a small, round, very dense nucleus undergoing pyknosis (Wright–Giemsa, 1,000× magnification).

lesion and suggest possible causes of the injury. This allows for more informed decisions about additional diagnostics and the medical therapy to pursue. In fact, in cases caused by pathogens, the inciting organism can often be directly identified cytologically.

CASES

CASE 1

Signalment/history

A 6-year-old, spayed female dog presented for a mucoid, bloody, vaginal discharge. An exploratory laparotomy was performed to remove potential ovarian remnants. The ovarian pedicles appeared grossly unremarkable. The tissue was excised and submitted for histopathology, and a smear of the vaginal discharge was submitted for cytology (Figures 2.48, 2.49).

Cytologic description

The sample was highly cellular. The majority of cells were degenerate neutrophils, most of which were filled with large numbers of bacterial cocci and fewer rods. Scattered mature squamous epithelial cells with abundant rounded to polygonal lightly basophilic cytoplasm and a small round nucleus were present.

Interpretation: septic suppurative inflammation.

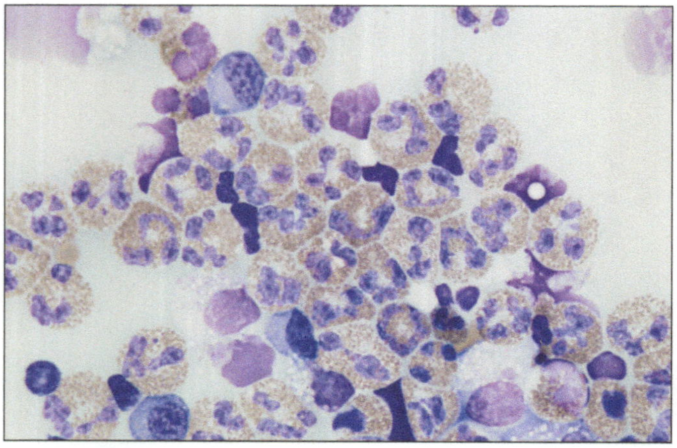
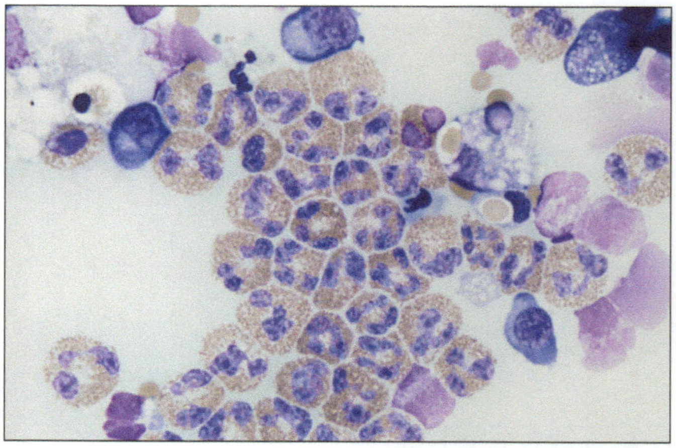

Figures 2.38, 2.39 Eosinophilic inflammation. Cytocentrifuged abdominal fluid from an 8-year-old, spayed female domestic shorthair cat with a history of vomiting and hypoalbuminemia. A thickened gastrointestinal wall and peritoneal effusion were detected ultrasonographically. Eosinophils are the predominant cell type. There are also low numbers of macrophages and plasma cells. Two small lymphocytes are present in 2.38 (Wright–Giemsa, 1,000× magnification).

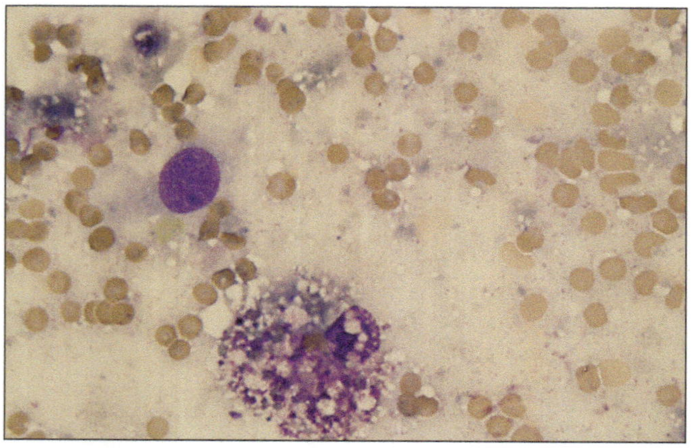

Figure 2.40 Granulomatous inflammation. FNA from a subcutaneous mass on the shoulder of a 3-year-old, spayed female domestic shorthair cat. A reactive macrophage (lower center) and a partially lysed cell (upper left) are shown. The macrophage has abundant, vacuolated cytoplasm and a round, eccentrically located nucleus with clumped chromatin (Wright–Giemsa, 1,000× magnification).

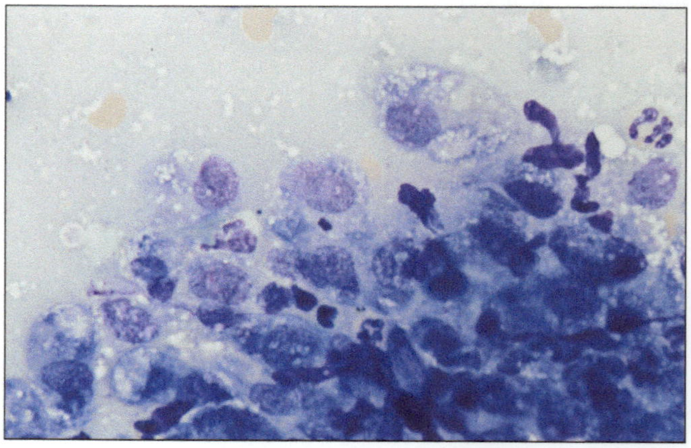

Figure 2.41 Granulomatous inflammation. FNA of a subcutaneous mass from a dog. There is an aggregate of macrophages with basophilic cytoplasm, small distinct cytoplasmic vacuoles, and a stippled nucleus. Often, macrophages that are arranged this closely together are termed 'epithelioid macrophages'. Low numbers of neutrophils also are present (Wright–Giemsa stain, 1,000× magnification).

Comment

Cornified epithelial cells are typically observed during proestrus and estrus; however, these cells may also come from the cervix or the labia. Given the large numbers of neutrophils and clear indication of infection, this sample is most consistent with bacterial vaginitis. Culture and sensitivity are recommended.

Discussion

It is important to be aware of the normal cytologic appearance of tissues in the area that was sampled before interpreting the data. In this case, low numbers of neutrophils and squamous epithelial cells are a normal finding in vaginal swabs, depending on when the sample was taken during the estrous cycle. However, squamous epithelial cells can come from several structures near the vagina and should be interpreted with caution in spayed females. The high numbers of neutrophils and intracellular organisms present supported a diagnosis of vaginitis rather than proestrus. Indeed, the histologic sections did not contain any ovarian tissue.

CASE 2

Signalment/history

A 10-year-old, intact female Husky presented for a subcutaneous mandibular mass. Six months prior, the patient had been diagnosed and treated for lymphoma. Fine needle aspirates of the right mandibular lymph node (Figure 2.50) and the mass (Figure 2.51) were submitted for cytology.

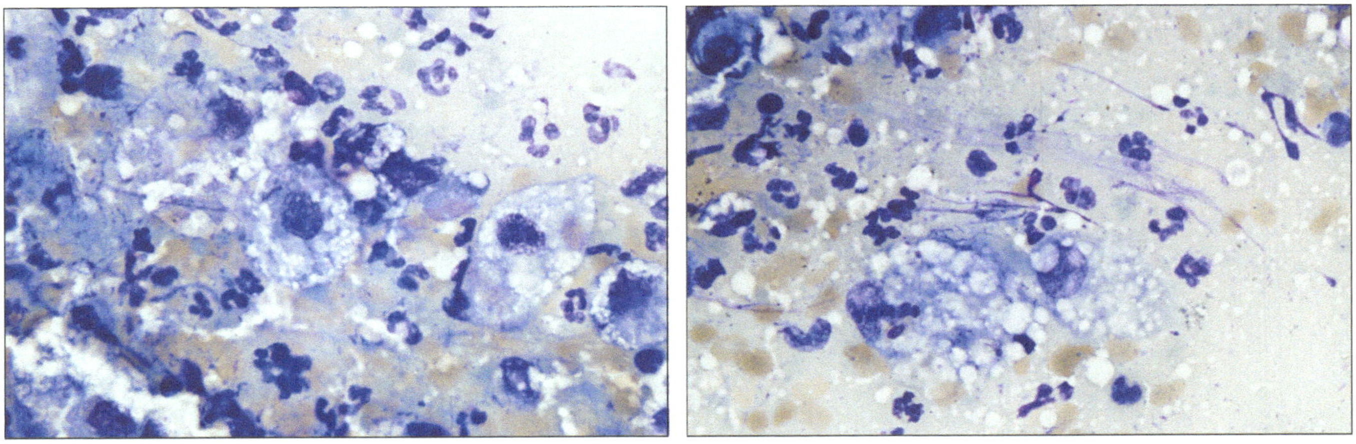

Figures 2.42, 2.43 Pyogranulomatous inflammation. FNA from a subcutaneous mandibular mass on a 14-year-old, neutered male mixed-breed dog. Degenerate neutrophils are present in large numbers. More than 20% of the cells are large macrophages. Many of the macrophages are vacuolated (Wright–Giemsa, 1,000× magnification).

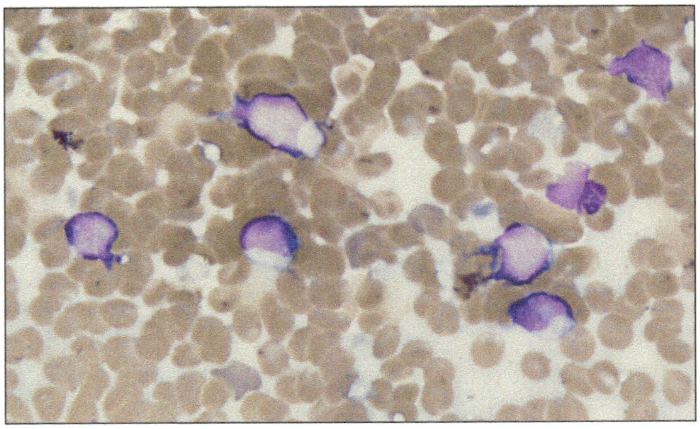

Figure 2.44 Lymphocytic inflammation. FNA of a dermal mass on the bridge of the nose of a 2-year-old, spayed female Border Collie. The sample contains moderate numbers of small to intermediate-sized lymphocytes with scant cytoplasm and a rounded nucleus with smooth chromatin. Large numbers of erythrocytes are present in the background (Wright–Giemsa, 1,000× magnification).

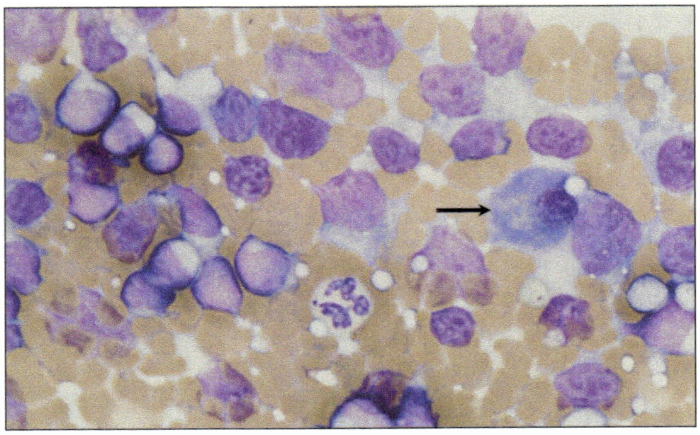

Figure 2.45 Lymphoplasmacytic inflammation. FNA from a firm, dermal lesion on the head of a cat. There are several erythrocytes and moderate numbers of lysed cells present. Intact small lymphocytes and fewer intermediate-sized lymphocytes and plasma cells (arrow) are observed. One neutrophil is present at the center of the image (Wright–Giemsa, 1,000× magnification).

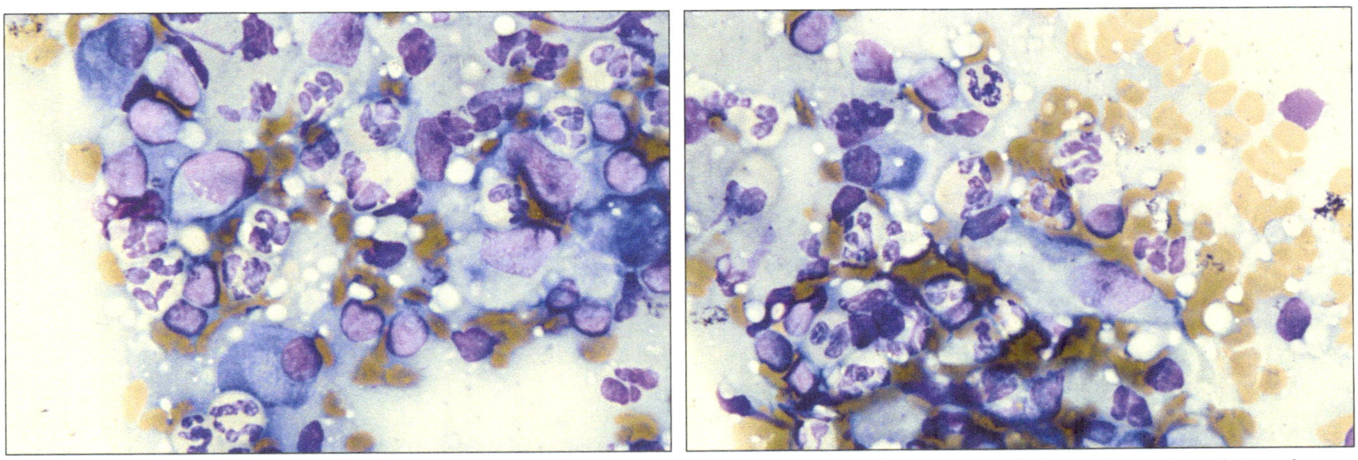

Figures 2.46, 2.47 Mixed inflammation. FNA of a raised dermal mass on the pinna of an 8-year-old, neutered male Boxer. A mixed population of neutrophils, macrophages, lymphocytes, and plasma cells is seen (Wright–Giemsa, 1,000× magnification).

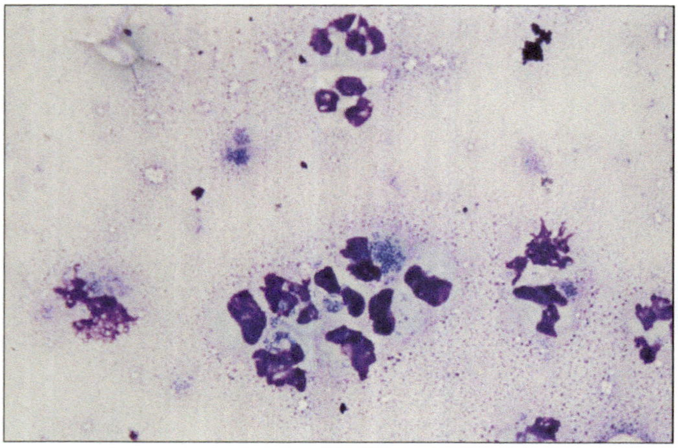

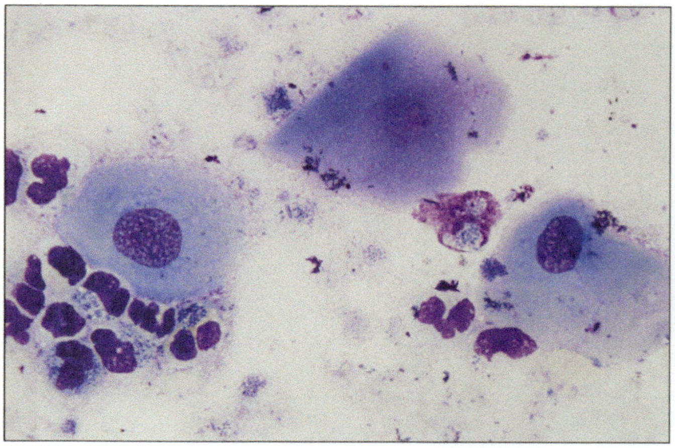

Figures 2.48, 2.49 Bacterial vaginitis. Vaginal smear from a 6-year-old, spayed female Labrador Retriever. Several degenerate neutrophils are present. Many neutrophils contain phagocytized bacterial cocci and rare bacterial rods. Additionally, three squamous epithelial cells are present in 2.49 (Wright–Giemsa, 1,000× magnification).

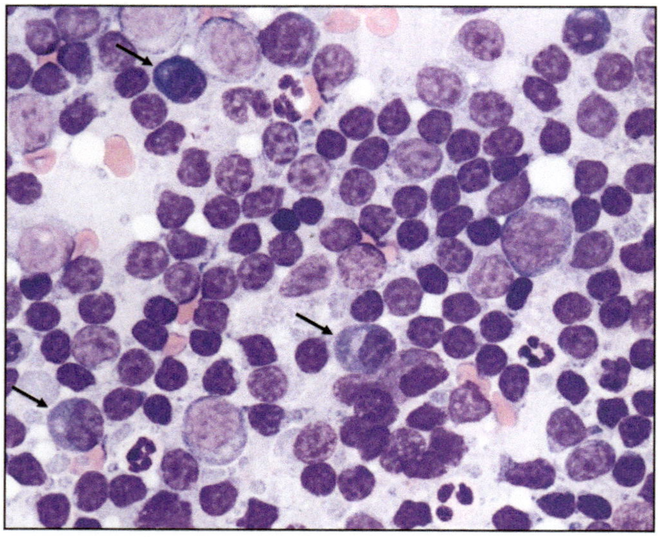

Figure 2.50 FNA of an enlarged right mandibular lymph node from a 10-year-old, intact female Husky. The majority of cells are small lymphocytes. There are moderate numbers of intermediate-sized and large lymphocytes. Increased numbers of plasma cells (arrows) are present (Wright–Giemsa, 1,000× magnification).

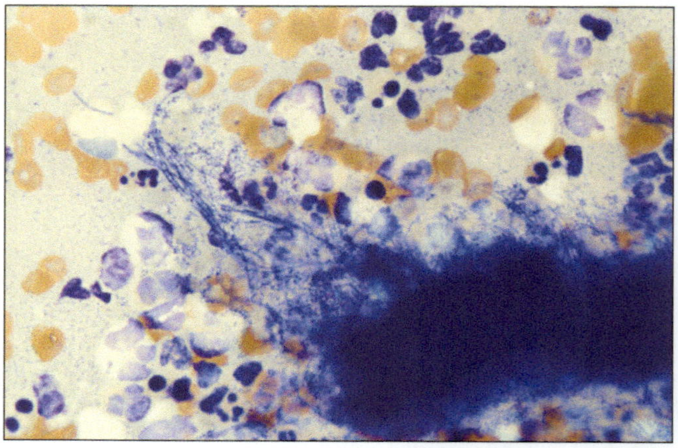

Figure 2.51 FNA from a subcutaneous mandibular mass on a 10-year-old, intact female Husky. Severely degenerate neutrophils are present in large numbers. Several bacterial organisms, including mats of filamentous bacterial organisms, are shown (Wright–Giemsa, 1,000× magnification).

Cytologic description

The lymph node aspirate contained moderate numbers of cells. Most cells were small to intermediate-sized lymphocytes. Few large lymphocytes were seen. There were occasional plasma cells, nondegenerate neutrophils, and eosinophils. The sample from the mass was highly cellular with a small amount of blood in the background. Large numbers of degenerate and nondegenerate neutrophils were present. Lower numbers of macrophages were seen. There were bacterial cocci and rods throughout the slide and within degenerate neutrophils. Large aggregates of filamentous bacteria surrounded by dying inflammatory cells were noted.

Interpretation: lymph node: lymphoid hyperplasia; mass: suppurative inflammation with mixed bacterial sepsis including filamentous bacteria.

Comment

Aerobic and anaerobic bacterial cultures of samples from the mass are recommended.

Discussion

Infection with filamentous bacteria is often associated with pyogranulomatous inflammation. In this case, the suppurative nature of the mass lesion suggests that this was an acute inflammatory process. It is

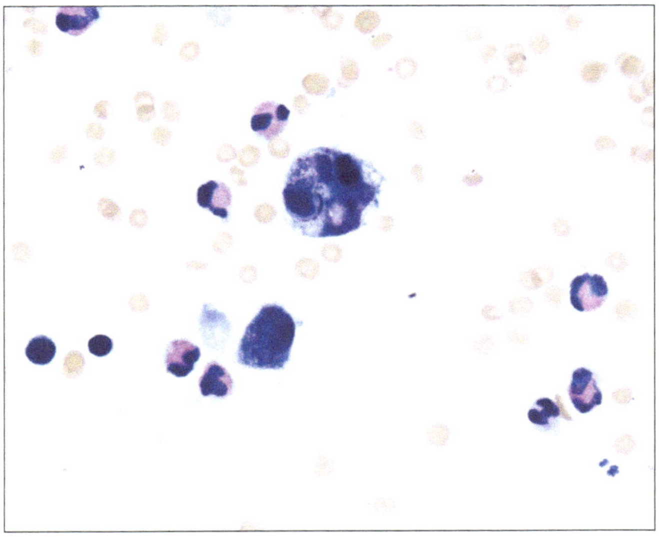

Figure 2.52 FNA of a swollen area on the right rear leg. Several eosinophils with segmented nuclei and pink cytoplasmic granules are shown. There are two macrophages near the center of the image. One macrophage contains phagocytized cellular debris. Two lymphocytes are present at the lower left of the image. A neutrophil is present at the lower right. There are scattered erythrocytes in the background (Wright–Giemsa, 1,000 × magnification).

likely that this lesion was identified quickly because the owners were sensitive to swelling in the mandibular area due to the recent diagnosis of lymphoma.

CASE 3

Signalment/history

A 7-year-old, male, neutered domestic short haired cat presented right rear leg swelling and alopecia that had persisted for 4 months. The swelling was firm and erythematous. Bacterial cultures were negative. An FNA of the lesion was performed (Figure 2.52).

Cytologic description

The mass aspirate was moderately to highly cellular with a small amount of peripheral blood. Most cells were eosinophils. Fewer macrophages were seen. Macrophages were arranged individually and in small aggregates. Several macrophages contained cytoplasmic vacuoles and/or phagocytized cellular debris. Occasional neutrophils, small lymphocytes, and intermediate-sized lymphocytes were observed. Rare plasma cells, basophils, and mast cells were noted. No infectious organisms or overtly neoplastic cells were seen.

Interpretation: mass: marked eosinophilic inflammation.

Comment

The clinical appearance of the mass along with the cytologic finding of eosinophilic inflammation supports a diagnosis of an eosinophilic granuloma complex. Biopsy with histopathology is recommended if clinically warranted.

Discussion

Eosinophilic granuloma complex lesions are often associated with underlying allergic and hypersensitivity reactions. Other diseases can cause similar lesions, including ringworm and mite infestation. Further evaluation of cats diagnosed with eosinophilic granuloma complex is critical for proper treatment of the lesions.

REFERENCES

Acharya K.R., Ackerman S.J. (2014) Eosinophil granule proteins: Form and function. *J Biol Chem 289*(*25*):17406–17415.

Argiles J.M., Lopez-Soriano F.J., Busquets S. (2012) Counteracting inflammation: A promising therapy in cachexia. *Crit Rev Oncogen 17*(*3*):253–262.

Baggiolini M., Clark-Lewis I. (1992) Interleukin-8, a chemotactic and inflammatory cytokine. *FEBS Lett 307*(*1*):97–101.

Bartz R.R., Piantadosi C.A. (2010) Clinical review: Oxygen as a signaling molecule. *Crit Care 14*(*5*):234.

Berlacher M.D., Vieth J.A., Heflin B.C. et al. (2013) FcγRIIa ligation induces platelet hypersensitivity to thrombotic stimuli. *Am J Pathol 182*(*1*):244–254.

Borriello F., Granata F., Marone G. (2014) Basophils and skin disorders. *J Invest Dermatol 134*(*5*):1202–1210.

Brady C.A., Otto C.M., Winkle T.J. et al. (2000) Severe sepsis in cats: 29 cases (1986–1998). *J Am Vet Med Assoc 217*:531–535.

Butler K.M., Baker C.J., Edwards M.S. (1987) Interaction of soluble fibronectin with group B streptococci. *Infect Immun 55*(*10*):2404–2408.

Choi E.Y., Santoso S., Chavakis T. (2009) Mechanisms of neutrophil transendothelial migration. *Front Biosci 14*:1596–1605.

Clarke E.V., Tenner A.J. (2014) Complement modulation of T cell immune responses during homeostasis and disease. *J Leukoc Biol 96*(*5*):745–756, https://doi.org/10.1189/jlb.3MR0214-109R

Dahlén S.E., Björk J., Hedqvist P. et al. (1981) Leukotrienes promote plasma leakage and leukocyte adhesion in postcapillary venules: In vivo effects with relevance to the acute inflammatory response. *Proc Natl Acad Sci USA 78*(*6*):3887–3891.

Del Rosso M., Fibbi G., Pucci M. et al. (2008) The plasminogen activation system in inflammation. *Front Biosci 13*:4667–4686.

Diefenbach A., Colonna M., Koyasu S. (2014) Development, differentiation, and diversity of innate lymphoid cells. *Immunity 41*(*3*):354–365.

Dimasi D., Sun W.Y., Bonder C.S. (2013) Neutrophil interactions with the vascular endothelium. *Int Immunopharmacol 17*(*4*):1167–1175.

Eckersall P.D., Bell R. (2010) Acute phase proteins: Biomarkers of infection and inflammation in veterinary medicine. *Vet J 185*(*1*):23–27.

Elizabeth V.C., Andrea J.T. (2014) Complement modulation of T cell immune responses during homeostasis and disease. *Journal of Leukocyte Biology 96*(*15*):745–756, https://doi.org/10.1189/jlb.3MR0214-109R.

Ferrante C.J., Leibovich S.J. (2012) Regulation of macrophage polarization and wound healing. *Adv Wound Care 1*(*1*):10–16.

Fukata M., Arditi M. (2013) The role of pattern recognition receptors in intestinal inflammation. *Mucosal Immunol 6*(*3*):451–463.

Gibbert K., Schlaak J.F., Yang D. (2013) IFN-a subtypes: Distinct biological activities in antiviral therapy. *Br J Pharmacol 168*(*5*):1048–1058.

Halin C., Mora J.R., Sumen C. et al. (2005) In vivo imaging of lymphocyte trafficking. *Ann Rev Cell Develop Biol 21*:581–603.

Hamad O.A., Nilsson P.H., Wouters D. et al. (2010) Complement component C3 binds to activated normal platelets without preceding proteolytic activation and promotes binding to complement receptor 1. *J Immunol 184*(*5*):2686–2692.

Hauptman J.G., Walshaw R., Olivier N.B. (1997) Evaluation of the sensitivity and specificity of diagnostic criteria for sepsis in dogs. *Vet Surg 26(5)*:393–397.

Hemmerich S., Bertozzi C.R., Leffler H. et al. (1994) Identification of the sulfated monosaccharides of GlyCAM-1, an endothelial-derived ligand for L-selectin. *Biochemistry 33(16)*:4820–4829.

Johnson E.E., Wessling-Resnick M. (2011) Iron metabolism and the innate immune response to infection. *Microbes Infect 14(3)*:207–216.

Johnson E.E., Wessling-Resnick M. (2012) Iron metabolism and the innate immune response to infection,Microbes Infect 289(3):207-216. ISSN 1286-4579, https://doi.org/10.1016/j.micinf.2011.10.001

Késmárky G., Kenyeres P., Rábai M. et al. (2008) Plasma viscosity: A forgotten variable. *Clin Hemorheol Microcirc 39(1–4)*:243–246.

Kokkonen J.O., Kovanen P.T. (1989) Proteolytic enzymes of mast cell granules degrade low density lipoproteins and promote their granule-mediated uptake by macrophages in vitro. *J Biolog Chem 264(18)*:10749–10755.

Leask A. (2013) Integrin β1: A mechanosignaling sensor essential for connective tissue deposition by fibroblasts. *Adv Wound Care 2(4)*:160–166.

Lee H., Lee I., Choue R. (2013) Obersity, inflammation, and diet. *Pediatr Gastroenterol Hepatol Nutr 16(3)*:143–152.

Lee H.N., Surh Y.J. (2012) Therapeutic potential of resolvins in the prevention and treatment of inflammatory disorders. *Biochem Pharmacol 84(10)*:1340–1350.

Martins-Green M., Petreaca M., Wang L. (2013) Chemokines and their receptors are key players in the orchestra that regulates wound healing. *Adv Wound Care 2(7)*:327–347.

Miyata N., Roman R.J. (2005) Role of 20-hydroxyeicosatetraenoic acid (20-HETE) in vascular system. *J Smooth Muscle Res 41(4)*:175–193.

Mosmann T.R., Li L., Sad S. (1997) Functions of CD8 T-cell subsets secreting different cytokine patterns. *Semin Immunol 9(2)*:87–92.

Nauseef W.M., Borregaard N. (2014) Neutrophils at work. *Nature Immunol 15(7)*:602–611.

Ogawa H., Binion D.G., Heidemann J. et al. (2005) Mechanisms of MAdCAM-1 gene expression in human intestinal microvascular endothelial cells. *Am J Physiol Cell Physiol 288(2)*:C272–281.

Panigrahy D., Kaipainen A., Greene E.R. et al. (2010) Cytochrome P450-derived eicosanoids: The neglected pathway in cancer. *Cancer Metast Rev 29(4)*:723–735. https://doi.org/10.1007/s10555-010-9264-x

Papayannopoulos V. (2018) Neutrophil extracellular traps in immunity and disease. *Nat Rev Immunol 18(2)*:134–147.

Pohlman L.M. (2010) Basophils, mast cells, and their disorders. In: *Schalm's Veterinary Hematology*, 6th edn. (eds. D.J. Weiss, K.J. Wardrop) John Wiley, Ames, p. 292.

Raphael I., Nalawade S., Eagar T.N. et al. (2014) T cell subsets and their signature cytokines in autoimmune and inflammatory diseases. *Cytokine* pii:S1043-4666(14)00539-0.

Rauch I., Müller M., Decker T. (2013) The regulation of inflammation by interferons and their STATs. *JAK-STAT 2(1)*:e23820.

Rossi A., Acquaviva A.M., Iuliano F. et al. (2005) Up-regulation of prostaglandin biosynthesis by leukotriene C4 in elicited mice peritoneal macrophages activated with lipopolysaccharide/interferon-γ. *J Leukoc Biol 78(4)*:985–991.

Rutkowski K., Dua S., Nasser S. (2012) Anaphylaxis: Current state of knowledge for the modern physician. *Postgrad Med J 88(1042)*:458–464.

Sacks S.H. (2010) Complement fragments C3a and C5a: The salt and pepper of the immune response. *Eur J Immunol 40(3)*:668–670.

Sadik C.D., Luster A.D. (2012) Lipid-cytokine-chemokine cascades orchestrate leukocyte recruitment in inflammation. *J Leukoc Biol 91(2)*:207–215.

Salazar F., Ghaemmaghami A.M. (2013) Allergen recognition by innate immune cells: Critical role of dendritic and epithelial cells. *Front Immunol 4*:356.

Schmaier A.H. (2008) The elusive physiologic role of Factor XII. *J Clin Invest 118(9)*:3006–3009.

Schulze-Topphoff U., Prat A., Bader M. et al. (2008) Roles of the kallikrein/kinin system in the adaptive immune system. *Int Immunopharmacol 8(2)*:155–160.

Serhan C.N., Chiang N., Van Dyke T.E. (2008a) Resolving inflammation: Dual anti-inflammatory and pro-resolution lipid mediators. *Nat Rev Immunol 8(5)*:349–361.

Serhan C.N., Yacoubian S., Yang R. (2008b) Anti-inflammatory and proresolving lipid mediators. *Ann Rev Pathol 3*:279–312.

Soehnlein O., Lindbom L., Weber C. (2009) Mechanisms underlying neutrophil-mediated monocyte recruitment. *Blood 114(21)*:4613–4623.

Stoffels J.M., Zhao C., Baron W. (2013) Fibronectin in tissue regeneration: Timely disassembly of the scaffold is necessary to complete the build. *Cell Mol Life Sci 70(22)*:4243–4253.

Takayama Y., Aoki R. (2012) Roles of lactoferrin on skin wound healing. *Biochem Cell Biol 90(3)*:497–503.

Terawaki K., Yokomizo T., Nagase T. et al. (2005) Absence of leukotriene B4 receptor 1 confers resistance to airway hyperresponsiveness and Th2-type immune responses. *J Immunol 175(7)*:4217–4225.

Tornhamre S., Sjölinder M., Lindberg A. et al. (1998) Demonstration of leukotriene-C4 synthase in platelets and species distribution of the enzyme activity. *Eur J Biochem 251(1–2)*:227–235.

Uhlig S., Göggel R., Engel S. (2005) Mechanisms of platelet-activating factor (PAF)-mediated responses in the lung. *Pharmacol Rep 57*:206–221.

van Kessel K.P., Bestebroer J., van Strijp J.A. (2014) Neutrophil-mediated phagocytosis of *Staphylococcus aureus*. *Front Immunol 5*:467.

Wang Y., Lindstedt K.A., Kovanen P.T. (1996) Phagocytosis of mast cell granule remnant-bound LDL by smooth muscle cells of synthetic phenotype: A scavenger receptor-mediated process that effectively stimulates cytoplasmic cholesteryl ester synthesis. *J Lipid Res 37(10)*:2155–2166.

Webb J.L., Latimer K.S. (2011a) Leukocytes. In: *Duncan & Prasse's Veterinary Laboratory Medicine Clinical Pathology*, 5th edn. (ed. K.S. Latimer) John Wiley, Ames, p. 68.

Webb J.L., Latimer K.S. (2011b) Leukocytes. In: *Duncan & Prasse's Veterinary Laboratory Medicine Clinical Pathology*, 5th edn. (ed. K.S. Latimer) John Wiley, Ames, p. 51.

Weiss D.J., Souza C.D. (2010) Monocytes and macrophages and their disorders. In: *Schalm's Veterinary Hematology*, 6th edn. (eds. D.J. Weiss, K.J. Wardrop) John Wiley, Ames, p. 303.

Weninger W., Biro M., Jain R. (2014) Leukocyte migration in the interstitial space of non-lymphoid organs. *Nat Rev Immunol 14(4)*:232–246.

Wyble C.W., Hynes K.L., Kuchibhotla J. et al. (1997) TNF-alpha and IL-1 upregulate membrane-bound and soluble E-selectin through a common pathway. *J Surg Res 73(2)*:107–112.

Zhang H., Park Y., Wu J. et al. (2009) Role of TNF-alpha in vascular dysfunction. *Clin Sci 116(3)*:219–230.

Zhao Y.O., Khaminets A., Hunn J.P., Howard J.C. (2009) Disruption of the *Toxoplasma gondii* parasitophorous vacuole by IFNγamma-inducible immunity-related GTPases (IRG proteins) triggers necrotic cell death. *PLoS Pathog 5(2)*:e1000288.

CHAPTER 3

CANCER BIOLOGY

Timothy M. Fan

INTRODUCTION

Cancer biology is the study of pathologic processes responsible for the genesis of rogue cells, and integrates multiple complementary scientific disciplines including genetics, epigenetics, and intracellular signaling. Being a disease that affects complex, multicellular organisms, various descriptive terms are used to describe unregulated cell growth including neoplasia, tumor, malignancy, and cancer. While these descriptive terms are not equivalent and connote nuanced differences, they are often used interchangeably by scientists and laypeople alike. Based on biologic behaviors operative locally and distantly, tumors can be categorized as benign or malignant in nature, and correspondingly have different prognoses. Benign tumors are transformed cell populations that grow locally and do not disseminate beyond the site of origination, and respect natural tissue boundaries such as the basement membrane. Conversely, malignant tumors are invasive and breach the normal tissue microenvironment and have the capacity to spread regionally and distantly through lymphatic or hematogenous routes, as well as by direct extension into body cavities.

With dramatic improvements in nutrition and preventative medicine practices instituted worldwide, coupled with the progressive age extension of the human and companion animal populations, cancer has risen to being one of the most common causes of mortality. In the USA and other developed countries worldwide, cancer remains the second leading cause of death, only exceeded by heart disease, with one out of four people dying because of uncontrolled cancer progression. Similarly, the most common pathophysiologic process causing deaths in adult dogs (>1 year old) is the development of cancer (Fleming *et al.*, 2011), with one out of three adult dogs dying from this single pathologic condition. Interestingly, the predisposition to develop cancer appears to be enriched in canines, and likely an unintended by-product of selective breeding practices for specific phenotypic traits. Based on the substantive fraction of human beings and companion animals that suffer and subsequently succumb to cancer, a strong and clinically warranted impetus exists for studying tumor biology. With focused initiatives that incorporate scientists and clinicians from diverse professional disciplines, it is anticipated that new knowledge will be generated that better elucidates the molecular underpinnings of cancer. Excitingly, over the past two decades, there has been continued prominence and scientific value ascribed to the discipline of comparative oncology, and pet dogs and cats are now viewed as valuable translational models for studying cancer biology and therapeutics (Oh & Cho, 2023; LeBlanc & Mazcko, 2020). Through the concerted efforts on both human and companion animal sides, rapid advances in knowledge are being made in cancer biology and promise to improve the prevention, diagnosis, and treatment of the most lethal cancer histologies.

TISSUE ORIGINS OF CANCER

Human beings and companion animals are complex, multicellular, eukaryotic organisms with a hierarchical organization of tissues that provide anatomic structure and specialized function. All nucleated cells that make up bodily tissues of chordates are derived from one of three primary germ cell layers – the endoderm, the mesoderm, and the ectoderm – within the developing embryo. The endoderm serves as the origin of cells that form the epithelial component of visceral organs, including the lining of the gastrointestinal and respiratory tracts, as well as endocrine glands such as the thyroid and pancreas. The mesoderm forms tissues responsible for anatomic structure and function and includes skeletal muscle, bone, connective tissue, heart, and the urogenital system, while the ectoderm gives rise to the outer components of the body including skin and hair, as well as some parts of the central nervous system (Solnica-Krezel & Sepich, 2012; Tam *et al.*, 2003).

Given that cancer is a disease of self-tissues, it is not surprising that the origins of cancer can also be traced back to specific embryonic cell layers, with human beings and companion animals exhibiting some divergence in the predominant tissue origins for the most commonly occurring cancers. In humans, most cancers (~80%) arise from the endoderm germ layer, which constitutes the epithelial linings and glandular tissues of the body. Cancers arising from the endoderm and most cancers of the ectoderm are classified as epithelial malignancies such as adenomas or carcinomas and are distinguished based on their respective biologic behaviors.Malignant epithelial tumors, termed carcinomas, account for more than 80% of the cancer-related deaths in the USA, and specifically as a result of metastatic disease. The most common carcinomas of endodermal tissues arise from the epithelial linings of the colon, lung, breast, and prostate; however, the most and least biologically aggressive carcinomas are of pancreas and thyroid origin, respectively (Ryan *et al.*, 2014; Schneider & Chen, 2013; Thota *et al.*, 2014). Carcinomas can be broadly segregated into two categories based on the major function

DOI: 10.1201/9781003258551-3

of epithelia. Epithelial cells that provide a protective and sealed anatomic barrier can give rise to squamous cell carcinomas, while epithelial cells with specialized secretory activities can develop into adenocarcinomas. While epithelial malignancies are less common in companion animals, some prominent problematic tumors include oral squamous cell carcinoma in felines and urothelial carcinomas in canines (Bilgic *et al.*, 2015; Knapp *et al.*, 2019).

The mesoderm serves as the predominant germ cell layer, which gives rise to nonepithelial malignancies in human beings and companion animals and can be broadly divided into two distinct categories. The first group of mesoderm-derived cancers develop from mesenchymal cell lineages and are termed sarcomas. In comparison with epithelial malignancies, sarcomas in humans constitute only a small percentage (1%) of adult tumors; however, they contribute to a substantive fraction (>20%) of tumors diagnosed in the pediatric population, primarily affecting the musculoskeletal system (osteosarcoma, Ewing's sarcoma) (Burningham *et al.*, 2012). For companion animals, the percentage of cancers classified as mesenchymal in origin is approximately equal to tumors derived from the endoderm germ cell layer (Dobson *et al.*, 2002). Connective tissue cells, including fibroblasts, adipocytes, osteoblasts, myoblasts, and endothelial cells, can give rise to the development of sarcomas. The mesoderm also serves as the origin of hematopoietic tissues, and the second category of cancers arising from this embryonic germ cell layer includes a diverse group of 'liquid' tumor histologies collectively referred to as hematopoietic malignancies. In companion animals, hematopoietic malignancies, such as diffuse, large B-cell lymphoma, make up the lion's share of 'liquid' cancers, with lymphoid leukemia and multiple myeloma comprising a smaller fraction of cancer types (Atherton & Mason, 2022).

Nervous tissues develop from the gastrulation and transplantation of the ectodermal germ cell layer with subsequent formation of the neuroectoderm, which can give rise to cancers of the central and peripheral nervous system including astrocytomas, neuroblastomas, schwannomas, oligodendrogliomas, and medulloblastomas (Pytel & Lukas, 2009). In addition to the three germ cell layers, migratory and multipotent cells derived from the neural crest, including melanocytes and neurosecretory cells, can malignantly transform to develop cancers including melanoma, small-cell lung carcinoma, and functional adrenal gland tumors. As mentioned previously, the emergence of comparative oncology has afforded unique opportunities to study companion animal tumors that are believed to have shared biology (Oh & Cho, 2023). The National Cancer Institute has identified six tumor types of comparative interest, being diffuse large B-cell lymphoma, mammary gland carcinoma, astrocytoma, osteosarcoma, urothelial carcinoma, and oral malignant melanoma.

CANCER IS A GENETIC DISEASE

The etiology of cancer has evolved over the past 50 years, with early theories in the late 20th century suggesting that tumor development could result from diverse causes including dysregulated cellular differentiation, infectious agents (viruses), and genetic mutations. Although these rival hypotheses were not mutually exclusive, the prevailing theory, which has gained the broadest scientific support, is the concept that altered cellular genetics, or altered expression (epigenetics), is responsible for cancer formation. Supporting the hypothesis that gene mutations might be incriminated in cancer development were the experiments conducted by Bruce Ames. Through an *in-vitro* screening test using histidine auxotrophic mutant strains of *Salmonella typhimurium*, Ames was able to characterize the mutagenic potential of different chemical compounds (Ames *et al.*, 1960, 1963). Derived from these seminal experiments, chemical agents identified as being mutagenic, i.e., having the capacity to alter the genetic code, were then correlated with their ability to act as carcinogens through the formation of cancer (Ames, 1979; Ames *et al.*, 1973). The foundational correlations documented by Ames yielded the compelling inference that the carcinogenic potential of chemical agents was derived from their ability to damage genes and thus the DNA of cells. While the foundations of cancer development still are hinged on 'altered' genetic messaging, in the era of epigenetics, it is now well accepted that altered gene transcription, in the absence of mutated genes, is enough to drive cancer development (Flavahan *et al.*, 2017).

CARCINOGENESIS

With the acceptance that cancer was a consequence of cellular genetic alterations, it became possible to explain how exposure to different mutagens might lead to cancer formation. Importantly, it was recognized that agents with mutagenic properties likely acted as carcinogens, i.e., agents that promote the development of cancer but do not necessarily cause gene mutations. However, not all carcinogens were necessarily mutagenic, but rather non-mutagenic carcinogens could favor the development of cancer through tumor promotion or epigenetic effects. Broadly, agents or conditions that alter DNA and promote the development of cancer can be categorized into three different carcinogenic categories: chemical, physical, or biological.

CHEMICAL CARCINOGENESIS

Early evidence for the potential of chemicals to act as carcinogens was first observed in the late 18th century by two scientists named John Hill and Percivall Potts, a botanist and surgeon by profession, respectively. First, Hill observed that the aristocratic elite in England who preferentially used ground powdered tobacco leaves as 'snuff', as opposed to the smoking of cigarettes by commoners, were more likely to develop symptoms of nasal cancer (Redmond, 1970). Shortly after, Potts reported an association between exposure to chimney soot and scrotal squamous cell carcinoma development in young boys who worked as chimney sweeps (Brown & Thornton, 1957). These two early clinical observations made by Hill and Potts supporting the potential for chemical carcinogenesis were later validated scientifically in the early 20th century through detailed studies by a Japanese pathologist named Katsusaburo Yamagiwa. In a series of *in-vivo* experiments, a highly reactive chemical species called benzo[*a*]pyrene, a polycyclic aromatic hydrocarbon found in coal tar, was topically painted onto the inner ear surface of rabbits chronically over a course of months, with the resultant development of squamous cell carcinoma (Yamagiwa & Ichikawa, 1977). Based on the experimental findings reported by Yamagiwa, a 'cause and effect' relationship was established between exposure to certain chemicals and the consequent development of cancer. These original seminal findings reported by Yamagiwa served as a foundation for establishing the National Toxicology Program under the US Department of Health and Human Services, which provides a current and cumulative list of 243 chemicals that have been identified as known carcinogens or reasonably anticipated to behave as carcinogens (National Toxicology Program, 2011). Building upon this infrastructure, the National Toxicology Program has launched Toxicology in the 21st Century (Tox21), an automated high throughput screen of potentially mutagenic compounds that are found in today's industrialized world (Jeong *et al.*, 2022).

In addition to the list of known chemical carcinogens, many reactive chemical agents derived exogenously or endogenously through the cellular metabolism of dietary nutrients have the potential to participate in chemical carcinogenesis. Despite the multiple sources of chemical agents, mechanistically chemical carcinogens share a common mode of action: the creation of electrophilic substrates that have the capacity to react with nucleophilic sites in the purine and pyrimidine rings of nucleic acids. Specifically, chemically reactive carcinogens exert their effects by adding functional groups that form covalent bonds with DNA. The resultant chemically modified bases, called DNA adducts, can distort the organized helical structure of DNA, which in turn can promote errors in DNA replication and consequent gene mutations (Chambers, 1985; Hemminki *et al.*, 1986; Rabes, 1986). Interestingly, the purposeful formation of DNA adducts is the basis for how some chemotherapeutic agents, such as alkylating agents, are used to fight cancer. Food and Drug Administration regulation of new alkylating agents includes the incidence of secondary malignancies, an unwanted side effect of persistent DNA adduct formation in normal tissues that can ultimately lead to cancer formation (Demoor-Goldschmidt & de Vathaire, 2019).

The ability of chemical carcinogens to act as electrophiles can be inherent (ultimate carcinogen) or require cellular metabolism with the consequent formation of reactive chemical species. Given that some xenobiotic chemicals require metabolic conversion prior to elimination, gene polymorphisms that influence activities of metabolic pathways, including the cytochrome P450 and other detoxification systems, have the potential to directly influence carcinogenic potency (Agundez, 2004, 2008; Bozina *et al.*, 2009). Similarly, endogenous and normal cellular reactions, including oxidative respiration and lipid peroxidation, can produce gene mutations in cells through the generation of reactive oxygen species, which can react with DNA to produce oxidized nucleic acid bases such as 8-oxo-2'-deoxyguanosine (Cooke *et al.*, 2003; Karihtala & Soini, 2007). The ability to form reactive oxygen species as a necessary by-product of cellular respiration suggests the risk of cancer formation is inextricably intertwined with the act of living.

PHYSICAL CARCINOGENESIS

Broadly, physical carcinogens comprise a diverse set of agents including electromagnetic radiation of differing energetic levels (ultraviolet and ionizing radiation), temperatures, mechanical trauma, and solid materials. Mechanistically, physical carcinogens have the capacity to damage cellular DNA either directly, as is the case with electromagnetic radiation, or through chronic trauma and non-specific irritation with consequent oxidative injury (Nelson, 1965; Spadari *et al.*, 1987). Although a vast body of scientific studies has characterized the mutagenic effects of various physical factors, clinical observations derived from human beings exposed to radiation or asbestos serve as foundational evidence for carcinogenesis induction through non-chemical mechanisms. While there is strong evidence linking cancer formation with physical carcinogens, the latency period for cancer formation can often be protracted, even in the range of several decades for humans.

With respect to radiation-induced carcinogenesis, differences in energy levels influence the type of DNA alteration. For ultraviolet radiation, a photochemical reaction occurs between intrastrand thymine or cytosine bases in DNA, resulting in molecular lesions termed pyrimidine dimers, which commonly include the formation of cyclobutane pyrimidine dimers and 6,4 photoproducts (Epstein, 1970; Granstein & Sober, 1982). The formation of pyrimidine dimers results in a conformational 'kink' in the three-dimensional helical structure of DNA, which requires repair to avert genetic alterations. At least two cellular mechanisms exist for the repair of pyrimidine dimers, including spontaneous photoactivation and repair by nucleotide excision repair mechanisms (Sinha & Hader, 2002). In human beings that have defective nucleotide excision repair, a genetic disease condition called xeroderma pigmentosum, exposure to normal sunlight increases the incidence of skin cancer formation by 1,000-fold (Takebe *et al.*, 1989). Higher energy electromagnetic radiation, such as ionizing radiation, directly causes damage to nucleotide bases, as well as inducing single- and double-strand breaks in the DNA structure (Ward, 1988). Additionally, ionizing radiation can interact with water molecules within a cell and result in the production of free radicals, which can also damage DNA. The generation of free radicals from ionizing radiation interaction with water is responsible for most (67%) DNA damage induced by radiation therapy. Collectively, the mutagenic and carcinogenic effects of ionizing radiation are principally a consequence of unrepaired or misrepaired double-strand breaks in DNA, which predispose to global genomic instability and chromosomal aberrations (Hoeijmakers, 2001a, 2001b).

Another well-studied physical carcinogen is asbestos exposure. Asbestos is a naturally occurring silicate mineral that exists as a fibrous crystalline with physical properties, including thermal resistance, which historically made asbestos suitable for the fabrication of building materials. The carcinogenic potential of chronic asbestos inhalation in humans, for the development of mesothelioma and bronchogenic carcinoma, has been recognized for over 50 years (Borow *et al.*, 1973). The potential mechanisms for asbestos's carcinogenic properties have been scientifically proposed and include three non-mutually exclusive theories: (1) oxidative stress theory, (2) chromosome tangling theory, and (3) adsorption theory (Barrett *et al.*, 1989; Toyokuni, 2009). The oxidative stress theory has gained the broadest scientific support, as the role of chronic irritation as a risk factor for carcinogenesis is well characterized (Ohshima & Bartsch, 1994). The oxidative stress theory postulates that free radicals are produced in the immediate microenvironment by asbestos fibers serving as substrates for the Fenton reaction or through the liberation of free radicals (oxidative burst) by tissue resident macrophages that engulf asbestos fibers. As such, asbestos acts as a physical carcinogen through the chronic production of reactive oxygen species and consequent mutagenic changes to the DNA of resident cells. These changes to DNA with the consequent manifestation of malignancy (mesothelioma) occur over long stretches of time, and the average latency period from asbestos exposure and cancer formation is several decades (Frost, 2013).

BIOLOGICAL CARCINOGENESIS

The role of infectious agents in the development of cancer was intensively studied during the 1970s, and mechanisms of carcinogenesis were delineated. Worldwide, less than 20% of all cancers are related to infectious agents; however, this minority cause of cancer is mostly preventable. Broadly, biological carcinogens can support tumor cell initiation and promotion either directly, as is the case for viral infections, or indirectly, such as with bacterial or parasitic infections that drive chronic inflammation and oxidative injury within the pathogen-host microenvironment. With respect to pathogens indirectly causing cancer in human beings, such as *Helicobacter pylori* and mucosa-associated lymphoid tissue lymphoma or *Schistosoma haematobium* and squamous cell carcinoma of the bladder, chronic inflammation with the consequent generation of reactive oxygen species strongly participates in the carcinogenic process (Ohshima & Bartsch, 1994). Similarly, in dogs, a strong association for esophageal sarcoma development because of chronic inflammation secondary to *Spirocerca lupi* infection has been reported by several independent investigations (Bailey, 1963; Dvir *et al.*, 2010; Ranen *et al.*, 2004; Ribelin and Bailey, 1958). Additionally, in felines, traumatic rupture of the eye orbit with the release of protected antigens has been reported to drive chronic inflammation and subsequent post-traumatic sarcoma development (Wood & Scott, 2019). Recently, some investigations have tried to link bartonellosis with the development of canine lymphoma and hemangiosarcoma, while *Bartonella* spp. DNA was identified in tumor tissues, a cause-and-effect could not be established and it remains uncertain what role arthropod vector diseases might play in malignant transformation or risk in dogs (Duncan *et al.*, 2008; Lashnits *et al.*, 2020).

Unlike other infectious agents, the oncologic pathogenesis of viral infections is not reliant on the generation of chronic inflammation, but rather on the direct integration of viral genetic information into susceptible host cells. Tumor viruses can be categorized as retroviruses or DNA viruses, with their mechanisms of carcinogenesis being distinct. Retroviruses can be categorized as acute transforming and late transforming, which depicts the expected latency period between viral infection and the development of cancer. Acute transforming retroviruses contain viral oncogenes (v-onc), and upon infection of susceptible cells, transcription of v-onc genes results in the immediate dysregulation of proto-oncogene functions (see Oncogenes) and consequent malignant transformation. Late transforming retroviruses do not carry viral oncogenes, and the dysregulation of normal proto-oncogene activities is through proviral insertional mutagenesis (see Oncogenes), which is driven by the strong promoter or enhancer activities of proviral long terminal repeat sequences. However, the latency for late transforming retrovirus-induced cancers can be protracted, as proviral insertion near a cellular oncogene tends to be random and require multiple rounds of cellular and viral replication before pathologic insertion can be achieved.

More relevant to the development of cancer in human beings are DNA viruses, which include Epstein–Barr virus, human herpesvirus 8, and human papillomavirus (Martin & Gutkind, 2008). Mechanistically, once integrated into the host cell genome, a DNA virus can transcribe viral-specific proteins, which promote the immortalization of infected cells. Of the oncogenic DNA viruses, the molecular pathogenesis of human papillomavirus-associated cancers is understood with greater certainty in comparison with other DNA viral-induced malignancies. Human papillomavirus codes for two viral-specific proteins, E6 and E7, which serve to disable tumor suppressor protein activities, specifically p53 and Rb, respectively. The E6 viral protein accelerates the proteasome degradation of p53 protein, while the E7 protein competitively binds to Rb with consequent release of E2F family transcription factors (Dyson *et al.*, 1989; Scheffner *et al.*, 1993). Biologic activities of both E6 and E7 proteins result in the dysregulation of cell cycle checkpoints, which consequently promotes unchecked cellular proliferation, genomic instability, and mutagenesis.

CELLULAR RESPONSES TO MUTAGENIC INJURY

Mutagens have the potential to cause DNA damage; however, most cells that acquire DNA damage do not pose a risk for cancer development in the host organism. One main reason why DNA damage does not always translate into tumor formation is that only 1.5% of the entire genome is responsible for coding proteins. As such, DNA mutations occurring in the remaining 98.5% of the genome will not directly lead to dysregulated protein synthesis. However, it is well recognized that non-coding DNA plays a critical role in gene expression through various mechanisms, including long non-coding RNA and microRNA (Lange *et al.*, 2021). In the event a mutation does occur in an exome region, control of the cell cycle is central to safeguarding against cancer development, and cells that acquire DNA alterations can induce cell cycle arrest, programmed cell death, or both. Dysregulation within these two key cellular programs (i.e., cell cycle arrest and apoptosis) predisposes to genomic instability and a consequent increased risk for tumor formation.

CELL CYCLE

The cell cycle is a coordinated sequence of molecular events that regulate normal cell division and is comprised of four discrete phases termed M phase, S phase, G1 phase, and G2 phase. Inclusive of these four active phases of cell division, there exists an additional quiescent phase known as G0 (Figure 3.1) (Golias *et al.*, 2004; Schafer, 1998). In tissues that undergo rapid cell division, referred to as labile tissues, including the bone marrow and intestinal epithelium, a substantive fraction of resident cells is actively recruited into the cell cycle. In contrast, cells derived from organs that rest in a homeostatic state, referred to as stable tissues, remain in the non-proliferative G0 phase, unless cell replication is stimulated through mitogenic signals that recruit cells into the G1 phase.

Coordinated progression through the cell cycle is mediated by molecular checkpoints under the control of enzymes called cyclin-dependent kinases (CDKs). The activities of specific CDKs are responsible for regulating the passage of cells through discrete phases of the cell cycle (Figure 3.1) (Grana & Reddy, 1995; Satyanarayana & Kaldis, 2009). Stringent control of the cell cycle is necessary to minimize the generation of heritable errors in DNA replication and the avoidance of genomic instability, and the activities of CDKs are tightly regulated through the following redundant molecular mechanisms:

- Full enzymatic activities of CDKs require the coupling/pairing of preferential cyclin proteins with specific CDK subunits. Although the transcription of CDK subunits is relatively constant throughout the cell cycle, the translational stability of cyclin proteins is highly variable (except for Cyclin D), and mediated by proteasome degradation pathways, and selective cyclin protein expressions are specific to different phases of the cell cycle. Given the cyclic nature of cyclin protein stability, the activities of CDKs can be tuned and regulated by cyclin expression. Specific couplings of cyclins and CDKs are listed below and their cell cycle regulating activities are summarized in Table 3.1.
  - D-type cyclins (D1, D2, and D3) partner with CDK4 or CDK6.
  - E-type cyclins (E1 and E2) partner with CDK2.
- A-type cyclins partner with CDK2 or CDK1.
  - B-type cyclins partner with CDK1.
- Phosphorylation positively and negatively regulates the activities of cyclin/CDK complexes. Full CDK kinase activity requires an activating phosphorylation and is performed by CDK-activating kinases. Dephosphorylation of inhibitory sites through the activity of phosphatases is necessary to fully activate cyclin/CDK complexes too. As such, phosphorylation and dephosphorylation serve as molecular switches to control cyclin/CDK activities.
- Activity of cyclin/CDK complexes is directly regulated by two discrete classes of inhibitory proteins known as CDK inhibitors (Harper, 1997), which include the following:
  - INK4 proteins. This family of proteins specifically binds to CDK4 monomers and distorts the cyclin-binding domain, reducing the affinity for CDK4 to bind with D-type cyclins (Carnero & Hannon, 1998). Specific proteins belonging to the INK4 family include $p16^{INK4A}$, $p15^{INK4B}$, $p18^{INK4C}$, and $p19^{INK4D}$. Given their binding to CDK4 monomers, INK4 proteins regulate cell cycle progression restricted to the G1 phase and principally regulated genomic integrity prior to the S phase of the cell cycle.
- CIP/KIP proteins. This family of proteins bind to cyclin/CDK heterodimers and obstruct the ATP-binding site in the catalytic cleft of CDKs (Hengst & Reed, 1998; Nakayama & Nakayama, 1998). Specific proteins belonging to the CIP/KIP family include $p21^{Cip1}$, $p27^{Kip1}$, and $p57^{Kip2}$. The CIP/KIP proteins are promiscuous with their binding to cyclin/CDK heterodimers, and therefore can regulate the cell cycle at all checkpoints, and are not restricted to being operative only in the G1 phase of the cell cycle like the INK4 family of proteins.

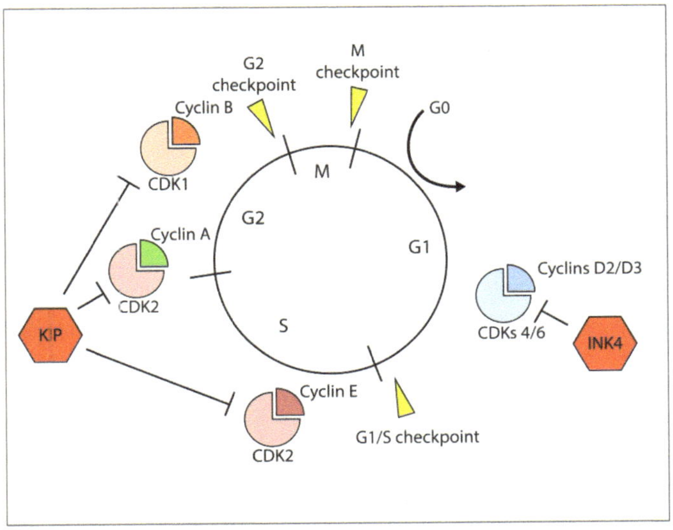

Figure 3.1 The cell cycle and regulatory control points. The cell cycle is divided into four phases (G1, S, G2, and M) and the inclusion of an additional quiescent phase (G0). Three cellular checkpoints (G1/S, G2, and M) ensure that DNA is replicated and segregated to daughter cells with high fidelity. Sequential and orderly procession through the cell cycle is regulated by activities mediated by cyclin-CDKs.

Table 3.1 Cell cycle and associated regulatory kinases

Cell cycle phase	Cyclin	Cyclin-dependent kinase
G0	C	CDK3
G1	D and E	CDK2, CDK4, and CDK6
S	A and E	CDK2
G2	A	CDK2 and CDK1
M	B	CDK1

In normal cells, the p53 protein is principally responsible for controlling cell cycle progression. Following DNA damage, p53 behaves as a transcription factor for scores of genes and promotes the gene expression of the CIP/KIP family of CDK inhibitors (Boulaire *et al.*, 2000; Gartel *et al.*, 1996). The multi-layered regulation of the cell cycle is critical for ensuring that cells harboring DNA damage will be arrested prior to DNA synthesis and permits the correction of aberrant genomic information through the activities of DNA repair systems. The regulatory checkpoints within the cell cycle minimize the chances for perpetuating heritable genome mutations (initiation phase of the malignant transformation cycle) that could be passed onto daughter cells and thus serve as a principal safeguard against the initiation and continued development of cancer.

PROGRAMMED CELL DEATH

Apoptosis is a normal cellular process executed through the activation of conserved cellular signaling pathways that lead to the orderly dismantling of damaged cells marked for death. Although most fundamental research has characterized differences between apoptosis and necrosis, it is now recognized that cell death can be executed by various pathways leading to the description and study of multiple divergent forms of cell death including ferroptosis, pyroptosis, immunogenic cell death, and necroptosis to name a few (Galluzzi *et al.*, 2018). Stimuli capable of inducing the apoptotic pathway include radiation, hypoxia, nutrient deprivation, and exposure to genotoxic agents (Haupt *et al.*, 2003). Cells undergoing apoptosis adopt characteristic morphologic changes including membrane blebbing, cell shrinkage, and chromatin condensation with orderly nuclear and chromosomal DNA fragmentation. Triggering of apoptosis can be achieved through extrinsic and intrinsic pathways, which converge on a common pathway mediated by executioner caspase enzymes (Figure 3.2) (Zimmermann *et al.*, 2001).

The extrinsic arm of the apoptosis pathway is mediated through cell surface receptor clustering mediated by ligand binding and consequent proximity activation of extrinsic initiator procaspases-8 and -10. Cell surface receptors involved in the initiation of the extrinsic cell death pathway include the FAS receptor and tumor necrosis factor-family death receptors (Elmore, 2007; Wang & El-Deiry, 2003; Waring & Mullbacher, 1999). Upon ligand/receptor binding, recruitment of procaspase-8 and -10 molecules to associated cytoplasmic death domains results in the proximity activation of these procaspases to active caspases (Figure 3.2, extrinsic pathway). Fully active extrinsic caspases then proceed to cleave and activate executioner procaspases-3, -6, and -7. Activated executioner caspases cleave multiple substrates, which leads to DNA fragmentation and cell death.

The intrinsic apoptotic pathway, also referred to as the mitochondrial pathway, is initiated following cellular stress or damage to DNA. Mediated predominantly by the DNA damage sensing properties of p53 and consequent transcription of pro-apoptotic proteins such as Bid, Bad, Bax, and Bak, mitochondrial permeability is increased and leads to the leakage of cytochrome c from the mitochondrial intermembrane space. Once cytochrome c is released, it binds with the cytosolic protein Apaf-1, forming a seven spoke-like wheel complex called the apoptosome (Figure 3.2, intrinsic pathway). Once formed, the apoptosome can recruit and bind with intrinsic initiator procaspase-9, with subsequent cleavage of procaspase-9 to caspase-9 through a proximity activation mechanism (Li & Yuan, 2008; Parrish *et al.*, 2013). Like the extrinsic pathway, caspase-9 consequently cleaves and activates executioner procaspases-3, -6, and -7 with the ultimate induction of DNA cleavage and cell death (Yuan & Akey, 2013). Hence, in normal cells when DNA is damaged and unable to be repaired, p53 protein is principally responsible for directing cells into programmed death through the upregulation and expression of proapoptotic proteins such as Bax and caspases, hence serving as a principal safeguard against the survival of cells harboring mutagenic DNA.

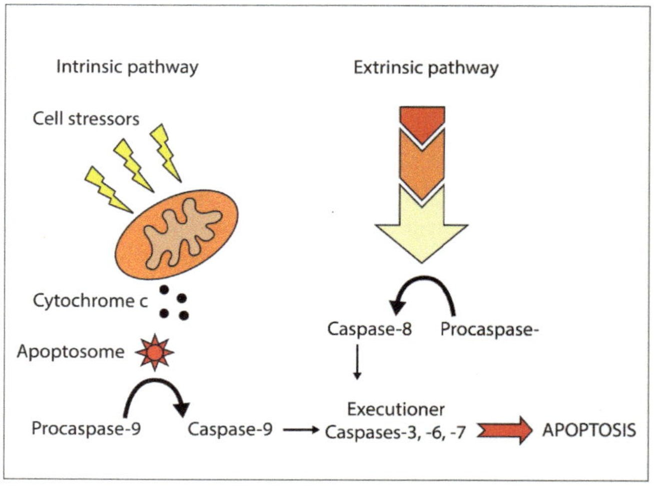

Figure 3.2 **Programmed cell death pathways. Initiation of apoptosis is mediated by two distinct yet overlapping pathways with communication between both arms through the generation of truncated Bid. Extrinsic activation is mediated by death receptor clustering, with subsequent proximity activation of extrinsic initiator procaspases (e.g., procaspase-8 activation to caspase-8). Intrinsic activation is stimulated by diverse cellular stressors, including radiation, chemotherapy, hypoxia, and nutrient deprivation, leading to cytochrome c release from the intermembrane space of the mitochondria. Cytosolic cytochrome c binds with Apaf-1 to form a complex called the apoptosome. Procaspase-9 is recruited to the apoptosome, with consequent proximity activation to initiator caspase-9. Active initiator caspases then cleave and activate executioner caspases-3, -6, and -7, resulting in DNA cleavage and cell death.**

MALIGNANT TRANSFORMATION: A MULTISTEP PROCESS

With the identification that carcinogens were responsible for the development of cancer, scientists were able to study the key cellular events leading to overt tumor formation. It became evident, particularly in the study of chemical carcinogenesis, that the maladaptation to a cancerous phenotype required an individual cell to acquire several concurrent genetic or epigenetic perturbations, and such 'steps' towards a malignant phenotype could be categorized into three distinct stages: initiation, promotion, and progression (Boyland, 1985; Foulds, 1954, 1965). The ultimate outcome of this multistep process is the development of cancer cells with invasive properties (Figure 3.3).

Initiation

The potential for tumor initiation starts with any mutagenic event leading to a change in cellular DNA, often a single base alteration,

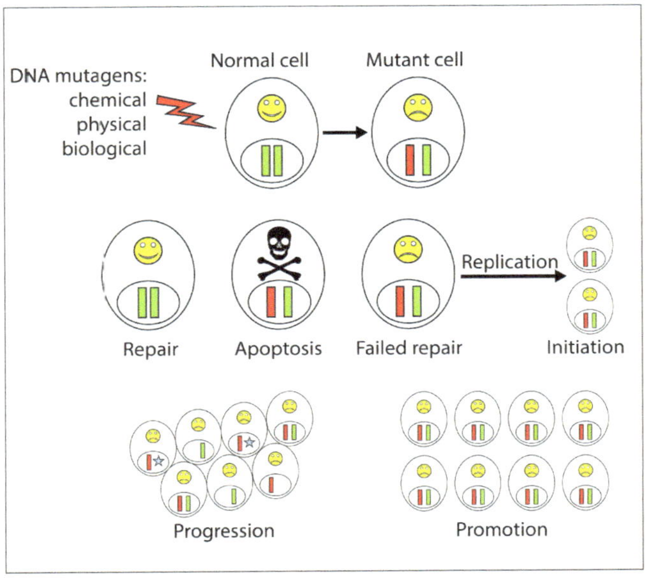

Figure 3.3 **Steps involved in cellular malignant transformation. Following a mutagenic event, normal cellular outcomes include cell cycle arrest with complete DNA repair, catastrophic and irreparable DNA damage leading to apoptosis, or failed DNA repair. Perpetuation of heritable genomic defects to daughter cells represents the initiation phase of malignant transformation. Clonal expansion of initiated cells and acquisition of additional genetic mutations represent the steps of tumor promotion and progression, respectively.**

in susceptible cells. Following the induction of DNA mutation, cellular outcomes include (1) programmed cell death, (2) cell cycle arrest with repair of DNA damage, or (3) failure to repair DNA damage. In cells undergoing apoptosis or successfully repairing DNA damage, the mutagenic event and potential for carcinogenesis are completely neutralized. However, in cells failing to repair DNA mutations and subsequent procession through DNA replication, the production of heritable genome changes becomes irreversible and constitutes the event of 'initiation'. However, not all initiated cells will proceed forward to establish cancer, as some initiated cells will harbor silent genetic mutations given that 98.5% of the genome is not responsible for protein coding. Additionally, the cellular outcomes of initiated cells can be dormancy or apoptosis. As such, an initiated cell is not synonymous with a tumor cell, as the genomic alterations of an initiated cell might remain undetectable throughout the life of the host organism unless additional genomic perturbations are acquired that further promote cell proliferation and genomic instability.

Promotion

During tumor promotion, initiated cells are provided with a selective growth advantage through transient increases in cell division, decrease in apoptosis, or a combination (Wright *et al.*, 1994). Clonal expansion of initiated cell populations can occur following exposure to non-genotoxic or weakly genotoxic agents and result in the formation of pre-malignant lesions (Slaga, 1983). Many chemicals have been identified that act as tumor promoters, with croton oil, tetradecanoyl phorbol acetate, and phenobarbital serving as examples. In addition to chemical agents, tumor promotion can be elicited by trauma or cell death, which results in inflammation and the release of growth, survival, and pro-angiogenic factors (Grivennikov & Karin, 2010; Rundhaug & Fischer, 2010). Real life examples that might be striking are the habit of drinking alcohol and smoking as a pastime, with combustion of cigarette smoke providing the carcinogens, and drinking alcohol serving as a promoting agent through the induction of gingival mucosal cell death and compensatory cell proliferation (Pelucchi *et al.*, 2006).

Progression

During the clonal expansion of initiated cell populations, pre-malignant cells have the potential to acquire additional genetic mutations, and a major hallmark of tumor progression is chromosomal instability (Loeb, 1991; Nowell, 1976). As a result of genetic instability, pre-malignant cells acquire additional karyotype alterations that allow for increased growth speed, invasiveness, and metastatic potential. Many of the chromosomal abnormalities that accumulate during tumor progression include mutations that inactivate tumor suppressor genes and activate oncogenes.

Tumor suppressor genes

Genes classified as tumor suppressors have the capacity to protect normal cells from malignant transformation. Classically, tumor suppressor genes have been described as acting recessively and as following the 'two-hit hypothesis', originally proposed by Alfred G. Knudson in 1971 (Knudson, 1971), which implies that both maternal and paternal alleles that encode a specific tumor suppressor gene must be affected before a deficient phenotype is produced. Despite the validity of the 'two-hit hypothesis' for many genes, altered phenotypes can be produced because of genetic change within one parental allele; such exceptions include haploinsufficiency and dominant negative mutations (Payne & Kemp, 2005), whereby the phenotype is blended and not dichotomous. Broadly, tumor suppressor genes can be categorized as 'gatekeepers' or 'caregivers', and more recently 'landscapers' based on their different mechanisms for minimizing heritable genomic changes (Deininger, 1999; Levitt & Hickson, 2002).

Gatekeepers

'Gatekeeper' genes function by directly controlling cell growth via cell cycle regulation or promote programmed cell death. Gatekeeper genes are principally responsible for protecting against tumor cell initiation, which is the first and critical step in the malignant transformation process. Mutations in gatekeeper genes can occur at both the somatic and germline levels, with sporadic tumors more frequently having somatic mutations and hereditary tumor syndromes driven by germline mutations in gatekeeper genes (Vogelstein & Kinzler, 2004). Li-Fraumeni syndrome and Retinoblastoma are examples of hereditary tumor syndromes in which germline mutations occur in

P53 and retinoblastoma (RB) genes, respectively (Strahm & Malkin, 2006).

The two most notable gatekeeper tumor suppressor genes are the P53 gene and the RB gene, both serving critical functions in regulating the cell cycle (Sager, 1992). Referred to as the 'Guardian', of the genome, the p53 protein is responsible for initiating multiple cellular programs that prevent malignant transformation, including the activation of DNA repair proteins, arrestment of the cell cycle at the G1/S checkpoint, and induction of apoptosis (Efeyan & Serrano, 2007). In parallel with the P53 gene, the RB gene serves as a master regulator of cell cycle progression in the G1 phase. Early in the G1 phase, Rb protein exists in a hypophosphorylated state and binds tightly with E2F family transcription factors (Cobrinik *et al.*, 1992). The association of Rb protein with E2F family transcription factors prevents the transcription of target genes required to progress past the G1/S checkpoint. Upon progressive phosphorylation of the Rb protein by active CDKs, E2F family transcription factors are released by the Rb protein, allowing cells to progress into the DNA synthesis phase of the cell cycle (Cobrinik *et al.*, 1992; Hamel *et al.*, 1992). Since the discovery of the P53 and RB genes as tumor suppressor genes, a multitude of additional gatekeeper tumor suppressor genes have been identified (Table 3.2).

Caregivers

'Caregiver' genes are another category of genes responsible for protecting the genome. These genes are involved in maintaining genomic stability, principally through regulation of DNA repair pathways, which reduces the mutational rate of the host genome (Goode *et al.*, 2002). Unlike gatekeeper genes, which are principally involved in protecting against tumor cell initiation, caregiver genes play a larger role in the tumor progression stage of malignant transformation. Mutations in caregiver genes have the potential to accelerate the multistep tumorigenic process simply because of enhanced genomic instability and consequent acquisition of additional genetic mutations. The importance of caregiver genes is highlighted by the increased likelihood for developing hereditary breast and ovarian cancer in women harboring *BRCA1* and *BRCA2* gene mutations (King *et al.*, 2003; Szabo & King, 1995). Mechanistically, BRCA1 and BRCA2 proteins participate in the formation of a large multi-subunit protein complex called BRCA1-associated genome surveillance complex, which is critical for the identification and repair of double-strand DNA breaks through homologous recombination (Liu & West, 2002). Ineffective repair of DNA breaks, in particular double-strand breaks, dramatically increases the risk for progressive genomic instability and cancer development (Karran, 2000; Moynahan *et al.*, 1999). In human cancer patients with BRCA1 and BRCA2 mutations, inhibitors of PARP have proved to be exceptionally effective in killing mutated cancer cells through a process known as 'synthetic lethality' (Helleday, 2011). Although not as extensive as gatekeeper genes, many tumor suppressor genes that function as caregivers and participate in cancer susceptibility have been identified and characterized (Table 3.2).

Table 3.2 **Abbreviated list of recognized tumor suppressor genes**

Major gatekeeper genes		
Gene	**Protein function**	**Associated tumors**
Major caregiver genes		
Gene	**Protein function**	**Associated tumors**
APC	Cell adhesion, signal transduction pathway	Colorectal cancer
VHL	Transcriptional elongation regulation	Schwannoma, meningioma, others
PTEN	Phosphatase	Hamartoma, glioma, others
RB1	Cell cycle control	Osteosarcoma, others
TP53	Cell cycle control, apoptosis	Sarcoma, leukemia, others
NF1	Ras GAP activity	Neurofibroma, sarcoma, others
CDKN2A	Cell cycle control	Melanoma, pancreatic cancer
WT1	Transcription factor	Nephroblastoma
BRCA1	DNA repair, cycle checkpoint control	Breast and ovarian cancer
BRCA2	DNA repair, cycle checkpoint control	Breast and ovarian cancer
ATM	DNA repair	Lymphoma
FANCA	DNA repair	Acute myeloid leukemia
MLH1	DNA mismatch repair	Lymphoma, sarcoma, others
NER	Nucleotide excision repair	Skin cancer

Landscaper genes

In addition to gatekeeper and caregiver tumor suppressor genes, a third category of genes with suppressive properties has been proposed and termed 'landscaper' genes. As suggested by their name, landscaper genes act on the microenvironment in which cells reside (Cooper & Giancotti, 2019). Interestingly, it is well accepted that cellular behaviors can be directly affected by the microenvironment, a process known as 'outside to inside' signaling, often mediated by integrins. Aberrations in landscaper genes that are responsible for mechanical properties of the extracellular matrix could result in changes in cellular behaviors, as well as alter microenvironmental cues including growth factors, cell adhesion molecules, and extracellular matrix properties, which in turn can influence the behavior of resident-initiated cells (Kinzler & Vogelstein, 1998).

Oncogenes

Proto-oncogenes code for normal cellular machinery involved in cell growth and differentiation, which includes growth factors, growth factor receptors, protein kinases, adaptor proteins, G-protein signaling transducers, and transcription factors (Table 3.3). Genetic alterations capable of dysregulating the expression or activity of proto-oncogenes can lead to dominant, gain-of-function mutations with the consequent generation of an active oncogene. Unlike tumor suppressor genes, conversion of a proto-oncogene to an oncogene necessitates only one parental allele to be transformed within a susceptible cell to obtain a phenotypic change. The conversion of proto-oncogenes to hyperactive oncogenes can

Table 3.3 **Abbreviated list of recognized oncogenes**

Gene	Protein function	Associated tumors
ALK	Receptor tyrosine kinase	Lymphoma
BCL-2	Anti-apoptotic protein	Lymphoma, leukemia
C-MYC	Transcription factor	Leukemia, carcinoma, others
EGFR	Cell surface receptor	Squamous cell carcinoma
GLI	Transcription factor	Glioblastoma
KIT	Receptor tyrosine kinase	Sarcoma, gastrointestinal stromal tumor, others
JUN	Transcription factor	Sarcoma
RAS	G-protein signal transduction	Carcinoma
RET	Receptor tyrosine kinase	Thyroid carcinoma, multiple endocrine neoplasia
SIS	Growth factor	Glioma, fibrosarcoma
SRC	Tyrosine kinase	Sarcoma
TRK	Receptor tyrosine kinase	Colon and thyroid carcinoma

be categorized into at least four mutagenic mechanisms: (1) point mutations, (2) gene amplification, (3) chromosomal translocation, and (4) viral insertions.

Point mutations can produce phenotypic changes either through the generation of proteins resistant to normal regulatory cues or through degradation pathways, resulting in constitutive activation or functional hyperactivation. The RAS oncogene transcribes a protein harboring a point mutation, which endows resistance to normal regulatory enzymatic activity (GTPase activity) and consequently allows for sustained and dysregulated intracellular signaling (Hamilton & Vogelstein, 1988).

The identification of homogeneously staining regions and double minutes are genetic hallmarks of gene amplification, which can result in the transformation of a proto-oncogene to an oncogene. The translational product of gene amplification is normal; however, the absolute quantities of protein can be log orders greater than normal given the dramatic increases in mRNA transcripts. The overexpression of human epidermal growth factor receptor 2 (HER2) in aggressive breast cancer is an example of gene amplification that serves as a drug target for improving cancer management using an antibody called Herceptin (Ross & Fletcher, 1999).

Chromosome translocations can result from the joining of different chromosome arms and have the potential to produce excessive levels of normal or novel proteins because of coupling strong promoter sequences upstream of proto-oncogene coding regions. As such, chromosomal translocation serves as one genetic mechanism responsible for the conversion of proto-oncogenes to oncogenes. Perhaps the most well studied and therapeutically targetable chromosomal translocation is the Philadelphia chromosome, which is a balanced chromosomal translocation between chromosomes 9 and 22 (Koretzky, 2007). The Philadelphia chromosome produces a novel BCR–ABL fusion gene capable of producing a protein with excessive tyrosine kinase activities and serves as the oncogenic mutation responsible for the development of chronic myeloid leukemia (Konopka & Witte, 1985; Westbrook, 1988). The drug Gleevec was engineered to inhibit the BCR–ABL fusion protein and is first-line therapy for human cancer patients diagnosed with chronic myelogenous leukemia (Iqbal & Iqbal, 2014).

Historically, the discovery and characterization of oncogenes were first described in studies of viruses with cancer forming properties. Mechanistically, retroviruses exert their oncogenic effects through a process termed insertional mutagenesis, whereby viral genetic material is inserted into the host cell's genome. Differences in penetrance and latency of tumor development following retroviral infection are associated with the type of retrovirus and classified as either acute or late transforming. Acute transforming retroviruses carry viral oncogenes (v-onc) within their genome, and on infection of host cells, the transcription of v-onc is driven by strong viral promoter sequences found within the 5′ long terminal repeat sequences. Consequently, malignant transformation occurs rapidly following infection with acute transforming retroviruses (Gray, 1991; Uren *et al.*, 2005). In contrast, late transforming retroviruses do not carry viral oncogenes within their genome, and therefore are not likely to induce rapid malignant transformation. Rather, late transforming retroviruses randomly insert into the host cell genome with the low incident possibility of being inserted in proximity to a normal cellular proto-oncogene. In these rare instances, strong viral promoters and enhancers of late transforming retroviruses are capable of hijacking the transcription of proximal cellular proto-oncogenes, resulting in gain-of-function activities (Gray, 1991; Uren *et al.*, 2005). Retroviral infection as a cause of malignancy in human beings is rare, with one example being human T-cell lymphotropic virus type 1, which is associated with the development of adult T-cell leukemia/lymphoma (Robert-Guroff *et al.*, 1985). In parallel, several retroviruses are responsible for the development of cancers in felines and include feline leukemia virus, feline immunodeficiency virus, and feline sarcoma virus (Beatty, 2014; Fujinaga & Green, 1971; Hoover & Mullins, 1991; Jarrett, 1975; Linenberger & Abkowitz, 1995; McDonough *et al.*, 1971).

TUMOR MASS HETEROGENEITY

Based on the malignant transformation paradigm, the origin of cancer arises from a single initiated cell and corresponds with the accepted clonal nature of cancer development (Wainscoat & Fey, 1990). However, during the processes of tumor promotion and progression, individual tumor cells can show distinct properties including differences in gene expression profiles, cellular morphologies, and biologic behaviors, which generate intratumoral heterogeneity. The development of tumor heterogeneity has the potential to compromise the successful treatment of cancer, not only in the context of tumor cell susceptibilities to anticancer therapeutics, but also the development of tumor cells with augmented invasive and metastatic capacities. Two main theories have been proposed to explain the development of tumor mass heterogeneity: (1) the clonal selection theory and (2) the cancer stem cell theory; both provide a conceptual framework for understanding the mechanisms of cancer progression.

Clonal selection theory

The concept for the clonal evolution of cancer was first proposed in the late 20th century and sought to explain the observation that tumors often become more aggressive in their biologic behaviors, such as growth rate, invasiveness, and metastatic capacity, as a function of time (Greaves & Maley, 2012; Nowell, 1986). Clonal evolution of individual cancer cells within a tumor mass represents the sequential selection of variants derived from a common malignantly transformed clone. In this Darwinian model, driver mechanisms for clonal evolution of cancer cells are believed to be from the combined effects of internal and external factors. Intrinsically, the genetic instability of tumor cells, known as a mutator phenotype, serves as a principal driver for clonal evolution. On repeated rounds of initiated cell proliferation, the probability of acquiring additional genetic mutations continually increases, and a small fraction of mutated cells will have the chance to acquire some additional growth advantages. Consequently, mutants with superior 'fitness' become the predominant subpopulations within a tumor mass. The co-existence of multiple 'fit' subpopulations provides the basis for tumor mass heterogeneity (Figure 3.4). In addition to the intrinsic genetic instability of tumor cells that contributes to clonal evolution, host factors that are operative within the tumor microenvironment are expected to exert selective pressures that drive the expansion of malignant clonal subpopulations. Host-derived factors involved in clonal evolution within the immediate tumor environment include immune surveillance, growth factors, and inflammation.

Cancer stem cell theory

Stem cells are pluripotent cells with the capacity for indefinite proliferation and differentiation, and they serve as an inexhaustible cell source for replenishing normal cell populations undergoing homeostatic programmed cell death. Cancer stem cells are tumor cells that possess stem cell properties. The stem cell theory of cancer proposes that tumor mass heterogeneity is driven by a small fraction of malignantly transformed stem cells with the capacity to (1) divide and expand the cancer stem cell pool and (2) differentiate into heterogeneous non-tumorigenic cancer cell types that constitute the bulk of cells within a tumor mass (Figure 3.4).

Cancer stem cell division can be asymmetric, with daughter cell progenies being either stem cell in nature or not. Non-cancer stem cell progeny are categorized as transit amplifying cells. The specific population of transit amplifying cells demonstrates limited replication potential yet constitutes the major proportion of cells within a tumor mass. In contrast with transit amplifying cells, cancer stem cells comprise only a small percentage of the tumor cell mass and generally remain divisionally silent for the majority of the time. Definitive evidence supporting the cancer stem cell theory was derived from

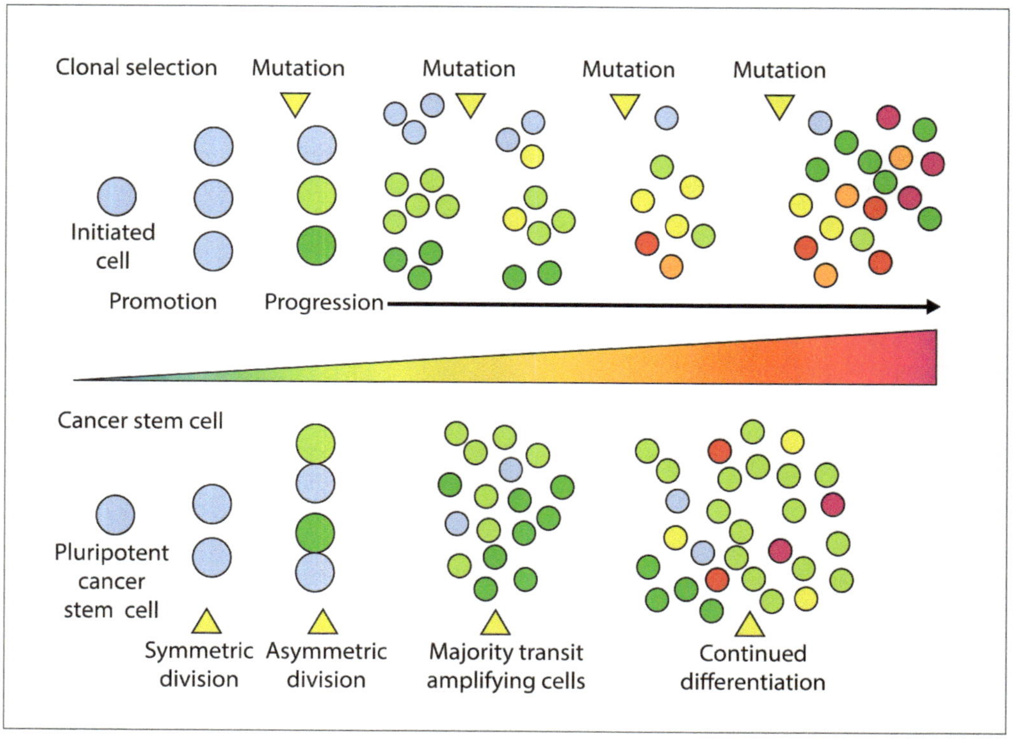

Figure 3.4 Different models for generating tumor heterogeneity. The clonal selection model suggests that genomic instability is the underlying mechanism for generating tumor heterogeneity. Genetic mutations that provide growth advantages will have the potential to drive the development of phenotypically different clonal subpopulations. The cancer stem cell model proposes that tumor heterogeneity is a consequence of a small number of pluripotent cancer stem cells capable of asymmetric division. Cancer stem cells give rise to transit amplifying populations, which are variably differentiated cancer cells with limited replicative potential.

studies of acute myelogenous leukemia, where a small population of $CD34^+CD38^-$ cells were capable of tumorigenesis and recapitulating tumor cell heterogeneity in a NOD/SCID murine preclinical model of leukemia (Bonnet & Dick, 1997). Shortly following the identification of cancer stem cells in hematologic malignancies, evidence for their existence in solid tumor histologies was first described in human glioma (Ignatova *et al.*, 2002). To date, ample scientific evidence has been gathered to support the existence of cancer stem cells across a diverse group of both hematopoietic and solid tumor histologies (Prager *et al.*, 2019).

The implications for the cancer stem cell theory are significant, as it indicates that only a small fraction of cancer cells within a tumor mass are fundamentally responsible for the genesis, maintenance, and recurrence of cancer. As such, thousands of scientific investigations have focused on understanding the properties of cancer stem cells with the intent of identifying the cellular behaviors and vulnerabilities that could be exploited for improving cancer prevention and treatment (Ju *et al.*, 2022).

Hallmarks of cancer

Given the genetic basis of cancer and the diverse mutagenic stimuli that a vast number of germline and somatic cells are exposed to routinely, it is remarkable that the generation of renegade cells and consequent development of macroscopic tumor masses are relatively infrequent events in complex, multicellular organisms. Largely by virtue of the inherent genetic safeguards such as cell cycle arrest, programmed cell death, and DNA repair mechanisms, host organisms survive for an entire lifetime without fatal cancer development. Nonetheless, in rare instances where all steps of malignant transformation are achieved, cells display conserved aberrant biologic behaviors that serve as foundational abnormalities shared by cancer cells. This constellation of deranged cellular activities and properties are considered the seminal hallmarks of cancer (Hanahan & Weinberg, 2000, 2011).

Self-sufficiency in growth signals

Normal cell growth and proliferation require the transcriptional activation of genes responsible for cell cycling. Such stimulatory intracellular signals can be derived from the binding of cell surface receptors with diffusible growth factors, extracellular matrix components, or cell-to-cell interactions. In the absence of external stimulation, normal cells will not proliferate, but rather remain quiescent in the G0 phase. In contrast, cancer cells acquire genetic mutations that do not have the requirement of exogenous stimulatory signals for cell replication and are deemed growth self-sufficient. The achievement of growth self-sufficiency can be accomplished by cancer cells through different genetic alterations that are most commonly are associated with oncogene activation. Classical oncogenic mutations leading to growth self-sufficiency include excessive growth factor production, overexpression of growth receptors, constitutive activation of signaling pathways, and disruption of negative feedback mechanisms responsible for terminating proliferative responses.

Insensitivity to antigrowth signals

Complementing the actions of growth self-sufficiency, cancer cells also exhibit insensitivity to antigrowth signals, and in combination, both properties promote and accelerate the unrestrained proliferation of cancer cells. Normal cells will obey signals derived from the immediate microenvironment, including cues provided by neighboring cells and extracellular matrix, to arrest from the cell cycle and terminally differentiate. However, genetic mutations in tumor suppressor genes, such as P53 and RB, can endow cancer cells with insensitivities to antigrowth signaling, with consequent unrestricted cell cycling and proliferation.

Evading apoptosis

Apoptosis is a form of programmed cell death and serves as a homeostatic mechanism to allow normal cells to be removed from the host organism. The apoptotic program involves hundreds of proteins; however, p53 serves as a master regulator. As such, mutations in the P53 gene can endow cancer cells with the ability to evade programmed cell death, even in the face of catastrophic genomic injury. Blocks in the apoptotic program in cancer cells are common and can be mediated through multiple mechanisms including downregulation of membrane death receptors, increased anti-apoptotic protein expression, and sequestration of initiator and executioner caspases.

Limitless replicative potential

Normal cells have a finite replicative potential, which is dictated by the rate of successive telomere length erosion following each round of DNA replication. Except for normal pluripotent stem cells, normal somatic cells following repeated cellular divisions will ultimately undergo a process called senescence and lose the capacity for further replication. Mechanistically, finite replication due to telomere erosion serves as a protective barrier to prevent highly mutagenic processes such as breakage–fusion–bridge cycling, which is the inadvertent fusion of sister chromatid pairs during mitosis. Cancer cells express telomerase, an enzyme typically used by pluripotent stem cells that allows for the maintenance of telomere length with consequent endowment of infinite replicative potential. The use of telomerase or other telomere lengthening strategies by cancer cells serves as a conserved mechanism allowing the achievement of cellular immortalization.

Sustained angiogenesis

Angiogenesis is the process by which new blood vessels are derived from pre-existing vasculature. Based on the limits of nutrient and oxygen diffusion, macroscopic tissue growth exceeding 1–2 mm in diameter requires the establishment of new blood vessels. The regulation of angiogenesis is complex and requires the coordinated interplay and balance between pro- and anti-angiogenic peptides that act on endothelial cells. Under normal physiological conditions, angiogenesis can be transient and reversible, as demonstrated in normal wound healing. However, cancer cells favor activation of the angiogenic switch, which shifts the balance to sustained new blood vessel formation and thereby allows for the continued macroscopic growth of tumor cell masses.

Tissue invasion and metastasis

The outgrowth of cancer can be biologically categorized as being benign or malignant and is dependent on behavior attributes of cancer cell populations. The most problematic tumor histologies are those that invade and involve distant organs through the process of metastasis. Tissue invasion is mediated by the increased directional motility of cancer cells in conjunction with the liberation of proteases capable of degrading the basement membrane and associated extracellular matrix proteins including collagen, fibronectin, and gelatin. Tumor cell metastasis is the progressive extension of localized tissue invasion, where individual or small numbers of tumor cells have entered the circulatory system, either a blood or lymphatic vessel, and proceeded to disseminate to distant organs. The specific steps of this metastatic cascade can be categorized into discrete processes: (1) detachment from the primary tumor, (2) migration and intravasation, (3) circulatory transport, (4) arrest and extravasation, (5) resistance to anoikis and colonization, and (6) angiogenesis.

Two emerging hallmarks of cancer

Since the first description of the hallmarks of cancer in 2000 (Hanahan & Weinberg, 2000), new investigations conducted over the last decade have suggested that two additional characteristics reflective of tumor behavior should be considered as emerging hallmarks. Specifically, cancer cells appear to universally demonstrate properties that allow for the reprogramming of energy metabolism and evading immune destruction (Hanahan & Weinberg, 2011). With regards to altered energy metabolism, the capacity of cancer cells to preferentially utilize aerobic glycolysis has been recognized for close to 100 years, and is termed the Warburg effect. The underlying mechanism for cancer cells to preferentially utilize glycolysis as a main energy source remains enigmatic; however, it has been hypothesized that increased glycolysis might allow for the diversion of glycolytic intermediates into biosynthetic pathways that support rapid cellular proliferation, and hence provide a growth advantage for cancer cells (Vander Heiden *et al.*, 2009). Addressing the capacity of tumor cells to evade immune destruction, substantive preclinical and epidemiologic evidence supports the important role of the immune system as a barrier to tumor formation and progression. As such, the presence of malignantly transformed cells, which progress to develop into macroscopic tumor burdens in immunocompetent hosts, would suggest that a conserved set of mechanisms are employed by cancer cells for immune system evasion.

SUMMARY AND FUTURE DIRECTIONS

With the exponential gains in our understanding of cancer biology and the wider acceptance of comparative oncology, it is hoped that new frontiers in the prevention, detection, and treatment of cancer will be discovered for humans and companion animals alike. Given the conservation of key tumor characteristics that define malignancy, fundamental advances made through the study of preclinical murine models, comparative oncology trials in pet dogs and cats with naturally occurring cancers, or by epidemiologic studies in human beings should provide the opportunity to co-advance our understanding of cancer. Focused efforts should be made by health professionals and comparative researchers to support synergistic discovery opportunities that have the potential to accelerate cancer research, which can benefit both people and companion animals.

REFERENCES

Agundez J.A. (2004) Cytochrome P450 gene polymorphism and cancer. *Curr Drug Metab 5*:211–224.

Agundez J.A. (2008) Polymorphisms of human N-acetyltransferases and cancer risk. *Curr Drug Metab 9*:520–531.

Ames B.N. (1979) Identifying environmental chemicals causing mutations and cancer. *Science 204*:587–593.

Ames B.N., Garry B., Herzenberg L.A. (1960) The genetic control of the enzymes of histidine biosynthesis in Salmonella typhimurium. *J Gen Microbiol 22*:369–378.

Ames B.N., Hartman P.E., Jacob F. (1963) Chromosomal alterations affecting the regulation of histidine biosynthetic enzymes in Salmonella. *J Mol Biol 7*:23–42.

Ames B.N., Lee F.D., Durston W.E. (1973) An improved bacterial test system for the detection and classification of mutagens and carcinogens. *Proc Natl Acad Sci U S A 70*:782–786.

Atherton M.J., Mason N.J. (2022) Bite-size introduction to canine hematologic malignancies. *Blood Adv 6*:4073–4084.

Bailey W.S. (1963) Parasites and cancer: Sarcoma in dogs associated with Spirocerca Lupi. *Ann N Y Acad Sci 108*:890–923.

Barrett J.C., Lamb P.W., Wiseman R.W. (1989) Multiple mechanisms for the carcinogenic effects of asbestos and other mineral fibers. *Environ Health Perspect 81*:81–89.

Beatty J. (2014) Viral causes of feline lymphoma: Retroviruses and beyond. *Vet J 201*:174–180.

Bilgic O., Duda L., Sanchez M.D. et al. (2015) Feline oral squamous cell carcinoma: Clinical manifestations and literature review. *J Vet Dent 32*:30–40.

Bonnet D., Dick J.E. (1997) Human acute myeloid leukemia is organized as a hierarchy that originates from a primitive hematopoietic cell. *Nat Med 3*:730–737.

Borow M., Conston A., Livornese L. et al. (1973) Mesothelioma following exposure to asbestos: A review of 72 cases. *Chest 64*:641–646.

Boulaire J., Fotedar A., Fotedar R. (2000) The functions of the cdk-cyclin kinase inhibitor p21WAF1. *Pathol Biol (Paris) 48*:190–202.

Boyland E. (1985) Tumour initiators, promoters, and complete carcinogens. *Br J Ind Med 42*:716–718.

Bozina N., Bradamante V., Lovric M. (2009) Genetic polymorphism of metabolic enzymes P450 (Cyp) as a susceptibility factor for drug response, toxicity, and cancer risk. *Arhiv Za Higijenu Rada I Toksikologiju-Archives of Industrial Hygiene and Toxicology 60*:217–242.

Brown J.R., Thornton J.L. (1957) Percivall Pott (1714–1788) and chimney sweepers' cancer of the scrotum. *Br J Ind Med 14*:68–70.

Burningham Z., Hashibe M., Spector L. et al. (2012) The epidemiology of sarcoma. *Clin Sarcoma Res 2*:14.

Carnero A., Hannon G.J. (1998) The INK4 family of CDK inhibitors. *Curr Top Microbiol Immunol 227*:43–55.

Chambers R.W. (1985) Chemical carcinogenesis: A biochemical overview. *Clin Biochem 18*:158–168.

Cobrinik D., Dowdy S.F., Hinds P.W. et al. (1992) The retinoblastoma protein and the regulation of cell cycling. *Trends Biochem Sci 17*:312–315.

Cooke M.S., Evans M.D., Dizdaroglu M. et al. (2003) Oxidative DNA damage: Mechanisms, mutation, and disease. *FASEB J 17*:1195–1214.

Cooper J., Giancotti F.G. (2019) Integrin signaling in cancer: Mechanotransduction, stemness, epithelial plasticity, and therapeutic resistance. *Cancer Cell 35*:347–367.

Deininger P. (1999) Genetic instability in cancer: Caretaker and gatekeeper genes. *Ochsner J 1*:206–209.

Demoor-Goldschmidt C., de Vathaire F. (2019) Review of risk factors of secondary cancers among cancer survivors. *Br J Radiol 92*:20180390.

Dobson J.M., Samuel S., Milstein H. et al. (2002) Canine neoplasia in the UK: Estimates of incidence rates from a population of insured dogs. *J Small Anim Pract 43*:240–246.

Duncan A.W., Marr H.S., Birkenheuer A.J. et al. (2008) Bartonella DNA in the blood and lymph nodes of Golden Retrievers with lymphoma and in healthy controls. *J Vet Intern Med 22*:89–95.

Dvir E., Clift S.J., Williams M.C. (2010) Proposed histological progression of the Spirocerca lupi-induced oesophageal lesion in dogs. *Vet Parasitol 168*:71–77.

Dyson N., Howley P.M., Munger K. et al. (1989) The human papilloma virus-16 E7 oncoprotein is able to bind to the retinoblastoma gene product. *Science 243*:934–937.

Efeyan A. (2007) Serrano M: p53: Guardian of the genome and policeman of the oncogenes. *Cell Cycle 6*:1006–1010.

Elmore S. (2007) Apoptosis: A review of programmed cell death. *Toxicol Pathol 35*:495–516.

Epstein J.H. (1970) Ultraviolet carcinogenesis. *Photophysiology 5*:235–273.

Flavahan W.A., Gaskell E., Bernstein B.E. (2017) Epigenetic plasticity and the hallmarks of cancer. *Science 357*.

Fleming J.M., Creevy K.E., Promislow D.E. (2011) Mortality in north American dogs from 1984 to 2004: An investigation into age-, size-, and breed-related causes of death. *J Vet Intern Med 25*:187–198.

Foulds L. (1954) The experimental study of tumor progression: A review. *Cancer Res 14*:327–339.

Foulds L. (1965) Multiple etiologic factors in neoplastic development. *Cancer Res 25*:1339–1347.

Frost G. (2013) The latency period of mesothelioma among a cohort of British asbestos workers (1978–2005). *Br J Cancer 109*:1965–1973.

Fujinaga K., Green M. (1971) Mechanism of carcinogenesis by RNA tumour viruses: The RNA-and DNA-dependent DNA polymerase activities of feline sarcoma virus. *J Gen Virol 12*:85–93.

Galluzzi L., Vitale I., Aaronson S.A. et al. (2018) Molecular mechanisms of cell death: Recommendations of the Nomenclature Committee on Cell Death 2018. *Cell Death Differ 25*:486–541.

Gartel A.L., Serfas M.S. (1996) Tyner AL: p21–Negative regulator of the cell cycle. *Proc Soc Exp Biol Med 213*:138–149.

Golias C.H., Charalabopoulos A., Charalabopoulos K. (2004) Cell proliferation and cell cycle control: A mini review. *Int J Clin Pract 58*:1134–1141.

Goode E.L., Ulrich C.M., Potter J.D. (2002) Polymorphisms in DNA repair genes and associations with cancer risk. *Cancer Epidemiol Biomarkers Prev 11*:1513–1530.

Grana X., Reddy E.P. (1995) Cell cycle control in mammalian cells: Role of cyclins, cyclin dependent kinases (CDKs), growth suppressor genes and cyclin-dependent kinase inhibitors (CKIs). *Oncogene 11*:211–219.

Granstein R.D., Sober A.J. (1982) Current concepts in ultraviolet carcinogenesis. *Proc Soc Exp Biol Med 170*:115–125.

Gray D.A. (1991) Insertional mutagenesis: Neoplasia arising from retroviral integration. *Cancer Invest 9*:295–304.

Greaves M., Maley C.C. (2012) Clonal evolution in cancer. *Nature 481*:306–313.

Grivennikov S.I., Karin M. (2010) Inflammation and oncogenesis: A vicious connection. *Curr Opin Genet Dev 20*:65–71.

Hamel P.A., Gallie B.L., Phillips R.A. (1992) The retinoblastoma protein and cell cycle regulation. *Trends Genet 8*:180–185.

Hamilton S.R., Vogelstein B. (1988) Point mutations in human neoplasia. *J Pathol 154*:205–206.

Hanahan D., Weinberg R.A. (2000) The hallmarks of cancer. *Cell 100*:57–70.

Hanahan D., Weinberg R.A. (2011) Hallmarks of cancer: The next generation. *Cell 144*:646–674.

Harper J.W. (1997) Cyclin dependent kinase inhibitors. *Cancer Surv 29*:91–107.

Haupt S., Berger M., Goldberg Z. et al. (2003) Apoptosis – The p53 network. *J Cell Sci 116*:4077–4085.

Hemminki K., Forsti A., Mustonen R. et al. (1986) DNA adducts in experimental cancer research. *J Cancer Res Clin Oncol 112*:181–188.

Hengst L., Reed S.I. (1998) Inhibitors of the Cip/Kip family. *Curr Top Microbiol Immunol 227*:25–41.

Helleday T. (2011) The underlying mechanism for the PARP and BRCA synthetic lethality: Clearing up the misunderstandings. *Mol Oncol 5*:387–393.

Hoeijmakers J.H. (2001a) Genome maintenance mechanisms for preventing cancer. *Nature 411*:366–374.

Hoeijmakers J.H. (2001b) DNA repair mechanisms. *Maturitas 38*:17–22; discussion 22–23.

Hoover E.A., Mullins J.I. (1991) Feline leukemia virus infection and diseases. *J Am Vet Med Assoc 199*:1287–1297.

Ignatova T.N., Kukekov V.G., Laywell E.D. et al. (2002) Human cortical glial tumors contain neural stem-like cells expressing astroglial and neuronal markers in vitro. *Glia 39*:193–206.

Iqbal N., Iqbal N. (2014) Imatinib: A breakthrough of targeted therapy in cancer. *Chemother Res Pract 2014*:357027.

Jarrett W.F. (1975) Cat leukemia and its viruses. *Adv Vet Sci Comp Med 19*:165–193.

Jeong J., Kim D., Choi J. (2022) Application of ToxCast/Tox21 data for toxicity mechanism-based evaluation and prioritization of environmental chemicals: Perspective and limitations. *Toxicol In Vitro 84*:105451.

Ju F., Atyah M.M., Horstmann N. et al. (2022) Characteristics of the cancer stem cell niche and therapeutic strategies. *Stem Cell Res Ther 13*:233.

Karihtala P., Soini Y. (2007) Reactive oxygen species and antioxidant mechanisms in human tissues and their relation to malignancies. *APMIS 115*:81–103.

Karran P. (2000) DNA double strand break repair in mammalian cells. *Curr Opin Genet Dev 10*:144–150.

King M.C., Marks J.H., Mandell J.B. et al. (2003) Breast and ovarian cancer risks due to inherited mutations in BRCA1 and BRCA2. *Science 302*:643–646.

Kinzler K.W., Vogelstein B. (1998) Landscaping the cancer terrain. *Science 280*:1036–1037.

Knapp D.W., Dhawan D., Ramos-Vara J.A. et al. (2019) Naturally-occurring invasive urothelial carcinoma in dogs, a unique model to drive advances in managing muscle invasive bladder cancer in humans. *Front Oncol 9*:1493.

Knudson A.G. Jr. (1971) Mutation and cancer: Statistical study of retinoblastoma. *Proc Natl Acad Sci U S A 68*:820–823.

Konopka J.B., Witte O.N. (1985) Activation of the abl oncogene in murine and human leukemias. *Biochim Biophys Acta 823*:1–17.

Koretzky G.A. (2007) The legacy of the Philadelphia chromosome. *J Clin Invest 117*:2030–2032.

Lange M., Begolli R., Giakountis A. (2021) Non-coding variants in cancer: Mechanistic insights and clinical potential for personalized medicine. *Noncoding RNA. 7*(3): 47.

Lashnits E., Neupane P., Bradley J.M. et al. (2020) Molecular prevalence of Bartonella, Babesia, and hemotropic Mycoplasma species in dogs with hemangiosarcoma from across the United States. *PLoS One 15*:e0227234.

LeBlanc A.K., Mazcko C.N. (2020) Improving human cancer therapy through the evaluation of pet dogs. *Nat Rev Cancer 20*:727–742.

Levitt N.C., Hickson I.D. (2002) Caretaker tumour suppressor genes that defend genome integrity. *Trends Mol Med 8*:179–186.

Li J., Yuan J. (2008) Caspases in apoptosis and beyond. *Oncogene 27*:6194–6206.

Linenberger M.L., Abkowitz J.L. (1995) Haematological disorders associated with feline retrovirus infections. *Baillieres Clin Haematol 8*:73–112.

Liu Y., West S.C. (2002) Distinct functions of BRCA1 and BRCA2 in double-strand break repair. *Breast Cancer Res 4*:9–13.

Loeb L.A. (1991) Mutator phenotype may be required for multistage carcinogenesis. *Cancer Res 51*:3075–3079.

Martin D., Gutkind J.S. (2008) Human tumor-associated viruses and new insights into the molecular mechanisms of cancer. *Oncogene 27*:S31–S42.

McDonough S.K., Larsen S., Brodey R.S. et al. (1971) A transmissible feline fibrosarcoma of viral origin. *Cancer Res 31*:953–956.

Moynahan M.E., Chiu J.W., Koller B.H. et al. (1999) Brca1 controls homology-directed DNA repair. *Mol Cell 4*:511–518.

Nakayama K., Nakayama K. (1998) Cip/Kip cyclin-dependent kinase inhibitors: Brakes of the cell cycle engine during development. *Bioessays 20*:1020–1029.

Nelson N. (1965) Formal discussion: Chemical and physical carcinogens. *Cancer Res 25*:1314–1316.

Nowell P.C. (1976) The clonal evolution of tumor cell populations. *Science 194*:23–28.

Nowell P.C. (1986) Mechanisms of tumor progression. *Cancer Res 46*:2203–2207.

Oh J.H., Cho J.Y. (2023) Comparative oncology: Overcoming human cancer through companion animal studies. *Exp Mol Med 55*:725–734.

Ohshima H., Bartsch H. (1994) Chronic infections and inflammatory processes as cancer risk factors: Possible role of nitric oxide in carcinogenesis. *Mutat Res 305*:253–264.

Parrish A.B., Freel C.D., Kornbluth S. (2013) Cellular mechanisms controlling caspase activation and function. *Cold Spring Harb Perspect Biol 5*.

Payne S.R., Kemp C.J. (2005) Tumor suppressor genetics. *Carcinogenesis 26*:2031–2045.

Pelucchi C., Gallus S., Garavello W. et al. (2006) Cancer risk associated with alcohol and tobacco use: Focus on upper aero-digestive tract and liver. *Alcohol Res Health 29*:193–198.

Prager B.C., Xie Q., Bao S. et al. (2019) Cancer stem cells: The architects of the tumor ecosystem. *Cell Stem Cell 24*:41–53.

Pytel P., Lukas R.V. (2009) Update on diagnostic practice: Tumors of the nervous system. *Arch Pathol Lab Med 133*:1062–1077.

Rabes H.M. (1986) DNA adducts and cell cycle. *J Cancer Res Clin Oncol 112*:189–195.

Ranen E., Lavy E., Aizenberg I. et al. (2004) Spirocercosis-associated esophageal sarcomas in dogs. A retrospective study of 17 cases (1997–2003). *Vet Parasitol 119*:209–221.

Redmond D.E. Jr. (1970) Tobacco and cancer: The first clinical report, 1761. *N Engl J Med 282*:18–23.

Ribelin W.E., Bailey W.S. (1958) Esophageal sarcomas associated with Spirocerca lupi infection in the dog. *Cancer 11*:1242–1246.

Robert-Guroff M., Markham P.D., Popovic M. et al. (1985) Isolation, characterization, and biological effects of the first human retroviruses: The human T-lymphotropic retrovirus family. *Curr Top Microbiol Immunol 115*:7–31.

Ross J.S., Fletcher J.A. (1999) HER-2/neu (c-erb-B2) gene and protein in breast cancer. *Am J Clin Pathol 112*:S53–S67.

Rundhaug J.E., Fischer S.M. (2010) Molecular mechanisms of mouse skin tumor promotion. *Cancers (Basel) 2*:436–482.

Ryan D.P., Hong T.S., Bardeesy N. (2014) Pancreatic adenocarcinoma. *N Engl J Med 371*:2140–2141.

Sager R. (1992) Tumor suppressor genes in the cell cycle. *Curr Opin Cell Biol 4*:155–160.

Satyanarayana A., Kaldis P. (2009) Mammalian cell-cycle regulation: Several Cdks, numerous cyclins and diverse compensatory mechanisms. *Oncogene 28*:2925–2939.

Schafer K.A. (1998) The cell cycle: A review. *Vet Pathol 35*:461–478.

Scheffner M., Huibregtse J.M., Vierstra R.D. et al. (1993) The HPV-16 E6 and E6-AP complex functions as a ubiquitin-protein ligase in the ubiquitination of p53. *Cell 75*:495–505.

Schneider D.F., Chen H. (2013) New developments in the diagnosis and treatment of thyroid cancer. *CA Cancer J Clin 63*:374–394.

Sinha R.P., Hader D.P. (2002) UV-induced DNA damage and repair: A review. *Photochem Photobiol Sci 1*:225–236.

Slaga T.J. (1983) Overview of tumor promotion in animals. *Environ Health Perspect 50*:3–14.

Solnica-Krezel L., Sepich D.S. (2012) Gastrulation: Making and shaping germ layers. *Annu Rev Cell Dev Biol 28*:687–717.

Spadari S., Sutherland B.M., Pedrali-Noy G. et al. (1987) Alteration of DNA tertiary structure by physical and chemical carcinogens: Involvement in DNA repair processes. *Toxicol Pathol 15*:82–87.

Strahm B., Malkin D. (2006) Hereditary cancer predisposition in children: Genetic basis and clinical implications. *Int J Cancer 119*:2001–2006.

Szabo C.I., King M.C. (1995) Inherited breast and ovarian cancer. *Hum Mol Genet 4*:1811–1817.

Takebe H., Nishigori C., Tatsumi K. (1989) Melanoma and other skin cancers in xeroderma pigmentosum patients and mutation in their cells. *J Invest Dermatol 92*:236S–238S.

Tam P.P., Kanai-Azuma M., Kanai Y. (2003) Early endoderm development in vertebrates: Lineage differentiation and morphogenetic function. *Curr Opin Genet Dev 13*:393–400.

Thota R., Pauff J.M., Berlin J.D. (2014) Treatment of metastatic pancreatic adenocarcinoma: A review. *Oncology (Williston Park) 28*:70–74.

Toyokuni S. (2009) Mechanisms of asbestos-induced carcinogenesis. *Nagoya J Med Sci 71*:1–10.

Uren A.G., Kool J., Berns A. et al. (2005) Retroviral insertional mutagenesis: Past, present and future. *Oncogene 24*:7656–7672.

Vander Heiden M.G., Cantley L.C., Thompson C.B. (2009) Understanding the Warburg effect: The metabolic requirements of cell proliferation. *Science 324*:1029–1033.

Vogelstein B., Kinzler K.W. (2004) Cancer genes and the pathways they control. *Nat Med 10*:789–799.

Wainscoat J.S., Fey M.F. (1990) Assessment of clonality in human tumors: A review. *Cancer Res 50*:1355–1360.

Wang S., El-Deiry W.S. (2003) TRAIL and apoptosis induction by TNF-family death receptors. *Oncogene 22*:8628–8633.

Ward J.F. (1988) DNA damage produced by ionizing radiation in mammalian cells: Identities, mechanisms of formation, and reparability. *Prog Nucleic Acid Res Mol Biol 35*:95–125.

Waring P., Mullbacher A. (1999) Cell death induced by the Fas/Fas ligand pathway and its role in pathology. *Immunol Cell Biol 77*:312–317.

Westbrook C.A. (1988) The ABL oncogene in human leukemias. *Blood Rev 2*:1–8.

Wood C., Scott E.M. (2019) Feline ocular post-traumatic sarcomas: Current understanding, treatment and monitoring. *J Feline Med Surg 21*:835–842.

Wright S.C., Zhong J., Larrick J.W. (1994) Inhibition of apoptosis as a mechanism of tumor promotion. *FASEB J 8*:654–660.

Yamagiwa K., Ichikawa K. (1977) Experimental study of the pathogenesis of carcinoma. *CA Cancer J Clin 27*:174–181.

Yuan S., Akey C.W. (2013) Apoptosome structure, assembly, and procaspase activation. *Structure 21*:501–515.

Zimmermann K.C., Bonzon C., Green D.R. (2001) The machinery of programmed cell death. *Pharmacol Ther 92*:57–70.

CHAPTER 4

CYTOLOGY OF SKIN AND SUBCUTANEOUS TISSUE

Indira Pargass and Samantha N. Schlemmer

INTRODUCTION

Lesions involving the skin and subcutaneous tissues are the most common samples collected for cytologic evaluation from companion animals. This is likely due to the fact that the lesions are clearly visible or palpable, so they are observed by owners and noted during routine physical examination. Their location makes them easy to aspirate or fenestrate, using a needle (i.e., fine needle aspirate or biopsy; henceforth referred to as FNA), without the need for more invasive techniques. Surface lesions of the skin also can be sampled for cytology using scrape, impression, hair-pluck, and tape collection techniques. This chapter will focus on FNA of skin and subcutaneous lesions and highlight some of the common/important superficial skin cytology lesions. More information about these types of collection methods and diseases associated with lesions on the surface of the skin can be found in Chapters 1 and 18 ('Sample Acquisition and Preparation' and 'Cytology of the Ear', respectively).

Cytology of cutaneous and subcutaneous lesions often provides a fast, accurate analysis of the underlying pathogenesis of disease. In one study, FNA cytologic samples were diagnostic in 83.2% (243/292) of cases from dogs and cats with cutaneous and subcutaneous masses (Ghisleni *et al.*, 2006). When compared with histologic diagnosis (gold standard), the sensitivity and specificity of cytology were extremely good (89.3% and 97.9%, respectively) and the positive predictive value was excellent (99.4%). The negative predictive value was somewhat low (68.7%), as expected from a technique that utilizes such a small amount of starting material, may not be representative of the entire lesion, and lacks tissue architecture. This study indicates that the limitations of cytology are minor for most lesions in the skin and subcutaneous tissues. Indeed, accurate cytologic information is often instrumental in guiding diagnostic planning and treatment strategies.

STRUCTURES OF THE INTEGUMENT

The integumentary system is the largest organ of the body and is an extremely important barrier to systemic injury and infection. It plays a key role in water and electrolyte homeostasis, temperature regulation, and production of vitamin D3, and acts as a sensitive sensory organ. It is composed of the epidermis, dermis, and hypodermis (subcutis) (Figure 4.1a). Specific areas of skin are specialized and may or may not contain hair follicles and glands. Numerous vascular, neural, and lymphatic structures are intimately associated with all components of the integument.

Epidermis

Epidermal cells comprise the outermost layer of the integument, which develops from the embryonic ectoderm. Most cells of the integument are stratified squamous epithelial cells, although simple cuboidal epithelial cells form the secretory and ductal components of glands. The distinct stratified layers of the integument are derived from the basal cell layer of the epidermis (Figure 4.1b). Basal cells and epidermal stem cells are present in the stratum basale at the deepest layer of the epidermis. They are attached to a basement membrane at the interface with the dermis. Melanocytes are also found in this layer, and in the outer root sheath of hair follicles, and produce melanin which gives color to skin and hair. Basal cells are small, cuboidal cells with very distinct cell junctions and a small round nucleus. As basal cells migrate toward the most superficial layer of the epidermis, they flatten and form the cells of the stratum spinosum. These cells are larger, have more cytoplasm, and are polyhedral in shape (Welle & Linder, 2021). These cells continue to migrate toward the surface. In the stratum granulosum, cells become layered upon each other and begin to produce keratohyalin granules (keratin precursors). Their nuclei begin to shrink and become pyknotic. In some specialized areas of the skin (nose, foot pads, teats), the next layer of skin (stratum ludicum) contains enough layers of cells that it can be visualized histologically. Cells of the stratum lucidum are pale, flattened cells that often lack a nucleus. Finally, the most superficial layer of cells forms the stratum corneum, which is made up of dead, keratinized, squamous epithelial cells that eventually slough off as the skin regenerates. These cells are typically polygonal with abundant keratinized cytoplasm and have a pyknotic nucleus or lack a nucleus altogether. Cytologically, keratin in cells is a light blue–green color and may have a glassy appearance when stained with Romanowsky-type stains. In most areas of the integument, the squamous epithelial cells at the surface become cornified and lack a nucleus. These cells are described as keratin flakes or keratinized or keratinaceous debris in cytology samples and are more angular and blue–green to pink–purple in color (Figures 4.2).

DOI: 10.1201/9781003258551-4

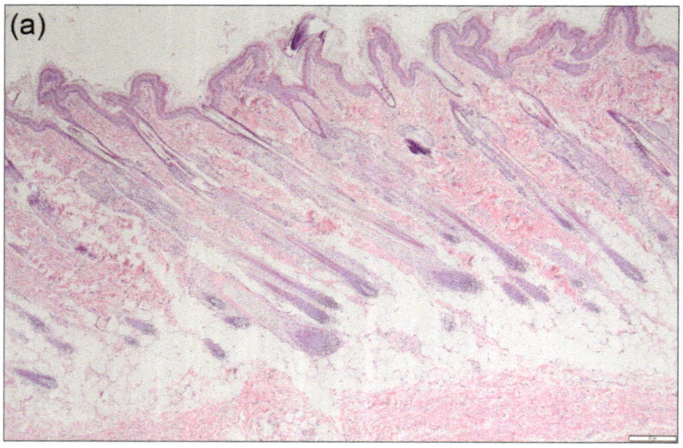

Figure 4.1a Integument histopathology. Section of skin from a 2-month-old Husky. The integument is composed of the epidermis, dermis, and subcutis. The epidermis is the most external layer (top; Figure 4.1b). The dermis lies just beneath the epidermis and is composed of collagen and elastin fibers, vasculature, and adnexal structures (including hair follicles and sebaceous glands, which are in longitudinal section in this specimen). The subcutis is composed of adipose tissue (round clear spaces) and collagen (bottom) (H&E, 50× magnification).

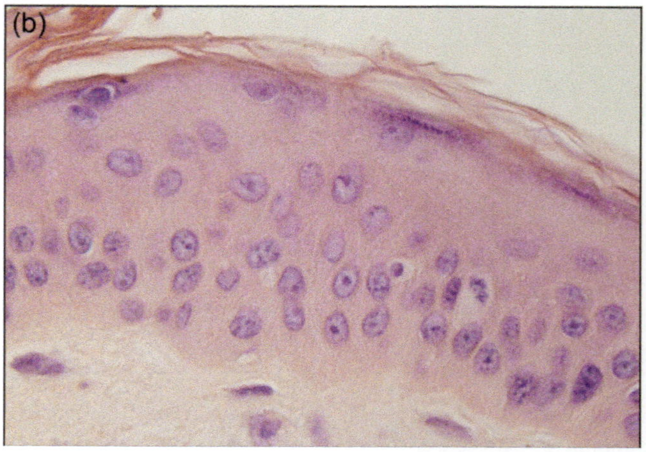

Figure 4.1b Epidermis histopathology. Section of skin from a 15-year-old domestic longhair cat. The pale cells at the bottom of the image make up the superficial dermis. Basal epithelial cells are the first layer of eosinophilic cells with large round nuclei just above the dermis. The next layer of nuclei in the middle of the eosinophilic cells is associated with the stratum spinosum. The stratum granulosum is the layer of cells that have very pale nuclei or have lost their nuclei. Some cells of the stratum granulosum just underneath the surface layer of keratinized cells contain basophilic granules. The stratum corneum is the bright pink, flaky, keratinized material at the top of the image (H&E, 1,000× magnification).

Dermis and adnexal structures

The dermis is made up of mesenchymal cells and collagenous fibers derived from the embryonic mesoderm. There are two zones within the dermis: the papillary zone (conforms to the stratum basale of the epidermis) and the reticular zone (deeper and contains more dense collagenous tissue). The dermis contains the epidermal appendages/derivatives (adnexal structures), vasculature, and nerves. Adnexal structures consist of hair follicles, arrector pili muscles, sweat glands, sebaceous glands, and other specialized structures. Hair follicles extend from the epidermis to the deep dermis or the subcutis, depending on the species (Welle & Linder, 2021).

Subcutaneous structures

Like the dermis, the tissue beneath the dermis originates from the embryonic mesoderm and is composed of mesenchymal cells and collagenous fibers, connecting the dermis to the underlying tissues. In many areas of the integument, there are large numbers of adipocytes in the subcutis that form the panniculus adiposus layer of the integument.

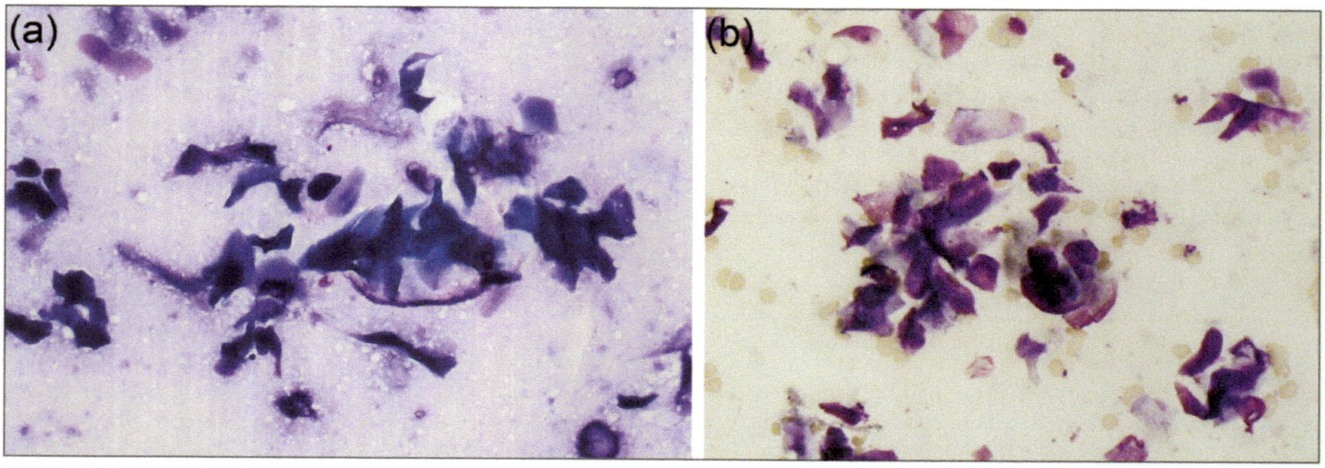

Figures 4.2a,b Superficial keratinocytes from the skin surface are large and angular or polygonal cells that stain somewhat variably with Wright–Giemsa stain. Cells may be aqua-blue to bright blue (a, 500× magnification) or eosinophilic to purple (b, 500× magnification). Importantly, superficial keratinocytes lack a nucleus.

Glandular structures

Sebaceous glands

Sebaceous glands are alveolar holocrine glands associated with hair follicles. They are also a component of the anal sac glands of cats. These glands produce sebum, which acts as a barrier against microbes, prevents loss of water, and maintains hair health. Sebaceous cells are round, highly vacuolated, have a low nuclear-to-cytoplasmic ratio, and occur in cohesive clusters. Meibomian glands are modified sebaceous glands which are found in the eyelid margin and produce meibum (the superficial lipid layer of the tear film) (Welle & Linder, 2021). The cells of the meibomian glands are arranged in parallel rows of lobules and their ducts are lined by keratinized stratified squamous epithelium (White & Bellnap, 2015). See Chapter 17 ('Ocular Cytology') for more information on meibomian glands and associated lesions.

Sweat glands

Sweat glands can be classified as epitrichial (ducts empty into the hair follicle, i.e. apocrine) or atrichial (ducts empty directly onto the skin surface, i.e. merocrine, eccrine) glands. Apocrine glands are derived from primary hair germ and are found in all haired skin usually deep to the sebaceous glands (Mauldin & Peters-Kennedy, 2016). They are the predominant type of sweat gland in domestic animals. Sweat gland secretory cells are columnar while ductal cells are more cuboidal. Specialized apocrine glands are present within the inner wall of the anal sacs. Ceruminous glands are modified apocrine glands which produce cerumen in the external ear canal [see Chapter 18 ('Cytology of the Ear') for discussion of the cytology of ceruminous glands and associated lesions]. Merocrine glands are found in canine foot pads, and they are made up of cuboidal secretory and ductal cells.

Mammary glands

The mammary glands are modified apocrine sweat glands composed of glandular tissue, an associated duct system, and connective tissue septae (Liebich, 2019). Aspiration of normal mammary gland tissue typically yields blood with few or no mammary gland cells. Mammary cells (if present) may include secretory cells (uniformly sized cells with round nuclei and basophilic cytoplasm, found in clumps or acini; Figures 4.3, 4.4), ductular cells (cells with basilar, ovoid nuclei and small amounts of cytoplasm, sometimes found in small sheets), and myoepithelial cells (Allison, 2020). The myoepithelial cells originate from the same stem cells as glandular epithelial cells but appear as spindle-shaped to stellate cells (Gudjonsson, 2005; Emanuelli *et al.*, 2020; Figure 4.5).

Cytology preparations of mammary lesions (both neoplastic and non-neoplastic) may also contain mammary secretions. These secretions are usually lowly cellular and contain lipid or proteinaceous secretory material, the latter of which typically appears as lakes of smooth, basophilic material (Figures 4.3, 4.4).

Foam cells may be found in mammary gland aspirates or in mammary secretions. These are round cells that resemble macrophages (Figure 4.6). They typically exhibit heavily vacuolated cytoplasm and may also contain basophilic secretory material. In humans, immunohistochemistry has shown that mammary foam cells are consistently positive for CD68 and are, therefore, of histiocytic/macrophage origin

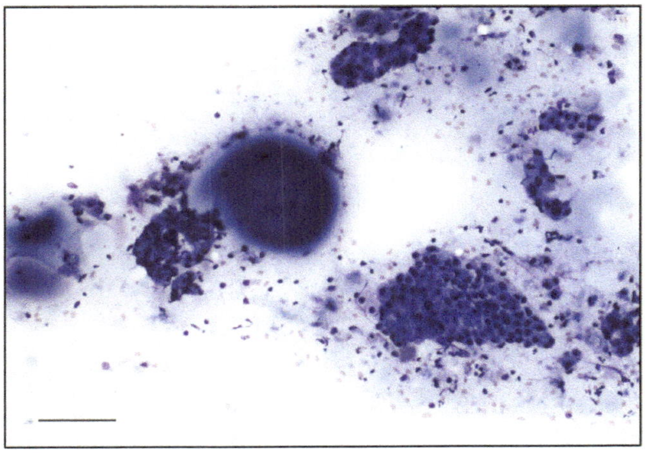

Figure 4.3 Clumps of epithelial cells and lakes of basophilic secretory material from a mammary mass in a 15-year-old, spayed female Pomeranian dog. These epithelial cells are relatively uniform in size and display few criteria of malignancy (Wright–Giemsa, scale bar = 100 μm).

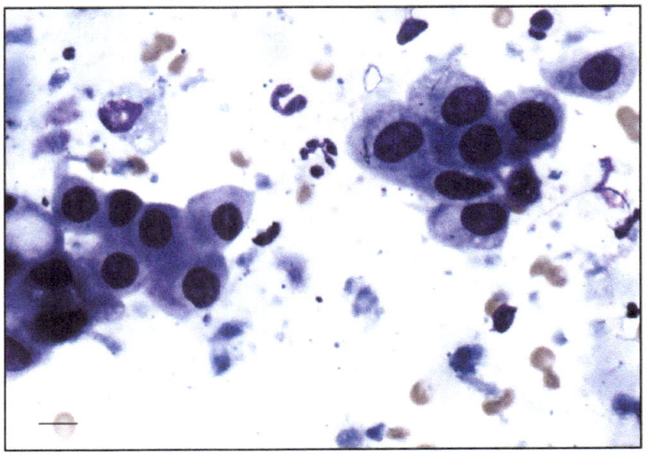

Figure 4.4 Higher magnification view of the same case as Figure 4.3, showing a clump of relatively uniform epithelial cells, a foam cell, and basophilic secretory material. Several neutrophils are also present, indicating inflammation or possibly necrosis associated with the lesion (Wright–Giemsa, scale bar = 10 μm).

(King *et al.*, 2002). Low numbers of macrophages and neutrophils may also be found in mammary aspirates.

Other subcutaneous glands

Please see Chapters 6 ('Oral Cavity Cytology') and 16 ('Cytology of Endocrine Tissues') for further information on salivary gland and thyroid and parathyroid gland cytology, respectively.

CYTOLOGIC APPEARANCE OF LESIONS IN SKIN AND SUBCUTANEOUS TISSUES

The cytologic appearance of aspirates from lesions in or under the skin can be grouped into very broad categories: acellular samples,

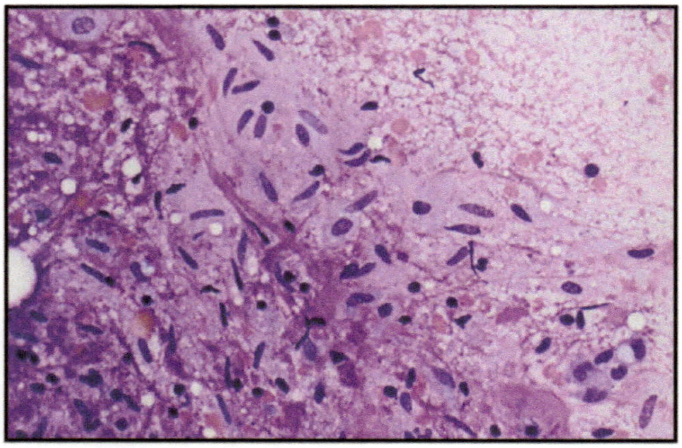

Figure 4.5 Spindloid cells admixed with granular to fibrillar pink extracellular matrix material and a few blood cells in an FNA from a mammary mass on a 7-year-old, spayed female Boxer. These cells appear most consistent with myoepithelial cells but could represent mesenchymal/stromal cells (Wright–Giemsa, 500× magnification).

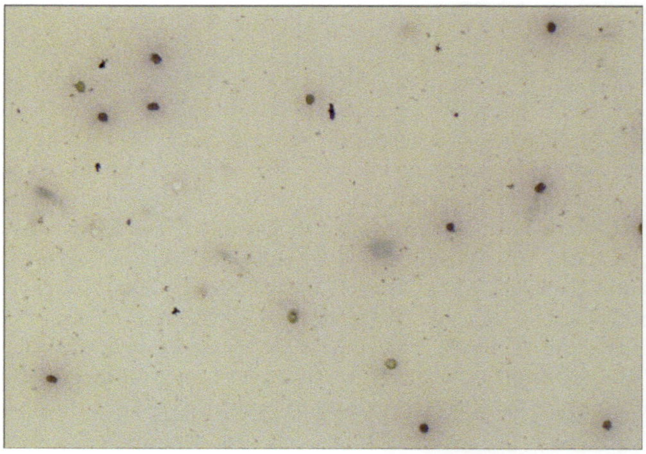

Figure 4.7 Cystic fluid in a skin mass from a 10-year-old domestic shorthair cat. There is a thin layer of proteinaceous material in the background of the slide. No nucleated cells are present. A few erythrocytes are seen (Wright–Giemsa, 500× magnification).

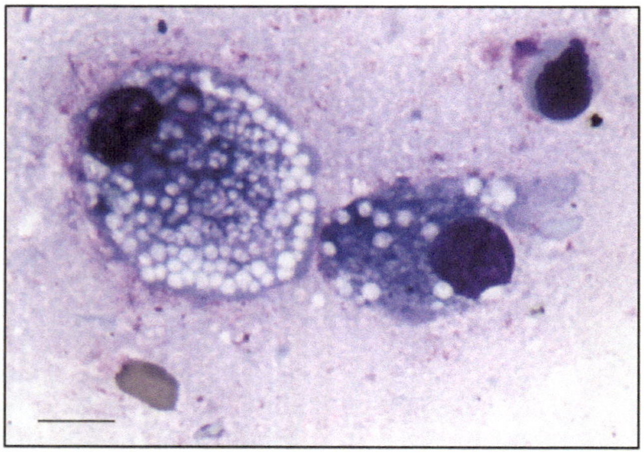

Figure 4.6 Foam cells from a mammary mass in a dog. These cells are often found in mammary gland or mammary masses and appear similar to macrophages (Wright–Giemsa, scale bar = 10 μm).

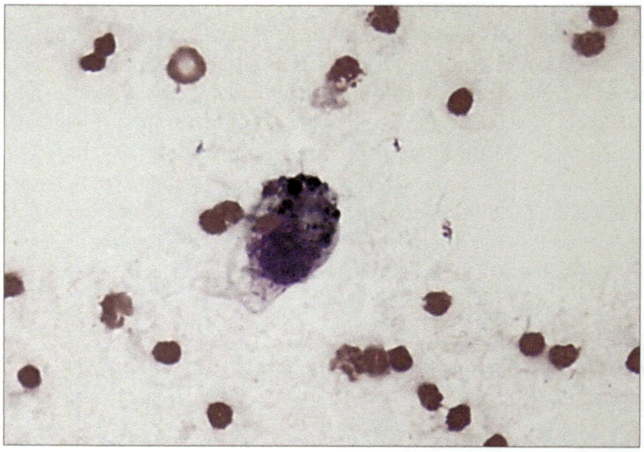

Figure 4.8 Hemosiderin-laden macrophage in an FNA of a hemorrhagic subcutaneous mass from a dog. The macrophage contains one visible erythrocyte and several variably sized, rounded, black pigment structures consistent with hemosiderin (Wright–Giemsa, 1,000× magnification).

samples containing cellular debris, bloody samples, inflammatory samples, or tissue samples (which may be normal, hyperplastic, or neoplastic). If the sample is pauci- or acellular, the diagnosis of a cyst should be considered (Figure 4.7). More commonly, an acellular sample indicates that the aspirate was inadequate and repeat aspiration (potentially with suction applied) or biopsy with histopathology would be recommended. Cellular debris may be present because cells have been damaged during collection or because the lesion is necrotic. These samples are often non-diagnostic because cellular morphology cannot be adequately assessed. Aspiration of different areas of the lesion may be beneficial in these cases.

If the sample contains intact cells, the cells need to be identified as peripheral blood cells, inflammatory cells, or cells representative of tissue/elements associated with the lesion. When there are large numbers of erythrocytes with low numbers of leukocytes and rare tissue cells, identification of the underlying pathologic process can be challenging. Hemorrhage can be diagnosed in properly processed samples that contain a large amount of blood if erythrophagocytic and/or hemosiderin-laden macrophages are seen (Figure 4.8). Platelets are not observed in lesions with acute or chronic hemorrhage but may be seen during peracute hemorrhage. In samples that lack these features and contain platelets, it may be helpful to analyze a peripheral blood smear and a bloody cytology sample concurrently to determine if inflammation is present or if the sample is mostly peripheral blood. If the leukocyte density in the tissue aspirate is higher than the peripheral blood nucleated cell count, inflammation should be suspected. The inflammatory processes discussed in Chapter 2 ('General Principles of Inflammation') apply to lesions of the skin and subcutaneous tissues. Common causes of inflammation in these lesions are expanded on later in this chapter. If noninflammatory cells are present, the tissue type that the cells originated from is determined on the basis of cellular morphology. Most noninflammatory (tissue) cell types can be classified as epithelial, mesenchymal, or round cells.

Epithelial cells typically are round or polygonal with distinct cell borders and round nuclei. They often are arranged in sheets or clusters with visible cell junctions (Figure 4.9). Cell junctions appear as distinct pale lines around the edges of adjacent cells. Mesenchymal cells are spindle-shaped or have wispy, indistinct cell borders with ovoid nuclei and usually are observed individually on the slide but may be aggregated together (Figure 4.10). Aggregates of mesenchymal cells lack cell–cell junctions and can appear intertwined, rather than being arranged next to each other, occasionally admixed with pink fibrillar extracellular matrix material. Mesenchymal cell aggregates can be difficult to distinguish from sheets of epithelial cells, which may prevent cytologic differentiation between tumor types. In these cases, clinical presentation, special stains, and biopsy with histopathology can help to determine the diagnosis (Andreasen *et al.*, 1988; Hoinghaus *et al.*, 2008). Finally, round cells are individualized cells with rounded cytoplasm and round nuclei. The major round cell tumors and their distinctive cytologic appearances are described later in this chapter.

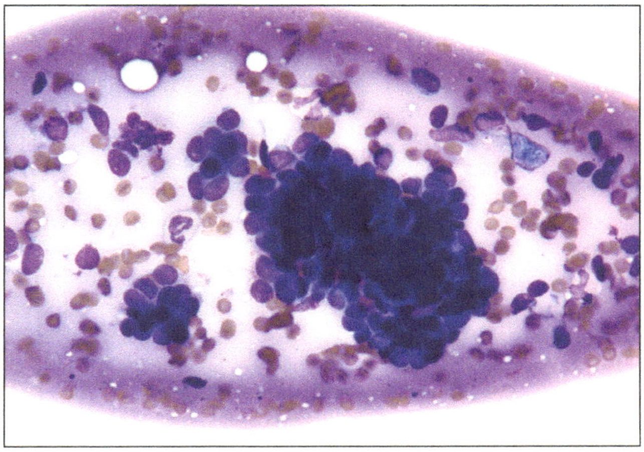

Figure 4.9 **Epithelial cells are often clustered together. Cell–cell junctions can be seen as a thin, clear line between neighboring cells (Wright–Giemsa, 500× magnification).**

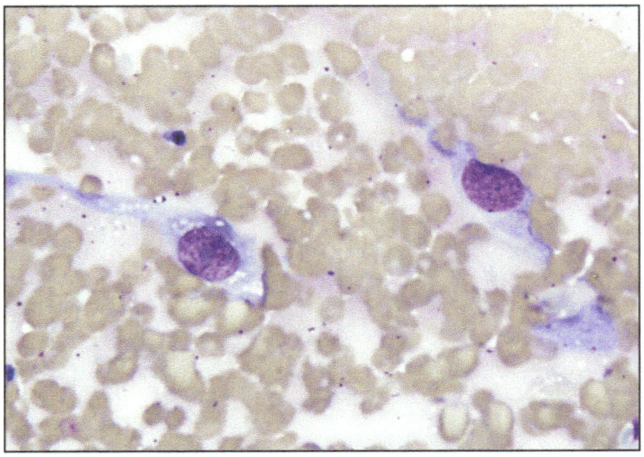

Figure 4.10 **Mesenchymal cells in an FNA of a subcutaneous mass on the prepuce of a dog. Cells are large with abundant, spindle-shaped, basophilic cytoplasm and an oval nucleus with coarsely stippled chromatin. Small, distinct, clear cytoplasmic vacuoles and a prominent nucleolus are visible in the cell to the left. This patient was diagnosed with hemangiosarcoma (Wright–Giemsa, 1,000× magnification).**

BENIGN VERSUS MALIGNANT LESIONS

When adequate numbers of tissue cells are present in a cytologic sample, morphologic characteristics are used to determine if the lesion could be benign or malignant. Characteristics of malignancy include anisocytosis, anisokaryosis, karyomegaly, binucleation, multinucleation, prominent or large nucleoli, multiple nucleoli, angular or elongated nucleoli, nuclear molding, abnormal nuclear shape, aberrant mitotic figures, atypical cytoplasmic vacuolation, increased nuclear to cytoplasmic (N:C) ratio, and dysmaturation of nuclear and cytoplasmic morphology (Figure 4.11). The characteristics of malignancy involving the nucleus are considered more reliable than the cytoplasmic characteristics. In most cancers, a diagnosis of malignancy can be made if there are three or more cytologic characteristics of malignancy present (Raskin, 2023; Meinkoth *et al.*, 2020).

It is important to note, however, that some lesions can appear cytologically benign but have a very aggressive biologic behavior. For example, some well-differentiated malignant neoplasms, such as

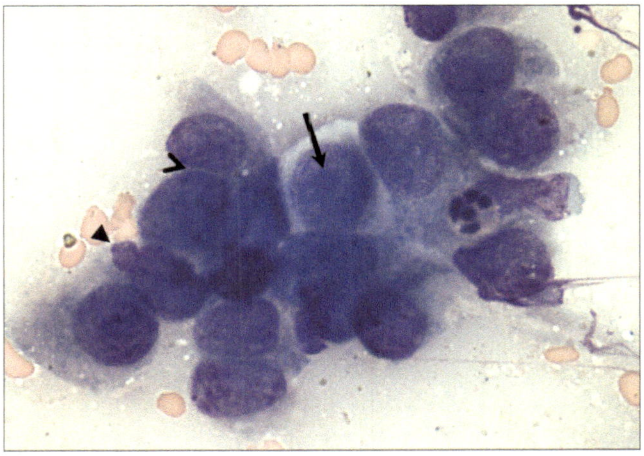

Figure 4.11 **Malignant cells from a canine mammary carcinoma. Cells are large with scant to abundant basophilic cytoplasm, a large round nucleus, and stippled chromatin. A large nucleolus can be seen in some of the cells (arrow). Characteristics of malignancy include anisocytosis, anisokaryosis, cytomegaly, increased nuclear to cytoplasmic ratio, nuclear molding (open arrowhead), binucleation, and nuclear blebbing (closed arrowhead) (Wright–Giemsa, 1,000× magnification).**

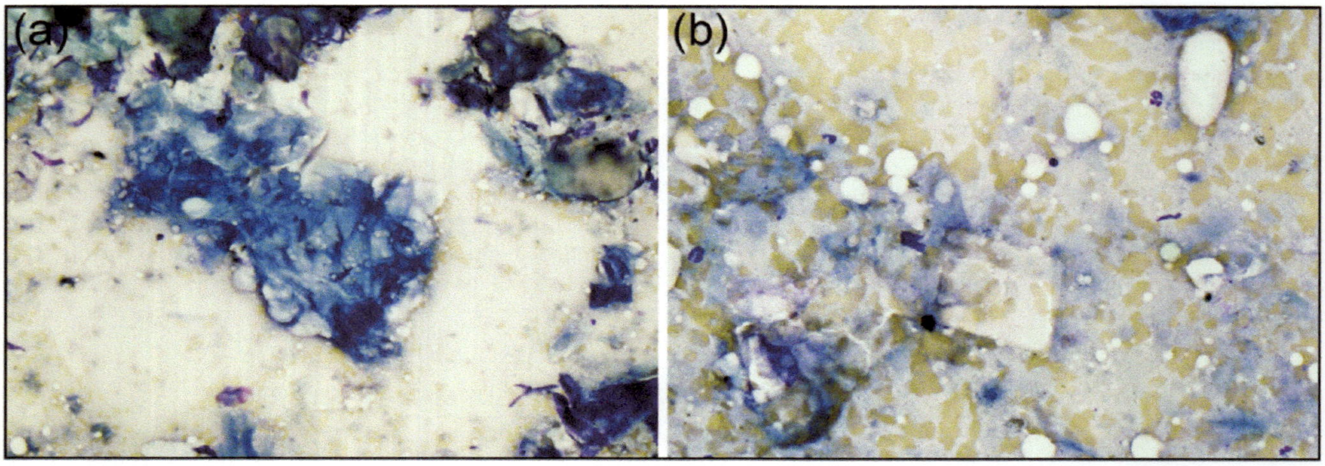

Figures 4.12 (a) FNA from a skin mass on the thorax of an 8-year-old dog. The sample is consistent with an epidermal inclusion cyst with a small amount of blood contamination. There are several polygonal blue anucleate keratinized epithelial cells. (b) Occasional cholesterol crystals (large rectangular nonstaining structures) also are observed (Wright–Giemsa: a, 200× magnification; b, 500× magnification).

perianal gland tumors and thyroid tumors, may lack sufficient cytologic criteria of malignancy and may be difficult to distinguish from hyperplasia or their benign counterparts. It is also critical to recognize that cells in some lesions have criteria of malignancy but are simply dysplastic. In cases that contain both inflammatory and noninflammatory (tissue) cell types, dysplastic changes can occur in tissue cells that mimic characteristics of malignancy. This finding is common in lesions that are ulcerated or necrotic. It can be extremely challenging to distinguish dysplastic changes from the anaplastic changes caused by neoplastic cell transformation. This is why the presence of inflammation often precludes a definitive diagnosis of cancer on cytology. In these cases, biopsy with histopathology or repeat aspiration is necessary if the mass persists after resolution of the inflammation or the clinical suspicion of neoplasia is high. Mammary masses, in particular, are an important example of lesions that may be difficult to diagnose on cytology (see 'Tumors of Glandular Structures – Mammary Masses' section).

POORLY CELLULAR, BUT DIAGNOSTIC, SAMPLES

Cysts

Cystic structures usually palpate as firm, round masses in the dermis or subcutis. They form when cellular secretions or debris become entrapped under the skin. Collection of a clear to creamy fluid is expected during aspiration of a cyst. Microscopically, the fluid appears as a thin basophilic or eosinophilic background in a cytologic sample (see Figure 4.7). Complete surgical removal of a cyst can be curative in dogs and cats.

Epidermal inclusion cysts (epidermoid, follicular, or infundibular cysts)

Epidermal inclusion cysts form when keratinized epithelial cells fail to exfoliate and become trapped under the superficial epidermis. Aspirates of follicular cysts tend to have a thick, chalky appearance. Keratin debris (often seen as clumps of amorphous sky-blue material) and large numbers of anucleate, keratinized, squamous epithelial cells are present in these samples (Figures 4.12a, b). Also, clear rectangular cholesterol crystals (formed from the breakdown of cell membranes) are often identified (Figure 4.13). If nucleated squamous epithelial and/or basal epithelial cells are also present, then a follicular tumor is a possibility, as these tumors can have cytological characteristics similar to epidermal inclusion cysts (see the 'Epidermal and Follicular Tumors' section later in this chapter).

When these cysts rupture and/or become inflamed or infected, neutrophilic to pyogranulomatous inflammation will be mixed in with the keratinized debris (Figure 4.14).

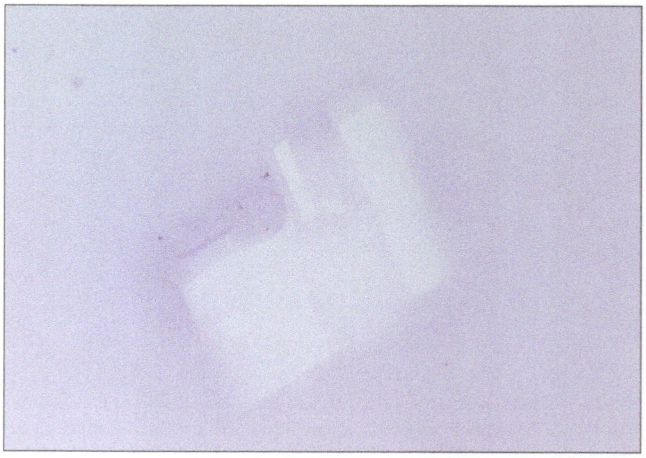

Figure 4.13 Cholesterol crystals can be found in epidermal inclusion cysts and lesions where cell degradation is occurring (Wright–Giemsa, 500× magnification).

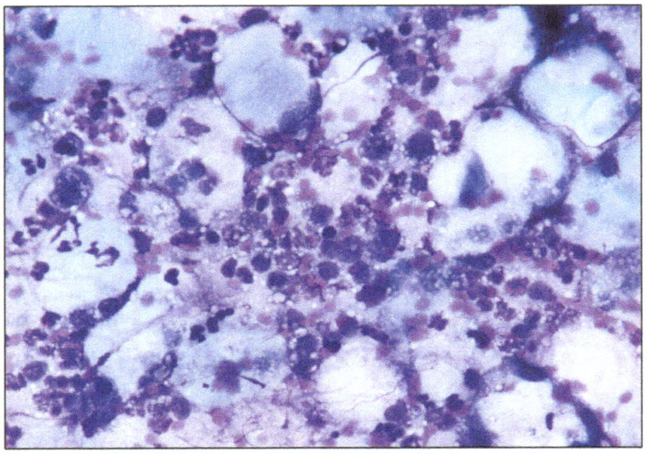

Figure 4.14 **Inflamed epidermal inclusion cyst with numerous variably degenerate neutrophils, vacuolated macrophages, and pale blue keratinized debris (Wright–Giemsa, 500× magnification).**

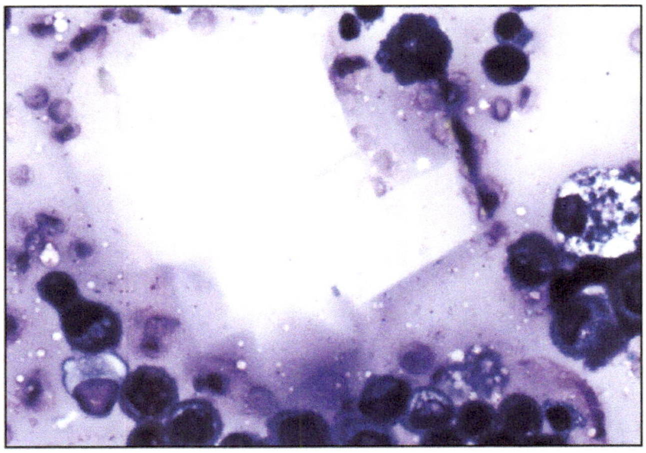

Figure 4.15 **Cholesterol crystals from a cystic area in a mammary carcinoma in a 12-year-old, spayed female Doberman Pinscher (same lesion as Figures 4.16a–c). Cholesterol crystals typically appear as clear, flat, rectangular structures, often with a notch in one or more corners of the rectangle. They often appear in mica-like stacks (Wright–Giemsa, scale bar = 10 μm).**

Sebaceous duct cysts

Sebaceous cysts form when proteinaceous product (keratin and sebum) is secreted into the center of a group of epithelial cells that line the mass. Grayish-white to brownish to yellowish cheese-like material can be released if the cyst becomes ruptured. Small clusters of benign-appearing epithelial cells that line the cyst may be present in the cytologic sample. If these cells are present, differential diagnoses include many of the, mostly benign, epithelial and adnexal tumors described later in this chapter.

Apocrine cysts

Occlusion of the sweat gland duct can lead to cyst formation. These can present as flocculant swellings and, when aspirated, can contain clear to brown-tinged fluid. Cytologically they are often acellular but can contain low numbers of cuboidal to columnar epithelial cells (Raskin & Conrado, 2023). These may be difficult to discern from cystic portions of an apocrine neoplasm.

Mammary cyst (mammary duct ectasia)

Mammary cysts may form as a result of dilated, distended ducts (Goldschmidt *et al.*, 2011). They can be a dysplastic, non-neoplastic condition (most common in middle-aged to older female dogs), or may also be associated with neoplastic lesions. These cystic lesions aspirate as fluid, which may be brownish, yellowish, or red in appearance. Slides prepared from the cystic fluid typically contain proteinaceous background material and may also contain mammary secretory material, blood cells, macrophages, and/or foam cells. Cholesterol crystals (large, transparent, flat, rectangular crystalline structures often with a notch in one or more corners) are a common finding in many cystic lesions, including mammary cysts (Figure 4.15). Clumps of epithelial cells may also be found in mammary cystic lesions. Benign and malignant mammary gland neoplasms may contain cystic areas (Figures 4.15, 4.16a–c), so if the lesion contains both solid areas and cystic areas, it is important to aspirate the solid portion to assess these more cellular areas for a potential neoplastic lesion.

Tissue injury

Poorly cellular cytologic samples from damaged tissue may reflect aspiration of a hematoma, hygroma, or seroma. These samples may need to be centrifuged to adequately concentrate and evaluate any cells present. Hematomas are bloody fluids with low numbers of macrophages that contain phagocytized erythrocytes, blue-black pigment consistent with hemosiderin (a breakdown product of erythrocytes; Figure 4.8), and/or hematoidin crystals (diamond-shaped/rhomboid golden crystals, also an erythrocyte breakdown product). A seroma is an accumulation of serous fluid within the skin, usually near a surgical incision site or area of previous trauma, and may contain low numbers of erythrocytes, occasional reactive macrophages with intracytoplasmic vacuoles, and rare to low numbers of neutrophils. No platelets are observed in hematomas or seromas, unless there is peracute hemorrhage or concurrent peripheral blood contamination. Hygromas are fluid-filled swellings that form over bony prominences (commonly the elbow) and pressure points, particularly in large-breed dogs. These lesions typically contain low numbers of macrophages and sometimes reactive fibrocytes (spindle-shaped mesenchymal cells).

Sialoceles may appear as soft, fluctuant swellings, most commonly in the cranial cervical area or mouth, and form due to leakage of saliva into surrounding tissues of the face due to trauma or obstruction of the salivary duct. Please see Chapter 6 ('Oral Cavity Cytology') for further information on salivary gland and associated lesions.

Fibroplasia and desmoplasia

Proliferative, reactive fibroblasts can be seen as a reparative response to trauma/wounds in addition to irritation from local inflammation, foreign body, or neoplasia (i.e., scirrhous reaction). Cytology of reactive fibroblasts typically yields low numbers of individualized spindle cells sometimes associated with pink fibrillar matrix material. Spindle cells have scant to moderate amounts of basophilic cytoplasm

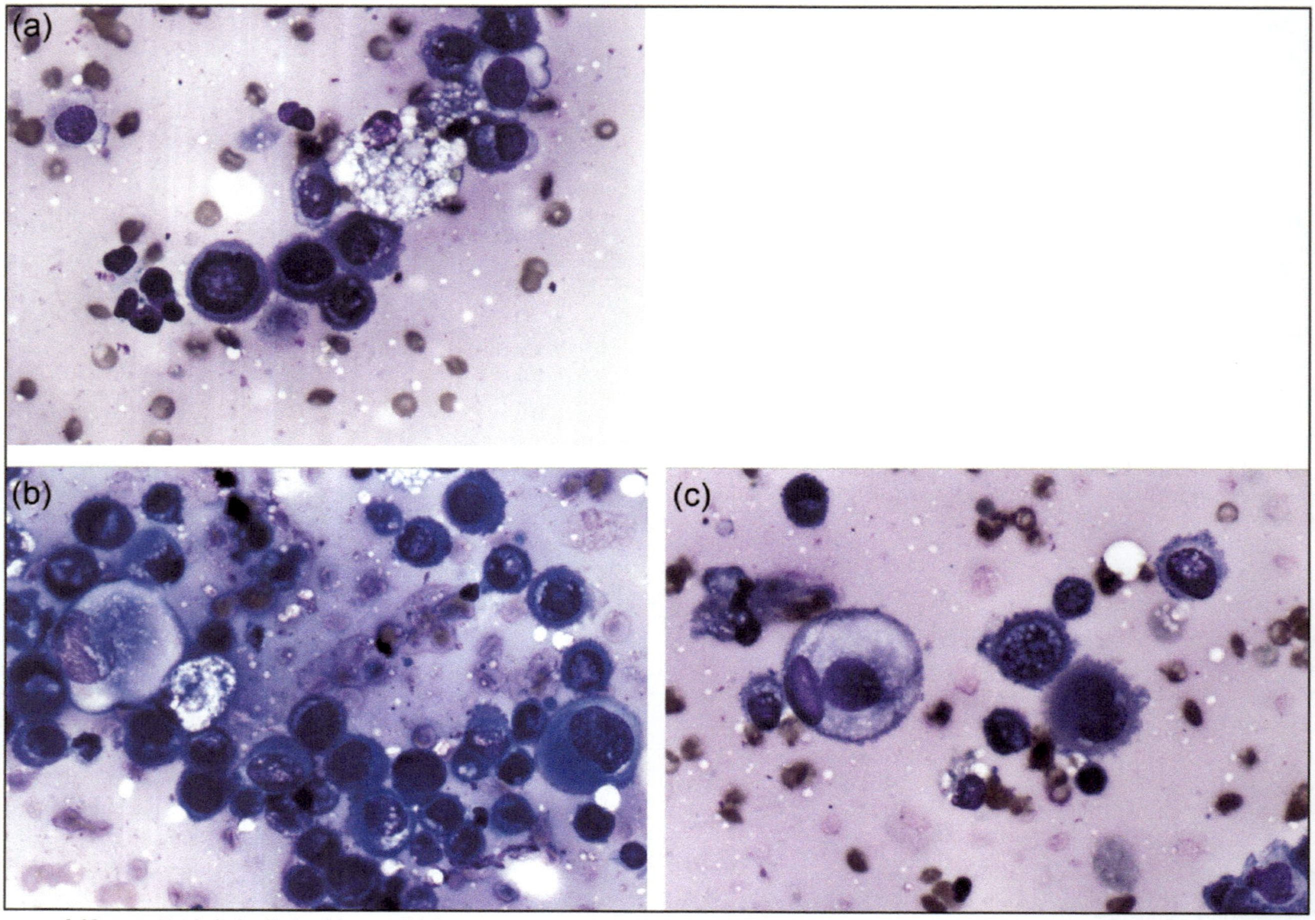

Figures 4.16a–c **Epithelial cells (and foam cells) from a mammary carcinoma in a 12-year-old, spayed female Doberman Pinscher. Note that the epithelial cells have several criteria of malignancy, including a mitotic figure (a), anisocytosis and anisokaryosis, binucleation (c), and prominent nucleoli. They also appear more rounded which may reflect dissociation or exfoliation into fluid or anaplasia. The cholesterol crystals in Figure 4.15 are from a cystic area within this lesion (Wright–Giemsa, scale bar = 10 µm).**

and an ovoid nucleus with an open chromatin pattern and often small nucleoli (Figure 4.17). Moderate anisocytosis and anisokaryosis can be present as well as occasional binucleation, making it challenging to distinguish from mesenchymal neoplasia. Low numbers of spindle cells in the sample, numerous inflammatory cells, and the presence of individually occurring spindle cells with a low degree of atypia were recently identified as cytologic features encountered in fibroplasia compared to mesenchymal neoplasia (Masserdotti & Drigo, 2022). Ultimately, correlation with clinical history and often histopathology are needed.

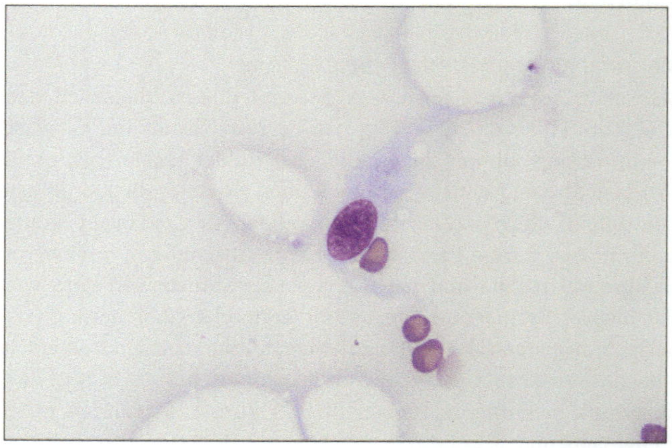

Figure 4.17 **Reactive fibroblast in an FNA of a firm subcutaneous nodule at a previous surgical excision site from a dog. The cell is slightly plump with an ovoid nucleus with lacy chromatin and faint punctate nucleoli, and low amounts of thin, lightly basophilic, spindle-shaped cytoplasm (Wright–Giemsa, 1,000× magnification).**

Calcinosis circumscripta and cutis

Minerals can be deposited in the skin secondary to trauma, mineral imbalances, and glucocorticoids (endogenous and exogenous). Calcinosis circumscripta can present as firm solitary lesions typically over joints, pressure points, bony prominences, or sites of previous trauma and are thought to be a result of dystrophic mineralization. Calcinosis cutis can present as gritty plaque-like lesions in the inguinal region as well as the dorsum and extremities, and it has been fairly

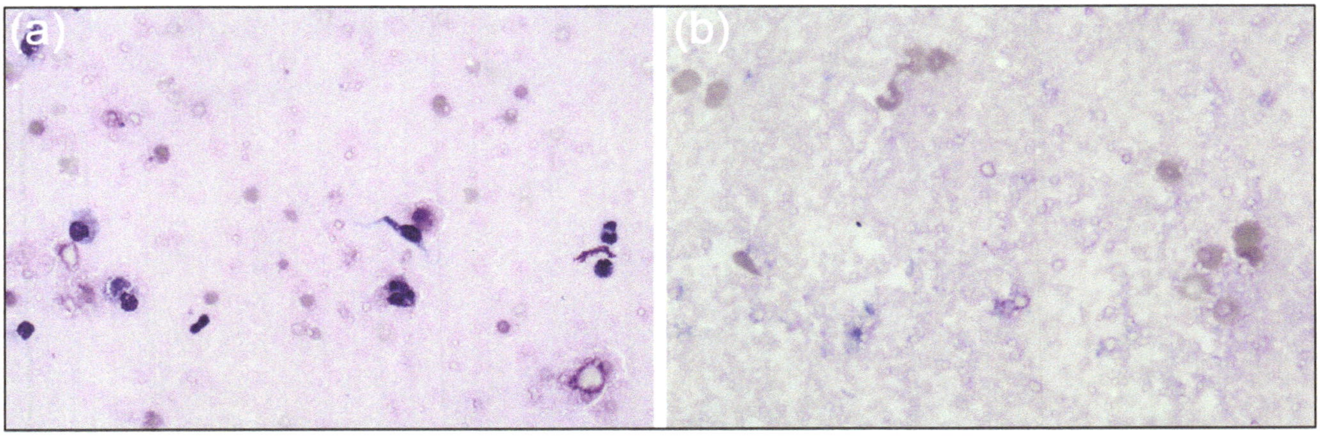

Figures 4.18a, b Calcinosis circumscripta. FNA of a 3–4 cm firm mass overlying the right scapula of a 9-month-old female intact Doberman Pinscher. There is abundant extracellular small rounded to irregular nonstaining crystalline material (mineral, a and b) with few erythrocytes and low numbers of vacuolated macrophages and rare mesenchymal cells (a) (Wright–Giemsa: a, 500× magnification; b, 1,000× magnification).

well recognized in dogs with hyperadrenocorticism. Chalky white, gritty to pasty material may be discharged from these lesions. Smears of this material consist of a thick dense layer of lightly staining to nonstaining granular crystalline material with low numbers of cells such as macrophages and fibroblasts (Figure 4.18a, b). Inflammatory cells such as neutrophils, lymphocytes, and plasma cells may also be seen.

INFLAMMATION AND INFLAMMATORY LESIONS

Neutrophils

If neutrophils are the predominant cell type observed (>85%) in a cytologic sample and other inflammatory cells are less prevalent, the lesion is diagnosed as 'neutrophilic inflammation'. The terms 'suppurative' or 'purulent' have also been used to describe this type of inflammation. The morphologic appearance of the neutrophils may aid in diagnosis of the underlying cause of the inflammation (Figure 4.19). Degenerate neutrophils have karyolytic nuclei with pale, swollen chromatin and are suggestive of an underlying bacterial or fungal infection (Figure 4.20), such as can be seen with an abscess. If the neutrophils are nondegenerate (i.e., they appear similar to neutrophils found in peripheral blood samples), a sterile inflammatory process may be more likely (Figure 4.21). Causes of sterile inflammation include immune-mediated disease (e.g., pemphigus, cutaneous adverse drug reactions – discussed later in this chapter), caustic injury, and trauma.

Karyorrhectic and pyknotic neutrophils (which have clumped, fragmented, and condensed chromatin) suggest a chronic inflammatory process (Figures 4.22a, b). Chronic inflammation is also suspected when low numbers of macrophages are observed along with large numbers of neutrophils. When an infectious organism can be identified within the cytoplasm of neutrophils or macrophages (intracellular), the lesion can be classified as 'septic' (Figure 4.23), not to be confused with sepsis and septicemia (unless identified in the blood). If

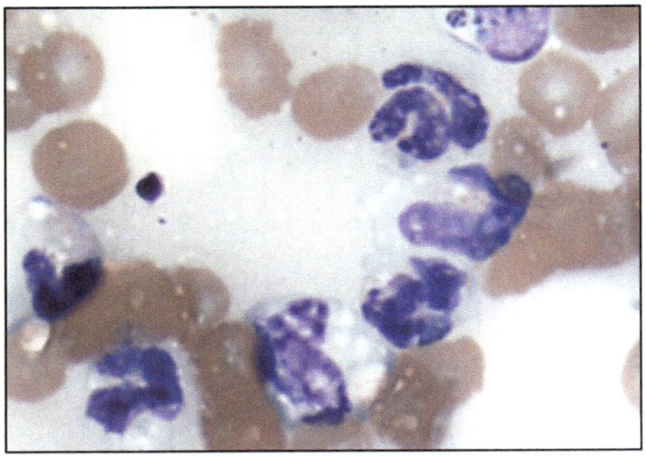

Figure 4.19 Degenerate neutrophils in a septic subcutaneous abscess from a dog. The nuclei of the segmented neutrophils are swollen and have a more open chromatin pattern than expected (Wright–Giemsa, 2,000× magnification).

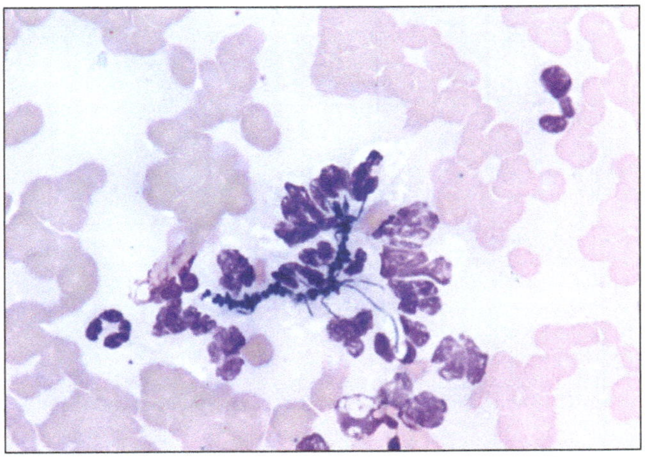

Figure 4.20 Degenerate neutrophils associated with *Dermatophilus congolensis* infection (Wright–Giemsa, 1,000× magnification).

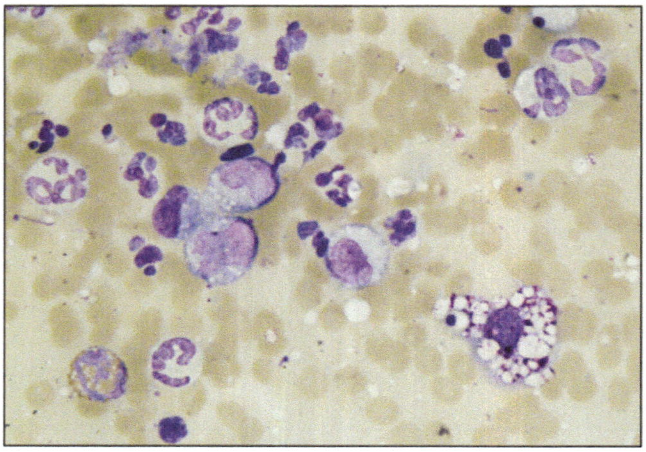

Figure 4.21 Mixed inflammatory reaction in a 1-cm mass on the left flank of a 9-month-old Bernese Mountain Dog. Several neutrophils and erythrocytes, lower numbers of macrophages, an eosinophil, and a lymphocyte are present. Nondegenerate neutrophils have nuclei that are dense with crisp edges, similar to neutrophils in peripheral blood smears (Wright–Giemsa, 1,000× magnification).

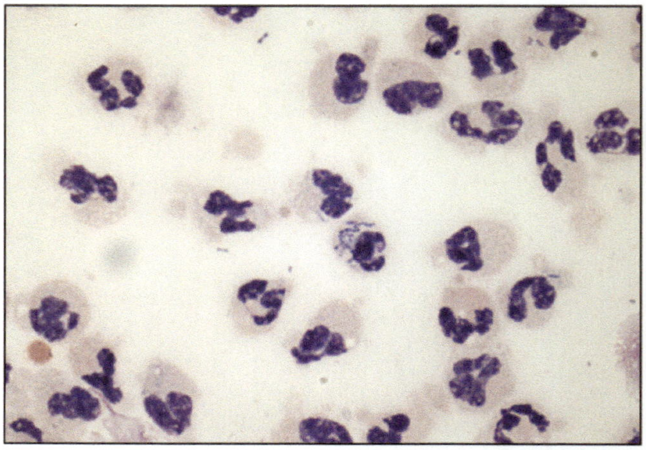

Figure 4.23 Septic suppurative inflammation. Several mildly degenerate neutrophils are present. One of the cells in the center contains several bacterial cocci and rare bacterial rods. A few extracellular bacteria can also be seen (Wright–Giemsa, 1,000× magnification).

an organism cannot be identified, the cause of disease is less certain. Recent or ongoing administration of antimicrobials can prevent the cytologic diagnosis of bacterial infection. If clinically relevant, bacterial and/or fungal culture should be performed when inflammation is observed even if the neutrophils appear nondegenerate.

Histiocytes

The term histiocyte is used generically to describe cells of the macrophage or dendritic (e.g. Langerhans cells (LC) and interstitial dendritic cells) lineage (Moore P.F., 2023). These cells are characterized as large mononuclear cells with modest amounts of basophilic cytoplasm that may contain vacuoles and a paracentric to eccentric rounded to lobulated nucleus.

Macrophages

When the majority of cells in a cytologic sample are macrophages, the lesion is diagnosed as 'macrophagic' or sometimes 'histiocytic' inflammation. On histopathology, the presence of these large mononuclear cells in conjunction with epithelioid macrophages (macrophages with a more rounded to polygonal appearance, resembling epithelial cells) with or without multinucleated giant cells is consistent with 'granulomatous' inflammation. Multinucleated giant cells in inflammatory lesions should not be interpreted as neoplastic cells (Figure 4.24). Causes of granuloma formation include foreign body

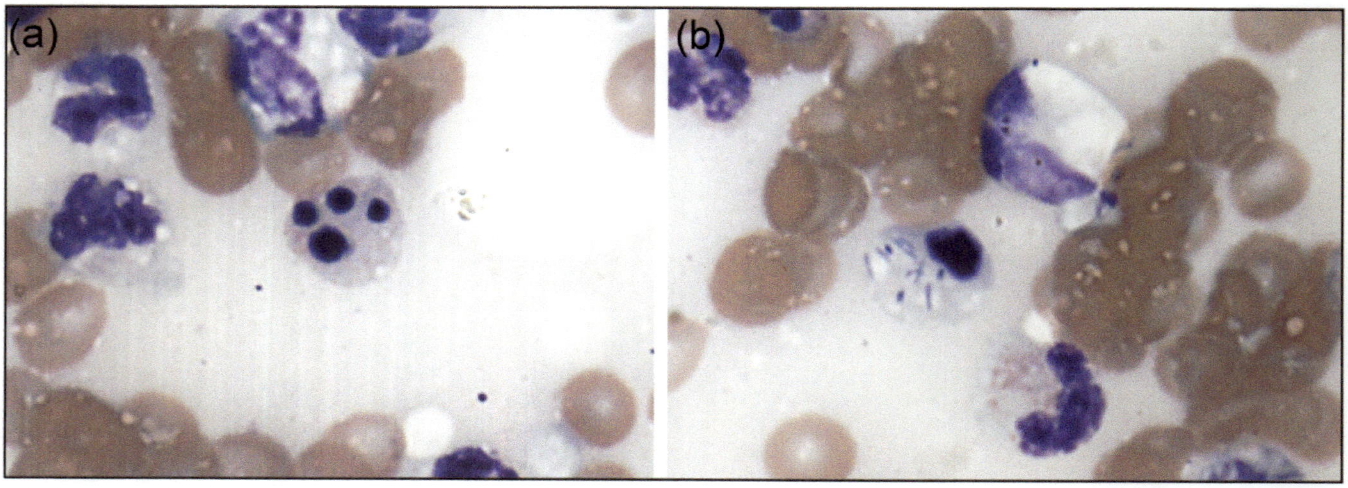

Figures 4.22a, b Chromatin condensation in cells in a septic subcutaneous abscess from a dog. (a) The nucleus of the cell in the center of the image with four areas of condensed chromatin is karyorrhectic. (b) A pyknotic cell with a single spot of condensed chromatin is shown at the center of the image. The cell contains several bacterial rods. Degenerate neutrophils are also present in both images (Wright–Giemsa, 2,000× magnification).

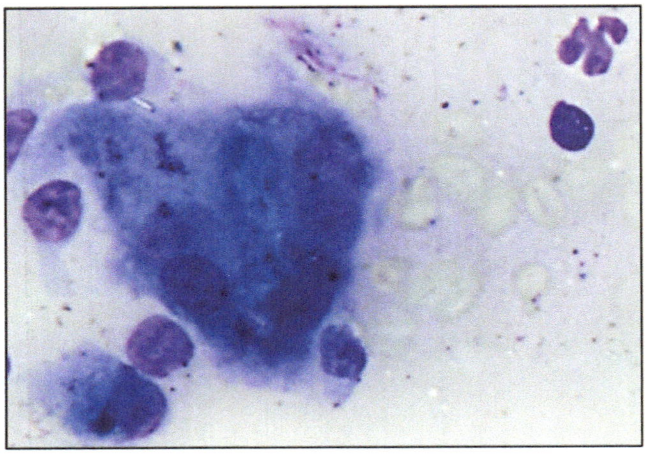

Figure 4.24 Multinucleated giant cell in an FNA from a subcutaneous granuloma in a dog. A large multinucleated macrophage is shown. Other cell types present include erythrocytes, macrophages, a degenerate neutrophil, and two lysed cells that lack cytoplasm (Wright–Giemsa, 2,000× magnification).

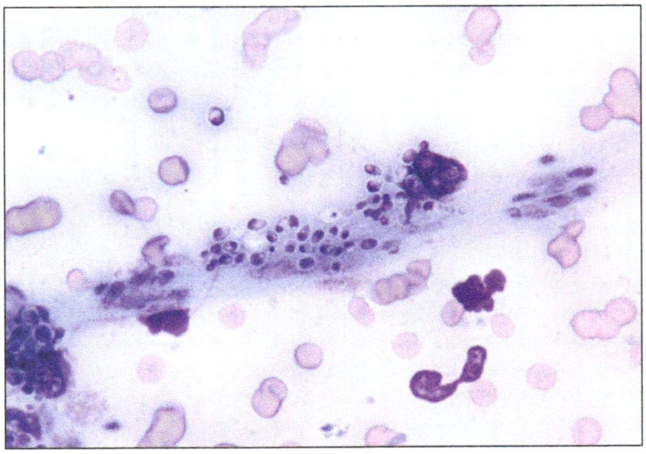

Figure 4.25 *Histoplasma capsulatum* organisms are small 1–2 μm diameter yeast structures with a thin distinct clear cell wall and often a crescent-shaped nucleus. The organisms in this image are associated with a ruptured cell but typically organisms are observed within macrophages (Wright–Giemsa, 1,000× magnification).

reaction, fungal infection, atypical bacterial infection, and chronic inflammation. Classic examples of diseases that induce granulomatous inflammation include histoplasmosis (Figure 4.25) and mycobacterial infections (Figures 4.26a, b).

Reactive histiocytoses

In dogs and cats, the majority of histiocytic disorders involve proliferations of cells of LC or interstitial dendritic cell lineage. There are several subtypes of histiocytic disorders (Affolter & Moore, 2000; Affolter & Moore, 2002; Moore *et al.*, 2006; Moore P.F., 2023). Currently, cutaneous histiocytosis (CH) and systemic histiocytosis (SH) are considered non-neoplastic, inflammatory diseases. CH and SH are referred to as the 'reactive histiocytoses' and have only been identified in dogs. Histiocytoma, canine cutaneous Langerhans cell histiocytosis (LCH), feline progressive histiocytosis, and histiocytic sarcoma are neoplastic diseases, discussed later in this chapter (see 'Histiocytic Neoplasms').

CH and SH are histiocyte and lymphocyte-rich inflammatory disorders associated with a degree of immune dysregulation and are due to abnormal accumulation of activated dermal interstitial dendritic cells (Moore, 2014; Moore P.F., 2023). Cells appear similar to macrophages and have abundant lightly basophilic cytoplasm and an ovoid nucleus with finely stippled chromatin. Neutrophils and small lymphocytes are also observed. If dermal dendritic cells form masses in the skin and subcutis, the disease is called 'cutaneous histiocytosis',

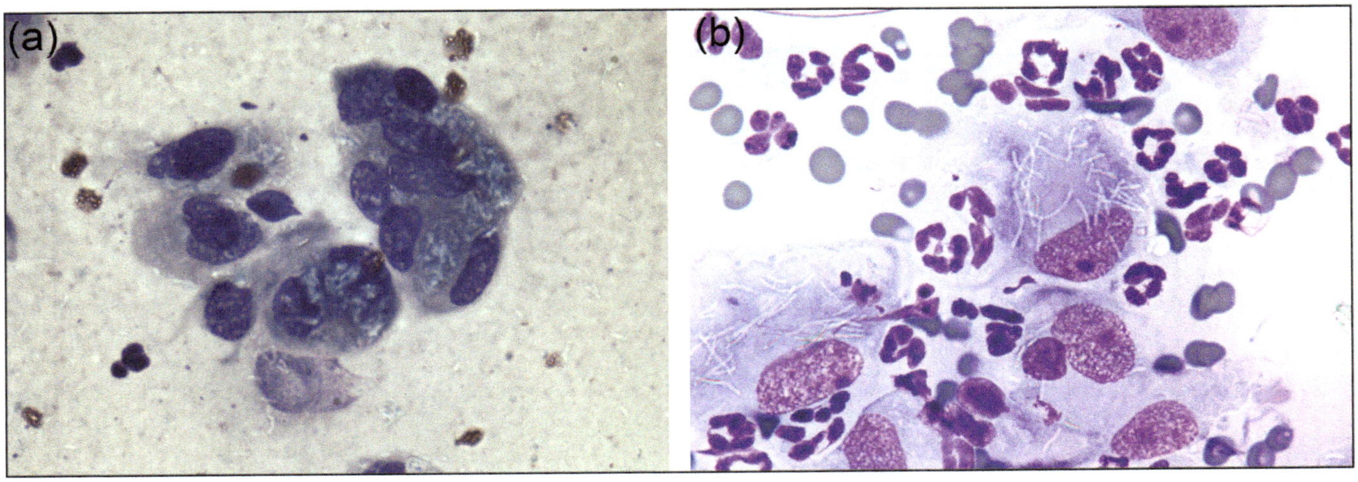

Figures 4.26a, b Mycobacterial infection. (a) FNA of a subcutaneous mass from a cat. The image shows several macrophages that contain nonstaining bacterial rods. A few partially intact neutrophils and rare erythrocytes also are present. Extracellular bacterial rods can be observed against the basophilic proteinaceous background of the sample. (b) FNA of a nasal mass from a cat. The image shows several macrophages that contain nonstaining bacterial rods. Several intact neutrophils and low numbers of erythrocytes also are present (Wright–Giemsa, 1,000× magnification).

and the local lymph nodes can also be affected. In systemic histiocytosis, the lesions are diffuse and are typically found in the skin, ocular and nasal mucosa, and sometimes the internal organs (Mays & Bergeron, 1986; Moore P.F., 2023). Affected animals have multiple skin lesions that wax and wane. Long-term immunosuppressive treatment is often needed for these patients (Coomer & Liptak, 2008).

Neutrophils and macrophages

When a lesion contains a mixed population of neutrophils and macrophages, it may be described as 'neutrophilic and macrophagic' or 'pyogranulomatous' inflammation. The macrophages associated with granulomatous and pyogranulomatous inflammation are often described as epithelioid because of their similar appearance to epithelial cells. The list of differential causes for pyogranulomatous inflammation is similar to the list for granulomatous inflammation (foreign body reaction, fungal infection, atypical bacterial infection, and chronic inflammation).

Close examination of these samples for fungal elements and filamentous bacteria is warranted. Examples of infectious organisms associated with pyogranulomatous inflammation include *Pythium insidiosum* (Figure 7.32 in Chapter 7, 'Cytology of the Gastrointestinal Tract'), *Lagenidium* spp., *Blastomyces dermatitidis* (Figure 4.27), *Coccidioides immitis* (Figure 12.16b in Chapter 12, 'Musculoskeletal Cytology'), *Histoplasma capsulatum* (Figure 4.25), *Sporothrix schenckii*, and *Nocardia* spp. (Figure 4.28). Special stains such as silver and periodic acid–Schiff stains can be helpful to highlight organisms if they are not seen using a routine Romanowsky-type stain (Figure 4.29).

Fungal organisms can be present as yeast (rounded to ovoid structures) and/or hyphae (linear structures, often with septations,

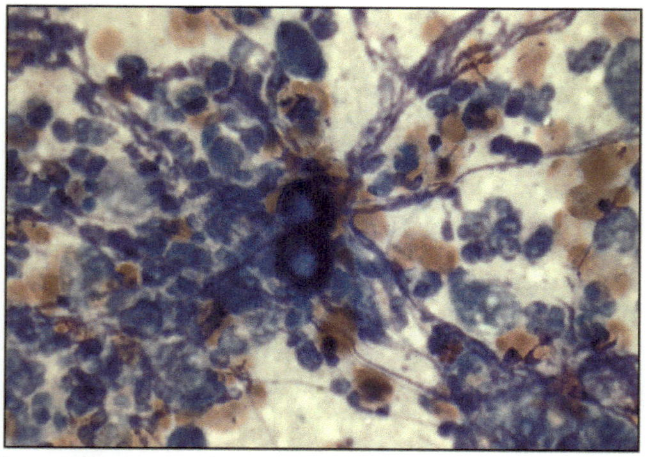

Figure 4.27 **Pyogranulomatous inflammation due to blastomycosis. Imprint cytology of a draining skin lesion from a dog. The sample contains several degenerate neutrophils, lower numbers of macrophages, and large (17–22 μm), round, yeast structures. The organism has a deeply basophilic nucleus, a distinctive double-contoured capsule, and exhibits broad-based budding consistent with *Blastomyces dermatitidis*. There is also nuclear streaming present (linear purple strands), not to be confused with fungal hyphae (Wright–Giemsa, 1,000× magnification).**

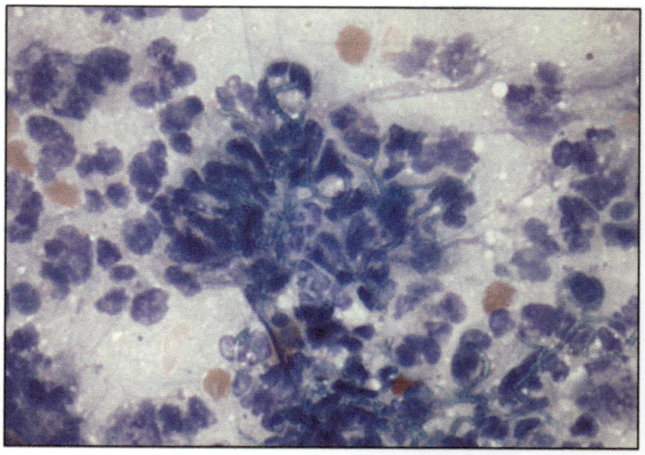

Figure 4.28 **Pyogranulomatous inflammation due to nocardial infection. Multiple subcutaneous masses from an immunosuppressed dog were aspirated. Several branching, thin, filamentous organisms were entrapped within large numbers of degenerate neutrophils and fewer macrophages. Culture for anaerobic bacterial and fungal organisms yielded *Nocardia abscessus* (Wright–Giemsa, 1,000× magnification).**

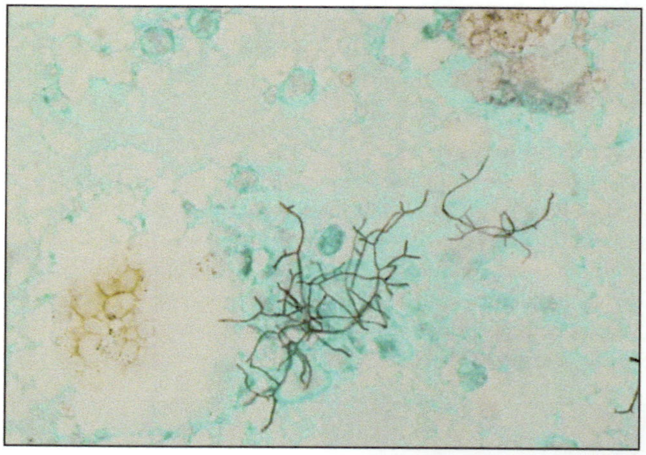

Figure 4.29 **FNA of a subcutaneous mass from a 4-year-old Bichon Frisé. The dark golden-brown branching structures are *Nocardia* spp. organisms. This stain would also highlight fungal elements (Grocott's methenamine silver, 100× magnification).**

occasionally branching), not to be confused with debris or nuclear streaming. Some organisms have distinct cytologic features. The yeast form of *Blastomyces dermatitidis* (Figure 4.27) ranges from 8 to 22 μm and has a double-contoured wall and broad-based budding. These organisms are deeply basophilic and easily identified in cytologic preparations. *Coccidioides immitis* organisms appear as variably sized, thick, basophilic spherules (20–200 μm) with a thick blue to purple wall and a granular internal structure (due to the presence of endospores). The endospores are round, 2–5 μm in diameter, and can be confused with *Histoplasma* spp. when seen extracellularly (Fisher, 2020; Raskin & Conrado, 2023). *Histoplasma capsulatum* (Figure 4.25) is a much smaller organism (approximately 2 μm) and is often phagocytized by macrophages. It is rounded, has a thin clear cell wall, and contains a crescent-shaped eosinophilic nuclear structure. *Sporothrix schenckii* can appear similar to *Histoplasma* spp.; however, some organisms have more of an elongate, fusiform shape. *Pythium insidiosum* and *Lagenidium* spp. are waterborne fungus-like organisms, and infection typically causes pyogranulomatous inflammation with an eosinophilic component in the gastrointestinal tract and less commonly in the skin (observed as cutaneous nodular ulcerated lesions). Cytology preparations show the presence of poorly staining, poorly septate, broad, branching hyphae (Fisher, 2020; Raskin & Conrado, 2023).

Neutrophilic and macrophagic inflammation can also be seen with reactive fat (panniculitis), where subcutaneous fat becomes inflamed secondary to trauma, foreign bodies, vaccines, infection, and idiopathic causes. Panniculitis presents as subcutaneous or deep cutaneous nodules. Aspirates consist of mature adipocytes, extracellular free lipid, lipid-laden rounded to spindled cells (macrophages and/or fibroblasts), and variable numbers of neutrophils. These cytological findings may be difficult to discern from an inflamed lipomatous mass.

Eosinophils

'Eosinophilic inflammation' is diagnosed in cytologic samples that contain >10% eosinophils (Figure 4.30). Eosinophils are not commonly seen in the blood or tissue; therefore, even low numbers of eosinophils are considered significant. Frequently, significant numbers of neutrophils and/or macrophages are also present in these lesions. This type of inflammation is associated with parasites, allergic diseases, type I hypersensitivity reactions (e.g., due to insect bites or stings), immune-mediated diseases, and paraneoplastic conditions. Eosinophilic inflammation is supportive of a diagnosis of eosinophilic granuloma, which is one of the most distinct and common manifestations of eosinophilic granuloma complex (EGC) in cats that have a raised, erythematous, alopecic mass. The other clinical presentations of ECG are eosinophilic plaques and indolent (rodent) ulcers. Some other differentials for eosinophilic plaque or granuloma are infectious agents (e.g., demodecosis, fungal and fungal-like infections) and a paraneoplastic response to certain tumors such as mast cell tumors, lymphomas, and carcinomas (Raskin & Conrado, 2023).

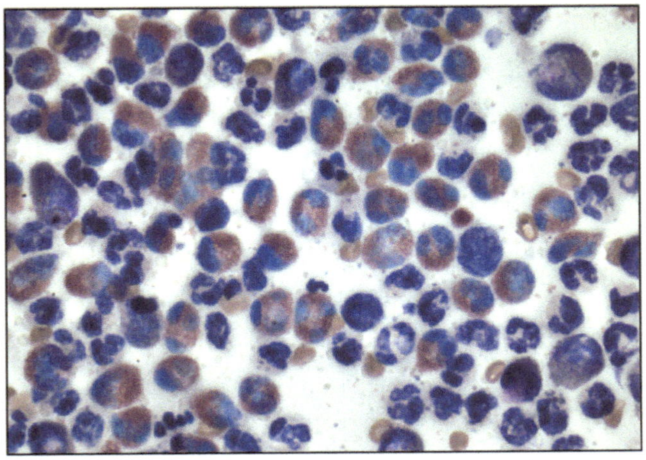

Figure 4.30 Eosinophilic inflammation in a hairless, raised, erythematous, dermal lesion from a cat. There are large numbers of eosinophils filled with eosinophilic cytoplasmic granules. Large numbers of neutrophils also are present (Wright–Giemsa, 1,000× magnification).

Lymphocytes

In lesions diagnosed as 'lymphocytic inflammation', the majority of cells are small, well-differentiated lymphocytes. Additionally, low numbers of intermediate-sized lymphocytes are expected to be present in these lesions. If plasma cells are also observed, the term 'plasmacytic–lymphocytic' or 'lymphoplasmacytic' inflammation is used (Figure 4.31). Antigenic stimulation is the most common cause of both lymphocytic and plasmacytic–lymphocytic inflammation. Examples of sources of antigen include insect bites, vaccines, and viral infections. Delayed (type IV) hypersensitivity reactions should be considered when lymphocytic or plasmacytic–lymphocytic inflammation is observed.

Mixed inflammation

Cytologic samples may contain large numbers of neutrophils, macrophages, and lymphocytes (with or without rare eosinophils). These lesions are diagnosed as 'mixed inflammation' to indicate that many inflammatory cell types are present. Chronic inflammation, acral lick dermatitis/lick granulomas, and vaccine reactions are commonly associated with a mixed inflammatory response. In vaccine reactions, brightly eosinophilic to magenta globular material can often be seen within macrophages (Figures 4.32a, b). Blue or blue-gray globular

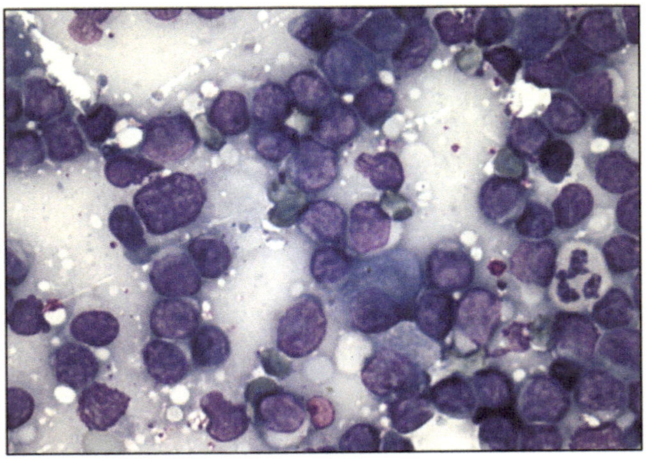

Figure 4.31 Plasmacytic–lymphocytic inflammation in an FNA of a small, firm, subcutaneous mass from a cat. The majority of cells are small lymphocytes with a nuclear diameter less than the diameter of the neutrophil. A few intermediate-sized lymphocytes with nuclei approximately the diameter of the neutrophil are present. One plasma cell also is shown at the center of the image (Wright–Giemsa, 1,000× magnification).

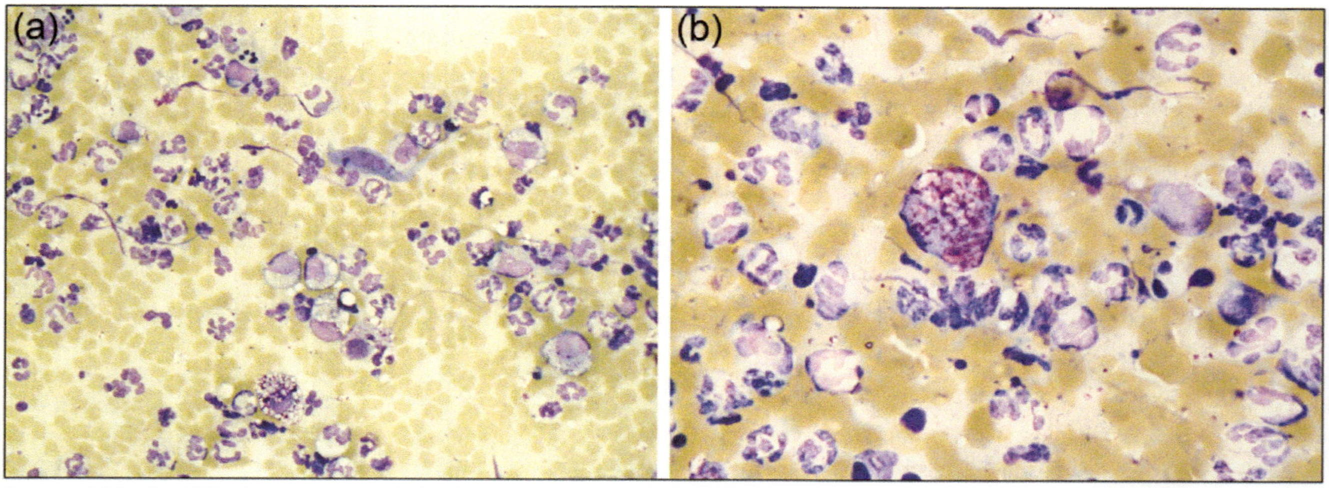

Figures 4.32a, b **FNA of a 1 cm mass on the left flank of a 9-month-old Bernese Mountain Dog. Several neutrophils, lower numbers of macrophages, rare lymphocytes and fibroblasts, and several erythrocytes are present. Some macrophages contain bright eosinophilic globular material consistent with vaccine adjuvant (Wright–Giemsa: a, 500× magnification; b, 1,000× magnification).**

material may also be seen within macrophages, and is associated with the use of vaccines that have a metal-containing adjuvant (e.g. certain rabies vaccines; Scruggs & LeBlanc, 2015).

With mastitis, cytological preparations of mammary secretions or aspirates contain predominantly neutrophils that may be degenerate, or variable numbers of neutrophils, lymphocytes, and macrophages depending on the causative agent. If due to an infection, organisms (most commonly bacteria) may be seen within neutrophils and macrophages (Fisher, 2020).

DERMATOLOGIC CYTOLOGY

This section provides a brief review of the common non-neoplastic dermatologic lesions, some of which are discussed in other parts in this chapter. These skin lesions can be infectious or noninfectious, inflammatory or noninflammatory, and can be evaluated via cytology using a variety of sample collection techniques such as needle aspirates, scrapes, swabs, and impression smears (see Chapter 1, 'Sample Acquisition and Preparation'). This review focuses on microbial overgrowth, dermatophytosis, mite infestation, and pemphigus foliaceus. Other noninfectious, inflammatory lesions, such as cutaneous adverse drug reactions, foreign body reactions, vaccine reactions, and acral lick dermatitis, are mentioned in the 'Mixed Inflammation' section. For additional dermatologic information, the readers are directed to the references.

Low numbers of bacteria and few fungi can be found on the skin surface in health, as part of the normal microbiota. Bacterial or fungal overgrowth and secondary skin infections can be seen when there is compromise of the skin barrier (e.g., trauma, inflammation) or immunosuppression, and affected patients can present with pruritus, erythema, and scaling (Albanese, 2017). Cytology samples of microbial overgrowth will have significantly increased numbers of microbes and may or may not contain inflammation

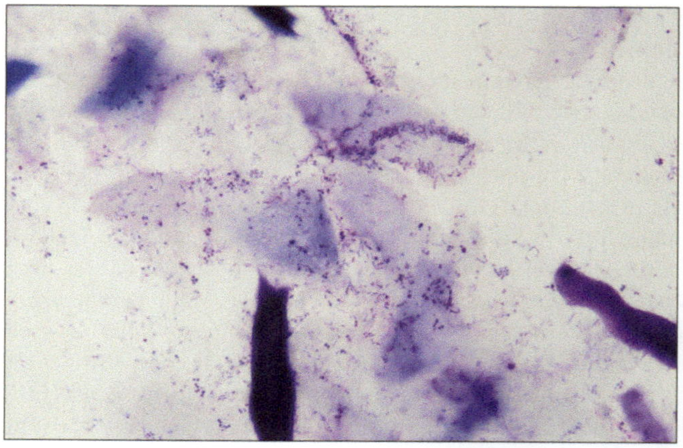

Figure 4.33 **Bacterial overgrowth. Three-year-old English Bulldog with moderate cutaneous erythema and exudate of tail fold skin. Impression smear cytology revealed numerous anucleate squamous epithelial cells, keratin, keratinaceous debris, and bacteria (paired cocci and rods) without inflammation. This patient was previously diagnosed with atopic dermatitis of unknown etiology (Diff-Quik®, 1,000× magnification).**

(Figure 4.33). When inflammation is present, it could represent pyoderma or an abscess. Superficial pyoderma commonly presents as cutaneous pustules, papules, erosions, moist exudation, crusts, and erythema, while deep pyodermas (e.g., bacterial folliculitis and furunculosis) can present as ulcers, swellings, nodules, and draining tracts. *Staphylococcus* spp. is most commonly involved. Other bacterial pathogens may also cause pyoderma, such as *Streptococcus* spp. and rods such as *Escherichia coli*, *Pseudomonas* species, or *Klebsiella* spp. (Welle & Linder, 2021). Neutrophilic inflammation or a mixed inflammatory response (neutrophils and macrophages +/– lymphocytes) is typically observed on cytology with pyoderma, and neutrophils may appear degenerate and contain phagocytized bacteria. Deeper pyodermas can also contain fragments of keratin extracellularly as well as within macrophages and sometimes few acantholytic keratinocytes. Bacterial abscesses typically have many degenerate neutrophils and bacteria may be seen extracellularly and within neutrophils (Figures 4.19, 4.22a–b, 4.23).

Cutaneous fungal overgrowth is more commonly attributed to *Malassezia* species than *Candida*. On cytology, *Malassezia* appears as small (3–8-µm) oval to peanut or foot-print shaped, broad-based budding organisms (Figures 18.2, 18.35 in Chapter 18, 'Cytology of the Ear'), which are extracellular or may be adhered to the surfaces of keratinized squamous epithelial cells. Finding greater than two organisms per high power field (100× oil objective) is suggestive of *Malassezia* overgrowth (Fisher, 2020). A mixed inflammatory response (lymphocytes and macrophages) may be seen with *Malassezia* dermatitis, in addition to neutrophils if secondary pyoderma develops (Raskin & Conrado, 2023). *Candida* is a commensal that is found in the GI tract and mucous membranes but can cause mucocutaneous or cutaneous disease, particularly in immunosuppressed animals. This organism can appear as small (2–10-µm) ovoid yeast organisms that bud or have elongate germ tube formation with pseudohyphae and sometimes true hyphae (Figures 6.14 and 7.30a–c in Chapters 6, 'Oral Cavity Cytology', and 7, 'Cytology of the Gastrointestinal Tract').

Other important dermatologic etiologic agents, some of which are zoonotic, include ringworm or dermatophytosis and mite infestation. Dermatophytosis can be diagnosed via trichogram (hair pluck, prepared with mineral oil or 10–20% potassium hydroxide solution); some lesions may also fluoresce with a Wood's lamp (UV light). On cytology, fungal arthrospores (small round to ovoid structures) may be visualized within hair shafts (endothrix, e.g., *Trichophyton mentagrophytes*; see Figure 4.69a) or on the hair shaft surface (ectothrix, e.g., *Microsporum canis* or *M. gypsum*); hyphae may also be seen. Mite infestation can be caused by *Demodex* (demodectic or follicular mange), *Sarcoptes* (canine scabies), *Notoedres* (feline scabies), and *Cheyletiella*. Low numbers of *Demodex* can be found in the skin but increases can result in clinical signs such as pruritus and alopecia. These organisms are found primarily within hair follicles, have an elongate cigar shape, eight legs (nymphs and adults; Figure 18.5 in Chapter 18, 'Cytology of the Ear'), and are best visualized on deep skin scrapes performed in the middle of the lesions. Demodecosis can have a cytologic appearance similar to deep pyoderma, as secondary bacterial infections can develop. Canine scabies is caused by *Sarcoptes scabei* var. *canis* and adults are ovoid and measure 200–400 µm in diameter with four paired short legs (Figure 4.34; Miller *et al.*, 2013). Lesions associated with infestation include papules, areas of erythema, crusting, and alopecia. Multiple superficial skin scrapes should be collected to increase the chance of detecting the mites in dogs with suspected scabies. Feline scabies is caused by *Notoedres cati*, which is similar in morphology but smaller than *Sarcoptes* (Miller *et al.*, 2013). Unlike canine scabies, often many mites are visualized on skin scrapes from cats with scabies. Cheyletiellosis is termed 'walking dandruff' because mites can be grossly seen moving along the skin of infected animals. They are highly contagious and can spread to other animals and humans. Animals may be asymptomatic or can have dry scaling (appears similar to dandruff) along the dorsum, alopecia, crusting, and pruritus. Tape impressions, examination of hair and scale samples, and flea combs are some methods used to identify mites, which have four pairs of legs with combs and characteristic accessory mouthparts that terminate in prominent hooks (Figure 4.35; Miller *et al.*, 2013). *Otodectes*, an aural mite, is discussed in Chapter 18 ('Cytology of the Ear'). Fleas can also incite an allergic dermatitis with gross lesions of papules, crusts, alopecia, and erythema (Albanese, 2017). Cytologically these lesions commonly contain mostly eosinophilic inflammation with variable numbers of mast cells, basophils, and macrophages. This cytologic pattern can also be seen with atopic dermatitis, food allergy, and other arthropod-bite/sting (e.g. mosquito).

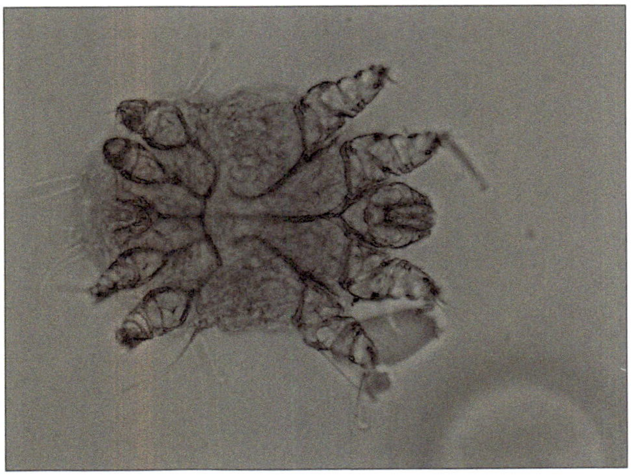

Figure 4.34 *Sarcoptes* spp. adult mite. (Unstained, 200× magnification; image courtesy of Dr. Roxanne Charles.)

Autoimmune skin disease is uncommon in dogs and cats and typically requires biopsy with histopathology for diagnosis. Two important autoimmune complexes include pemphigus and lupus. Pemphigus complex includes pustular and blistering disorders – pemphigus foliaceus, pemphigus vulgaris, pemphigus vegetans, and pemphigus erythematosus. Within this complex, pemphigus foliaceus is the most common, and typically presents as pustules that eventually progress to form crusts. Cytology of these lesions contains non-degenerate neutrophils and many acantholytic cells (individually occurring keratinocytes that are round/oval to polygonal in shape, have deeply basophilic cytoplasm, and a round centrally located nucleus) are observed (Figure 4.36). Eosinophils may also be seen with this disease (Albanese, 2017). While acantholytic cells can be supportive of pemphigus, they can also be seen (albeit in lower numbers) with bacterial pyoderma and dermatophytosis, so thorough examination for infectious agents is recommended. The lupus complex includes discoid lupus erythematosus (DLE) and systemic lupus erythematosus, with DLE primarily affecting the skin. DLE lesions typically involve the face (around the nose and eyes) and footpads and may include erythema, depigmentation, ulceration, or erosion (Miller *et al.*, 2013). Biopsy is considered the diagnostic method of choice, coupled with clinical signs and antinuclear antibody testing. Additional discussion on SLE can be found in Chapter 12 ('Musculoskeletal Cytology').

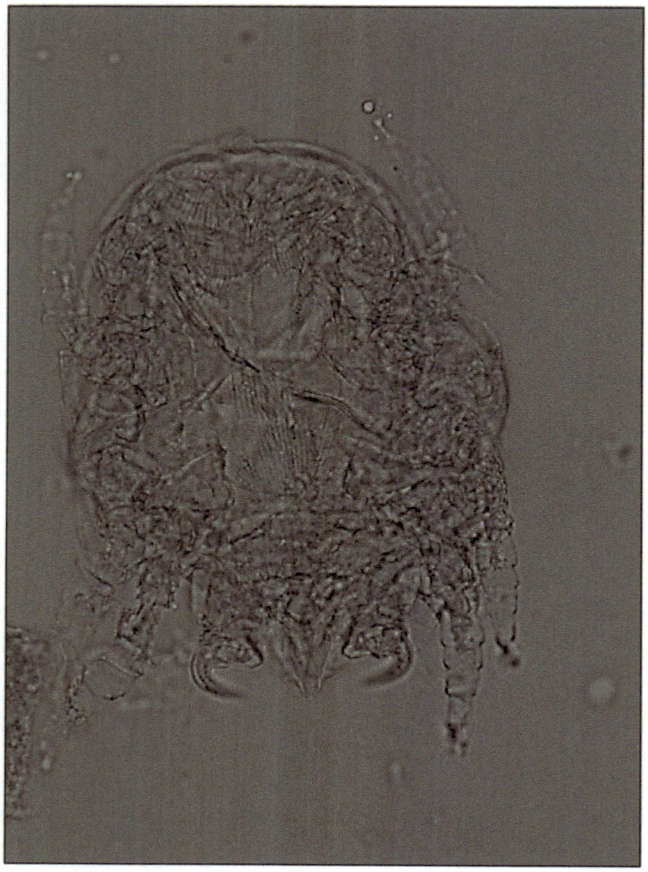

Figure 4.35 *Cheyletiella* spp. adult mite. (Unstained, 200× magnification; image courtesy of Dr. Roxanne Charles.)

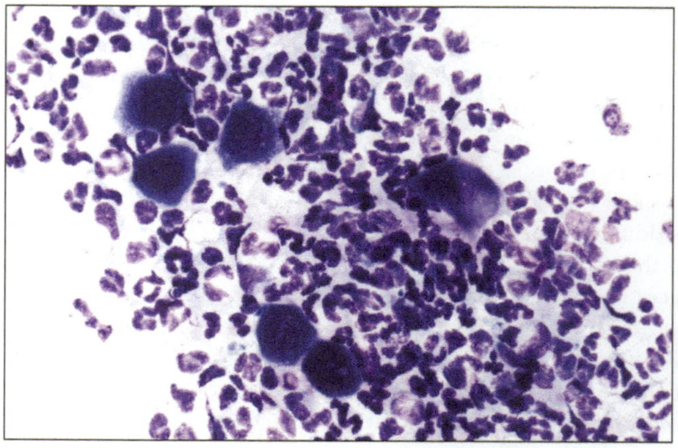

Figure 4.36 Pemphigus foliaceus. Impression smear of moist erythematous lesions under cutaneous crusts in a 13-year-old Miniature Schnauzer with diffuse dermatitis. There are numerous variably degenerate neutrophils and modest numbers of individualized squamous epithelial cells. Several epithelial cells appear acantholytic with a more rounded appearance and deeper blue cytoplasm (Diff-Quik®, 500× magnification).

EPIDERMAL AND FOLLICULAR TUMORS

Basal epithelial cells

Epidermal and follicular tumors may contain basal epithelial cells, which are found at the deepest level of the epidermis. These basal cells appear cuboidal with scant, lightly basophilic cytoplasm and a small, round nucleus with a dense chromatin pattern (Figures 4.37a, b). Sheets of basal cells have a cobblestone appearance due to very distinct cell junctions. In dogs with cutaneous tumors containing basal epithelial cells, a short list of differential diagnoses may be reported including follicular tumors and adnexal tumors. Follicular tumors include infundibular keratinizing acanthoma, trichoblastoma, warty dyskeratoma, trichofolliculoma, trichoepithelioma, tricholemmoma,

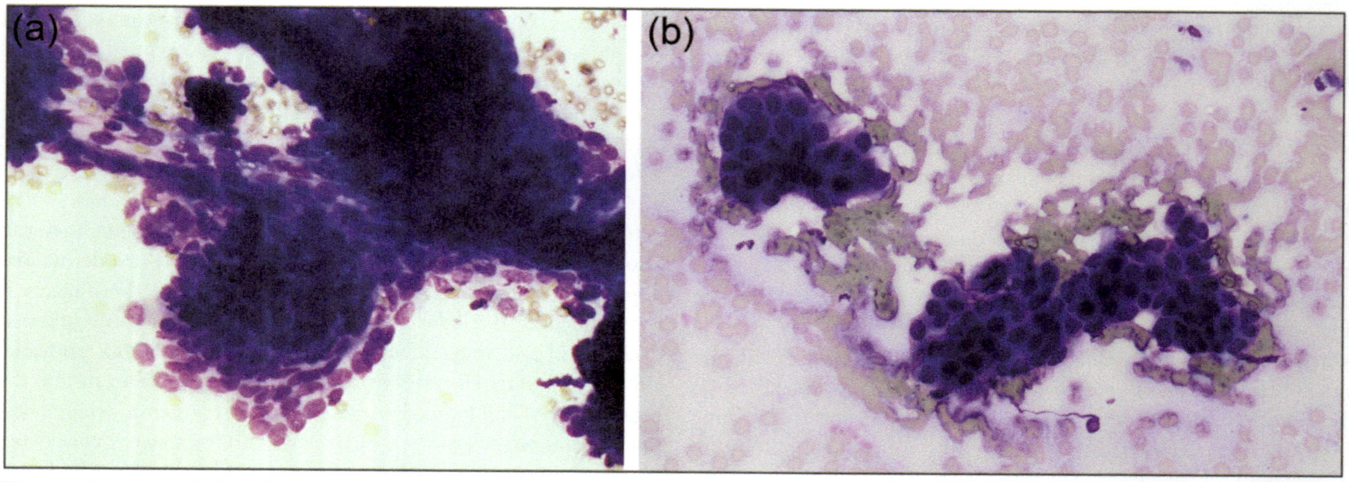

Figures 4.37a, b (a) FNA of a cutaneous mass from a 10-year-old Malamute. (b) FNA of a cutaneous mass from a 10-year-old mixed breed dog. Basal epithelial cells are present. Cells are small and cohesive with scant pale cytoplasm and a small rounded dense nucleus. Distinct cell junctions can be observed (Wright–Giemsa, 500× magnification).

and pilomatricoma, the majority of which are benign. These cutaneous basilar epithelial neoplasms often appear similar on cytology, and histopathologic examination is necessary to evaluate the arrangement of neoplastic cells within the mass and the degree of epithelial, trichofollicular epithelial, sweat gland, or sebaceous gland differentiation (Goldschmidt *et al.*, 2020; Gross *et al.*, 2005; Bohn *et al.*, 2006). There are, however, certain features of trichoblastomas that may aid in distinguishing them from the other types of cutaneous follicular lesions on cytology, such as the presence of a pink matrix, very low numbers of spindle cells, and clusters of uniformly sized basaloid epithelial cells (Adedeji, 2017). Malignant basal cell tumors are relatively common in cats but are rare in dogs. Basal cell carcinoma is diagnosed if there are enough characteristics of malignancy observed in the basal cell population without squamous or adnexal differentiation. The cytologic diagnosis of basal cell carcinoma should be confirmed by histology, as markedly dysplastic benign tumors have been reported (Bohn *et al.*, 2006).

Squamous epithelial cells

Cutaneous papilloma (wart)

This is common in dogs and rare in cats. It can be virus-induced (most common and due to papillomavirus infection) or less commonly occur as a spontaneous lesion of non-viral origin. On cytology, the cells typically resemble normal squamous epithelial cells, with mature forms predominating (Figure 4.38). The cells are nucleated to anucleate. Larger ovoid to fusiform nucleated cells with large eccentrically located nuclei and vacuolated/foamy or stippled pink to purple cytoplasm may also be seen. These are thought to represent hypertrophied keratinocytes (koilocytes), a feature of papillomavirus infection (Fisher, 2020).

Squamous cell carcinoma

Squamous cell carcinomas in cats and dogs have an aggressive biologic behavior. They often develop in the nonpigmented skin near mucous membranes and metastasize to the draining lymph nodes. When squamous cell carcinomas become ulcerated, secondary infection with bacteria and marked neutrophilic inflammation are observed. This may complicate the cytologic diagnosis of squamous cell carcinoma. The neoplastic cells can occur individually and in sheets or cohesive clusters, and in well-differentiated tumors, the cells are often angular in shape and keratinized. Most neoplastic squamous epithelial cells have several distinctive characteristics of malignancy. Classic changes in cellular morphology include abnormal cytoplasmic vacuolation, which gives the cells a signet-ring appearance (Figure 4.39a), aberrant keratinization (Figure 4.39b), or perinuclear vacuolization (Figure 4.39b). Tadpole-shaped cells, cells with an increased N:C ratio (Figure 4.39c, d), and asynchrony of nuclear and cytoplasmic maturation are also common findings (Figure 4.39b). Emperipolesis can be seen, a process where neutrophils and malignant cells traffic through larger malignant cells (Raskin & Conrado, 2023). In cases of poorly differentiated squamous cell carcinoma, these distinctive characteristics are not observed and tumors may simply be diagnosed as carcinomas. Squamous cell carcinomas can invade bone and occasionally osteoclasts can be observed in cytologic aspiration of cutaneous masses (Figure 4.39e).

DERMAL AND SUBCUTANEOUS MESENCHYMAL TUMORS

As previously mentioned, the dermis and subcutis contain supportive, connective tissues made up of resident mesenchymal/spindle cells and extracellular fibrillar and matrix materials. These resident cells include fibrocytes/fibroblasts, adipocytes, endothelial cells, nerves,

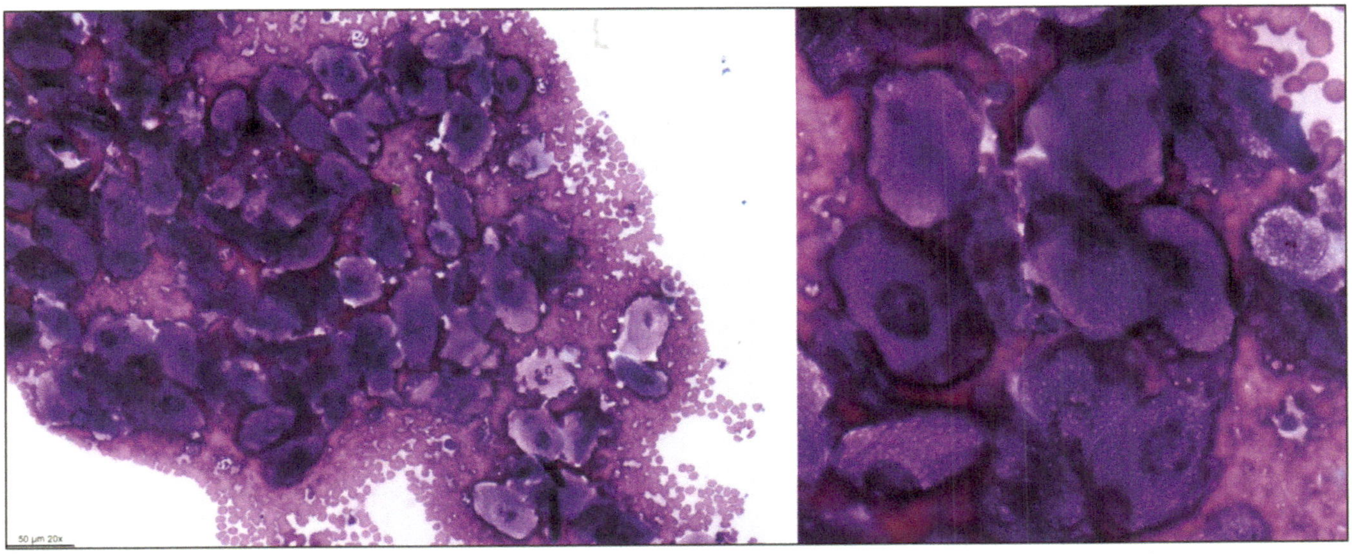

Figures 4.38 Cutaneous papilloma. FNA of a verrucous growth on the surface of the right paw of a 2-year-old mixed breed dog. There are numerous squamous epithelial cells that display mild atypia and some of which display a finely vacuolated keratinizing cytoplasm resembling koilocytes (Wright–Giemsa: Left, 200× magnification; Right, 500× magnification; images courtesy of Dr. Carolina Azevedo, obtained on the Vetscan Imagyst®, DAL-16056, DAL-16057).

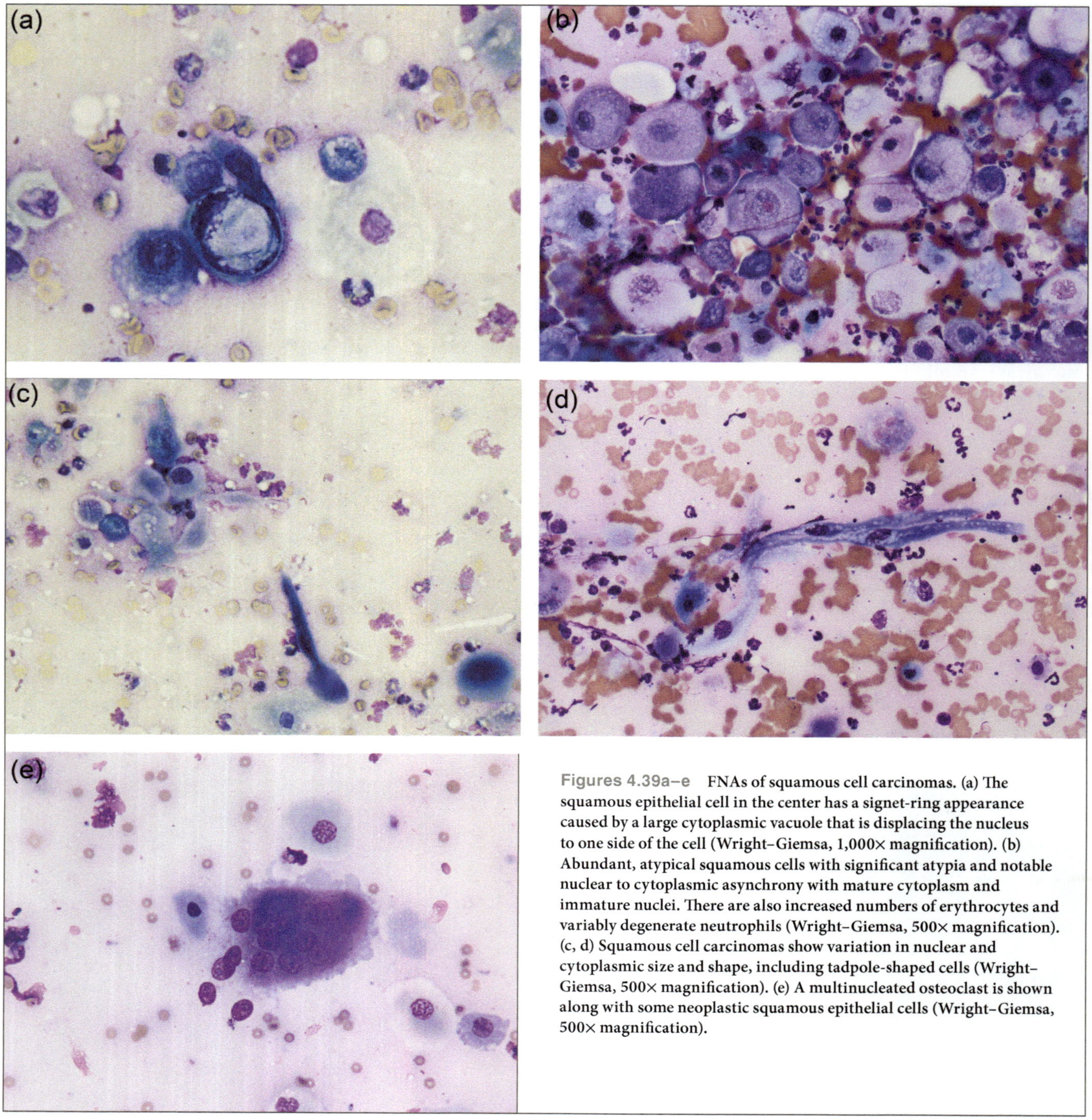

Figures 4.39a–e FNAs of squamous cell carcinomas. (a) The squamous epithelial cell in the center has a signet-ring appearance caused by a large cytoplasmic vacuole that is displacing the nucleus to one side of the cell (Wright-Giemsa, 1,000× magnification). (b) Abundant, atypical squamous cells with significant atypia and notable nuclear to cytoplasmic asynchrony with mature cytoplasm and immature nuclei. There are also increased numbers of erythrocytes and variably degenerate neutrophils (Wright-Giemsa, 500× magnification). (c, d) Squamous cell carcinomas show variation in nuclear and cytoplasmic size and shape, including tadpole-shaped cells (Wright-Giemsa, 500× magnification). (e) A multinucleated osteoclast is shown along with some neoplastic squamous epithelial cells (Wright-Giemsa, 500× magnification).

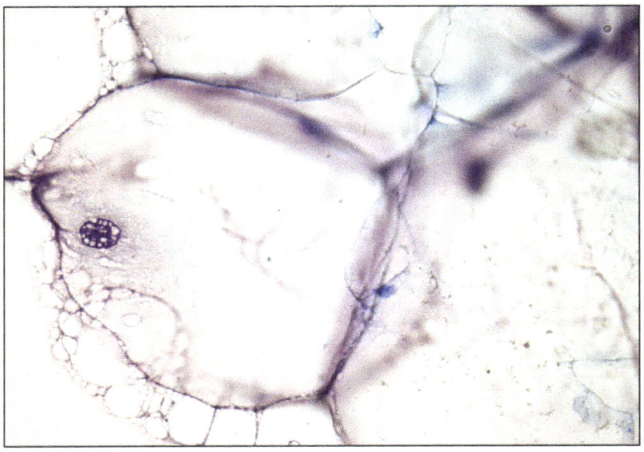

Figure 4.40 Aggregate of adipocytes in an FNA of a large, flocculent, subcutaneous mass from a dog. Cells are large and markedly distended by a single, clear, cytoplasmic vacuole. A small rounded vesicular nucleus can be seen in one of the cells (Wright–Giemsa stain, 500× magnification).

and muscle-associated cells, such as pericytes and myofibroblasts, which can be sites of tumor formation.

Lipoma

Lipomas are one of the most common benign mesenchymal tumors in dogs and cats. Cytologic specimens of lipomatous masses are often grossly oily when material is prepared on a glass slide after FNA. They are also commonly acellular because the specimen can wash off during the staining process. When adipocytes from the lesion remain on the slide, they can appear individually and/or as small aggregates of cells with clear cytoplasm and large, clear vacuoles. The vacuoles cause marked distension of the cytoplasm and displace the small oval nucleus to the edge of the cell (Figure 4.40). Adipocytes from lipomas are cytologically identical to normal subcutaneous fat. Therefore, a diagnosis of lipoma can be supported by the clinical finding of a large, flocculent, subcutaneous mass coupled with the aforementioned FNA gross and cytologic findings.

Soft tissue tumors

When spindle cells are present in increased numbers and display mild to marked atypia, there is increased concern for a spindle cell soft tissue tumor, particularly when there is an absence of inflammation (Masserdotti & Drigo, 2022). Soft tissue tumors comprise a heterogeneous population of neoplasms that range from benign to malignant and are often difficult to distinguish on cytology alone, requiring histopathology for grading (to predict biologic behavior) as well as immunohistochemical staining (for subclassification by tissue of origin and/or phenotype) (Avallone *et al.*, 2007; Roccabianca *et al.*, 2020).

Examples of more benign soft tissue tumors (Figures 4.41a, b) include fibroma, myxoma, perivascular wall tumor, and some nerve-sheath tumors (i.e., neurofibroma). Some of these lesions have distinct cytologic features that may suggest the tumor type. For example, myxomas usually contain a thick, eosinophilic, proteinaceous matrix that entraps the spindle cells, which are a monomorphic population with relatively scant basophilic cytoplasm and a small oval nucleus (Figure 4.42); linear arrangements of cells in the specimen (windrowing) can also be seen due to the increased viscosity of the myxoid matrix. Cells from perivascular wall tumors and peripheral nerve sheath tumors often have very elongated, wispy cytoplasmic extensions, small and distinct cytoplasmic vacuoles, and a large oval nucleus (Figure 4.43a, b). Perivascular wall tumors can also contain multinucleate 'crown' cells (Figure 4.43b).

Classically, we have considered lesions composed of abundant neoplastic spindle cells that display mild to moderate criteria of malignancy in the integument as 'soft tissue sarcomas' because most of them display similar biologic behavior (locally invasive with low to

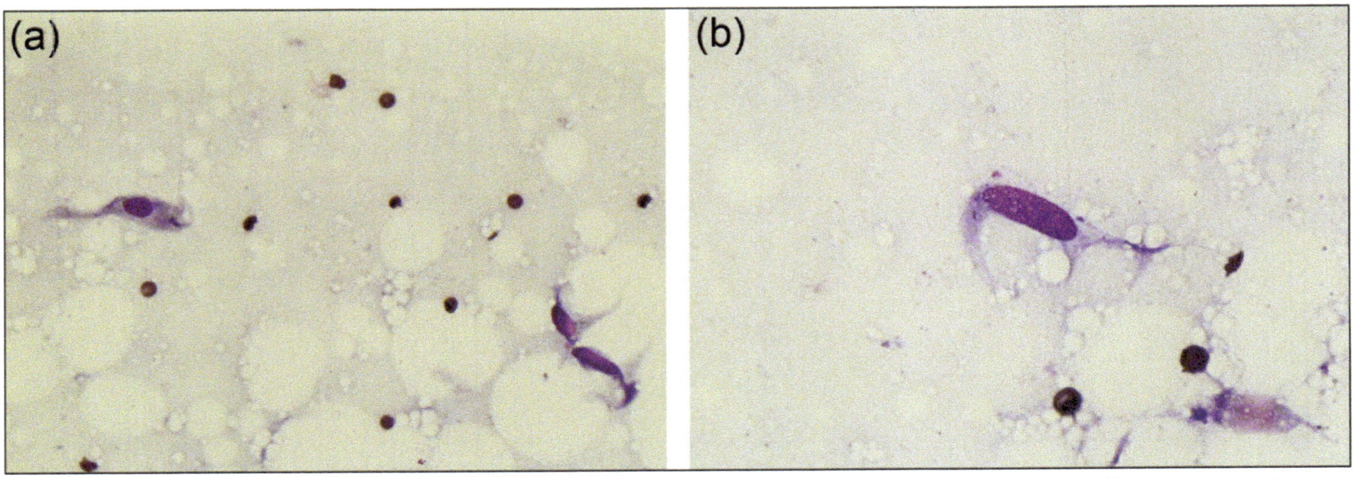

Figures 4.41a, b FNA of a subcutaneous mass on the sacrum from a 7-year-old Boxer. Small individualized mesenchymal cells are present with low numbers of erythrocytes in a thin basophilic proteinaceous background. Cells are small and spindle-shaped with light blue cytoplasm and a thin oval nucleus, most consistent with a benign mesenchymal tumor (Wright–Giemsa: a, 500× magnification; b, 1,000× magnification).

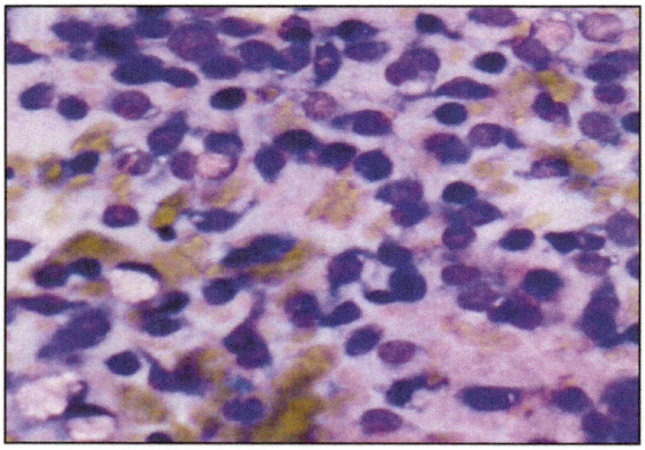

Figure 4.42 FNA of a subcutaneous mass on the right shoulder of an 11-year-old German Shorthaired Pointer. Individualized spindle-shaped cells are entrapped in a thick eosinophilic proteinaceous extracellular matrix suggestive of a myxoma (Wright–Giemsa, 600× magnification).

moderate recurrence rate and low metastatic rate); however, there is increasing evidence that differences in presentations and outcomes may exist among the different types of soft tissue sarcomas (Roccabianca *et al.*, 2020).

Sarcomas

Cytology samples from sarcomas contain spindle cells with more significant criteria of malignancy (Figure 4.44). Examples of malignant spindle cell tumors that can occur in the subcutis include fibrosarcoma, myxosarcoma, liposarcoma, osteosarcoma, and hemangiosarcoma. These sarcoma subtypes have different biologic behaviors and can require different treatment strategies. As with the more benign spindle cell tumors, most sarcomas cannot be differentiated from one another cytologically, but sometimes distinctive characteristics are present that allow pathologists to provide a more specific provisional diagnosis, some of which are discussed below. Histiocytic sarcoma is described with the round cell tumors.

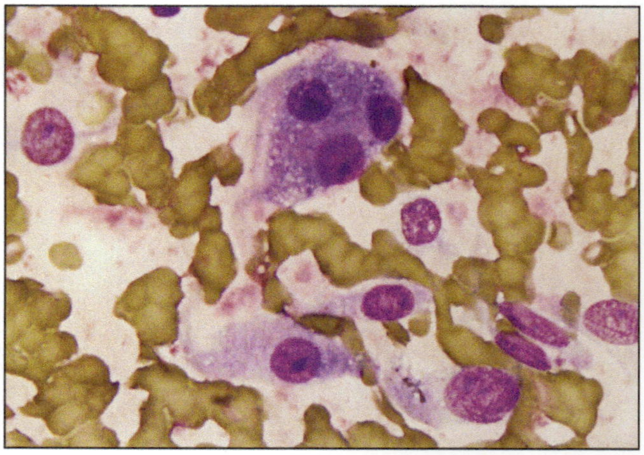

Figure 4.44 FNA of a subcutaneous mass on the hindlimb of a 9-year-old Labrador Retriever. There are moderate numbers of individualized spindle-shaped cells and moderate numbers of erythrocytes in a thin eosinophilic extracellular matrix. Cells have variable amounts of lightly basophilic cytoplasm and one or more large ovoid nuclei. Nuclei have stippled chromatin with one to two prominent nucleoli. A trinucleate cell is shown. Marked anisocytosis and anisokaryosis were noted. This sample is most suggestive of a sarcoma (Wright–Giemsa, 1,000× magnification).

Fibrosarcoma and myxosarcoma

Cytologic samples from fibrosarcomas have atypical mesenchymal cells frequently admixed with variably thick fibrillar pink matrix material (collagen) (Evans *et al.*, 2018b). Occasional multinucleate tumor cells may also be seen. Keloid fibroma/fibrosarcoma is an uncommon variant in which the neoplastic cells occur in association with abundant amounts of eosinophilic, glassy, thick bands of

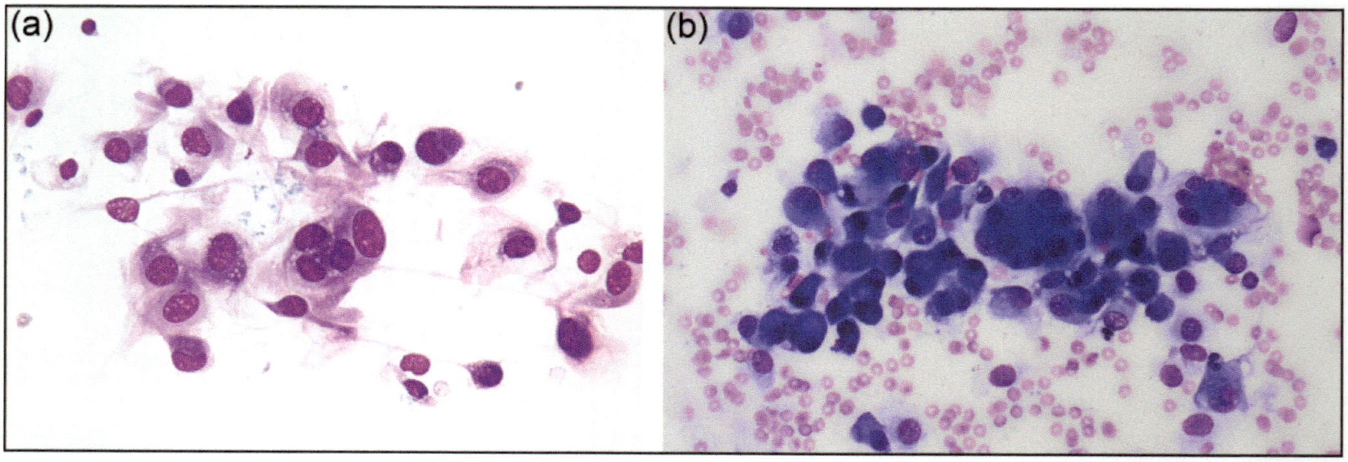

Figures 4.43a, b FNAs of perivascular wall tumors. (a) Several wispy individualized mesenchymal cells are present. Cells have a moderate amount of lightly basophilic cytoplasm and an ovoid nucleus. Nuclei have dense chromatin. Small distinct cytoplasmic vacuoles are present in a few of the cells. Mild to moderate anisocytosis and anisokaryosis are observed (Wright–Giemsa, 1,000× magnification). (b) Multinucleate neoplastic cells have nuclei forming a ring around the periphery of the cell, consistent with 'crown' cells (Wright–Giemsa, 500× magnification).

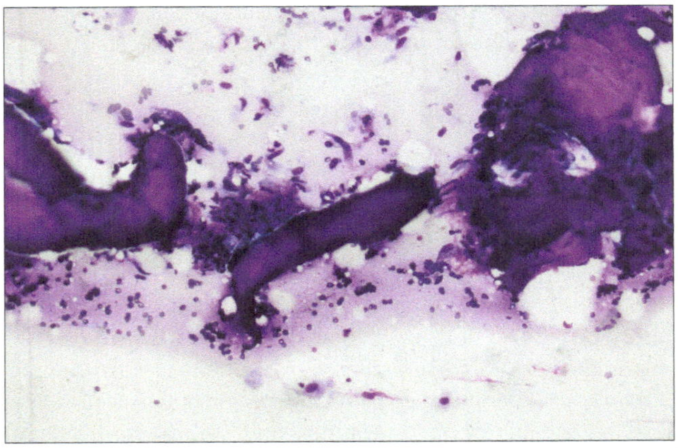

Figure 4.45 **FNA of a mass near the hip of an adult dog. There are several individualized to aggregated spindle-shaped cells that display mild to moderate atypia and are often adhered to thick eosinophilic material (most consistent with keloid) (Wright–Giemsa, 500× magnification).**

hyalinized collagen (Raskin & Conrado, 2023; Figure 4.45). The myxoid variant of fibrosarcoma (myxosarcoma) can have similar thick proteinaceous background material and windrowing of cells as in myxomas (Figure 4.42). Samples from myxosarcomas contain large, spindle-shaped, mesenchymal cells with an oval nucleus and exhibit several characteristics of malignancy (Figures 4.46a, b). The myxoid matrix material is Alcian blue (pH 2.5) positive (Roccabianca *et al.*, 2020).

Liposarcoma

Liposarcomas are rare tumors of adipose tissue that contain cells with deeply basophilic cytoplasm, clear (often punctate) lipid-filled vacuoles, a large ovoid nucleus, and many characteristics of malignancy (Figures 4.47a, b). Hibernoma (brown fat tumor) can have a similar appearance to liposarcoma and staining with UCP-1 may help discern these two entities (Piccione & Dial, 2020). Other cytologic differentials could include xanthoma, balloon cell melanoma, meibomian or sebaceous adenocarcinoma, clear cell carcinoma, rhabdomyoma/rhabdomyosarcoma, granular cell tumor, and oncocytoma (Piccione & Dial, 2020; Sebastian *et al.*, 2021). Positive Oil-Red-O staining can be used to help confirm adipocyte/lipocyte origin (Masserdotti *et al.*, 2006).

Osteosarcoma

Osteosarcomas can occur as de novo extraskeletal tumors secondary to trauma, foreign body, injections, certain infections, idiopathic, as well as metastatic tumors. This tumor often exfoliates well and contains several anaplastic osteoblasts: large ovoid to spindle-shaped cells with abundant basophilic cytoplasm, an ovoid nucleus, and one to three prominent nucleoli. In the more oval-shaped cells, the nucleus is eccentrically located and a perinuclear clear zone may be visible, resembling plasma cells. Neoplastic cells sometimes contain small, angular, eosinophilic, cytoplasmic granules (Figure 4.48a). Less commonly, erythrophagocytosis is seen in the osteoblasts (Barger *et al.*, 2012). Many criteria of malignancy can be seen, including multinucleation and mitotic figures. There may be osteoclasts present (large multinucleated cells with an eosinophilic hue to the cytoplasm; Figure 4.48b). Bright, smooth, eosinophilic extracellular matrix (e.g., osteoid) may also be seen (Figure 4.48c).

Depending on the degree of cellularity and atypia, it can sometimes be challenging to distinguish osteosarcoma from osteoma or heterotopic ossification, such as can occur with ossifying myositis or osseous metaplasia of another epithelial or mesenchymal neoplasm, necessitating biopsy for further characterization (Roccabianca *et al.*, 2020). Alkaline phosphatase staining can be useful in the diagnosis of osteosarcoma on cytologic preparations, where it is highly sensitive and specific when expressed by atypical spindle cells; however, it does

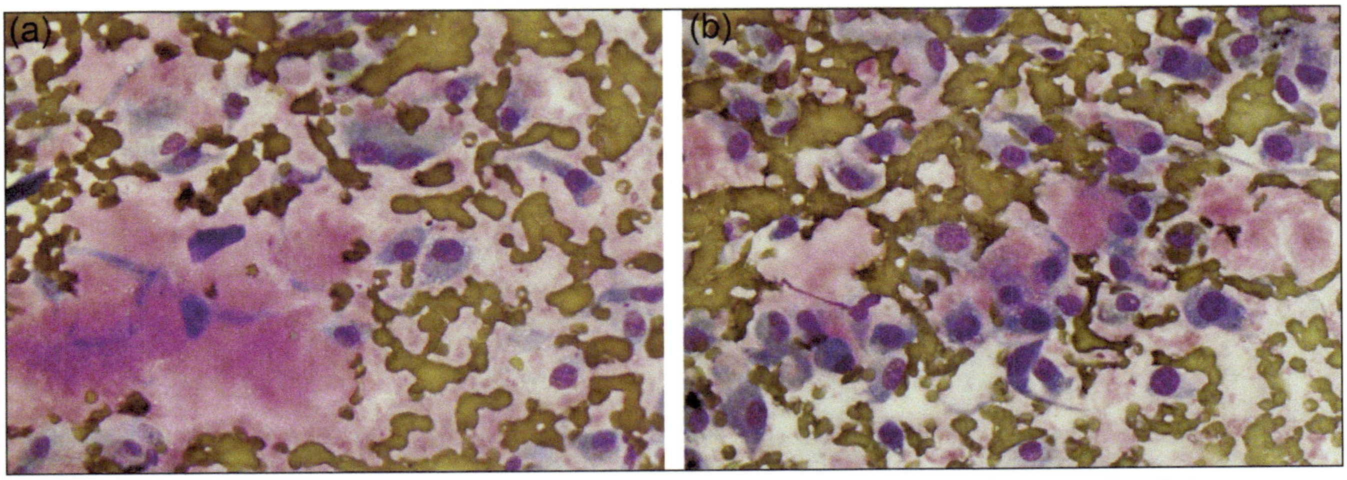

Figures 4.46a, b **FNA from a subcutaneous mass on the third digit of the right hind foot of a 5-year-old Labrador Retriever. Several wispy individualized mesenchymal cells are associated with a thick eosinophilic extracellular matrix. Cells have a variable amount of lightly basophilic cytoplasm and an ovoid nucleus. Nuclei have stippled chromatin and one or more prominent nucleoli. Moderate anisocytosis and anisokaryosis are observed. A binucleate cell is present in 4.46a. The sample is most consistent with a myxosarcoma (Wright–Giemsa, 500× magnification).**

not discern between reactive and neoplastic osteoblasts and is rarely expressed by non-osteoblastic tumors (Barger *et al.*, 2005; Ryseff & Bohn, 2012).

Hemangiosarcoma and lymphangiosarcoma

Hemangiosarcomas typically contain abundant blood with low numbers of very large, spindle-shaped, neoplastic, mesenchymal cells with an oval nucleus. The cells often contain small, distinct cytoplasmic vacuoles and may exhibit erythrophagia or contain blue–black pigment consistent with hemosiderin (Barger *et al.*, 2012; Figures 4.49a, b). Some samples can have erythroid precursors and/or aggregates of blood leukocytes due to pooling in abnormal vasculature. Blood contamination of another sarcoma or hemangioma could appear similar cytologically. Lymphangiosarcoma is another rare neoplasm of the lymphatic vasculature that can occur anywhere on the body, but a common location is the ventral abdomen of cats. These lesions can have increased proportions of lymphocytes and atypical rounded to spindled cells (Azevedo *et al.*, 2020). Endothelial cells should express CD31, while lymphatic cells can be distinguished using PROX-1 on immunocytochemistry (Roccabianca *et al.*, 2020).

Injection-site sarcoma

More commonly reported in cats, but also rarely seen in dogs, are sarcomas secondary to injection or vaccination, often attributable to adjuvanted vaccines (such as rabies). The lesion is believed to arise from pluripotent mesenchymal stem cells, and histopathology commonly reveals fibrosarcoma but other sarcomas have also been documented (Roccabianca *et al.*, 2020). Cytologic appearance, therefore, varies based on the type of sarcoma but contains atypical spindle cells with frequent multinucleation and rarely blue, blue–gray, or magenta adjuvant material. Current monitoring recommendations for injection-site sarcoma in cats involve the '3-2-1' rule, whereby biopsy/excision of the lesion should be performed if a mass-lesion is present 3 months after injection, becomes >2-cm in diameter, or increases in size 1 month after injection (Hartmann *et al.*, 2015).

TUMORS OF GLANDULAR STRUCTURES

Sebaceous gland tumors

Neoplasia of the sebaceous gland can arise from germinative cells (basaloid reserve cells), sebocytes (sebaceous cells), or ductal cells. Tumors of the basaloid reserve cells include sebaceous epithelioma and epitheliomatous sebaceous carcinoma, and tumors of the sebocytes (and ductal cells) include nodular sebaceous hyperplasia, sebaceous (ductal) adenoma, and sebaceous carcinoma. Nodular sebaceous hyperplasia is the most common type of sebaceous tumor in dogs (Albanese, 2017; Mauldin & Peters-Kennedy, 2016).

Lesions composed of sebaceous epithelial cells are usually benign in dogs and cats. Sebaceous hyperplasia and sebaceous adenomas appear cytologically similar. They contain cohesive clusters of round cells with abundant, highly vacuolated, basophilic cytoplasm and a small, centrally located, round nucleus with dense chromatin (Figure 4.50a, b). Sebaceous epithelial cells tend to be arranged in thick clumps, which create a kaleidoscope of vacuoles when the fine focus is adjusted on the microscope. Basaloid reserve cells may also be seen. These are small cells with small round nuclei and scant amounts of basophilic cytoplasm (Albanese, 2017). Sebaceous epitheliomas consist of a mixture of clusters of basaloid epithelial cells and scattered clusters of well-differentiated sebaceous epithelial cells (Figure 4.50b). Low numbers of well-differentiated squamous epithelial cells may also be seen (Raskin & Conrado, 2023). Sebaceous carcinomas are rare in dogs and cats and typically have several cytologic characteristics of malignancy.

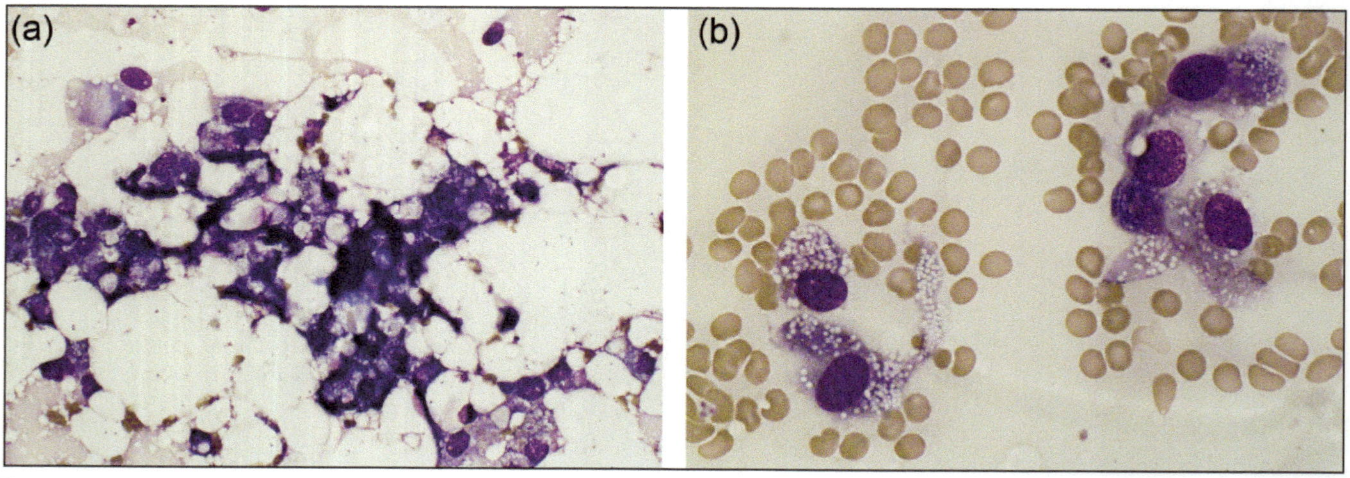

Figures 4.47a, b FNA of a mass on the right lumbar region of a 1-year-old dog, suggestive of liposarcoma. (a) Spindle-shaped cells are closely associated with clear, round spaces consistent with lipid vacuoles. Binucleate cells, anisocytosis, and anisokaryosis are observed. (b) Cells have abundant basophilic cytoplasm filled with small, distinct, clear vacuoles. Nuclei are large and ovoid with stippled chromatin. A large prominent nucleolus is seen in some of the cells (Wright–Giemsa: a, 500× magnification; b, 1,000× magnification).

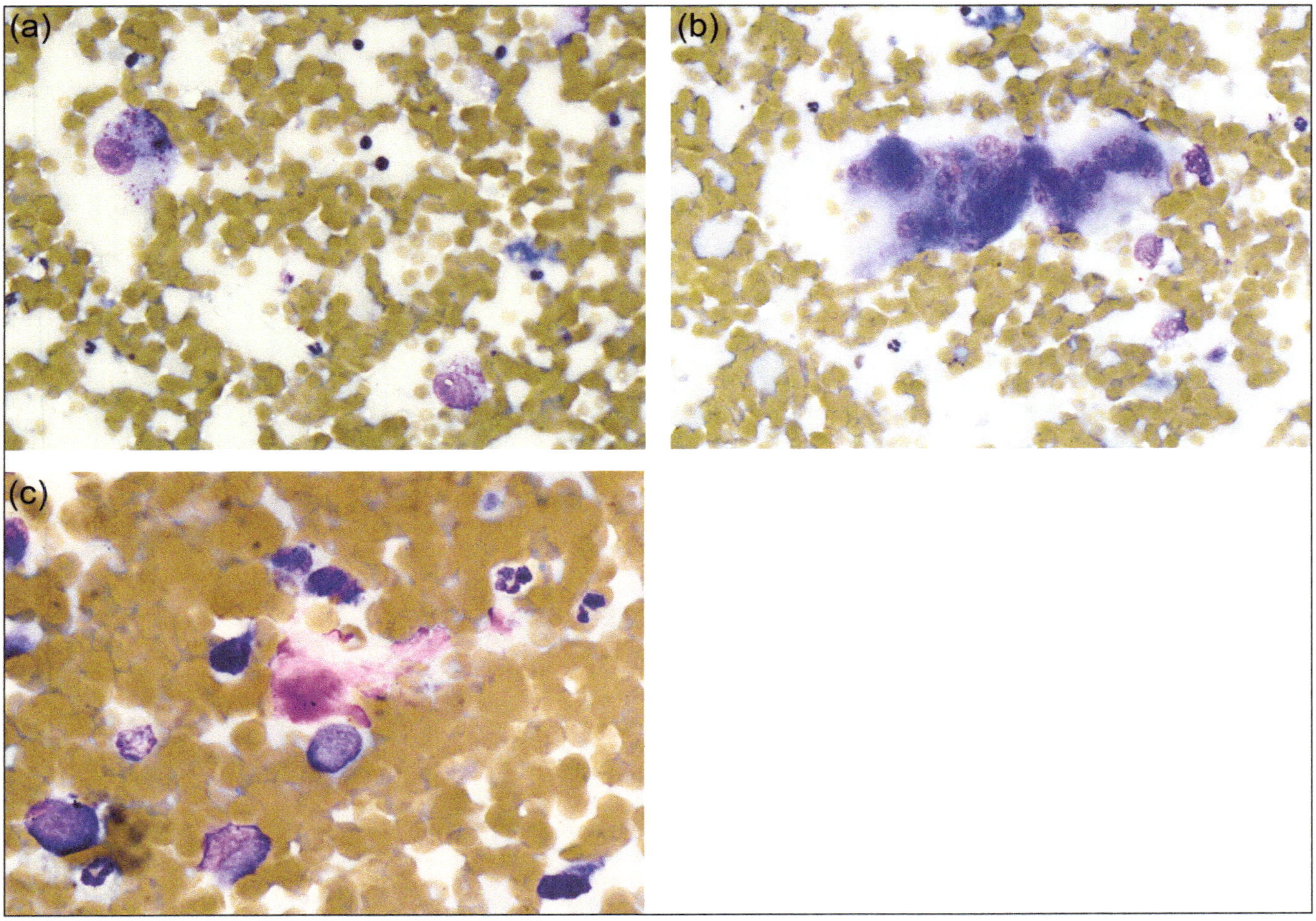

Figures 4.48a–c FNA of a subcutaneous mass on the left shoulder of an 8-year-old Rottweiler. (a) Two large osteoblasts are shown with abundant basophilic cytoplasm and an eccentrically located oval nucleus. Nuclei have stippled chromatin and a large prominent oval nucleolus. Cells contain several small irregular eosinophilic cytoplasmic granules. There is a moderate amount of blood in the background of the sample. (b) Two multinucleated osteoclasts are shown in a moderate amount of blood. (c) Bright eosinophilic extracellular material consistent with osteoid is often present in aspirates of osteosarcomas (Wright–Giemsa: a & b, 500× magnification; c, 1,000× magnification).

Perianal gland tumors

Perianal gland tumors (also known as hepatoid gland or circumanal gland tumors) are common tumors in dogs, particularly intact males, and can be responsive to androgens. They originate from modified sebaceous gland epithelium within the dermis. These tumors can occur anywhere on the caudal half of the animal but are most frequently encountered around the tail and hindlimbs. Cytologically, tumor cells are present in clusters and resemble hepatocytes (hence the term hepatoid) with rounded, abundant, lightly basophilic cytoplasm that has an eosinophilic hue, and a round nucleus with a single prominent nucleolus (Figure 4.51a). Smaller numbers of epithelial cells with a high nuclear-to-cytoplasm ratio, scant cytoplasm, round nucleus with dense chromatin pattern (basal cell appearance, called reserve cells) are often closely associated with the clusters of perianal gland cells (Figures 4.51b, c). While increased numbers of reserve cells could be seen with perianal gland epitheliomas, the proportion of reserve cells does not appear to correlate with malignancy among perianal gland tumors (Evans *et al.*, 2018a). Perianal gland adenocarcinomas are rarely reported and can appear well-differentiated to pleomorphic on cytology (McCourt *et al.*, 2018). Therefore, histopathology is recommended to discern perianal gland hyperplasia and benign and malignant tumors (Goldschmidt & Hendrick, 2002). Due to androgen responsiveness, castration can help reduce perianal gland tumor size, potentially simplifying surgical removal.

Apocrine gland tumors

Apocrine gland anal sac adenocarcinoma (AGASACA) is an important aggressive, malignant tumor in dogs and rarely reported in cats. This tumor is often not detected until palpated during a rectal

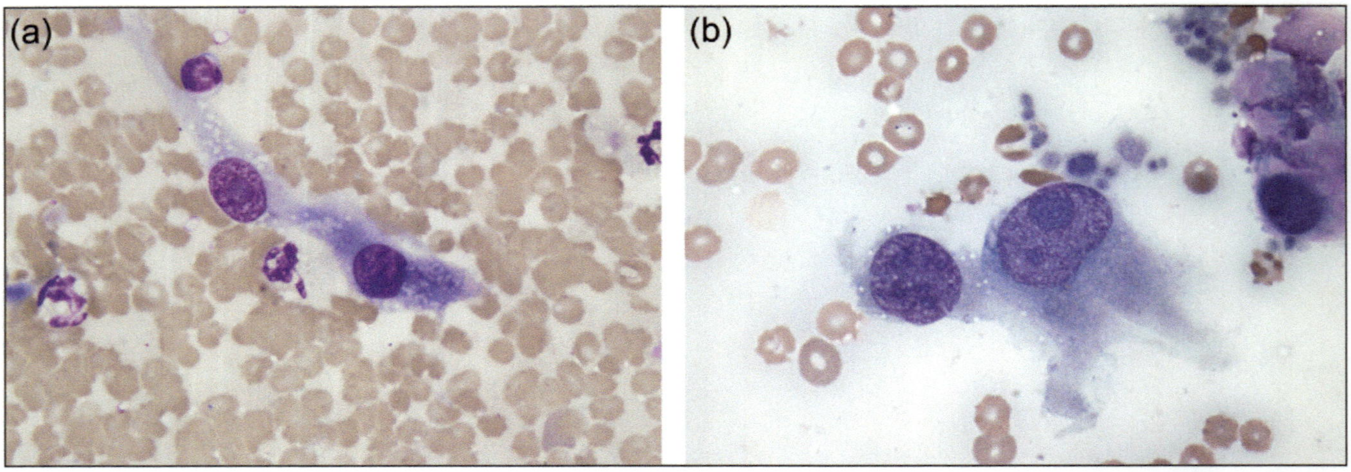

Figures 4.49a, b Hemangiosarcoma. FNAs of a subcutaneous mass on the prepuce of a dog. (a) Mesenchymal cells are large with abundant, spindle-shaped, basophilic cytoplasm and an oval nucleus with coarsely stippled chromatin. Small, distinct, clear cytoplasmic vacuoles and a prominent nucleolus are visible. Three neutrophils, a lymphocyte, and several erythrocytes are present in the background. (b) Marked characteristics of malignancy are observed within the mesenchymal cells in this sample. Anisocytosis, anisokaryosis, atypical nuclear shape, stippled chromatin, multiple prominent nucleoli, and variably sized nucleoli are shown. Erythrocytes, platelets, and a small amount of extracellular eosinophilic matrix (upper right) are present in the background (Wright–Giemsa, 1,000× magnification).

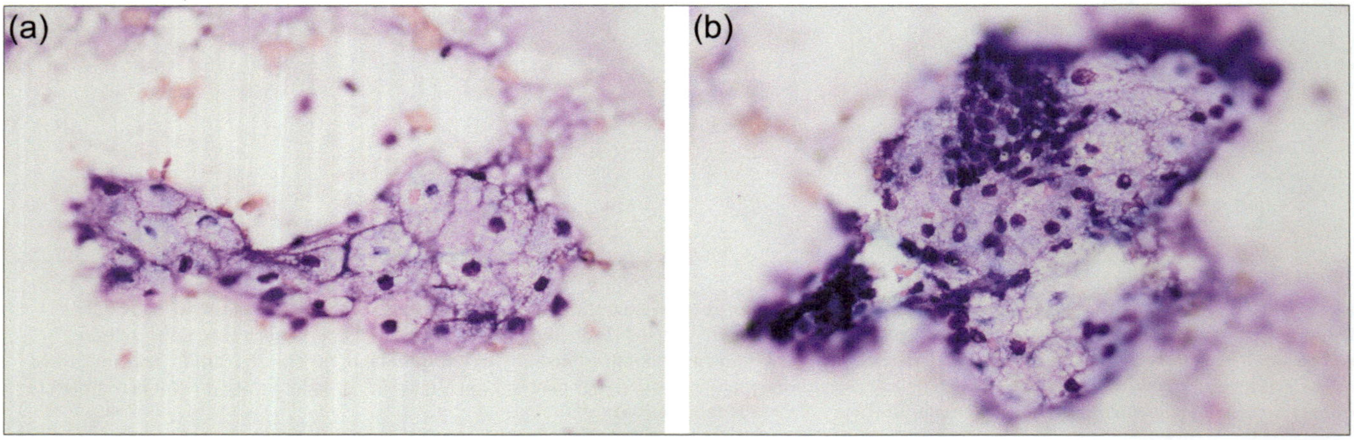

Figures 4.50a, b (a) Sebaceous epithelial cells have abundant vacuolated cytoplasm and a small round nucleus with dense chromatin. Distinct basophilic cellular junctions are present (Wright–Giemsa, 1,000× magnification). (b) Sebaceous epithelioma with larger vacuolated sebaceous epithelial cells mixed with smaller, more basilar epithelial cells with scant cytoplasm (top and left) (Wright–Giemsa, 500× magnification).

examination. It frequently metastasizes and can cause significant hypercalcemia due to the production of parathyroid hormone-related protein (Meuten *et al.*, 1981; Rosol *et al.*, 1990). On cytology, this tumor has a neuroendocrine appearance, characterized by numerous free nuclei within a lightly basophilic background of lysed cytoplasm (Figures 4.52a–c), which can be helpful in discerning an AGASACA from a perianal gland tumor; location of the mass is also very important in this distinction. Of note, AGASACA typically does not display significant criteria of malignancy on cytology despite its aggressive biologic behavior. Patients with suspected AGASACA should undergo staging, including abdominal ultrasound and evaluation of draining or enlarged lymph nodes, in addition to serum biochemical analysis for hypercalcemia (total and ionized, free calcium).

Apocrine tumors of the sweat gland can also occur elsewhere in the skin of dogs and cats (Conroy & Breen, 1972; Simko *et al.*, 2003; Haziroglu *et al.*, 2014). Apocrine gland adenomas are somewhat common in dogs but rare in cats, while apocrine gland carcinomas are relatively uncommon in both species. They can present as solitary, nodular lesions on the head, limbs, and abdomen. Adenocarcinomas are also rarely reported and less common sites include the clitoris, the vulva, and the eyelid in dogs (Hirai *et al.*, 1997; Neihaus *et al.*, 2010; Rout *et al.*, 2016). Aspirates of apocrine gland tumors often contain clusters of columnar to cuboidal cells, occasionally with intracytoplasmic blue-gray secretory material, and sometimes basilar (ductal) cells. These lesions can have cystic portions (see 'Apocrine cysts').

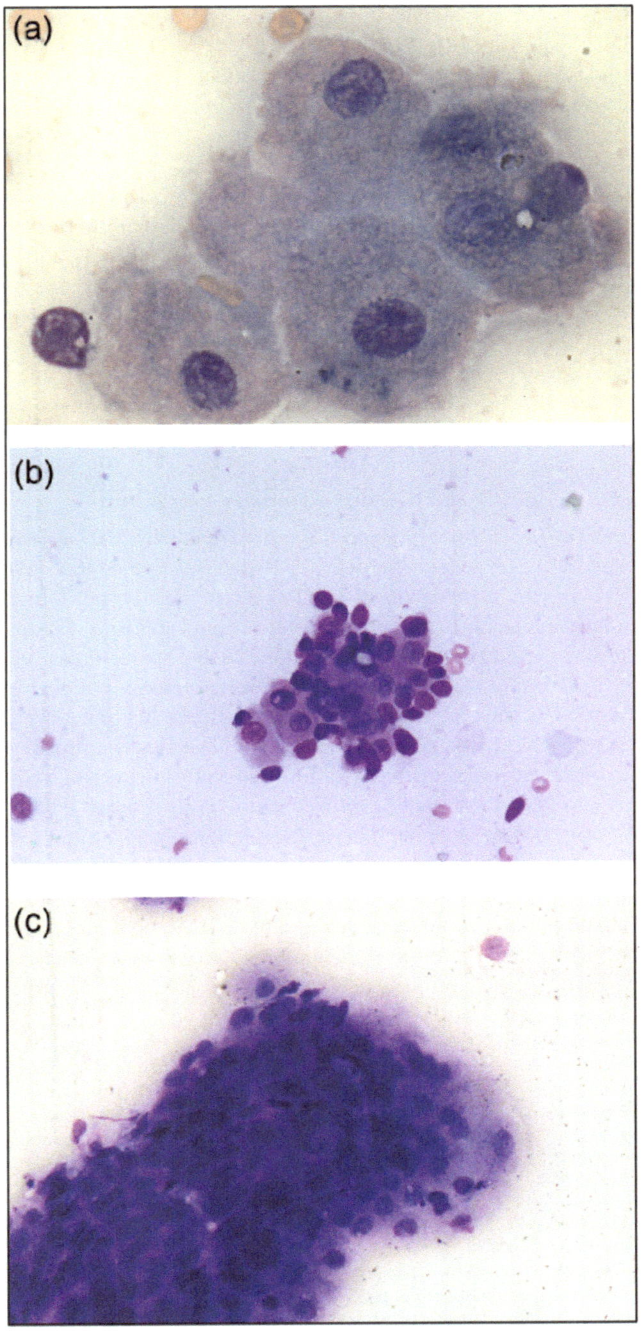

Figures 4.51a–c FNA of a skin mass from the tail base of a dog. (a) Perianal gland tumor cells are large, uniform, hepatoid cells with abundant cytoplasm that is lightly basophilic and stippled with pale eosinophilic material. The nuclei are large with a single prominent nucleolus. The cell to the right of the image is binucleate. One free nucleus from a lysed cell is present to the far left of the image (Wright–Giemsa, 1,000× magnification). (b, c) Perianal gland tumor cells are closely associated with smaller reserve cells that have more rounded and condensed nuclei with scant cytoplasm (Wright–Giemsa, 500× magnification).

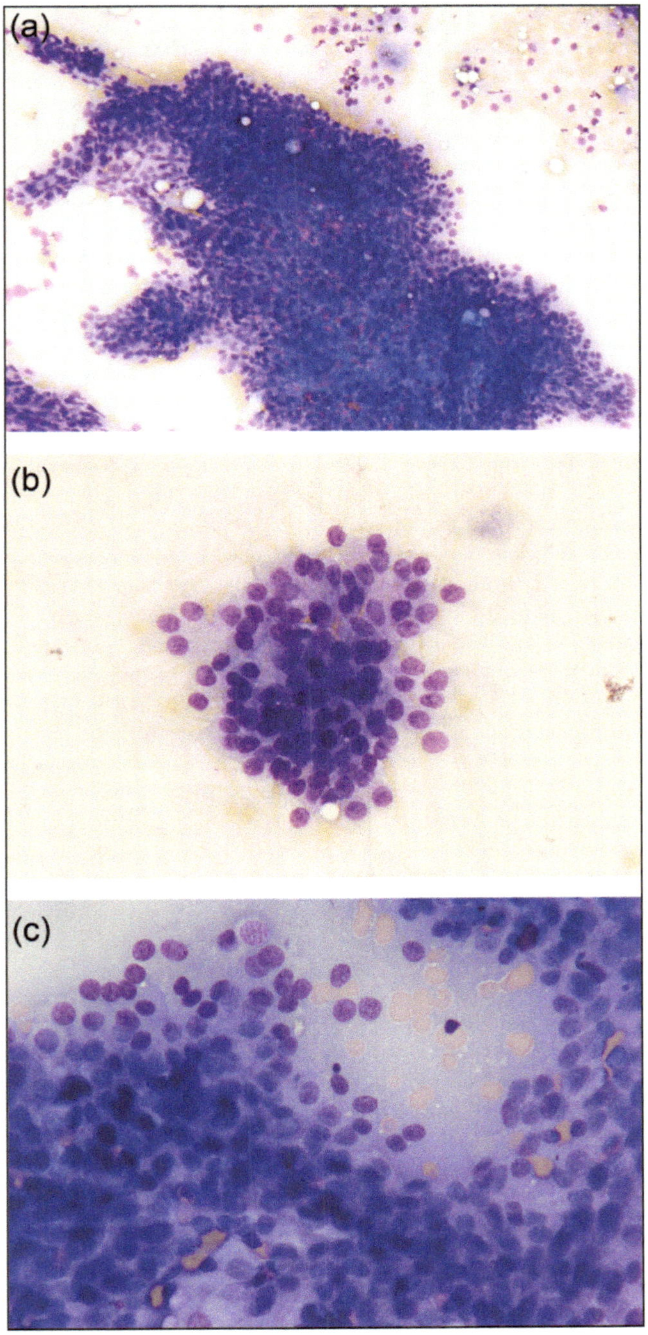

Figures 4.52a–c (a, b) FNA from a left anal gland mass of a 12-year-old Nova Scotia Duck Tolling Retriever. The sample contains large sheets of cells with indistinct cell junctions and a small round nucleus. Given the location of this mass, it is consistent with an adenocarcinoma of the apocrine gland of the anal sac. (b) Nuclei are arranged in small circles (acinar-like structures) in a few clusters of cells. (c) A second example of the sheets of cells that are observed in an apocrine gland tumor (Wright–Giemsa: a, 200× magnification; b & c, 500× magnification).

Mammary masses

Mammary masses are common lesions in both the dog and the cat, particularly intact animals or those neutered later in life. Possible causes for mammary masses include cysts, inflammation/infection (i.e., mastitis), hyperplasia, and benign and malignant neoplasms. Cytology of mammary lesions can be challenging because they can have multiple components including cystic regions, inflammation, and neoplasia all in the same lesion, and even neoplastic lesions can contain both epithelial and mesenchymal elements (mixed tumors and carcinosarcomas). In addition, benign mammary epithelial neoplasia or hyperplasia may not be easily distinguished from carcinoma. In some cases, epithelial cells aspirated from malignant tumors/carcinomas may not have sufficient cytologic criteria of malignancy for an unequivocal cytologic diagnosis of malignancy. On the other hand, some tumors may display multiple criteria of malignancy in an FNA sample (appearing consistent with a carcinoma), and yet be diagnosed as benign tumors on histopathologic evaluation. Furthermore, aspirates from tumors with both epithelial and mesenchymal cells may not contain sufficient numbers of the different cell types for recognition of the mixed nature of the neoplasm. Cytology also cannot detect factors that are useful in histopathologic diagnosis of malignancy, such as invasion into lymphatic structures and enumeration of mitoses. Due to these factors, excisional biopsy and histopathologic evaluation are often recommended for mammary tumors where malignancy is suspected (such as feline mammary neoplasms or large masses). However, cytology of mammary lesions can be a good screening test to detect infection versus neoplasia or epithelial *vs.* mesenchymal *vs.* round cell tumor. Approximately 30–50% of canine mammary tumors and 80–90% of feline mammary tumors are malignant (Brodey *et al.*, 1983; Goldschmidt *et al.*, 2017; Seixas *et al.*, 2011), and complete tumor removal with resection of the entire mammary chain and draining lymph nodes is indicated in many dogs and nearly all cats.

Canine mammary masses

Mammary gland tumors are the most common neoplasms diagnosed in intact female dogs (Dorn *et al.*, 1968; Goldschmidt *et al.*, 2017). Early ovariohysterectomy will reduce the chance of developing mammary neoplasia. Dogs spayed prior to their first estrus are much less likely to develop mammary neoplasia (0.5% chance during their lifetime), with an increasing chance of developing tumors in those dogs spayed after their first cycle (8% before the second estrus, and 26% before the third cycle, with no significant protective effect after the third cycle or after 4 years of age; Schneider *et al.*, 1969; Sorenmo *et al.*, 2020). Treatment with hormones also increases the risk of mammary gland tumor development, and treatment with low-dose progestins alone can result in an increased risk of benign tumors while combinations of estrogens and progestins have an increased risk of malignant tumors (Sorenmo *et al.*, 2020). Mammary tumors are much less common in male dogs than in females (62 times more common in females), and mammary tumors in male dogs are usually benign lesions (Saba *et al.*, 2007). Mammary tumors are most common in middle-aged or older dogs, with an increasing incidence from approximately 7 to 13 years of age (Sorenmo *et al.*, 2020). Breeds with an increased risk of mammary tumors include Boxers, Poodles, Chihuahuas, Yorkshire Terriers, Maltese, English Springer Spaniels, Brittany Spaniels, English Setters, German Shepherds, Pointers, and Doberman Pinschers (Sorenmo *et al.*, 2020).

Mammary gland tumors may arise from secretory or ductular cells, myoepithelial cells, or stromal cells. While cytology of mammary lesions has been previously reported to have good sensitivity, specificity, and correlation with histopathology, other studies have reported much lower diagnostic utility (Simon *et al.*, 2009, Griffiths *et al.*, 1984; Allen *et al.*, 1986). Therefore, it is generally believed that in dogs, cytology cannot reliably distinguish between benign and malignant mammary neoplasia, and histopathology is still recommended if a mammary neoplasm is suspected. It can be useful, however, if mastitis or another neoplasm is occurring in the region of the mammary gland (i.e. round cell tumor).

Canine epithelial and complex mammary neoplasms

Tumors of the mammary gland may arise from epithelial (secretory or ductular) or myoepithelial cells. Epithelial cells can appear cuboidal, columnar, or rounded and may be present in clumps or forming papillary, trabecular, or even acinar-like arrangements (if glandular origin) on cytology (Allison & Walton, 2020). Myoepithelial cells can vary from rounded to cuboidal to more commonly spindled and should be differentiated from mesenchymal cells (Emanuelli *et al.*, 2020). Cytologic criteria of malignancy (anisocytosis, anisokaryosis, prominent nucleoli, binucleation and multinucleation, and/or increased N:C ratio) may be utilized in the evaluation of epithelial cells from aspirates of mammary tumors (Figures 4.16a–c and 4.53–4.55a, b), but this can be problematic, as some malignant tumors lack significant criteria of malignancy for a definitive cytologic diagnosis of carcinoma, while some benign epithelial tumors may exhibit mild to moderate criteria of malignancy. The cytologic criteria of malignancy that have been statistically associated with mammary

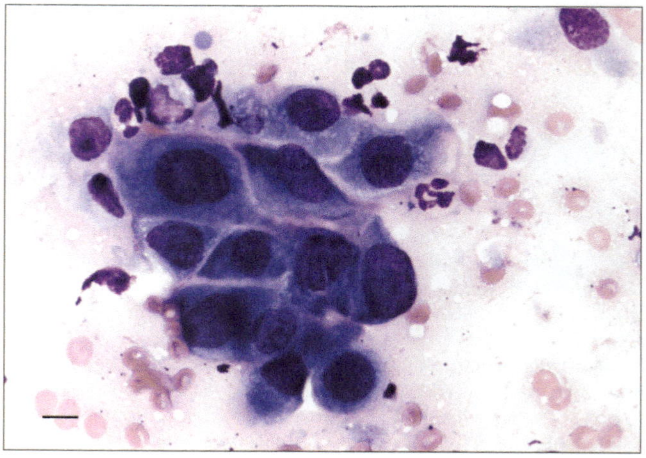

Figure 4.53 Epithelial cells from a mammary carcinoma in a dog. These are large, polygonal cells that exhibit several criteria of malignancy (anisocytosis, anisokaryosis, coarse chromatin, nucleoli, and binucleation with nuclear molding) (Wright–Giemsa, scale bar = 10 μm).

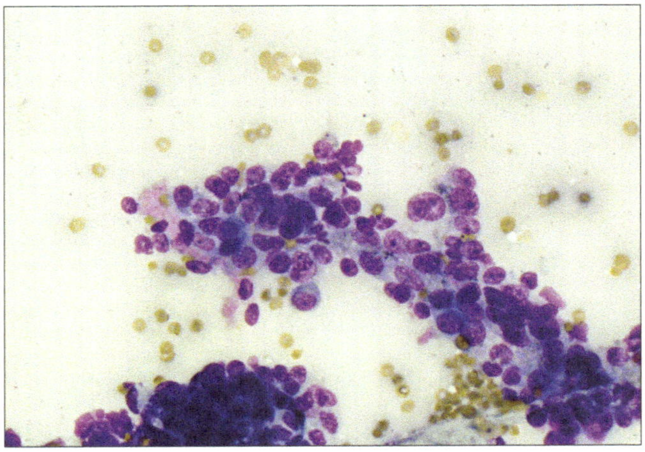

Figure 4.54 Small neoplastic epithelial cells from a 3 × 5 cm firm fixed mass associated with the left fifth mammary gland of an intact female Miniature Poodle. The cells are densely clustered and have a high nuclear to cytoplasmic ratio, rounded nuclei, stippled chromatin, and a prominent nucleolus. Some irregularly shaped nuclei are noted. Moderate anisokaryosis is present. There is a small amount of eosinophilic extracellular matrix associated with the cells (Wright–Giemsa, 500× magnification).

carcinoma include variable nuclear size (anisokaryosis), nuclear giant forms, high N:C ratio, variable or abnormally shaped nucleoli, and macronucleoli (Allen *et al.*, 1986). Simple mammary tumors consist of neoplastic epithelial cells (either epithelial or myoepithelial), while complex tumors consist of both epithelial and myoepithelial cells. Benign mammary gland epithelial neoplasms in the dog include adenoma (simple and complex or adenomyoepithelioma), myoepithelioma, duct adenoma, and duct papilloma (intraductal papillary adenoma) (Sorenmo *et al.*, 2020). Malignant mammary gland epithelial neoplasms are namely carcinomas, including simple, complex, squamous cell, among others.

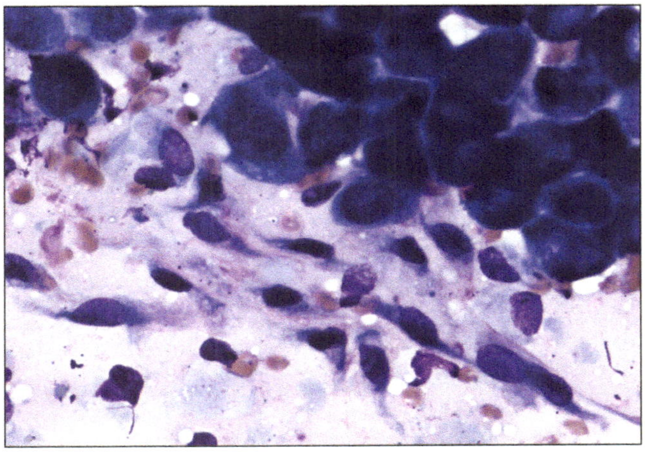

Figure 4.56 Epithelial cells and spindle cells from a mixed mammary tumor in a dog. The spindle cells are associated with pink matrix material. The epithelial cells exhibit several criteria of malignancy, including anisocytosis, anisokaryosis, prominent nucleoli, and coarse chromatin, concerning for a malignant lesion (Wright–Giemsa, scale bar = 10 μm).

Canine mixed mammary tumors

Mixed mammary tumors exhibit proliferation of both epithelial and/or myoepithelial and stromal (mesenchymal) cells with usually cartilage and/or bone production (Im *et al.*, 2014). Mixed tumors include benign mixed tumor and malignant mixed tumor (carcinosarcoma; Goldschmidt *et al.*, 2011; Sorenmo *et al.*, 2020). FNA cytology of mixed tumors will typically yield clumps of epithelial cells along with spindle cells, which may be associated with matrix material (Figures 4.56, 4.57a–d). Osteoclasts may be found in mixed tumors with bone formation or in mammary osteosarcomas (Figure 4.58).

Canine mammary gland sarcomas

Mesenchymal neoplasms of the canine mammary gland can include fibrosarcoma, osteosarcoma, chondrosarcoma, and hemangiosarcoma,

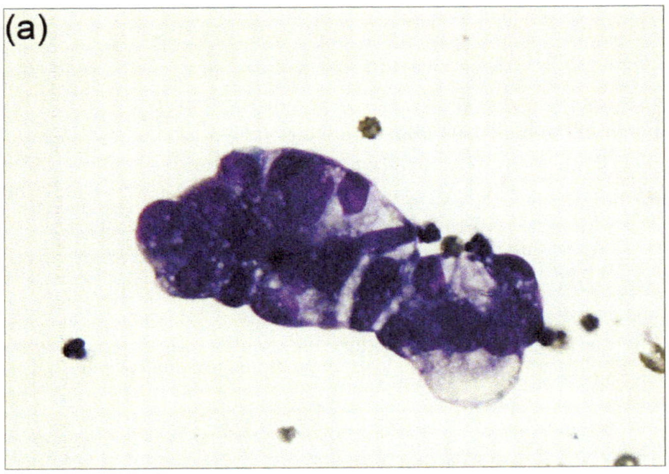

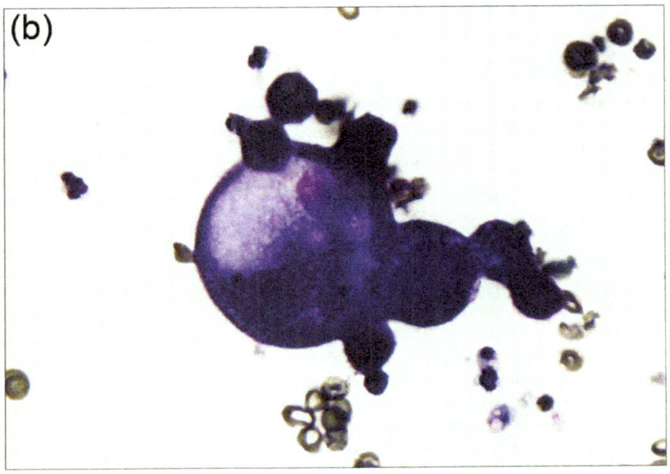

Figures 4.55a, b FNA from a 2 × 5 cm mass associated with the left fifth mammary gland of an intact female Golden Retriever. Poorly organized clusters of large, vacuolated epithelial cells with distended, deeply basophilic cytoplasm and a variably sized, round nucleus are seen. The sample is suspicious for a malignant mammary tumor (Wright–Giemsa, 1,000× magnification).

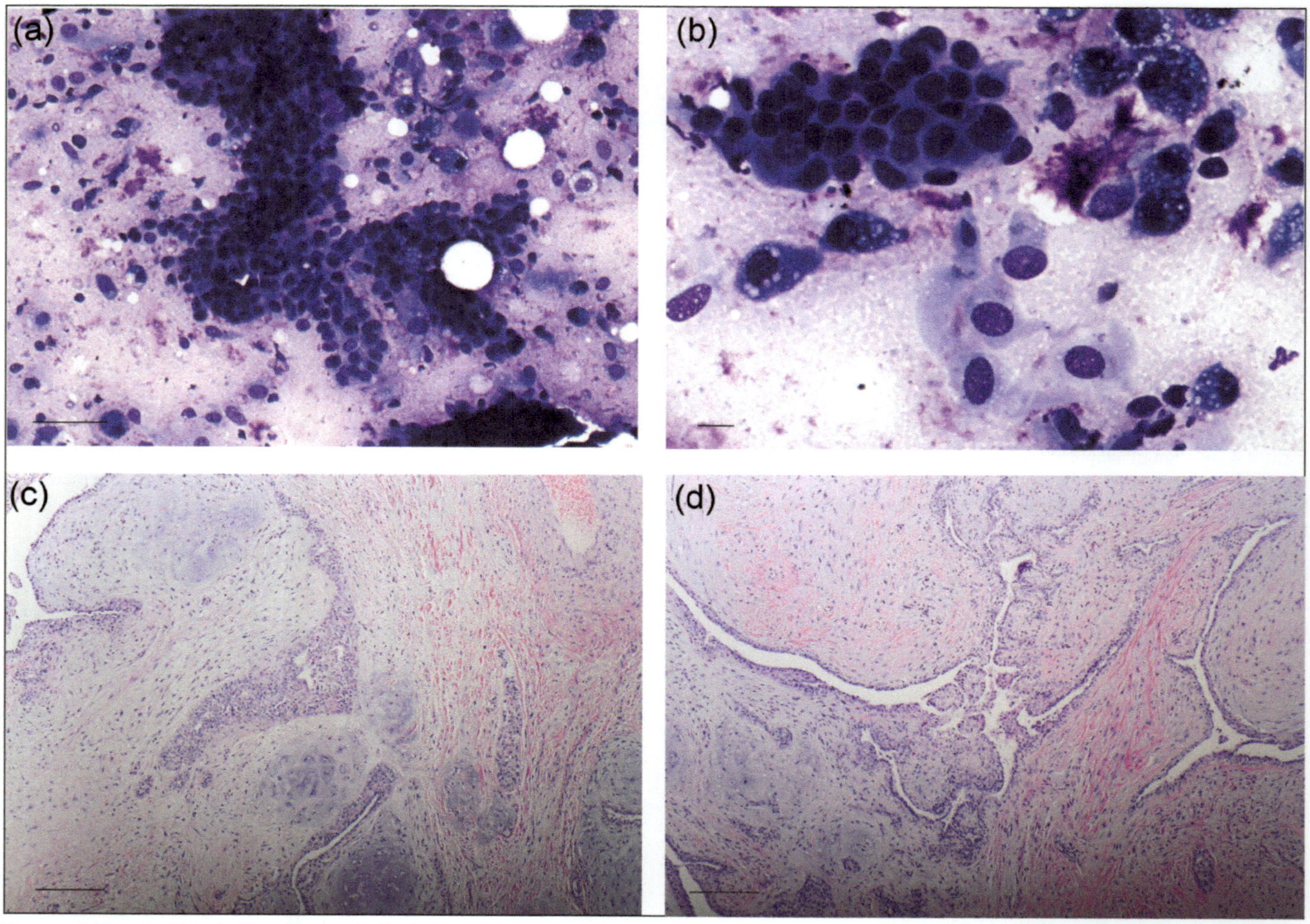

Figures 4.57a–d FNA (a, b) and biopsy (c, d) of a mammary mass in a 13-year-old, male Labrador Retriever. (a) The aspirates revealed numerous clumps of small epithelial cells with mild anisocytosis and anisokaryosis, along with a population of spindle cells and associated pink-staining matrix material (Wright-Giemsa, scale bar = 50 µm). (b) A higher magnification view of the FNA of the mass. This field includes epithelial cells, spindle cells, and foam cells (Wright-Giemsa, scale bar = 10 µm). (c, d) Histopathology of the mammary mass. Both epithelial and spindle cell elements are present as well as smooth, basophilic material, indicating production of cartilage within the lesion. The histologic diagnosis was benign mixed mammary tumor (H&E, scale bar = 100 µm).

with osteosarcoma being the most commonly diagnosed sarcoma (Goldschmidt *et al.*, 2011; Sorenmo *et al.*, 2020). Aspirates from these lesions will appear similar to these tumors in other tissues. These may sometimes be difficult to distinguish from mixed mammary tumors with FNA cytology, particularly in mixed mammary tumors where large numbers of epithelial cells are not aspirated.

Feline mammary lesions

Mammary gland tumors are less commonly encountered in cats than dogs and, similar to dogs, occur more frequently in intact females; however, unlike dogs, the majority of mammary tumors (85–95%) in cats are malignant (Hayes *et al.*, 1981; Allen, 1973; Seixas *et al.*, 2011). Mammary tumor risk has been reported to decrease by 91% if spayed before 6 months, by 86% between 7 and 12 months, and by 11% between 13 and 24 months, with no protective effect after 24 months (Sorenmo *et al.*, 2020). Progestin use can also increase relative risk (overall 3.4, 5.3 for benign, and 2.8 for malignant tumors; Sorenmo *et al.*, 2020). Mammary tumors are much less common in male cats than in females (Hayes *et al.*, 1981; Viste *et al.*, 2002). Mammary neoplasia is seen predominantly in middle-aged to older cats with a mean age at diagnosis of 10–12 years old (Zappuli *et al.*, 2015). Epidemiologic studies have demonstrated an increased incidence of mammary carcinoma in the Siamese breed, with Siamese cats having twice the risk of developing carcinoma compared with other breeds (Hayes *et al.*, 1981; Ito *et al.*, 1996). There are too few studies comparing cytologic diagnosis of mammary tumors with histopathology results to discern the diagnostic utility of FNA in felines at this time.

Feline fibroadenomatous change

Fibroadenomatous change (feline mammary hypertrophy/fibro-adenoma complex, feline fibroepithelial hypertrophy) is the most

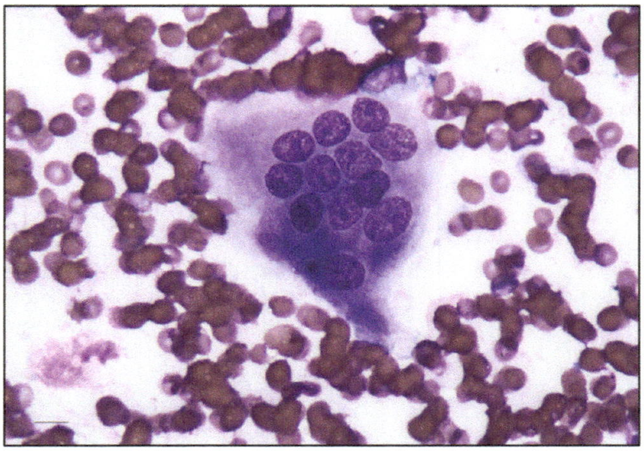

Figure 4.58 **An osteoclast found in an aspirate of a mammary mass. Osteoclasts are large cells with multiple, uniformly sized nuclei and moderate to large amounts of basophilic cytoplasm with faint pink granulation. They may be found in tumors with osseous differentiation, such as mixed mammary tumors or osteosarcoma (Wright–Giemsa, scale bar = 10 μm).**

common cause of benign mammary tumors in cats (Allen *et al.*, 1973). These hyperplastic lesions are the result of endogenous or exogenous progestin-induced proliferation of epithelial and stromal cells. Cats with fibroadenomatous hyperplasia have one or more enlarged (sometimes markedly enlarged) mammary glands. It is most common in young (up to 2 years old), intact, cycling queens or in pregnant cats (Rutteman & Misdorp, 1993). Neutered female cats with ovarian remnants can also develop fibroadenomatous change, and this condition has been documented in neutered female cats or in male cats that have been treated with progestins (megestrol acetate; Hayden *et al.*, 1981; MacDougall, 2003). Fibroadenomatous change is a benign condition, and the masses will often regress spontaneously, after ovariohysterectomy, or termination of progestin treatment (Rutteman & Misdorp, 1993; Giménez *et al.*, 2010). If FNA cytology is performed on these lesions, findings should include clusters of uniformly sized, cuboidal epithelial cells, as well as a population of spindle-shaped stromal cells with associated pink-staining matrix (Solano-Gallego & Masserdotti, 2023).

Feline epithelial mammary neoplasms

Mammary epithelial neoplasms in the cat typically arise from epithelial cells with very rare proliferations of myoepithelial cells encountered. Benign neoplasms of the feline mammary gland are uncommon and could include adenoma, ductal adenoma, and duct papilloma (intraductal papillary adenoma) (Zappuli *et al.*, 2020). The majority of feline mammary neoplasms are malignant and represent carcinomas of various histotypes, such as simple, solid, tubular, tubulopapillary, among others. Squamous cell carcinoma or carcinomas with squamous differentiation may also be found (Sorenmo *et al.*, 2020). Considering the relatively high percentage of feline mammary neoplasms that are malignant, excisional biopsy and histopathologic evaluation are often recommended, even if the epithelial cells appear benign when examined by FNA cytology. Aspiration of regional lymph nodes to check for metastasis is recommended, as well as assessment of thoracic radiographs for metastatic lesions, because metastasis would indicate a shorter survival time (Ito *et al.*, 1996; Seixas *et al.*, 2011). Tumor size has been correlated with the prognosis of feline mammary neoplasms (Weijer & Hart, 1983; MacEwen *et al.*, 1984; Ito *et al.*, 1996). Cats with large tumors (>3 cm in diameter) were found to have a median survival time of approximately 6 months, while cats with tumors 2–3 cm in diameter had a median survival time of 2 years (MacEwen *et al.*, 1984).

Feline mammary gland sarcomas

Mesenchymal neoplasms of the mammary gland are very rare, but the most common in the cat are fibrosarcoma and hemangiosarcoma (Zappuli *et al.*, 2020). Again, these will appear cytologically similar to these tumors in other tissues.

ROUND CELL TUMORS

Round cell tumors affecting dogs and cats include lymphoma, plasmacytoma, and mast cell tumor, while histiocytoma and transmissible venereal tumor only occur in dogs. Cats can, however, develop a distinct cutaneous histiocytic neoplasm known as feline progressive histiocytosis (described below). Round cell tumors typically exfoliate well, are highly cellular, and can display distinctive cytologic characteristics that often allow for a definitive diagnosis to be made from an FNA. Immunocytochemical staining can be used to confirm the diagnosis or to reach a definitive diagnosis if classic cytologic characteristics of the tumor are not present (Fernandez *et al.*, 2005).

Lymphoma

Cutaneous lymphoma can appear as plaque-like or nodular lesions and often multiple lesions are noted. They contain a monomorphic population of small, intermediate, or large lymphocytes. When composed of large lymphocytes, a diagnosis of lymphoma can be made on cytologic evaluation. Large lymphocytes have variable amounts of basophilic cytoplasm, a nucleus larger than a neutrophil in diameter, and one or more prominent nucleoli. Intermediate-sized lymphocytes have nuclei that are approximately the size of a neutrophil with scant to modest amounts of basophilic cytoplasm and a round or irregular nucleus with open chromatin and variably prominent nucleoli (Figure 4.59). Small-cell lymphomas are composed of small lymphocytes with condensed chromatin and can be difficult to distinguish from lymphocytic inflammation. Histopathology is important in discerning epitheliotropic (neoplastic lymphocytes infiltrate the epidermis and/or adnexa) and nonepitheliotropic cutaneous lymphoma (neoplastic lymphocytes infiltrate the dermis and/or subcutis), in addition to determination of phenotype with IHC, PCR for antigen receptor rearrangement, and/or flow cytometry. Most cutaneous lymphomas are T-cell lymphomas (Day, 1995). If a cutaneous lesion consists of

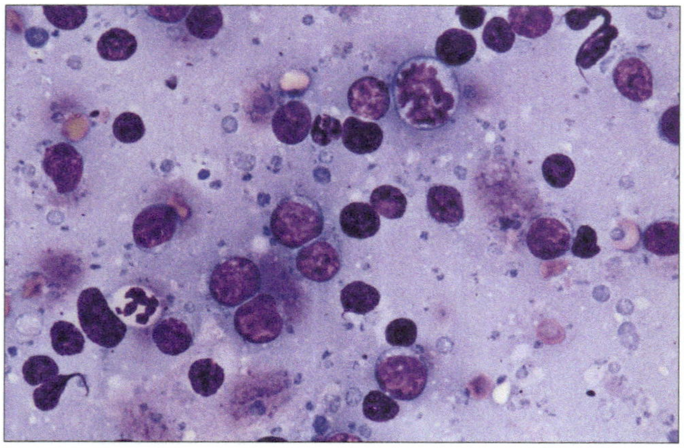

Figure 4.59 Cutaneous lymphoma. FNA of a dermal mass from a 10-year-old German Shepherd dog. The majority of the intact cells are intermediate to large lymphocytes, measuring approximately the same diameter as or slightly larger than a neutrophil. These cells have scant cytoplasm with more open chromatin and variably distinct nucleoli. There is a mitotic figure pictured (top off-center) and several lysed cells/bare nuclei and round basophilic cytoplasmic fragments. The size of the lymphoid population and homogeneity support a diagnosis of cutaneous lymphoma (Wright–Giemsa, 1,000× magnification).

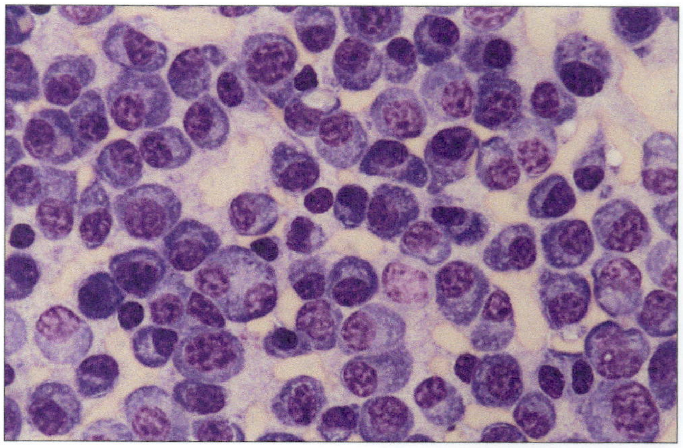

Figure 4.60 Plasma cell tumor. FNA of a dermal mass from a dog. The sample contains large numbers of individualized round cells and moderate numbers of erythrocytes. The round cells have a moderate amount of basophilic cytoplasm and frequently a pale perinuclear Golgi zone. They have an eccentrically placed rounded nucleus. A larger, binucleate cell is present (Wright–Giemsa, 500× magnification).

mostly small to intermediate-sized lymphocytes, cutaneous lymphocytosis may be another consideration. This is a very rare lymphoproliferative disease more commonly reported in cats than dogs, and it is still unknown whether it represents a reactive or neoplastic disease but it does share clinical and histopathologic similarities to cutaneous lymphoma. Biopsy with IHC and clonality testing may be helpful in making this distinction (Albanese, 2022).

Plasma cell tumor

Most cutaneous plasma cell tumors (plasmacytomas) of dogs and cats present as firm, raised dermal lesions and are benign neoplasms. FNA samples contain several round cells with abundant, basophilic cytoplasm, a perinuclear clearing in the area of the Golgi zone, and a round, eccentrically placed nucleus. Multinucleation (namely binucleation) is a common finding and a distinguishing characteristic of this tumor (Figure 4.60). Although rare, erythrophagocytosis has been reported in cases of plasmacytoma (Yearley *et al.*, 2007). Malignant plasma cell tumors usually have several characteristics of malignancy. When multiple cutaneous plasma cell tumors are present, it may represent a more aggressive disease process (similar to multiple myeloma), and advanced diagnostics, such as serum and urine protein electrophoresis, assessment for lytic lesions, and bone marrow infiltration may be considered for staging (Moore A.R., 2023).

Mast cell tumor

The clinical appearance of mast cell tumors is variable. They can present as a firm, erythematous, cutaneous nodule, a deep, flocculent, subcutaneous mass, or anything in between. Mast cell tumors are composed of round cells with a rounded, centrally located nucleus

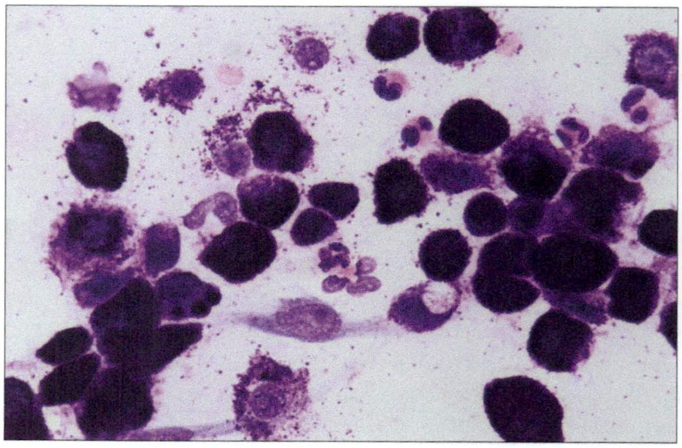

Figure 4.61 Mast cell tumor. Fenestration of a flocculent, subcutaneous mass from a dog. The sample contains large numbers of individualized round cells filled with numerous metachromatic, cytoplasmic granules. Anisocytosis is moderate. The nucleus is round, pale, and often obscured by the cytoplasmic granules. There are also a few eosinophils and reactive fibroblasts (Wright–Giemsa, 1,000× magnification).

that is often difficult to visualize because it is obscured by several small, distinct, metachromatic, cytoplasmic granules (Figure 4.61). Rarely, mast cells contain phagocytized erythrocytes (Barger *et al.*, 2012). Eosinophils and/or large reactive fibroblasts may be present in large numbers and are more commonly observed in dogs compared with cats (Figure 4.61). In lesions with large numbers of fibroblasts, cords of extracellular eosinophilic matrix (collagen) are often observed.

The distinguishing feature of this tumor is the cytoplasmic granulation. However, mast cell granules do not always stain with Diff-Quik® stain, which may prevent diagnosis of the tumor (Figure 4.62). A mast cell tumor should be suspected in lesions with large numbers

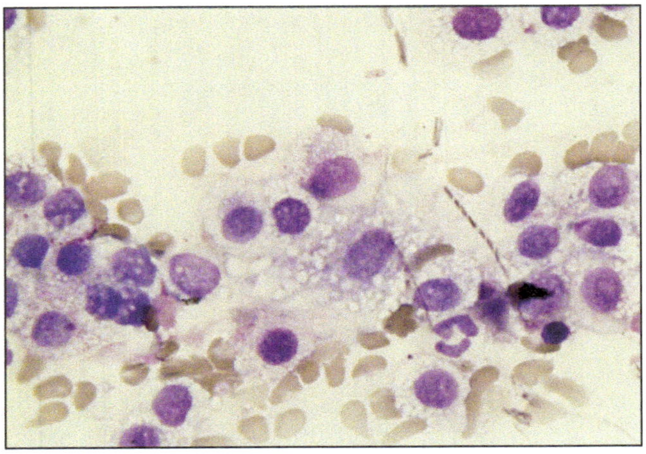

Figure 4.62 Mast cell tumor. FNA of a subcutaneous mass from a dog. There are several rounded cells with abundant cytoplasm and a centrally located round nucleus. Cells appear to contain vacuoles; however, a few metachromatic granules can be seen in some of the cells, allowing the diagnosis of a mast cell tumor to be made (Diff-Quik®, 1,000× magnification).

of round cells that are associated with an eosinophilic infiltrate. Submission of an unstained slide to a diagnostic laboratory for Wright–Giemsa staining can confirm suspicion of a mast cell tumor.

Histopathologic grading is regarded as the most consistent and reliable prognostic assessment in canine cutaneous mast cell tumors. Recently cytologic grading of Wright–Giemsa-stained slides has been attempted using some histologic criteria of malignancy. Cytologic findings associated with a poor outcome included poor granularity of the tumor cells or the presence of two or more atypical features, including anisokaryosis, mitotic figures, binucleation/multinucleation, nuclear pleomorphism, and reduced numbers of fibroblasts/collagen fibrils (Camus *et al.*, 2016; Scarpa *et al.*, 2016; Paes *et al.*, 2022). Clinical stage is also important in assessing prognosis and can be achieved through cytologic evaluation of draining lymph nodes, spleen, and liver, although disease may be missed due to the small sample size of an FNA. Histopathologic evaluation of draining lymph nodes can also be assessed for a histologic node grade that has been shown to correlate with survival (Weishaar *et al.*, 2014). Dogs with tumors affecting the prepuce, scrotum, and mucous membranes have been noted to experience a worse prognosis, while subcutaneous tumors seem to have a better prognosis (London & Thamm, 2020).

In cats, mast cell tumors often present as small, solitary, raised, white, hairless nodules. If solitary, these are typically benign and complete surgical removal is curative. However, if multiple are present or there is suspicion of splenomegaly, evaluation of splenic mast cell neoplasia would be warranted as this would carry a worse prognosis (London & Thamm, 2020). Atypical cutaneous mast cell tumors have been reported in young cats <4 years of age. The cells in these patients appear anaplastic, but the tumors have been reported to resolve on their own (Henry & Herrera, 2013). As with dogs, feline mast cell tumors with an increased mitotic index in histologic sections correlate with a poor prognosis (Strefezzi *et al.*, 2003; Romansik *et al.*, 2007; Elston *et al.*, 2009; Sabattini & Bettini, 2010; Sabattini & Bettini, 2019).

Histiocytic neoplasms

Histiocytoma

Histiocytoma is a common benign neoplasm of dogs. Tumors often are described as smooth, round, raised, mildly erythematous, cutaneous nodules with alopecia. Typically, the tumors spontaneously regress within a few months of diagnosis, although inflammation or infection can delay this. Surgical removal is recommended if the lesion persists to prevent progression to a malignant histiocytic neoplasm. These tumors are made up of Langerhans dendritic cells, which cytologically appear as round cells with lightly basophilic cytoplasm that becomes paler toward the edges of the cell. Nuclei are ovoid or bean-shaped and tend to be eccentrically placed with or without an indistinct nucleolus. Mitotic figures can be seen and there is a basophilic proteinaceous background. An infiltrate of small lymphocytes is seen as these tumors begin to regress and helps distinguish histiocytomas from plasma cell tumors or poorly granular mast cell tumors (Figures 4.63a, b). This infiltrate can become the predominant cell type and may complicate the diagnosis of histiocytoma.

Cutaneous Langerhans cell histiocytosis

Cutaneous Langerhans cell histiocytosis is a rare condition of dogs (the Shar Pei breed is overrepresented) in which multiple cutaneous histiocytomas occur in the skin at the same site or at distant sites. It can also progress into a multisystemic disease involving the lymph nodes, lungs, and other internal organs. The cells are morphologically similar and have the same immunophenotype as those found in cutaneous histiocytoma (Sharma *et al.*, 2021; Moore P.F., 2023). Animals present with multiple skin lesions that may respond to treatment with lomustine (CCNU), but they typically recur (Moore, 2014). The overall prognosis of these diseases is guarded due to lesion ulceration and recurrence. Immunocytochemistry can be used to help differentiate these lesions from cutaneous lymphomas.

Histiocytic sarcoma

Histiocytic sarcomas (HS) originate from neoplastic histiocytes (usually interstitial dendritic cells), and in the skin they occur within the dermis or subcutis. On cytology, the cells can be round and/or spindle-shaped, and marked atypia can be observed (Figures 4.64a, b). The cells have lightly basophilic cytoplasm, an ovoid to round nucleus which is often indented, and multiple, prominent nucleoli (Affolter & Moore, 2002; Albanese, 2017; Moore P.F., 2023). This tumor typically displays marked criteria of malignancy including frequent multinucleation and mitotic figures (Figures 4.64b). Phagocytized erythrocytes or cellular debris may be observed in the neoplastic cells (Barger *et al.*, 2012). When spindle cells with marked cytologic atypia predominate in lesions, HS can appear similar to other high-grade sarcomas and undifferentiated pleomorphic sarcoma (also known as anaplastic sarcoma with giant cells, giant cell tumor of soft parts, and malignant fibrous histiocytoma), and immunophenotyping can

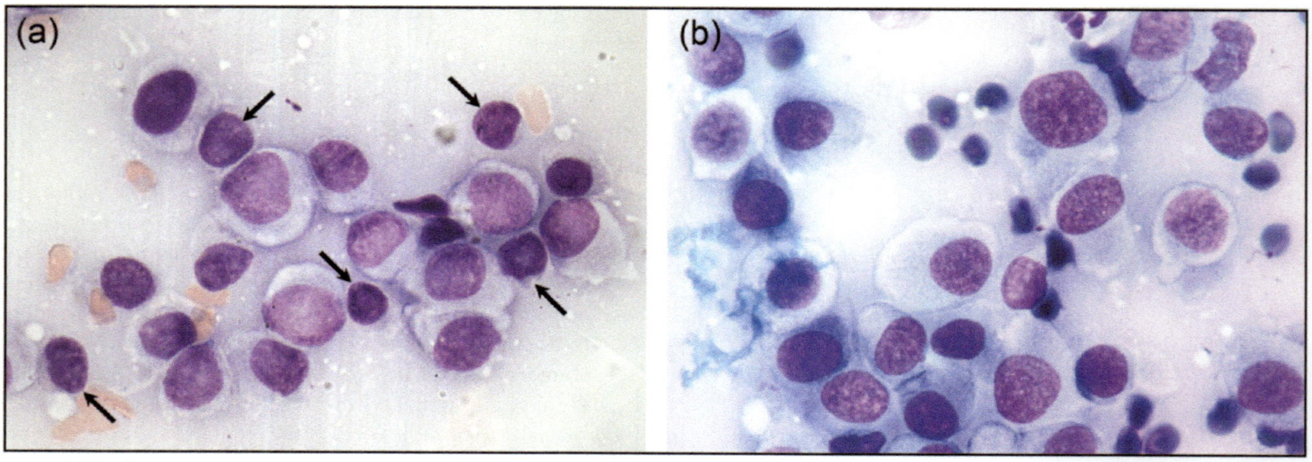

Figures 4.63a, b Histiocytoma. FNAs of hairless, raised, dermal lesions on the distal extremities from two dogs. The cells are individually arranged. They are rounded with abundant, lightly basophilic cytoplasm that becomes wispy and paler at the outer edge of the cell. Cells have a large ovoid nucleus that is often eccentrically located and has a slightly open chromatin pattern. The samples also have a basophilic proteinaceous material and contain low numbers of erythrocytes. (a) Several small lymphocytes are present (arrows) (Wright–Giemsa, 1,000× magnification).

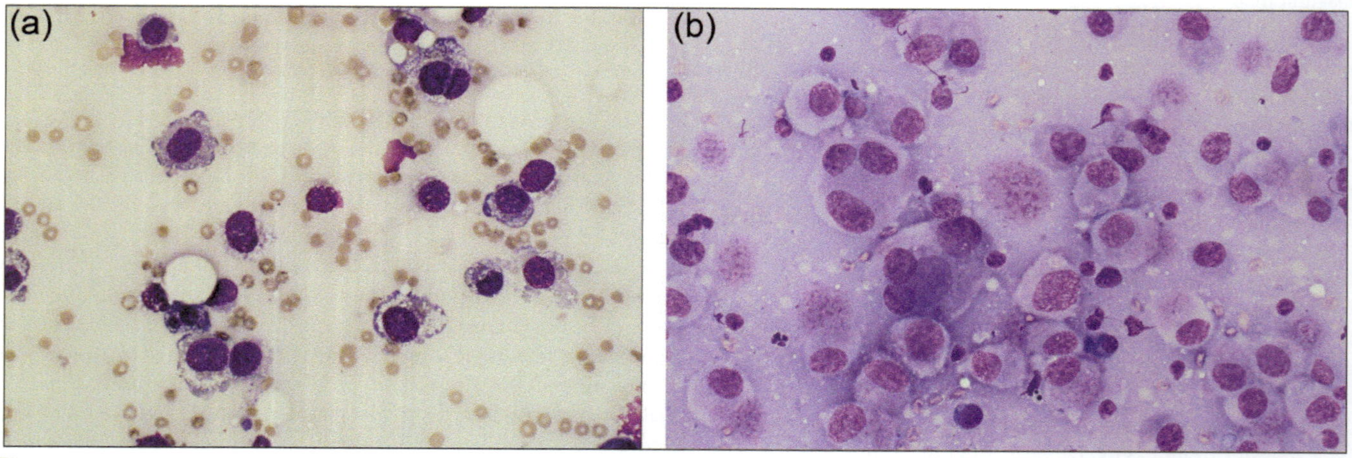

Figures 4.64a, b FNAs of histiocytic sarcomas. (a) FNA of a subcutaneous mass from a 12-year-old dog. Cells are rounded with abundant basophilic cytoplasm. Cytoplasmic vacuoles are observed. Nuclei are ovoid with coarsely stippled chromatin. Binucleate cells and anisokaryosis are noted. Multiple small, dark, prominent nucleoli are present in most of the cells (Wright–Giemsa, 500× magnification). (b) FNA of a mass on the right lateral thigh of a 9-year-old dog. Neoplastic cells display marked atypia including multinucleation, anisokaryosis, and karyomegaly (Wright–Giemsa, 500× magnification).

be used to differentiate. Immunochemical identification of ionized calcium-binding adaptor molecule 1 (Iba1), lysozyme, vimentin, major histocompatibility (MHC) class II, CD11b, CD18, and CD204 expression by the neoplastic cells supports a diagnosis of histiocytic sarcoma (Yamazaki *et al.*, 2014). Histiocytic sarcoma is the cause of death in approximately 14% of Bernese Mountain Dogs and Flat-Coated Retrievers (Erich *et al.*, 2013). In cases of localized histiocytic sarcoma, cutaneous lesions on the limbs are frequently reported. Primary histiocytic sarcoma has also been reported in the spleen, lymph nodes, lungs, joints, and central nervous system.

Feline progressive histiocytosis

In cats, there is a distinct entity of neoplastic dermal interstitial dendritic cells that can present as single or multiple cutaneous nodules and plaques, often found on the head or distal limbs. This can behave as a low-grade histiocytic sarcoma whereby lesions are typically slowly progressive and can spread systemically in the terminal stage (Affolter & Moore, 2006; Moore, 2014; Moore P.F., 2023). Cells have a histiocytic appearance with abundant lightly basophilic cytoplasm and an ovoid nucleus with stippled chromatin and are admixed with small T lymphocytes and neutrophils (Pinto da Cunha *et al.*, 2014); cellular pleomorphism can increase with disease progression. Immunocytochemistry with CD1 is used in the diagnosis of this disease.

Transmissible venereal tumor

Transmissible venereal tumors (TVTs) are common in dogs from tropical and subtropical areas of the world. Cells that make up these tumors

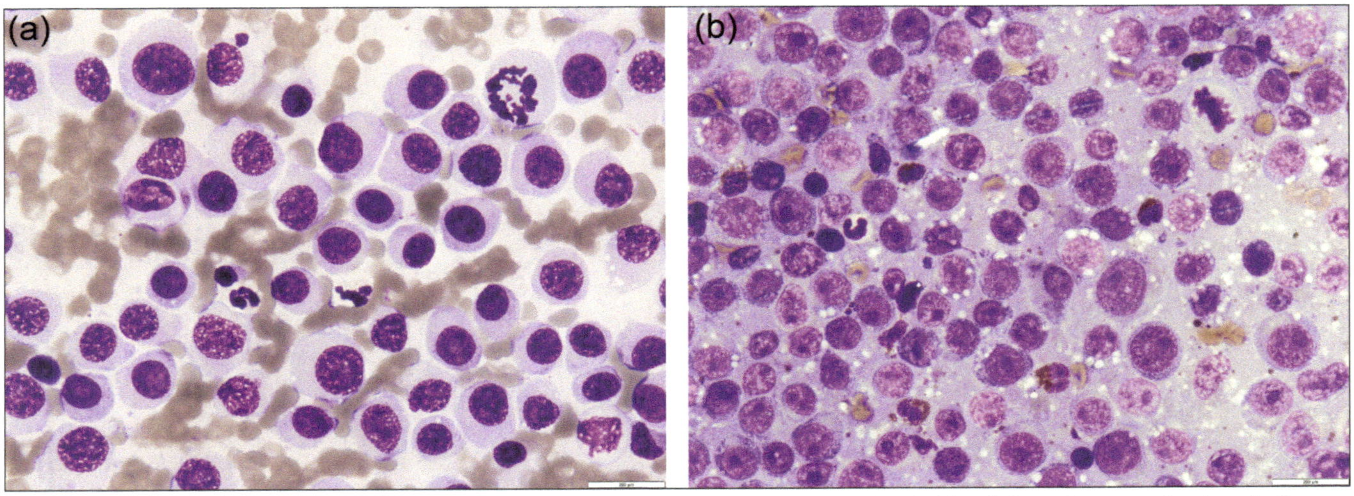

Figures 4.65a, b **Transmissible venereal tumors. (a) FNA of a vaginal mass from a dog. The sample is highly cellular and consists of nucleated cells present in a bloody background. There are numerous individually occurring round cells with distinct cell borders and scant to moderate amounts of light basophilic cytoplasm. Low numbers of cells contain a few small distinct intracytoplasmic vacuoles. The nuclei are round and have a smooth to reticular to coarse chromatin pattern. Moderate anisocytosis and anisokaryosis are noted. A few neutrophils and small lymphocytes and occasional mitotic figures are also seen (Wright–Giemsa, 1,000× magnification). (b) FNA of a preputial mass from a dog. The sample is highly cellular and consists of nucleated cells present in a vacuolated background containing low numbers of red blood cells. There are high numbers of individually occurring round cells with distinct cell borders and scant to moderate amounts of light basophilic cytoplasm, often containing low numbers of small distinct intracytoplasmic vacuoles. The nuclei are round, have a reticular to coarse chromatin pattern and a single distinct nucleolus. Moderate anisocytosis and anisokaryosis are noted. A few neutrophils and small lymphocytes and occasional mitotic figures are also seen (Wright–Giemsa, 1,000× magnification).**

are canine-derived cells that have an aberrant number of chromosomes and contain a long interspersed nuclear element insertion near the oncogene c-myc (Murgia *et al.*, 2006). The neoplastic disease can spread from affected to unaffected animals and is often observed around the genitals and muzzle. TVTs may become large, but they regress if there is an effective humoral immune response to the neoplastic cells (Goldschmidt & Hendrick, 2002). TVT cytology samples contain round cells that have moderate to abundant, lightly basophilic cytoplasm and a round, centrally located nucleus. Punctate, round, clear, distinct cytoplasmic vacuoles are the distinguishing feature of this tumor (Figure 4.65). A lymphocyte infiltrate (typically small lymphocytes) may also be seen and is reflective of an immune response to the tumor cells.

MELANOMAS

Melanomas originate from melanocytes in the skin and can occur in the skin, mucosa, and even the anal sac. The morphology of melanocytes can be spindle-shaped or round with a round to variably shaped nucleus. Cells may be individualized or aggregated on the slide. The distinguishing characteristic of melanocytes is the presence of round or rice-shaped, brown–black to blue–gray, melanin granules (Figures 4.66a, b). Small, well-circumscribed, well-differentiated, melanotic melanomas (sometimes referred to as melanocytomas) typically are benign in cats and dogs unless they are near a mucous membrane or a nail bed. Amelanotic melanomas are much more difficult to diagnose; because of the pleomorphism of melanocytes, there is virtually no morphologic indicator of cell type unless melanin granules are seen. Immunocytochemical stains, such as S-100 or Melan-A, can aid in making a diagnosis of amelanotic melanoma (Smith *et al.*, 2002). Malignant melanomas, including most amelanotic melanomas, are very aggressive tumors that rapidly spread to draining lymph nodes. Cells tend to be large and pleomorphic with several criteria of malignancy. They may contain a somewhat distinctive, large, round, prominent nucleolus that takes up the majority of the nucleus, termed 'owl's eye' nucleoli (Figure 4.67). Aspiration of draining lymph nodes and thoracic imaging is recommended whenever a malignant melanoma is diagnosed.

CASES

CASE 1

Signalment/history

A 15-year-old, spayed female domestic shorthair cat presented for a mass in the left mandibular area. FNAs of the mass were submitted for cytologic evaluation.

Cytologic description

The sample was highly cellular with low numbers of erythrocytes and neutrophils in the background. The majority of cells were large

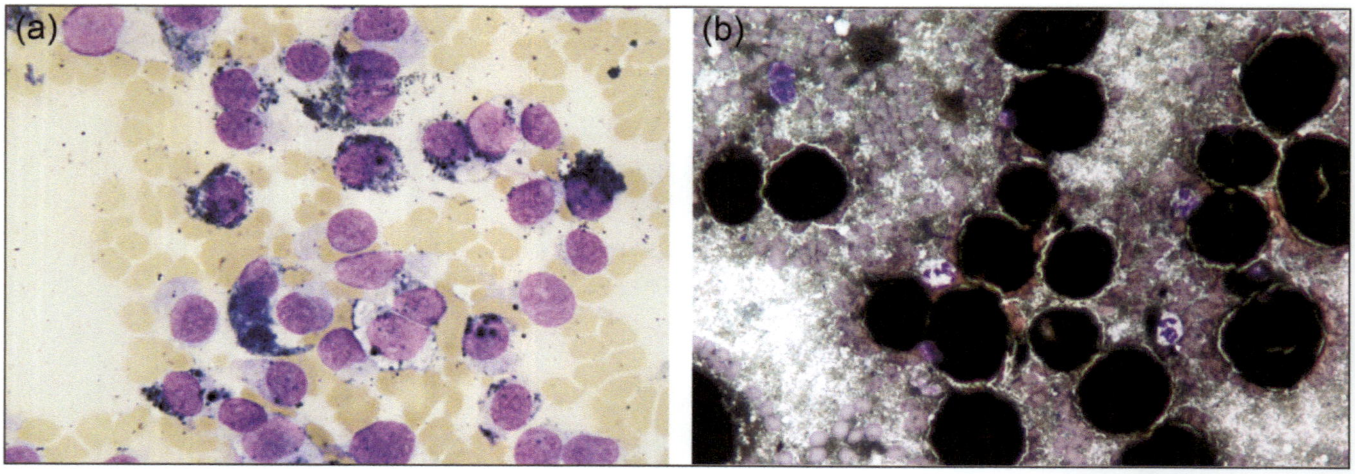

Figures 4.66a,b Melanomas. (a) FNA of a 1-cm black mass on the right pinna of a 4-year-old Labrador Retriever. The sample contained several individualized rounded to spindle-shaped cells with scant lightly basophilic cytoplasm, variable numbers of pinpoint black cytoplasmic granules, and a large round to ovoid nucleus with finely stippled chromatin. (b) FNA of a mass from an adult domestic shorthair cat. Cells in this sample are rounded and filled with black granules that obscure the morphology of the nucleus. Large numbers of black granules are present in the background of the sample (Wright–Giemsa, 1,000× magnification).

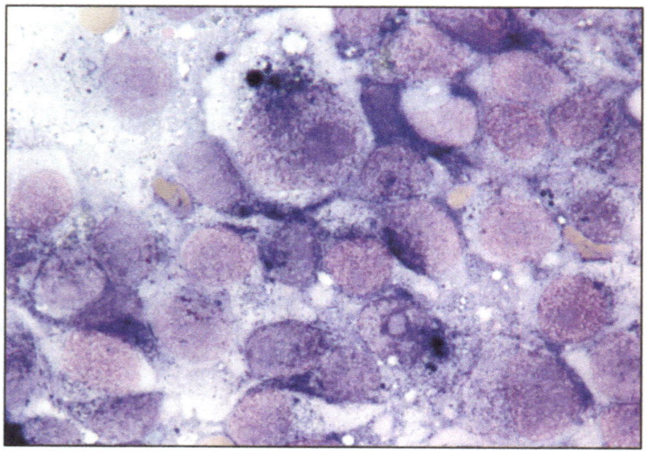

Figure 4.67 FNA of a dermal mass from a dog. Malignant melanocytes exhibit marked anisocytosis and anisokaryosis. They have a variable amount of lightly basophilic cytoplasm and an ovoid nucleus with stippled chromatin and a prominent nucleolus. A few variably sized black granules are seen in some of the cells. The cell at the top center of the image has a very large 'owl's eye' nucleolus (Wright–Giemsa stain, 1,000× magnification).

rounded cells with abundant basophilic cytoplasm, a large round nucleus, stippled chromatin, and one to two large prominent nucleoli (Figures 4.68a, b). Very large 'owl's eye' nucleoli were present in several cells. Marked anisocytosis and anisokaryosis were observed. There were several binucleate cells and aberrant mitotic figures. Low numbers of cells contained small black pigment consistent with melanin (Figure 4.68c).

Interpretation: Amelanotic melanoma.

Discussion

Amelanotic melanomas can be difficult to diagnose unless a few melanin granules can be found. This diagnosis should be suspected in cases where it is difficult to determine if the neoplastic cells are round, epithelial, or mesenchymal cells.

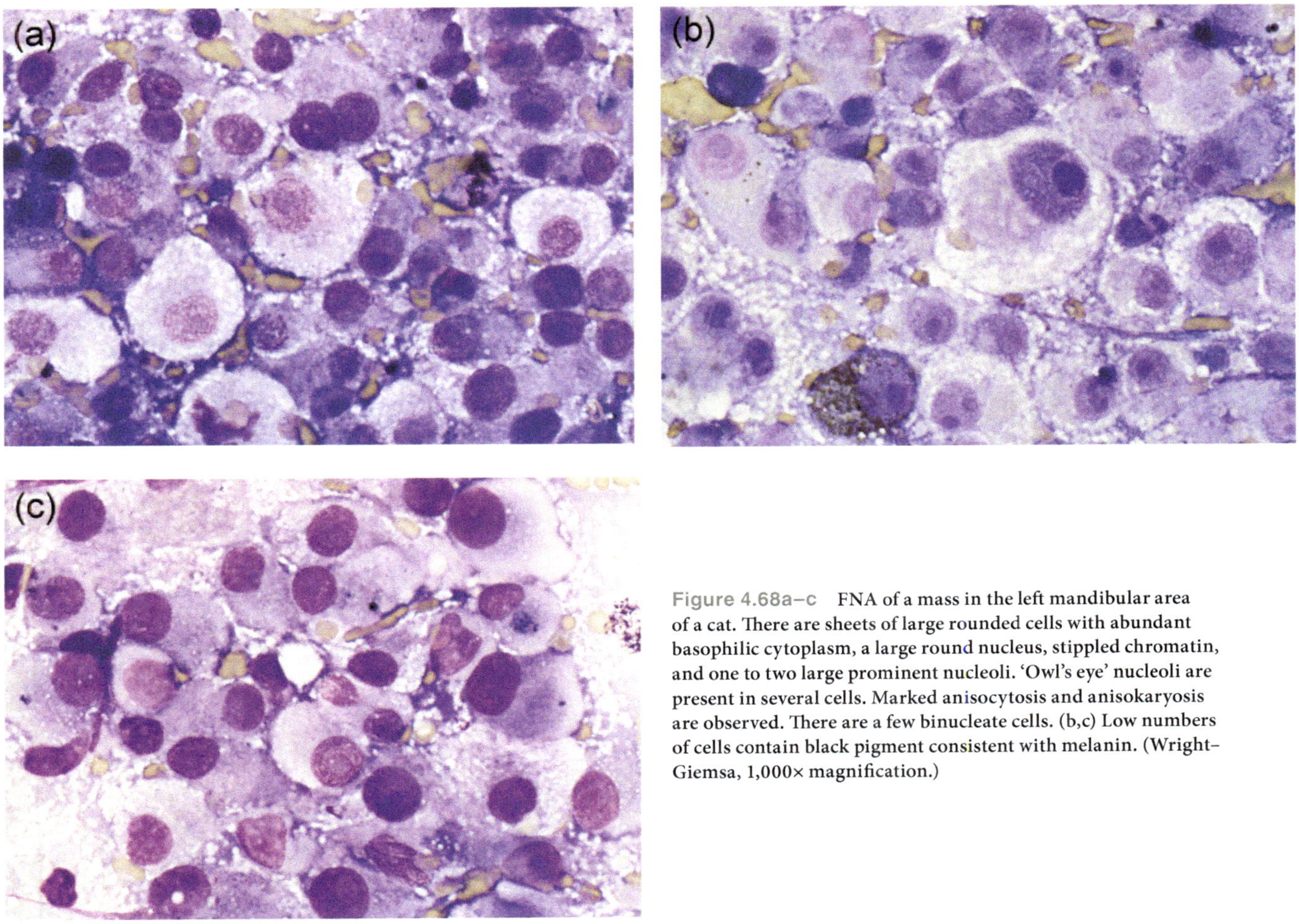

Figure 4.68a–c FNA of a mass in the left mandibular area of a cat. There are sheets of large rounded cells with abundant basophilic cytoplasm, a large round nucleus, stippled chromatin, and one to two large prominent nucleoli. 'Owl's eye' nucleoli are present in several cells. Marked anisocytosis and anisokaryosis are observed. There are a few binucleate cells. (b,c) Low numbers of cells contain black pigment consistent with melanin. (Wright–Giemsa, 1,000× magnification.)

CASE 2

Signalment/history

A 1-year-old, spayed female German Shorthair Pointer presented with a crusty skin lesion. A skin scraping was performed and submitted for cytologic evaluation.

Cytologic description

Slides were highly cellular with minimal peripheral blood contamination. They contained a mixed inflammatory cell population predominated by degenerate neutrophils with fewer macrophages and eosinophils. Small 3–6 µm diameter round deeply basophilic yeast-like structures were present individually and in clusters. Some septate branching hyphal structures were also observed (Figure 4.69a). Fungal organisms were seen extracellularly and within macrophages (Figures 4.69b, c). Rarely, short rod-shaped bacterial organisms were seen within neutrophils (Figure 4.69d). Many mature squamous epithelial cells were present (Figure 4.69e). The background of the sample consisted of moderate cellular debris and basophilic proteinaceous material.

Interpretation: Marked septic mixed inflammation with evidence of fungal (most suggestive of a dermatophyte) and bacterial organisms.

Discussion

Unstained slides were submitted for DNA isolation and polymerase chain reaction to determine the identity of the fungal organisms. The DNA sequence had 99% homology with *Trichophyton mentagrophytes*.

CASE 3

Signalment/history

A 3-year-old, female, domestic shorthair cat (indoor/outdoor) presented for a swollen nose and multiple, variably sized, small, hairless masses on both ears. An FNA of one of the ear masses was submitted for cytological evaluation.

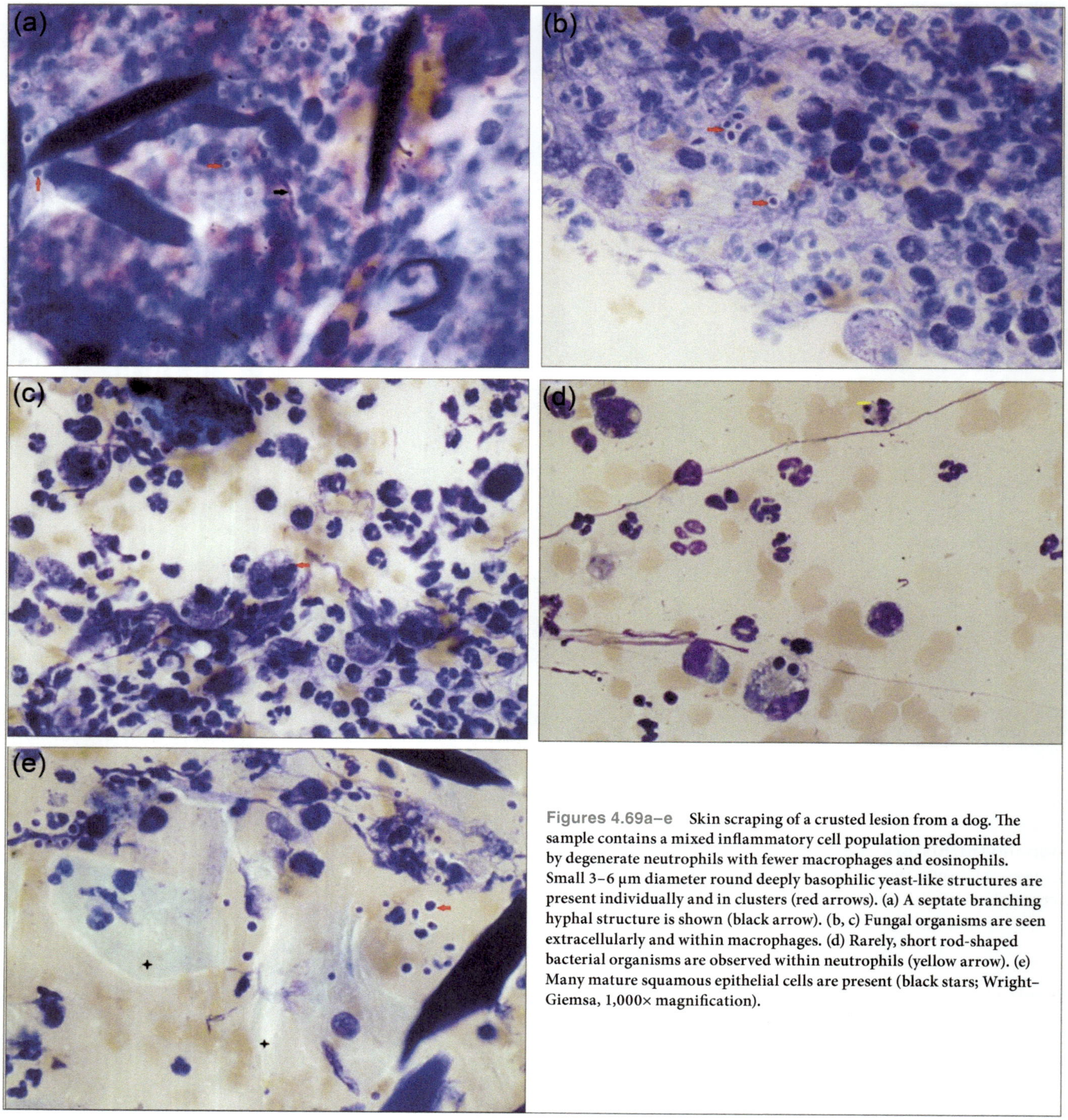

Figures 4.69a–e Skin scraping of a crusted lesion from a dog. The sample contains a mixed inflammatory cell population predominated by degenerate neutrophils with fewer macrophages and eosinophils. Small 3–6 µm diameter round deeply basophilic yeast-like structures are present individually and in clusters (red arrows). (a) A septate branching hyphal structure is shown (black arrow). (b, c) Fungal organisms are seen extracellularly and within macrophages. (d) Rarely, short rod-shaped bacterial organisms are observed within neutrophils (yellow arrow). (e) Many mature squamous epithelial cells are present (black stars; Wright-Giemsa, 1,000× magnification).

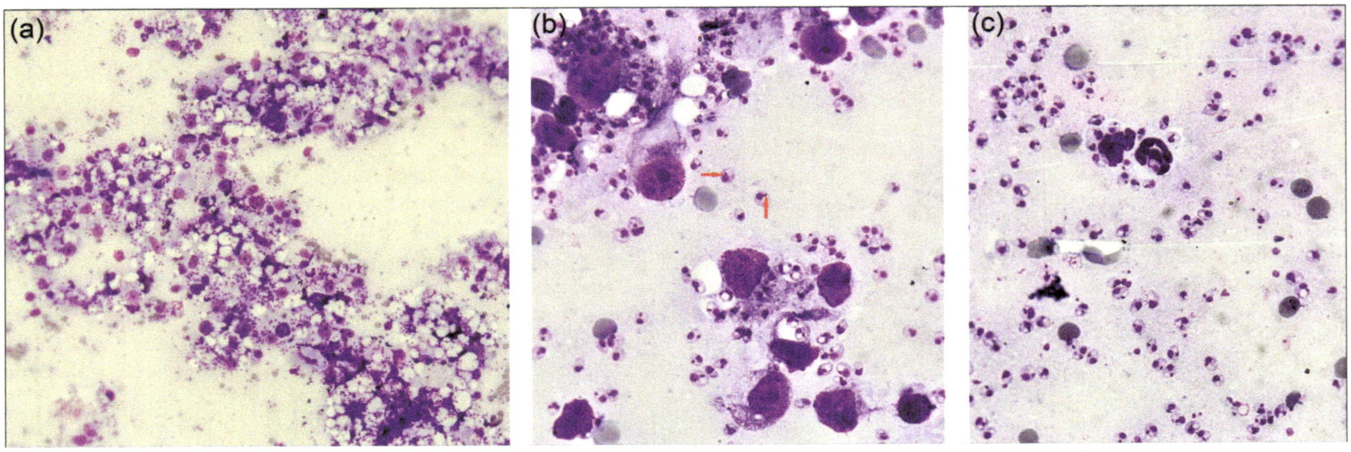

Figures 4.70a–c FNA of ear masses from a cat. The sample contains high numbers of extracellular and intracellular, small, round to oval organisms and high numbers of a mixture of inflammatory cells, with macrophages predominating (a). The organisms are round to oval, 2–3 µm in diameter, have an eccentrically located, round, purple staining nucleus and a small rod-shaped kinetoplast that has a perpendicular orientation (b, red arrows). They are present intracellularly within macrophages (b) and neutrophils (c), and extracellularly in very high numbers (Wright–Giemsa 200× magnification, A; 1,000× magnification, b and c). (a) High numbers of inflammatory cells (predominantly macrophages) and numerous extracellular and intracellular small, round to oval organisms. (b) The organisms are present extracellularly and within macrophages. The organisms contain an eccentrically located nucleus and a small rod-shaped kinetoplast that has a perpendicular orientation (red arrows). (c) Organisms are present extracellularly and within neutrophils.

Cytologic description

The slides were highly cellular and consisted of nucleated cells present in a background containing high numbers of red blood cells, low amounts of nuclear debris, and high numbers of small extracellular organisms (Figures 4.70a–c). There were high numbers of macrophages and lower numbers of neutrophils, and many contained low to high numbers of the same organisms. These were round to oval, approximately 2–3 µm in diameter, and contained a round purple-staining nucleus and a perpendicularly oriented small rod-shaped kinetoplast (Figure 4.70b). The organisms were also sometimes present in large variably sized phagocytic vacuoles within the macrophages, and were consistent with *Leishmania* amastigotes. Low numbers of bi-nucleated macrophages and multinucleated giant cells were also observed.

Interpretation: Marked mixed inflammation (predominantly macrophagic) with *Leishmania* amastigotes present.

Discussion

Unstained slides were submitted for PCR and DNA sequencing analysis to determine the species of *Leishmania* present. Results revealed the presence of *Leishmania amazonensis*.

REFERENCES

Adedeji A.O., Affolter V.K., Christopher M.M. (2017) Cytologic features of cutaneous follicular tumors and cysts in dogs. *Vet Clin Pathol 46*:143–150.

Affolter V.K., Moore P.F. (2000) Canine cutaneous and systemic histiocytosis: Reactive histiocytosis of dermal dendritic cells. *Am J Dermatopathol 22*:40–48.

Affolter V.K., Moore P.F. (2002) Localized and disseminated histiocytic sarcoma of dendritic cell origin in dogs. *Vet Pathol 39*:74–83.

Affolter V.K., Moore P.F. (2006) Feline progressive histiocytosis. *Vet Pathol 43*(*5*):646–655.

Albanese F. (2017) Cytology of canine and feline non-neoplastic skin diseases. In: *Canine and Feline Skin Cytology*, 1st edn. Springer Cham, Switzerland, pg 132.

Albanese F., Abramo F., Marino M., Massaro M., Marconato L., Minoli L., Martini V., Aresu L. (2022) Feline and canine cutaneous lymphocytosis: Reactive process or indolent neoplastic disease? *Vet Sci 9*(*1*):26.

Allen H.L. (1973) Feline mammary hypertrophy. *Vet Pathol 10*:501–508.

Allen S.W., Prasse K.W., Mahaffey E.A. (1986) Cytologic differentiation of benign from malignant canine mammary tumors. *Vet Pathol 23*(*6*):649–655.

Allison R.W., Walton R.M. (2020) Subcutaneous glandular tissue: Mammary, salivary, thyroid, and parathyroid. In: *Cowell and Tyler's Diagnostic Cytology and Hematology of the Dog and Cat*, 5th edn. (eds. A.C. Valenciano, R.L. Cowell) Elsevier, St. Louis, p. 102.

Andreasen C.B., MaHaffey E.A., Duncan J.R. (1988) Intermediate filament staining in the cytologic and histologic diagnosis of canine skin and soft tissue tumors. *Vet Pathol 25*:343–349.

Avallone G., Helmbold P., Caniatti M. et al. (2007) The spectrum of canine cutaneous perivascular wall tumors: Morphologic, phenotypic and clinical characterization. *Vet Pathol 44*:607–620.

Azevedo C.N., Sterman A.A., Stranahan L.W. et al. (2020) Pathologic and flow cytometric features of a case of canine ventral cervical lymphangiosarcoma. *J Vet Diag Invest 32*(*3*):476–480.

Barger A., Graca R., Bailey K., Messick J., de Lorimier L.P., Fan T., Hoffmann W. (2005) Use of alkaline phosphatase staining to differentiate canine osteosarcoma from other vimentin-positive tumors. *Vet Pathol 42*(*2*):161–165.

Barger A.M., Skowronski M.C., MacNeill A.L. (2012) Cytologic identification of erythrophagocytic neoplasms. *Vet Clin Pathol 41*(*4*):587–589.

Bohn A.A., Wills T., Caplazi P. (2006) Basal cell tumor or cutaneous basilar epithelial neoplasm? Rethinking the cytologic diagnosis of basal cell tumors. *Vet Clin Pathol 35*:449–453.

Brodey R.S., Goldschmidt M.H., Roszel J.R. (1983) Canine mammary gland neoplasms. *J Am Anim Hosp Assoc 19*:61–81.

Camus M.S., Priest H.L., Koehler J.W. et al. (2016) Cytologic criteria for mast cell tumor grading in dogs with evaluation of clinical outcome. *Vet Pathol 53(6)*:1117–1123.

Conroy J.D., Breen P.T. (1972) Apocrine sweat gland carcinoma with lymphatic invasion in a dog. *Vet Clin North Am Small Anim Pract 67(3)*:297–298.

Coomer A.R., Liptak J.M. (2008) Canine histiocytic diseases. *Comp Contin Educ Pract Vet 30(4)*:202–204.

Day M.J. (1995) Immunophenotypic characterization of cutaneous lymphoid neoplasia in the dog and cat. *J Comp Pathol 112*:79–96.

Dorn C.R., Taylor D.O., Frye F.L. et al. (1968) Survey of animal neoplasms in Alameda and Contra Costa Counties, California. I. Methodology and description of cases. *J Natl Cancer Inst 40(2)*:295–305.

Elston L., Sueiro F.A., Cavalcanti J. et al. (2009) The importance of the mitotic index as a prognostic factor for canine cutaneous mast cell tumors: A validation study. *Vet Pathol 46(2)*:362–364.

Emanuelli M.P., Kommers G.D., Antoniazzi A.Q., Bernardes F.C.S., Lopes S.T.A., Fighera R.A. (2020) Myoepithelial cells and extracellular matrix in the cytologic differentiation of canine mammary tumors. *Vet Clin Pathol. 49*:451–458.

Erich S.A., Rutteman G.R., Teske E. (2013) Causes of death and the impact of histiocytic sarcoma on the life expectancy of the Dutch population of Bernese mountain dogs and Flat-coated retrievers. *Vet J 198(3)*:678–683.

Evans S.J.M., Connolly S.L., Schaffer P.A., Vieson M.D., Stiles A., Moore A.R. (2018a) Basal cell enumeration does not predict malignancy in canine perianal gland tumor cytology. *Vet Clin Pathol 47*:634–637.

Evans S.J.M., Frank C.B., Avery P.R., Moore A.R. (2018b) What is your diagnosis? Subcutaneous mass on a dog. *Vet Clin Pathol 47*:160–161.

Fernandez N.J., West K.H., Jackson M.L. et al. (2005) Immunohistochemical and histochemical stains for differentiating canine cutaneous round cell tumors. *Vet Pathol 42*:437–445.

Fisher D.J. (2020) Cutaneous and subcutaneous lesions. In: *Cowell and Tyler's Diagnostic Cytology and Hematology of the Dog and Cat*, 5th edn. (eds. A.C. Valenciano, R.L. Cowell) Elsvier, St Louis, pp. 74–100.

Ghisleni G., Roccabianca P., Ceruti R. et al. (2006) Correlation between fine-needle aspiration cytology and histopathology in the evaluation of cutaneous and subcutaneous masses from dogs and cats. *Vet Clin Pathol 35*:24–30.

Giménez F., Hecht S., Craig L.E. et al. (2010) Optimizing the management of feline mammary masses: Early detection, aggressive therapy. *J Feline Med Surg 12(3)*:214–224.

Goldschmidt M., Munday J.S., Scruggs J.L., Klopfleisch R., Kiupel M. (2020) *Surgical Pathology of Tumors of Domestic Animals: Volume 1: Epithelial Tumors of the Skin* (ed. M. Kiupel) Davis-Thompson DVM Foundation.

Goldschmidt M., Pena L., Rasotto R. et al. (2011) Classification and grading of canine mammary tumors. *Vet Pathol 48*:117–131.

Goldschmidt M.H., Hendrick M.J. (2002) Tumors of the skin and soft tissues. In: *Tumors in Domestic Animals*, 4th edn. (ed. D.J. Meuten) Blackwell, Ames, pp. 45–118.

Goldschmidt M.H., Pena L., Zappulli V. (2017) Tumors of the mammary gland. In: *Tumors in Domestic Animals*, 5th edn. (ed. D.J. Meuten) John Wiley & Sons, Ames, pp. 575–606.

Griffiths G.L., Lumsden J.H., Valli V.E. (1984) Fine needle aspiration cytology and histologic correlation in canine tumors. *Vet Clin Pathol 13(1)*:13–17.

Gross T.L., Ihrke P.J., Walder E.J. et al. (2005) *Skin Diseases of the Dog and Cat: Clinical and Histopathologic Diagnosis*, 2nd edn. Blackwell, Oxford, pp. 562–694.

Gudjonsson T., Adriance M.C., Sternlicht M.D. et al. (2005) Myoepithelial cells: Their origin and function in breast morphogenesis and neoplasia. *J Mammary Gland Biol 10(3)*:261–272.

Hartmann K., Day M.J., Thiry E. et al. (2015) Feline injection-site sarcoma: ABCD guidelines on prevention and management. *J Feline Med Surg 17(7)*:606–613.

Hayden D.W., Johnston S.D., Kiang D.T. et al. (1981) Feline mammary hypertrophy/fibroadenoma complex: Clinical and hormonal aspects. *Am J Vet Res 42*:1699–1703.

Hayes H.M. Jr, Milne K.L., Mandell C.P. (1981) Epidemiological features of feline mammary carcinoma. *Vet Rec 108(22)*:476–479.

Haziroglu R., Haligur M., Keles H. (2014) Histopathological and immunohistochemical studies of apocrine sweat gland adenocarcinomas in cats. *Vet Comp Oncol 12(1)*:85–90.

Henry C., Herrera C. (2013) Mast cell tumors in cats: Clinical update and possible new treatment avenues. *J Feline Med Surg 15*:41–47.

Hirai T., Mubarak M., Kimura T. et al. (1997) Apocrine gland tumor of the eyelid in a dog. *Vet Pathol 34(3)*:232–234.

Hoinghaus R., Hewicker-Trautwein M., Mischke R. (2008) Immunocytochemical differentiation of canine mesenchymal tumors in cytologic imprint preparations. *Vet Clin Pathol 37*:104–111.

Im K.S., Kim N.H., Lim H.Y. et al. (2014) Analysis of a new histological and molecular-based classification of canine mammary neoplasia. *Vet Pathol 51(3)*:549–559.

Ito T., Kadosawa T., Mochizuki M. et al. (1996) Prognosis of malignant mammary tumor in 53 cats. *J Vet Med Sci 58(8)*:723–726.

King B.L., Crisi G.M., Tsai S.C., Haffty B.G., Phillips R.F., Rimm D.L. (2002) Immunocytochemical analysis of breast cells obtained by ductal lavage. *Cancer 96*:244–249.

Liebich H. (2019) Common integument. In: *Veterinary Histology of Domestic Mammals and Birds*, 5th edn. 5M Publishing Ltd, Sheffield, p. 336.

London C.A., Thamm D.H. (2020) Mast cell tumors. In: *Withrow & MacEwen's Small Animal Clinical Oncology*, 6th edn. (eds. D.M. Vail, D.H. Thamm, J.M. Liptak) Elsevier, St. Louis, p. 604.

MacDougall L.D. (2003) Mammary fibroadenomatous hyperplasia in a young cat attributed to treatment with megestrol acetate. *Can Vet J 44(3)*:227–229.

MacEwen E.G., Hayes A.A., Harvey H.J. et al. (1984) Prognostic factors for feline mammary tumors. *J Am Vet Med Assoc 185(2)*:201–204.

Masserdotti C., Bonfanti U., De Lorenzi D. et al. (2006) Use of Oil Red O stain in the cytologic diagnosis of canine liposarcoma. *Vet Clin Pathol 35*:37–41.

Masserdotti C., Drigo M. (2022) Cytologic features of reactive fibroplasia in cutaneous and subcutaneous lesions of dogs: A retrospective study. *Vet Clin Pathol 51*:244–251.

Mauldin E.A., Peters-Kennedy J. (2016) Integumentary system. In: *Jubb, Kennedy and Palmer's Pathology of Domestic Animals*, 6th edn. (ed. M.G. Maxie) Elsevier, St Louis, pp. 509–736.

Mays M.B., Bergeron J.A. (1986) Cutaneous histiocytosis in dogs. *J Am Vet Med Assoc 188*:377–381.

McCourt M.R., Levine G.M., Breshears M.A., Wall C.R., Meinkoth J.H. (2018) Metastatic disease in a dog with a well-differentiated perianal gland tumor. *Vet Clin Pathol 47*:649–653.

Meinkoth J.H., Cowell R.L., Tyler R.D. (2020) Cell types and criteria of malignancy. In: *Cowell and Tyler's Diagnostic Cytology and Hematology of the Dog and Cat*, 5th edn. (eds. A.C. Valenciano, R.L. Cowell) Elsevier, St. Louis, p. 18.

Meuten D.J., Cooper B.U., Capen C.C. et al. (1981) Hypercalcemia associated with an adenocarcinoma derived from the apocrine glands of the anal sac. *Vet Pathol 18*:454–471.

Miller W.H., Griffin C.E., Campbell K.L. (2013) Parasitic skin disease. In: *Muller and Kirk's Small Animal Dermatology*, 7th edn. (eds W.H. Miller, C.E. Griffin, K.L. Campbell) Elsevier, St. Louis, p. 296–320.

Moore A.R. (2023) Diagnosing multiple myeloma and related disorders. *Vet Clin North Am Small Anim Pract 53(1)*:101–120.

Moore P.F. (2014) A review of histiocytic diseases of dogs and cats. *Vet Pathol 51(1)*:167–184.

Moore P.F. (2023) Histiocytic diseases. *Vet Clin North Am Small Anim Pract 53(1)*:121–140.

Moore P.F., Affolter V.K., Vernau W. (2006) Canine hemophagocytic histiocytic sarcoma: A proliferative disorder of CD11d+ macrophages. *Vet Pathol 43*:632–645.

Murgia C., Pritchard J.K., Kim S.Y. et al. (2006) Clonal origin and evolution of a transmissible cancer. *Cell 126*:477–487.

Neihaus S.A., Winter J.E., Goring R.L. et al. (2010) Primary clitoral adenocarcinoma with secondary hypercalcemia of malignancy in a dog. *J Am Anim Hosp Assoc 46(3)*:193–196.

Paes P.R., Horta R.S., Luza L.C., Pierezan F., Costa M.P., Lavalle G.E. (2022) Inclusion of fibroblasts and collagen fibrils in the cytologic grading of canine cutaneous mast cell tumors. *Vet Clin Pathol 51*:339–348.

Piccione J., Dial S.M. (2020) Cytologic appearance of hibernoma in two dogs. *Vet Clin Pathol. 49*:125–129.

Pinto da Cunha N., Ghisleni G., Scarampella F., Fabbrini F., Sforna M., Cornegliani L., Caniatti M., Avallone G., Moore P., Roccabianca P. (2014) Cytologic and immunocytochemical characterization of feline progressive histiocytosis. *Vet Clin Pathol 43*:428–436.

Raskin R.E. (2023) General categories of cytologic interpretation. In: *Canine and Feline Cytopathology: A Color Atlas and Interpretation Guide*, 4th edn. (eds. R.E. Raskin, D.J. Meyer, K.M. Boes) Elsevier, St. Louis, p. 15.

Raskin R.E., Conrado F.O. (2023) Integumentary system. In: *Canine and Feline Cytopathology: A Color Atlas and Interpretation Guide*, 4th edn. (eds. R.E. Raskin, D.J. Meyer, K.M. Boes) Elsevier, St. Louis, p. 35.

Roccabianca P., Schulman F.Y., Avallone G., Foster R.A., Scruggs J.L., Dittmer K. et al. (2020) *Surgical Pathology of Tumors of Domestic Animals: Volume 3: Tumors of Soft Tissue* (ed. M. Kiupel) Davis-Thompson DVM Foundation.

Romansik E.M., Reilly C.M., Kass P.H. et al. (2007) Mitotic index is predictive for survival for canine cutaneous mast cell tumors. *Vet Pathol 44*:335–341.

Rosol T.J., Capen C.C., Danks J.A. et al. (1990) Identification of parathyroid hormone-related protein in canine apocrine adenocarcinomas of the anal sac. *Vet Pathol 27*:89–95.

Rout E.D., Hoon-Hanks L.L., Gustafson T.L. et al. (2016) What is your diagnosis? Clitoral mass in a dog. *Vet Clin Pathol 45*:197–198.

Rutteman G.R., Misdorp W. (1993) Hormonal background of canine and feline mammary tumours. *J Reprod Fertil 47*:483–487.

Ryseff J.K., Bohn A.A. (2012) Detection of alkaline phosphatase in canine cells previously stained with Wright–Giemsa and its utility in differentiating osteosarcoma from other mesenchymal tumors. *Vet Clin Pathol 41*:391–395.

Saba C.F., Rogers K.S., Newman S.J. et al. (2007) Mammary gland tumors in male dogs. *J Vet Intern Med 21(5)*:1056–1059.

Sabattini S., Bettini G. (2010) Prognostic value of histologic and immunohistochemical features in feline cutaneous mast cell tumors. *Vet Pathol 47*:643–653.

Sabattini S, Bettini G. (2019) Grading cutaneous mast cell tumors in cats. *Vet Pathol 56(1)*:43–49.

Scarpa F., Sabattini S., Bettini G. (2016) Cytological grading of canine cutaneous mast cell tumours. *Vet Comp Oncol 14*:245–251.

Schneider R., Dorn C.R., Taylor D.O. (1969) Factors influencing canine mammary cancer development and postsurgical survival. *J Natl Cancer Inst 43*:1249–1261.

Scruggs J.L., LeBlanc C.J. (2015) Identification of blue staining vaccine-derived material in inflammatory lesions using cultured canine macrophages. *Vet Clin Pathol 44*:152–156.

Sebastian K.N., Magestro L., Kiupel M., Radin M.J. (2021) What is your diagnosis? Lingual mass aspirate from a dog. *Vet Clin Pathol 50*:615–617.

Seixas F., Palmeira C., Pires M.A. et al. (2011) Grade is an independent prognostic factor for feline mammary carcinomas: A clinicopathological and survival analysis. *Vet J 187*:65–71.

Sharma D., Goldschmidt M.H., Vernau W., Dusick A.F. (2021) What is your diagnosis? Dermal nodules in a dog. *Vet Clin Pathol 50*:81–83.

Simko E., Wilcock B.P., Yager J.A. (2003) A retrospective study of 44 canine apocrine sweat gland adenocarcinomas. *Can Vet J 44(1)*:38–42.

Simon D., Schoenrock E., Nolte I. et al. (2009) Cytologic examination of fine-needle aspirates from mammary gland tumors in the dog: Diagnostic accuracy with comparison to histopathology and association with postoperative outcome. *Vet Clin Pathol 38*:521–528.

Smith A.H., Goldschmidt M.H., McManus P.M. (2002) A comparative review of melanocytic neoplasms. *Vet Pathol 39*:651–678.

Solano-Gallego L., Masserdotti C. (2023) Reproductive system. In: *Canine and Feline Cytopathology: A Color Atlas and Interpretation Guide*, 4th edn. (eds. R.E. Raskin, D.J. Meyer, K.M. Boes) Elsevier, St. Louis, p. 440.

Sorenmo K.U., Worley D.R., Goldschmidt M.H. (2020) Tumors of the mammary gland. In: *Withrow & MacEwen's Small Animal Clinical Oncology*, 6th edn. (eds. D.M. Vail, D.H. Thamm, J.M. Liptak) Elsevier, St. Louis, p. 604.

Strefezzi R.D.F., Xavier J.G., Catão-Dias J.L. (2003) Morphometry of canine cutaneous mast cell tumors. *Vet Pathol 40*:268–275.

Viste J.R., Myers S.L., Singh B. et al. (2002) Feline mammary adenocarcinoma: Tumor size as a prognostic indicator. *Can Vet J 43(1)*:33–37.

Weijer K., Hart A.A. (1983) Prognostic factors in feline mammary carcinoma. *J Natl Cancer Inst 70(4)*:709–716.

Weishaar K.M., Thamm D.H., Worley D.R., Kamstock D.A. (2014) Correlation of nodal mast cells with clinical outcome in dogs with mast cell tumour and a proposed classification system for the evaluation of node metastasis. *J Comp Pathol 151(4)*:329–338.

Welle M., Linder K. (2021) The Integument. In: *Pathological Basis of Veterinary Disease*, 7th edn. (ed. J.F. Zachary) Elsevier, St Louis, pp. 1095–1262.

White B., Bellnap E. (2015) Clinical approach to canine eyelid disease: Blepharitis. *Today's Veterinary Practice 5(4)*:74–79.

Yamazaki H., Takagi S., Oh N. et al. (2014) Comparative analysis of mRNA expression of surface antigens between histiocytic and nonhistiocytic sarcoma in dogs. *J Vet Intern Med 28*:204–210.

Yearley J.H., Stanton C., Olivry T. (2007) Phagocytic plasmacytoma in a dog. *Vet Clin Pathol 3*:293–296.

Zappulli V., Rasotto R., Caliari D., Mainenti M., Peña L., Goldschmidt M. H., Kiupel M. (2015) Prognostic evaluation of feline mammary carcinomas: A review of the literature. *Vet Pathol 52(1)*:46–60.

Zappulli V., Pena L., Rasotto R., Goldschmidt M., Gama A., Scruggs J.L. et al. (2020) *Surgical Pathology of Tumors of Domestic Animals: Volume 2: Mammary Tumors* (ed. M. Kiupel) Davis-Thompson DVM Foundation.

CHAPTER 5

CYTOLOGY OF LYMPHOID TISSUES

Stefano Comazzi and Amy L. MacNeill

LYMPH NODE

Indications for sampling

Lymph node aspiration is extremely safe, rapid, easy to perform, and is recommended for all enlarged lymph nodes (both in cases of isolated and generalized lymphadenomegaly). In addition, lymph node cytology is indicated in many cases with minimally enlarged lymph nodes to evaluate if there is an underlying infectious disease (e.g. *Leishmania* spp., *Toxoplasma* spp., yeast), to provide material for molecular diagnostics, or to stage malignant neoplastic diseases. The specific lymph nodes that are draining an area where a primary lesion is located should be sampled to evaluate the patient for spread of disease. The identification of the sentinel lymph node (i.e. the first node draining a lesion) is challenging in veterinary medicine and often requires mapping via vital dyes. Sampling multiple lymph nodes in the draining area is suggested in order to check early tumor dissemination. Sampling multiple lymph nodes should also be performed when a systemic disease is suspected, as cytologic features may vary among different nodes.

SAMPLING TECHNIQUES

The most appropriate sampling technique depends on the site and the gross appearance of the node to be sampled as well as the tests being performed on the sample. For cytologic evaluation of lymph nodes, fine needle aspiration (FNA) or fenestration is performed as described for other solid tissues (see Chapter 1). As with large masses, aspiration of peripheral areas of the node is preferred, since the center of a large node could be entirely necrotic. Alternatively, impression smears can be prepared following surgical excision of a lymph node and may provide useful diagnostic information due to the extreme rapidity and morphologic details of cytologic impressions. It is recommended that multiple slides are prepared and a subset is stained with a Romanowsky-type stain for microscopic evaluation. Previously stained slides can be used in some immunocytochemistry (ICC) protocols; others require unstained slides. Stained or unstained cytology slides can be submitted for polymerase chain reaction (PCR)-based diagnostics. Samples collected for analysis by flow cytometry should be placed into a suspension medium (e.g. Roswell Park Memorial Institute (RPMI) 1640, phosphate buffered saline, or other physiologic saline solution with the addition of 10% of serum of the same animal). An aliquot of the sample collected into suspension medium can be processed for use in PCR assays or cytocentrifuged at approximately 100 g for 3 minutes for microscopic examination. If microbiology cultures are required, a portion of the sample should be placed into a sterile tube.

SAMPLE STABILITY

Fixed smears may be stored at room temperature for several days before staining and if ICC is requested, they can be fixed in methanol-acetone, wrapped in foil, and stored at −20°C. Immunoreactivity is stable for several months. For flow cytometry, cells should be suspended in a liquid medium at a final concentration of 10^6 cells/ml, kept refrigerated, and processed within 24 hours. Some specific preservatives or freezing techniques may also be used, but immunoreactivity may be affected, therefore fresh samples are preferred. One or more cytologic slides should always accompany samples for flow cytometry, because they are necessary for correct evaluation of flow cytometric results. For molecular biology (e.g. PCR for analysis of T- and B-cell receptor gene rearrangements or detection of infectious diseases), tubes containing cell suspensions can be stored at −80°C. Also, stained or unstained cytology slides can be submitted for PCR analysis after being stored for extended periods of time.

Cytologic features related to sampling

Often, FNAs of lymph nodes are unsuccessful and tissue surrounding or near the lymph node is aspirated instead. Mandibular nodes are in close proximity to salivary glands. Thus, aspiration of salivary epithelial cells is not uncommon (Figure 5.1). Samples from the salivary gland are cellular and viscous. They contain a proteinaceous (mucinous) background that causes windrowing of cells in the sample. Typically, most cells are glandular epithelial cells with abundant vacuolated cytoplasm and a small rounded nucleus with dense chromatin. Occasional clusters of ductal epithelial cells forming small tubular structures may be observed. These cells have scant, lightly basophilic cytoplasm, distinct cell junctions, and a round nucleus. Variable numbers of small lymphocytes may be seen if the lymph node was concurrently aspirated, but lymphoglandular bodies are generally scarce. Neutrophils and other inflammatory cell types are not expected unless there is an ongoing disease process causing sialadenitis. Many lymph nodes (popliteal for instance) are surrounded by adipose

DOI: 10.1201/9781003258551-5

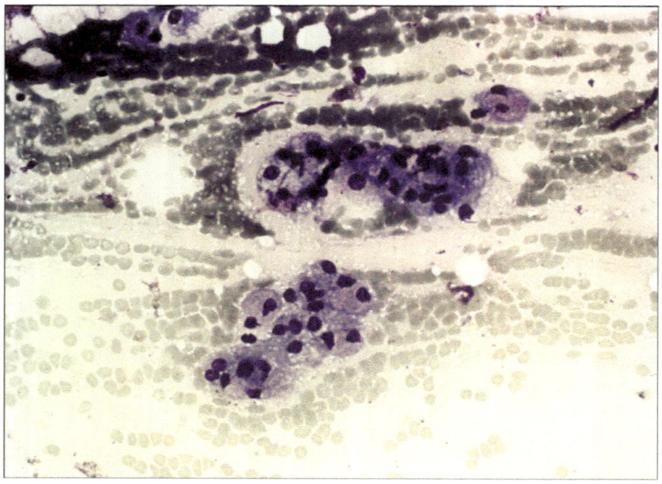

Figure 5.1 Dog, mandibular lymph node, FNA. Large clusters of glandular epithelial cells, likely from the salivary gland adjacent to the lymph node (May–Grünwald–Giemsa, 400× magnification).

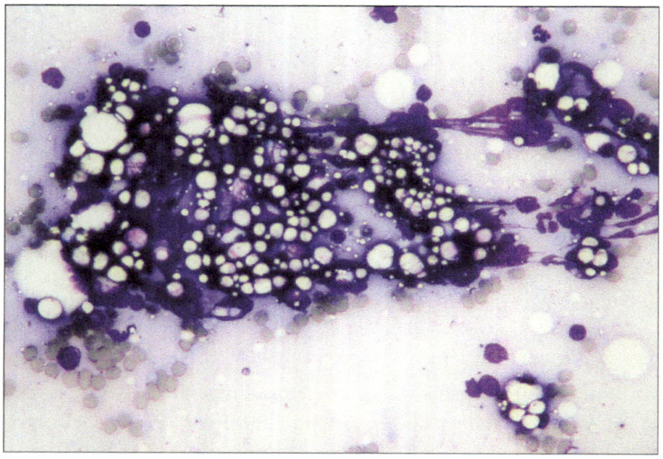

Figure 5.2 Dog, popliteal lymph node, FNA. Presence of lipid droplets and aggregate adipocytes from the adjacent adipose tissue intermingled with lymphoid cells (May–Grünwald–Giemsa, 600× magnification).

tissue, so samples from these nodes frequently show a scarce cellularity and an abundant population of normal adipocytes (Figure 5.2). Sampling internal lymph nodes is usually ultrasound guided. Ultrasound gel may be found on the smear (Figure 5.3) and should not be confused with metachromatic/azurophilic granules or microorganisms.

Necrosis and disrupted cells are frequent if a very large lymph node is sampled.

Additional techniques to refine cytologic diagnosis

IMMUNOPHENOTYPING

Due to the different prognoses associated with T- and B-cell lymphomas, immunophenotyping of neoplastic cells is routinely performed to subtype lymphoma in the dog (Marconato et al., 2013a).

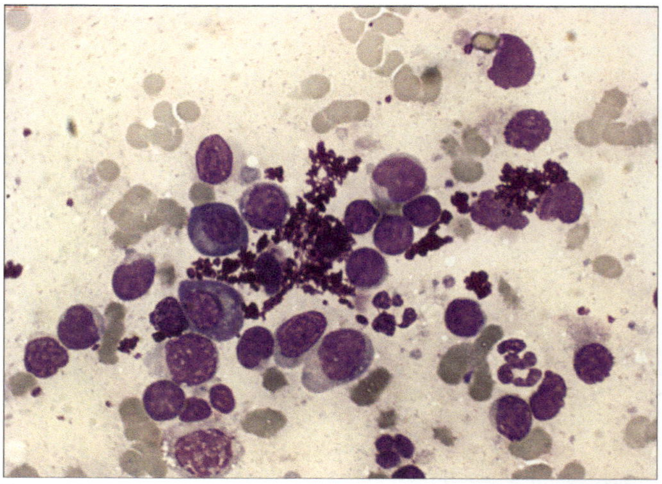

Figure 5.3 Cat, intestinal lymph node, FNA. Abundant purple granular material referable to ultrasound gel, among lymphoid and plasma cells from the reactive lymph node (May–Grünwald–Giemsa, 1,000× magnification).

A large panel of specific antibodies is now available for both dogs and cats (Table 5.1) and may work both in ICC and flow cytometry protocols. Each immunophenotyping technique has some pros and cons. One advantage of ICC is that immunolabeling can be performed on stored smears (months after sampling if smears are adequately fixed and frozen). Another advantage is that relatively low numbers of cells are required to determine if cells are positive for a given antigen (Caniatti et al., 1996). Labeling for more than one antigen can be performed on a single slide using multiple fluorescent secondary antibodies or chromogens, but more commonly, one slide is needed for each antigen detected by ICC. Also, ICC is moderately time-consuming and the number of cells evaluated is low in comparison with flow cytometry, possibly affecting the final diagnosis if a mixed population of cells is present. Flow cytometry has several advantages: (1) analysis of very large numbers of cells, which allows for resolution of poorly represented populations of cells (such as in mixed populations, residual disease, or initial disease); (2) detection of multiple cell markers on a single cell; (3) accurate quantitation of positive cells; (4) high reproducibility and accuracy; and (5) extreme rapidity, with results already available in few hours from sampling. As a disadvantage, flow cytometry requires fresh samples and a minimum of 2×10^6 cells. The issue of storage may be partly overcome by using specific preservatives or freezing media, but these are poorly standardized in veterinary medicine and a fresh sample is preferable (Comazzi & Gelain, 2011).

PCR to detect antigen receptor rearrangements (PARR) and specific PCR techniques for diagnosis of infectious diseases may help to solve differentials among neoplastic and reactive diseases (Lana et al., 2006a). Recent papers identified 100% sensitivity and specificity of PARR for known cases of lymphoma *vs.* non-lymphoma diagnosed using fine needle aspirates from dogs (Ehrhart et al., 2018). For feline lymphoma some authors reported 78% sensitivity and 81% accuracy for B-cell lymphoma (Welter et al., 2021) but undetermined specificity for T-cell lymphoma (Moore et al., 2005). Therefore, the lineage

Table 5.1 **List of the most common antibodies validated for immunophenotyping canine and feline hematopoietic diseases. Different antibodies and clones show different immunoreactivity in different sample and fixation type**

Immunophenotypic marker	Cell type identified	Validated in
CD1	Dendritic cells, histiocytes	Dog
CD3ε (T cell receptor)	T cells	Dog, cat
CD4	T helper cells, T regulatory cells (Tregs), neutrophils (dogs)	Dog, cat
CD5 (scavenger receptor)	T cell	Dog, cat
CD8	Cytotoxic T cells	Dog, cat
CD11b	Myeloid lineage	Dog, cat
CD11d	Neutrophils, macrophages, splenic T lymphocytes, granular lymphocytes	Dog, cat
CD14 (LPS-BP receptor)	Monocytes, macrophages	Dog, cat
CD18 (integrin β2)	All leukocytes (higher in granulocytes and monocytes)	Dog, cat
CD19	B cells	Dog
CD20	B cells	Dog
CD21 (complement receptor)	Mature B cells	Dog, cat
CD22	Mature B cells	Dog
CD25 (IL-2RA)	Activated lymphocytes	Dog
CD3 (CD62L)	Hematopoietic precursor cells	Dog
CD41/61 (GPIIb/IIIa)	Platelets and megakaryocytes	Dog
CD44	All leukocytes, erythrocyte precursors	Dog
CD45 (common leukocyte antigen)	All leukocytes	Dog
CD79a (Igα of the B-cell receptor)	B cells	Dog, cat
CD117 (c-Kit)	Mastocytes, some hematopoietic precursor cells	Dog
CD204 (scavenger receptor)	Myeloid cells, histiocytes	Dog
FoxP3	Activated lymphocytes, Tregs	Dog
Ionized calcium-binding adapter molecule 1 (IBA1)	Macrophages	Dog
IgE	Mastocytes, B cells	Dog
MHC class II	Monocytes, macrophages, B cells, some T cell subsets	Dog
Pax5	B cells	Dog, cat
Surface immunoglobulin (IgG or IgM)	Mature B cells	Dog
TCRαβ	Most T cells	Dog
TCRγδ	Splenic or intestinal T cells	Dog

of neoplastic lymphocytes is assessed by PARR with a sufficient reliability, even though immunophenotyping techniques are the method of choice and provide a higher accuracy rate (Thaleim et al., 2013). If necessary, DNA for PCR techniques may be extracted from stained cytologic smears or from paraffin embedded biopsies. Unfortunately, PCR is time-consuming and expensive and results should be interpreted with caution since false-positive and false-negative results are reported in many different conditions.

MICROBIOLOGY

Culture via standard microbiology techniques is rarely performed using lymph node aspirates and is generally limited to selected bacterial diseases. The main advantage is that these techniques can also provide data about antibiotic susceptibility, which is clinically useful.

Normal anatomy and cytology

The lymph node parenchyma is surrounded by a connective tissue capsule extending inwards in fibrous septae. Subcapsular sinuses drain lymph from the periphery into the cortical sinuses and sinusoids. The cortex of a lymph node is formed by primary and secondary follicles. Primary follicles are mainly composed of small, resting B lymphocytes. The secondary follicles develop after antigenic stimulation (Figure 5.4). In histologic sections of lymph nodes, areas of B lymphocyte development can be identified by a central, pale-staining area, representing the germinal center where differentiation occurs, and a thin peripheral rim of more intensely basophilic cells where clonal expansion occurs. Low numbers of macrophages and dendritic cells are also present in germinal centers. The germinal center is surrounded by a dark layer of small B memory cells with clumped chromatin called the mantle cell zone. In the dog, there is a thin layer of light colored, medium-sized macronucleolated cells

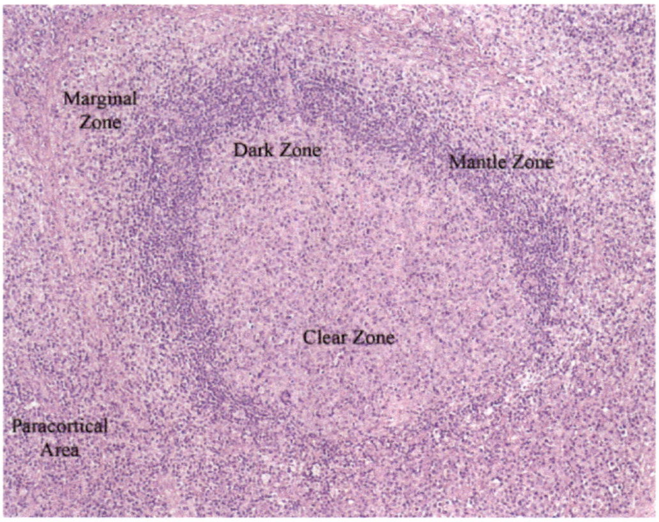

Figure 5.4 Dog, peripheral lymph node, histology. A secondary follicle with central germinal center (clear and dark zone) surrounded by an inner rim of mantle cells and an outer rim called the marginal zone (H&E, 100× magnification) (courtesy L. Aresu).

around the follicles termed the marginal zone. The paracortex is the interfollicular tissue and is composed mainly of small T lymphocytes, rare T immunoblasts, interdigitating cells, and macrophages. Lastly, the medullary cords are comprised mainly of plasma cells, mature lymphocytes, and macrophages, which are adjacent to sinus spaces.

The main cytologic appearances of the different cells present in normal lymph node aspirates are described in Figure 5.5 and Table 5.2. Although these cell types can be identified, it is the ratio of small, intermediate, and large lymphocytes that is most important to assess cytologically. In a normal lymph node aspirate, approximately 80% of cells are small lymphocytes, 15% are intermediate-sized lymphocytes, and 5% are large lymphocytes. Small percentages of other cell types (plasma cells, macrophages/histiocytes, neutrophils, mast cells, and eosinophils) also may be observed in normal lymphoid tissue. Phagocytized cellular remains are often seen in the cytoplasm of lymph node macrophages (also named tingible body macrophages). Interspersed among the cells, a moderate number of small, round, gray-blue cytoplasmic fragments (lymphoglandular bodies) are normally recognized in cytologic smears. They may increase if cellular fragility is increased, particularly in lymphoma cases, but also in non-neoplastic conditions.

Lymph node hyperplasia

No precise morphologic distinction between normal and hyperplastic cytologic lymphocyte populations exists. However, lymph node hyperplasia is suspected when node enlargement is present and lymph node cytology is normal without detectable inflammatory or neoplastic cells. Subtypes of lymphoid hyperplasia that may be recognized histologically are listed in Table 5.3. Follicular hyperplasia can be difficult to differentiate from lymphoma in cats in cytologic samples (Figure 5.6). Paracortical hyperplasia is less often confused with lymphoma, as small lymphocytes predominate (Figures 5.7,

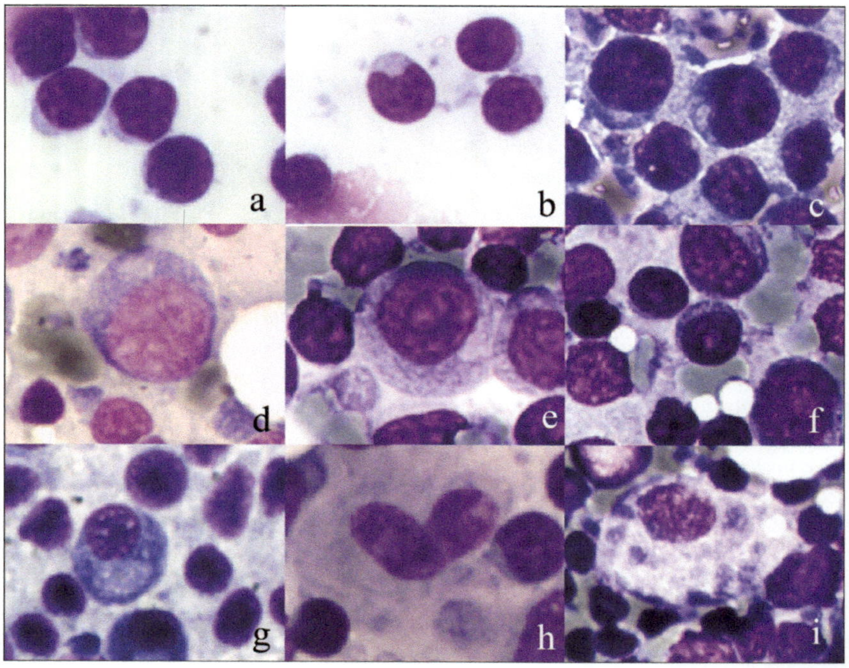

Figure 5.5 Dog, peripheral lymph node, FNA. Cell populations that may be found in a normal lymph node. a, small lymphocytes; b, centrocytes; c, lymphoblast; d, centroblast; e, immunoblast; f, medium-sized macronucleolated cells (marginal zone); g, plasma cells; h, interdigitating cells; i, macrophage with tingible bodies. See text for description (May–Grünwald–Giemsa, 1,000× magnification).

Table 5.2 **Subtypes of cells that may be identified in cytologically normal canine lymph node samples**

Cell subtype	% expected	Cytologic description	Origin
Small lymphocytes	>80%	Small lymphocytes; nuclear diameter 7–10 μm; scarce rim of basophilic cytoplasm; round or slightly indented nucleus; clumped chromatin; no visible nucleolus	B or T lymphocytes
Centrocytes	5–10%	Small to intermediate-sized lymphocytes; nuclear diameter 10–14 μm; moderate amount of clear cytoplasm; cleaved nucleus; dense, unclumped chromatin; no visible nucleolus	Follicular B cells
Centroblasts	1–5%	Intermediate to large lymphocytes; nuclear diameter 14–21 μm; moderate amount of deeply basophilic cytoplasm; occasional cytoplasmic vacuoles; eccentric, round nucleus; decondensed, finely stippled chromatin; multiple, often peripheral, nucleoli	Follicular B cells
Immunoblasts	1–5%	Large lymphocytes; nuclear diameter up to 28 μm; abundant, deeply basophilic cytoplasm; occasional cytoplasmic vacuoles; round nucleus; finely stippled chromatin; one central prominent nucleolus	B or T lymphocytes
Lymphoblasts	<1%	Small lymphoid precursors; nuclear diameter 7–14 μm; scarce, clear cytoplasm; irregular nuclear margins; often clear perinuclear halo; fine chromatin; poorly distinguishable nucleoli	B or T lymphocytes
Medium-sized macronucleolated cells	<1% (Absent in cats)	Small to intermediate lymphocytes; nuclear diameter 10–14 μm; abundant, deeply basophilic cytoplasm; round nucleus; single, centrally located, prominent nucleolus	Marginal zone B cells (Fournel-Fleury et al., 1997)
Plasma cells	<2%	Mature lymphocytes; nuclear diameter 7–14 μm; abundant deeply basophilic cytoplasm; often contains a perinuclear clear halo (Golgi zone); eccentric, round nucleus; clumped	Medullary cord B
Flame cells	<1%	Plasma cells with brightly eosinophilic cytoplasmic borders	Medullary cord B cells
Mott cells	<1%	Plasma cells containing several clear, distinct cytoplasmic vacuoles (Russell bodies)	Medullary cord B cells
Dendritic cells	<1%	Poorly defined cytoplasm with thin prolongations; one or more oval nuclei	Follicular histiocytes
Interdigitating cells	<1%	Abundant, pale cytoplasm with poorly defined margins; convoluted to twisted nucleus; pale chromatin	Paracortical histiocytes
Macrophages	<2%	Abundant, pale cytoplasm; often phagocytic with tingible bodies; oval to convoluted nucleus; may form multinucleated giant cells if reactive	Paracortical and medullary cord histiocytes
Inflammatory cells	<5%	Neutrophils	Hematopoietic cells
	<3%	Eosinophils	
	<3%	Mast cells	

Table 5.3 **Classifications of lymph node hyperplasia**

Histologic classification	Histologic description	Cytologic description	Cytologic differentials
Follicular hyperplasia (Figure 5.6)	Prominent germinal center with well-defined polarity	Increased centroblasts (15–20%) increased centrocytes; increased mitoses; plasma cells	Lymphoma; reactive lymph node
Paracortical hyperplasia (Figures 5.7, 5.8)	Paracortical expansion with many small lymphocytes, variable T immunoblasts and several interdigitating cells	Increased numbers of small lymphocytes, some immunoblasts	Lymphoma

5.8). Importantly when atypical lymphoid hyperplasia is listed as a cytologic interpretation, lymphoma should remain a differential for lymph node enlargement (Figure 5.9). Atypical hyperplasia indicates that, although cell subsets are not present in abnormal numbers, the small or intermediate-sized lymphocytes have a remarkably uniform morphology or a slightly atypical morphology (e.g. decreased nuclear to cytoplasmic ratio, cleaved nuclei, hand mirror appearance) that raises suspicion for neoplastic transformation. In these cases, molecular diagnostics (PARR or flow cytometry) may provide additional information about the underlying disease process. Transitory lymphoid hyperplasia in young cats can have cytologic features that

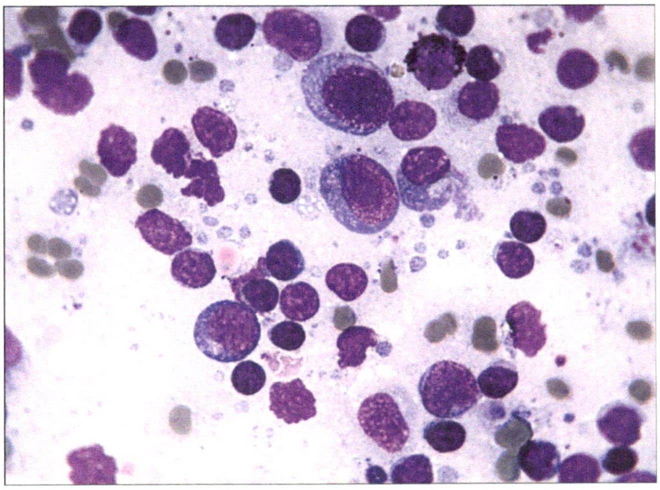

Figure 5.6 Cat, enlarged subcutaneous lymph node, FNA. Follicular hyperplasia. An admixed population of small lymphocytes, large blast cells, a plasma cell, and a mast cell. The presence of a continuum of lymphoid cells at different maturation stages and some plasma cells may help to differentiate follicular hyperplasia from an early phase of follicular lymphoma (May-Grünwald-Giemsa, 1,000× magnification).

strongly mimic lymphoma, being composed of a high prevalence of medium to large blasts, with fewer small lymphocytes and plasma cells (Figure 5.6). This condition is likely correlated to active infection

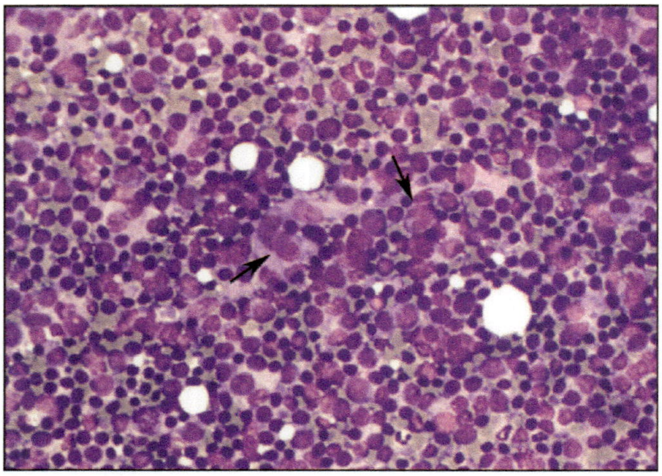

Figure 5.7 Dog, enlarged peripheral lymph node, FNA. Paracortical hyperplasia. Two large interdigitating cells (arrows) in a mixed lymphoid population are evident (May–Grünwald–Giemsa, 400× magnification).

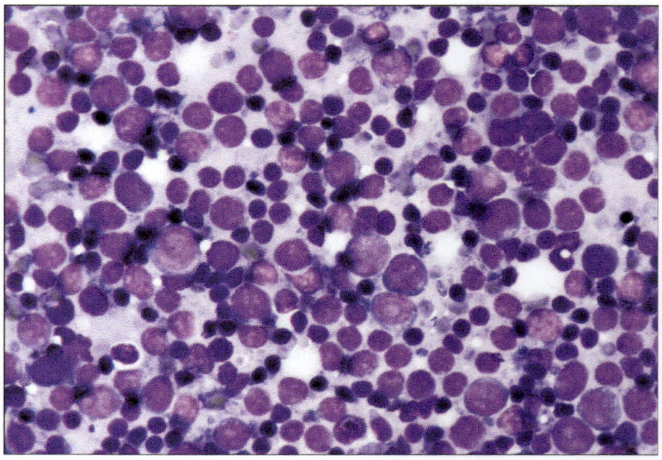

Figure 5.9 Cat, peripheral lymph node, FNB. Atypical lymphoid hyperplasia (distinctive peripheral lymph node hyperplasia). Increase of large blast cells mimicking lymphoma and residual small lymphocytes (May–Grünwald–Giemsa, 600 × magnification).

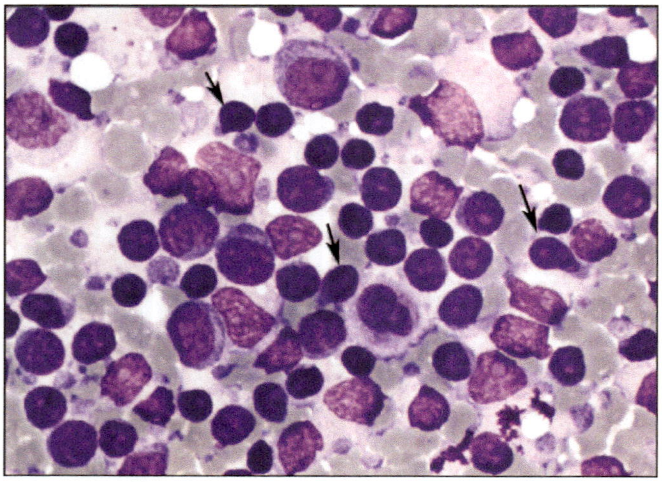

Figure 5.8 Dog, enlarged peripheral lymph node, FNA. Paracortical hyperplasia. A mixed population of lymphoid cells at different maturation stages and one interdigitating cell. Three 'hand-mirror'-shaped cells, likely of T cell origin, are indicated by the arrows (May–Grünwald–Giemsa, 1,000× magnification).

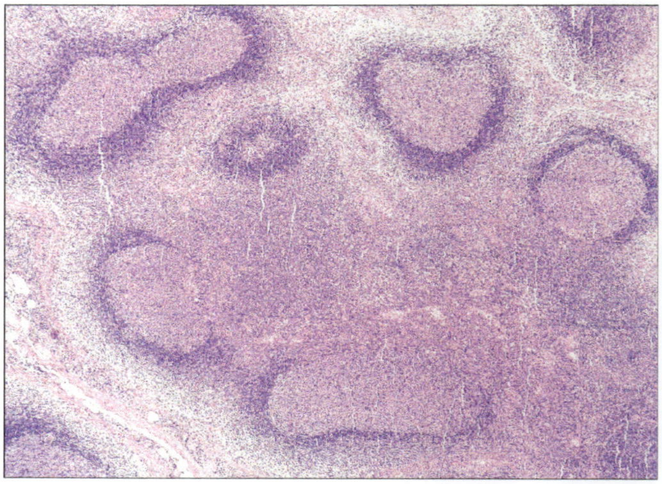

Figure 5.10 Dog, peripheral lymph node, histology. Reactive hyperplasia. Follicles are characterized by expansion of germinal centers, uniform mantle zones, and a well-defined marginal zone hyperplasia (H&E, 50× magnification) (courtesy L. Aresu).

with feline immunodeficiency virus or other infectious disease and generally regresses spontaneously within 2–3 months (Moore et al., 1986).

Lymphoid reactivity

Lymphoid reactivity is a common cause of lymphadenopathy. Histologically, there is an expansion of secondary follicles with increased numbers of plasma cells (Figure 5.10). Cytology samples from reactive lymph nodes are predominated by small lymphocytes, with mildly increased numbers of intermediate-sized lymphocytes and lymphoblasts, and increased numbers of plasma cells (>2% of the overall cell population) (Figures 5.11, 5.12). There may also be increased macrophages with tingible bodies. Plasma cell hyperplasia linked to cutaneous diseases with scaling and skin damage may be classified as dermatopathic lymphadenopathy (Figure 5.13). Dermatopathic lymphadenopathy is further characterized by several macrophages and abundant brown–black pigment (melanin granules) phagocytized by macrophages or scattered in the background. Scattered eosinophils, neutrophils, and mast cells also may be present.

If plasma cell hyperplasia is severe, plasma cell neoplasms should be considered as a differential. Typically, neoplastic plasma cells will have characteristics of malignancy, including bi- and multinucleation,

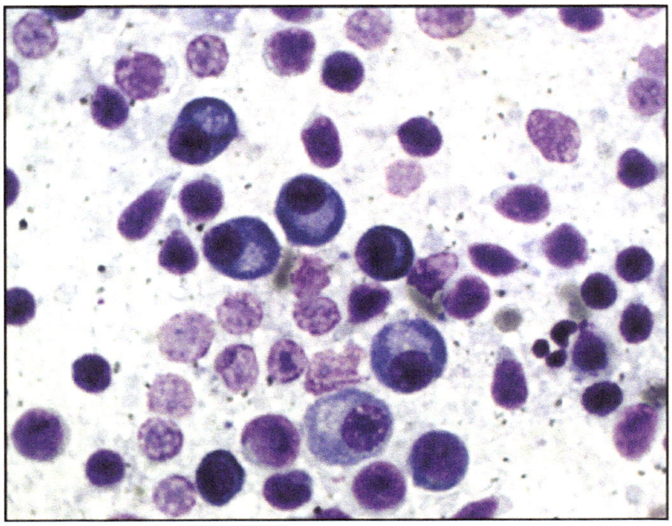
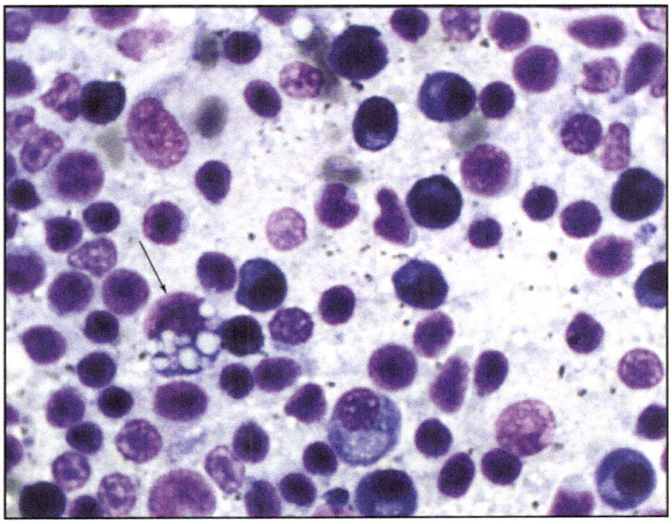

Figures 5.11, 5.12 Dog, peripheral lymph node, FNA. Plasma cell hyperplasia. Increased numbers of plasma cells are admixed with lymphocytes. A Mott cell with large clear vacuoles (Russell bodies) is indicated by the arrow (May–Grünwald–Giemsa, 1,000× magnification).

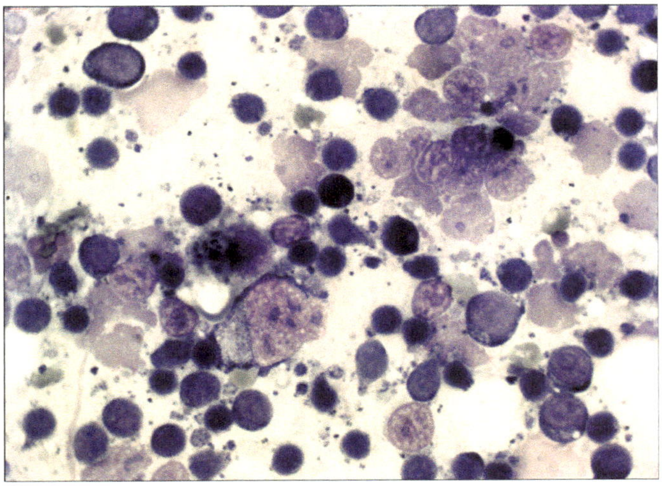

Figure 5.13 Dog, axillary lymph node, FNA. Dermatopathic lymphadenopathy. In the context of a plasma cell hyperplasia, small black melanin granules are found free in the background or phagocytized by macrophages. This feature is suggestive of the retention of melanin pigment from a cutaneous lesion (May–Grünwald–Giemsa, 1,000× magnification).

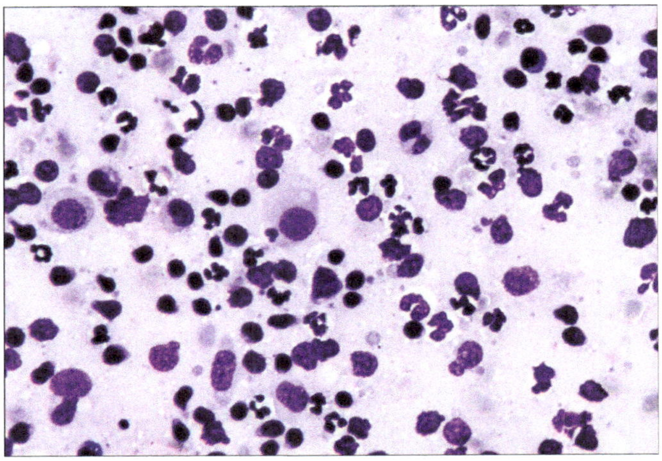

Figure 5.14 Dog, mandibular lymph node, FNA. Neutrophilic lymphadenitis. Numerous mildly degenerated neutrophil granulocytes in a background of residual lymph node (May–Grünwald–Giemsa, 600× magnification).

marked anisocytosis and anisokaryosis, and immature chromatin patterns. Ancillary tests, such as serum protein electrophoresis and radiographic screening for bony lysis, may be useful to differentiate between marked lymphoid reactivity and plasma cell neoplasms.

Lymphadenitis

Lymphadenitis is characterized by a conspicuous number of inflammatory cells, although the lymphoid population is generally prevalent, and may be associated with some degree of lymphoid hyperplasia or reactivity. Three different lymphadenitis types are defined according to the main characteristic inflammatory population.

Neutrophilic lymphadenitis

Suppurative (purulent) lymphadenitis is diagnosed when more than 5% of cells in the sample are neutrophils, which may be degenerate and/or contain bacteria (Figure 5.14). Occasionally, the lymphoid population is almost completely substituted by neutrophils. Bacterial infections are the most common cause, but neoplastic or immune-mediated diseases may lead to such a feature. In severe cases, necrosis may be present. As the disease process becomes more chronic,

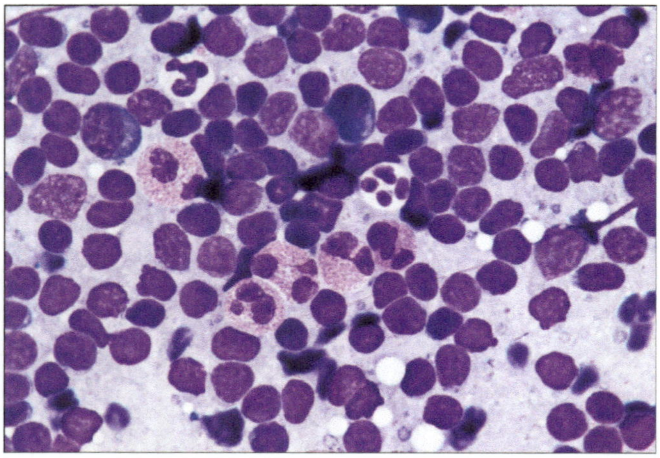

Figure 5.15 Cat, peripheral lymph node, FNA. Eosinophilic lymphadenitis. Several eosinophils are evident in a background of resident lymphoid cells. Neutrophils and a plasma cell are also present (May-Grünwald-Giemsa, 1,000× magnification).

increased numbers of macrophages will infiltrate the lymph node and a diagnosis of pyogranulomatous lymphadenitis should be made. Chronic bacterial and fungal infections are commonly associated with the development of pyogranulomatous lymphadenitis.

Eosinophilic lymphadenitis

In cases of eosinophilic lymphadenitis, more than 3% of cells are eosinophils (Figure 5.15). Diseases associated with eosinophilic lymphadenitis include parasitic infections (endoparasites or ectoparasites), hypersensitivity reactions (particularly allergic dermatitis), and paraneoplastic inflammation. Feline eosinophilic granuloma complex or hypereosinophilic syndrome could also cause eosinophilic lymphadenitis. Peripheral blood should be evaluated to rule out the possibility that the eosinophils in the aspirate are a component of blood contamination, rather than an infiltrating cell population in the lymphoid tissue.

Granulomatous lymphadenitis

Granulomatous lymphadenitis is characterized by an increased number (>3%) of histiocytic cells or macrophages (Figures 5.16, 5.17). Epithelioid macrophages or multinucleated giant cells may also be present. In some cases, the causative agent may be detected. Systemic fungal infections, including aspergillosis (Figure 5.18),

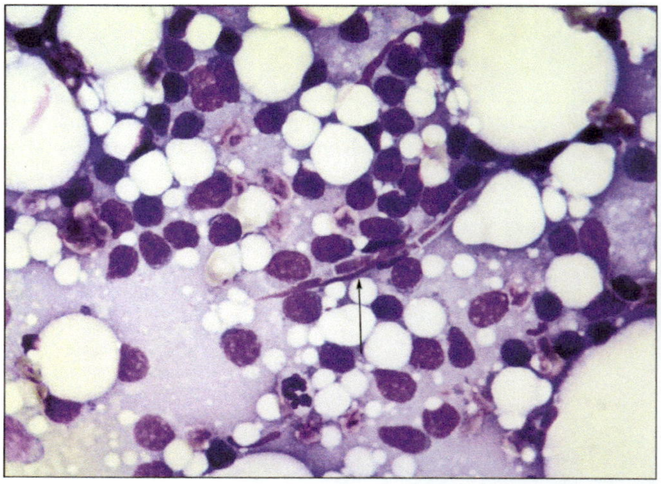

Figure 5.18 Dog, peripheral lymph node, FNA. Aspergillosis. A septated hypha is indicated by the arrow (May-Grünwald-Giemsa, 1,000× magnification) (courtesy U. Bonfanti).

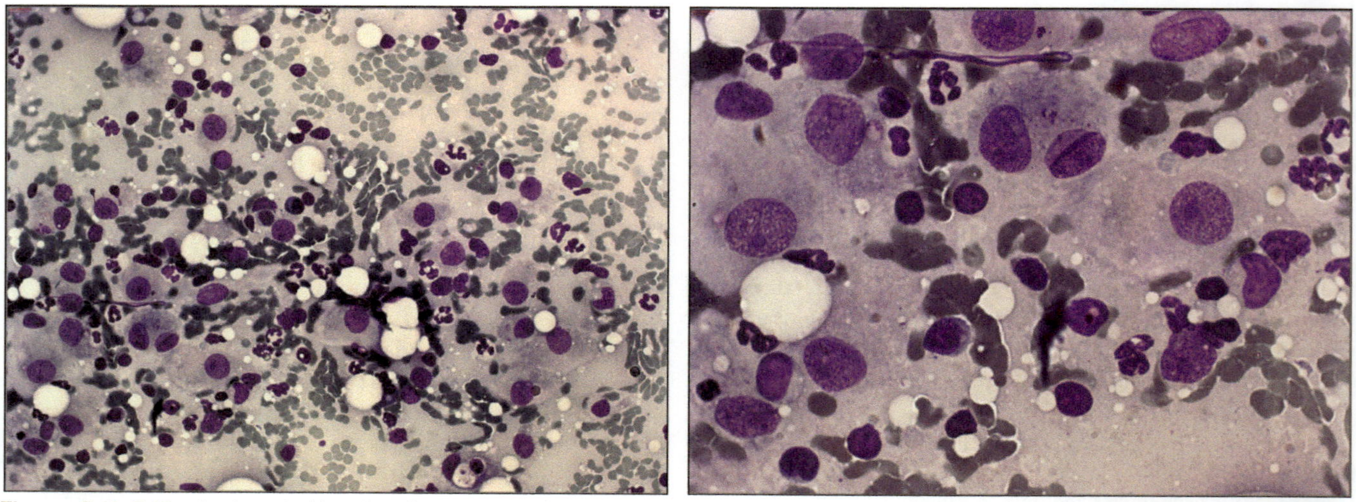

Figures 5.16, 5.17 Cat, intestinal lymph node, FNA. Granulomatous lymphadenitis. (5.16) Several large epithelioid macrophages and some neutrophils are found among lymphoid cells (May-Grünwald-Giemsa, 400× magnification). (5.17) Particularly large epithelioid cells and a binucleated cell (May-Grünwald-Giemsa, 1,000× magnification).

blastomycosis (Figure 5.19), cryptococcosis (Figures 5.20, 5.21), histoplasmosis (Figure 5.22), coccidioidomycosis, mycobacteriosis (Figure 5.23), salmon fluke poisoning disease (*Neorickettsia helminthoeca*; Figure 5.24), protothecosis (Figure 5.25), cytauxzoonosis (Figure 5.26), and toxoplasmosis (Figure 5.27) may be accompanied by granulomatous or pyogranulomatous lymphadenitis. Leishmaniosis may also lead to granulomatous or pyogranulomatous lymphadenitis and concurrent plasma cell hyperplasia is commonly seen (Figure 5.28). Organisms may be identifiable by standard stain or may appear as negative impressions in the cytoplasm of phagocytes, as with *Mycobacterium* spp. (Figure 5.23). Cytological diagnosis of certain organisms may be improved using special stains

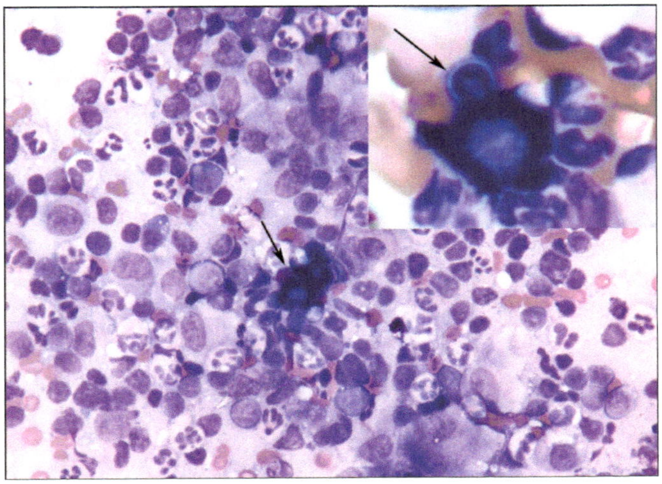

Figure 5.19 Dog, peripheral lymph node, FNA. Blastomycosis. Yeast structures (arrows) are surrounded by a pyogranulomatous inflammation (Wright-Giemsa, 1,000× magnification). Inset: a budding yeast is recognizable at high magnification (Wright-Giemsa, approximately 3,000× magnification) (courtesy A. Barger).

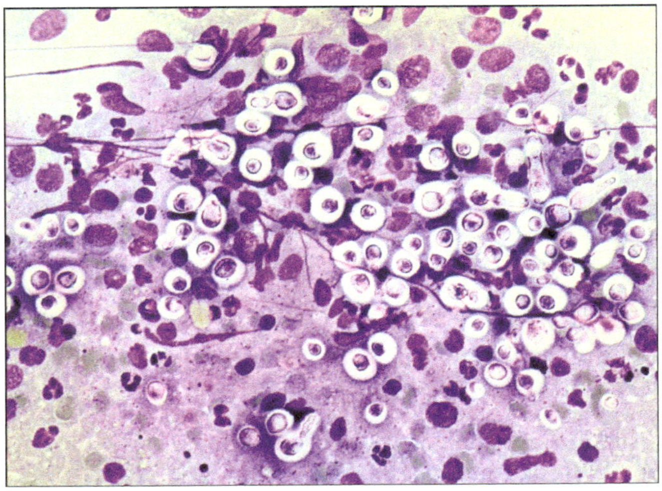

Figure 5.20 Dog, lymph node, FNA. Cryptococcosis. Several yeast forms surrounded by a thick clear halo representing the capsule, in a background of necrotic debris (May-Grünwald-Giemsa, 1,000× magnification) (courtesy U. Bonfanti).

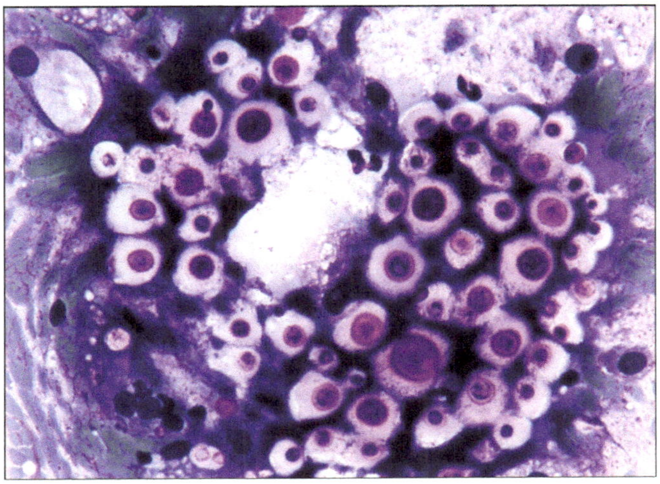

Figure 5.21 Dog, peripheral lymph node, FNA. Cryptococcosis. An islet of pleomorphic yeasts at different maturation stages and occasionally showing budding (Wright-Giemsa, 1,000× magnification) (courtesy A. Barger).

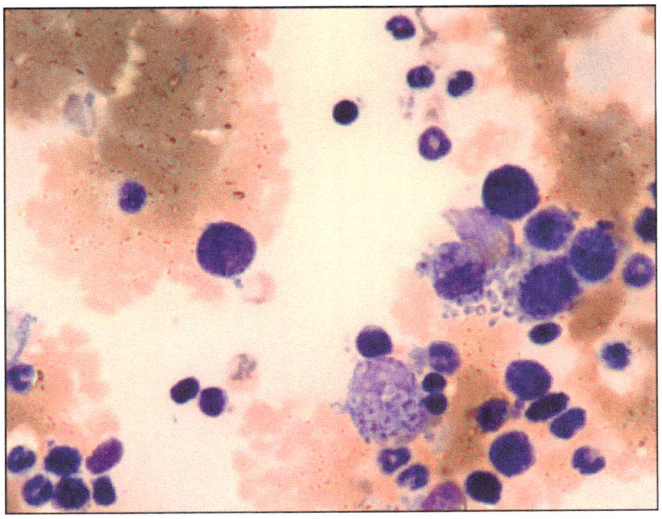

Figure 5.22 Dog, peripheral lymph node, FNA. Histoplasmosis. Numerous yeast forms are found in the macrophages or in the background (Wright-Giemsa, 1,000× magnification) (courtesy A. Barger).

such as Ziehl-Neelsen for *Mycobacterium* spp. (Figure 5.29), periodic acid-Shiff or silver stains for fungi and *Prototheca* spp., and ink stain for *Cryptococcus* spp.

Extramedullary hematopoiesis

Extramedullary hematopoiesis (EMH, myeloid metaplasia) limited to one hematopoietic lineage or to a mixture of erythroid, myeloid, and megakaryocytic lineages may occur within lymphoid tissues. Strong regeneration due to hemolytic anemia, leukemoid reactions, or megakaryocytic hyperplasia may induce EMH. Immature hematopoietic cells at all stages of maturation may be identified and are

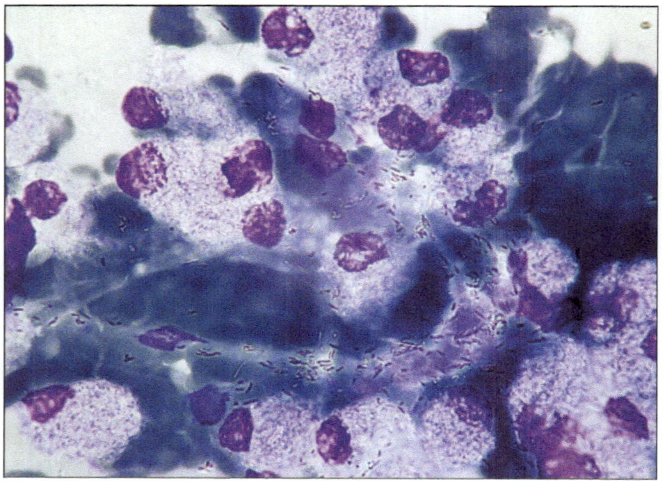

Figure 5.23 Cat, peripheral lymph node, FNA. Mycobacteriosis. Several negatively stained rods are found in the macrophages, and more rarely, free in the background (May–Grünwald–Giemsa, 1,000× magnification) (courtesy W. Bertazzolo).

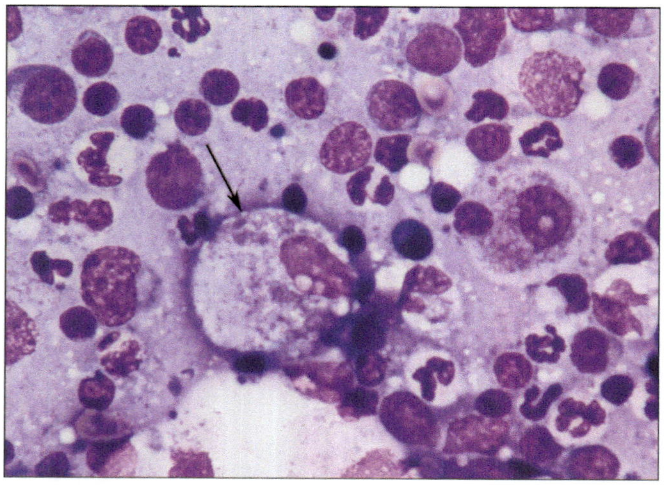

Figure 5.24 Dog, peripheral lymph node, FNA. Salmon fluke poisoning disease. Several small gray to pink granules (arrow), referable to *Neorickettsia helminthoeca* within macrophages, in a background of a pyogranulomatous lymphadenitis (Wright–Giemsa, 1,000× magnification) (courtesy A. Barger).

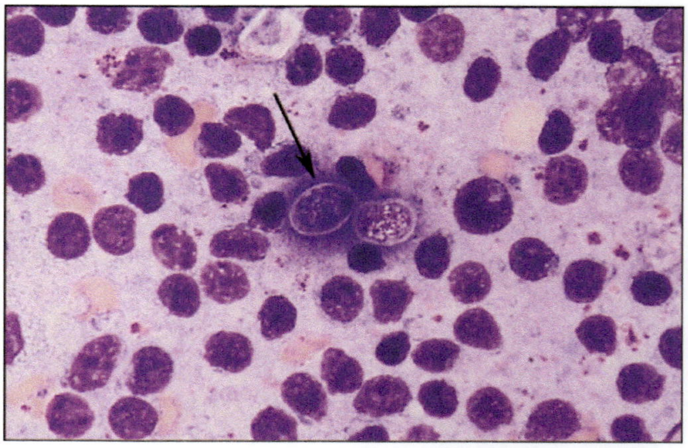

Figure 5.25 Dog, intestinal lymph node, FNA. Protothecosis. Two oval structures with thin clear walls, referable to endospores of *Prototheca* (arrow), are identifiable in the background of a necrotic lymph node (May–Grünwald–Giemsa, 1,000× magnification) (courtesy C. Masserdotti).

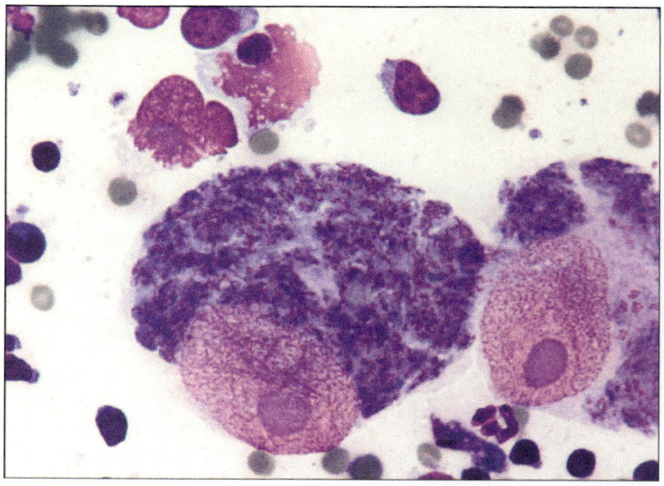

Figure 5.26 Cat, peripheral lymph node, FNA. Cytauxzoonosis. Two large schizonts engulfing mononuclear phagocytes. The schizonts are composed of several small merozoites (small piroplasms), which are released with the rupture of the schizont and represent the infective form for the erythrocytes (Wright–Giemsa, 1,000× magnification) (courtesy A. Barger).

often associated with plasma cell hyperplasia. The presence of hematopoietic precursors in multiple stages of maturation enables cytologists to differentiate EMH from infiltration of acute myeloid leukemia (AML). In AML, the majority of myeloid cells are myeloblasts. If myeloblasts are the predominant non-lymphoid cell in the sample, cytologic evaluation of a peripheral blood smear and a bone marrow aspirate is recommended.

Lymphoma

Lymphoma (previously also called 'lymphosarcoma' or 'malignant lymphoma') occurs in approximately 20 out of 100,000 dogs and accounts for 50–90% of hematopoietic neoplasms in cats, but the overall incidence of lymphoma in cats is unknown (Vail, 2013). The etiology of lymphoma is likely multifactorial (environmental exposure to carcinogens, immunologic causes, genetic factors). In cats retroviral infections (FeLV and FIV) and passive exposure to tobacco smoking have been demonstrated as possible predisposing factors. Genetic factors are thought to include germline and somatic mutations, altered oncogene and tumor suppressor gene expression, epigenetic changes, and disrupted signal transduction and apoptosis pathways (Thomas et al., 2001).

The role of cytology in the diagnosis of canine lymphoma has been considered crucial due to: (1) the high prevalence of diffuse, overtly nodular lymphomas in dogs, thus increasing the accuracy of cytologic aspiration; (2) the minimal invasiveness of cytologic sampling

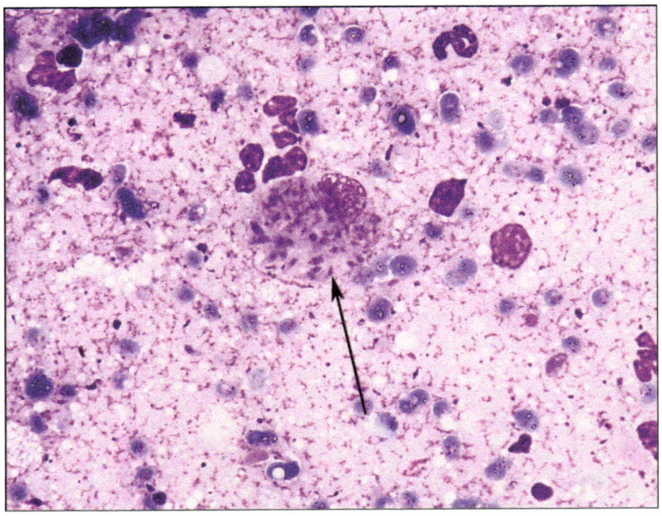

Figure 5.27 Cat, peripheral lymph node, FNA. Toxoplasmosis. Macrophage containing several 'banana-shaped' tachyzoites (arrow) in a necrotic background (May–Grünwald–Giemsa, 1,000× magnification) (courtesy C. Masserdotti).

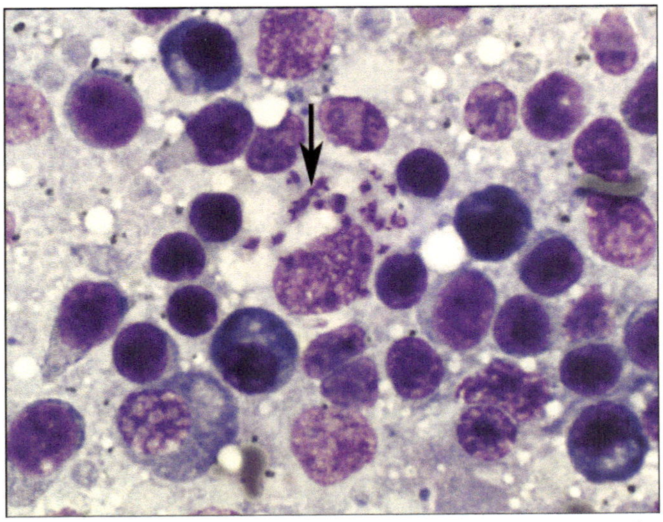

Figure 5.28 Dog, peripheral lymph node, FNA. Leishmaniosis. Several *Leishmania* amastigotes (arrow) in the cytoplasm of a macrophage in the context of a plasma cell hyperplastic lymph node. Note the mixed population composed of plasma cells, small lymphocytes, and hand-mirror-shaped T-lymphoid cells (May–Grünwald–Giemsa, 2,000× magnification).

compared with histologic biopsies, that encourages owner compliance; and (3) the limited use of subtype-specific therapeutic protocols, which discourages the use of invasive techniques in the diagnostic work up. On the other hand, the role of cytology in feline lymphoma is more challenging since: (1) feline lymphomas are often limited to internal organs or lymph nodes, thus sampling may be difficult and often requires sedation; (2) lymphoma classification schemes used in dogs are not easily applicable to cats; and (3) the presence of lymphoma subtypes composed of small lymphocytes and of hyperplastic conditions that strongly resemble lymphoma.

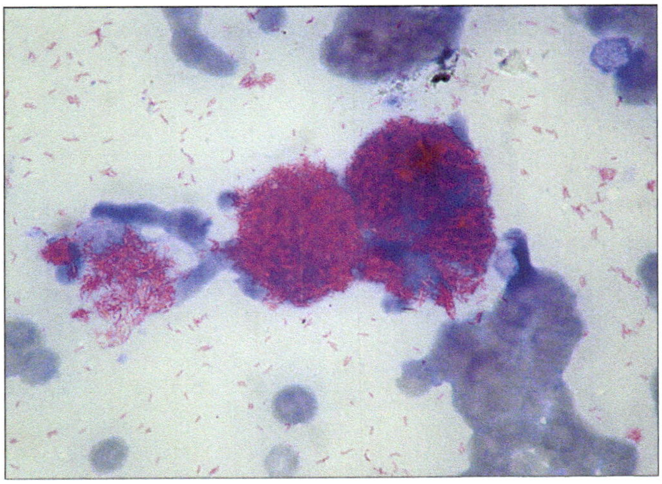

Figure 5.29 Same case as Figure 5.23. Mycobacteriosis. The free and intracellular rods stain intensely with Ziehl–Neelsen, supporting acid resistance (courtesy W. Bertazzolo).

In a survey among veterinarians (Regan et al., 2013), the use of cytology in the diagnostic algorithm for lymphoma widely exceeded that of histologic biopsy (88% versus 28%). In the authors' opinion, cytology plays a central role in the diagnostic approach to canine lymphadenopathy since it allows veterinarians to easily differentiate lymphoid reactivity from lymphoma in the great majority of cases. In a recent study, cytology had a 92.6% sensitivity and 89.4% specificity in distinguishing lymphoma *vs.* non-lymphoma in dogs (Martini et al., 2021). The immunophenotype of the lymphoma can also be determined from a cytologic sample if flow cytometry or ICC is added (Comazzi & Gelain, 2011). However, cytology alone shows variable diagnostic performances in immunophenotyping and grading, ranging from more than 80% sensitivity and 95% specificity for low-grade T-cell lymphoma to less than 20% sensitivity for low-grade B-cell lymphoma and about 60% specificity for high-grade B-cell lymphoma (Martini et al, 2022). Immunophenotyping via flow cytometry or immunocytochemistry likely improve these performances but histology and immunohistochemistry of a whole lymph node are suggested to definitively diagnose subtype and grade or to solve differentials in selected, challenging cases. Cytological criteria used in dogs to predict immunophenotyping are not useful in immunophenotyping feline nodal lymphoma (Gambini et al., 2021).

Classification of lymphoma

Classification of lymphomas has been widely revised during the last 50 years both in human and in veterinary medicine. Until recently, the most suitable classification schemes were the modified Kiel classification (Fournel-Fleury et al., 1997), which is based on morphologic abnormalities in lymphoid cells and was partially linked to specific biological behavior of lymphomas in dogs (Ponce et al., 2004), and the World Health Organization (WHO) classification (Valli et al, 2011), which is focused on histopathology and immunophenotype. Some

Table 5.4 **Classifications and cytologic descriptions of lymphomas in dogs and cats**

World Health Organization classification (modified)	Comparable classifications	Cytologic description	Additional clinical information
Anaplastic large-cell lymphoma	Anaplastic lymphoma	Very large lymphocytes; abundant, deeply basophilic cytoplasm; binucleated or multinucleated cells; anisokaryosis	B-cell, T-cell, and undifferentiated immunophenotypes exist
Precursor lymphomas	B lymphoblastic lymphoma; T lymphoblastic lymphoma	Small lymphocytes (CD34+); scant unipolar cytoplasm; round or often indented nucleus; irregular nuclear margins; fine chromatin; poorly visible nucleoli; high mitotic index (Figure 5.30)	B lymphoblastic lymphoma has an aggressive clinical behavior (Raskin, 2010). T lymphoblastic lymphoma has a longer survival time than B lymphoblastic lymphoma (Lurie et al., 2008), often has a mediastinal location, and may induce hypercalcemia
Selected B-cell lymphomas			
Burkitt's lymphoma	Burkitt's-type lymphoma, high grade	Small/intermediate lymphocytes; deeply basophilic cytoplasm, often vacuolized; round, non-cleaved nucleus; variably condensed chromatin; multiple nucleoli; high mitotic index; tingible body macrophages (Figure 5.31)	Very aggressive behavior in dogs (Ponce et al., 2004). Genetic translocations demonstrated in dogs (Breen & Modiano, 2008)
Small lymphocytic lymphoma	Small B-cell lymphoma, low grade	Small lymphocytes; thin rim of cytoplasm; rounded nucleus; clumped chromatin; low mitotic index	Generally a good prognosis
Lymphoplasmacytic lymphoma	Small B-cell lymphoma, low grade	Abundant cytoplasm; Golgi zone; eccentric nucleus	Accounts for 4.9% of feline lymphoproliferative diseases and 3.4% of canine lymphomas (Valli, 2007)
Marginal zone lymphoma	Marginal lymphoma, low grade	Medium-sized macronucleolated cells; rare centroblasts; rare immunoblasts; low to moderate mitotic index (Figure 5.32)	Nodal form may show expansion of marginal zone or may be diffuse and progress to diffuse large B-cell lymphoma. Localized splenic form is less aggressive with a good prognosis after splenectomy (Stefanello et al., 2011; O'Brien et al., 2013)
Follicular lymphoma	Follicular lymphoma, low grade	Centrocytes and small lymphocytes; variable number of centroblasts affecting grade and prognosis; low mitotic index (Figures 5.33, 5.34)	Histopathology or molecular biology is generally necessary to differentiate from follicular hyperplasia
Diffuse large B-cell lymphoma	Large B-cell lymphomas, high grade; T-cell-rich large B-cell lymphoma; centroblastic lymphoma; immunoblastic lymphoma; plasmacytoid lymphoma; anaplastic lymphoma	Centroblastic lymphoma Intermediate/large centroblasts; few immunoblasts; few medium-sized macronucleolated cells; residual small lymphocytes; moderate to high mitotic index (Figures 5.35, 5.36) Imunoblastic lymphoma >80% large immunoblasts; high mitotic index (Figure 5.37) Plasmacytoid lymphoma; small/intermediate lymphocytes; pale Golgi zone; eccentric, round nucleus; clumped chromatin; frequent binucleation (Figure 5.38)	The centroblastic cytologic appearance accounts for 60–80% of lymphomas in dogs (Vail et al., 2013). Germinal center and activated B-cell subtypes were identified using gene expression profile analysis in the dog (Richards et al., 2013). Histopathology is shown (Figure 5.39)
Selected T-cell lymphomas			
T-cell lymphomas	High-grade T-cell lymphomas; pleomorphic mixed small and large cell lymphoma; pleomorphic large-cell lymphoma; plasmacytoid T-cell lymphoma; T immunoblastic lymphoma	Pleomorphic mixed small and large-cell lymphoma >90% pleomorphic lymphocytes; moderately abundant, lightly basophilic cytoplasm; indented or 'flower-like' nucleus; smooth chromatin; one or more poorly visible nucleoli; moderate to high mitotic index (Figures 5.40, 5.41) Pleomorphic large-cell lymphoma (Fournel-Fleury et al., 2002). Intermediate to large cells; very high mitotic index (Figures 5.42, 5.43) Plasmacytoid T-cell lymphoma (Ponce et al., 2010). Small/intermediate lymphocytes; pale Golgi zone; eccentric, round nucleus; clumped chromatin; frequent binucleation; high mitotic index T immunoblastic lymphoma; high mitotic index	Generally aggressive with a lower rate of complete remission to chemotherapy and a shorter survival time than high-grade B-cell lymphomas (Vail et al., 2013)
Mature nodal T-cell (T-zone) lymphoma	Low-grade T-cell lymphomas; small clear cell lymphoma; pleomorphic small-cell lymphoma	Small clear cell lymphoma Small/intermediate lymphocytes; moderately abundant, clear cytoplasm often with a hand-mirror shape; round nucleus; condensed chromatin; scarcely visible nucleolus; low mitotic index (Figures 5.44, 5.45)	Immunophenotype: CD3+/CD5+/CD21+/CD45 low (Martini et al., 2015; Seelig et al., 2014). Generally have an indolent behavior
Large granular lymphocyte lymphoma	Large granular lymphocyte lymphoma	Intermediate/large lymphocytes; clear to deeply basophilic cytoplasm; often vacuolated cytoplasm; round to indented nucleus; single, central, prominent nucleolus; high mitotic index (Figures 5.46, 5.47)	Often alimentary in cats. Typically involves the spleen in dogs

attempts to identify correlations among the two different classification schemes have been made (Ponce et al., 2010; Table 5.4), but we are still far from a definitive classification scheme. The ability to predict WHO classification subtype via cytology alone has been evaluated in a recent study (Martini et al., 2022) and results showed variable accuracy depending on the subtype with the higher in T zone lymphoma and the lower in peripheral T-cell lymphoma (PTCL). The main diagnostic issues were differentiation among B-cell lymphoma subtypes

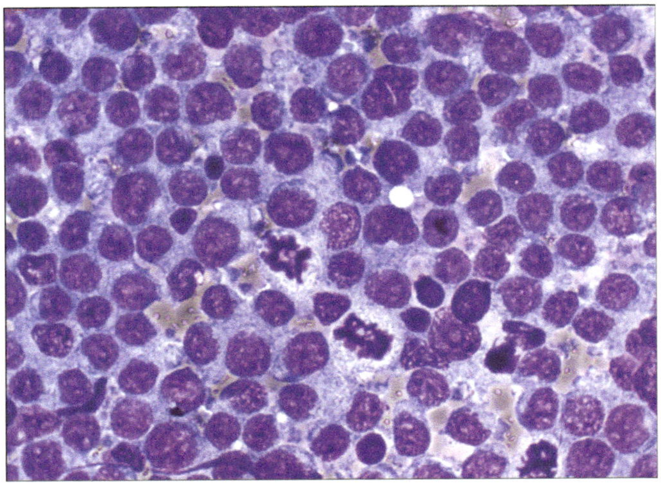

Figure 5.30 Dog, peripheral lymph node, FNA. Lymphoblastic lymphoma. Highly prevalent population of small/medium lymphoid cells with scarce, basophilic cytoplasm, round to indented nucleus, and poorly visible nucleoli. Several mitosis are also present (May–Grünwald–Giemsa, 1,000× magnification).

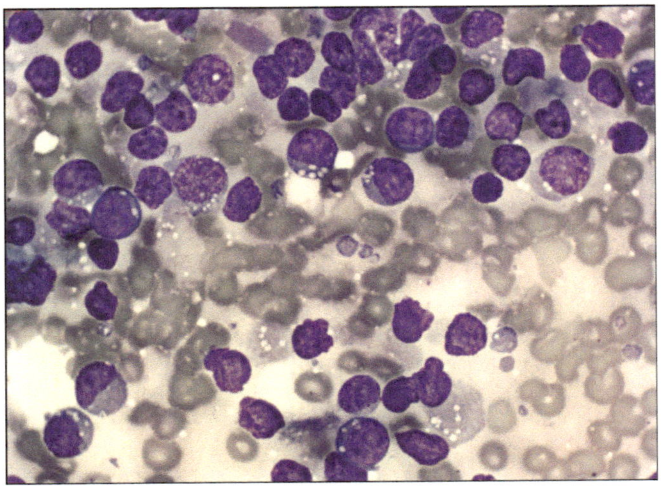

Figure 5.31 Dog, peripheral lymph node, FNA. Burkitt-type lymphoma. Single population of small/medium cells with cytoplasm vacuoles, round, noncleaved nucleus, and visible nucleoli (May–Grünwald–Giemsa, 1,000× magnification).

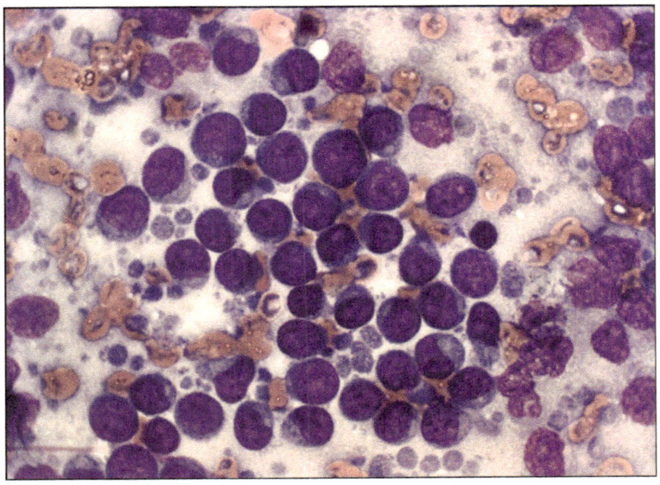

Figure 5.32 Dog, peripheral lymph node, FNA. Marginal lymphoma. Single population of medium-sized blast cells with round nucleus and prominent central nucleolus (May–Grünwald–Giemsa, 1,000× magnification).

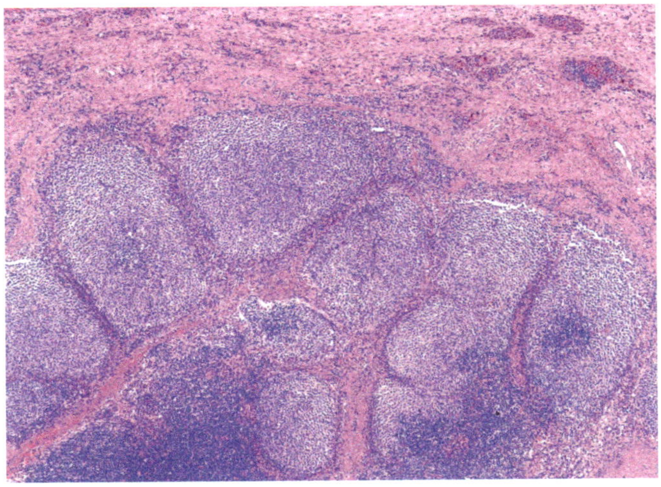

Figure 5.33 Dog, peripheral lymph node, histology. Follicular lymphoma. Neoplastic expansion of follicles associated with fading of mantle cell cuffs and peculiar inverse follicular pattern (H&E, 50× magnification). (Courtesy L. Aresu.)

and overestimation of PTCL with inclusion of many B-cell lymphoma subtypes. Addition of immunophenotyping via flow cytometry likely increases the accuracy of cytological diagnosis but research on this aspect is still ongoing. More recently, gene expression profile analysis was used to group specific morphologic subtypes into three different entities, which may have prognostic relevance in canine lymphomas (Frantz et al., 2013); however, additional studies are needed to confirm these results.

New diagnostic techniques have identified new subtypes of lymphoma, but in order for classification schemes to be clinically relevant, they need to reflect biological behavior, median survival times, and response to tailored therapy. Recently, a WHO subtype has been described as an aggressive B-cell lymphoma and provisionally named diffuse small B-cell lymphoma, (DSBCL, Hughes et al, 2021). This entity is characterized by small cells, with scarce cytoplasm, round nuclei with condensed chromatin and indistinct nucleoli but a high number of mitosis are present. Flow cytometry confirms a prevalence of B cells with low forward scatter properties (suggesting small size). Further studies are still needed to define and validate the diagnostic approach for DSBCL and to identify potential prognostic factors.

Currently, cytologic evaluation is a very powerful tool to diagnose lymphoma, but often is insufficient for further characterization of the disease. Immunophenotyping is highly recommended and additional diagnostics, including histologic subtyping, are needed to predict

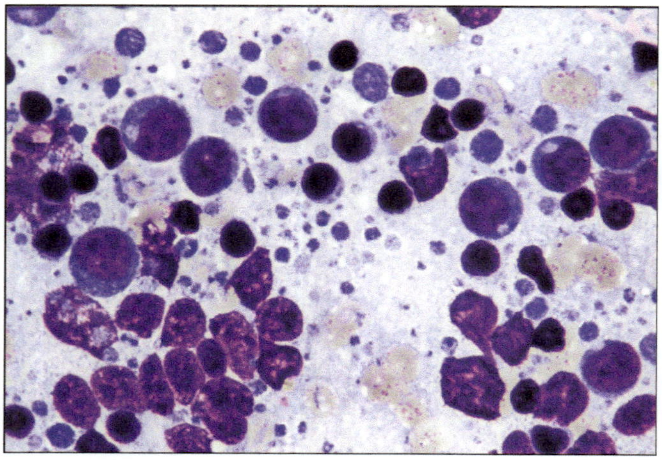

Figure 5.34 Dog, peripheral lymph node, FNA. Follicular lymphoma. A mixed population of center-follicular cells (small lymphoid cells and large centroblasts) is identified. Cytology alone does not allow differentiation of follicular lymphoma from follicular hyperplasia, but the lack of a continuum in lymphoid maturation and of plasma cells supports lymphoma (May–Grünwald–Giemsa, 1,000× magnification).

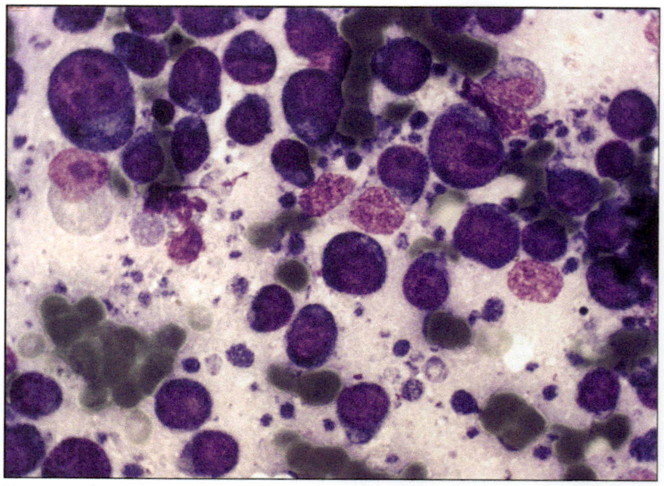

Figure 5.36 Dog, peripheral lymph node, FNA. Large B-cell lymphoma, centroblastic pleomorphic. A mixed population of large centroblasts (upper left), immunoblasts, and medium-sized macronucleolated cells is identifiable (May–Grünwald–Giemsa, 1,000× magnification).

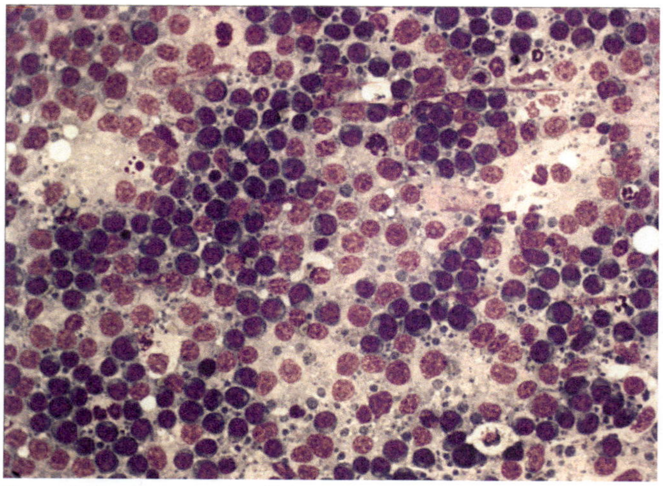

Figure 5.35 Dog, peripheral lymph node, FNA. Large B-cell lymphoma, centroblastic monomorphic. A prevalent population of medium/large blast cells, some mitoses, and macrophages with tingible bodies, giving a 'starry-sky appearance', are seen (May–Grünwald–Giemsa, 400× magnification).

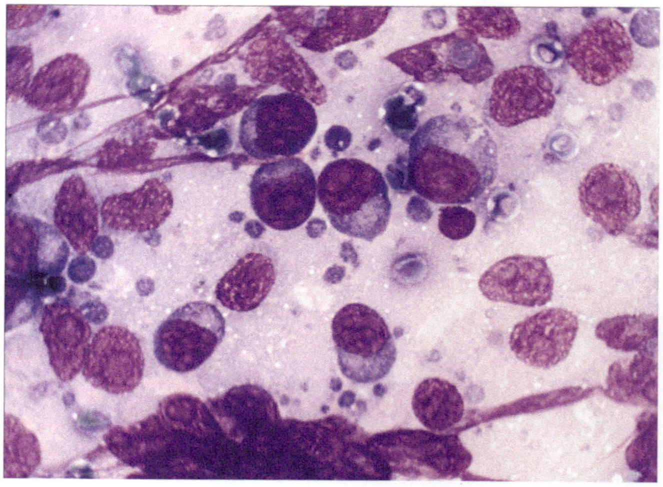

Figure 5.37 Dog, peripheral lymph node, FNA. Large B-cell lymphoma, immunoblastic. Some large blasts with moderately abundant cytoplasm, round nuclei with fine chromatin, and one or more prominent central nucleoli (May–Grünwald–Giemsa, 1,000× magnification).

clinical outcomes. Diagnostic staging of lymphoma relies heavily on localization of the neoplastic cells and clinical signs of disease. The WHO guideline for clinical staging of lymphoma in domestic animals is summarized in Table 5.5 (Owen, 1980). In dogs, prognostic factors with a strong association with response to chemotherapy and/or survival include: (1) location of the lymphoid neoplasm; (2) clinical stage; (3) WHO substage; (4) histologic grade; and (5) immunophenotype. For example, a poor prognosis is warranted for patients with mediastinal lymphomas, high-grade B-cell lymphomas with bone marrow infiltration (Marconato et al., 2013b), WHO substage b classification, high-grade T-cell tumors, B-cell tumors with low expression of major histocompatibility complex (MHC) class II or of CD21 (Rout et al. 2020) or high expression of CD25 by flow cytometry or high percentage of Ki67 positive cells, and lymphoma patients with concurrent non-regenerative anemia. Histology may provide information about treatment response as well as overall prognosis. For example, patients with high-grade lymphomas tend to have a better initial response to therapy but have worse median survival times, whereas patients with indolent lymphomas have prolonged survival times. More than 80% of dogs present with stage III or IV lymphoma (Vail et al., 2013). Most

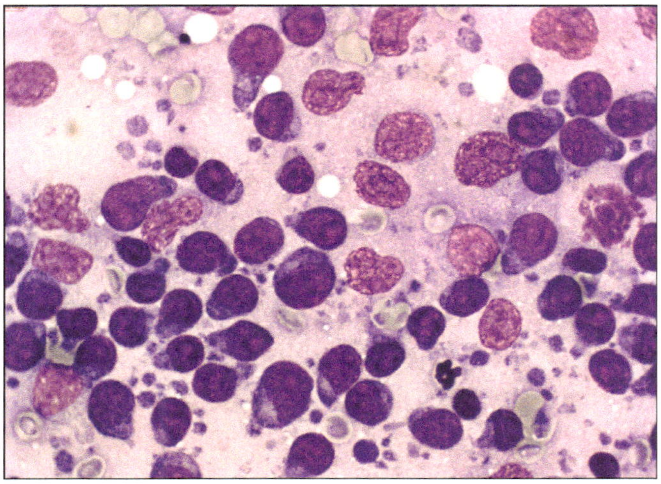

Figure 5.38 Dog, peripheral lymph node, FNA. Large B-cell lymphoma, plasmacytoid. Several large blasts with unipolar elongated cytoplasm and prominent nucleolus (May–Grünwald–Giemsa, 1,000× magnification).

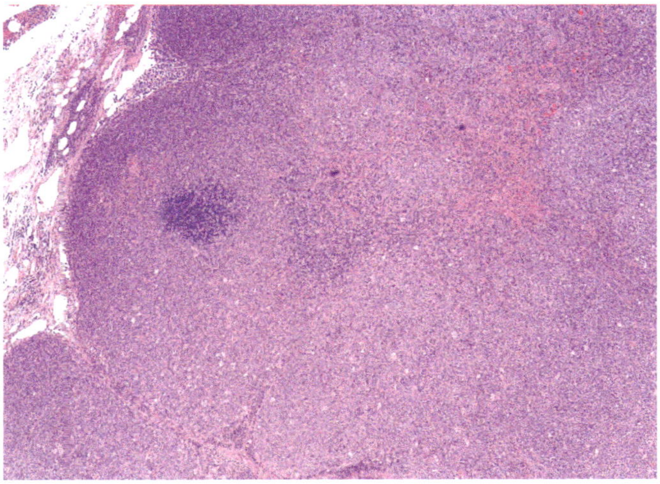

Figure 5.39 Dog, peripheral lymph node, histology. Diffuse large B-cell lymphoma. Diffuse growth of the neoplastic lymphocytes with loss of normal node structure (H&E, 50× magnification). (Courtesy L. Aresu.)

cats present with low-grade T-cell lymphomas of the alimentary tract, which generally have a good prognosis (Vail, 2013).

Cytological criteria for diagnosis of lymphoma

Lymphoma should be a differential diagnosis in dogs with generalized peripheral lymphadenopathy (84% of canine cases are multicentric lymphomas) and in cats with signs of gastrointestinal disease or an enlarged internal lymph node (Vail et al., 2013). In most cases of canine lymphoma, the disease is easily diagnosed by cytologic samples that contain a high percentage (often >50%) of large lymphoid cells with a nuclear diameter >15 micrometers (larger than a neutrophil) and one or more prominent nucleoli. Nucleoli are very distinctive in hematopoietic cells, including lymphoid cells, and appear as a ring of clumped chromatin around a central, clear area. Mitosis, also atypical, may be present and suggestive of high grade (Figure 5.48) but mitotic index may be quite variable among different histotypes. Lower numbers of small and intermediate-sized lymphocytes can be present. Plasma cells and inflammatory leukocytes should be rare. In cases where 30–50% of lymphoid cells are large lymphocytes and plasma cells are virtually absent, lymphoma is likely. Lymphomas comprised of small -or intermediate-sized lymphocytes are generally more difficult to definitively diagnose cytologically. If nearly all the cells in a sample are small or intermediate-sized and have a uniform morphology, lymphoma should be suspected and additional diagnostics recommended.

LYMPHOMA SUBTYPES WITH DISTINCTIVE CYTOLOGIC MORPHOLOGY

Large granular lymphocyte lymphoma

Large granular lymphocyte (LGL) lymphoma is a specific lymphoma subtype that may be observed in cats, mainly in alimentary lymphoma, and occasionally occurs in dogs, often with splenic or hepatic involvement. In cats with LGL lymphoma, response to therapy and survival are generally very poor; median survival time is approximately 1.5 months (Krick et al., 2008; Moore et al., 2012). However, a recent paper reported a small percentage (about 7%) of cats having LGL lymphoma with long survival (Finotello et al., 2018). In dogs, prognosis varies with the degree of organ and bone marrow involvement. Most neoplastic LGL lymphomas exhibit a cytotoxic T-cell immunophenotype ($CD3^+CD8^+$) and are often positive for the aβ-T-cell receptor. More rarely, a natural killer cell phenotype ($CD3^-$) is diagnosed (McDonough & Moore, 2000; Roccabianca et al., 2006). Note that canine patients with chronic lymphoid leukemias often have circulating granular lymphocytes (Tasca et al., 2009), but this disease process is not equivalent to LGL lymphoma and does not carry the same prognosis (Workman & Vernau, 2003).

Cytology is characterized by medium-sized lymphoid cells with moderately abundant gray or light blue cytoplasm containing azurophilic magenta granules, often located in a perinuclear area. The granule size may vary from pinpoint to >2 micrometers in diameter (Figure 5.46) and may be surrounded by a clear halo in the cat (Figure 5.47). The nucleus is round to indented and may be condensed without visible nucleoli (in more differentiated forms) or smooth with prominent nucleoli in less differentiated tumors. Care must be taken to distinguish LGL lymphoma from poorly granulated mast cell tumors, in which granules are often homogeneously distributed throughout the cytoplasm.

Hodgkin-like lymphoma

Hodgkin-like lymphoma is a rare lymphoma subtype occasionally reported in the cat (Valli, 2007; Steinberg & Keating, 2008). This disease generally involves one or a few lymph nodes, mainly in the head or neck region, and is considered an indolent disease with survival

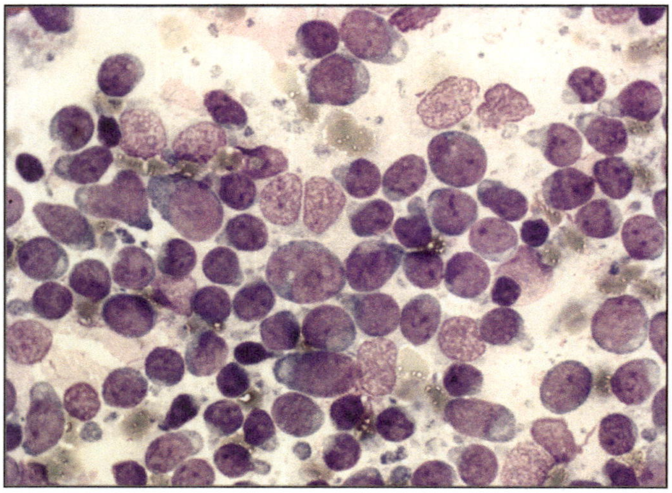

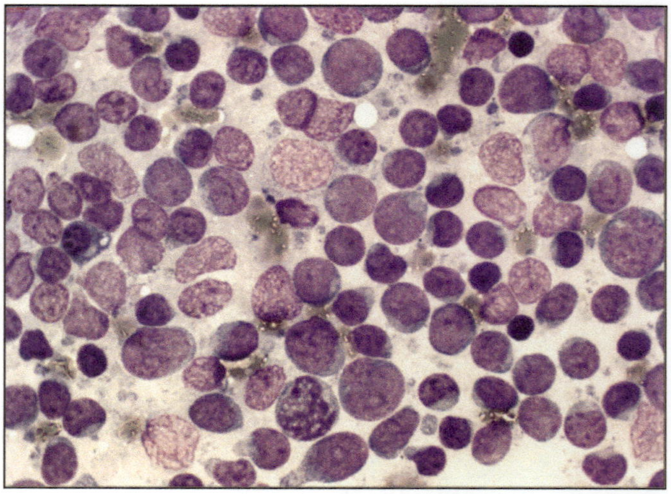

Dog, peripheral lymph node, FNA. High-grade T-cell lymphoma, pleomorphic mixed small and large. (May–Grunwald–Giemsa, 1,000× magnification).

Figure 5.40 A mixed population of small cells and pleomorphic medium/large blasts with moderately abundant, mildly basophilic cytoplasm, indented to convoluted nuclei with smooth chromatin and rare nucleoli.

Figure 5.41 High-grade T-cell lymphoma, pleomorphic mixed small and large. Note the mixed population of cells and the presence of occasional plasma cells.

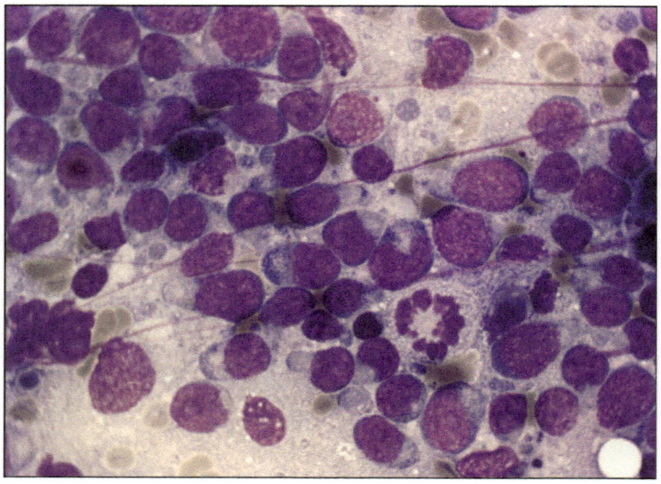

Figure 5.42 Dog, peripheral lymph node, FNA. High-grade T-cell lymphoma, pleomorphic large. A prevalent population of large blast cells is found. Mitotic figures are frequent (May–Grünwald–Giemsa, 1,000× magnification).

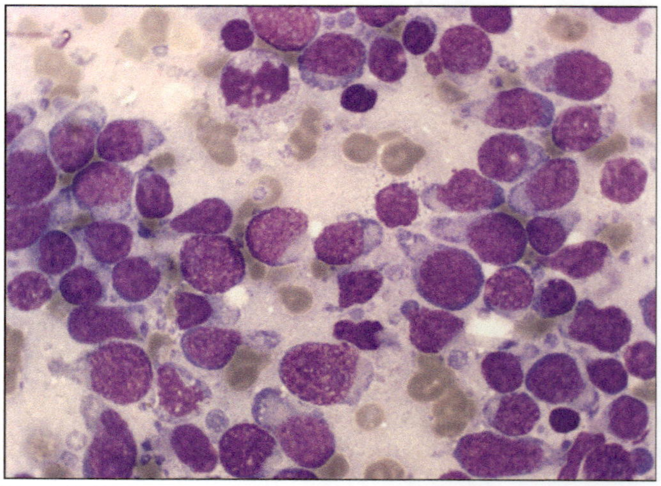

Figure 5.43 Dog, peripheral lymph node, FNA. High-grade T-cell lymphoma, pleomorphic large. Many of the cells have moderately abundant unipolar cytoplasm (May–Grünwald–Giemsa, 1,000× magnification).

times of 1 year or more (Vail, 2013). Cytology shows a very heterogeneous population of cells predominated by small lymphocytes or cells with a plasmacytoid appearance. Large macrophages containing cellular debris are frequent. Immunophenotyping shows a prevalent population of small reactive T cells, although the neoplastic population is assumed to be of B cell origin (T-cell rich, large B-cell lymphoma). Occasionally, some Reed–Sternberg cells (popcorn-like cells) may be found. These are large cells with pale cytoplasm, often binucleated with round to ovoid nuclei and prominent large nucleoli (Figures 5.49, 5.50) and may have a histiocytoid appearance, although Reed–Sternberg cells generally are negative for both B- and T-cell markers (CD79a and CD3, respectively) as well as for dendritic and macrophage markers. These cells are quite distinctive and strongly suggest Hodgkin-like lymphoma, although they are not pathognomonic and histopathology plus immunohistochemistry is mandatory to confirm the diagnosis.

T-zone lymphoma

T-zone lymphoma is an indolent lymphoma subtype reported in dogs (Valli et al., 2013). T-zone lymphomas often arise in mandibular lymph nodes and are definitively diagnosed using immunohistochemistry to

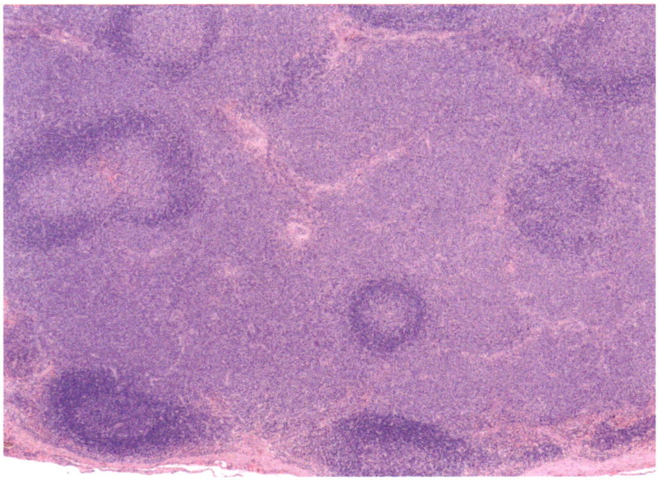

Figure 5.44 Dog, peripheral lymph node, histology. T-zone lymphoma. Neoplastic expansion of paracortex and compression of residual follicles (H&E, 50× magnification). (Courtesy L. Aresu.)

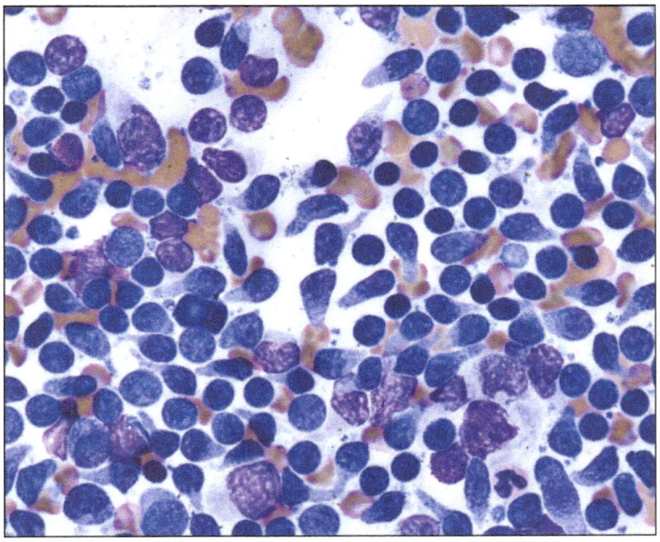

Figure 5.45 Dog, mandibular lymph node, FNA. Possible T-zone lymphoma. There is a marked expansion of intermediate-sized lymphocytes that often have 'hand-mirror' morphology (Wright–Giemsa, 1,000× magnification).

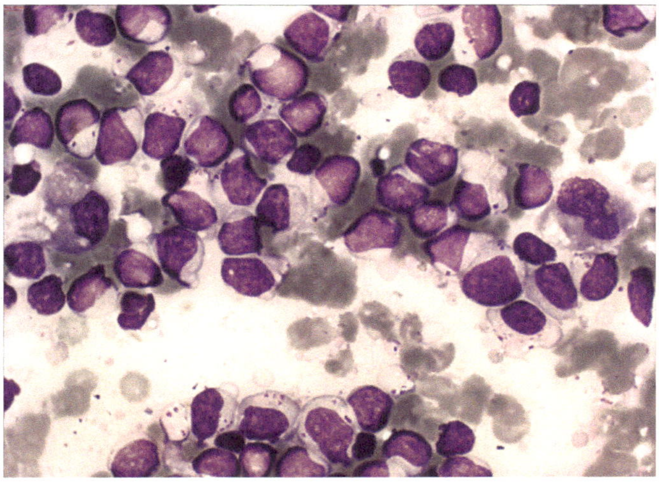

Figure 5.46 Dog, peripheral lymph node, FNA. Large granular lymphocyte lymphoma. Prevalent population of medium-sized cells with clear cytoplasm and variable azurophilic cytoplasmic granules (May–Grünwald–Giemsa, 1,000× magnification).

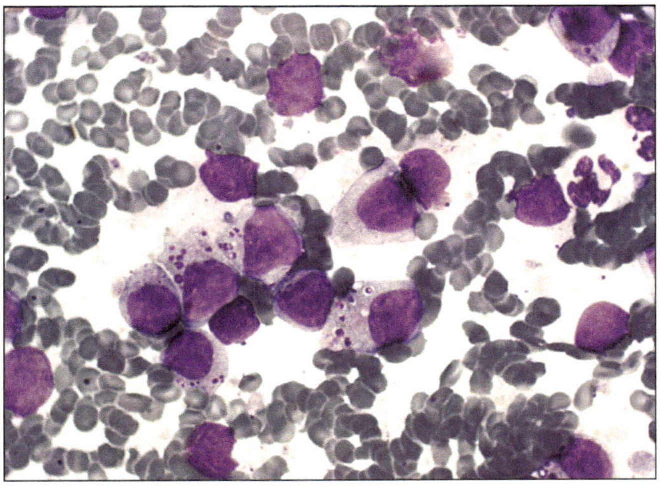

Figure 5.47 Cat, intestinal lymph node, FNA. Large granular lymphocyte lymphoma. Neoplastic cells often contain large azurophilic granules surrounded by a clear halo, resembling a capsule (May–Grünwald–Giemsa, 1,000× magnification).

Table 5.5 **World Health Organization clinical staging of lymphomas in dogs and cats**

Localization of neoplasm	Stage	Substage
A: Generalized	I: Lymphoma in a single lymph node or organ (except bone marrow)	a: Without systemic disease
B: Alimentary	II: Lymphoma in ≥2 lymph nodes in one region of the body	b: With systemic disease
C: Thymic	III: Lymphoma in several lymph nodes (generalized disease)	
D: Skin	IV: Stage III + liver and/or splenic lymphoma	
E: Leukemia	V: Lymphoma with bone marrow infiltration	
F: Other		

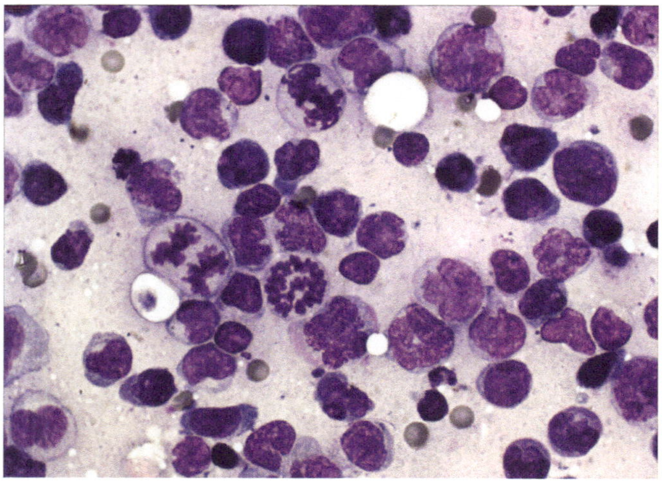

Figure 5.48 Cat, peripheral lymph node, FNA. High-grade lymphoma. Prevalent population of pleomorphic large cells with indented to convoluted nuclei. Several mitotic figures, also atypical, are found (May–Grünwald–Giemsa, 1,000× magnification).

identify a neoplastic population of $CD3^+$ cells expanding the paracortical zones of a lymph node. In most cases of T-zone lymphoma, the neoplastic cells are negative for CD45 (Seelig et al., 2014; Martini et al., 2015; Stein et al., 2021; Kojima et al., 2022). Cytologically, neoplastic lymphocytes associated with T-zone lymphomas often have a 'hand-mirror' or 'tadpole' appearance (Valli et al., 2013). The lymphocytes are intermediate-sized with a moderate amount of basophilic cytoplasm that extends away from a round nucleus. The nuclear chromatin is commonly smooth to finely stippled. The extensions of cytoplasm are wide close to the nucleus and taper slightly further away from the nucleus. Unlike samples where cell morphology is artificially altered by a poor smearing technique, 'hand-mirror' lymphocytes have cytoplasm that extends away from the nucleus in random directions, relative to each other, on the slide (Figure 5.45). If this cytologic morphology is observed, additional diagnostics (e.g. flow cytometric or immunohistochemical analyses) are recommended to determine if the atypical lymphocytes are $CD3^+CD45^-$ cells. If this is the case, an indolent T-zone lymphoma is likely.

Metastatic neoplasia

Metastatic disease is suspected if atypical cells are detected in cytologic smears of lymph node aspirates. Suspected neoplastic cells should be carefully evaluated for features of malignancy to ensure the cells have not simply been aspirated from tissue located close to the lymph node. Lymph nodes affected by metastatic diseases often show concurrent hyperplasia.

When superimposed lymph node hyperplasia is present, a benign, mixed lymphoid population is observed with increased numbers of reactive plasma cells and/or macrophages. Lymph node cytology has high specificity but low sensitivity for metastatic disease due to the small sample size of a cytology aspirate; false-negative results occur if neoplastic cells are not aspirated. Histology and immunohistochemistry should be performed before excluding lymph node metastasis.

Epithelial tumors metastasize to regional lymph nodes relatively frequently. Detection of neoplastic cells in lymph nodes is not rare with adenocarcinomas (Figure 5.51) and squamous cell carcinomas (Figure 5.52), and this finding affects prognosis. Neoplastic cells may be observed individually or in small clusters and they are easily distinguishable from the lymphoid population due to the large size and the morphologic appearance of the neoplastic cells. However, neoplastic cells from anaplastic carcinomas may metastasize singularly and are more difficult to differentiate from large lymphoid blasts or reactive macrophages.

Nonepithelial neoplasms metastasize through lymphatic vessels less commonly than epithelial tumors, but in some cases lymph node metastases may be found. Oral melanoma has a high tendency to

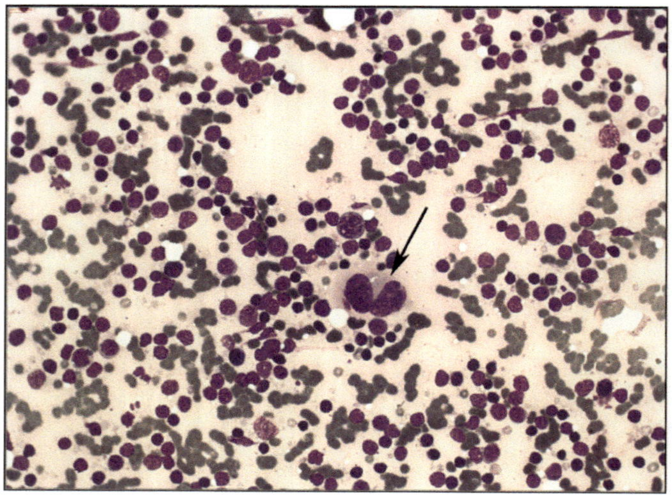

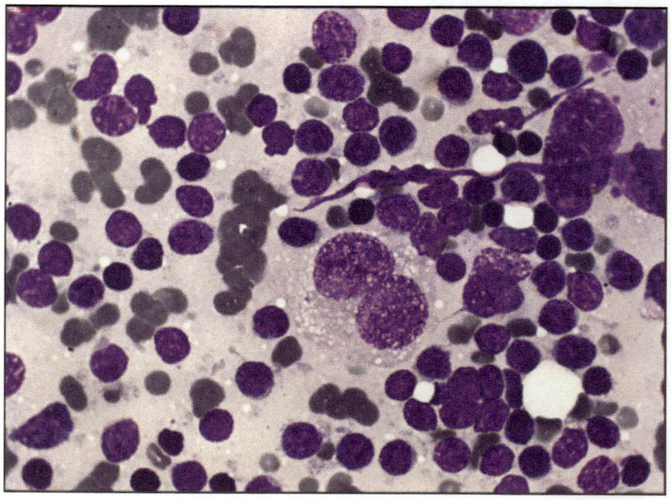

Cat, prescapular lymph node, FNA. Hodgkin-like lymphoma.

Figure 5.49 A large histiocytoid binucleated cell (Reed–Sternberg cell, arrow) is evident in the background of small lymphocytes (May–Grünwald–Giemsa, 400× magnification).

Figure 5.50 The Reed–Sternberg cell at higher magnification (May–Grünwald–Giemsa, 1,000× magnification).

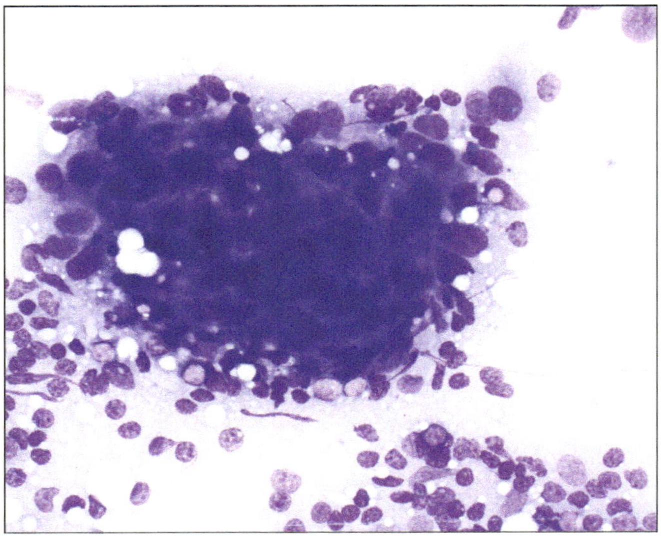

Figure 5.51 Dog, prescapular lymph node, FNA. A large cluster of epithelial cells is found among several small lymphocytes. Fewer intermediate and large lymphocytes as well as mildly increased numbers of plasma cells were present (not shown). Previously, this patient was diagnosed with a mammary carcinoma, suggesting metastasis from the mammary tumor (Wright-Giemsa, 500× magnification).

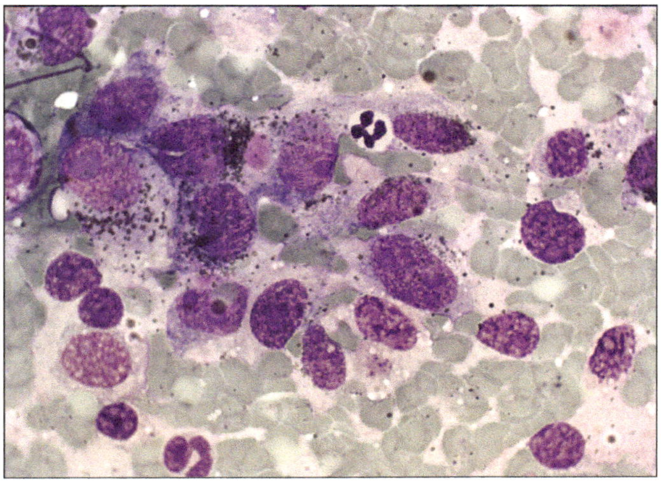

Figure 5.53 Dog, mandibular lymph node, FNA. Several large spindle cells, often cont aining fine black granules, indicating a metastasis from an oral malignant melanoma (May-Grünwald-Giemsa, 1,000× magnification).

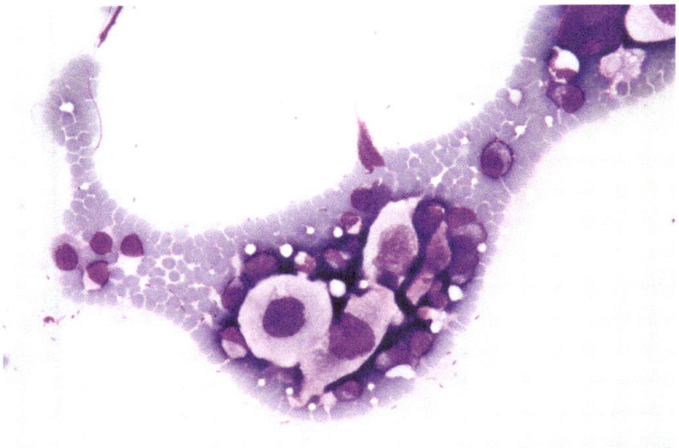

Figure 5.52 Cat, mandibular lymph node, FNA. Voluminous atypical epithelial cells with abundant clear cytoplasm and angular margins suggesting metastasis from an oral squamous cell carcinoma (May-Grünwald-Giemsa, 600× magnification).

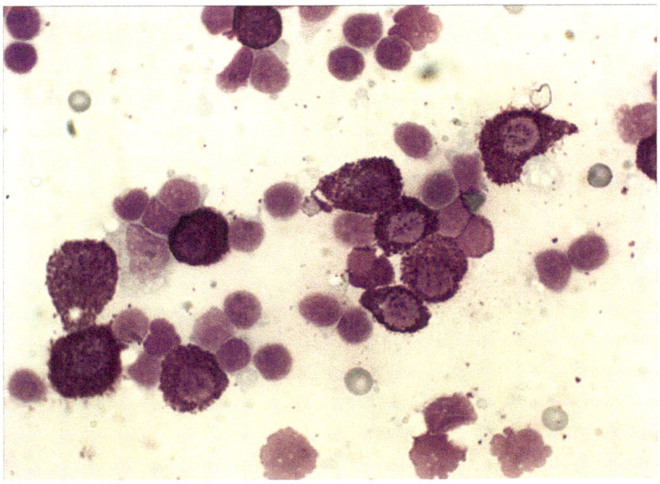

Figure 5.54 Dog, peripheral lymph node, FNA. Mast cell tumor. Many well-differentiated, granulated mast cells are found in the draining lymph node from a dog with cutaneous mastocytoma (May-Grünwald-Giemsa, 1,000× magnification).

metastasize to submandibular lymph nodes. Neoplastic cells may be spindle-shaped to oval to round and may occasionally be found in small clusters. Fine brown/black granules may be observed (Figure 5.53), but are lacking in aspirates from amelanotic melanomas, making this tumor type much more difficult to identify. Neoplastic melanocytes must be differentiated from melanin laden macrophages (melanophages) that may accompany melanocytic tumors or reactive conditions. Granules in melanophages are generally more variable in size and larger than seen in melanocytes, and cytoplasmic vacuoles are frequently found. Hemangiosarcoma may also metastasize to lymph nodes. Neoplastic cells are generally individualized, spindle-shaped, large, and may contain phagocytized erythrocytes, blue-black hemosiderin pigment, or small vacuoles.

Metastasis of round cell tumors also occurs frequently. Lymph node aspirates may be a part of the staging procedure for mast cell tumors. Since detection of mast cells in lymph nodes may be a normal feature, the issue of the percentage of mast cells in a lymph node aspirate must be considered if metastasis is suspected. Generally, a percentage higher than 3% mast cells with atypical morphologic characteristics (e.g. poorly granulated cells, binucleation) is suggestive of lymph node infiltration (Figure 5.54). The presence of foci of aggregated mast cells may strongly support the hypothesis of metastatic disease, as this feature is rarely recognized in normal cytologic aspirates. Eosinophilic infiltration accompanying the primary neoplasia may also be present. Less frequently, transmissible venereal tumors (TVTs) invade lymph nodes. Cells from TVTs are round with gray cytoplasm, often vacuolated, and have a round nucleus with coarse chromatin. Plasma cell tumors (multiple myeloma and plasmacytoma) do not typically invade lymph nodes, but in some cases neoplastic plasma cells may be found (Figure 5.55). It may be difficult to differentiate severe plasma cell hyperplasia from a metastatic plasma cell tumor. In these cases, bone marrow aspirates and serum protein electrophoresis are recommended.

Extranodal lymphoid neoplasms including cutaneous epitheliotropic lymphoma, chronic lymphoid leukemia, and acute lymphoid leukemia may infiltrate lymph nodes. Cutaneous epitheliotropic lymphoma (mycosis fungoides) cells are variable in size, with moderately abundant, lightly basophilic cytoplasm, sometimes with fine purple granules, and an indented nucleus that is occasionally cerebriform (Sezary cell-type) and poorly visible nucleoli (Figure 5.56). These cells generally exhibit a T CD8$^+$ phenotype, which may be useful for tracking the infiltration in the lymph nodes and in the bone marrow. Leukemias that infiltrate lymph nodes generally cause mild to moderate lymphadenomegaly and only rarely efface the normal

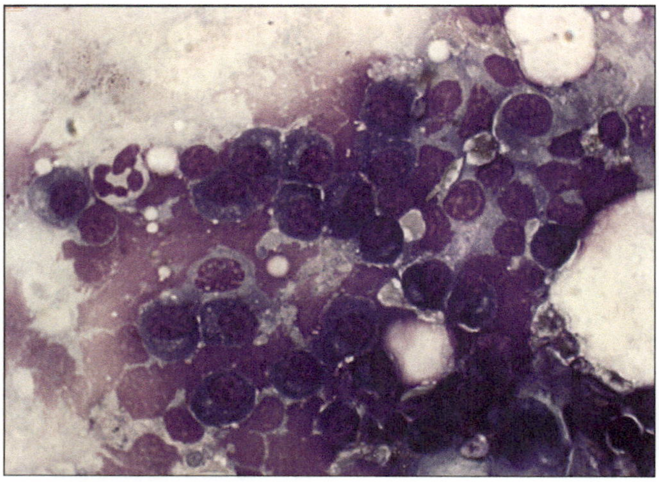

Figure 5.55 Dog, peripheral lymph node, FNA. Plasma cell tumor. Several plasma cells with mild signs of malignancy. The high percentage of cells in spite of the minimal atypia supports the diagnosis of a well-differentiated plasma cell tumor (May–Grünwald–Giemsa, 400× magnification).

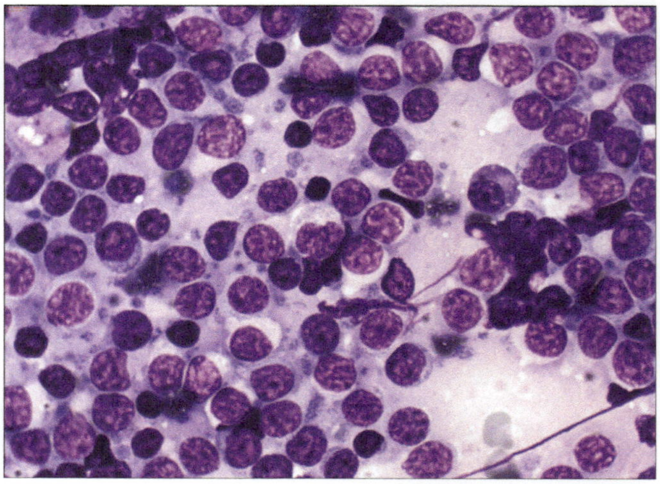

Figure 5.57 Dog, peripheral lymph node, FNA. Chronic lymphocytic leukemia. Presence of many neoplastic small lymphoid cells with clear cytoplasm admixed with resident and reactive lymph nodal population (May–Grünwald–Giemsa, 1,000× magnification).

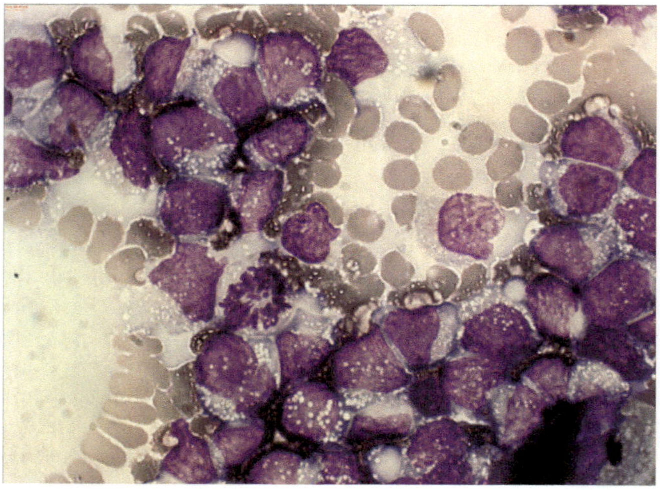

Figure 5.56 Dog, axillary lymph node, FNA. Mycosis fungoides. Several large lymphoid cells with mildly basophilic cytoplasm, several vacuoles, oval or indented nuclei, and several mitotic figures. This feature is suggestive of lymph node metastasis from cutaneous epitheliotropic lymphoma (May–Grünwald–Giemsa, 1,000× magnification).

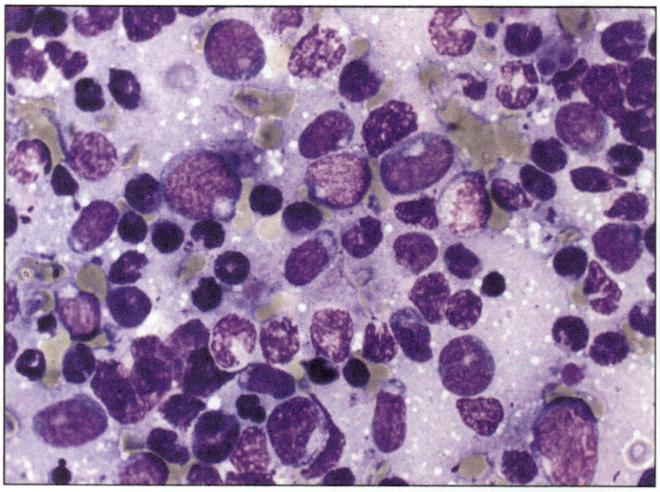

Figure 5.58 Dog, peripheral lymph node, FNA. Acute myeloid leukemia. Large blast cells with an indented nucleus and clear perinuclear halo (resembling monoblasts) are admixed with resident and reactive lymph nodal population; some neutrophils are also evident. Flow cytometry confirmed the monoblastic origin of the neoplastic cells (May–Grünwald–Giemsa, 1,000× magnification).

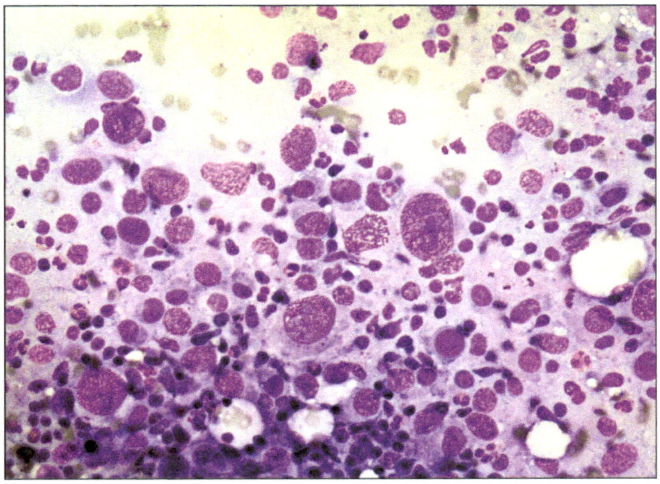

Figure 5.59 **Dog, peripheral lymph node, FNA. Disseminated histiocytic sarcoma. Several large, pleomorphic histiocytoid cells, isolated or in clusters, with several malignancy signs, replace most of the resident lymphoid population (May–Grünwald–Giemsa, 400× magnification) (courtesy Ugo Bonfanti).**

resident lymphoid population (Figures 5.57, 5.58). Complete blood count (CBC), examination of peripheral blood smears, and bone marrow aspiration cytology are needed to fully characterize infiltrative leukemias. Molecular testing is often needed to definitively diagnose the presence of metastatic lymphoid cells within a lymph node.

Histiocytic diseases (mainly disseminated histiocytic sarcoma and malignant histiocytosis) frequently metastasize to lymph node. Tumor cells may be identified by their large size and pleomorphism (Figure 5.59). Malignant histiocytes often have abundant cytoplasm that is lightly basophilic and vacuolated; in some subtypes, erythrophagocytosis may be found. Nuclei are bean-shaped or convoluted, with prominent nucleoli, and are frequently multinucleated. Although hystiocytic lineage-specific markers are lacking, immunostaining for CD18, CD45, CD11c, CD11d, CD1, and MHC class II may help to confirm cytologic suspicion and define the subtype of the disease (Moore, 2014).

SPLEEN

Indications for sampling

Sampling for splenic cytology by fine needle biopsy, preferably without aspiration, is indicated in cases of splenomegaly and when changes in ultrasonographic aspects of the spleen have been identified. In addition, the spleen may be investigated in staging procedures for mast cell tumors, lymphoma, and histiocytic diseases. Book et al. (2011) reported splenic infiltration as a prognostic factor predicting survival in dogs with mast cell tumors. However, a study that evaluated healthy dogs and dogs with cutaneous mastocytoma concluded that the significance of finding increased numbers of mast cells in splenic aspirates, without any concurrent ultrasonographic changes, is too low to support splenic aspiration as a staging tool (Finora et al., 2006). A recent paper reported more than 30% false-negative results in staging cutaneous mast cell tumors via cytology when compared to histology (Ku et al., 2017). Some authors suggest that care should be taken in performing aspiration from splenic masses because of the possible dissemination of neoplastic cells along the needle tract or the rupture of blood-filled masses (Osborne et al., 1974; Johnson et al., 1989). However, several studies (Ballegeer et al., 2007, Watson et al. 2011; Christiansen et al., 2016) reported percutaneous ultrasound-guided FNA as sufficiently safe and accurate, providing a high agreement with histologic biopsies.

Sampling

FNA or fenestration may be performed without general anesthesia, but ultrasound-guided sampling is highly recommended. Dogs should be placed in right lateral or dorsal recumbency and surgical disinfection of the skin should be performed. Body movement should be carefully avoided by sedation or restraint, particularly if thrombocytopenia is present. Whichever technique is employed, a 21–23-gauge needle should be used to minimize hemodilution and reduce complications. Fine needle fenestration is the preferred method of collecting splenic cytology samples because it allows for minimal hemodilution and adequate cellularity (Leblanc et al., 2009). Collection of a sample for ancillary techniques (flow cytometry and molecular biology) requires FNA; coating of the syringe and needle with 4% EDTA helps to avoid clotting. Regardless of the sampling technique, smears should be prepared in the same manner as blood films to minimize rupture of splenic cells and erythrocytes. If splenectomy is performed, impression smears can be prepared so that an immediate diagnosis may be made. The fresh cut tissue should be gently blotted onto absorbent paper before making imprints to remove excess blood and tissue fluids. Staining techniques are similar to those used for other lymphoid tissues and, if necessary, ancillary staining can be performed.

Cytologic features related to sampling

Ultrasound gel is often found in smears of splenic aspirates and should not be confused with granules from LGLs or mast cells. Blood contamination severely affects many cytologic smears by masking the relevant cell population. In addition to erythrocytes, cells from circulating blood may affect interpretation if severe leukocytosis is present, and may lead to a false interpretation of splenitis. Platelet clumps are another common component of peripheral blood in the sample. Extra- or perisplenic cells may be collected in the needle during sampling. In particular, mesothelial cells may be found isolated or in small clusters with a honeycomb appearance (Figure 5.60). This finding is considered incidental.

Normal anatomy and cytology

The spleen is surrounded by a thick capsule composed of fibroelastic tissue and smooth muscle cells. The capsule is covered by peritoneum and extends into the splenic parenchyma in trabeculae. The parenchyma is divided into red pulp, mainly composed of erythrocytes intermingled with a reticular stroma, blood vessels, and endothelial sinuses, and white pulp, composed of periarterial lymphatic sheets

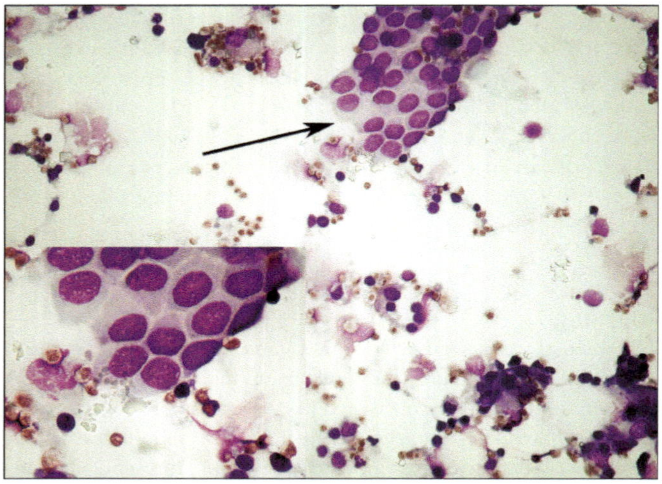

Figure 5.60 Dog, spleen, FNA. Large sheet of mesothelial cells (arrow) with honeycomb appearance (inset). This feature is suggestive of sampling contamination and does not have any pathological meaning (May–Grünwald–Giemsa, 400× magnification) (courtesy U. Bonfanti).

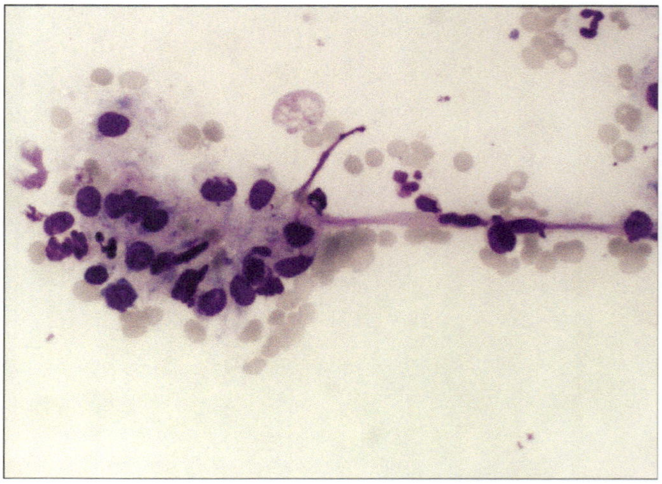

Figure 5.61 Dog, spleen, FNA. Macrophages embedded in fine reticular fibers surrounding a capillary structure. This feature is consistent with ellipsoids and does not have any pathological meaning (May–Grünwald–Giemsa, 400× magnification).

and lymphatic nodules supported by the reticular stroma. Splenic nodules may resemble primary or secondary follicles according to their activation status. The splenic artery enters the hilus of the organ and branches in an arterial tree, continuing in fine pulp capillaries, often surrounded by pericapillary macrophage sheets supported by reticular fibers (ellipsoids). The capillaries end in a terminal capillary that opens into the reticular stroma of the red pulp or into venous sinuses.

Erythrocytes and lymphoid cells are the prevalent cell populations in splenic cytology samples. Their proportion may vary according to the area sampled and blood contamination. Lymphoid cells are mainly composed of mature small lymphocytes but, if germinal centers are sampled, blasts may be present in high percentages. Immunophenotyping of splenic lymphoid cells showed that T cells predominate (52%) in adult dogs, being mainly composed of T helper (CD4+) cells (32%). Approximately 25% of cells are B cells in adult dogs, but they may be the prevalent population (52%) in newborn puppies (Faldyna et al., 2005). In addition to erythrocytes and lymphocytes, a few macrophages and plasma cells may be found. Due to the normal activity of removal of damaged red blood cells, splenic macrophages may contain hemosiderin pigment (staining blue–black) or hematoidin crystals (golden yellow). Other cells that may normally be found at low percentages are mast cells, neutrophils, endothelial cells, and fibrocytes. The presence of aggregates of connective reticular tissue, often surrounded by macrophages (ellipsoids) or containing endothelial cells, fibrocytes, and lymphoid cells, is a normal cytologic feature (Figure 5.61).

Extramedullary hematopoiesis

The spleen is a major hematopoietic organ in fetal life. This function decreases after birth but it remains potentially inducible in cases of bone marrow failure or ineffective hematopoiesis. EMH is the most common cytologic finding in splenic aspirates, being present in approximately 24% of samples from dogs (O'Keefe & Couto, 1987). Often, clinical disease associated with EMH cannot be detected in these patients. Myelolipoma is a rare benign condition characterized by a marked EMH in the context of several lipid droplets and small clusters of normal appearing adipocytes (Figure 5.62). This disease process needs to be confirmed histologically. Severe EMH has been associated with chronic hemolytic anemia, myelo- and lymphoproliferative disorders, nonregenerative anemias with bone marrow failure, and splenic hemangiosarcoma (Bertazzolo et al., 2005). Detection of excessive numbers of macrophages with erythrophagocytosis may support a diagnosis of immune-mediated anemia. Evaluation of

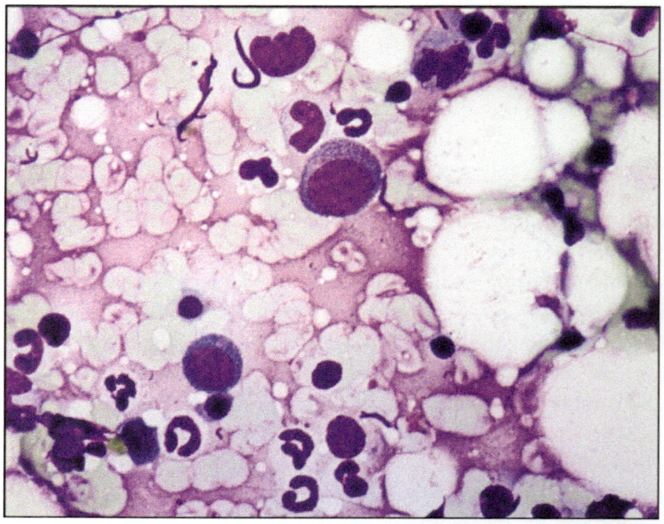

Figure 5.62 Dog, spleen, FNA. Myelolipoma. Myeloid and erythroid precursors and immature cells supporting extramedullary hematopoiesis, several lipid droplets, and normal adipocytes (May–Grünwald–Giemsa, 1,000× magnification).

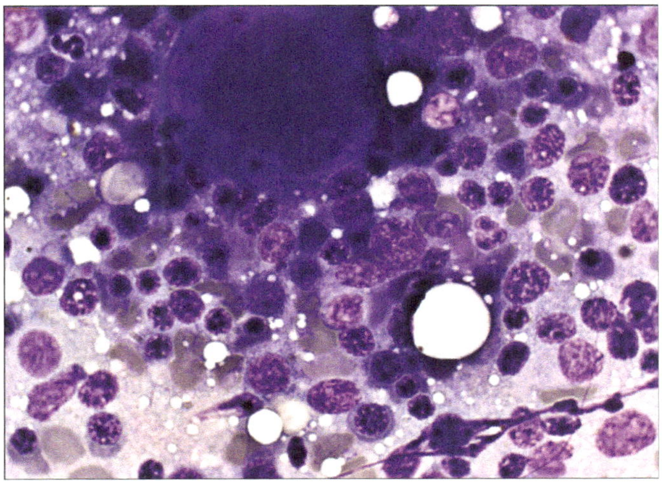

Figure 5.63 Dog, spleen, FNA. Extramedullary hematopoiesis. A large megakaryoblast and several erythroid immature cells are evident (May–Grünwald–Giemsa, 1,000× magnification).

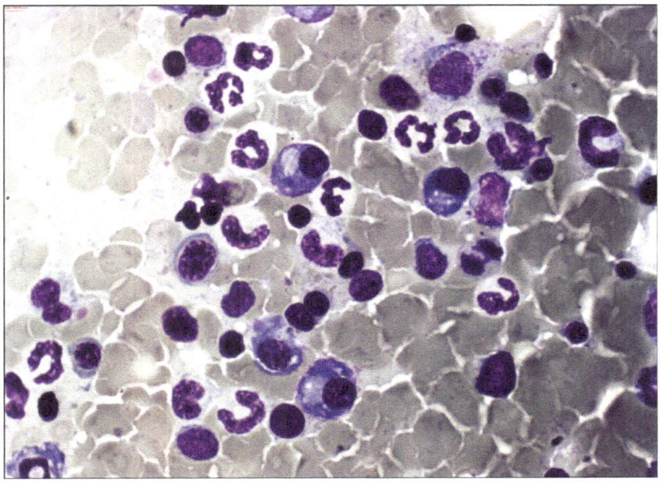

Figure 5.64 Dog, spleen, FNA. Reactive hyperplasia and extramedullary hematopoiesis. Several plasma cells and hematopoietic immature cells are found (May–Grünwald–Giemsa, 1,000× magnification).

CBC data and a bone marrow aspirate are recommended if underlying disease is suspected. Splenomegaly is uncommon in animals with EMH, but hypoechoic nodules may be found. The detection of erythroid, myeloid, and megakaryocytic precursors is diagnostic for EMH (Figure 5.63). Sometimes, islets of immature erythroid cells surrounding macrophages (nurse cells) may be found.

Reactive hyperplasia

The term splenic hyperplasia may be related to a variety of non-neoplastic conditions that lead to a diffuse enlargement of the spleen or to nodular focal lesions. Reactive hyperplastic spleen has an increase in the numbers of macrophages and plasma cells (Figure 5.64). Small lymphocytes are still the predominant lymphoid population, but medium to large lymphocytes frequently are increased. Mast cells may also be increased and are often associated with sheets of reticular fibers and capillaries. Neutrophils may be found and support possible concurrent inflammation.

Splenitis

Splenitis may be due to infectious or noninfectious diseases including immune-mediated diseases and malignancies. Concurrent peripheral blood evaluation is mandatory to determine if inflammatory cells are a component of the peripheral blood or a true infiltrate. Although detection of organisms may be challenging with infectious etiologies, splenic cytology may increase the sensitivity of peripheral blood smear examination alone. Leishmaniasis, histoplasmosis, cytauxzoonosis, babesiosis (Figure 5.65), hepatozoonosis (Figure 5.66), erhlichiosis, and anaplasmosis may cause histiocytic splenitis.

The term hemophagocytic syndrome is used to describe a wide range of different conditions characterized by an increased number of macrophages showing erythrophagocytosis and concurrent peripheral cytopenias. This condition is not rare in dogs, whereas it is quite rare in cats. Hemophagocytic syndrome may be idiopathic or associated with immune-mediated, infectious, or neoplastic diseases (Weiss, 2007). The distinction between reactive hemophagocytic syndrome and neoplastic hemophagocytic histiocytic sarcoma is often difficult.

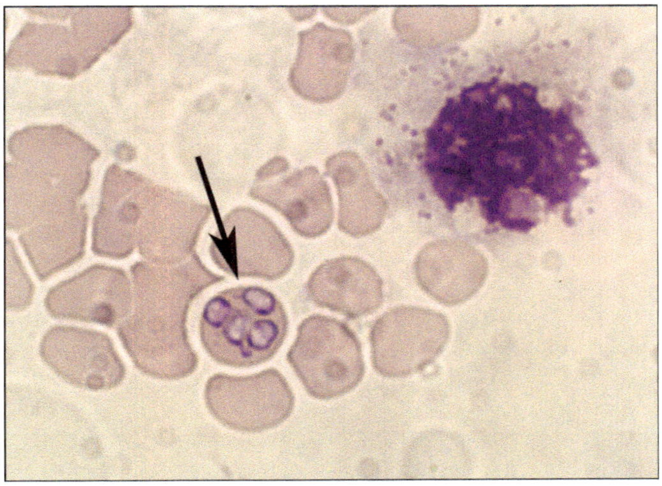

Figure 5.65 Dog, spleen, FNA. Babesiosis. Four round to piriform merozoites of *B. canis* are found in an erythrocyte (arrow) (May–Grünwald–Giemsa, 2,000× magnification).

Non-hematopoietic neoplasia

Neoplastic conditions commonly affect the spleen. Neoplastic diseases were present in approximately half of the samples from splenectomized dogs (Neer, 1996); this percentage was slightly lower (37%) in cats (Spangler & Culbertson, 1992). Hemangiosarcoma is the most common neoplasm of the spleen. Hemangiosarcoma has a poor prognosis since it tends to metastasize rapidly via blood flow or rupture of the primary splenic lesion. In a cytologic study on a cohort of 19 dogs with hemangiosarcoma, cytologic features were very variable (Bertazzolo

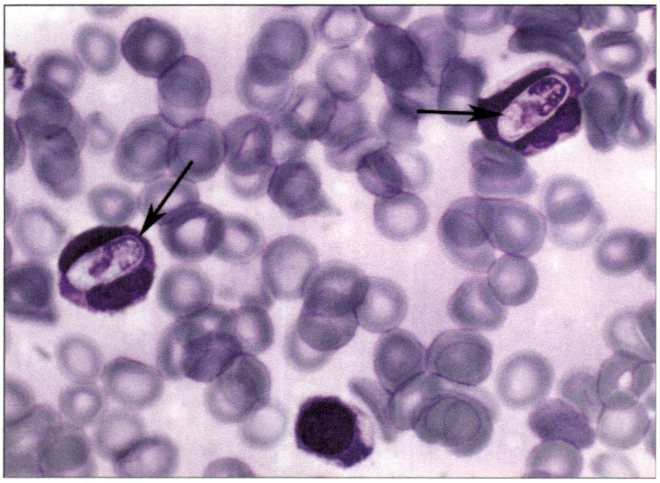

Figure 5.66 Dog spleen, FNA. Hepatozoonosis. Large cigar-shaped gamonts are visible in two neutrophils (arrows) (May–Grünwald–Giemsa, 2,000× magnification).

et al., 2005). However, there are some common features that can lead to suspicion of hemangiosarcoma in an FNA or an impression smear. Blood contamination is often abundant and acute erythophagocytosis or hemosiderin-laden macrophages are frequent findings. Cellularity may be variable, likely depending more on the histologic subtype than on the sampling technique used. Cells may exfoliate singly or in loose clusters, or may aggregate in epithelioid-like nests mimicking epithelial architecture (Figure 5.67). Neoplastic cells are large, ranging from spindle to stellate to oval, with moderately abundant basophilic cytoplasm, sometimes with multiple punctate vacuoles (Figure 5.68). The nucleus is ovoid with coarse chromatin and one or more prominent nucleoli. Anisocytosis and anisokaryosis are common features. Binucleated and multinucleated cells are often found. Cytologic diagnosis of poorly differentiated hemangiosarcomas may be challenging. Immunophenotyping for positivity to factor VIII-related antigen and CD31 supports a diagnosis of hemangiosarcoma.

Other primary mesenchymal tumors are rare in the spleen, but fibrosarcoma, leiomiosarcoma, osteosarcoma, liposarcoma, myxosarcoma, and pleomorphic undifferentiated sarcoma have been reported (Spangler et al., 1994). Cytologic aspects of these tumors are not different from those in other tissues. As in other lymphoid tissues, metastases of many tumor types may be found in the spleen.

Hematopoietic neoplasia

Primary or metastatic hematopoietic tumors may occur in the spleen. In many cases, splenic aspiration is a part of the staging procedure following a diagnosis of mastocytoma, lymphoma, or histiocytic diseases. In other cases, the spleen is the only organ involved and ultrasound-guided FNA is performed to investigate ultrasonic abnormalities or focal lesions.

LYMPHOMA

The distinction between primary splenic lymphoma and metastatic lymphoma is not always possible, but a high percentage of primary splenic lymphomas are low-grade B-cell lymphomas often arising from the marginal or the mantle zone, and systemic involvement is limited. Detection of an increased percentage of blasts should be interpreted with care, since blasts are increased in hyperplastic and reactive conditions. Detection of more than 40% blasts in a splenic FNB is suggestive of lymphoid neoplasia. If necessary, PARR may help reach a more definitive diagnosis (Williams et al., 2006). Other papers suggest considering a splenic involvement when there are >5% blasts in dogs with a previous diagnosis of multicentric lymphoma (Nerschbach et al., 2016).

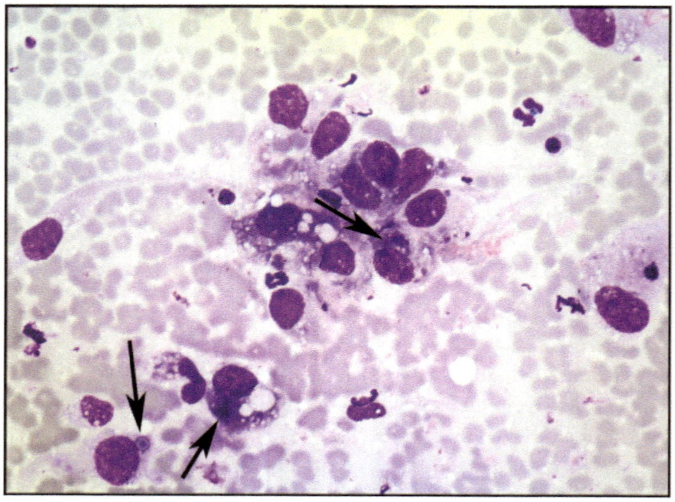

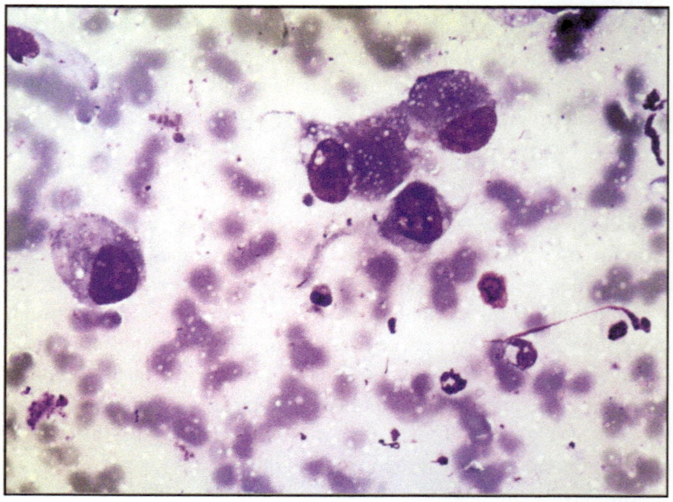

Dog, spleen, FNA. Hemangiosarcoma.

Figure 5.67 Clusters of pleomorphic mesenchymal cells varying from polygonal to spindle. Erythrophagocytosis (arrows) is a common feature.

Figure 5.68 Large globoid, to stellate hemangioblasts, with deeply basophilic cytoplasm, and several microvacuoles (May–Grünwald–Giemsa, 600× magnification) (courtesy U. Bonfanti).

Histology is necessary to further subtype lymphomas of the spleen and may provide some prognostic information. Marginal zone lymphomas are nodular (Figures 5.69, 5.70) or diffuse and have a more favorable prognosis in dogs than marginal zone lymphoma in the lymph node (Stefanello et al., 2011). Mantle cell lymphomas have been reported in spleen from both dogs and cats and have a good prognosis (Valli, 2007). Hepatosplenic lymphoma is a rare and aggressive T cell lymphoma variant described cytologically as medium-/large-sized cells that often have fine magenta cytoplasmic granules and variably shaped nuclei. High-grade, diffuse large B-cell lymphoma commonly infiltrates the spleen and progresses from multifocal to coalescing lesions, with variable response to therapy (Valli, 2007). In dogs, T-cell chronic lymphocytic leukemia (CLL) often arises from the spleen (McDonough & Moore, 2000; Workman & Vernau, 2003). These cells often have an LGL appearance (Figure 5.71), with moderately abundant, clear cytoplasm with fine, azurophilic, perinuclear granules, and express CD8 by flow cytometry (McDonough & Moore, 2000). Concurrent leukocytosis may be found, but bone marrow infiltration is not a constant feature with T-cell CLL. T-cell CLL may be an indolent disease and survival may often exceed 2–3 years. CLL of B cell origin is less frequent in the dog and likely derives from the bone marrow.

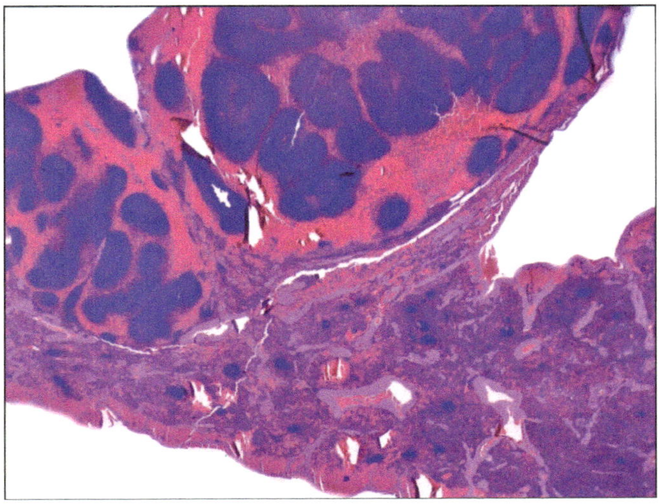
Figure 5.69 Dog, spleen, histology. Portion of spleen with marginal zone lymphoma (H&E, 50× magnification) (courtesy L. Aresu).

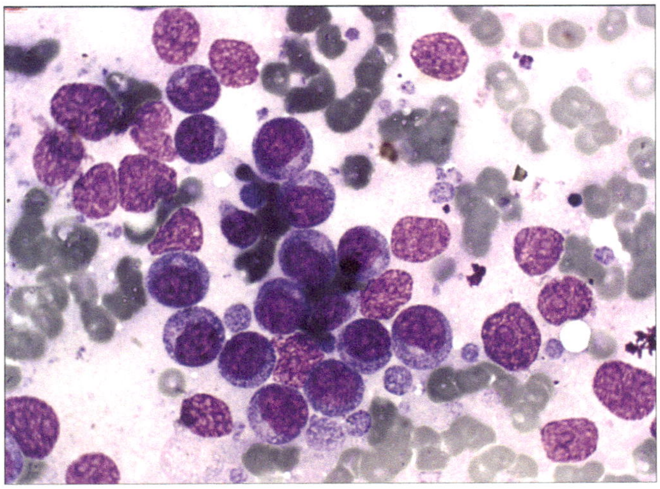
Figure 5.70 Dog, spleen, FNA, Marginal lymphoma. A single, prevalent population of medium-sized macronucleolated cells is recognizable (May-Grünwald-Giemsa, 1,000× magnification).

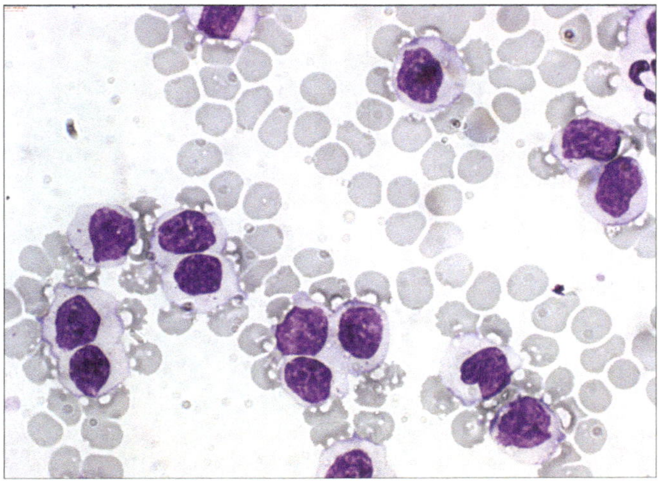
Figure 5.71 Dog, spleen, FNA. Chronic lymphocytic leukemia. A single population of mature neoplastic lymphoid cells with moderately abundant clear cytoplasm, sometimes containing fine azurophilic granules, is recognizable (May-Grünwald-Giemsa, 1,000× magnification).

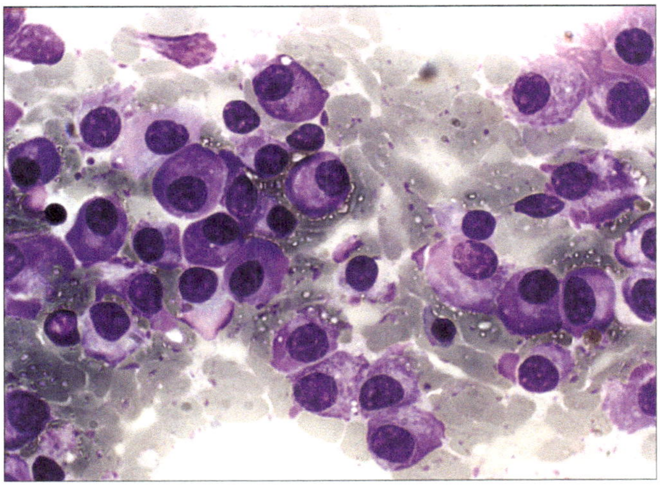
Figure 5.72 Dog, spleen, FNA. Plasma cell tumor. A prevalent population of medium-sized round cells with abundant cytoplasm, often irregularly eosinophilic, eccentric round nuclei with coarse to clumped chromatin and no visible nucleoli (May-Grünwald-Giemsa, 1,000× magnification).

PLASMA CELL TUMORS

Plasma cell tumors in the spleen include multiple myelomas (mainly in cats) and extramedullary plasmacytomas. Diffuse enlargement of

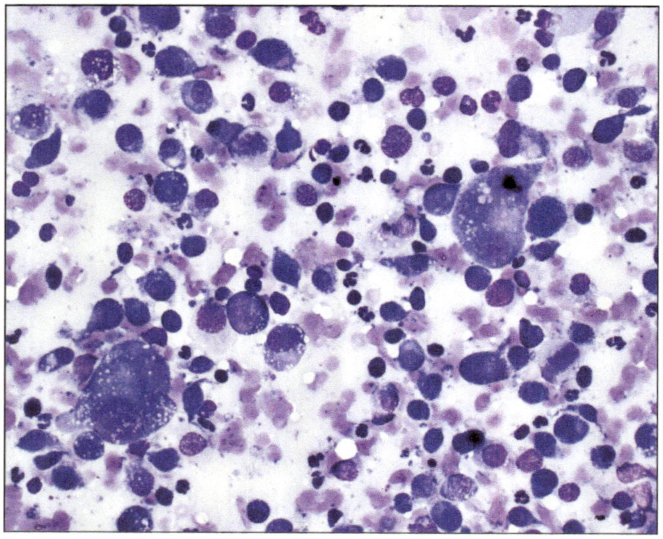

Figure 5.73 Dog, spleen, FNA. Disseminated histiocytic sarcoma. Large histiocytoid cells, with vacuolated cytoplasm intermingled with lymphoid cells and neutrophils (Wright–Giemsa, 500× magnification).

spleen and a massive presence of plasma cells at different stages of differentiation are the main features. Cells may exhibit characteristics of malignancy and binucleated cells are frequent (Figure 5.72). Monoclonal increases in globulin concentration may be detected by serum protein electrophoresis.

Histiocytic disorders

The spleen is a common site of malignant histiocytic tumors. Two different types of histiocytic sarcomas may be distinguished based on cytomorphology and immunoreactivity. Disseminated histiocytic sarcoma derives from a clonal expansion of splenic dendritic cells with a $CD1^+$, $CD11c^+$, $CD11d^-$, $MHC\text{-}II^+$ immunophenotype (Affolter & Moore, 2002). Neoplastic cells are large and discrete, often with abundant, clear cytoplasm, indistinct cell borders, and cytoplasmic vacuoles. The nucleus is oval to convoluted with finely reticulated or irregularly clumped chromatin (Figures 5.73). Binucleated and multinucleated giant cells are frequent and characteristics of malignancy are prominent including severe anisocytosis and anisokaryosis. Hemophagocytic histiocytic sarcoma derives from macrophages that are immunopositive for CD11d, while expression of CD1 and MHC-II is low and CD11c is generally negative (Moore et al., 2006). This neoplasm has a poor prognosis. A mild to moderate anemia is often present. Neoplastic cells are large with foamy cytoplasm and contain phagocytized erythrocytes and/or hemosiderin (Figures 5.74–5.76). The detection of erythrophagocytosis in neoplastic cells supports the diagnosis of hemophagocytic histiocytic sarcoma; however, several other round cell tumors (mastocytoma, lymphoma, plasma cell tumors, osteosarcoma, megakaryocytic leukemia; Figures 5.77–5.79) and some sarcomas (e.g., hemangiosarcoma, osteosarcoma) have been demonstrated to occasionally exhibit erythrophagocytosis (Barger et al., 2012); thus this feature must be interpreted with caution.

Mast cell tumors

Although mast cells are a normal resident cell population in spleen, their percentage may increase in reactive conditions and with metastatic mast cell tumors. The detection of a high number of mast cells in the spleen of either dogs or cats with mast cell tumors is associated with a worse prognosis (Book et al., 2011). Splenic infiltration from cutaneous mastocytoma is generally associated with splenomegaly and has been reported in 37% of a cohort of 19 dogs (Book et al., 2011) and even more commonly in feline mast cell tumors (Spangler & Culbertson, 1992). Determining if the number of mast cells in a splenic aspirate is increased can be difficult. Stefanello et al. (2009) suggested the following aspects to define splenic infiltration: (1)

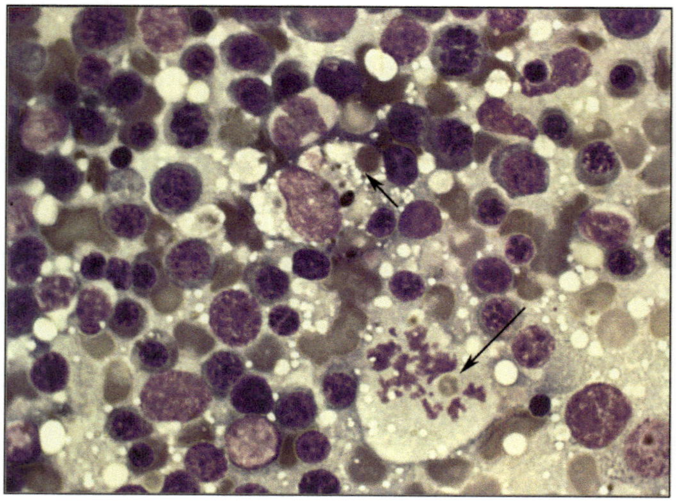

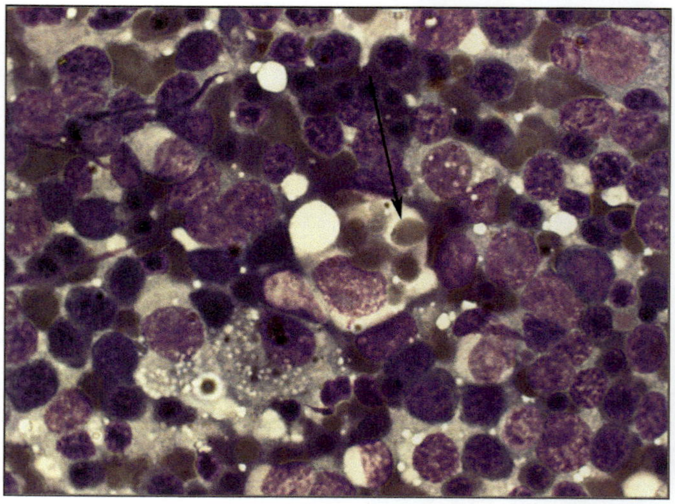

Dog, spleen, FNA. Hemophagocytic histiocytic sarcoma.

Figure 5.74 Large histiocytoid neoplastic cells and a huge atypical mitotic figure are found in a background of severe extramedullary hematopoiesis and erythrophagocytosis (arrows).

Figure 5.75 Intense recent erythrophagocytosis (arrows) in a neoplastic macrophage. Some histiocytoid cells are also seen (May–Grünwald–Giemsa, 1,000× magnification).

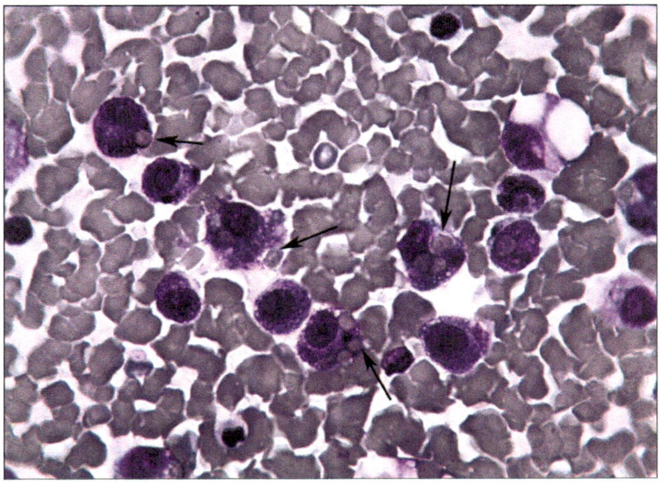

Figure 5.76 Cat, spleen, FNA. Mast cell tumor with erythrophagocytosis (arrows) (May–Grünwald–Giemsa, 1,000× magnification) (courtesy M. Gelain).

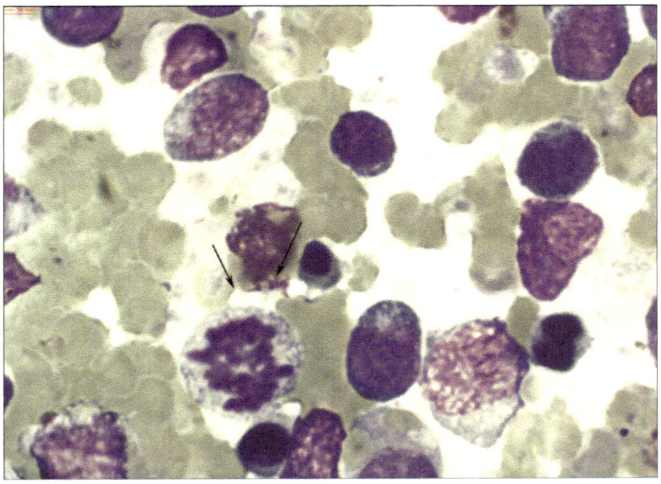

Figure 5.77 Dog, spleen, FNA. Diffuse large B-cell lymphoma. Recent erythrophagocytosis (arrows) in a neoplastic blast cell (May–Grünwald–Giemsa, 2,000× magnification).

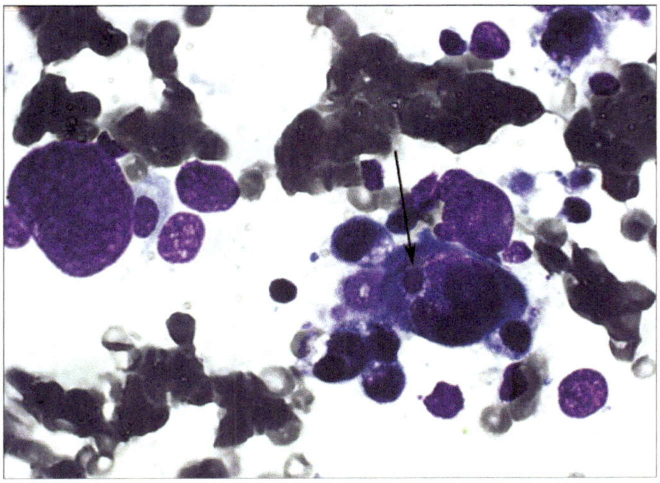

Figure 5.78 Dog, spleen, FNA. Acute megakaryoblastic leukemia. Recent erythrophagocytosis (arrow) in a neoplastic cell (May–Grünwald–Giemsa, 1,000× magnification).

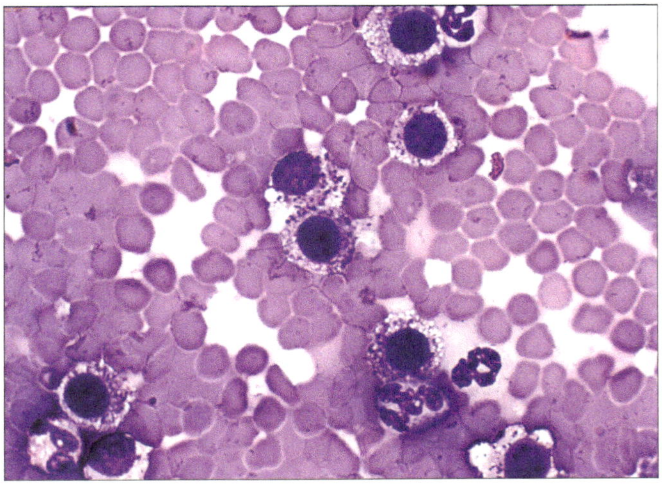

Figure 5.79 Dog, spleen, FNA. Well-differentiated mast cell tumor. Presence of an abundant population of well-differentiated mast cells (Diff-Quik®, 1,000× magnification) (courtesy D.M. Lupi).

presence of aggregates of well-differentiated mast cells; (2) presence of a large number of well-differentiated mast cells (Figure 5.79); or (3) presence of mast cells with atypical morphology (poor granulation or pleomorphism). Poorly granulated mast cells may be frequently found in cats, mainly when visceral mastocytosis is present. In these cases, care should be taken to differentiate neoplastic mast cells from other round cell tumors.

ACUTE LEUKEMIAS

Infiltration of spleen leading to splenomegaly is a common feature in acute leukemias. Detection of medium to large blast cells is the main cytologic finding. In most cases, immunophenotyping is mandatory to define the neoplastic cell lineage. However, morphology may help to suggest cellular origin in some specific acute myeloid leukemias, such as erythroleukemia or megakaryocytic leukemia (Figure 5.80).

THYMUS

Normal thymus is not usually accessible for aspiration. Impression smears contain large numbers of small, well-differentiated lymphocytes. Thymic epithelium can be observed. Other features include Hassall's corpuscles, which are tight clusters of epithelioid macrophages with cell junctions, and moderate numbers of mast cells.

Thymic enlargements may be the result of some different neoplastic and non-neoplastic conditions. Thymic hemorrhage is a rare

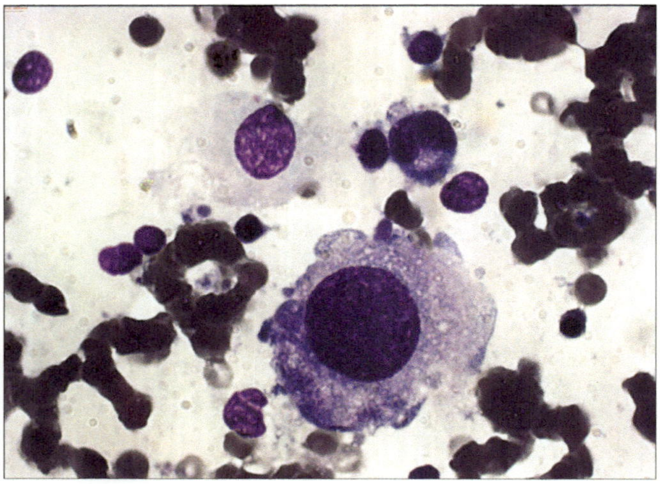

Figure 5.80 Same case as Figure 8.78. Megakaryoblastic leukemia. A large neoplastic megakaryoblast (May–Grünwald–Giemsa, 1,000× magnification).

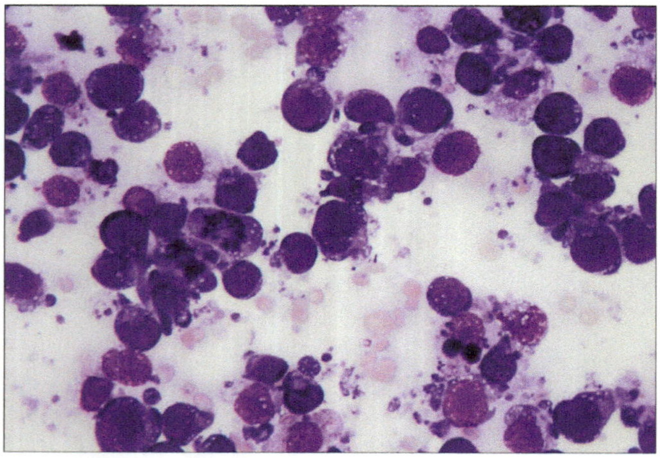

Figure 5.81 Cat, FNA from a mediastinal mass. Presence of a single population of large lymphoid blasts with prominent nucleoli consistent with high-grade thymic lymphoma. Phagocyting macrophages and mitosis are also present (Wright–Giemsa, 600× magnification).

non-neoplastic disease condition that may lead to severe transitory enlargement of thymus due to blood accumulation in the context of thymus. FNAs allow collection of a highly hemodiluted sample with an admixed population of mature T lymphocytes and fewer blasts showing different immunophenotypes via flow cytometry. Among neoplastic diseases thymic (mediastinal) lymphoma and thymoma are the most frequent and should be differentiated also in light of different therapeutic approaches (chemotherapy *vs.* surgery) and prognosis.

Thymic lymphomas are frequent in young cats and are often related to feline leukemia virus infection (Vail, 2013). The main lymphoid population is often composed of small to intermediate lymphocytes with cleaved nuclei with or without a prominent nucleolus. Occasionally, large blasts may be the prevalent lymphoid population and help to differentiate lymphoma from other lymphocytic-rich

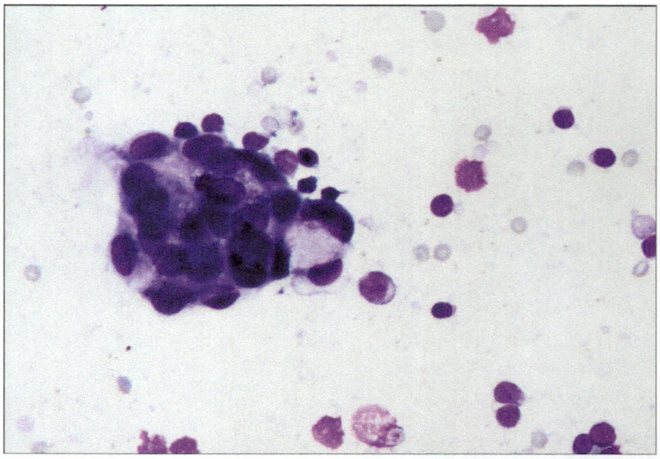

Figure 5.82 Dog, FNA from a mediastinal mass. Presence of a mixed lymphoid population with a single cluster of epithelial cells consistent with thymoma (Wright–Giemsa, 1,000× magnification).

neoplasms (Figure 5.81). Paraneoplastic hypercalcemia may be seen. Prognosis with thymic lymphoma is generally poor, with a median survival time of 2–3 months in cats (Vail, 2013).

Thymoma is also a cause of thymus enlargement. Thymic epithelial cells with some characteristics of malignancy may be observed. Cytologically, a thymoma consists of small lymphocytes with few large lymphocytes, mast cells, and occasional clusters of thymic epithelium (Figure 5.82). The ratio between lymphocytes and epithelial cells in histologic sections may be highly variable and is used to define different thymoma subtypes. Paraneoplastic conditions associated with thymoma include myasthenia gravis, hypercalcemia, megaesophagus, pemphigus foliaceous, superficial necrolytic dermatitis, exfoliative dermatitis, and pure red cell aplasia. Flow cytometric detection of double positive ($CD4^{+}CD8^{+}$) lymphocytes indicates the cells arose from a thymic mass, rather than an enlarged mediastinal lymph node. In dogs, finding a highly prevalent population of double-positive ($CD4^{+}CD8^{+}$) thymocytes is strongly suggestive of thymoma (Lana et al., 2006b). In cats, a high percentage of thymic lymphomas shows a double positive ($CD4^{+}CD8^{+}$) immunophenotype (Bernardi et al., 2020). Thus flow cytometric results do not help differentiate thymic lymphoma from thymoma. If clinically warranted, PARR is recommended to determine if the lymphocytes are neoplastic.

CASES

CASE 1

Signalment/history

A 7-month-old, male German Shepherd Dog presented for generalized lymphadenomegaly.

Clinical examination

The dog appeared alert and in good clinical condition. CBC and clinical chemistry were unremarkable except for a mild hyperproteinemia

(8.63 g/dl [86.3 g/l]). The dog had not traveled outside of southern Italy. FNAs were taken from the popliteal lymph node.

Cytologic description of the popliteal lymph node aspirate

Figure 5.83 shows a mixed lymphoid population composed of small lymphocytes, a plasma cell, and few large blasts. Closer magnification (Figure 5.84) reveals a mixed population of small lymphocytes, some with a unipolar cytoplasmic tail (red arrows) suggestive of a T cell origin. Several plasma cells (black arrows) and a large blast are visible. Note the black pigment in the background suggestive of melanin.

Cytologic interpretation

Based on the young age, the presence of a plasma cell, hyperplasia, hyperproteinemia, and location (southern Italy), a tentative diagnosis of canine leishmaniasis was made. Bone marrow was aspirated to search for the causative agent (Figure 5.85).

Cytologic description of the bone marrow aspirate

Two large macrophages containing several *Leishmania* amastigotes are found. Myeloid hyperplasia is visible in the background.

Cytologic interpretation

The final diagnosis was canine leishmaniasis.

Outcome

The dog was treated for leishmaniasis with allopurinol and meglumine antimoniate. Lymphadenomegaly, after a mild remission, persisted. Three months after the first admission, lymphadenomegaly increased

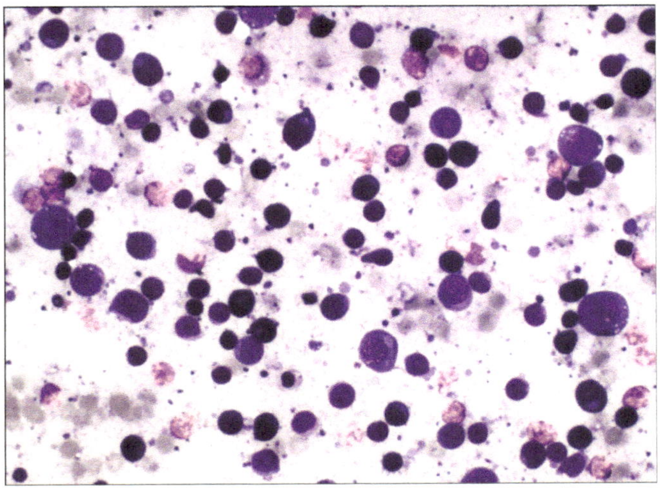

Figure 5.83 Dog, FNA from the popliteal lymph node. Presence of a mixed population composed of small lymphocytes, plasma cells, and few large blasts (May–Grünwald–Giemsa, 400× magnification).

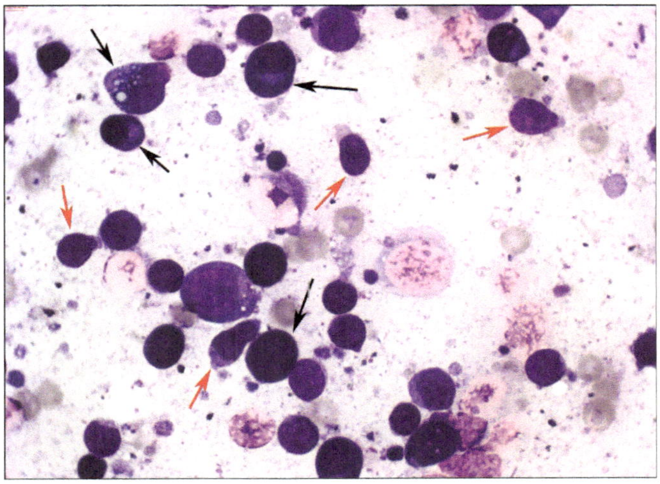

Figure 5.84 Dog, FNA from the popliteal lymph node. A mixed population of small lymphocytes, some with a unipolar cytoplasmic tail (red arrows) suggesting a T cell origin, several plasma cells (black arrows), and a large blast are visible. Note the black pigment in the background suggesting melanin (dermatopathic lymph node) (May–Grünwald–Giemsa, 1,000× magnification).

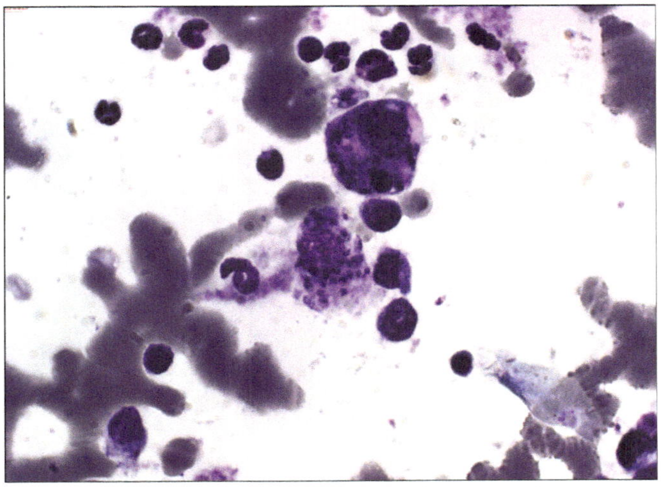

Figure 5.85 Dog, bone marrow aspirate. Two large macrophages containing several *Leishmania* amastigotes are found. Myeloid hyperplasia is visible in the background (May–Grünwald–Giemsa, 1,000× magnification).

and a subcutaneous nodule on the back appeared. An FNA was performed from the nodule and the enlarged lymph nodes (Figure 5.86).

Cytologic description of an enlarged lymph node

There are several large blast cells with abundant deeply basophilic cytoplasm, often vacuolated, oval to indented nuclei with smooth chromatin and several prominent nucleoli. Some fine pink/purple granules are visible in the juxtanuclear area. The same cells are found in the cutaneous lesion.

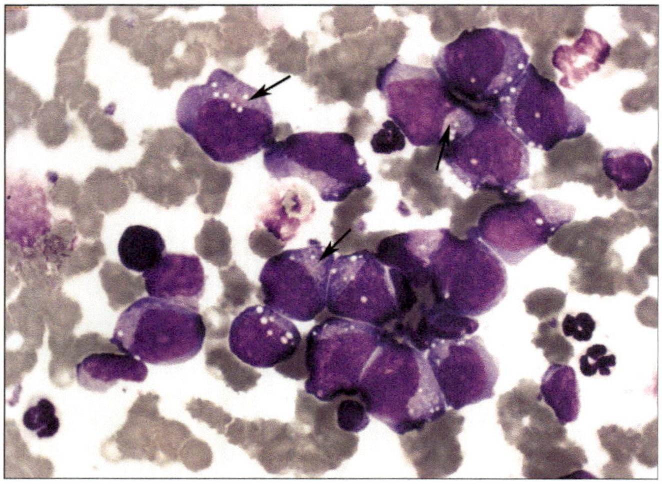

Figure 5.86 Dog, lymph node, FNA. There were several large blast cells with abundant deeply basophilic cytoplasm, often vacuolated, oval to indented nuclei with smooth chromatin, and several prominent nucleoli. Some fine pink/purple granules are visible in the juxtanuclear area (arrows). The same cells were found in the cutaneous lesion (May–Grünwald–Giemsa, 1,000× magnification).

Cytologic interpretation

A final diagnosis of high-grade lymphoma was made. Immunophenotyping was not performed but the morphologic aspect of the cells (abundant cytoplasm, indented nuclei, juxtanuclear azurophilic granules) suggests a possible T-cell lineage.

Discussion

Due to the rapid deterioration of the dog's condition, the owners elected for euthanasia.

The association between canine leishmaniasis and canine lymphoma is not rare in endemic areas (Foglia Manzillo et al., 2008) but reports are anecdotal and there are no specific studies to clarify if a higher prevalence of lymphoma is present in dogs with leishmaniasis. Possible pathogenic mechanisms for this are debated since either canine leishmaniasis could lead to persistent immune stimulation, thus promoting neoplastic transformation, or lymphoma could induce immunosuppression, which might promote the onset of leishmaniasis (Kopterides et al., 2007). In the present case, after a re-evaluation of the slides, a few neoplastic cells were already present in the first cytologic smear; therefore concurrent occurrence of the two diseases being merely coincidental cannot be excluded. The two cytologic patterns were superimposed in the first presentation and the detection of the causative agent directed therapy toward the infectious disease. The antiprotozoal therapy could have exacerbated the underlying lymphoma.

CASE 2

Signalment/history

A 6-year-old, male Boxer was brought to a private veterinary clinic with a huge wound in the cervical area.

Clinical examination

The dog appeared alert and generalized lymphadenomegaly was detected. Blood samples for CBC and clinical chemistry revealed a moderate nonregenerative, normocytic normochromic anemia (PCV = 25.4% [0.25 l/l]), and a moderate neutrophilia (PMNs = $14 \times 10^3/\mu l$) with a left shift. Circulating lymphocytes were within reference intervals ($4.2 \times 10^3/\mu l$). Clinical chemistry was unremarkable.

Diagnosis and initial treatment

A diagnosis of septic suppurative pyodermatitis, probably due to trauma, was made and antibiotic therapy was administered with

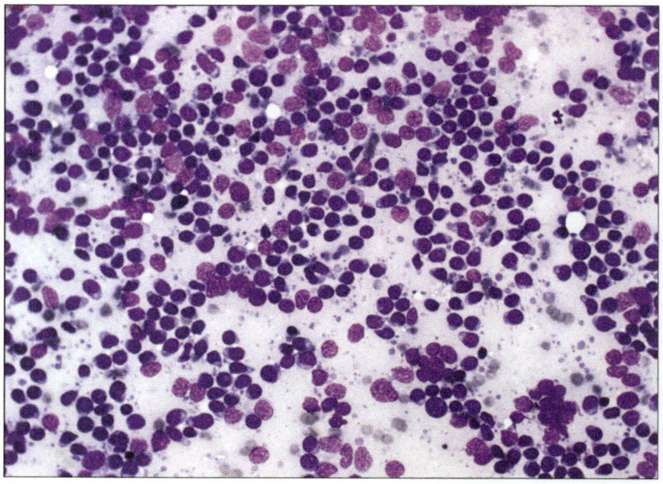

Figure 5.87 Dog, prescapular lymph node, FNA. Homogeneous population composed of small/medium lymphoid cells is found. Some ruptured cells are also seen in the background, suggesting increased fragility. Note the absence of mitotic figures (May–Grünwald–Giemsa, 400× magnification).

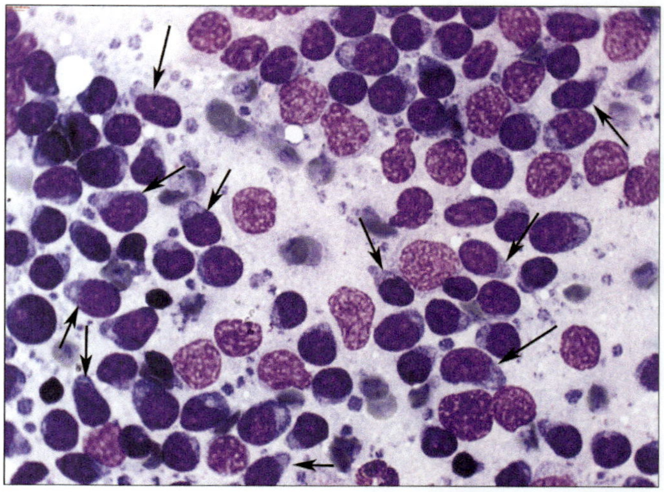

Figure 5.88 Dog, prescapular lymph node, FNA. Many of the cells (arrows) show small, unipolar cytoplasmic tails giving the characteristic hand-mirror shape (May–Grünwald–Giemsa, 1,000× magnification).

amoxycillin and clavulanic acid. After 15 days, the clinical condition improved and the neutrophil count returned to within the reference interval, but lymphadenomegaly persisted and the lymphocyte count increased to 7.1 × $10^3/\mu l$. Peripheral lymph nodes (prescapular and popliteal) were biopsied using an FNA technique (Figures 5.87 and 5.88).

Cytologic description

The sample from the prescapular lymph node contains a homogeneous population of small/medium lymphoid cells. Some ruptured cells are also seen in the background, suggesting increased fragility. Note the absence of mitotic figures. At higher magnification, most of the cells show a small, unipolar cytoplasmic tail, giving the characteristic hand-mirror shape.

Cytologic interpretation

Based on the cytologic appearance, a diagnosis of possible low-grade T-cell lymphoma (small clear cell lymphoma) was made. Differentials include paracortical hyperplasia. FNA biopsy was performed and the material collected was put in 1 ml RPMI 1640 medium for flow cytometry. Peripheral blood and a bone marrow aspirate were sampled for staging potentially neoplastic cells. Histologic biopsy via tru-cut was also taken.

Figure 5.89 shows histograms from multicolor flow cytometry of the lymph node aspirate. A prevalent population of medium-sized lymphoid cells scored positive for CD3, CD5, CD21, CD8, and CD4 and negative for CD45. This pattern is considered conclusive of low-grade T-cell lymphoma (T-zone). Peripheral blood was infiltrated by 35% of $CD5^+CD45^-$ cells. Neoplastic cells were also found at a high percentage in bone marrow (28%) but, since severe blood contamination was present, it was impossible to define correctly the percentage of infiltration.

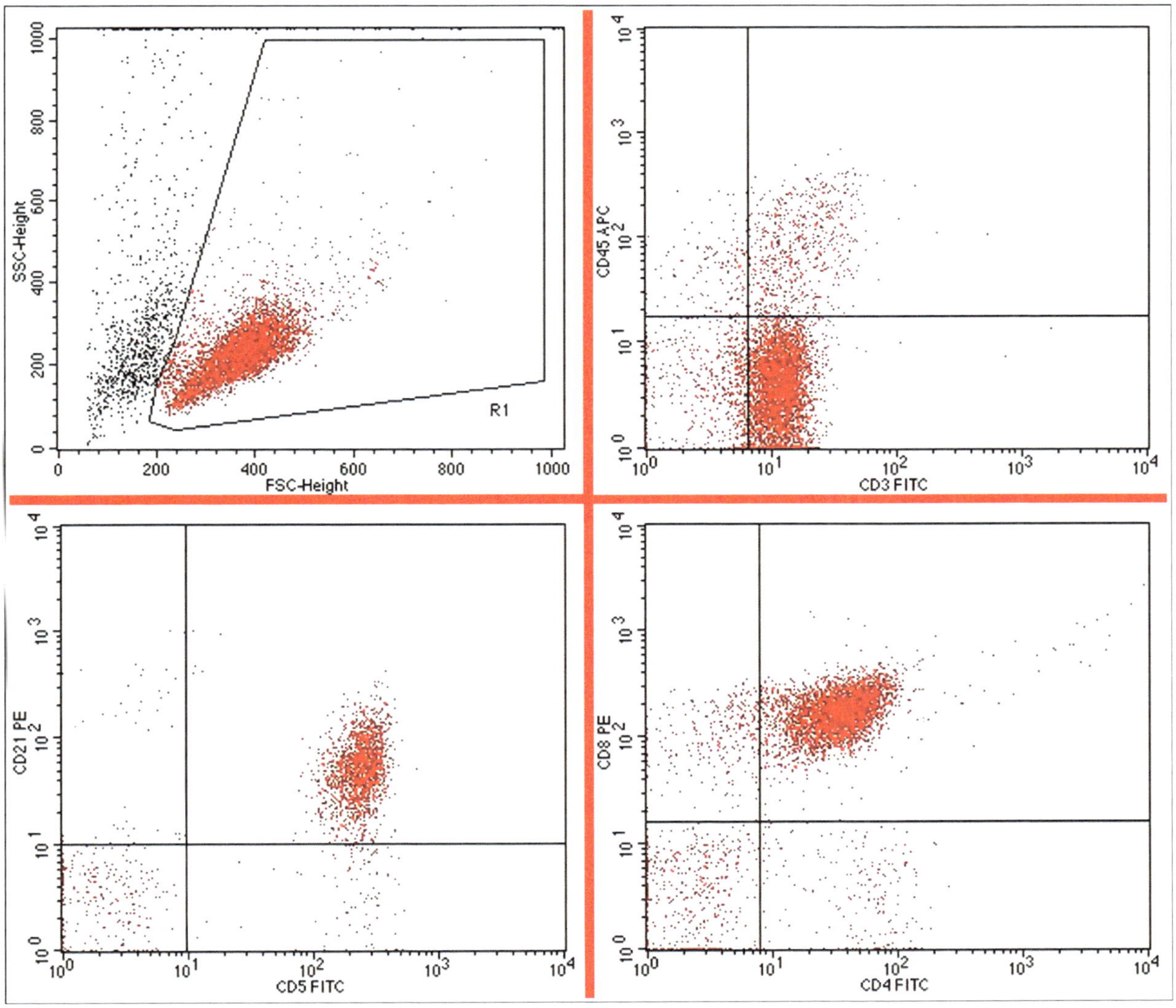

Figure 5.89 Multicolor flow cytometry of the lymph node aspirate. A prevalent population of medium-sized lymphoid cells scored positive for CD3, CD5, CD21, CD8, and CD4 and negative for CD45. This pattern is considered conclusive of low-grade T-cell lymphoma (T-zone). Peripheral blood was infiltrated by 35% of CD5+CD45− cells. Neoplastic cells were also found at a high percentage in bone marrow (28%) but, since severe blood contamination was present, it was impossible to define correctly the percentage infiltration.

Outcome

A final diagnosis of low-grade T-cell (small clear cell) lymphoma, corresponding to T-zone lymphoma in the WHO classification, was made. Histopathology confirmed the T-zone pattern and the dog was treated with chlorambucil and prednisone. Lymphadenomegaly resolved and the dog was alive and in good health 3 months after admission (complete remission).

Discussion

Low-grade T-cell lymphoma is a quite common lymphoma subtype arising from the T-zone. Cytology samples show a classical pattern of small cells with slightly basophilic cytoplasm (small clear cell), low mitotic index, and rare plasma cells. Neoplastic cells often show unipolar cytoplasm (hand-mirror shape). Cytology alone cannot differentiate this lymphoma subtype from paracortical hyperplasia and histology is typically suggested. Recently, a characteristic flow cytometric pattern has been described and this could help to differentiate this subtype on fine needle biopsy (Martini et al., 2015; Seelig et al., 2014). Neoplastic cells showed an aberrant lack of CD45 (pan leukocyte marker), a classical T-cell signature ($CD3^{+}CD5^{+}$), and aberrant expression of CD21, generally considered a B-cell marker. This aberrant expression has been also demonstrated via gene expression profiling (Frantz et al., 2013). T-zone lymphoma is generally considered an indolent lymphoma with a long survival (Ponce et al., 2004; Valli et al., 2006) but this may be influenced by staging and clinical condition.

CASE 3

Signalment/history

A domestic shorthair, female spayed, 5-year-old cat was presented to clinical visit with depression and occasional regurgitation.

Clinical examination

The cat appeared depressed but alert. A moderate dyspnoea was found. Complete blood cell count (CBC) and clinical biochemistry were unremarkable. Serology for feline leukemia virus (FeLV) and feline immunodeficiency virus (FIV) scored negative. Imaging revealed a huge mass in the cranial mediastinum compressing mainly the left lung. A moderate pleural effusion was also present. Effusion was collected in EDTA and submitted for cytology (Figure 5.90). Fine needle aspiration biopsy was taken and used to prepare some cytologic slides (Figure 5.91) and put in RPMI-1640 medium for flow cytometry (Figure 5.92).

Cytologic description

Pleural effusion showed a good cellularity (3,500 wbc/ul) composed by a mixed population of medium/small lymphocytes, sometimes with scarce cytoplasm and fine cytoplastic tails and several macrophages, often in cytophagia. Occasional mitosis, sometimes also atypical, were found in lymphoid cells (Figure 5.91).

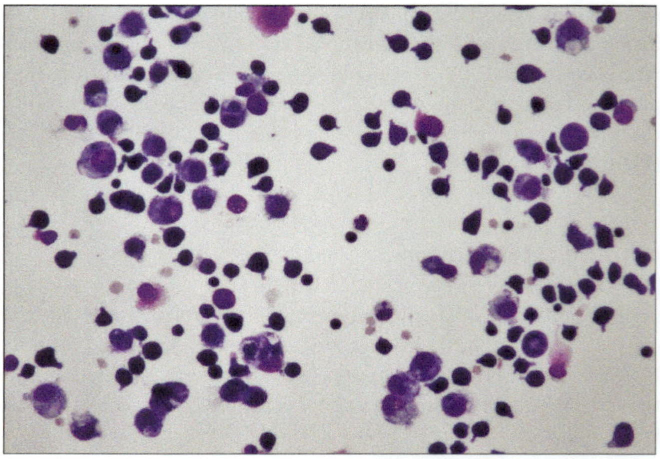

Figure 5.90 **Cat, pleural effusion, cytocentrifuged sample. The predominant cells are small to medium-sized lymphocytes (May-Grunwald-Giemsa, 400x magnification).**

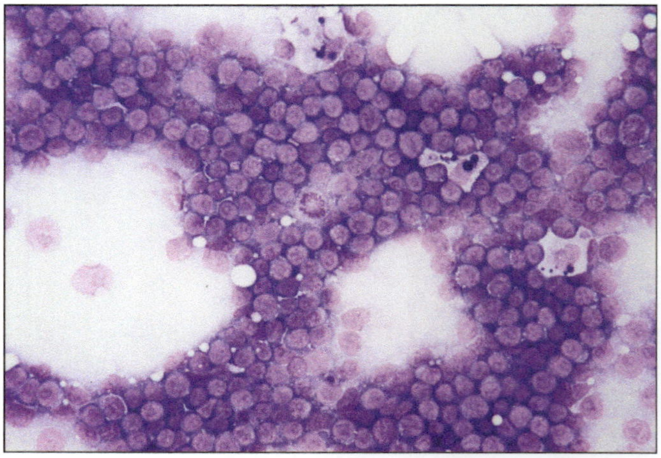

Figure 5.91 **Cat, cranial mediastinal mass, FNA. Many medium-lymphocytes and low numbers of phagocytic macrophages are present (May-Grunwald-Giemsa, 400x magnification).**

Cytology of the mediastinal mass showed a highly cellular sample composed by a prevalent population of medium-sized lymphoid cells, with scarce cytoplasm, round nuclei with decondensed chromatin and often a visible single nucleolus. Mitosis were often visible. Several macrophages, often in phagocytosis of cellular debris, were also visible (Figure 5.91).

Flow cytometry revealed a homogeneous population of T cells composed showing in more than 80% a double positive $CD4^{+}CD8^{+}$ phenotype (Figure 5.92).

Cytologic and flow cytometric interpretation

Effusion and mediastinal mass revealed a highly prevalent population composed by small to medium lymphocytes showing a double positive $CD4^{+}CD8^{+}$ T phenotype. This population may be consistent with either neoplastic T lymphomatous cells or normal thymocytes in the context

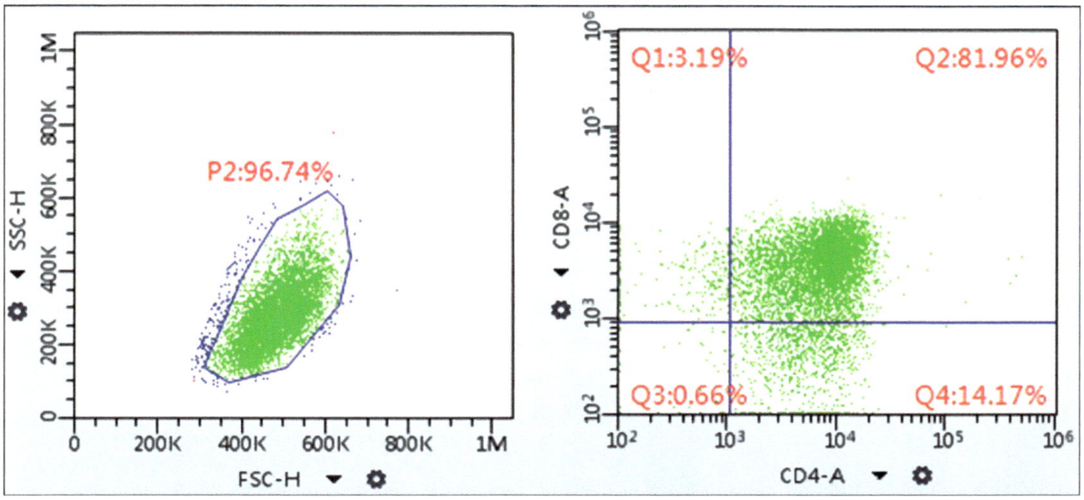

Figure 5.92 Flow cytometric analysis of cells from a cranial mediastinal mass in a cat. Over 80% of the lymphocytes are double positive for CD4 and CD8 (Q2).

of a non-lymphoid neoplasia. Main differential includes T mediastinal lymphoma and thymoma. Other T cell subpopulations (double negative CD4⁻CD8⁻ thymocytes, CD4⁺CD8⁻ T-helper, or CD4⁻CD8⁺ T-cytotoxic) were scarce and represent less than 20% of cells.

Outcome

PARR and histopathology were suggested for differential diagnosis. The owners refused further sampling for histology but allowed PARR on the cytological slides already available. Unfortunately, due to the rapid deterioration of symptoms, they elected for euthanasia few days later before receiving the results of PARR analysis. Necropsy was not permitted. PARR analysis revealed a monoclonal rearrangement for T cells consistent with T-cell lymphoma.

Discussion

Lymphoma and thymoma are the main differential for large masses in the mediastinum in cats and dogs. In lymphoma the neoplastic expansion is due to lymphoid component, likely from the thymus or the mediastinal lymph nodes, while in thymoma neoplastic cells often derived from the epithelial component of thymus and lymphoid population represent a non-neoplastic polyclonal component often accompanying some subtypes of the tumor. Finding just a population of small to medium lymphocytes with minimal atypia is not a rare event and cannot differentiate between the two diseases. However, clinical and therapeutic approaches strongly differ between lymphoma (chemotherapy) and thymoma (surgery and eventually radiotherapy). In dogs the majority of mediastinal lymphoma show a clonal expansion of T-helper ($CD4^+CD8^-$) or T-cytotoxic ($CD4^-CD8^+$) lymphocytes. Occasionally also double negative ($CD4^-CD8^-$) or B-cell lymphomas may be found while double positive ($CD4^+CD8^+$) lymphomas are quite rare. Flow cytometry using double labeling for CD4/CD8 may assist the differential diagnosis between canine mediastinal lymphoma and thymoma by demonstrating an expansion of one of the above mentioned lymphocyte subsets. According to some studies (Lana et al., 2006b) finding more than 10% of double positive $CD4^+CD8^+$ thymocytes is highly supportive of canine thymoma, but this approach is unfortunately useless in cats, since most feline mediastinal lymphomas show a double positive phenotype (Bernardi et al., 2020). PARR and histopathology are mandatory to solve differential in cats, however some cytological and immunophenotypic aspects may help to drive diagnosis of lymphoma vs thymoma:

1) Finding more than 60% lymphoid cells with a phenotype other than double positive $CD4^+CD8^+$ is diagnostic of lymphoma.
2) Finding a prevalence of large-sized cells, irrespectively from the phenotype is suggestive of lymphoma.
3) Finding a mixed population of T lymphoid cells with different phenotypes ($CD4^+$,$CD8^+$, $CD4^+CD8^+$, and $CD4^-CD8^-$) is suggestive of thymoma.

CASE 4

Signalment/history

A 6-year-old, male neutered domestic short-haired cat was evaluated for a history of weight loss and vomiting.

Clinical examination

The cat was bright, alert, and responsive. He was mildly dehydrated but no other abnormalities were detected during physical examination. CBC and clinical chemistry data were unremarkable. He tested negative for feline leukemia and immunodeficiency viruses (FeLV/FIV). An abdominal ultrasound detected a 7 cm × 5 cm mass in the stomach with loss of gastric wall layering. A FNA biopsy was collected from the mass.

Cytologic description

Most slides contained low to large numbers of lysed nuclei and a large amount of blood. One of the more highly cellular slides contained

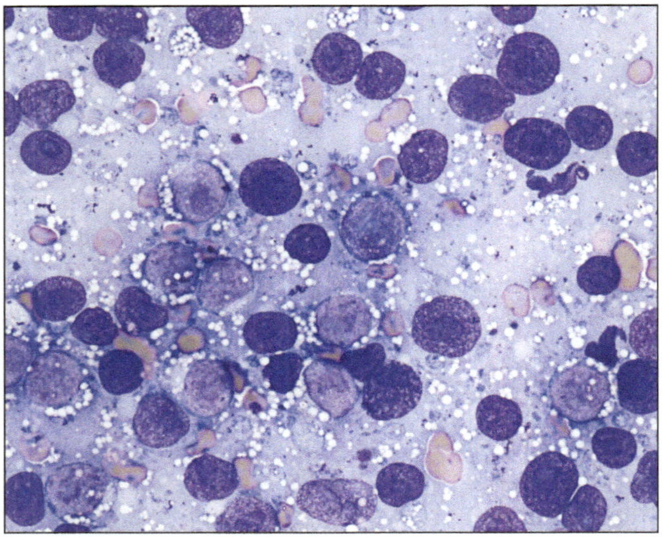

Figure 5.93 FNA from a gastric mass in a 6-year-old, male neutered, domestic short-haired cat. Several ruptured cells are present. The majority of intact cells are large lymphocytes with scant basophilic cytoplasm that contains several small, clear, cytoplasmic vacuoles (Wright–Giemsa, 1,000× magnification).

moderate numbers of intact large lymphocytes (Figure 5.93). The large lymphocytes had a scant to small amount of basophilic cytoplasm and often contained several small, clear, distinct, cytoplasmic vacuoles. The nucleus was eccentrically located and round with stippled chromatin and a large, prominent nucleolus. Nuclei were approximately 20 micrometers in diameter. Low numbers of nondegenerate neutrophils and macrophages were present. Rare small lymphocytes were seen. No gastric epithelial cells were observed.

Cytologic interpretation

The FNA is consistent with lymphoma. Immunophenotyping was recommended. Flow cytometric analysis could have been used for immunophenotyping if a new sample was obtained and placed in media; however the owner was reluctant to place the cat under anesthesia to collect a fresh sample. Immunocytochemistry was not recommended due to the paucity of intact cells in the slides that were evaluated cytologically. Therefore, PARR was performed.

Outcome

PARR results indicated T-cell receptor gene amplification was polyclonal and B cell receptor gene amplification was clonal. Therefore, there was a clonal population of large B cells in the sample, supportive of a diagnosis of large B-cell lymphoma in this cat.

Discussion

The most common gastric tumor in cats is lymphoma (Gualtieri et al., 1999). The majority of cats with gastric lymphoma also have neoplastic lymphocytes in other organs and/or abdominal lymph nodes. Most cats with gastric lymphoma that do not have involvement of other sites are diagnosed with a high-grade, large B-cell lymphoma (Gustafson et al., 2014). In a retrospective study of 16 cats with gastric lymphoma (Gustafson et al., 2014), the median age of diagnosis was 12.8 years. Dehydration and vomiting were the most common clinical signs. The CBC and chemistry data were often unremarkable and cats were negative for FeLV/FIV. The median overall survival time in cats receiving varied forms of chemotherapy was 171 days, whereas cats that did not respond to chemotherapy had an extremely short median survival time (33 days). In contrast, cats with low-grade, small-cell lymphoma involving the gastrointestinal tract typically respond better to chemotherapy and have significantly longer survival times (Lingard et al., 2009).

Large B cells with a distinctive vacuolated morphology are not uncommon to observe in FNAs from cats with lymphoma. Subjectively, this morphology tends to occur in aspirates from affected organs (e.g. renal and gastrointestinal lymphomas) more than aspirates from enlarged lymph nodes.

REFERENCES

Affolter V.K., Moore P.F. (2002) Localized and disseminated histiocytic sarcoma of dendritic cell origin in dogs. *Vet Pathol 39(1)*:74–83.

Ballegeer E.A., Forrest L.J., Dickinson L.M. et al. (2007) Correlation of ultrasonographic appearance of lesions and cytologic and histologic diagnoses in splenic aspirates from dogs and cats: 32 cases (2002–2005). *J Am Vet Med Assoc 230*:690–696.

Barger A.M., Skowronski M.C., MacNeill A.L. (2012) Cytologic identification of erythrophagocytic neoplasms in dogs. *Vet Clin Pathol 41*(*4*):587–589.

Bernardi S., Martini V., Perfetto S. et al. (2020) Flow cytometric analysis of mediastinal masses in cats: A retrospective study. *Front Vet Sci 7*:444.

Bertazzolo W., Dell'Orco M., Bonfanti U. et al. (2005) Canine angiosarcoma: Cytologic, histologic, and immunohistochemical correlations. *Vet Clin Pathol 34*(*1*):28–34.

Book A.P., Fidel J., Wills T. et al. (2011) Correlation of ultrasound findings, liver and spleen cytology, and prognosis in the clinical staging of high metastatic risk canine mast cell tumors. *Vet Radiol Ultrasound 52*(*5*):548–554.

Breen M., Modiano J.F. (2008) Evolutionary conserved cytogenetic changes in hematological malignancies of dogs and humans: Man and his best friend share more than companionship. *Chromosome Res 16*(*1*):145–154.

Caniatti M., Roccabianca P., Scanziani E. et al. (1996) Canine lymphoma: Immunocytochemical analysis of fine-needle aspiration biopsy. *Vet Pathol 33*(*2*):204–212.

Christiansen S.M., Hingerbuhler S.O., Mischke R. (2016) Relevance of cytology in canine spleen: A retrospective study. *Prakt Tierarzt 97*:668–679.

Comazzi S., Gelain M.E. (2011) Use of flow cytometric immunophenotyping to refine the cytological diagnosis of canine lymphoma. *Vet J 188*:149–155.

Comazzi S., Gelain M.E., Martini V. et al. (2011) Immunophenotype predicts survival time in dogs with chronic lymphocytic leukemia. *J Vet Intern Med 25*:100–106.

Ehrhart E.J., Wong S., Richter K. et al. (2018) Polymerase chain reaction for antigen receptor rearrangement: Benchmarking performances of a lymphoid clonality assay in diverse canine sample type. *J Vet Intern Med 33*:1392–1402.

Faldyna M., Sinkora J., Knotigova P. et al. (2005) Lymphatic organ development in dogs: Major lymphocyte subsets and activity. *Vet Immunol Immunopathol 104*(*3–4*):239–247.

Fincra K., Leibman N.F., Fettman M.J. et al. (2006) Cytological comparison of fine-needle aspirates of liver and spleen of normal dogs and of dogs with cutaneous mast cell tumors and an ultrasonographically normal appearing liver and spleen. *Vet Comp Oncol 4(3)*:178–183.

Finotello R., Vasconi M.E., Sabattini S. et al. (2018) Feline large granular lymphocyte lymphoma: An Italian Society of Veterinary Oncology (SIONCOV) retrospective study. *Vet Comp Oncol 16*:159–166.

Foglia Manzillo V., Pagano A., Guglielmino R. et al. (2008) Extranodal gamma-delta T-cell lymphoma in a dog with leishmaniasis. *Vet Clin Pathol 37(3)*:298–301.

Fournel-Fleury C., Magnol J.P., Bricaire P. et al. (1997) Cytohistological and immunological classification of canine malignant lymphomas: Comparison with human non-Hodgkin's lymphomas. *J Comp Pathol 117(1)*:35–59.

Fournel-Fleury C., Ponce F., Felman P. et al. (2002) Canine T-cell lymphomas: A morphological, immunological, and clinical study of 46 new cases. *Vet Pathol 39(1)*:92–109.

Frantz A.M., Sarver A.L., Ito D. et al. (2013) Molecular profiling reveals prognostically significant subtypes of canine lymphoma. *Vet Pathol 50(4)*:693–703.

Gambini M., Martini V., Bernardi S. Caniatti M., Gelain M.E., Roccabianca P., Comazzi S. (2021) Cytology of feline nodal lymphoma: Low interobserver agreement and variable accuracy in immunophenotype prediction. *J Comp Path 184*:1–6.

Gualtieri M., Monzeglio M.G., Scanziani E. (1999) Gastric neoplasia. *Vet Clin North Am Small Anim Pract 29(2)*:415–440.

Gustafson T.L., Villamil A., Taylor B.E., Flory A. (2014) A retrospective study of feline gastric lymphoma in 16 chemotherapy-treated cats. *J Am Anim Hosp Assoc 50(1)*:46–52.

Hughes K.L., Ehrhart E.J., Rout E.D., Harris L.J., Fernandez M., Yoshimoto J.A., Avery A. (2021) Diffuse small B-cell lymphoma: A high-grade malignancy. *Vet Pathol 58(5)*:912–922.

Johnson K.A., Powers B.E., Withrow S.J. et al. (1989) Splenomegaly in dogs. Predictors of neoplasia and survival after splenectomy. *J Vet Intern Med 3(3)*:160–166.

Kojima K., Chambers J.K., Mizuno T., Uchida K. (2022) Nodal T-zone lymphoma and T-zone hyperplasia in dogs. *Vet Pathol 59(5)*:733–739.

Kopterides P., Mourtzoukou E.G., Skopelitis E. et al. (2007) Aspects of the association between leishmaniasis and malignant disorders. *Trans Royal Soc Trop Med Hyg 101(12)*:1181–1189.

Krick E.L., Little L., Patel R. et al. (2008) Description of clinical and pathological findings, treatment and outcome of feline large granular lymphocyte lymphoma (1996–2004). *Vet Comp Oncol 6(2)*:102–110.

Ku C., Kass P.H , Christopher M.M. (2017) Cytologic-histologic concordance in the diagnosis of neoplasia in canine and feline lymph nodes: A retrospective study of 367 cases. *Vet Comp Oncol 15*:1206–1217.

Lana S.E., Jackson T.L., Burnett R.C. et al. (2006a) Utility of polymerase chain reaction for analysis of antigen receptor rearrangement in staging and predicting prognosis in dogs with lymphoma. *J Vet Intern Med 20(2)*:329–334.

Lana S., Plaza S., Hampe K. et al. (2006b) Diagnosis of mediastinal masses in dogs by flow cytometry. *J Vet Intern Med 20(5)*:1161–1165.

Leblanc C.J., Head L.L., Fry M.M. (2009) Comparison of aspiration and nonaspiration techniques for obtaining cytologic samples from the canine and feline spleen. *Vet Clin Pathol 38(2)*:242–246.

Lingard A.E., Briscoe K., Beatty J.A., Moore A.S., Crowley A.M., Krockenberger M., Churcher R.K., Canfield P.J., Barrs V.R. (2009) Low-grade alimentary lymphoma: Clinicopathological findings and response to treatment in 17 cases. *J Feline Med Surg 8*:692–700.

Lurie D.M., Milner R.J., Suter S.E. et al. (2008) Immunophenotypic and cytomorphologic subclassification of T-cell lymphoma in the boxer breed. *Vet Immunol Immunopathol 125(1–2)*:102–110.

Marconato L., Gelain M.E., Comazzi S. (2013a) The dog as a possible animal model for human non-Hodgkin lymphoma: A review. *Hematol Oncol 31(1)*:1–9.

Marconato L., Martini V., Aresu L. et al. (2013b) Assessment of bone marrow infiltration diagnosed by flow cytometry in canine large B cell lymphoma: Prognostic significance and proposal of a cut-off value. *Vet J 197(3)*:776–781.

Martini V., Marano G., Aresu L. et al. (2022) Performance of lymph node cytopathology in diagnosis and characterization of lymphoma in dogs. *J Vet Intern Med 36*:204–214.

Martini V., Poggi A., Riondato F. et al. (2015) Flow-cytometric detection of phenotypic aberrancies in canine small clear cell lymphoma. *Vet Comp Oncol 3(3)*:281–287.

McDonough S.P., Moore P.F. (2000) Clinical, hematologic, and immunophenotypic characterization of canine large granular lymphocytosis. *Vet Pathol 37(6)*:637–646.

Moore F.M., Emerson W.E., Cotter S.M. et al. (1986) Distinctive peripheral lymph node hyperplasia of young cats. *Vet Pathol 23(4)*:386–391.

Moore P.F. (2014) A review of histiocytic diseases of dogs and cats. *Vet Pathol 51(1)*:167–184.

Moore P.F., Affolter V.K., Vernau W. (2006) Canine hemophagocytic histiocytic sarcoma: A proliferative disorder of CD11d+ macrophages. *Vet Pathol 43(5)*:632–645.

Moore P.F., Rodriguez-Bertos A., Kass P.H. (2012) Feline gastrointestinal lymphoma: Mucosal architecture, immunophenotype, and molecular clonality. *Vet Pathol 49(4)*:658–668.

Moore P.F., Woo J.C., Vernau W. et al. (2005) Characterization of feline T cell receptor gamma (TCRG) variable region genes for the molecular diagnosis of feline intestinal T cell lymphoma. *Vet Immunol Immunopathol 106(3–4)*:167–178.

Neer T.M. (1996) Clinical approach to splenomegaly in dogs and cats. *Compend Cont Educ Pract 18*:35–46.

Nerschbach V., Eberle N., Joetzke A.E. et al. (2016) Splenic and hepatic ultrasound and cytology in canine lymphoma: Effects of findings on stage migration and assessment of prognosis. *Vet Comp Oncol 14*:82–94.

O'Brien D., Moore P.F., Vernau W. et al. (2013) Clinical characteristics and outcome in dogs with splenic marginal zone lymphoma. *J Vet Intern Med 27(4)*:949–954.

O'Keefe D.A., Couto C.G. (1987) Fine-needle aspiration of the spleen as an aid in the diagnosis of splenomegaly. *J Vet Intern Med 1(3)*:102–109.

Osborne C.A., Perman V., Stevens J.B. (1974) Needle biopsy of the spleen. *Vet Clin North Am Small Anim Pract 4(2)*:311–316.

Owen L.N., editor (1980) *Tumor-Node-Metastasis (TNM) Classification of Tumours in Domestic Animals*, 1st edn. World Health Organization, Geneva.

Ponce F., Magnol J.P., Ledieu D. et al. (2004) Prognostic significance of morphological subtypes in canine malignant lymphomas during chemotherapy. *Vet J 167(2)*:158–166.

Ponce F., Marchal T., Magnol J.P. et al. (2010) A morphological study of 608 cases of canine malignant lymphoma in France with a focus on comparative similarities between canine and human lymphoma morphology. *Vet Pathol 47(3)*:414–433.

Raskin R.E. (2010) Lymphoid system. In: *Canine and Feline Cytology: A Color Atlas and Interpretation Guide*, 2nd edn. (eds. R.E. Raskin, D.J. Meyer) Saunders Elsevier, St. Louis, pp. 77–122.

Regan R.C., Kaplan M.S., Bailey D.B. (2013) Diagnostic evaluation and treatment recommendations for dogs with substage-a high-grade multicentric lymphoma: Results of a survey of veterinarians. *Vet Comp Oncol 11(4)*:287–295.

Richards K.L., Motsinger-Reif A.A., Chen H.W. et al. (2013) Gene profiling of canine B-cell lymphoma reveals germinal center and postgerminal center subtypes with different survival times, modeling human DLBCL. *Cancer Res 73(16)*:5029–5039.

Roccabianca P., Vernau W., Caniatti M. Moore P.F. (2006) Feline large granular lymphocyte (LGL) lymphoma with secondary leukemia: Primary intestinal origin with predominance of a CD3/CD8αα phenotype. *Vet Pathol 43(1)*:15–28.

Rout E.D., Fernandez M., Yoshimoto J.A. et al. (2022) Clinical outcome and Ki67 evaluation in dogs with nodal small cell B-cell lymphoma diagnosed by flow cytometry. *J Vet Intern Med 36*:1770–1781.

Seelig D., Avery A.C., Webb T. et al. (2014) Canine T-zone lymphoma: Unique immunophenotypic features, outcome, and population characteristics. *J Vet Intern Med 28(3)*:878–886.

Spangler W.L., Culbertson M.R. (1992) Prevalence and type of splenic diseases in cats: 455 cases (1985–1991). *J Am Vet Med Assoc 201(5)*:773–776.

Spangler W.L., Culbertson M.R., Kass P.H. (1994) Primary mesenchymal (nonangiomatous/nonlymphomatous) neoplasms occurring in the canine spleen: Anatomic classification, immunohistochemistry, and mitotic activity correlated with patient survival. *Vet Pathol 31(1)*:37–47.

Stefanello D., Valenti P., Faverzani S. et al. (2009) Ultrasound-guided cytology of spleen and liver: A prognostic tool in canine cutaneous mast cell tumor. *J Vet Intern Med 23(5)*:1051–1057.

Stefanello D., Valenti P., Zini E. et al. (2011) Splenic marginal zone lymphoma in 5 dogs (2001–2008). *J Vet Intern Med 25(1)*:90–93.

Stein L., Bacmeister C., Kiupel M. (2021) Immunophenotypic characterization of canine nodal T-zone lymphoma. *Vet Pathol 58(2)*:288–292.

Steinberg J.D., Keating J.H. (2008) What is your diagnosis? Cervical mass in a cat. *Vet Clin Pathol 37(3)*:323–327.

Tasca S., Carli E., Caldin M. Menegazzo L., Furlanello T., Gallego L.S. (2009) Hematologic abnormalities and flow cytometric immunophenotyping results in dogs with hematopoietic neoplasia: 2010 cases (2002–2006). *Vet Clin Pathol 38(1)*:2–12.

Thalheim L., Williams L.E., Borst L.B. et al. (2013) Lymphoma immunophenotype of dogs determined by immunohistochemistry, flow cytometry, and polymerase chain reaction for antigen receptor rearrangements. *J Vet Intern Med 27(6)*:1509–1516.

Thomas R., Smith K.C., Gould R. et al. (2001) Molecular cytogenetic analysis of a novel high-grade canine T-lymphoblastic lymphoma demonstrating co-expression of CD3 and CD79a cell markers. *Chromosome Res 9(8)*:649–657.

Vail D.M. (2013) Feline lymphoma and leukemia. In: *Withrow and MacEwen's Small Animal Clinical Oncology*, 5th edn. (eds. S.J. Withrow, D.M. Vail, R.L. Page) Elsevier Saunders, St. Louis, pp. 638–649.

Vail D.M., Pinkerton M.E., Young K.M. (2013) Canine lymphoma and lymphoid leukemias. In: *Withrow and MacEwen's Small Animal Clinical Oncology*, 5th edn. (eds. S.J. Withrow, D.M. Vail, R.L. Page) Elsevier Saunders, St. Louis, pp. 611–628.

Valli V.E., Kass P.H., Myint M.S. Scott F. (2013) Canine lymphomas: Association of classification type, disease stage, tumor subtype, mitotic rate, and treatment with survival *Vet Pathol 50(5)*: 738–748.

Valli V.E.O. (2007) B-cell neoplasms. In: *Veterinary Comparative Hematopathology* (ed. V.E.O. Valli) Blackwell Publishing, Ames, pp. 207–273.

Valli V.E., San Miynth M., Barthel A. et al. (2011) Classification of canine malignant lymphomas according to the World Health Organization criteria. *Vet Pathol 48(1)*:198–211.

Valli V.E., Vernau W., de Lorimier L.P. et al. (2006) Canine indolent nodular lymphoma. *Vet Pathol 43(3)*:241–256.

Watson A.T., Penninck D., Knoll J.S. et al. (2011) Safety and correlation of test results of combined ultrasound-guided fine-needle aspiration and needle core biopsy of the canine spleen. *Vet Radiol Ultrasound 52(3)*:317–322.

Weiss D.J. (2007) Hemophagocytic syndrome in dogs: 24 cases (1996–2005). *J Am Vet Med Assoc 230(5)*:697–701.

Welter J., Dockova T., Groiss S. et al. (2021) Revisiting lymphocyte clonality testing for feline B cell lymphoma. *Vet Immunol Immunopathol 242*:110350.

Williams M., Avery A., Olver C.S. (2006) Diagnosing lymphoid hyperplasia vs lymphoma in canine splenic aspirates. *Vet Pathol 43*:809.

Workman H.C., Vernau W. (2003) Chronic lymphocytic leukemia in dogs and cats: The veterinary perspective. *Vet Clin North Am Small Anim Pract 33(6)*:1379–1399.

CHAPTER 6

ORAL CAVITY CYTOLOGY

Melinda S. Camus

INTRODUCTION

The oral cavity is the entry point of the gastrointestinal tract (GIT). It is where digestion begins with mastication of ingesta, which is mixed with salivary enzymes and passed through the oropharynx to the esophagus. The oral cavity is sampled most commonly due to the presence of ulcerative lesions and/or masses. Sampling techniques, including brushings, aspirates, and impression smears, similar to those utilized elsewhere, can be employed. Care should be taken to ensure sampling at a depth appropriate to the lesion. Superficial sampling, particularly of ulcerated lesions, is often unrewarding.

In health, the mouth, including the oropharynx, is lined by stratified squamous epithelium, which is fully keratinized on the tongue, hard palate, and cheeks and may be in various stages of keratinization elsewhere in the oral cavity. The feline tongue is covered with numerous papillae, which are composed of abundant amounts of connective tissue and keratin spines (Figure 6.1). The type and distribution of these papillae vary with life stage and potentially with environment, as papillae are believed to change with feeding behaviors (Haddad, 2019). Food is moistened by salivary secretions that come from numerous salivary glands, which produce mucous and serous secretions. Carnivores, including cats, are unique in that their saliva contains minimal α-amylase, which, in non-carnivores, initiates carbohydrate digestion in the oral cavity (Gelberg, 2021). Histologically, the mouth lacks a muscularis mucosae, submucosa, and muscularis externa, which are present in other sections of the GIT (Figure 6.2; Bacha & Bacha, 2012).

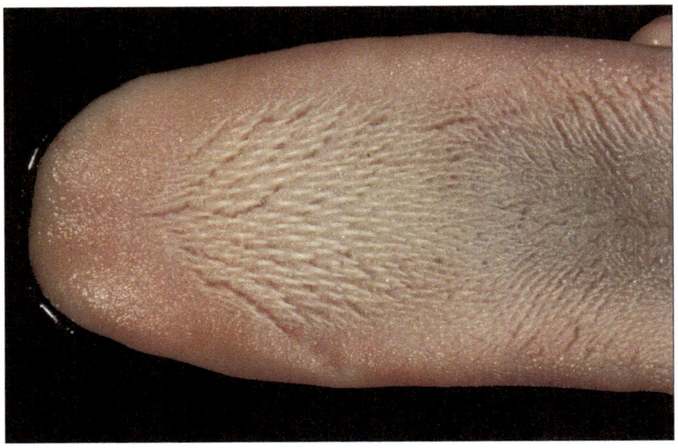

Figure 6.1 Feline tongue with keratin spines. (Courtesy Dr. Raquel Rech.)

'NORMAL' FINDINGS

Mixed populations of bacterial organisms, including *Actinomyces* spp., *Fusobacterium* spp., and spirochetes, normally inhabit the oral cavity and serve as a defense mechanism, occupying entry/attachment sites of potential pathogens. *Conchiformibius* (formerly *Simonsiella*) spp. are morphologically distinct bacteria that normally populate the oral cavity of warm-blooded vertebrates (Figure 6.3). *Conchiformibius* spp. form large aggregates that consist of individual organisms (approximately 1.5–6.5 µm long) that 'slide' along filaments composed of eight or more cells. Cells on the ends of the filaments can be curved, resulting in a crescent-shaped appearance. Occasionally 'super filaments' greater than 50 µm in length result when multiple cells remain attached (Figure 6.4). The presence of *Conchiformibius* spp. in cytologic specimens is indicative of sampling of or contamination from the oropharyngeal region (Hostetter, 2023).

In addition to indigenous aerobic and anaerobic bacterial flora, saliva serves as a barrier to pathogenic bacterial colonization, since it can flush microorganisms from the oral cavity and it contains antibacterial compounds (e.g., hydrogen peroxide and thiocyanate), numerous antimicrobial enzymes, and immunoglobulin A (Gelberg,

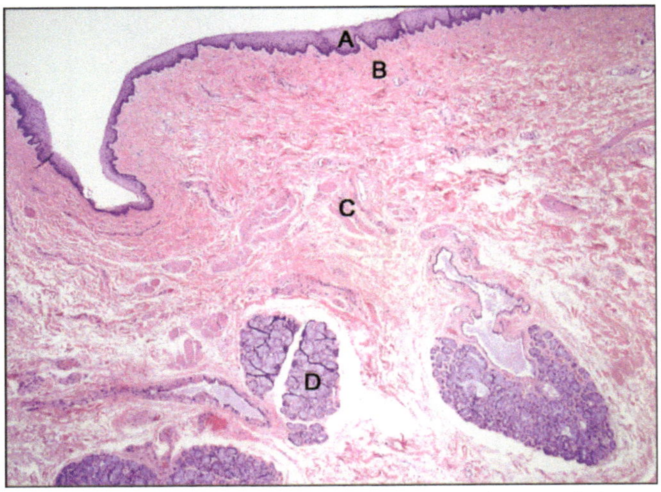

Figure 6.2 Histologic section of the oropharynx of a dog. Stratified, squamous epithelium, keratinized (A); lamina propria (B); skeletal muscle (C); mixed (mucous and serous) salivary gland (D) (H&E, 40× magnification).

DOI: 10.1201/9781003258551-6

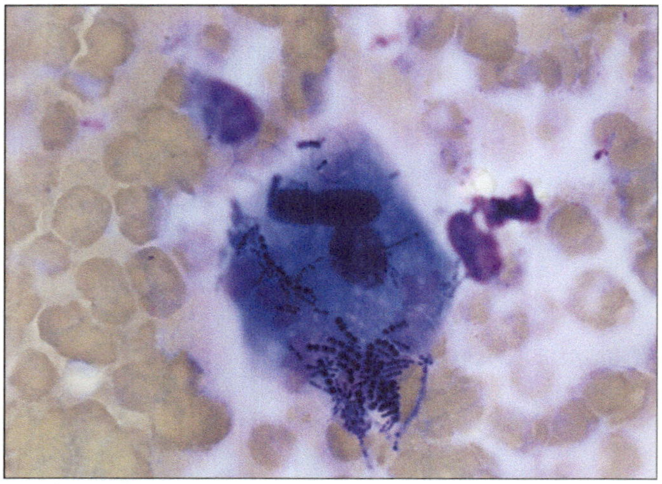

Figure 6.3 Oral cavity from a dog. Keratinizing squamous epithelial cell with adherent mixed bacteria, including *Conchiformibius* (formerly *Simonsiella*) spp. (modified Wright's, 1,000× magnification).

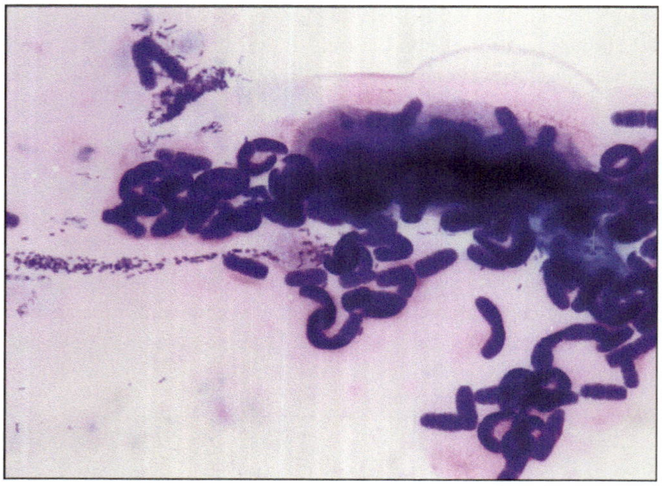

Figure 6.4 Oral cavity from a dog. *Conchiformibius* (formerly *Simonsiella*) spp. bacteria, including occasional 'superfilaments' (>50 μm long). A mixed population of bacterial rods and cocci is present in the background (modified Wright's, 1,000× magnification).

2021). Salivary glands, which arise from oral ectoderm, are located throughout the head and neck regions and drain into the oral cavity. In addition to the parotid, mandibular, and sublingual salivary glands found in all species, carnivores have an additional zygomatic salivary gland. Numerous small salivary glands, primarily named by their location (e.g. buccal, labial, lingual, palatine), are present throughout the oral cavity and can exhibit pathology (see Case 1; Gelberg, 2021). Salivary glands are often sampled accidentally with attempted aspiration of submandibular lymph nodes.

Cytologic samples from salivary glands are typified by a thick background of stippled eosinophilic mucus, which often exhibits 'windrowing', where cells are aligned linearly (Figure 6.5). This

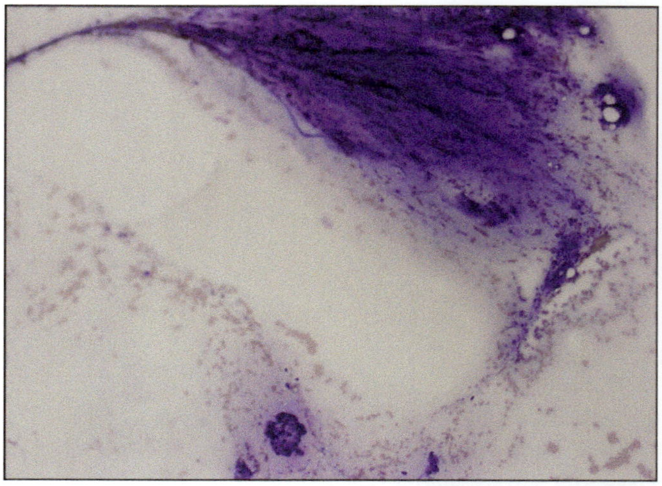

Figure 6.5 Salivary gland from a dog. Basophilic saliva strands admixed with blood in a linear ('windrowed') pattern. Small clusters of cohesive, vacuolated salivary epithelial cells (modified Wright's, 200× magnification).

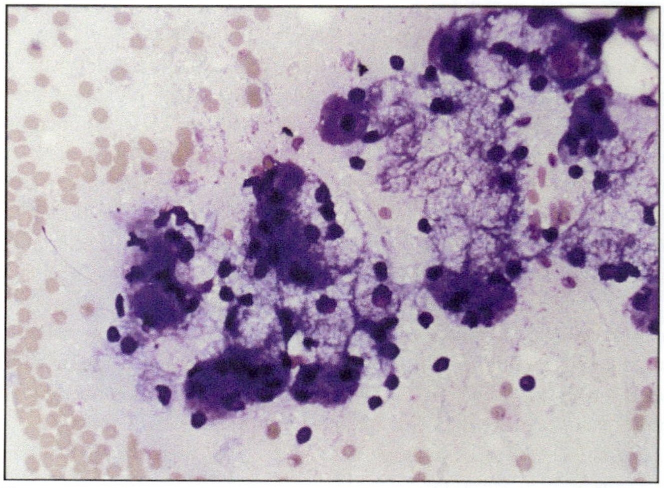

Figure 6.6 Salivary gland from a dog. Clusters of cohesive, uniform, round to polygonal epithelial cells with an abundant amount of basophilic cytoplasm. Most cells contain secretory product, appearing as nonstaining vacuoles. The less vacuolated cells are basal reserve cells (modified Wright's, 500× magnification).

pattern, also commonly observed with synovial fluid samples, results from preparation of the thick, viscous specimen. Salivary glands are composed of secretory epithelial cells. Aspirates typically yield cohesive clusters of foamy epithelial cells, often surrounded by more basilar epithelial cells with a high nuclear to cytoplasmic (N:C) ratio (Figure 6.6). Occasionally, amorphous, basophilic mucus droplets are noted both free and within the cytoplasm of the secretory epithelial cells (Figure 6.7).

Lymphoid tissue in carnivores is found bilaterally in crypts in the dorsolateral aspect of the oropharynx, referred to as palatine tonsils. Dogs and cats typically possess only palatine tonsils, unlike other

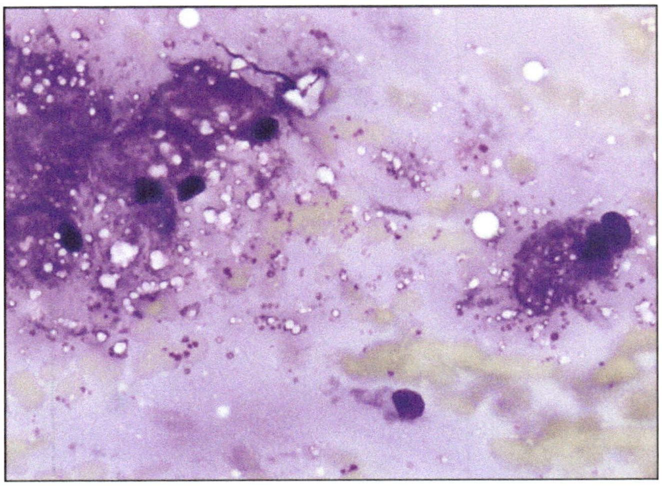

Figure 6.7 Salivary gland from a dog. Individualized salivary epithelial cells releasing amorphous, basophilic mucus globules, which are present both within the cytoplasm and free in the background (modified Wright's, 1,000× magnification).

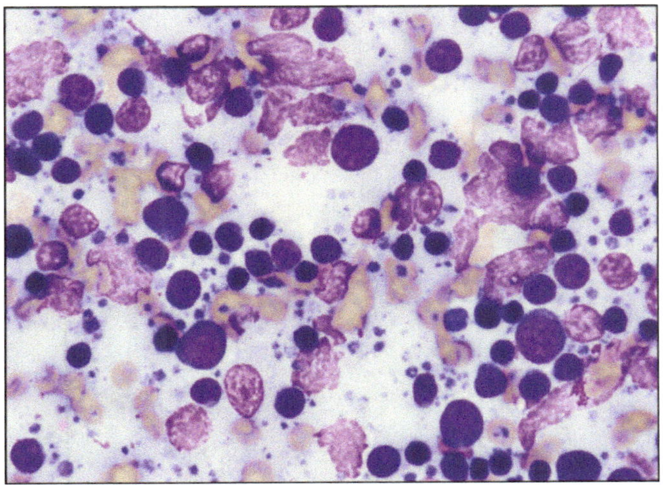

Figure 6.8 Tonsil from a dog. A heterogeneous lymphoid population composed of small, medium, and large lymphocytes. Numerous broken cells and resultant free nuclei are present, along with abundant lymphoglandular bodies (cytoplasmic fragments) (modified Wright's, 1,000× magnification).

species that often have tonsillar tissue adjacent to the tongue. Tonsils are covered by stratified squamous epithelium and contain a heterogeneous lymphoid population composed primarily of small lymphocytes with fewer medium and large lymphocytes. Small amounts of extracellular iron are commonly seen (Figure 6.8). Care must be taken not to confuse the presence of well-differentiated squamous epithelial cells in various stages of keratinization from tonsillar aspirates with neoplastic squamous cells, because the tonsils are covered by squamous epithelial cells (Figure 6.9). Unlike other lymphoid tissues, tonsils lack afferent lymphatic vessels and, therefore, do not drain the oral cavity. Their exact role in the immune process is uncertain, and it is speculated that they serve a role in lymphocyte production,

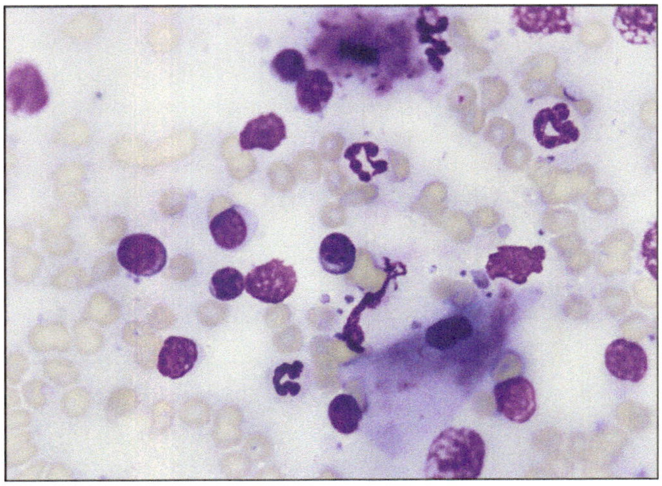

Figure 6.9 Tonsil from a dog. A heterogeneous lymphoid population with blood, lymphoglandular bodies (cytoplasmic fragments), and nuclear material in the background. Extracellular bacteria, including *Conchiformibius* spp., are noted. A single, keratinizing, nucleated squamous epithelial cell is noted (modified Wright's, 1,000× magnification).

antibody formation, and in the innate immune system, as sites of antigen sampling (Weise et al., 2002; Gelberg, 2021).

INFLAMMATION

Neutrophilic inflammation of the oral cavity is often associated with the gingiva (gingivitis), tongue (glossitis), pharynx (pharyngitis), or tonsils (tonsillitis; Figure 6.10). The term 'stomatitis' (from the Greek '*stoma*', meaning opening) is a general term for inflammation within the mouth. The presence of neutrophils in cytologic specimens from the mouth can be difficult to interpret, because neutrophils at the end

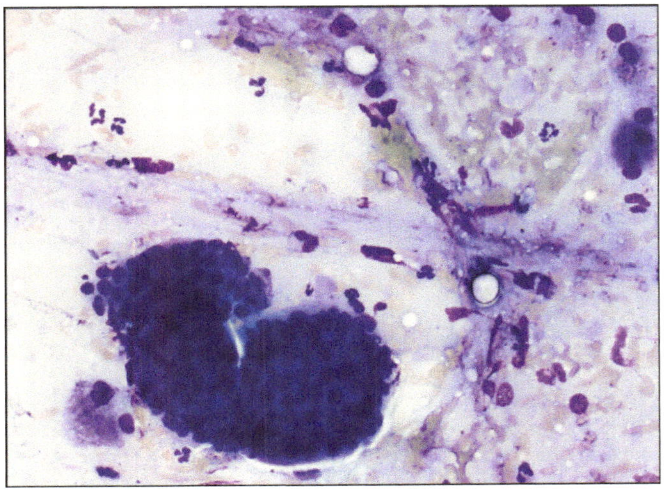

Figure 6.10 Salivary gland from a dog. Cluster of basilar salivary epithelial cells with scattered neutrophils, increased above the amount of blood contamination (modified Wright's, 500× magnification).

of their lifespan are removed via migration through the GIT, including the mouth (Gelberg, 2021). Additionally, as with any cytologic specimen, the contribution of neutrophils from the peripheral blood must be considered. Inflammation can arise secondary to numerous causes, including the presence of bacterial, fungal, and protozoal pathogens and/or foreign material, the latter of which may have a concurrent granulomatous inflammatory response (Figures 6.11–6.14) (Bochnakian *et al.*, 2018).

Eosinophilic inflammation is also nonspecific and can be seen with numerous etiologies, including hypersensitivity reactions, parasites, fungal infections, secondary to neoplasia (paraneoplastic), and foreign bodies. Most commonly in cats, but also reported in dogs, are lesions of the 'eosinophilic granuloma complex' (Figure 6.15). These lesions, historically termed 'rodent ulcers', are of unknown etiology, but may be linked to immune-mediated hypersensitivity. Free, fibrillar collagen strands are often noted within these lesions, due to the presence of collagenolytic factors within eosinophil granules (Figure 6.16; Gelberg, 2021).

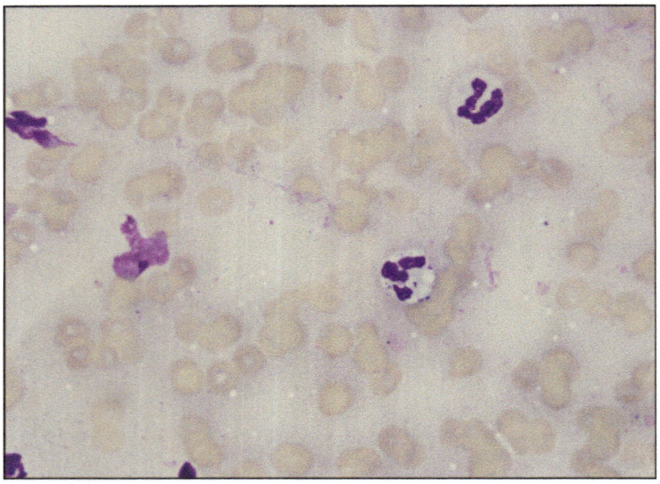

Figure 6.11 **Laryngeal polyp from a dog. Thick, basophilic proteinaceous background with blood and broken cells. Two intact segmented neutrophils. Central neutrophil contains small intracellular bacterial cocci (modified Wright's, 1,000× magnification).**

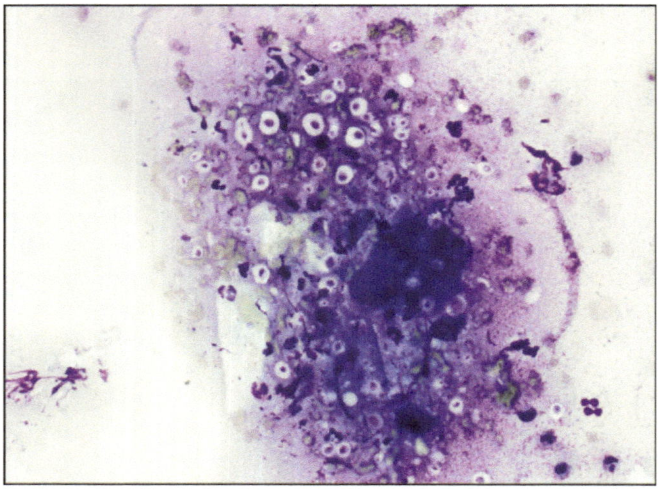

Figure 6.12 **Tongue mass from a cat. Keratinized, anucleate squamous epithelial cells with scattered nondegenerate neutrophils and numerous, variably sized basophilic fungal organisms surrounded by a thick, nonstaining capsule, morphologically most compatible with *Cryptococcus* spp. Culture confirmed *Cryptococcus neoformans* (modified Wright's, 500× magnification).**

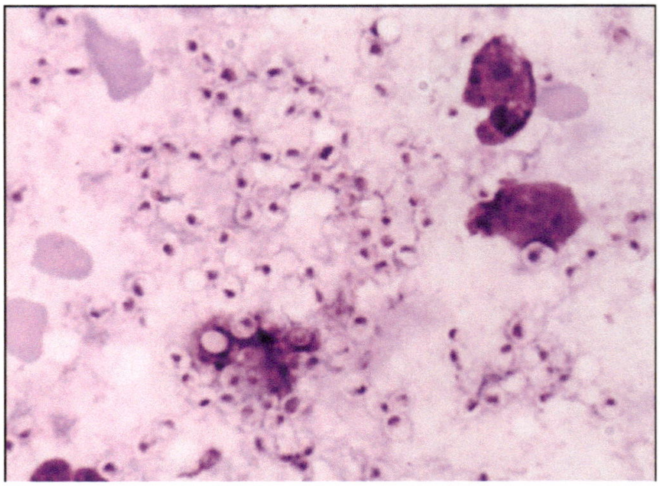

Figure 6.13 **Oral plaque from a cat. Numerous 2–4 μm diameter ovoid yeasts with a basophilic, polar nucleus and a clear halo, morphologically compatible with *Histoplasma capsulatum*. Scattered disrupted inflammatory cells are present. This organism can occasionally be found in tissue drainage and morphologically resembles *Sporthrix schecknii*, from which it must be distinguished (Wright–Giemsa, 1,000× magnification).**

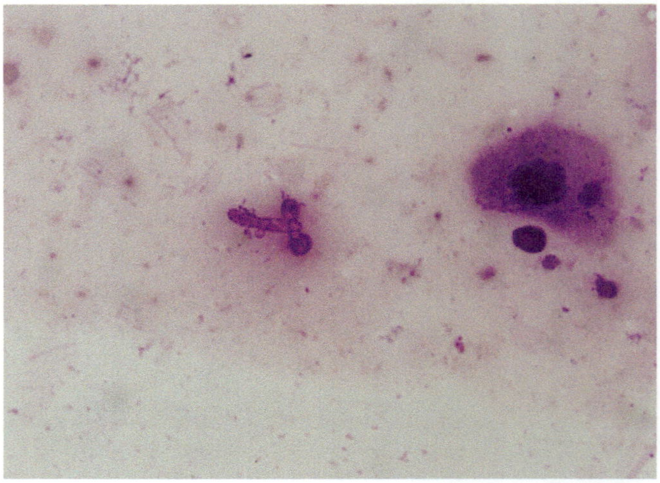

Figure 6.14 **Oral plaque from a dog. Fungal pseudohyphal fragment with roughly right-angle branching and bulbous ends, morphologically most compatible with *Candida* spp. A single nucleated, angular squamous epithelial cell is present (modified Wright's, 1,000× magnification).**

Lymphocytic, granulomatous, and mixed inflammation can also occur within the oral cavity and have similar significance as elsewhere in the body. Mixed inflammation is often seen with calcinosis circumscripta (dystrophic mineralization), which occasionally

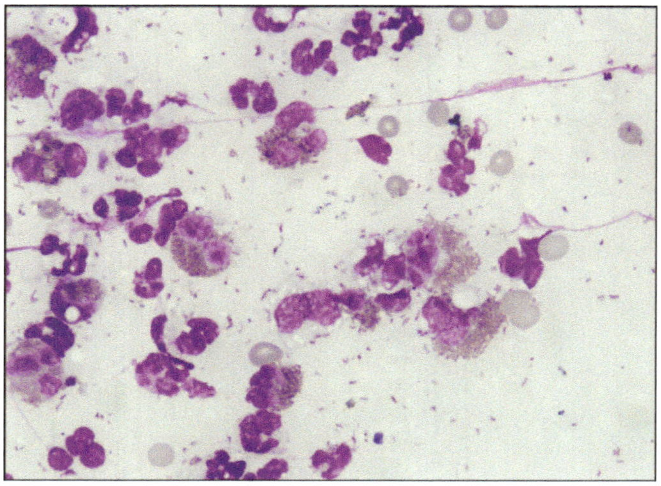

Figure 6.15 Ulcerated lip lesion in a cat. Numerous intact and broken eosinophils with fewer neutrophils. Abundant rice-grain shaped free eosinophil granules are noted in the background (modified Wright's, 1,000× magnification).

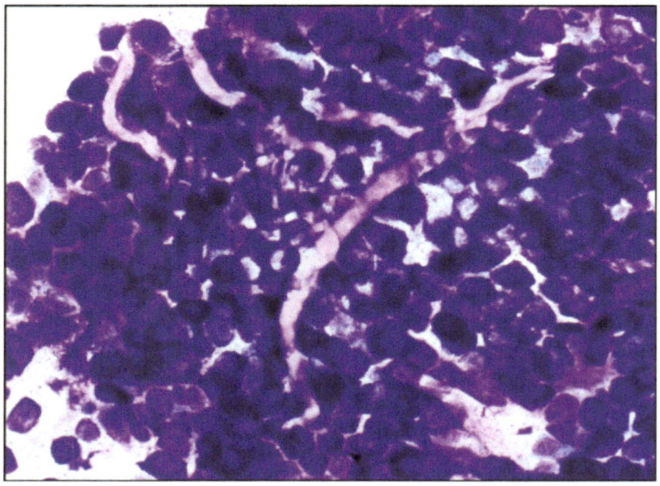

Figure 6.16 Mass aspirate from a cat. Irregularly branching bands of brightly eosinophilic to nonstaining collagen coursing through heavily granulated mast cells (mast cell tumor) (modified Wright's, 500× magnification).

presents as hard raised lesions under the tongue (Figure 6.17). Specific causes of this lesion are diverse and include trauma and the presence of foreign material (e.g. suture material) (Gelberg, 2021).

NEOPLASIA

The presence of oral masses is one of the most common reasons for cytologic examination of the oral cavity. Oral neoplasia accounts for approximately 5% of all canine neoplasms and approximately 6–10% of all feline cancers (Munday *et al.*, 2016). Many are discovered when a patient is presented for reluctance to eat, excessive salivation,

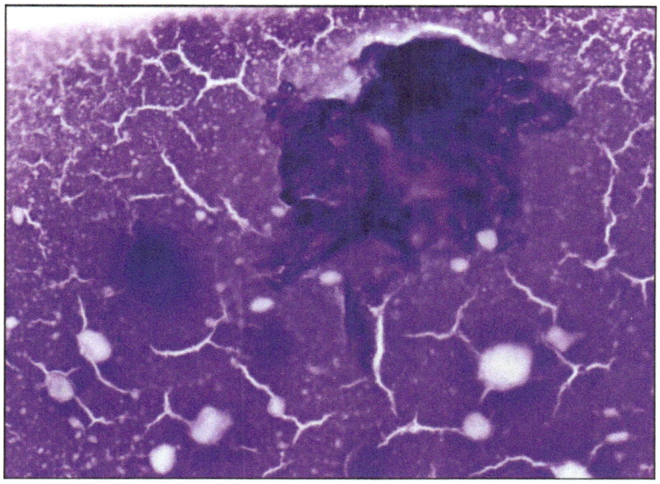

Figure 6.17 Tongue from a dog. Calcinosis circumscripta. Amorphous basophilic mineralized material and a single, poorly distinguishable aggregate of presumed macrophages (Diff-Quik®, 500× magnification).

or periodontal disease. A review of oral masses revealed that while they grossly appear similar to neoplasms, many of the mass-like oral lesions in both dogs and cats were hyperplasic and/or inflammatory, demonstrating that microscopy and/or advanced diagnostics are needed for characterization and that a presumption of neoplasia is inappropriate in the absence of other supporting signs (Mikiewicz *et al.*, 2019; Wingo 2018). Cytologic correlation with histologic diagnosis of oral neoplasms is high (Bonfanti *et al.*, 2015). While many types of neoplasia can occur in the oral cavity, some of the most common and/or unique are described below. As with any location, in lesions with evidence for concurrent inflammation, dysplastic change induced by the presence of inflammatory cytokines should not be confused with neoplastic change.

Melanoma

Melanoma is the most common malignant oral tumor of the dog, and melanocytic neoplasms comprise 30–40% of all canine oral tumors (Liptak, 2020; Smedley *et al.*, 2022). The neoplastic cells are of neural crest origin and, as such, can have a pleomorphic appearance, exhibiting morphologic features of both epithelial and mesenchymal cells. These cells are readily identifiable when they are heavily pigmented and contain abundant green–black, seed-shaped, intracytoplasmic melanin granules. However, in poorly differentiated, amelanotic melanomas, these neoplasms can be misidentified easily. Nuclei are typically round to ovoid and often contain two similarly sized round nucleoli, giving the nucleus the appearance of a 'pig's nose' or an 'owl's eye' (Figures 6.18, 6.19, 6.20). Immunostaining with immunocytochemistry using antibodies against cytokeratin, vimentin, and Melan A protein or immunohistochemistry with a panel of antibodies containing Melan-A, PNL-2, TRP-1, and TRP-2 may be helpful in identifying these neoplasms but may be cost prohibitive (Prześdziecki *et al.*, 2015; Smedley *et al.*, 2022). Although not all melanomas are malignant, those associated with the oral cavity are often biologically

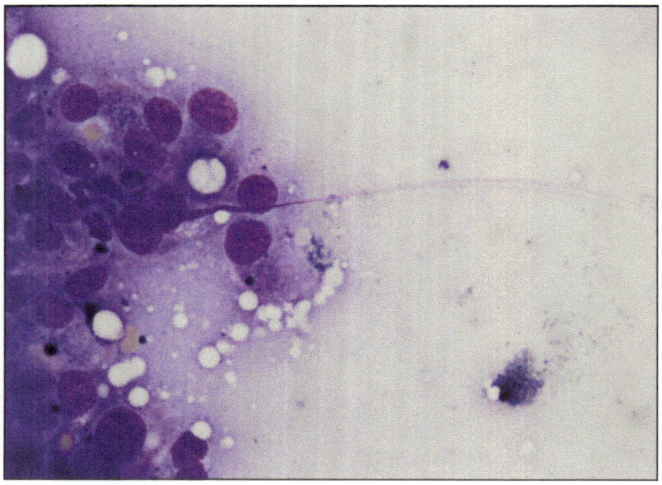

Figure 6.18 Oral mass from a dog. Melanoma. Multiple nuclei contain two prominent nucleoli, giving the appearance of a 'pig's nose. Low numbers of cells contain a faint black pigment dusting, and occasional aggregates of extracellular melanin granules are present. Cytoplasmic streaming from a disrupted nucleus is shown (modified Wright's, 1,000× magnification).

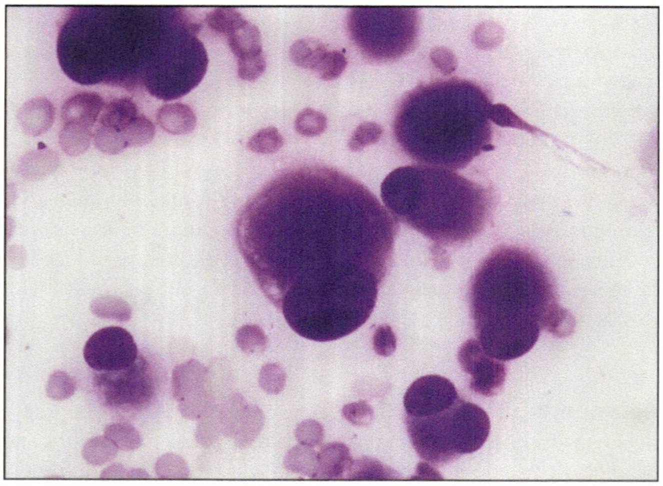

Figure 6.19 Oral mass from a dog. Amelanotic melanoma, confirmed with histopathology. Individualized round cells have an abundant amount of magenta-colored cytoplasm, which often stains lighter toward the periphery. Nuclei are ovoid and peripherally located typically with a single, prominent, deeply basophilic nucleolus. Two binucleated cells are seen. Anisocytosis and anisokaryosis are moderate to marked. No overt melanin granules are observed (Diff-Quik®, 1,000× magnification).

aggressive with frequent metastasis to the regional lymph nodes and lungs and with a metastatic rate dependent on site, size, and clinical stage (Liptak, 2020). Histologic examination of architecture is advised for prognostication (Smedley *et al.*, 2022).

Squamous cell carcinoma

Squamous cell carcinoma (SCC) is the second most common oral neoplasm in dogs and the most common oral cancer in cats, where it often occurs in the frenulum of the tongue (Andreasen *et al.*, 2016; Liptak,

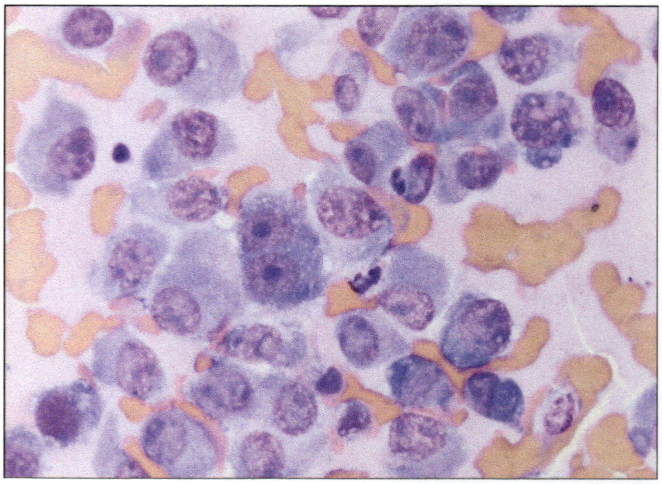

Figure 6.20 Oral mass from a dog. Amelanotic melanoma. Individualized spindle-shaped cells with moderate amounts of basophilic cytoplasm, that occasionally contains punctate vacuoles. Nuclei are round to ovoid with coarse chromatin and often one or more prominent, deeply basophilic nucleoli. A binculeated cell resembling 'eyes' is noted centrally. No overt melanin granules are observed (modified Wright's, 1,000x magnification).

2020). Squamous epithelial cells are present throughout the oral cavity, as they cover most surfaces in the mouth, including the tonsil. Neoplastic squamous cells typically exhibit numerous criteria of malignancy. An increased N:C ratio can be difficult to detect, as 'normal' squamous epithelial cells typically contain an abundant amount of cytoplasm relative to nuclear size. As squamous cells mature, they lose their nucleus in conjunction with the keratinization process. Fully keratinized squamous cells stain bright blue with Romanowsky stain and the presence of a nucleus in a keratinized cell is indicative of nuclear to cytoplasmic maturation asynchrony, which is often associated with a neoplastic process. Additionally, neoplastic squamous cells often contain numerous distinct, nonstaining vacuoles, which occasionally aggregate, forming a 'beard' around the nucleus with an aggregate of vacuoles on one nuclear pole. Bizarre cell shapes, including round, angular, and 'tadpole-shaped' cells, are noted commonly (Figures 6.21–6.24). The cytologic diagnosis of neoplasia can be complicated by the fact that intralesional keratin often incites a marked neutrophilic inflammatory response, which might be interpreted erroneously as inciting dysplastic rather than neoplastic change in the epithelial population (Figure 6.25).The prognosis in dogs with SCC varies, depending on type and location. Subtypes of non-tonsillar SCC have been developed in dogs, based on the World Health Organization (WHO) classification system, with a suggestion that the papillary subtype has a lower rate of distant metastasis and, therefore, a more favorable prognosis, than other types of non-tonsillar oral SCC (Thaiwong *et al.*, 2017). Tonsillar tumors and lesions at the base of the tongue carry a worse prognosis than SCCs at other oral locations.The prognosis in cats with SCC is poor, due to the aggressive nature of local lesions and the metastatic potential (Liptak, 2020). Tonsillar SCC are reportedly 10 times more common in animals living in cities versus in rural areas, implying that environmental pollutants may play a role in tumor development (Reif & Cohen, 1971).

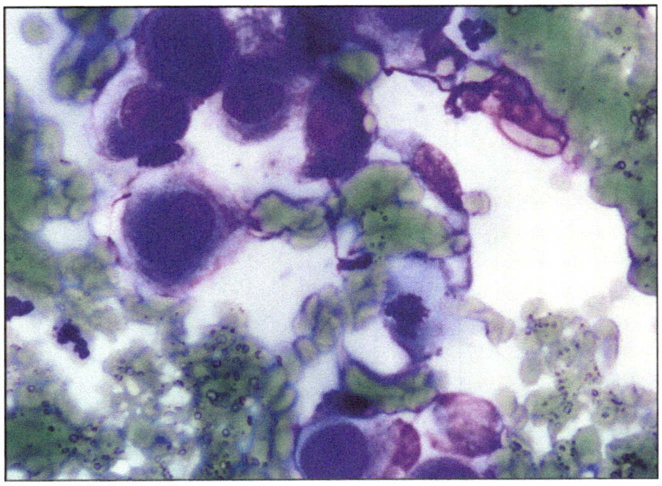

Figure 6.21 Mass at the base of a mandibular canine tooth from a dog. Squamous cell carcinoma. Individualized round to polygonal cells with a high N:C ratio. Nuclei are round to ovoid with coarsely clumped chromatin and one or more prominent nucleoli. Cytoplasm is deeply basophilic, consistent with keratinization. One mitotic figure is present. Anisocytosis and anisokaryosis are moderate (Diff-Quik®, 1,000× magnification).

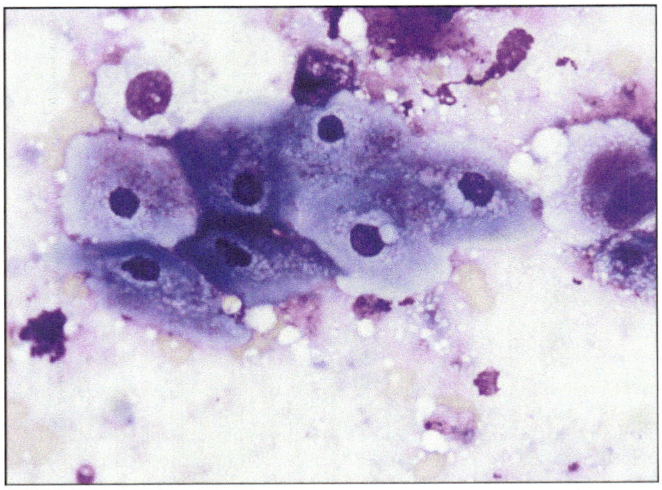

Figure 6.22 Mass on the zygomatic arch of a dog. Squamous cell carcinoma. Cohesive angular squamous epithelial cells exhibiting nuclear to cytoplasmic asynchrony, as keratinized cells should be anucleate. Aggregates of variably sized, nonstaining vacuoles surround the nucleus, forming a nuclear 'beard' (modified Wright's, 1,000× magnification).

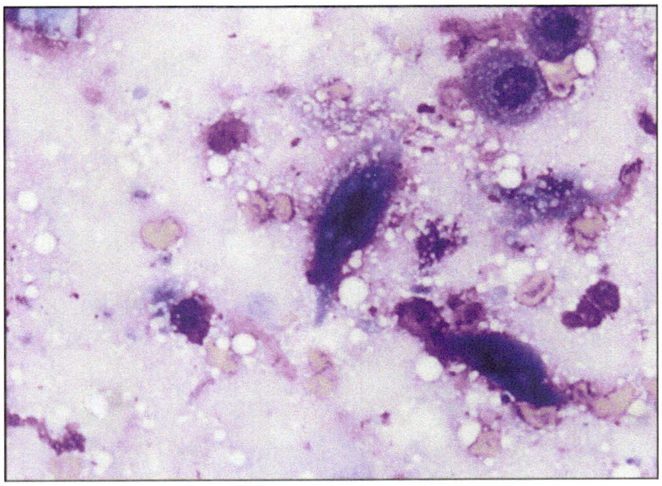

Figure 6.23 Oral mass from a dog. Squamous cell carcinoma. Individualized round to angular squamous epithelial cells exhibiting nuclear to cytoplasmic asynchrony are noted. The cell in the middle of the image tapers at one end, morphologically resembling a 'tadpole' (modified Wright's, 1,000× magnification).

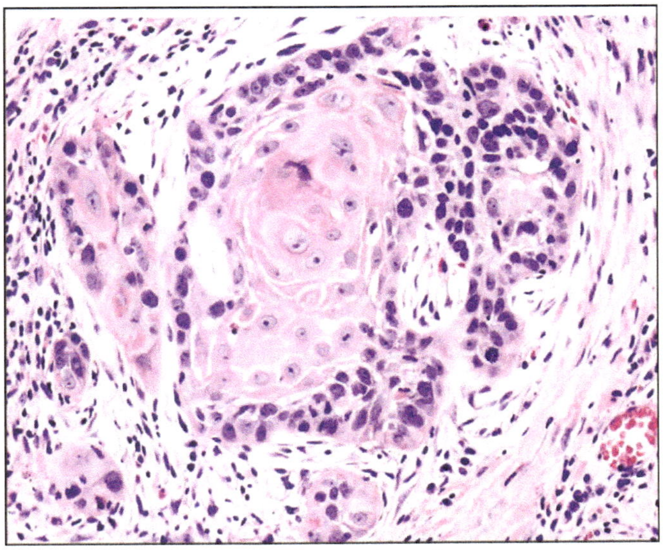

Figure 6.24 Histologic section of an oral mass from a cat. Squamous cell carcinoma. Nests of pleomorphic squamous epithelial cells (keratin pearls) are surrounded by more basilar epithelium, adipose tissue, and fibrovascular stroma (H&E, 400× magnification).

Fibrosarcoma

Oral fibrosarcoma is the third most common oral tumor of the dog and the second most common oral tumor of the cat (Liptak, 2020). This neoplasm often appears on the hard palate and, like other mesenchymal tumors, often exfoliates poorly, resulting in minimally cellular cytologic specimens. Therefore, a biopsy is often needed for diagnosis. When cells are present for evaluation, they typically have wispy cytoplasm with indistinct cellular borders, making assessment of anisocytosis and N:C ratio difficult. Nuclei are often ovoid with a coarse, open, chromatin pattern. There is a subset of oral fibrosarcomas with relatively benign looking morphology, exhibiting few criteria of malignancy, which are shown to be very biologically aggressive, with aggressive local invasion and a 30% metastatic rate (Cieckot *et al*., 1994; Munday *et al*., 2016). Therefore, even with minimal criteria of malignancy, there is suspicion for an aggressive lesion with the presence of proliferative mesenchymal cells (Figure 6.26).

Lesions formerly known as epulides

Epulis (plural = epulides) is a nonspecific term used to refer to a growth of the gingiva. Epulides cannot readily be distinguished cytologically

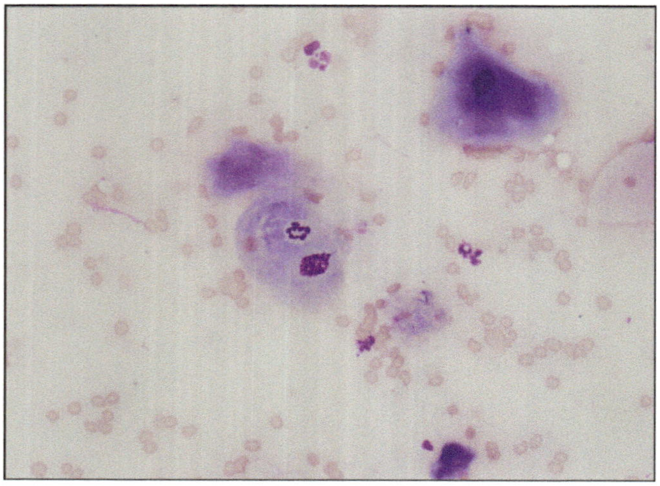

Figure 6.25 Digital mass from a cat. Squamous cell carcinoma. Squamous epithelial cells with blood and poorly preserved neutrophils. Either on or within (emperipolesis) the central squamous epithelial cell is a nondegenerate neutrophil (modified Wright's, 500× magnification).

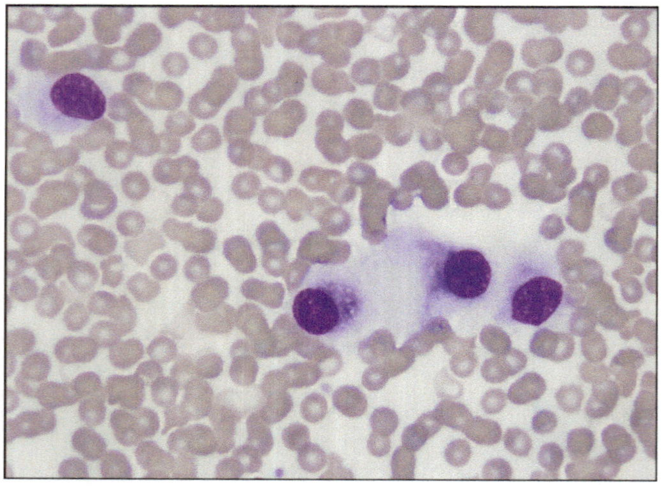

Figure 6.26 Mass on thorax of a dog. Fibrosarcoma. A poorly exfoliating neoplasm with a large amount of blood. Individual cells have wispy, indistinct, basophilic cytoplasm. Nuclei are round to ovoid with a coarse chromatin pattern and indistinct nucleoli (modified Wright's, 1,000× magnification).

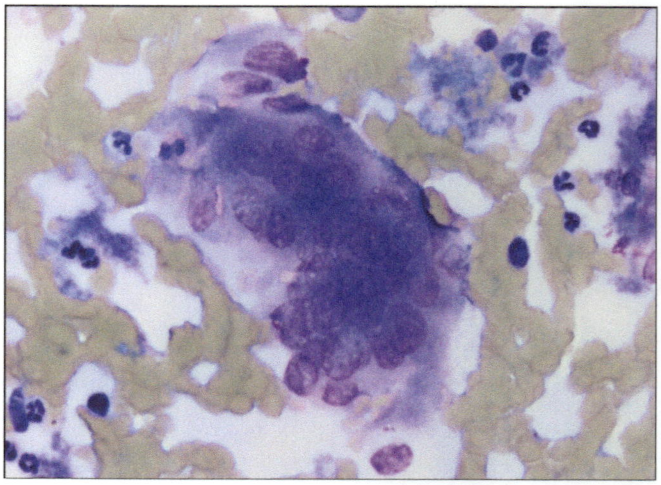

Figure 6.27 Hard palate mass from a dog. There is a single, large multinucleated cell, morphologically compatible with an osteoclast.

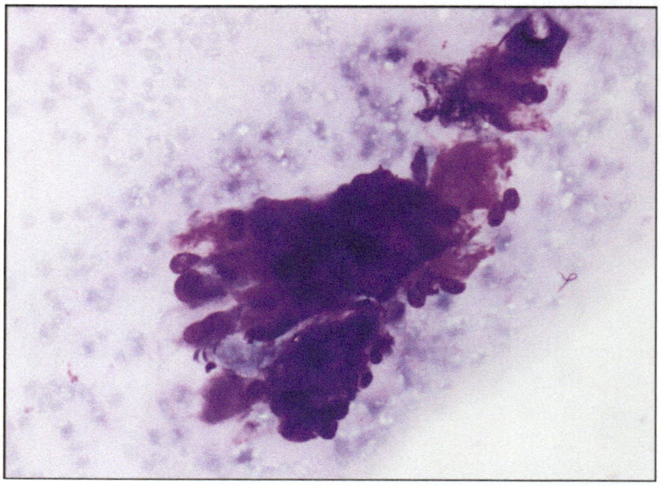

Figure 6.28 Gum mass from a dog. Peripheral odontogenic fibroma (formerly fibromatous epulis). Clusters of uniform, tightly cohesive, round-shaped epithelial cells with high N:C ratios and indistinct cell borders. Abundant brightly eosinophilic matrix material surrounds more pleomorphic, wispy, mesenchymal cells (modified Wright's, 500× magnification).

from gingival hyperplasia (Munday *et al.*, 2016; Gelberg, 2021). Historically, at least four types of epulides (acanthomatous, fibromatous, giant cell, ossifying) were recognized; some of these lesions contain inflammatory cells and/or osteoclasts, making interpretation difficult (Figure 6.27). Classification of these tumors has been simplified. Lesions formerly classified as acanthomatous epulides, which arise from the remnants of dental lamina in the gingiva (rests of Serres), are now termed acanthomatous ameloblastomas whereas all other subtypes are termed peripheral odontogenic fibromas (Wingo, 2018; Liptak, 2020). Bone in peripheral odontogenic fibromas is consistent with osseous metaplasia, eliminating the need for the term 'ossifying epulis' (Munday *et al.*, 2016). As squamous epithelial cells cover the mesenchymal gingiva, cells of mixed morphology are often noted in these lesions (Figure 6.28). Histologic examination of architecture is needed to characterize and further classify these lesions. While most exhibit benign biological behavior, acanthomatous ameloblastomas are often locally aggressive and invade the underlying bone of the maxilla or mandible. There is no report of distant metastasis, often allowing for management with aggressive local therapy (Liptak, 2013).

Viral papillomatosis

Lesions associated with viral papillomatosis are horizontally transmitted between dogs and are caused by the DNA virus canine

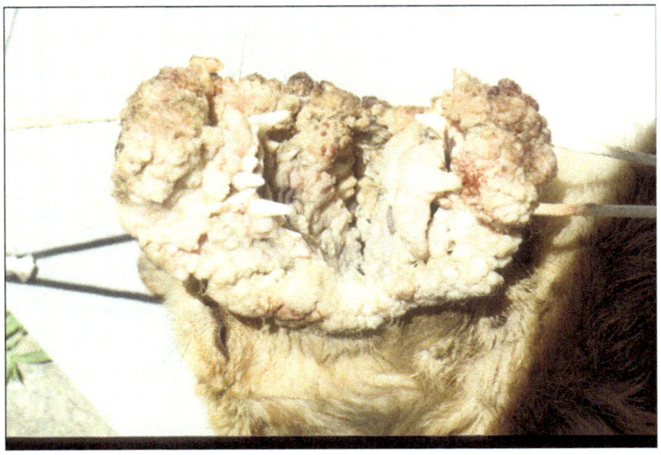

Figure 6.29 Canine viral papillomatosis. Numerous verrucous masses covering the tongue, the lips, the labial tissue, and the hard palate (courtesy Dr. David Driemeier).

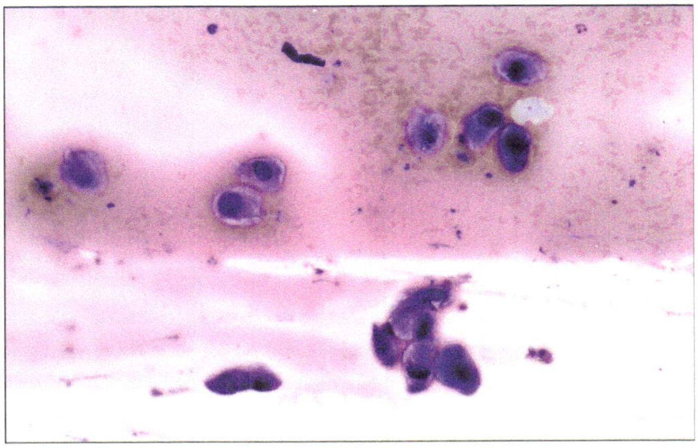

Figure 6.30 Toe mass from a dog. Canine papillomatosis. Aggregates of variably sized round to angular squamous epithelial cells with variable N:C ratios embedded in a brightly eosinophilic extracellular material (modified Wright's, 100× magnification) (courtesy Dr. Elena Gorman).

papillomavirus (CPV)-1 (Newkirk *et al.*, 2021; Liptak, 2020). Multiple viral-associated masses often arise on the tongue, lips, or oropharynx and exhibit a verrucous appearance (Figure 6.29). They occur most commonly in young dogs (less than 1 year old) and typically regress spontaneously within 1–2 months, although spread to other bodily locations, including the esophagus and haired skin, can occur (Higgins et al., 2001; Munday et al, 2016). These lesions are composed superficially of various stages of squamous epithelial cells overlying a mesenchymal (stromal) core, resulting in heterogeneous aspirates (Figure 6.30). Cytoplasmic viral inclusions can be seen occasionally. Papillomavirus-induced lesions in cats are rare, although sublingual masses in cats have been associated with the presence of *Felis catus* papillomavirus 1 (FcaPV-1) DNA (Munday, 2015a,b).

Granular cell tumor

Granular cell tumors are relatively uncommon, typically benign neoplasms and may appear on the larynx, tongue, lips, palate, and gingiva (Munday *et al.*, 2016). They have also been reported on the skin and in the central nervous system (Gross *et al.*, 2005). The term 'granular cell tumor' is descriptive, as the cell of origin is unknown (Munday *et al.*, 2016). Cytologically, granular cell tumors typically contain individualized round to polygonal cells with abundant pale pink cytoplasm, which contains numerous small, distinct, eosinophilic granules (Figure 6.31). Transmission electron microscopy has demonstrated that the granules are large, membrane-bound lysosomes. Granules are diastase resistant with periodic acid–Schiff stain (Figure 6.32; Higgins et al., 2001; Liptak, 2020). Nuclei are generally small and round and may be obscured by the granules. Occasionally, a spindloid

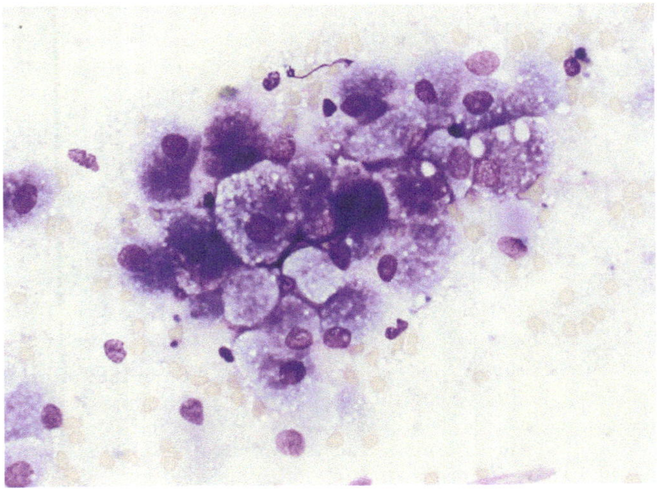

Figure 6.31 Laryngeal mass from a dog. Granular cell tumor. Cluster of loosely cohesive round-shaped to angular cells with an abundant amount of basophilic, vacuolated cytoplasm that typically contains a faint dusting of eosinophilic granules. Nuclei are round and centrally located with fine granular chromatin (modified Wright's, 500× magnification).

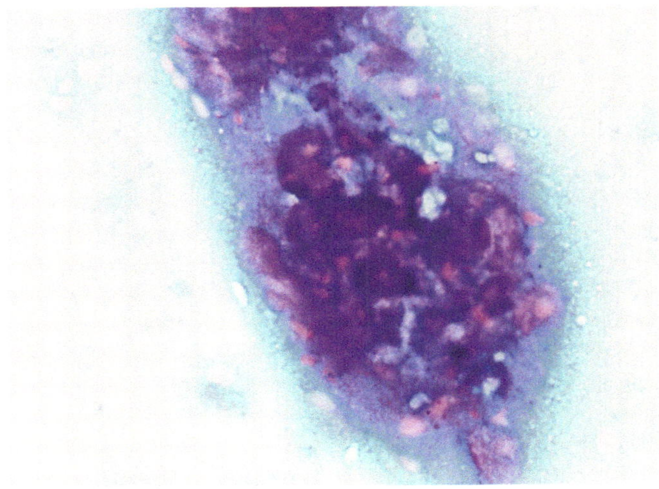

Figure 6.32 Cells from granular cell tumor in Figure 6.31 staining for periodic acid–Schiff (PAS) are brightly eosinophilic. (PAS, 500× magnification)

morphology is observed. Biological behavior is unpredictable, but lesions are often locally aggressive (Higgins et al., 2001, 2016).

Other tumors

Many other malignancies have been reported in the oral cavity and lesion location in the mouth should not preclude an appropriate cytologic diagnosis (Figure 6.33). Lymphoma, morphologically identical to that diagnosed at other locations, is the most common tonsillar neoplasm (Figure 6.34). Mast cell tumors, plasma cell tumors, and transmissible venereal tumors, with their distinct morphologic features, can be diagnosed in the mouth and on surrounding mucous membranes (Figures 6.35–6.37; Hostetter, 2023). Dental tumors (e.g., odontomas) may arise and typically surround or replace the dental arcade. These tumors are named based on their cell or tissue of origin and the degree of odontogenesis, and appropriately applying naming conventions requires experience examining these lesions (Gelberg, 2021).

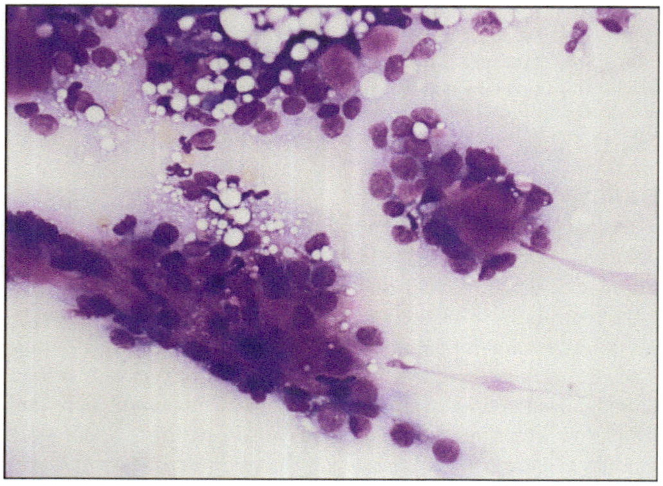

Figure 6.33 Salivary gland mass from a dog. Adenocarcinoma. Basilar-type salivary epithelial cells with high N:C ratios often form clusters and acini surrounding a bright eosinophilic extracellular secretory product. Anisocytosis and anisokaryosis are mild, making histologic confirmation necessary (modified Wright's, 500× magnification).

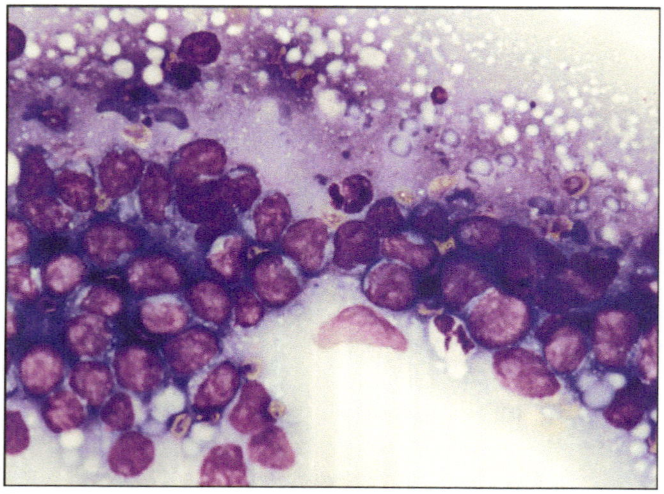

Figure 6.34 Laryngeal mass from a cat. Lymphoma. There is a monomorphic population of large lymphocytes with occasional indistinct nucleolar rings. Scattered lymphoglandular bodies are present in the background (modified Wright's, 1,000× magnification).

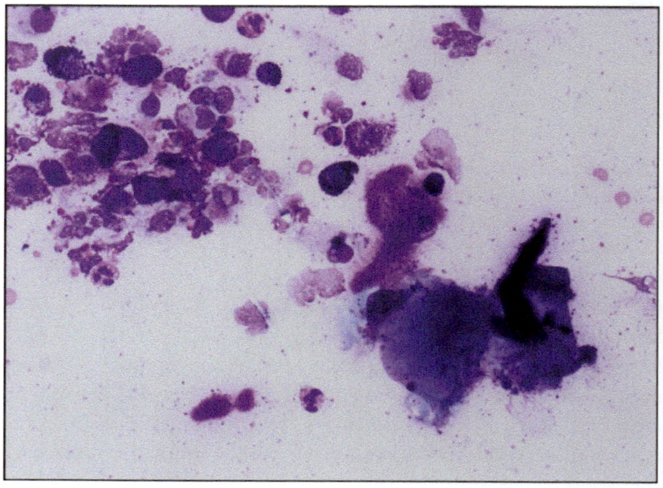

Figure 6.35 Oral mass from a dog. Mast cell tumor. Individualized round cells with abundant metachromatic intracytoplasmic granules. Nuclei are round and often do not take up stain. Eosinophils and free mast cell granules are in the background. Keratinized squamous epithelial cells with adherent *Conchiformibius* spp. organisms indicate oropharyngeal origin or contamination (modified Wright's, 500× magnification).

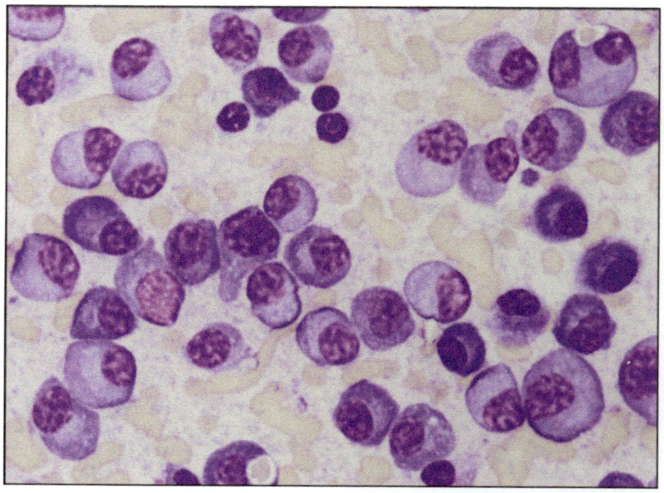

Figure 6.36 Lip mass from a cat. Plasmacytoma. Individualized round cells with a moderate to large amount of deeply basophilic cytoplasm that exhibits a perinuclear clear zone. Nuclei are peripheralized with a coarsely granular chromatin pattern. Occasional binucleated cells are seen and low numbers of erythrophagocytic plasma cells are present. Anisocytosis and anisokaryosis are mild (modified Wright's, 1,000× magnification).

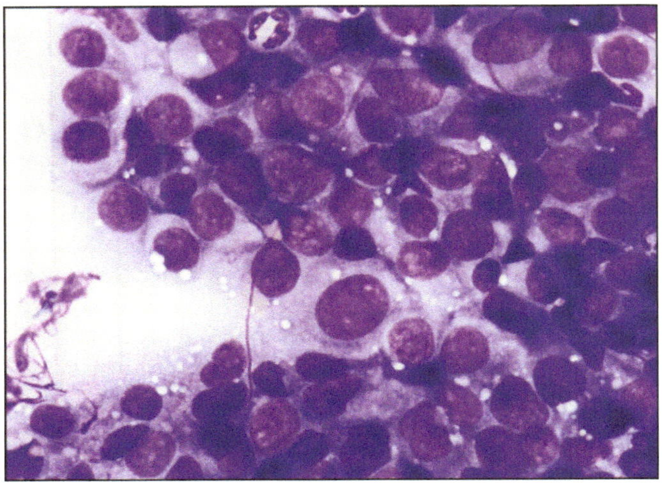

Figure 6.37 Labial mass from a dog. Transmissible venereal tumor. Aggregate of individualized round cells with pale, basophilic cytoplasm that occasionally contains discrete, nonstaining vacuoles. Nuclei are round to ovoid with finely granular chromatin. Anisocytosis and anisokaryosis are mild to moderate (modified Wright's, 1,000× magnification).

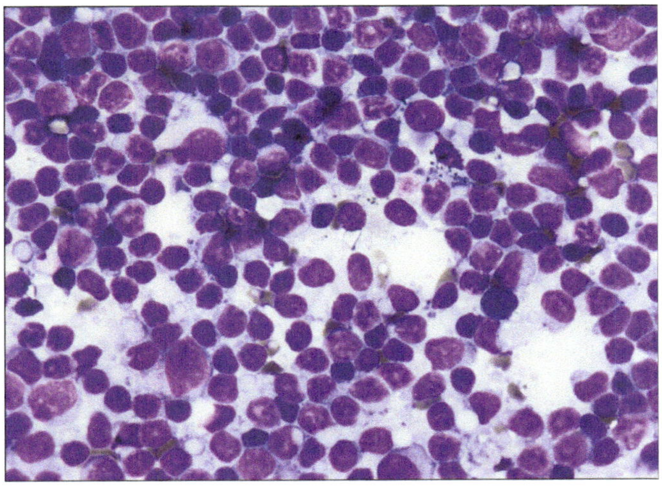

Figure 6.38 Lymph node. A heterogeneous lymphoid population, composed primarily of small lymphocytes with fewer medium and large lymphocytes. A small amount of hemosiderin and abundant lymphoglandular bodies are present in the background (modified Wright's, 500× magnification).

CASES

CASE 1

Signalment/history

An 11-year-old spayed female Labrador Retriever. The animal presented to the orthopedic surgery service for a 12-week recheck after a tibial plateau leveling osteotomy (TPLO) to correct a ruptured cruciate ligament. She was reportedly doing well at home, with minimal evidence of orthopedic pain.

Clinical examination

The examining clinician noticed a 3-cm, freely movable, subcutaneous mass on the left side of the neck, in the area of the left submandibular lymph node. Three aspirates were obtained and submitted for cytologic examination.

Cytologic description

One of the aspirates contained a heterogeneous lymphoid population, composed primarily of small lymphocytes, with fewer medium and large lymphocytes, and rare plasma cells. This aspirate was most compatible with aspiration of a cytologically unremarkable lymph node (Figure 6.38). The other two aspirates contained a large amount of blood, which aligned in a 'windrowing' pattern. Occasional individualized foamy round cells, interpreted as either macrophages or individualized secretory epithelial cells, were observed. Low numbers of angular yellow hematoidin crystals, indicative of prior hemorrhage, were also noted within the cytoplasm of low numbers of these cells. Free in the background were abundant amorphous collections of eosinophilic to amphophilic material, cytologically most compatible with saliva.

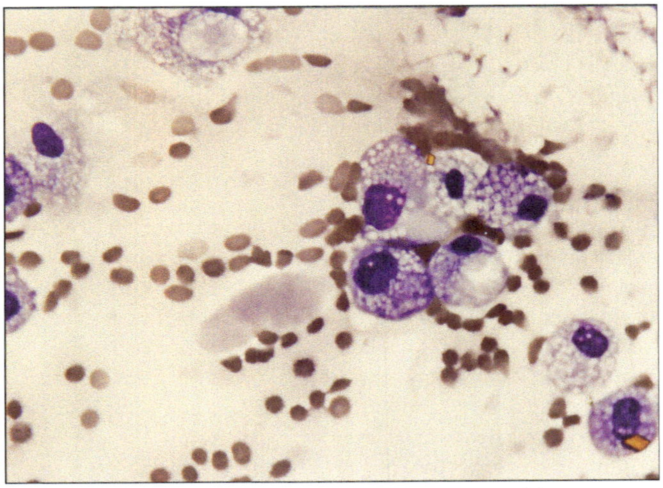

Figure 6.39 Facial swelling. Free blood in the background forms occasional linear structures ('windrows'). Individualized to very loosely cohesive round shaped cells (either macrophages or secretory epithelial cells) are present. Two 'mustard yellow' rhomboid hematoidin crystals are shown. Morphologically compatible with a sialocele (modified Wright's, 1,000× magnification).

Cytologic interpretation

The overall cytomorphology of this lesion was most compatible with a sialocele with previous hemorrhage (Figure 6.39).

Management

The owner elected to pursue surgical removal of the lesion, as repeated drainage simply resulted in lesion recurrence. Histologic examination of the architecture revealed abundant amounts of granulation tissue extending from the superficial dermis to the subcutis, which displaced

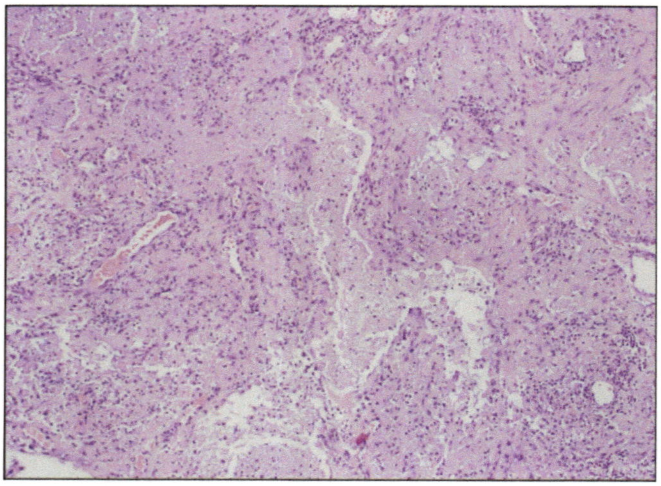

Figure 6.40 **Histologic section of tissue from facial swelling. Plump, organizing fibroblasts (granulation tissue) surrounding a central mass of amphophilic flocculent material (saliva). Morphologic diagnosis: sialocele (H&E, 100× magnification).**

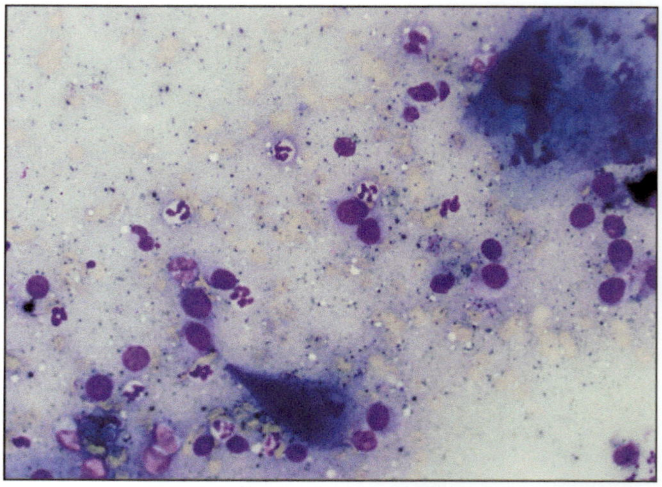

Figure 6.41 **Scattered, individualized, round-shaped to spindloid cells are present with high N:C ratios and a scant amount of lightly basophilic cytoplasm. Nuclei are round to ovoid. Abundant black melanin granules are free in the background. Occasional deeply basophilic, anucleate squamous epithelial cells are present with adherent *Conchiformibius* spp. organisms, indicative of origin or contamination from the oral cavity. Morphologically most compatible with melanoma (modified Wright's, 500× magnification).**

adjacent adnexa. A focally extensive area of pyogranulomatous inflammation was admixed with abundant amounts of amphophilic, flocculent material (saliva) and cellular debris. Scattered lymphocytes and plasma cells and multifocal areas of hemorrhage were noted. A morphologic diagnosis of sialocele was made (Figure 6.40).

Discussion

Sialoceles, also called salivary mucoceles, are accumulations of saliva in subcutaneous tissues with secondary purulent to pyogranulomatous inflammation. These lesions differ from ranulas (distensions of an epithelial lined salivary gland or duct) in that they are not lined by an epithelial lining. The exact cause of these lesions is unknown. However, it is likely that sialoceles are secondary to trauma, with disruption of a salivary duct resulting in leakage and encapsulation of saliva by connective tissue (Hostetter, 2023).

At the time of this patient's TPLO surgery, 12 weeks prior to presentation, there was reportedly a malfunctioning pulse oximeter used for surgical monitoring. This resulted in much manipulation of the tongue throughout the anesthetic procedure, which may have caused rupture of the duct of the sublingual salivary gland.

CASE 2

Signalment/history

An 8-year-old, neutered male Newfoundland presented for hematemesis and weakness. His owners brought in a tennis ball-sized structure that they found in his vomitus and believed to be a rubber ball.

Physical examination

Closer examination of the structure revealed that it was a solid piece of tissue. The tissue was bisected, and impression smears were made and submitted for cytologic evaluation. The patient was resistant to oral examination, and the owners elected not to sedate the animal to allow for proper restraint.

Cytologic/histologic evaluation

The impression smears were highly cellular and revealed a population of pleomorphic round-shaped to spindloid cells with abundant black, intracytoplasmic pigment granules. Nuclei were round to ovoid with coarsely granular chromatin and an occasional indistinct nucleolus. Low numbers of binucleated cells were seen. These findings were compatible with a cytologic diagnosis of melanoma (Figure 6.41). Scattered keratinized, anucleate squamous epithelial cells with adherent *Conchiformibius* spp. organisms were noted. The exact origin of the tumor was uncertain.

The tissue from which the impression smears were made was submitted for histologic examination (Figure 6.42). Histologic examination revealed a poorly demarcated, unencapsulated, infiltrative, densely cellular neoplasm composed of neoplastic melanocytes. Cells were arranged in sheets and interlacing streams supported by abundant fibrovascular stroma. Individual cells were pleomorphic, ranging from round to polygonal to spindloid, with variably distinct cell borders and scant to moderate amounts of eosinophilic cytoplasm containing variable numbers of melanin granules. Nuclei were centrally placed, ovoid to elongate, with vesiculated chromatin and one distinct, eosinophilic nucleolus. There were occasional karyomegaly and frequent binucleation. Anisocytosis and anisokaryosis were marked. There were 3 mitoses per 10 microscopic fields at 400× magnification. The melanoma was covered by moderately hyperplastic squamous epithelium with moderate parakeratotic hyperkeratosis, suggestive of gingival, buccal, or palatine origin.

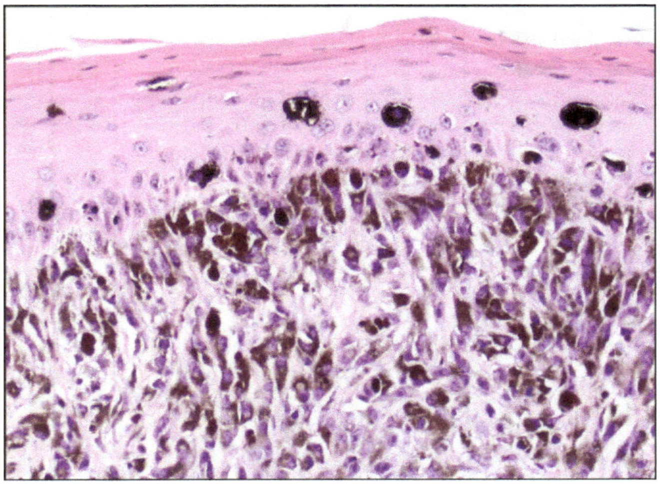

Figure 6.42 **Streams of spindloid to polygonal cells with abundant brown intracytoplasmic pigment granules dorsally displace the epithelium, which is covered with parakeratotic squamous epithelium. Morphologic diagnosis: melanoma (H&E, 400 magnification).**

Management/outcome

On receiving a diagnosis of melanoma, the owners allowed sedation, and oral examination revealed a large, ulcerated mass emanating from the soft palate. It is believed that the 'vomited' portion of the mass came from this location and that the dog was likely vomiting due to nausea induced by swallowing large amounts of blood arising from the tumor. Surgical debulking was attempted, and complete margins were unattainable. The patient died within 2 weeks of diagnosis.

CASE 3

Signalment/history

A 10-year-old neutered male domestic short-haired cat presented with a history of excessive salivation.

Clinical examination

The examining clinician noted a large, ulcerated mass beneath the tongue. Aspirates were obtained with sedation.

Cytologic description

The aspirates contained a pleomorphic population of individualized to minimally cohesive squamous epithelial cells, in varying stages of keratinization. Individual cells were large and round-shaped to angular, with abundant cytoplasm, often containing a large perinuclear clearing, typical of squamous epithelium. Occasional mitotic figures were noted. Anisocytosis was marked, with mild to moderate anisokaryosis. The number of neutrophils was increased over the amount of blood (Figure 6.43).

Cytologic interpretation

This lesion is consistent with a squamous cell carcinoma with neutrophilic inflammation. After biopsy, the diagnosis was confirmed with histologic examination of tissue architecture.

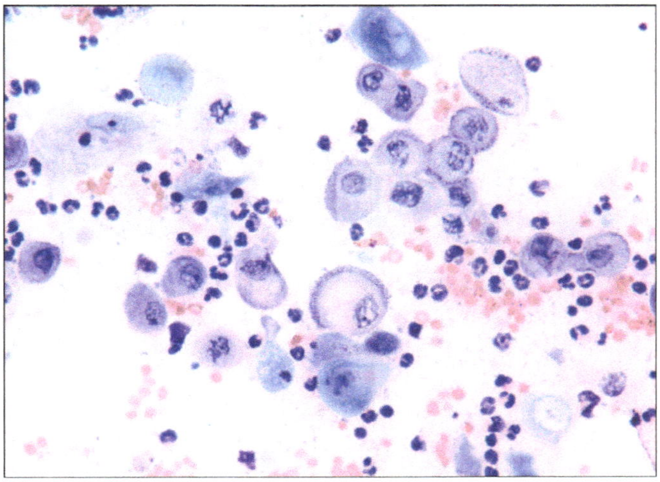

Figure 6.43 **Sublingual mass. A pleomorphic population of individualized to minimally cohesive squamous epithelial cells in varying stages of keratinization, which exhibit marked anisocytosis and mild to moderate anisokaryosis. The number of neutrophils is increased over the amount of blood. (Courtesy Dr. Anne Barger.)**

Management/outcome

The owners elected palliative care and euthanasia was elected one month after diagnosis, due to progression of symptoms and diminished quality of life.

REFERENCES

Andreasen S., Bjørndal K., Agander T.K., Wessel I., & Homøe P. (2016) Tumors of the sublingual gland: A national clinicopathologic study of 29 cases. *Eur Arch Otorhinolaryngol 273*:3847–3856.

Bacha W.J. Jr., Bacha L.M. (2012) Digestive system. In: *Color Atlas of Veterinary Histology*, 3rd edn. (eds. W.J. Bacha, L.M. Bacha) John Wiley & Sons, Ames, pp. 139–342.

Bochnakian M.S., Bezerra J.A.B., Fernandes K.S.B.R., Barros V.R., Paula V.V., Santos J.P.S., Filgueira K.D. (2018) Oral lesions secondary to visceral leishmaniasis in a dog with endogenous hyperadrenocorticism: Case report. *Arq Bras Med Vet Zootec 70*(*4*):1115–1119.

Bonfanti U., Bertazzolo W., Gracis M. et al. (2015) Diagnostic value of cytological analysis of tumours and tumour-like lesions of the oral cavity in dogs and cats: A prospective study on 114 cases. *Vet J 205*(*2*):322–327.

Cieckot P.A., Powers B.A., Withrow S.J. et al. (1994) Histologically low grade yet biologically high grade fibrosarcomas of the mandible and maxilla of 25 dogs (1982–1991). *J Am Vet Med Assoc 204*:610–615.

Gelberg H.B. (2021) Alimentary system and the peritoneum, omentum, mesentery, and peritoneal cavity. In: *Pathologic Basis of Veterinary Disease*, 7th edn. (ed. J.F. Zachary) Mosby Elsevier, St. Louis, pp. 322–336.

Gross T.L., Ihrke P.J., Walder E.J. et al. (2005) Melanocytic tumors. In: *Skin Diseases of the Dog and Cat: Clinical and Histopathological Diagnosis*, 2nd edn. (ed. T.L. Gross) Blackwell Publishing, Oxford, p. 832.

Haddad S., Noreldin A.E., Kamal B. et al. (2019) Morphological and functional comparison of lingual papillae in suckling and adult feral cats: Forensic evidence. *Anat Histol Embryol 48*:404–414.

Higgins R.J., Lecouteur R.A., Bollen, A.W. (2001) Granular cell tumor of the canine central nervous system: two cases. *Vet Pathol 38*(6):620–627.

Hostetter S.J. (2023) Oral cavity, gastrointestinal tract, and associated structures. In: *Canine and Feline Cytology: A Color Atlas and Interpretation Guide*, 2nd edn. (eds. R.E. Raskin, D.J. Meyer, K.M. Boes) Saunders Elsevier, St. Louis, pp. 287–296.

Liptak J.M., Withrow S.J. (2020) Cancer of the gastrointestinal tract. In: *Withrow & MacEwen's Small Animal Clinical Oncology*, 6th edn. (eds. D.M. Vail, D.H. Thamm, J. Liptak) Elsevier Saunders, St. Louis, pp. 381–445.

Mikiewicz M., Paździor-Czapula K., Gesek M. et al. (2019) Canine and feline oral cavity tumours and tumour-like lesions: A retrospective study of 486 cases (2015–2017). *J Comp Path 172*:80–87.

Munday J.S., Fairley R.A., Mills H. et al. (2015a) Oral papillomas associated with *Felis catus* papillomavirus type 1 in 2 domestic cats. *Vet Pathol 52*(6):1187–1190.

Munday J.S., French A.F. (2015b) Felis catus papillomavirus types 1 and 4 are rarely present in neoplastic and inflammatory oral lesions of cats. *Res Vet Sci 100*:220–222.

Munday J.S., Lőhr C.V., Kiupel M. (2016). Tumors of the alimentary tract. In: *Tumors in Domestic Animals*, 5th edn. (ed. D.J. Meuten) John Wiley & Sons, Ames, pp. 499–601.

Newkirk K.M., Brannick E.M., Kusewitt D.F. (2021) Neoplasia and tumor biology. In: *Pathologic Basis of Veterinary Disease*, 7th edn. (ed. J.F. Zachary) Mosby Elsevier, St. Louis, pp. 287–289.

Przeździecki R., Czopowicz M., Sapierayński R. (2015) Accuracy of routine cytology and immunohistochemistry in preoperative diagnosis of oral amelanotic melanomas in dogs. *Vet Clin Path 44*(*4*):597–604.

Reif J.S., Cohen D. (1971) The environmental distribution of canine respiratory tract neoplasms. *Arch Environ Health 22(1)*:136–140.

Smedley R.C., Sebastian K., Kiupel M. (2022) Diagosis and prognosis of canine melanocytic neoplasms. *Vet Sci 9*:175.

Thaiwong T., Sledge D.G., Collins-Webb A. et al. (2017) Immunohistochemical characterization of canine oral papillary squamous cell carcinoma. *Vet Pathol 55*(*2*):224–232.

Weise J.B., Meyer J.E., Helmer H. et al. (2002) A newly discovered function of palatine tonsils in immune defence: The expression of defensins. *Pol J Otolaryngol 56*:409–413.

Wingo K. (2018) Histopathologic diagnoses from biopsies of the oral cavity in 403 dogs and 73 cats. *J Vet Dent 35*(*1*):7–17.

CHAPTER 7

CYTOLOGY OF THE GASTROINTESTINAL TRACT

Elena Gorman

NORMAL GASTROINTESTINAL CYTOLOGY

The alimentary or gastrointestinal tract (GIT) in mammals is broken up into four major sections: the esophagus, the stomach, the small intestine, and the large intestine/colon and rectum. It is essentially a muscular tube lined by a mucous membrane. The cellular constituents making up the normal architecture of each section are specific and related to the function of each in order to aid in the passage and digestion of food while assisting in protection against ingested pathogens. All sections are comprised of four distinct layers of tissue: the mucosal layer at the luminal surface, a submucosal layer, a layer of smooth muscle, and an outer serosal/adventitial layer. These 'tunics' are designed for optimal protection, passage, absorption of water and nutrients, and excretion of waste (Figure 7.1).

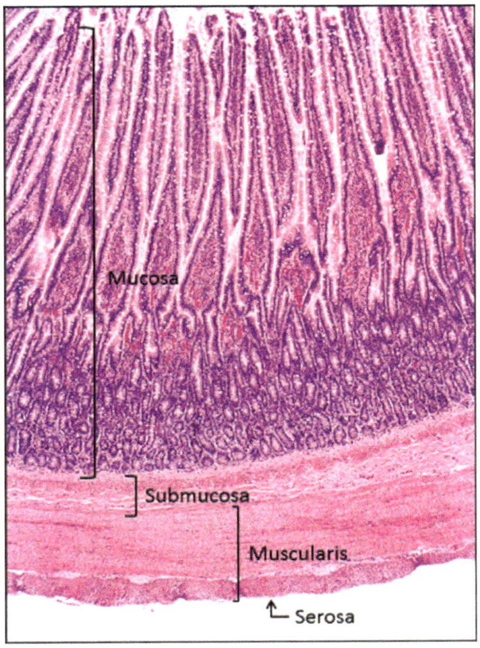

Figure 7.1 Histologic section of the intestine. Four distinct layers make up the intestinal 'tunics': mucosa, submucosa, muscularis, and serosa (H&E, 40× magnification) (courtesy Linda Meola).

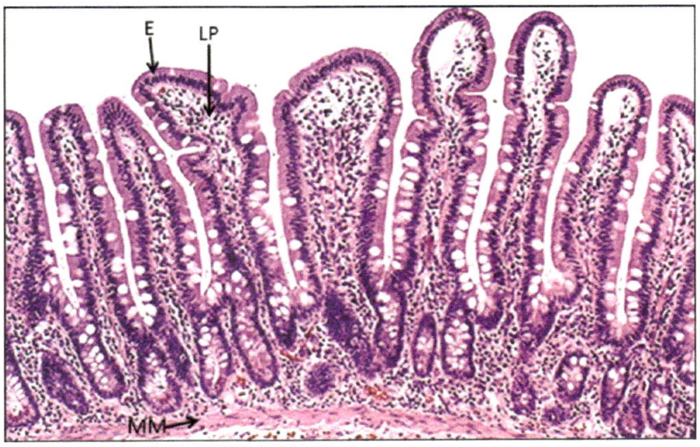

Figure 7.2 Histologic section of gastrointestinal mucosa. The mucosa is comprised of three layers from outer to inner: the epithelial layer (E), the lamina propria (LP), and the muscularis mucosae (MM) (H&E, 200× magnification).

Tunica mucosa

The epithelial mucosa lines the GI lumen and is divided into three distinct layers (Figure 7.2): the epithelial lining (lamina epithelialis), which is unique in each section of the intestine; a lamina propria layer, which contains lymphoid cells to assist in local immunity (Figure 7.3); and a thin layer of smooth muscle, the muscularis mucosae, which provides for local movement. Aggregates of lymphoid cells are found throughout the length of the GIT making up the 'gut-associated lymphoid tissue' (GALT) (Figure 7.4).

Tunica submucosa

The submucosal layer is comprised of loose collagenous connective tissue, which contains blood and lymphatic vessels and nerves for support of the mucosa.

Tunica muscularis

The muscular tunic is comprised of smooth muscle layers organized perpendicularly to each other for peristaltic activity.

DOI: 10.1201/9781003258551-7

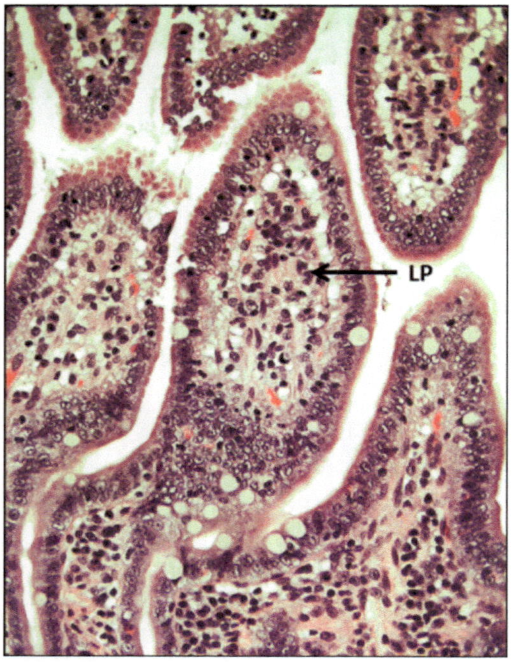

Figure 7.3 **Histologic section of small intestinal mucosa, feline. Lymphoid cells comprise the primary immune cell population of the lamina propria (LP, arrow) (H&E, 400× magnification).**

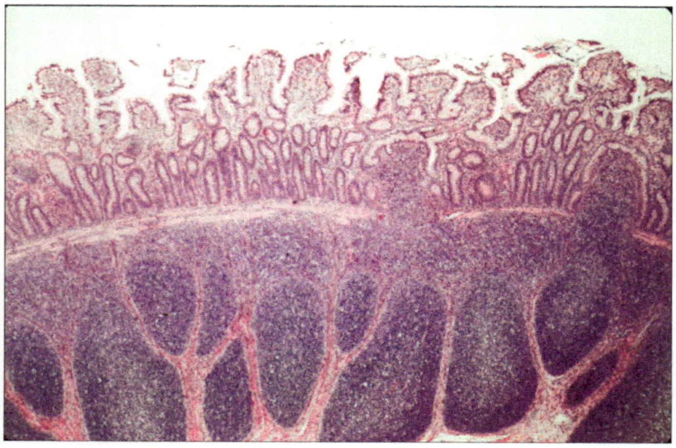

Figure 7.4 **Histologic section of the intestinal mucosa, canine. Lymphoid follicles (GALT) in the mucosa of the gastrointestinal tract (H&E, 40× magnification) (courtesy Barry Cooper).**

Tunica serosa/adventitia

The outer layer of the alimentary tract consists of loose supporting tissue and adipose with associated vessels and nerves. Within the abdominal cavity, this layer is referred to as the serosal layer and is lined by simple squamous epithelium (mesothelium).

SAMPLING THE GASTROINTESTINAL TRACT

Cytologic evaluation of GIT lesions is often performed in animals to aid diagnosis of solid masses or infiltrative GI disease. Even with concerns for devitalized tissue, complications from sampling are rare but can include bleeding, infection, and acute pancreatitis (Karadsheh & Al-Haddad, 2014). Several factors can influence the diagnostic yield of a sample including presence of necrosis, secondary inflammation, hemodilution, cell rupture, or poor exfoliation (Rivers *et al.*, 1997; Bonfanti *et al.*, 2006; von Babo *et al.*, 2012). Certain lesions affecting the GIT, such as chronic enteropathy, low-grade lymphoma, and poorly differentiated tumors, can be difficult to diagnose by cytology alone, and histology is typically needed for architecture and special staining. However, many GI lesions can be preliminarily or even definitively diagnosed by cytology of fine needle aspirates (FNAs), impression smears, or exfoliative cytology and rectal scrapes (Jergens *et al.*, 1998; Dell'Orco *et al.*, 2005; Bonfanti *et al.*, 2006; Maeda *et al.*, 2017).

Impression smears

Touch imprints from tissue samples acquired by endoscopic or full-thickness biopsies are excellent for the diagnosis of GI lesions. Touch imprints are often performed for quick interpretation of a lesion in order to begin initial treatment prior to obtaining final histopathology results. Care must be taken to avoid crushing the tissue or applying too much pressure while making impression smears, as cell rupture may confound the diagnosis.

Fine needle aspiration

Many reports have recognized the benefit of the co-utilization of imaging modalities such as endoscopy and ultrasound-guided FNA. Effective techniques to improve cell yield and minimize cell destruction have been proposed for cytologic samples. For obtaining diagnostic samples via FNA, factors such as needle size, aspiration/suction versus nonaspiration techniques, and lesion location have all been evaluated (Karadsheh & Al-Haddad, 2014). With regard to needle size, most studies show no difference between the use of 22-gauge versus 25-gauge needles. Aspiration may be superior for obtaining cells, particularly from fibrotic lesions or mesenchymal tumors. However, aspiration may result in increased hemorrhage or, in the case of lymphoproliferative lesions, increased cell rupture (Karadsheh & Al-Haddad, 2014).

Exfoliative cytology

In addition to FNA or impression smears post-biopsy of lesions in the GIT, exfoliative techniques such as brush cytology and rectal scrapings may be employed. (Rectal scraping is discussed further under 'Large Intestine [Cecum, Colon, and Rectum'].) In brush cytology, samples are acquired via endoscopy using a disposable guarded cytology brush instrument, which is passed through the accessory channel of the endoscope. The brush is extended beyond the protective sheath and rubbed or twirled vigorously over the mucosa to dislodge cells, then retracted back into its sheath and withdrawn. After removal, the brush is rolled across a slide to transfer the material for subsequent staining (Jergens *et al.*, 1998).

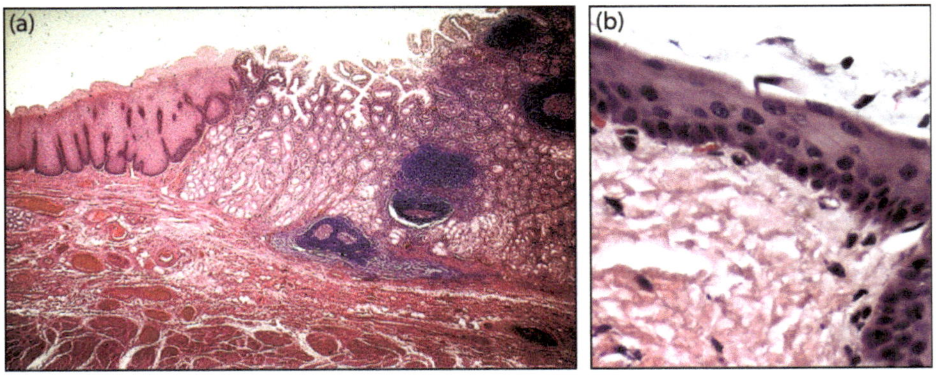

Figures 7.5a, b Histologic sections of the esophagus, canine. (a) Low-power (40x) magnification showing the gastroesophageal junction and the transition from stratified squamous epithelial mucosa to the glandular mucosa of the stomach. (b) Magnification of the esophageal mucosa showing the nonkeratinized squamous mucosal layer (H&E, 500× magnification).

Regardless of the technique utilized to obtain a sample, care should be taken to avoid excessive pressure during transfer and spreading of material onto a slide, as excessive pressure often results in cell rupture (Jergens *et al.*, 1998). Preparations made by FNA, impression smears, and brush exfoliation from endoscopic tissue biopsy have all been compared with histologic diagnosis for GI lesions (Rivers *et al.*, 1997; Jergens *et al.*, 1998; Bonfanti *et al.*, 2006; von Babo *et al.*, 2012; Karadsheh Al-Haddad, 2014). In most reports, despite the pitfalls mentioned above, good accordance has been shown, particularly for impression smears of tissue samples (Bonfanti *et al.*, 2006; von Babo *et al.*, 2012); therefore cytology remains a good technique to evaluate lesions, particularly neoplasms, in the GIT.

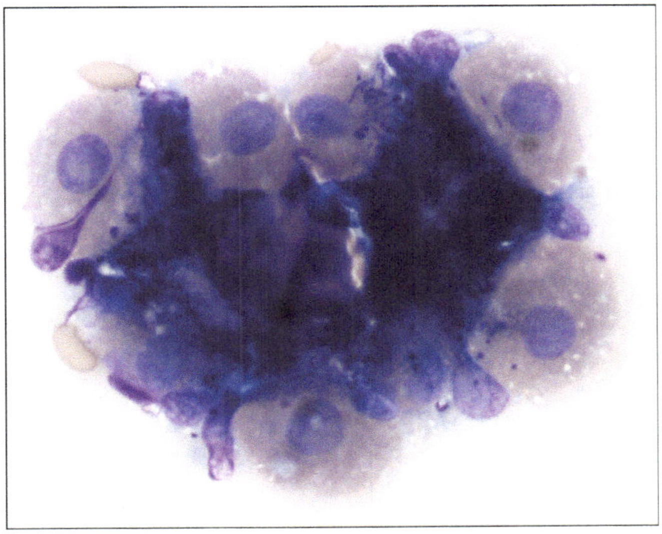

Figure 7.6 Cytology of normal esophageal squamous epithelial cells with overlying debris. These cells were obtained during endoscopic examination of the upper intestine and found adjacent to normal duodenal epithelium (see Figure 7.16a). The round shape with a single nucleus and eosinophilic cytoplasm gives these cells a 'fried egg' appearance typical for intermediate squamous epithelial cells (Wright–Giemsa, 500× magnification).

ESOPHAGUS

Normal

The esophagus is designed for the passage of macerated food and liquid into the stomach for further digestion. The luminal surface is therefore lined with a layer of stratified squamous epithelial cells, which protect the esophagus from damage (Figures 7.5a,b). Epithelial cells are not keratinized throughout the majority of the esophagus and are usually round in shape with a single nucleus and low nuclear to cytoplasmic (N:C) ratio (Figure 7.6). The esophageal submucosa contains mucous glands to aid lubrication. The muscularis layer is thick and contains skeletal muscle (except very near the stomach) (Bacha & Bacha, 2012).

Hyperplastic lesions

In hyperplastic lesions of the GIT, diagnosis is usually presumptively based on diagnostic imaging and the identification of uniform populations of epithelial cells. In the esophagus, squamous hyperplasia has been described with disorders such as chronic regurgitation and reflux gastroesophagitis. This may rarely result in a condition referred to as 'Barrett's esophagus' where chronic inflammation induces intestinal metaplasia and development of columnar epithelium in the esophagus. Full characterization of this disorder is reliant on endoscopic imaging and biopsy (Sellon & Willard, 2003).

Inflammatory lesions

As animals frequently ingest coarse materials, damage to the esophagus occasionally occurs and can result in signs of dysphagia, coughing, retching, hemoptysis, repeated swallowing, and occasionally

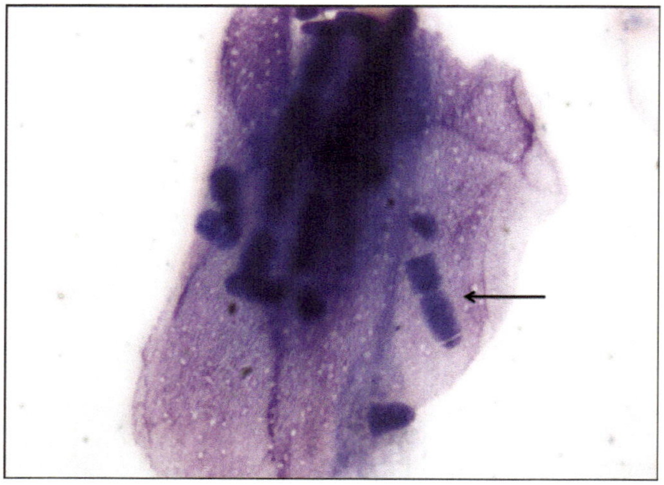

Figure 7.7 Mixed bacteria consistent with oral flora. Note the presence of large bacterial rods consistent with *Conchiformibius* (previously *Simonsiella*) spp. overlying a squamous epithelial cell (arrow) (Wright-Giemsa, 1,000× magnification).

ptyalism. In more chronic lesions, such as those caused by foreign bodies or esophageal parasites, anorexia and weight loss may be evident (Sellon & Willard, 2003). Inflammation is variable depending on the underlying disease. Esophageal infections may occur and are usually secondary to trauma. It is important to recognize the presence of normal oropharyngeal flora when interpreting the presence of bacteria in an upper GIT sample (Figure 7.7).

There are few infectious organisms that localize to the esophagus. The esophageal worm *Spirocerca lupi* is a nematode found in tropical and subtropical regions including the southeastern region of the United States. Infection follows ingestion of an intermediate host (coprophagous beetle). Larvae follow a specific migratory route, penetrating the gastric mucosa of the host, migrating along arteries, maturing in the thoracic aorta before eventually moving to the caudal esophagus. In the esophagus, the worm develops in large nodules (Figures 7.8a, b) and passes larvated eggs in feces that can be detected using zinc sulfate fecal flotation. Chronic lesions have been associated with the development of sarcomas in up to 25% of infected dogs (Porras-Silesky *et al.*, 2021).

Neoplastic lesions of the GIT are typically associated with clinical signs based on their localization. In the esophagus, masses may result in dysphagia, ptyalism, regurgitation, anorexia, and progressive weight loss.

Neoplasms of the esophagus

Epithelial tumors

Benign epithelial tumors of the alimentary tract are generally uncommon in small animals (Willard, 2012; Munday *et al.*, 2017). Few cases of primary esophageal carcinomas, most commonly squamous cell carcinoma (SCC), have been described in dogs and cats (Munday *et al.*, 2017). Prognosis in these lesions is guarded due to the difficulty in adequate removal and the metastatic tendency (Willard, 2012). Locally invasive tumors such as thyroid carcinomas or oral SCCs may invade into the esophagus. These are identified based on their similarity to cytologic appearance in other sites.

Stromal/spindle cell tumors

Stromal tumors of the esophagus are infrequently reported in dogs. Smooth muscle tumors, leiomyomas, and leiomyosarcomas have been reported in the esophagus (Frost *et al.*, 2003). These are usually nodular masses situated at the gastroesophageal junction in older animals (Munday *et al.*, 2017). Sarcomas, including fibrosarcomas and osteosarcomas, can develop secondary to infection with *Spirocerca lupi* (Porras-Silesky *et al.*, 2021).

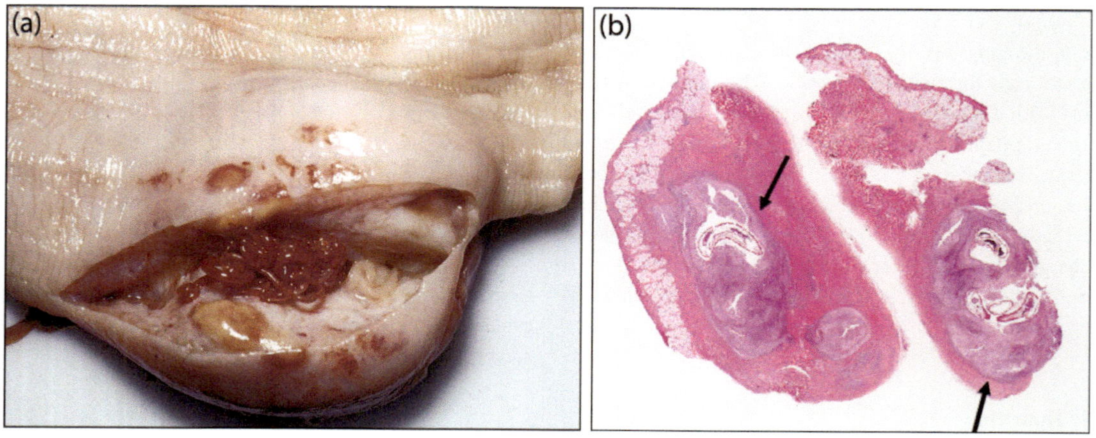

Figures 7.8a, b (a) Gross image of *Spirocerca lupi* infection in a dog. In the caudal esophagus, the worm develops in nodules and passes larvated eggs in feces, which can be detected via fecal flotation. (b) Histologic image of *Spirocerca* infection in the same dog. Note the marked inflammatory infiltrate surrounding the larva (cross-section) (arrows) (H&E, 20× magnification) (courtesy Roger J. Panciera).

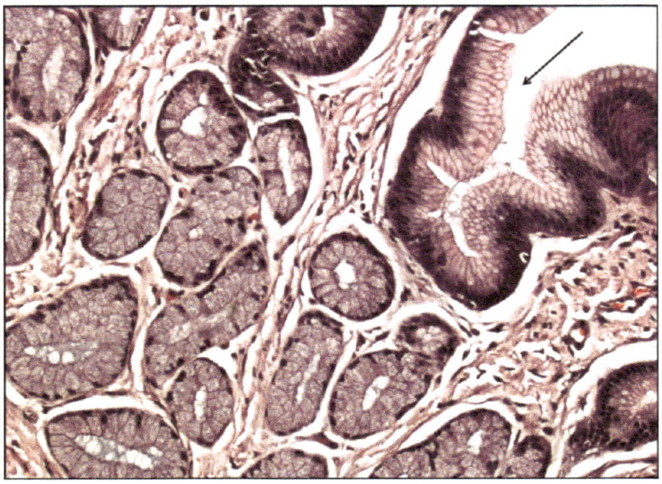

Figure 7.9 **Histology section of normal canine gastric epithelium. Note the presence of mucin-containing columnar epithelial cells. Fundic glands, present in cross-section, contain chief cells and parietal cells (H&E, 200× magnification).**

STOMACH

Normal

The mucosal layer in dogs and cats is comprised of glandular epithelial cells, which typically exfoliate well, particularly with impression smears from biopsy samples (Figure 7.9). In the fundus of the stomach, two populations of epithelial cells are present: the parietal cells and the chief cells. On cytology, mucosal epithelial cells are usually found in dense aggregates of uniform columnar cells with round nuclei and moderate amounts of basophilic cytoplasm. They often contain apical mucin-containing vacuoles (Figures 7.10a–c).

Hyperplastic lesions

As in other locations, hyperplastic lesions of the stomach are usually presumptively based on diagnostic imaging and the identification of uniform populations of epithelial cells. Mucin production may be increased in some regions and is generally identified as eosinophilic globular material and often found extracellularly. Cytologic samples may appear unremarkable or may be confounded by inflammation; therefore, definitive diagnosis usually requires additional histopathology and investigation for an underlying disorder.

Inflammatory lesions

Infectious gastritis

Helicobacter-associated gastroenteritis has been described in dogs and cats (Neiger & Simpson, 2000; Sapierzyńiski *et al.*, 2006; Jergens *et al.*, 2009). Most research is focused on the incidence of *Helicobacter pylori*, which is uncommonly identified in the stomach of dogs and cats, although when present it may be associated with more severe clinical signs than infection with other *Helicobacter* spp. (Neiger Simpson, 2000). The pathogenic role of *Helicobacter* in dogs and cats is not clear (Rossi *et al.*, 2008; Taillieu *et al.*, 2022). Signs of gastritis can include vomiting, abdominal pain, and inappetence (Sapierzyńiski *et al.*, 2006). Changes to the epithelial mucosa include fibrosis in the lamina propria, degenerative changes in the gastric glands, and hyperplasia of the parietal cells and lymphoid follicles. Cytologically, *Helicobacter* spp. are identified as spiral-shaped bacterial organisms in gastric samples (Figure 7.11). Evidence of associated inflammation and hyperplasia may be present on impression smears from the gastric mucosa. Organisms are small (approximately 2–4 μm); thus special staining is often necessary to fully identify their presence in tissue sections (Figures 7.12a, b). Speciation requires culture, polymerase chain reaction (PCR) or fluorescence *in situ* hybridization of biopsy specimens (Jergens *et al.*, 2009). Urea breath and blood tests or serology can be used to diagnose *Helicobacter* spp. noninvasively but as with other bacterial organisms, presence does not always correlate with signs of disease.

Gastric neoplasms

Epithelial tumors

Epithelial neoplasms of the stomach are uncommon in companion animals and are nearly always malignant. Rare cases of benign adenomas and hyperplastic polyps have been reported in dogs and cats, with

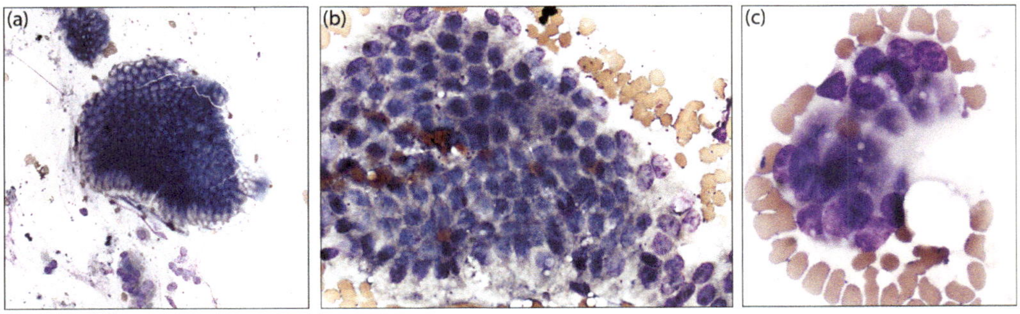

Figures 7.10a–c **Normal stomach cytology, canine. (a) Cohesive aggregates of columnar epithelial cells form well-delineated sheets. The cytoplasm is deeply basophilic and often appears vacuolated due to mucin production. (b) Eosinophilic mucin granules are frequently present in aspirates. (c) Small cluster of cells showing normal columnar shape (Wright–Giemsa: a, 200× magnification; b, 500× magnification; and c, 800× magnification).**

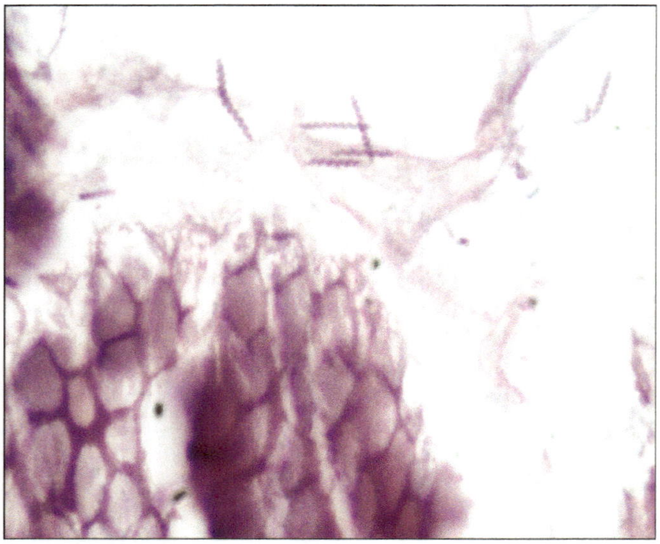

Figure 7.11 Stomach, canine. Tissue section from a gastric biopsy acquired endoscopically. Spiral-shaped bacteria consistent with *Helicobacter* spp. are present (H&E, 500× magnification).

brachycephalic breeds being overrepresented in some canine studies (Gualtieri *et al.*, 1999; Kuan *et al.*, 2009; Kehl *et al.*, 2022). Signalment is typically a young dog with a history of vomiting or regurgitation and weight loss consistent with a pyloric outflow obstruction. Similar to hyperplastic lesions, these usually appear cytologically as normal epithelium, and definitive diagnosis requires histopathology.

Malignant epithelial tumors, carcinomas and adenocarcinomas, uncommonly occur in the stomach of dogs and cats (Gualtieri *et al.*, 1999; Bonfanti *et al.*, 2006; von Babo *et al.*, 2012; Willard, 2012; Munday *et al.*, 2017). In humans, social and environmental factors, such as chronic infection with *Helicobacter* spp., have been associated with the development of gastric carcinoma. In dogs and cats, the etiology of this neoplasm is not known; however, a hereditary component is reported. Increased incidence of gastric carcinomas is described in specific canine breeds including Chow chows, Belgian shepherd dogs, Bouvier des Flandres, Collies, Standard poodles, and Dutch Tervuren shepherds (Lubbes *et al.*, 2009; Willard, 2012; Seim-Wikse *et al.*, 2013; Koterbay *et al.*, 2020). Similarly, a breed predisposition has been proposed for Persian and Siamese cats (Dennis *et al.*, 2006).

The most successful results for cytologic interpretation appear to be obtained by impression smears from biopsy specimens (Bonfanti *et al.*, 2006); however, FNA is usually successful in carcinomas due to the generally good exfoliation of tumor cells (Figure 7.13). An epithelial origin is usually apparent due to cohesion between cells, which may otherwise bear little resemblance to normal gastric epithelium (Figure 7.10). Further description of the cytologic features of these tumors can be found below in the intestinal sections.

Stromal/spindle cell tumors

Spindle cell tumors in the stomach are uncommon. Cytologically and histologically, these appear very similar; therefore most were historically, and often erroneously, diagnosed as smooth muscle tumors (leiomyomas and leiomyosarcomas). However, the utilization of immunohistochemical techniques to further classify these lesions has shown that many of these tumors are, in fact, gastrointestinal stromal tumors (GISTs), requiring reclassification of many of those masses (Maas *et al.*, 2007). Several studies have shown distinct localization and prognostic differences between these neoplasms and, therefore, further differentiation by use of specific markers including KIT (tyrosine kinase receptor), smooth muscle actin (SMA), and desmin (a myocellular cytoskeletal element) is often recommended.

In general, spindle cell tumors are usually diagnosed as smooth muscle origin (both leiomyosarcoma and leiomyoma) in the stomach in dogs (Frost *et al.*, 2003; Russell *et al.*, 2007; Gillespie *et al.*, 2011; Hayes *et al.*, 2013). GISTs have uncommonly been identified in the stomach of dogs (Frost *et al.*, 2003; Russell *et al.*, 2007). Rare cases of GIST are reported in the stomach of cats (Morini *et al.*, 2011). Other sarcomas such as osteosarcoma, histiocytic sarcoma, hemangiosarcoma, and undifferentiated sarcoma have rarely been described in the stomachs of dogs and cats. These latter tumors are typically metastases from primary sites and immunohistochemical staining is usually

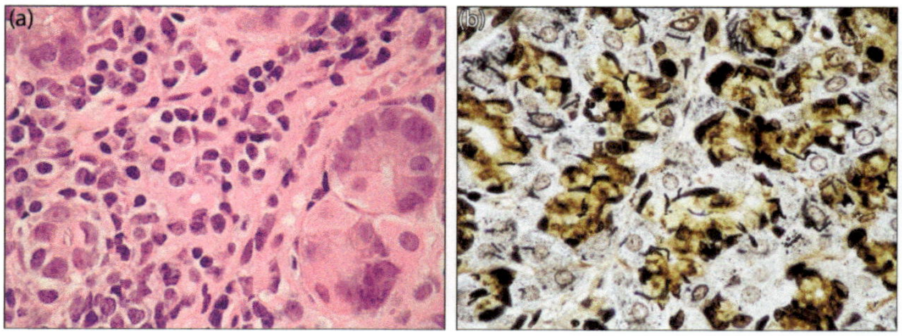

Figures 7.12a,b (a) Severe lymphoplasmacytic inflammation is present (H&E, 1,000× magnification). (b) Warthin-Starry silver stain highlights spirochetes (*Helicobacter* spp.) in the lamina propria (1,000× magnification) (7.12a courtesy Al Jergens; 7.12b from Jergens AE, Pressel M, Crandell J *et al.* (2009). Fluorescence in-situ hybridization confirms clearance of visible *Helicobacter* spp. associated with gastritis in dogs and cats. *J Vet Intern Med* 23(1):16–23. Reprinted with permission.)

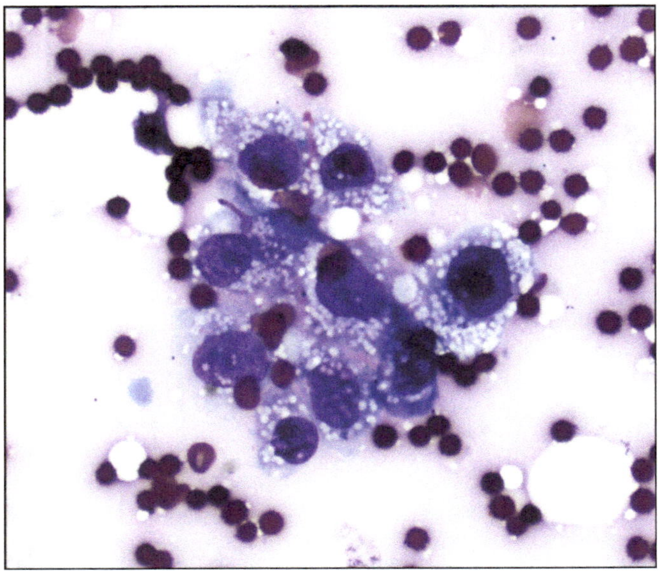

Figure 7.13 Cytology of an FNA of a gastric carcinoma from a cat. A small cohesive cluster of neoplastic epithelial cells displaying criteria for malignancy is present (Wright–Giemsa, 500× magnification).

necessary for full characterization of these tumor types (Patnaik, 1990; LaRock Ginn, 1997; Cruz-Arámbulo *et al.*, 2004; Bonfanti *et al.*, 2006; Shor *et al.*, 2009).

Identification of stromal/spindle cell tumors in the stomach can be accomplished by cytology, although studies report limited sensitivity with aspiration alone. Alternatively, impression smears have been shown to increase detection from approximately 44% to 100% (Bonfanti, 2006). Therefore, due to a tendency for poor exfoliation of stromal tumors, negative or equivocal results post-aspiration appear to be relatively common. A more detailed description of the cytologic appearance of these tumors can be found below in the intestinal sections.

Round cell tumors

Lymphoma

In cats, lymphoma is the most common neoplasm of the GIT including the stomach (Bonfanti *et al.*, 2006; Willard, 2012). Although lymphoma is also found in the canine GIT, gastric localization of lymphoma in dogs is infrequently described (Bonfanti *et al.*, 2006; Frank *et al.*, 2007).

The cause of gastric lymphoma is unknown; however, recent data suggest an association of alimentary lymphoma with infectious diseases such as *Helicobacter* spp. (Bridgeford *et al.*, 2008). Although feline leukemia virus (FeLV) infection has been associated with other forms of lymphoma, it has not been consistently linked to the development of the alimentary form in cats (Louwerens *et al.*, 2005; Krick *et al.*, 2008; Lingard *et al.*, 2009; Freiche *et al.*, 2021). A breed predilection in cats may exist as Siamese cats are overrepresented in some studies of feline lymphoma, including primary gastric tumors

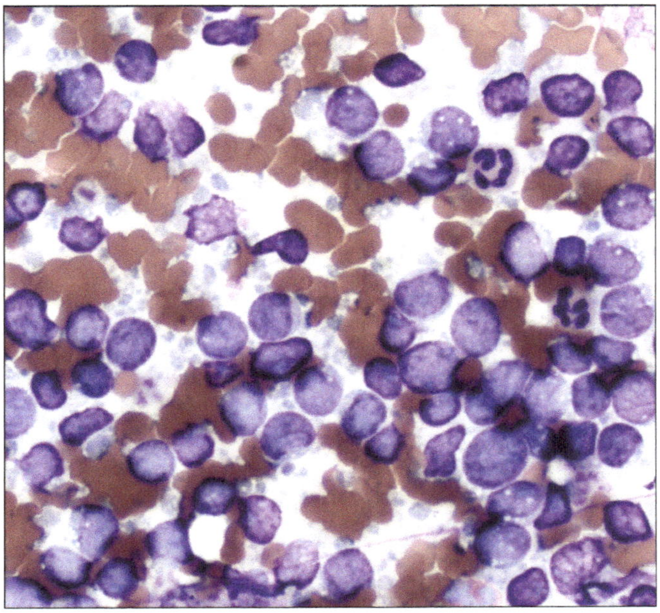

Figure 7.14 Feline, gastric mass. Large lymphocytes typically found in the gastric form of lymphoma. Small, discrete cytoplasmic vacuoles are commonly seen in feline large-cell lymphomas (Wright–Giemsa, 500× magnification).

(Bonfanti *et al.*, 2006; Rissetto *et al.*, 2011). Breed associations occur in dogs as well, although these are most typically noted in intestinal disease as primary gastric lymphoma appears rare in dogs.

FNA and cytology have been shown to be excellent for definitively diagnosing lymphoma in dogs and cats (Bonfanti *et al.*, 2006; Maeda *et al.*, 2017). Primary gastric lymphoma is typically comprised of a homogeneous population of large round lymphoid cells (Figures 7.14 and 7.15). Cells are often fragile and tumor cell rupture is common. Immunophenotyping of lymphoma has proven useful in predicting behavior in this tumor in most species. Although different morphologic variants of lymphoma are described in both dogs and cats, gastric lymphomas in cats are most likely to be of large B-cell (also called 'lymphoblastic') type (Figure 7.14) and typically are associated with aggressive behavior (Vezzali *et al.*, 2010; Moore *et al.*, 2012; Willard, 2012). More discussion on the features and diagnosis of lymphoma is provided in the following section under small intestinal lymphoma.

Mast cell neoplasia

Mast cell tumors may occur in the stomach of cats but are more common in the intestines in this species. In dogs, GI mast cell neoplasia, including gastric tumors, are only rarely described (Ozaki *et al.*, 2002) and usually associated with multifocal masses. Cytologically, they may appear similar to mast cells in other locations but can be variable in appearance. These are discussed more fully in the following section under small intestinal round cell tumors.

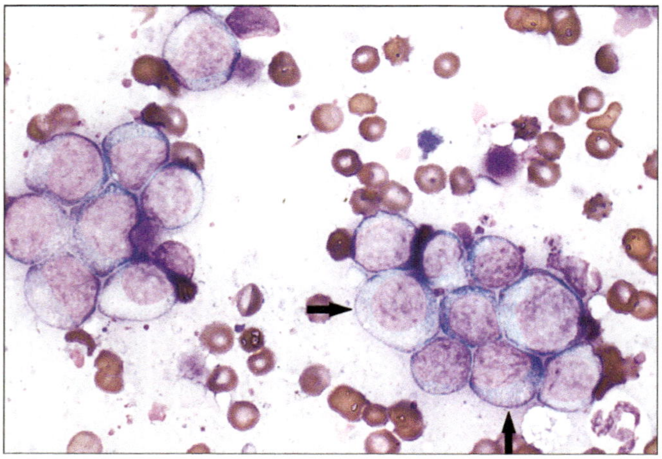

Figure 7.15 Canine, gastric mass. Large, atypical lymphocytes with increased amounts of cytoplasm are found in this patient's tumor. Small, fine eosinophilic granules (arrows) are identified in several cells characteristic of granular lymphoma, likely of cytotoxic T-cell (CD3+/CD8+) phenotype (Wright–Giemsa, 1,000× magnification).

SMALL INTESTINE (DUODENUM, JEJUNUM, AND ILEUM)

Normal

The epithelial layer is comprised of tall simple columnar epithelial cells with microvilli that function in absorption of nutrients (Figures 7.16a–c). Goblet cells are present and may be visualized in histologic and, occasionally, cytologic preparations. The lamina propria layer contains lymphoid cells along with occasional globular leukocytes and Paneth cells, which participate in primary defense. Therefore, few lymphocytes and mononuclear cells may be present when sampling the intestine.

Hyperplastic lesions

In hyperplastic lesions of the intestine, diagnosis is usually presumptive and based on clinical history, diagnostic imaging, and identification of uniform populations of epithelial cells. Some cellular atypia may be present due to associated lesions such as inflammation, including chronic enteropathy (CE), or underlying neoplasia (Figure 7.17). Lymphoid follicular hyperplasia is also common and may occur secondary to infectious disease. Lymphoid hyperplasia of mucosal lymphoid tissue may even form mass-like lesions and thus be mistaken for lymphoma or CE (Figure 7.18). Therefore, similar to hyperplastic lesions of the stomach, intestinal hyperplasia is not a cytologic diagnosis and usually requires additional histopathology and investigation for an underlying disorder.

Inflammatory lesions

In most inflammatory disorders of the GIT, diagnosis is a multistep process and typically includes additional diagnostics including fecal analysis, PCR or other assays for underlying infectious organisms, and, usually, tissue biopsy.

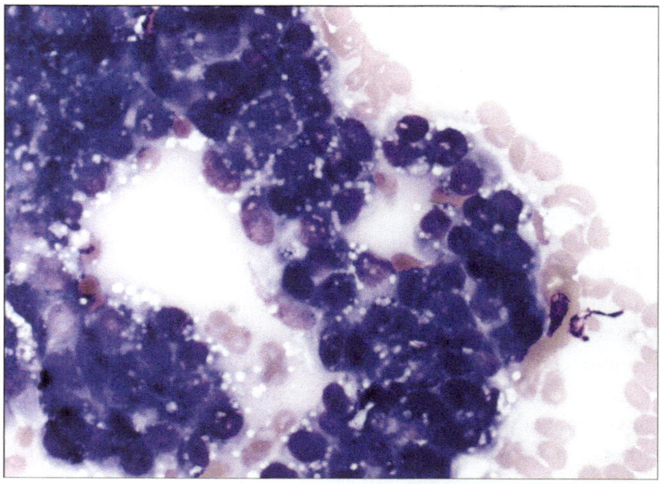

Figure 7.17 Small intestine, canine. Cytology of an FNA of intestinal epithelium overlying a sarcoma (same dog as in Figure 7.37). Note the epithelial cells display moderate atypia including basophilia and more prominent nucleoli but are still generally uniform in shape and size. These changes were interpreted as dysplastic based on additional findings (Wright–Giemsa, 500× magnification).

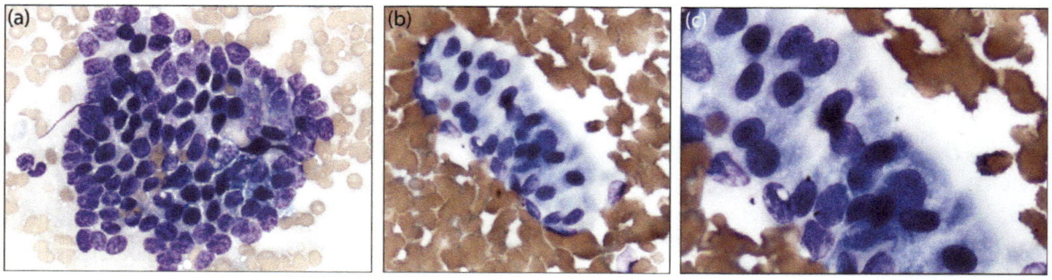

Figures 7.16a–c Normal small intestinal cytology, canine. (a) Duodenum; 500× magnification. (b) Jejunum; a row of uniform columnar epithelial cells with fine cilia; 500× magnification. (c) Jejunum; 1,000× magnification (Wright–Giemsa).

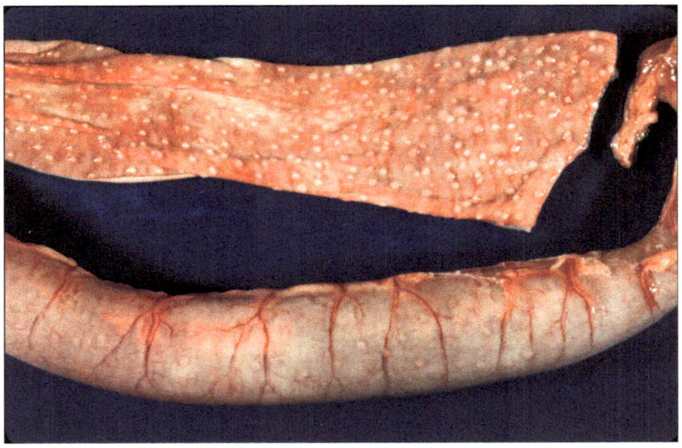

Figure 7.18 **Gross image showing marked lymphoid hyperplasia in the intestine of a dog. (Courtesy Barry Cooper.)**

Foreign body reactions

Like foreign bodies at other sites, intestinal foreign bodies are usually diagnosed by a history of exposure or noted ingestion of an object along with diagnostic imaging. Cytology is usually only performed in lesions where no known history of foreign object ingestion is present and/or imaging is equivocal for an obstruction. Cytology may show the presence of chronic, usually pyogranulomatous, inflammation or may be unrewarding if significant fibrosis is present. Bacteria and clinical evidence of sepsis may be present.

Chronic enteropathy/chronic inflammatory enteropathy

Chronic enteropathies (CE) are a spectrum of disorders with three current categories recognized based upon response to treatment: immunosuppressive- (steroid) responsive (also called idiopathic inflammatory bowel disease), food-responsive, and antibiotic-responsive enteropathy (Dandrieux & Mansfield, 2019). The pathogenesis of these disorders is complex and likely involves immune system dysregulation, environmental factors, and genetic predisposition (Jergens & Heilmann, 2022).

Idiopathic, immunosuppressive-responsive CE is an immune-mediated disease process characterized by infiltration of inflammatory cells into the lamina propria layer (see Figure 7.3) of the intestine. The pathogenesis of the disease is proposed to involve a loss of immunologic tolerance to normal antigens causing abnormal T-cell immune reactivity in the gut leading to chronic inflammation and injury (Cave, 2003). Inherited disorders are identified in numerous dog breeds including immunoproliferative enteropathy of Basenjis, familial protein-losing enteropathy and nephropathy in Soft-Coated Wheaten Terriers, and eosinophilic enteritis and granulomas in Siberian Huskies (German *et al.*, 2003). In cats, heritable gastroenteropathies are questionable, although some studies have shown increased incidence in purebred cats (Dennis *et al.*, 1992; Jergens *et al.*, 1992).

Food responsive CE in dogs and cats is evidenced by positive results of elimination diets (Guilford *et al.*, 2001; Makielski *et al.*, 2019). Affected dogs tend to be younger and may have less severe clinical signs than with other causes for CE (Jergens & Heilmann, 2022). Familial causes for these disorders include gluten-sensitive enteropathy in Irish Setters.

Antibiotic-responsive diarrhea (ARD; previously called small intestinal bacterial overgrowth) results in chronic GI signs in dogs. Idiopathic ARD has not been definitively identified in cats, although mild chronic enteropathy in cats may be controlled with antibiotic therapy alone. It is a diagnosis of exclusion where no underlying cause can be found but which is completely responsive to antibiotic treatment. However, this condition is currently debated as, despite initial response to antimicrobials, most patients will relapse post-discontinuation of treatment (Jergens & Heilmann, 2022). Additionally, overuse of antibiotics may also allow for disruption of normal enteric microbiota resulting in overgrowth of normal commensal organisms and resultant dysbiosis (Suchodolski, 2022). Affected dogs are typically young, large breeds, with German Shepherd dogs being overrepresented in many studies (Hall, 2011; Dandrieux & Mansfield, 2019). Clinical signs are typically due to chronic or recurrent small bowel diarrhea, although some dogs show signs of colitis. Microscopic evaluation of fecal samples from affected animals usually shows a mixed population of commensal bacteria although indication of changes in the normal microbiota (AKA dysbiosis) may be noted cytologically by apparent overgrowth of a particular population. Culture of fecal bacteria does not always correlate with bacterial numbers or species in the intestines, nor does culture indicate if bacterial toxins are produced (Weese, 2011; Suchodolski, 2022). Culture has therefore been largely replaced by molecular methods for organism detection. However, lack of standardization and variability in methodology between labs can make interpretation of results difficult (Suchodolski, 2022).

Lymphoplasmacytic gastroenteritis

Regardless of the underlying cause, lymphoplasmacytic gastroenteritis (LPE) is the most common histopathologic finding for CE in both dogs and cats (Jergens, 1999; German *et al.*, 2001; Maeda *et al.*, 2017; Makielski *et al.*, 2019). In LPE, the distribution of disease is primarily diffusely mucosal, with the lamina propria most severely affected. T cells predominate, but variable numbers of B cells, including plasma cells, can be identified (Figures 7.19a, b). Thus, CE is definitively diagnosed by histologic characterization, and full-thickness biopsy specimens are recommended to rule out underlying disorders causing secondary inflammation (Kleinschmidt *et al.*, 2009; Freiche *et al.*, 2021). However, infiltrates of inflammatory cells can be identified cytologically by aspiration of thickened mucosa or discrete lesions (Figure 7.20a, b). More severe forms may lead to ulceration and mixed inflammatory infiltrates, and multifocal disease is common. A concern exists that more severe lesions may progress to neoplasia. Indeed, lymphoma has been documented in both dogs and cats with a history of LPE (Jacobs *et al.*, 1990; Hart *et al.*, 1994; Roccabianca *et al.*, 2006; Lingard *et al.*, 2009). Furthermore, differentiating between a diagnosis of severe lymphoplasmacytic inflammation and low-grade, small-cell lymphoma is often difficult; therefore, a multistep approach incorporating histology, immunochemistry, and PCR analysis for

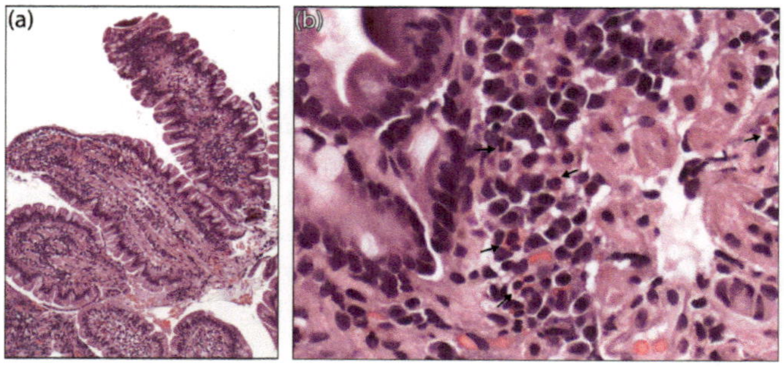

Figures 7.19a,b Small intestine, canine. Histologic section from a dog diagnosed with lymphoplasmacytic enteritis. (a) Note the marked expansion of lymphocytes in the lamina propria layer of the intestinal villi (H&E, 100× magnification). (b) At higher magnification, plasma cells, lymphocytes, and eosinophils (arrows) are more readily seen (H&E, 500× magnification).

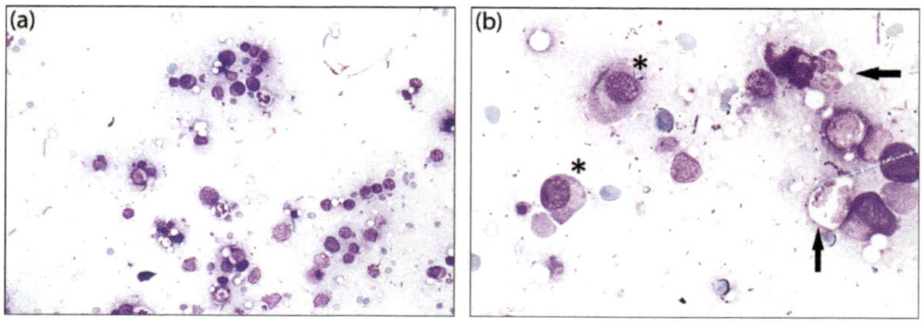

Figures 7.20a,b Intestine, feline. Aspirate from a thickened portion of ileum in a cat with lymphoplasmacytic gastroenteritis. (a) Mixed inflammation is present. Few erythrocytes and mixed bacteria are also present among eosinophilic proteinaceous background material (Wright–Giemsa, 400× magnification). (b) Small lymphocytes and numerous plasma cells (asterisks) and occasional neutrophils (arrows) are identified at higher magnification (Wright–Giemsa, 1000× magnification).

antigen receptor rearrangement (PARR) is usually recommended to aid histologic diagnosis of both entities (Kiupel *et al.*, 2011) (Figure 7.21).

Eosinophilic gastroenteritis

Eosinophilic inflammation can be seen with some underlying infectious causes (e.g. pythiosis and parasites described below) and as a paraneoplastic infiltrate secondary to neoplasia (see discussion under lymphoma below). However, primary idiopathic eosinophilic disease remains relatively uncommon in both dogs and cats. In cats, the disorder is poorly characterized. It may be associated with hypereosinophilic syndrome or food allergies, but often only mild increases in eosinophils are identified in the GIT of cats, even with food-responsive enteropathy (Guilford *et al.*, 2001) (Figures 7.22a, b, 7.23). When present, however, clinical signs are often more severe, clinicopathologic and histopathologic changes are more evident, and peritonitis may even be present (Figure 7.24) (Tucker *et al.*, 2014). A unique condition, 'feline gastrointestinal eosinophilic sclerosing fibroplasia', is described (Craig *et al.*, 2009; Weissman *et al.*, 2013; Linton *et al.*, 2015). Affected cats typically develop a focal, ulcerated intramural mass at the pyloric sphincter, ileocecocolic junction, or colon. Lesions

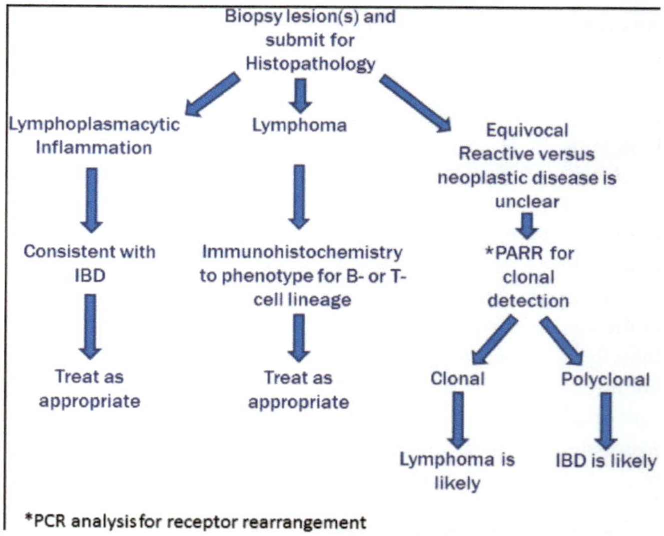

Figure 7.21 Diagnostic approach for lymphoproliferative disease in the gastrointestinal tract. Adapted from Kiupel M, Smedley RC, Pfent C *et al.* (2011) Diagnostic algorithm to differentiate lymphoma from inflammation in feline small intestinal biopsy samples. *Vet Pathol* 48(1):212–222.

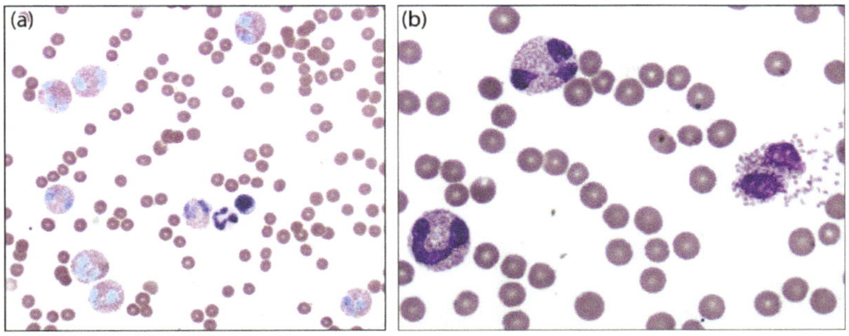

Figures 7.22a, b Jejunum, feline. Aspirate of a thickened region of intestine. Marked eosinophil infiltration is present (Wright–Giemsa: a, 500× magnification; b, 1,000× magnification).

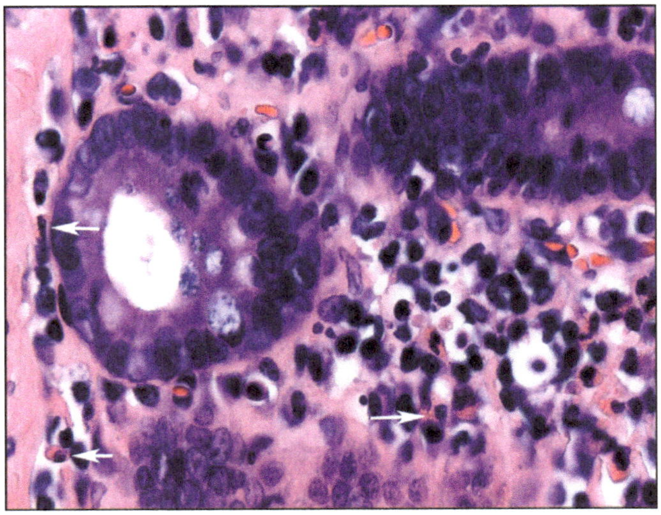

Figure 7.23 Histologic section from a cat with eosinophilic enteritis. Eosinophils are indicated by the arrows (H&E, 1,000× magnification).

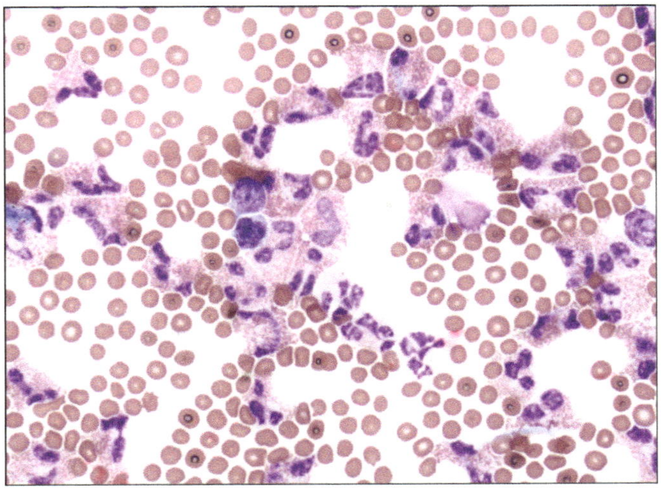

Figure 7.24 Peritoneal fluid, feline. Mixed inflammatory cells predominated by eosinophils are found in the abdominal effusion from a cat diagnosed with eosinophilic gastroenteritis (Wright–Giemsa, 700× magnification).

are characterized by eosinophilic inflammation and fibrosis and cats may also have eosinophilic lymphadenitis and peripheral eosinophilia. Lesions are often associated with microabscesses and bacterial infection. On histopathology, mast cells are also seen but this is not consistently reported in cytologic specimens (Linton *et al.*, 2015). Furthermore, aspiration of these lesions may be unrewarding due to fibrosis. The cause of this disorder is unknown.

In dogs, breed-associated eosinophilic disease has been described in the Rottweiler and Cavalier King Charles Spaniel (German *et al.*, 2002; Lyles *et al.*, 2009). This disorder may be associated with granulomas in the esophagus, stomach, and small and large intestines (see Figure 7.52). The pathogenesis of these lesions is unknown, but several pathogenic mechanisms are speculated, including parasitic and allergic reactions (Johnson, 1992; Lyles *et al.*, 2009).

Infectious causes of enteritis

Like primary gastric infections, small intestinal bacterial infections are relatively uncommon in dogs and cats. *Mycobacterium* spp. are well-known pathogens that typically result in systemic disease. Both classic tuberculosis (including *M. tuberculosis*, *M. bovis*, and *M. microti*) and opportunistic mycobacteriosis (including *M. fortuitum*) have been described in dogs and cats, although clinical disease is inconsistently reported in these species (Kukanich *et al.*, 2013; Pesciaroli *et al.*, 2014). In animals infected with *M. avium* subspecies *paratuberculosis* (MAP), chronic enteritis and colitis are common clinical signs. However, MAP-specific DNA can be identified within the intestinal and nodal tissue of dogs and cats that do not have pathologic lesions or clinical signs of GI disease (Glanemann *et al.*, 2008; Kukanich *et al.*, 2013). In clinically affected animals, infection with MAP typically induces granulomatous inflammatory infiltrates with variable degrees of lymphocytic and/or suppurative inflammation. The organism can usually be identified as nonstaining linear structures both in macrophages and extracellularly on Romanowsky-stained slides (Figures 7.25a–c). The organisms can further be visualized with the use of an acid-fast stain (Figure 7.25d). PCR for MAP DNA is necessary for speciation of the organism (Glanemann *et al.*, 2008).

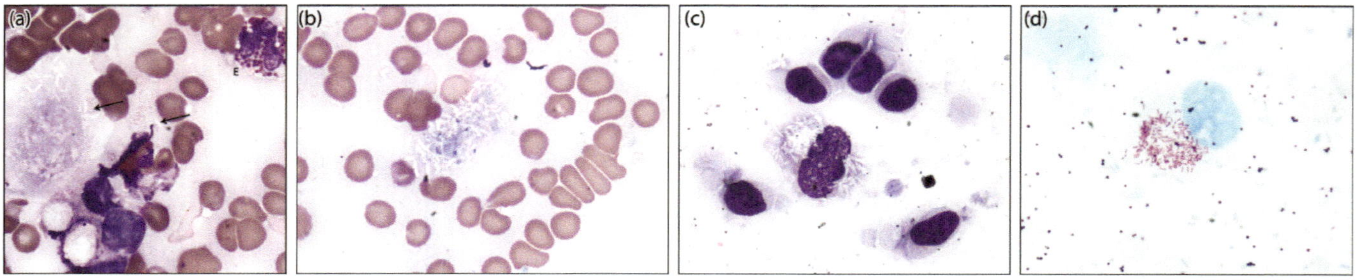

Figures 7.25a–d FNA from a region of intestinal thickening in a dog. (a, b) A mixed inflammatory infiltrate is present with numerous negative-staining linear structures (arrows) consistent with Mycobacterium spp. found in the macrophages (a) and throughout the background of the sample (b) (Wright–Giemsa, 1,000× magnification). (c) Same patient with organisms identified in an associated abdominal lymph node (Wright–Giemsa, 1,000× magnification). (d) Organisms stain red with an acid-fast stain (Ziehl–Neelsen, 2,000× magnification).

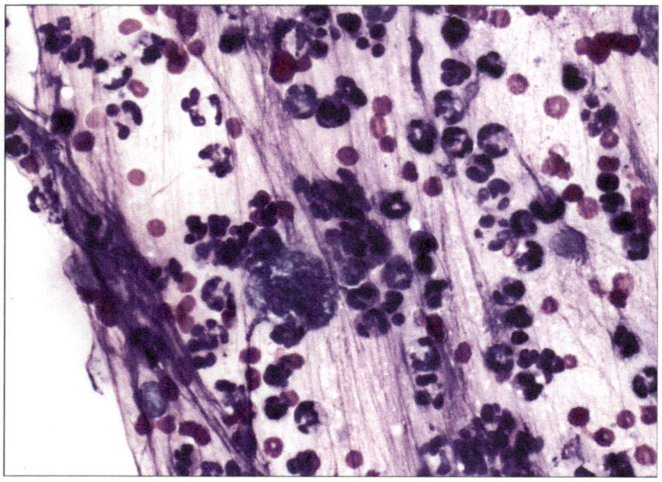

Figure 7.26 FNA from a mass in the intestine of a cat with feline infectious peritonitis (FIP) (confirmed post-mortem). Large numbers of nondegenerative neutrophils and occasional macrophages are found among thick fibrillar, eosinophilic, proteinaceous background material. The presence of granulomatous or pyogranulomatous inflammation without visible infectious organisms may be noted in lesions associated with FIP (Wright–Giemsa, 500× magnification).

Viral gastroenteritis

Numerous viral organisms are implicated in the development of gastroenteritis in dogs and cats. These include viruses that cause direct mucosal injury (e.g. parvovirus and coronavirus), as well as organisms that cause enteric signs secondary to immunosuppression (e.g. FIV) from T-cell infiltration and/or disruption of normal regulatory cell populations (Hartmann, 2011). Although histology of GIT biopsies may be diagnostic for some viral infections, cytology is rarely useful and antemortem diagnoses are usually reliant on viral ELISAs, serology, and PCR. An exception may be lesions induced by feline infectious peritonitis, where aspiration of large granulomas or infiltrated tissues (e.g. kidney or liver) may be useful in supporting a diagnosis in clinically affected cats (Figure 7.26) (Giordano *et al.*, 2005).

Fungal gastroenteritis

Fungal infections of the GIT are generally less common than bacterial or viral infections. A few dimorphic fungi may colonize the GIT in specific environmental regions. *Histoplasma capsulatum*, for example, is commonly associated with chronic enteritis and colitis in infected individuals (Brömel & Sykes, 2005). *Histoplasma* spp. are small, 2–4-µm diameter yeasts with a central body surrounded by a thin clear capsule. Organisms may be identified via impression smears or aspiration of masses and/or associated lymph nodes (Figures 7.27a, b). Impression smears from endoscopic or full-thickness biopsies are also diagnostic for identifying organisms in infected tissues (Figures 7.28a–c).

Occasionally, infection by environmental fungi or overgrowth of commensal species may develop in individuals with compromised GI health. Some studies analyzing the small intestinal content from healthy and diseased dogs from different geographic locations have detected a high prevalence and diversity of fungal DNA in both healthy dogs and dogs with chronic enteropathies. In cases of fungal-associated disease, the organisms are highly antigenic and typically result in marked granulomatous and pyogranulomatous

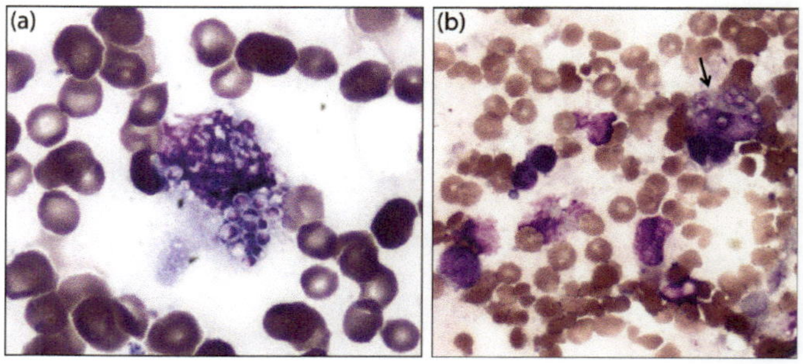

Figures 7.27a, b FNA of a region of thickened intestine from a dog with chronic diarrhea and weight loss. (a) Numerous small yeast organisms are identified in a degenerating macrophage. The yeasts are consistent with *Histoplasma capsulatum*. (Wright–Giemsa, 1,000× magnification). (b) Organisms (arrow) are also identified in an adjacent abdominal lymph node. (Wright–Giemsa, 500× magnification).

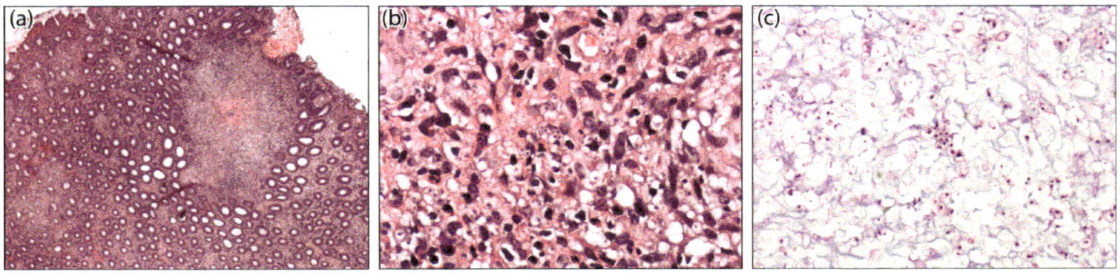

Figures 7.28a–c Histologic section from the intestine from the same dog as in Figure 7.27. (a) The intestinal mucosa is thickened by infiltrating macrophages with lesser numbers of neutrophils and a large granuloma (H&E, 100× magnification). (b) Severe granulomatous to pyogranulomatous inflammation is present secondary to large numbers of intralesional yeast identified as *Histoplasma capsulatum* (H&E, 700× magnification). (c) Periodic acid–Schiff stain assists identification of small intralesional yeast (700× magnification).

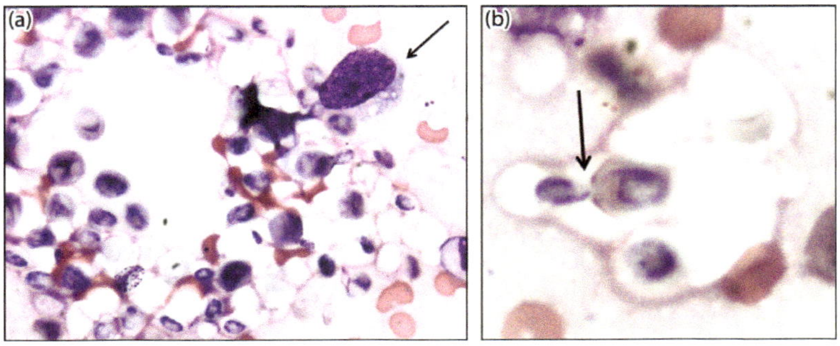

Figures 7.29a,b FNA from an intestinal mass in a cat diagnosed with cryptococcosis. (a) Extracellular round yeast organisms (approx. 5–15 in diameter) surrounded by variably thick clear-staining capsules are present along with a single macrophage (arrow). (b) Organism showing characteristic narrow-based budding (arrow) typical of Cryptococcus spp. (Wright–Giemsa, 1,000× magnification).

inflammatory infiltrates. Eosinophils may also be noted in some patients. Depending on the infection, spores, yeast, or hyphae may be identified in fecal smears, often surrounded by degenerating cellular constituents. Evidence of associated bacterial overgrowth may also be noted.

Candida, *Cryptococcus*, and *Aspergillus* spp. have all been reported to cause GI disease in animals (Schultz *et al.*, 2008; Suchodolski *et al.*, 2008; Uchiumi *et al.*, 2014; Johnston *et al.*, 2021). *Cryptococcus* spp. is ubiquitous and can result in disseminated disease in animals. It is found as large budding yeast surrounded by a thick nonstaining capsule (Figures 7.29a, b). As seen with other fungal infections, inflammation is usually granulomatous to pyogranulomatous in nature.

In human and veterinary medicine, the role of *Candida* spp. in antibiotic-associated diarrhea is controversial. Since *Candida* spp. exist physiologically in the GIT, the presence of small numbers of these organisms in stool is considered normal and, therefore, nonpathogenic. Individuals at risk for serious disseminated disease are more likely to be immunosuppressed, such as patients with cancer or secondary to GI perforation (Bradford *et al.*, 2013). In tissue samples, *Candida* spp. are recognized as small, oval to elongated, segmentally constricted pseudohyphae with occasional buds (Figures 7.30a–c).

Like candidiasis, disseminated aspergillosis has been linked to immunosuppression. The German Shepherd dog is overrepresented in most studies, which may be attributed to dysfunction of normal mucosal immunity in this breed (Schultz *et al.*, 2008; Olsson *et al.*, 2014). Organisms are found as septate and branching hyphae in infected tissue and, like other fungal infections, are associated with marked inflammation and cellular degeneration (Figure 7.31). Therefore, in most cases of fungal-associated gastroenteritis, evidence of systemic illness and chronic debilitation is usually present.

'Pseudofungi'

Algae and oomycetes such as *Prototheca*, *Pythium*, and *Lagenidium* spp. are often referred to as 'pseudofungi' based on their morphologic appearance and tendency to induce marked pyogranulomatous inflammatory infiltrates.

Protothecosis in animals is due to infection with a unicellular achlorophyllic algal organism (Masuda *et al.*, 2021). These organisms are opportunistic pathogens, which are ubiquitous soil saprophytes and typically found in moist environments in manure, water, and sewage. Despite worldwide distribution and prevalence in nature, they only rarely cause clinical signs of disease. Like opportunistic fungal infections, protothecosis has been linked to both localized and systemic disease in canine and feline patients. GI signs, usually colitis, are more common in dogs and are attributed to infection with *Prototheca zopfii* (Masuda *et al.*, 2021). More discussion on the identification and diagnosis of protothecosis is provided under large intestinal inflammatory disorders (see Figure 7.56).

Pythium insidiosum is a pathogenic oomycete found mainly in tropical and subtropical regions. Infection occurs mainly in horses,

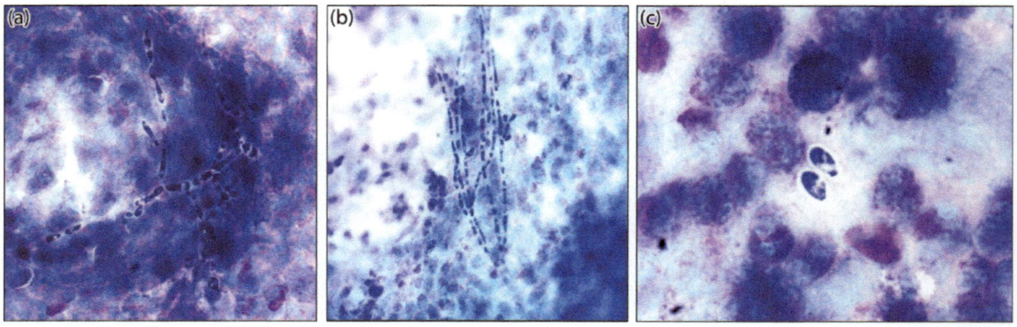

Figures 7.30a–c FNA of a mass associated with the ileum of a dog with candidiasis (C. albicans confirmed by culture). (a) Neutrophils, eosinophils, and a few macrophages are noted along with degenerating cellular debris. (b) Moderate numbers of fungal hyphae/pseudohyphae are present. Organisms are septate and branching with thin nonparallel walls. (c) Budding and spores are frequently seen (Wright–Giemsa, 1,000× magnification).

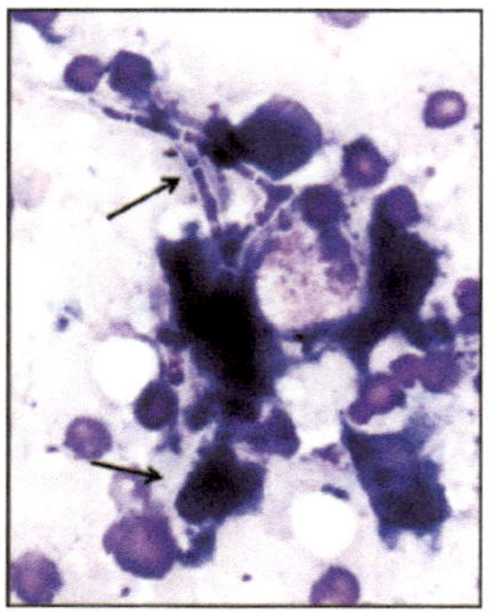

Figure 7.31 *Aspergillus* spp. infection in a dog. Long fungal hyphae (arrows) are found with associated pyogranulomatous inflammation and cellular degeneration in an intestinal lesion near the pancreas. Hyphae are septate and branching with thin clear cell walls. Disseminated disease was present in this patient (Wright–Giemsa, 1,000× magnification).

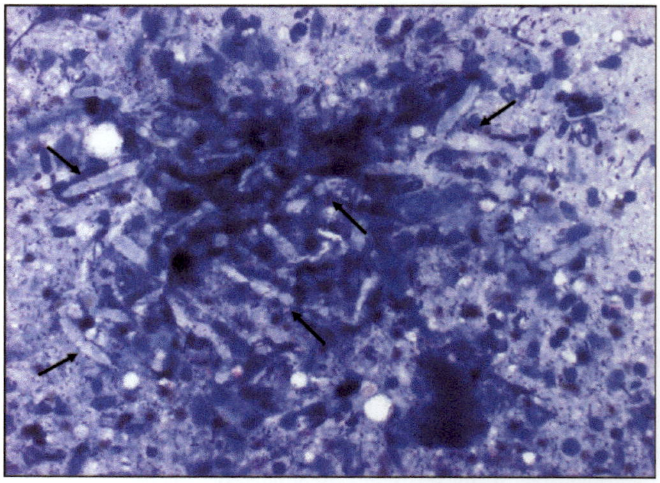

Figure 7.32 Impression smear from a gastrointestinal lesion from a dog with confirmed pythiosis. Aggregates of nonstaining hyphal structures with blunt rounded ends (arrows) are present among degenerating leukocytes (Wright–Giemsa, 700× magnification) (courtesy Mark Dunbar).

dogs, and humans and is rare in cats. The organism invades through small wounds via contact with water that contains motile zoospores or hyphae. Depending on the site of entry, infection can lead to different forms of disease including a cutaneous, vascular, ocular, GI, and, rarely, a systemic form (Gaastra *et al.*, 2010). Signs of enteritis are common in dogs with pythiosis. Vomiting, weight loss, intermittent diarrhea, and palpable abdominal masses are frequently described. Peripheral eosinophilia and hyperglobulinemia have also been identified in infected dogs (Berryessa *et al.*, 2008). Cytologically (and histologically), *Pythium* spp. can be challenging to detect. They form nonseptate, branched hyphae with irregular cell walls and stain poorly with Romanowsky stains (Figure 7.32). The infection frequently results in pyogranulomatous infiltrates similar to other fungal and algal organisms.

Lagenidium spp. are oomycetes closely related to *Pythium*. The pathogenic forms of lagenidiosis (L. *caninum* or *L. karlingii*) have clinical, epidemiologic, and cytologic characteristics similar to those of pythiosis in dogs, making them difficult to differentiate (Figure 7.33). Although enteric disease may occur with systemic infections, GI lesions are uncommon in animals infected with *Lagenidium* spp. (Grooters, 2003). The use of organism-specific antibodies or PCR is necessary for definitive diagnosis.

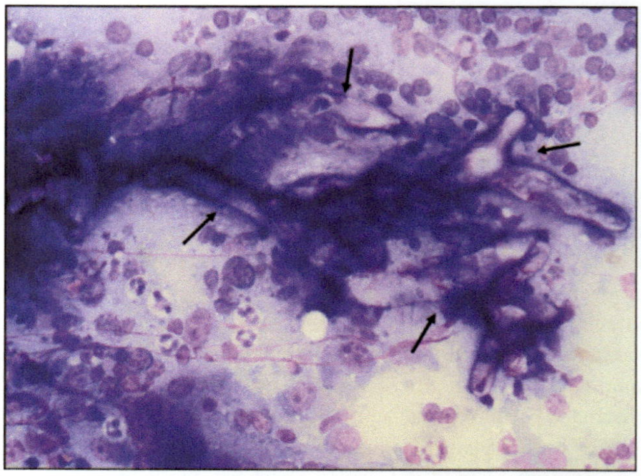

Figure 7.33 Gastrointestinal lesion from a dog. Similar to *Pythium*, *Lagenidium* spp. (arrows) stain poorly with Romanowsky stains (Wright–Giemsa, 700× magnification) (courtesy Mark Dunbar).

Neoplasms of the small intestine

Numerous tumor types are described in the intestinal tract of animals. Clinical signs are usually similar with vomiting, diarrhea, and/or anorexia frequently reported. On physical examination, poor body condition, a palpable mid-abdominal mass, pain, and thickened intestinal loops and/or ascites may be noted. Radiologic features of intestinal masses may reveal focal or diffuse changes depending on the tissue of origin. Many exhibit similar changes such as hypoechoic thickening of the intestinal wall, which may be noncircumferential and eccentric or circumferential, asymmetric, and eccentric (Laurenson *et al.*, 2011; Willard, 2012; Freiche *et al.*, 2021).

Epithelial tumors

Benign epithelial tumors of the small intestine are very rare in small animal patients. Malignant tumors, carcinomas and adenocarcinomas, are more commonly diagnosed in dogs and cats (Willard, 2012; Munday *et al.*, 2017). In cats, adenocarcinomas are the second most common neoplasm of the GIT comprising approximately 7% of reported cases. They are most often found in the mid-lower small intestine. Siamese and male cats are overrepresented in many studies (Slawienski *et al.*, 1997; Rissetto *et al.*, 2011; Munday *et al.*, 2017). Tumors frequently result in annular stenosis of a focal region of the intestine, but they may be more diffuse with circumferential thickening of the bowel. Metastasis to local lymph nodes and peritoneal surfaces is common in both species (see Case 1).

As described above, for the diagnosis of gastric tumors, the most successful results appear to be obtained by impression smears from biopsy specimens; however, FNA is usually successful as carcinomas typically exfoliate well. Carcinomas in all locations often appear similar. They are usually identified as cohesive clusters of atypical epithelial cells that display little resemblance to normal mucosa (Figure 7.16). Tumor cells frequently lose their normal columnar shape and often become more rounded to polygonal and frequently are found in 'piled' aggregates, indicating a loss of normal mucosal architecture. The cytoplasm is often deeply basophilic and the N:C ratio is typically increased, although cells may form variably sized cytoplasmic vacuoles which distort the cell. Nuclei often contain prominent nucleoli and nuclear molding may be observed. Moderate anisocytosis and anisokaryosis are usually present, and mitoses are often difficult to discern due to crowding (Figure 7.34).

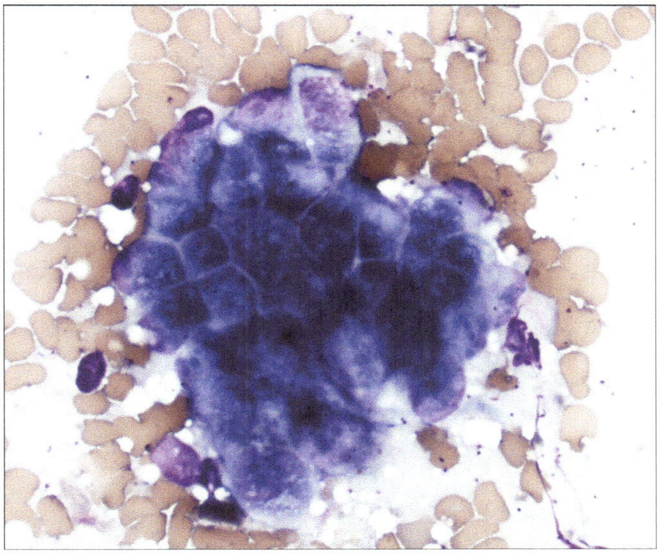

Figure 7.34 FNA from a mid-intestinal mass in a cat. A dense aggregate of neoplastic epithelial cells is present. Individual cells exhibit high N:C ratios, cytoplasmic basophilia, and prominent nucleoli characteristically found in intestinal adenocarcinomas (Wright–Giemsa, 500× magnification).

Stromal/spindle cell tumors

Spindle cell tumors of the intestinal tract are generally uncommon in small animals, comprising approximately 10–30% of intestinal tumors in dogs (Russell *et al.*, 2007). As noted above in the stomach, most spindle cell tumors were erroneously diagnosed as smooth muscle tumors (leiomyomas and leiomyosarcomas) prior to immunostaining techniques (see the examples of these tumors in the colon – Figures 7.61, 7.62). In dogs, spindle cell tumors located in the small intestine are most commonly diagnosed as GISTs; however, smooth muscle tumors are also reported in the small intestines (Frost *et al.*, 2003; Russell *et al.*, 2007; Gillespie *et al.*, 2011; Hayes *et al.*, 2013; Del Alcazar *et al.*, 2021). In cats, intestinal smooth muscle tumors and GISTs are quite rare and typically limited to case reports and small case series (Barrand & Scudamore, 1999; Rissetto *et al.*, 2011; Suwa & Shimoda, 2017).

Microscopically, leiomyomas and leiomyosarcomas are comprised of spindle-shaped cells with oval to cigar-shaped nuclei often forming bundles and streams (Figures 7.35a, b). Metastasis is uncommon but tumors can be locally invasive if poorly differentiated. GISTs are derived from the interstitial cells of Cajal (pacemaker cells) but cytologically often appear very similar to smooth muscle tumors (Figures 7.36a, b). Histologically, these are nonencapsulated cellular masses comprised of streams and short interlacing bundles of spindloid ('storiform' or 'palisading') to epithelioid cells. GISTs localize in the submucosa and muscularis but often expand transmurally and invade into the lamina propria. They are often associated with hemorrhage and necrosis. Metastasis to the liver, lymph nodes, and omentum may be more common with GISTs (Frost *et al.*, 2003; Hayes *et al.*, 2013).

Spindle cell tumors have variable exfoliation; therefore, FNA may result in limited cellularity. Cytologically, most appear similar with variable malignant criteria. Loose, noncohesive aggregates are also common with all forms including sarcomas; thus, more malignant forms may mimic poorly differentiated carcinomas (Figures 7.37a, b). As in all regions of the GIT, other sarcomas can occur in the small intestine and are usually metastatic lesions from other sites. These must be fully characterized by biopsy and immunohistochemical staining (Patnaik, 1990; LaRock & Ginn, 1997; Bonfanti *et al.*, 2006; Rissetto *et al.*, 2011).

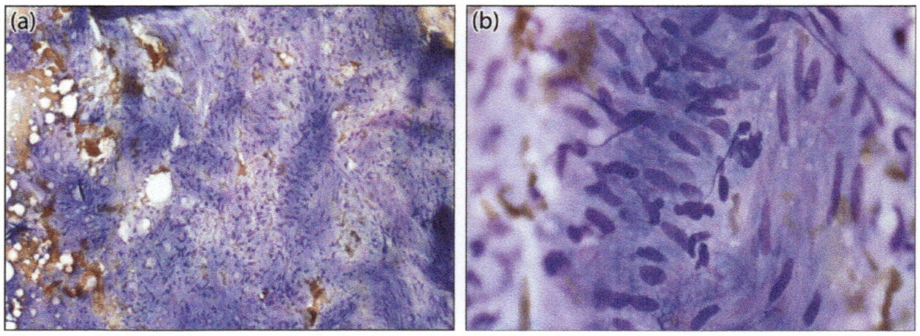

Figures 7.35a, b FNA of an intestinal mass in a dog diagnosed as a leiomyoma. A dense aggregate of relatively uniform, spindle-shaped cells is found entrapped within eosinophilic matrix material. Individual cells have elongated nuclei and indistinct cell borders (Wright–Giemsa: a, 100× magnification; b, 500× magnification).

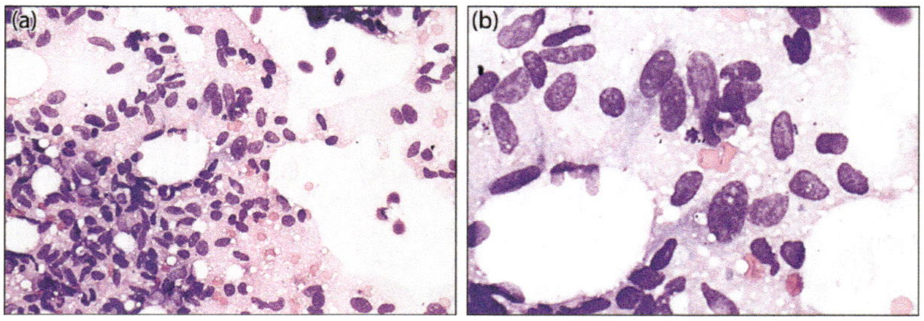

Figures 7.36a, b Cytology of a spindle cell tumor from the mid-intestinal tract of a dog. (a) Numerous disrupted spindle-shaped cells are identified at low magnification. This tumor was definitively diagnosed as a gastrointestinal stromal tumor via histology (Wright–Giemsa, 200× magnification). (b) At higher magnification (500×), spindle cells display only mild criteria for malignancy.

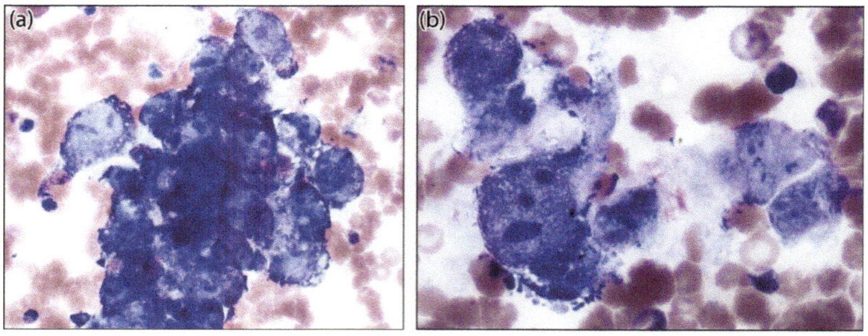

Figures 7.37a, b FNA of a mid-intestinal mass in a dog. Spindle to more oval-shaped cells are found in loose aggregates as well as individualized. Tumor cells in this lesion display marked malignant criteria including anaplasia. Hemangiosarcoma was suspected although not histologically confirmed (Wright–Giemsa: a, 500× magnification; b, 1,000× magnification).

Round cell tumors

Lymphoma

Lymphoma is the most common neoplasm of the feline GIT (Willard, 2012). Up to 70% of cats with lymphoma have GI involvement (Gabor *et al.*, 1998; Richter, 2003; Louwerens *et al.*, 2005) and small intestine location appears to be most common (Rissetto *et al.*, 2011). Although lymphoma is considered the most common or second most common neoplasm in the canine GIT, it occurs less frequently in dogs than in cats, accounting for only 7% of all cases of canine lymphoma (Rassnick *et al.*, 2009; Willard, 2012). In dogs, it is typically confined to the intestine but may rarely occur as a progressive stage of multicentric lymphoma (Frank *et al.*, 2007).

As in other anatomic locations, the cause of intestinal lymphoma is unknown. A genetic influence based on clear breed predilections for certain subtypes of lymphoma has been reported. For example, Boxers are predisposed to T-cell lymphoma, while Miniature Dachshunds develop more B-cell lymphomas including alimentary forms in both breeds (Lurie *et al.*, 2008; Pastor *et al.*, 2009; Rimpo *et al.*, 2022). Siamese cats are also overrepresented in some studies (Rissetto *et al.*, 2011). Neoplastic transformation of lymphocytes in patients with lymphoplasmacytic enteritis has been reported (Jacobs *et al.*, 1990; Hart *et al.*, 1994; Roccabianca *et al.*, 2006). As with the gastric form, infection with FeLV is not linked to formation of intestinal lymphoma

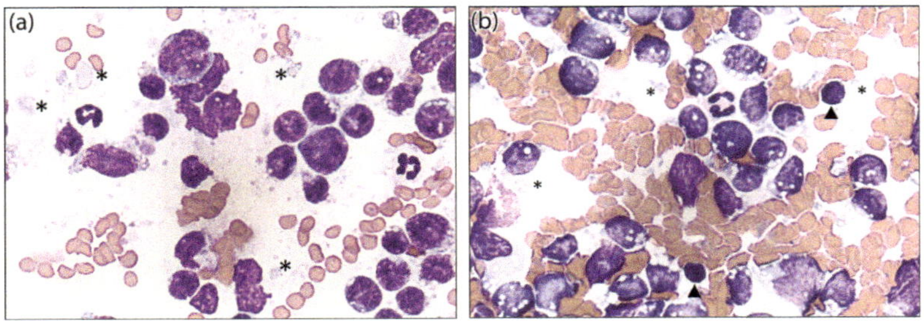

Figures 7.38a, b **Cytology of intestinal lymphoma from a cat stained with both quick stain and Wright–Giemsa. A predominance of intermediate to large-sized lymphoid cells is identified via both staining modalities with frequent cytoplasmic fragments (asterisks) due to cell rupture. (a) Diff-Quik®, 1,000× magnification. (b) Few small, mature lymphocytes are present for size comparison (arrow heads) (Wright–Giemsa, 1,000× magnification).**

in cats (Louwerens *et al.*, 2005; Krick *et al.*, 2008; Lingard *et al.*, 2009; Freiche *et al.*, 2021).

Clinical signs of intestinal lymphoma are similar to signs seen in other chronic disorders of the GIT. Hypoalbuminemia is a common biochemical abnormality (Frank *et al.*, 2007; Couto *et al.*, 2018; Freiche *et al.*, 2021). Hypercalcemia is uncommon (Willard, 2012).

Different morphologic variants of lymphoma, including the intestinal forms, have been described in dogs and cats (Vezzali *et al.*, 2010). These features, along with differentiation of the immunologic phenotype, have been shown to be important predictors of tumor behavior, progression of disease, response to therapy, and overall median survival time. For example, in both species, large T-cell lymphoma, also referred to as enteropathy-associated T-cell lymphoma (EATL) type 1, tends to be aggressive, quickly growing, and produces severe, progressive clinical signs (Willard, 2012). Low-grade intestinal, small-cell (EATL-type 2) lymphoma also occurs and is described most commonly in cats (Lingard *et al.*, 2009; Briscoe *et al.*, 2011; Moore *et al.*, 2012). Dogs may uncommonly develop this latter, low-grade form (Couto *et al.*, 2018; Lane *et al.*, 2018). In both species, this small-cell variant appears to have a more favorable outcome with greater survival times post-therapy (Lingard *et al.*, 2009; Couto *et al.*, 2018; Lane *et al.*, 2018; Freiche *et al.*, 2021). Staging post-diagnosis is also an important prognostic step in intestinal lymphoma as, regardless of phenotype, metastatic spread is common.

Cytologic evaluation of an FNA is a commonly used and valuable method for diagnosing lymphoma in the intestine. The diagnostic accuracy of this method is high, provided the smear preparations are of good quality (Bonfanti *et al.*, 2006; Ballegeer *et al.*, 2007; Maeda *et al.*, 2017). Although lymphocyte morphology may differ between variants, lymphoma is generally diagnosed by identifying a predominance of atypical lymphocytes associated with aspiration of a mass or thickened intestinal mucosa. Homogeneity, or a preponderance of one type of lymphoid population (e.g. large or intermediate-sized atypical lymphocytes), is highly suggestive of lymphoma (Figure 7.38 a, b). Diagnosis may be hindered by cell rupture, which is common in lymphoid disease in all locations due to fragility of lymphocytes. This is particularly true of large, immature lymphocytes where slides commonly contain numerous bare nuclei and cytoplasmic fragments (Figure 7.38 a, b). Predominance of granular lymphocytes may be identified in a variant of intestinal epitheliotropic lymphoma (Krick *et al.*, 2008; Roccabianca *et al.*, 2006) (Figure 7.39). While uncommon, paraneoplastic infiltration of eosinophils can be seen in some forms of T-cell lymphoma and is typically associated with more severe clinical disease (Figure 7.40).

Differentiation of low-grade alimentary lymphoma from lymphoplasmacytic enteritis can be challenging cytologically and even by endoscopic intestinal biopsies, which sample only the mucosa and submucosa (Kiupel *et al.*, 2011; Barrs & Beatty, 2012). Therefore, a multistep approach incorporating histology, immunochemistry, and PARR can be utilized to aid in the diagnosis of cases of suspected GI lymphoma in cats (Figure 7.21).

Determination of the immunophenotype of lymphoma cannot be reliably predicted by morphology of tumor cells alone; however, there are trends to suggest that most small to intermediate-sized variants of lymphoma tend to be of T-cell origin while large-cell, 'lymphoblastic'

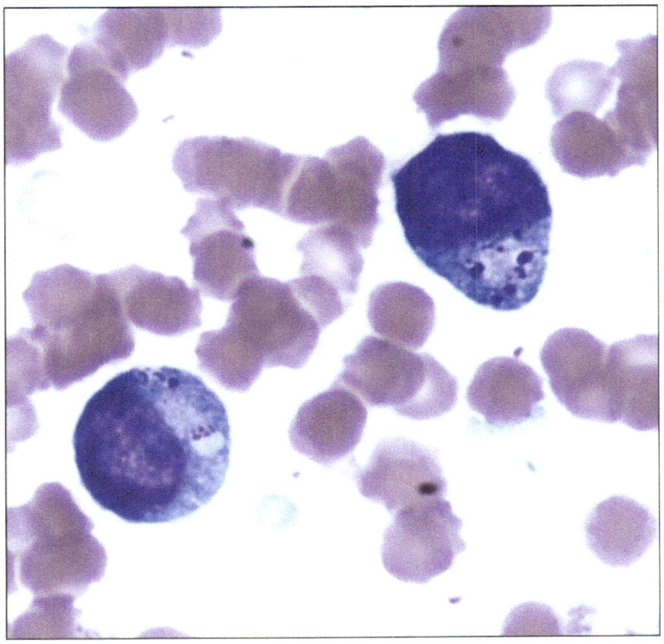

Figure 7.39 **Cytology of an intestinal mass from a cat with granular lymphoma. Note the eosinophilic granules packeted on one side of the cell (Wright–Giemsa, 1,000× magnification).**

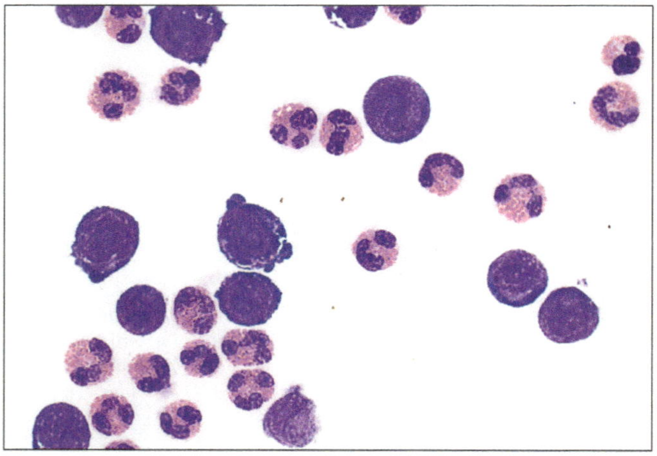

Figure 7.40 Cytology of abdominal fluid from a cat with large-cell lymphoma and paraneoplastic eosinophil infiltration. The cell count in the fluid was over 50,000/μL. Neoplastic cells are immature in appearance with large nucleoli (Wright–Giemsa, 500× magnification).

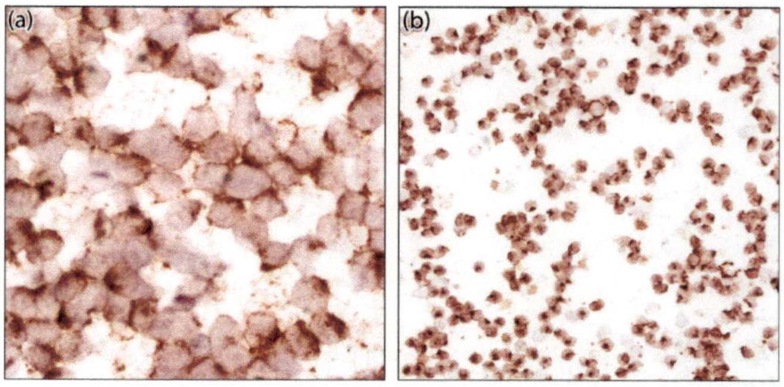

Figures 7.41a, b (a) Anti-CD79a antibody consistent with B-cell phenotype. (b) Anti-CD3 antibody consistent with T-cell phenotype (HRP polymer anti-rabbit IgG with Nova Red chromogen and hematoxylin counterstain: a, 1,000× magnification; b, 500× magnification).

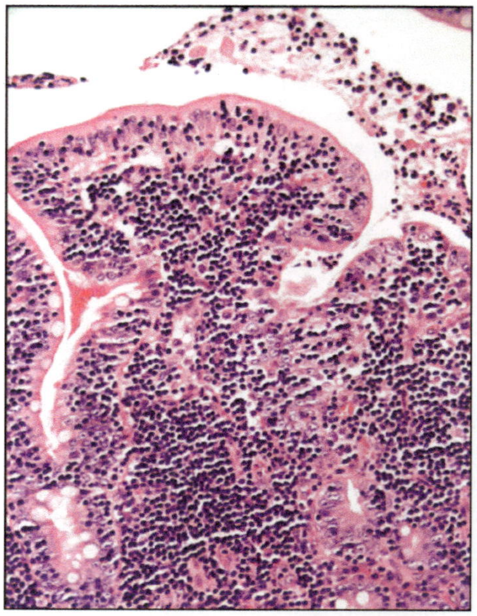

Figure 7.42 Histologic section of intestinal mucosa from a cat with lymphoma. Note the marked increase in lymphocytes within the lamina propria (H&E, 200× magnification).

types can include both T- and B-cell phenotypes (Gabor *et al.*, 1999; Sözmen *et al.*, 2005). In cases of intestinal granular lymphomas (Figure 7.39), immunophenotypic analysis has shown that these are typically $CD8^+/CD3^+$ (cytotoxic T-cell) neoplasms (Roccabianca *et al.*, 2006). There is some evidence that tumor location is predictive of both phenotype and prognosis in cats. For example, alimentary lymphomas are more likely to be of T-cell lineage when localized to the small intestine (Moore *et al.*, 2012). Furthermore, small intestinal T-cell tumors may have a better long-term prognosis than B-cell tumors in cats (Lingard *et al.*, 2009; Moore *et al.*, 2012). In comparison, large-cell ('lymphoblastic') lymphoma and granular lymphoma are aggressive neoplasms with a poorer long-term prognosis in both dogs and cats regardless of location (Krick *et al.*, 2008; Lurie *et al.*, 2008; Willard, 2012).

Immunophenotyping can usually be accomplished by supplying good quality, unstained cytology samples, preferably on positively charged slides (Caniatti *et al.*, 1996) (Figures 7.41a, b). Alternatively, aspirates from the lesion may be placed into an EDTA tube with a milliliter of saline and submitted to the diagnostic laboratory within 48 hours for processing for either immunocytochemical staining or flow cytometry (Caniatti *et al.*, 1996; Gibson *et al.*, 2004; Sözmen *et al.*, 2005). In cases of equivocal results due to a heterogeneous population of cells, a low cell yield, or low-grade lymphoma, additional diagnostic modalities may be necessary. This may include biopsy, where full-thickness biopsy is preferred to endoscopically acquired samples (Figure 7.42), and/or PARR (Avery, 2009; Kiupel *et al.*, 2011; Barrs & Beatty, 2012). Indeed, PARR has been shown to be highly sensitive for detection of neoplastic (versus reactive) proliferation of lymphocytes and may even assist in staging and predicting prognosis of disease (Keller et al., 2004; Lana *et al.*, 2006). However, clonal analysis alone may be misleading in some cases of lymphoma as both B- and T-cell receptors are frequently clonally rearranged but actual biphenotypic expression is less common (Sato *et al.*, 2011; Weiss *et al.*, 2011). Therefore, multimodal diagnostics are often necessary for full characterization of lymphoproliferative disorders, particularly in the GIT (see Case 2).

Enteric mast cell tumors

Feline intestinal mast cell neoplasia is recognized as the third most common intestinal tumor in cats (Rissetto *et al.*, 2011). Unlike lymphoma and adenocarcinoma, there are no breed predilections identified for the enteric form of this tumor (Rissetto *et al.*, 2011. Barrett *et al.*, 2018). Cytologically these tumors can display variable differentiation including poor granulation (Barrett *et al.*, 2018; London &

Thamm, 2020). Based on ultrastructural and histochemical features, enteric mast cell tumor is considered to be a separate entity from other visceral (e.g. splenic) mast cell neoplasms of cats. Tumors may occur anywhere along the intestinal tract; however, proximal and mid-intestinal locations are more frequently reported, whereas distal and large intestinal tumors appear to be less common. Interestingly, cats may also have concurrent intestinal lymphoma (Laurenson *et al.*, 2011). A unique variant of feline intestinal mast cell tumor characterized by moderate to marked eosinophilic infiltrates and sclerosis has recently been described. This variant is commonly associated with lymph node and hepatic metastases and a high mortality rate (Halsey *et al.*, 2010). Regardless of the variant, all cats with visceral mast cell neoplasia should be staged, as metastasis is common (Laurenson *et al.*, 2011; Barrett *et al.*, 2018; London & Thamm, 2020).

Clinical signs are typically vomiting, inappetence, and signs similar to other GI tumors. Anemia secondary to inflammation, chronic hemorrhage, or erythrophagocytosis by neoplastic mast cells is frequently identified (Figure 7.43).

In dogs, high-grade cutaneous mast cell tumors frequently exhibit metastasis, particularly to the spleen, liver, and regional lymph nodes (Stefanello *et al.*, 2009). Primary mucosal (including intestinal) mast cell tumors, however, are rare in dogs with only a few reports characterizing this disease (Takahashi *et al.*, 2000; Ozaki *et al.*, 2002; Kobayashi *et al.*, 2012). Purebred male dogs of miniature breeds appear to have a higher prevalence of intestinal mast cell tumors. These are frequently of high grade and the prognosis is extremely poor (Takahashi *et al.*, 2000).

Definitive diagnosis of intestinal mast cell neoplasia can usually be accomplished via cytologic evaluation of an FNA of the mass. Cells readily exfoliate and typically contain metachromatic granules. In cats, these granules are often smaller than those seen in other species and may not stain well with Diff-Quik® (Figure 7.44). However, caution is required when aspirating suspected visceral tumors, as mast cell degranulation may occur; therefore, pre-treatment with antihistamines is recommended (London & Thamm, 2020).

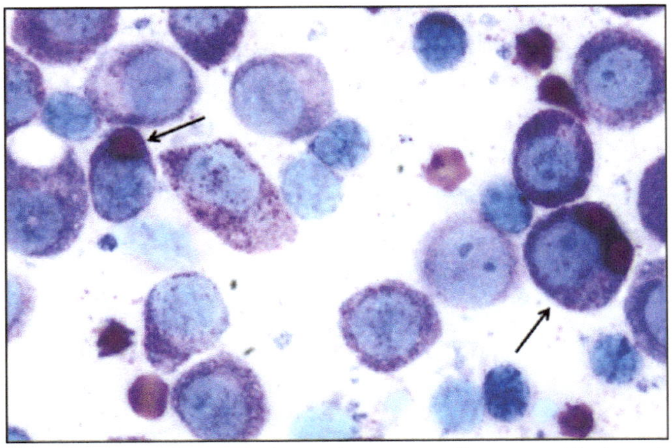

Figure 7.43 **Erythrophagia by neoplastic mast cells in a cat with visceral mast cell tumor (arrows) (Wright–Giemsa, 1,000× magnification).**

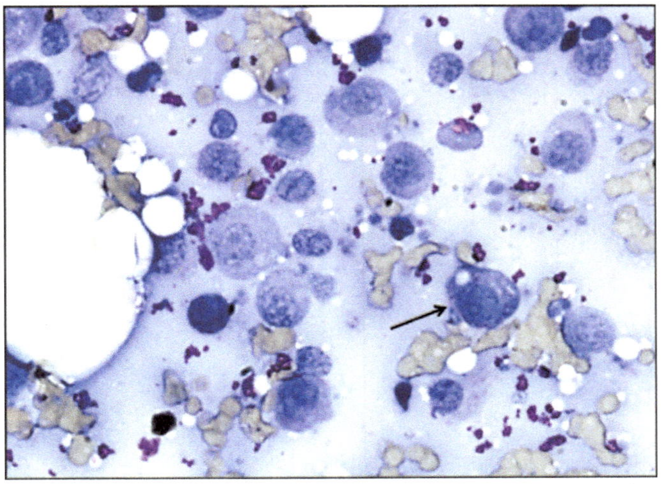

Figure 7.44 **Enteric mast cell tumor in a cat. Faint eosinophilic granules can be made out in a few of the cells (arrow). The globular extracellular eosinophilic material is likely ultrasound gel (Diff-Quik®, 500× magnification).**

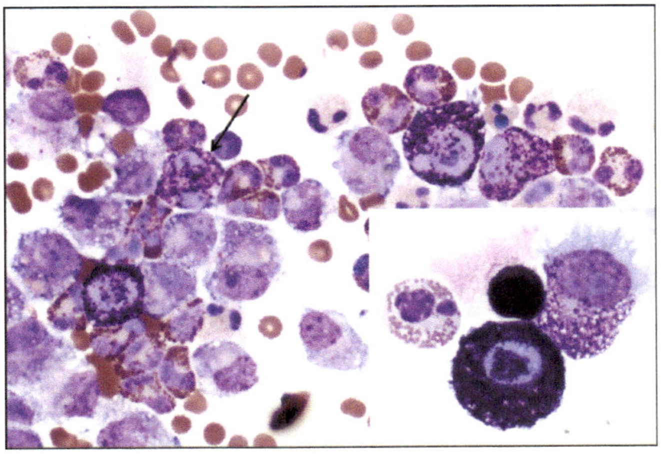

Figure 7.45 **Eosinophils and neoplastic mast cells in peritoneal effusion from a dog with visceral mast cell neoplasia (Wright–Giemsa, 500× magnification; inset 1,000× magnification).**

Peritoneal effusions, occasionally containing eosinophils, along with a peripheral eosinophilia, have been documented as paraneoplastic syndromes associated with visceral mast cell disease in dogs (Figure 7.45) and cats (Peaston & Griffey, 1994). Mast cell tumors may, therefore, be misdiagnosed (even by biopsy) as eosinophilic enteritis (Howl & Petersen, 1995). Thus, the presence of eosinophils should remain as a potential indicator for underlying mast cell disease.

LARGE INTESTINE (CECUM, COLON, AND RECTUM)

Normal

The colon contains larger numbers of goblet cells relative to the small intestine (Figures 7.46a, b, 7.47a, b). Villi are absent, and crypts are

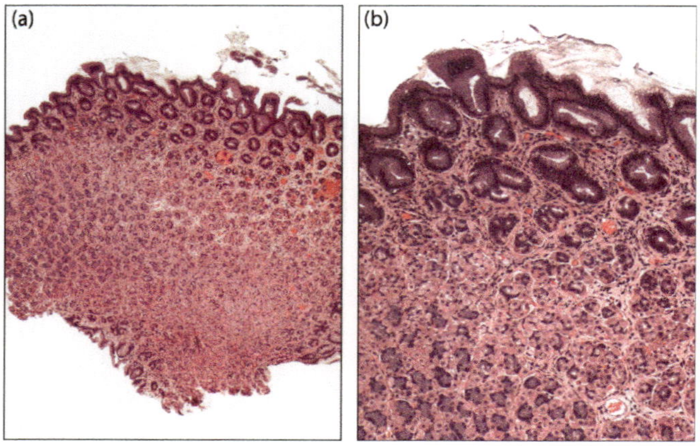

Figures 7.46a, b Histologic sections of normal colonic epithelium from a dog obtained by colonoscopic biopsy (H&E; a, 40× magnification; b, 100× magnification).

longer than in the small intestine (Bacha & Bacha, 2012). The rectum is lined by stratified squamous epithelium, which becomes progressively keratinized in the posterior portion as it approaches the anal canal. Apocrine anal glands occur in the submucosa and muscularis of the anal canal in both dogs and cats. Circumanal glands occur in the subcutis around the anus of the dog. These are modified sebaceous glands that resemble hepatocytes and thus are often referred to as 'hepatoid' glands. Diseases affecting these latter structures are described in Chapter 4.

Sampling of the large intestine may be accomplished by FNA or impression smears of affected tissue or masses similar to other lesions along the GIT. Additionally, endoscopic brush cytology (described above) and rectal scraping may assist in the detection of certain disease conditions such as infiltrative neoplasms or intestinal infections (e.g. histoplasmosis or protothecosis). Some fecal parasites may also be identified via rectal scrapings (see 'Intestinal Parasites' below). As the intent of a rectal scrape is to sample a larger concentration of cells directly from the colonic mucosa, tools such as a moistened cotton swab, fecal loop, or spatula are often used to gently dislodge cells. Additionally, gentle scraping of the rectal mucosa with a gloved fingertip usually results in good exfoliation of cells. Although judicious use of gel lubricant is helpful for rectal palpation, it is important to remember that the presence of this material can obscure cellular details and render cytologic assessment useless (Figure 7.48). Therefore, it is generally recommended to avoid the use of lubricants when obtaining a sample by rectal scrape.

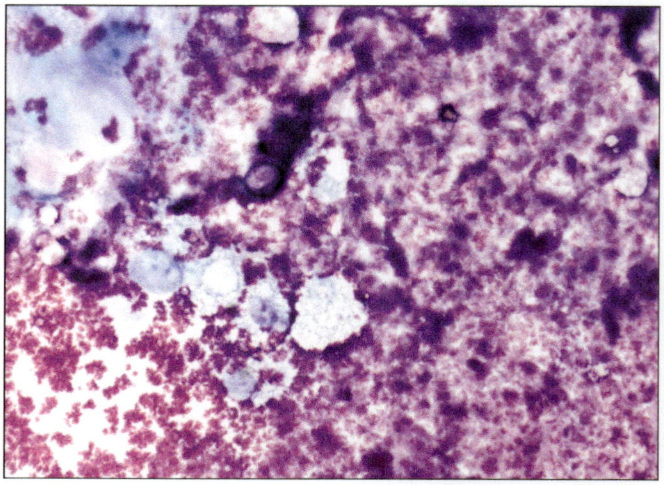

Figure 7.48 Rectal scraping from a dog. The cytologic constituents of the sample are obscured by the presence of amorphous, eosinophilic globular material consistent with gel lubricant (Wright–Giemsa, 500× magnification).

Hyperplastic lesions

Colonic hyperplasia is described uncommonly in animals and typically associated with primary inflammatory disease. The formation of colorectal polyps has been recognized as a cause for large bowel diarrhea in dachshunds in Japan (Uchida *et al.*, 2016). As hyperplastic epithelium cannot be differentiated from either normal colonic epithelium or adenomatous polyps, definitive diagnosis requires biopsy and histopathologic interpretation (see Figures 7.47).

Inflammatory lesions

Recent studies have speculated that chronic diarrhea in dogs is more often associated with lifestyle and behavioral (e.g. pica) factors than specific pathogens (Berset-Istratescu *et al.*, 2014). *Campylobacter* spp. (Figure 7.49) and *Clostridium* spp. (Figure 7.50) have both been cultured from the feces of dogs with and without diarrhea; therefore, the

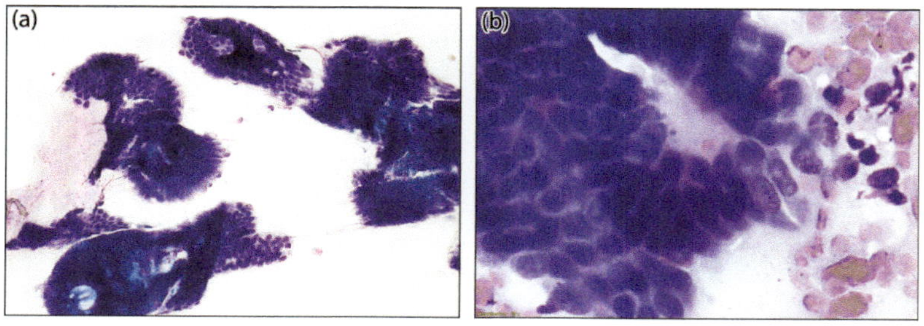

Figures 7.47a, b Cytology of normal colonic epithelium from a dog (Wright–Giemsa, a, 400× magnification; b, 1,000× magnification).

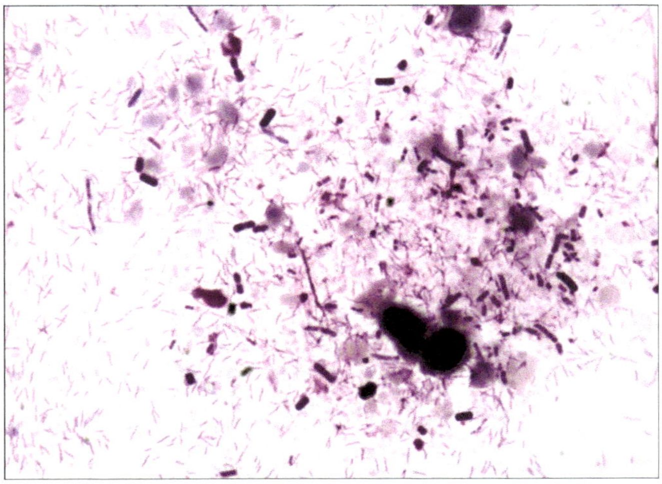

Figure 7.49 Fecal smear from a dog with diarrhea. Apparent overgrowth of spiral-shaped bacteria consistent with *Campylobacter* spp. (Wright–Giemsa, 1,500× magnification).

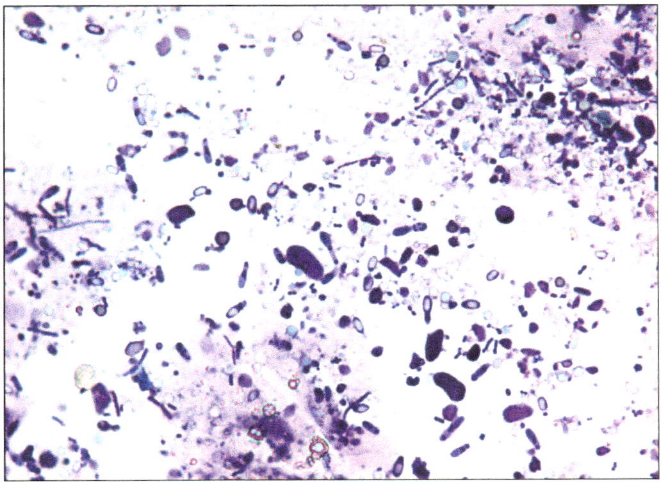

Figure 7.50 Fecal smear from a dog with diarrhea. Apparent overgrowth of bacterial rods consistent with *Clostridium* spp. (Wright–Giemsa, 1,500× magnification) (courtesy Anne Barger).

identification of these organisms in feces does not always correlate with the clinical status of the patient (Rossi *et al.*, 2008; Weese, 2011; Berset-Istratescu *et al.*, 2014).

Although chronic inflammatory GI disorders frequently cause multifocal GI lesions, primary colitis may be seen. Similar to other forms of CE, hereditary conditions have been documented in dogs, including histiocytic ulcerative colitis in Boxers (Figure 7.51a–c) and French Bulldogs (German *et al.*, 2003; Manchester *et al.*, 2013; Sims *et al.*, 2022) or eosinophilic granulomas in Rottweilers (Figure 7.52). Idiopathic colitis can also affect cats, although breed association is not described (Figure 7.53). Mixed inflammatory infiltrates may be seen on direct aspiration of focal lesions or rectal scraping. However, final, definitive diagnosis requires histopathology.

Fungal and 'pseudofungal' infections

Many fungal and algal organisms are associated with large intestinal lesions. Overgrowth of normal commensal and ingested organisms such as *Cyniclomyces guttulatus* may occur, resulting in diarrhea (Figure 7.54a, b). *Histoplasma capsulatum*, as described above, is commonly associated with chronic enteritis and, more often, colitis in infected individuals (Brömel & Sykes, 2005). *Histoplasma* spp. organisms may be identified on rectal scrapes or aspiration of mass lesions in the large intestine or associated lymph nodes, as dissemination is common (Figure 7.27, Case 3). Rarely, other pathogenic fungi such as *Cryptococcus* spp. can be found via rectal scrapes and/or fecal analysis (Figures 7.55a). Biopsies are also diagnostic for identifying organisms in infected tissues (Figure 7.55b).

As described for algal lesions found in the small intestinal tract, GI disease, particularly colitis, is more common in dogs infected with *Prototheca zopfii* (Masuda *et al.*, 2021). Rectal scrapes may be useful for identifying *Prototheca* spp., but definitive identification is often difficult as the organism is pleomorphic and may appear similar to commensal yeast in feces (Figures 7.56a–b). Organisms vary in size, depending on the species and stage of development, ranging from 1.3 to 13.4 µm in diameter. They have thin nonstaining cell walls, basophilic granular cytoplasm, small centrally placed nuclei, and reproduce by endosporulation. While morphologic features of the organisms may provide a preliminary diagnosis of protothecosis, definitive diagnosis and speciation require molecular analysis.

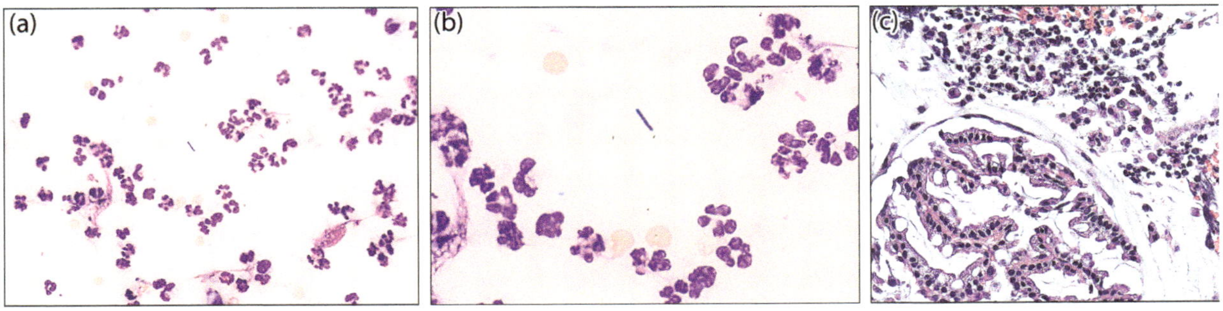

Figures 7.51a–c Colon, canine. Cytology from a rectal scrape from a 1-year-old Boxer dog with chronic hematochezia and large bowel diarrhea due to ulcerative colitis. (a) Mixed inflammatory cells including neutrophils and macrophages are present. (b) Intralesional bacterial rods are also found (Wright–Giemsa: a, 500× magnification; b, 1000× magnification). (c) Histology of the lesion shows hyperplastic epithelium associated with the inflammatory population (H&E, 400× magnification).

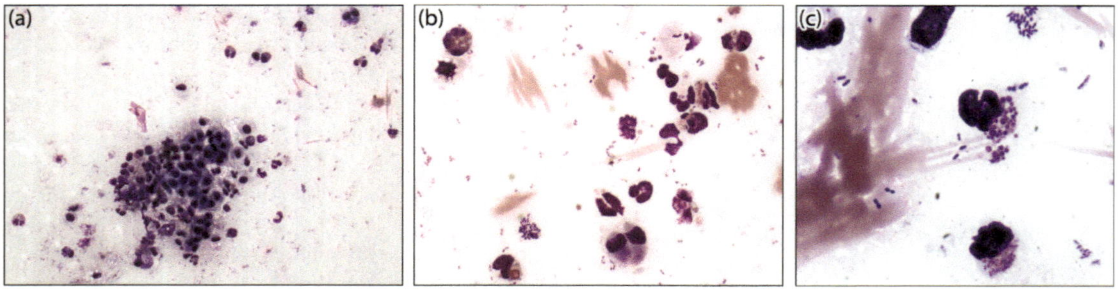

Figures 7.52a–c Colon, canine. Cytology from a rectal scrape from a dog with eosinophilic colitis. (a) Clusters of uniform colonic epithelial cells is found among scattered eosinophils with few neutrophils. (b) Eosinophils are more readily identified at higher magnification. (c) Canine eosinophil granules are often variably sized and may coalesce (Wright–Giemsa: a, 300× magnification; b, 700× magnification; c, 1,000× magnification).

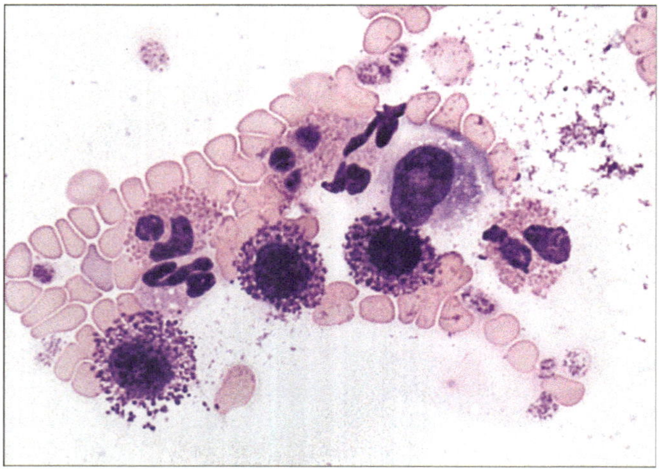

Figures 7.53 Colon, feline. Cytology from an aspirate from a 10-year-old cat with chronic large bowel diarrhea due to idiopathic eosinophilic colitis. Mast cells can be found admixed with eosinophils in several slides, which may mimic underlying mast cell neoplasia (Wright–Giemsa: 500× magnification).

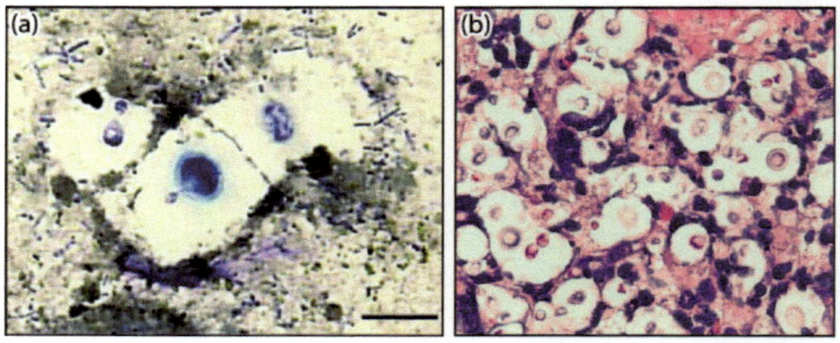

Figures 7.55a, b Direct fecal smear from a dog with systemic cryptococcosis. (a) Encapsulated, narrow-based budding organisms consistent with *Cryptococcus* are seen (Wright–Giemsa, bar = 20 μm). (b) Histologic section of colon from the same dog with systemic cryptococcosis. Numerous encapsulated organisms are seen in the colonic mucosa and submucosa (H&E, 1,000× magnification). (From Graves TK, Barger AM, Adams B *et al.* (2005) Diagnosis of systemic cryptococcosis by fecal cytology in a dog. *Vet Clin Pathol* 34(4):409–412. Reprinted with permission.)

Intestinal parasites

Rectal scrapings and fecal analysis are frequently performed for the diagnosis of parasites in dogs and cats. The list of infective organisms is long, with the sensitivity of detection being based on the mode of acquisition (Table 7.1). Rectal scrapings and direct smears of feces are often useful for detecting protozoan pathogens such as *Giardia* and *Tritrichomonas* spp. (Figures 7.57, 7.58, respectively), while other organisms may require more refined flotation, sedimentation, and centrifugation methods. Occasionally, parasite ova may be identified on stained smears of feces (Figure 7.59).

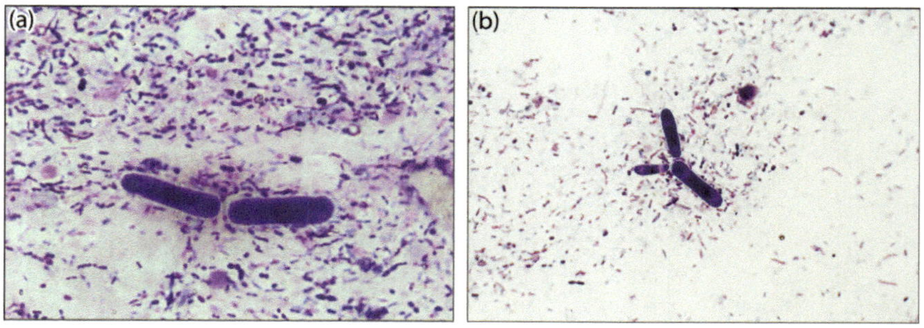

Figures 7.54a, b Fecal sample from a French Bulldog with chronic large-bowel diarrhea. The sample contains numerous large cigar-shaped yeast organisms, consistent with *C. guttulatus*, among mixed bacteria. Organisms are found individually, (a) in short chains, and (b) branching in the sample (Wright–Giemsa, 1,000× magnification).

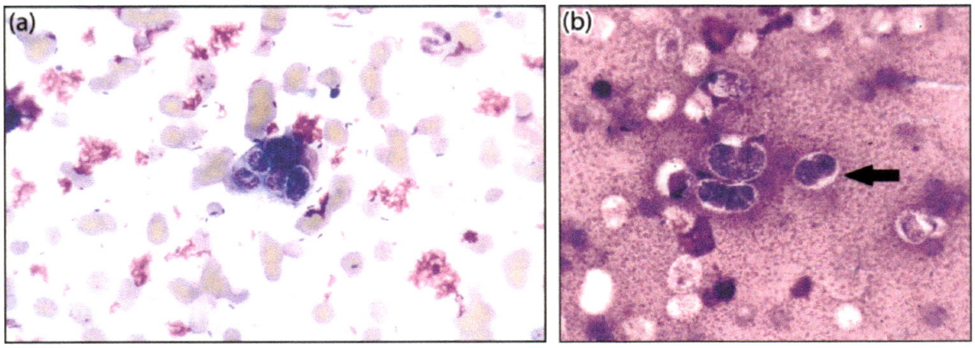

Figures 7.56a–b Rectal scrapes from two dogs with chronic colitis due to *Prototheca* infection. (a) Small numbers of oval organisms with thin clear cell walls and granular basophilic contents are found among a background of erythrocytes. The flocculant magenta material is consistent with gel-lubricant. (b) Organisms are variable in size. Note the presence of endosporulation (arrow) (Wright–Giemsa, 100× magnification) (7.56a courtesy Mary Christopher; 7.56b courtesy William Vernau).

Table 7.1 **Selected parasites causing signs of gastrointestinal disease in dogs and cats**

Organism	Common name	Examples in dogs and cats	Diagnosis
Nematodes	Roundworms (aka: ascarids)	*Toxocara canis, Toxascaris leonina*	Sugar flotation
	Hookworms	*Ancylostoma caninum, Uncinaria stenocephala*	Sugar flotation
	Whipworms	*Trichuris vulpis*	Sugar flotation
	Threadworm	*Strongyloides stercoralis*	Flotation (fresh feces)
	Esophageal worm	*Spirocerca lupi*	$NaNO_3$ [specific gravity 1.36] or sugar flotation
Protozoa	Flagellates	*Giardia lamblia*	Fluorescent antibody stain; fecal smear; stained smears or culture
	Coccidia	*Tritrichomonas foetus*	Sugar flotation; PCR or culture
		Eimeria spp.	
		Isospora sp.	Sugar flotation
Trematodes Cestodes	Flukes Tapeworms	*Nanophyetus salmincola*	Sedimentation or fecal smear; flotation, but less reliable
Cestodes	Tapeworms	*Taenia* spp. *Dipylidium caninum* *Echinococcus* spp.	Flotation or identification of segments around anus PCR for speciation

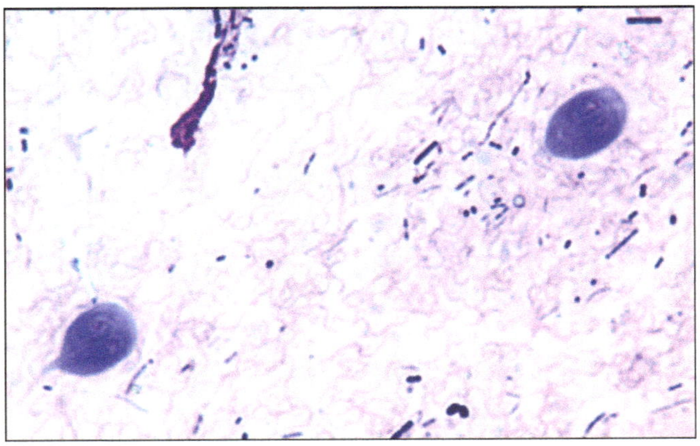

Figure 7.57 Fecal sample from a dog with *Giardia* spp. (Wright–Giemsa, 1,800× magnification) (courtesy Anne Barger)

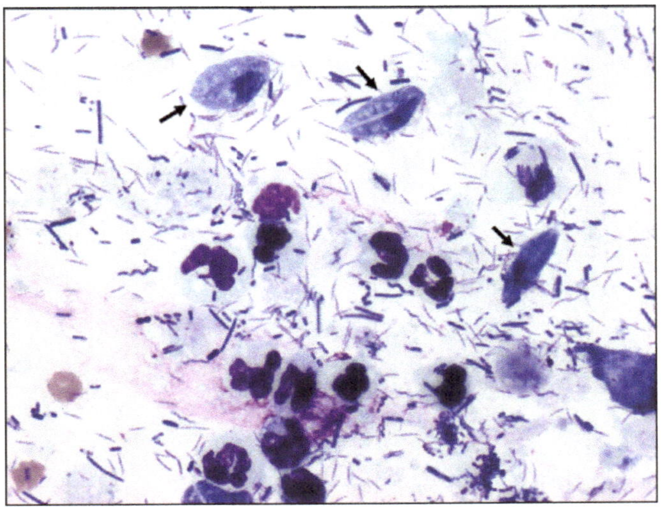

Figure 7.58 Fecal sample from a cat with *Tritrichomonas foetus* (arrows) (Wright–Giemsa, 800× magnification) (courtesy Mark Dunbar).

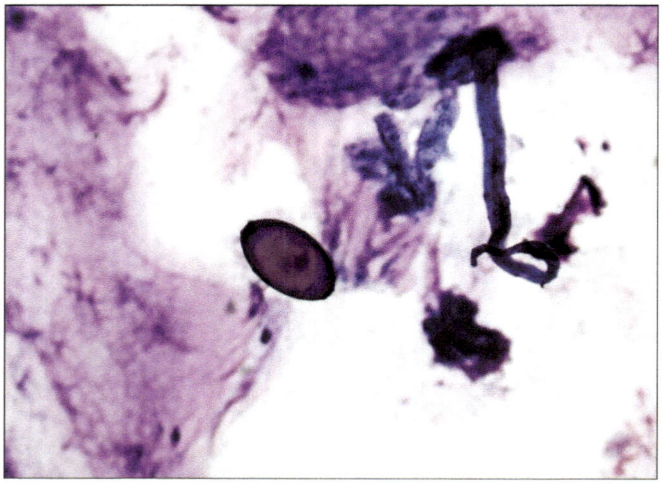

Figure 7.59 Rectal scrape from a dog with colitis. A large double-operculated ovum consistent with *Trichuris vulpis* is present (Wright–Giemsa, 200× magnification).

Neoplasms of the large intestines

Epithelial tumors

In the rectum, benign tumors are more frequently reported than at other locations within the GIT. Indeed, benign epithelial tumors appear to occur with equal frequency to malignant tumors in dogs. In cats, however, only a few reports of benign epithelial proliferations are found (Kehl *et al.*, 2022). Benign epithelial tumors include adenomatous polyps, which are described as sessile, raised, pedunculated, single, or multiple mass lesions. Diagnosis of benign tumors by cytology can be difficult as differentiation from hyperplastic proliferation is often not possible. Therefore, the definitive diagnosis of such lesions usually necessitates surgical biopsy and histopathology (Valerius *et al.*, 1997; Danova *et al.*, 2006; Willard, 2012; Munday *et al.*, 2017).

Adenocarcinomas of the intestines are generally more common in cats than in dogs. In dogs, however, they tend to be located in the colon and rectum. Unlike cats, where Siamese cats are overrepresented, a breed predisposition is not consistently seen in dogs; however, progression from benign polyps to adenocarcinoma is speculated (Slawienski *et al.*, 1997; Saito *et al.*, 2018). Cytologically, colonic carcinomas/adenocarcinomas are similar to tumors at other locations and are described more fully above (Figures 7.60a, b).

Stromal/spindle cell tumors

As previously stated, smooth muscle tumors (leiomyosarcoma, leiomyoma) appear to occur more commonly in the stomach and throughout the small intestine in dogs; however, GISTs are more commonly reported in the large intestines (Frost *et al.*, 2003; Russell *et*

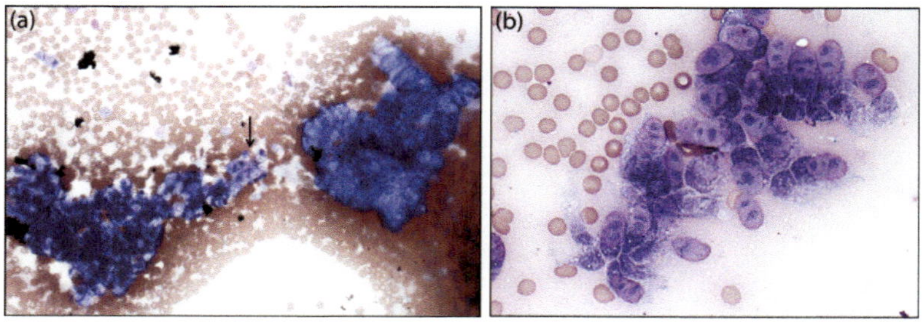

Figures 7.60a, b Cytology obtained from an FNA of a colonic lesion from a dog. (a) Two large aggregates of epithelial cells are present. At 200× magnification, criteria for malignancy are already apparent. Note the deep basophilia and multiple nucleoli (arrow). (b) Epithelial cells often maintain some semblance of normal shape but exhibit criteria for malignancy consistent with adenocarcinoma (Wright–Giemsa; a, 200× magnification; b, 600× magnification).

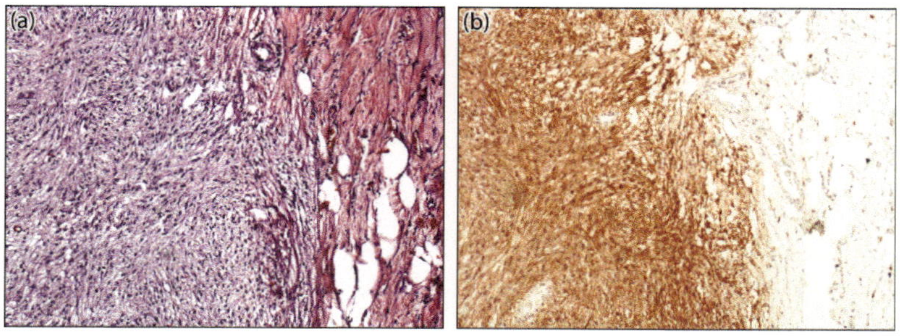

Figures 7.61a, b Gastrointestinal stromal tumor in the cecum of a dog. (a) Histology section of the tumor shows interlacing neoplastic spindle cells adjacent to normal tissue (H&E, 100× magnification). (b) Tumor cells show marked reactivity for KIT expression (HRP polymer anti-rabbit IgG with Nova Red chromogen and hematoxylin counter stain, 100× magnification).

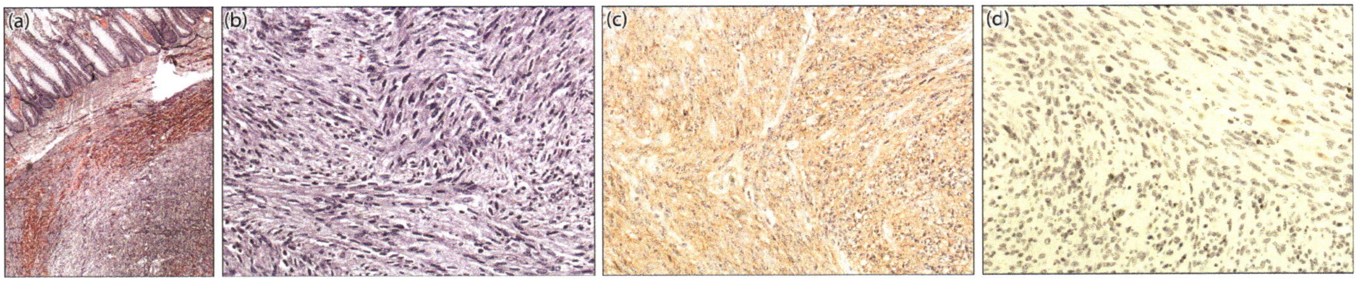

Figures 7.62a–d Histologic section of a leiomyosarcoma in the colon of a dog. (a) A large expansile mass is found invading into the submucosa (H&E, 40× magnification). (b) Tumor cells are spindle-shaped and found in streams (H&E, 200× magnification). (c) Tumor cells are positive for smooth muscle actin (HRP polymer anti-rabbit IgG with Nova Red chromogen and hematoxylin counter stain, 200× magnification). (d) Tumor cells are negative for KIT expression (HRP polymer anti-rabbit IgG with Nova Red chromogen and hematoxylin counter stain, 200× magnification).

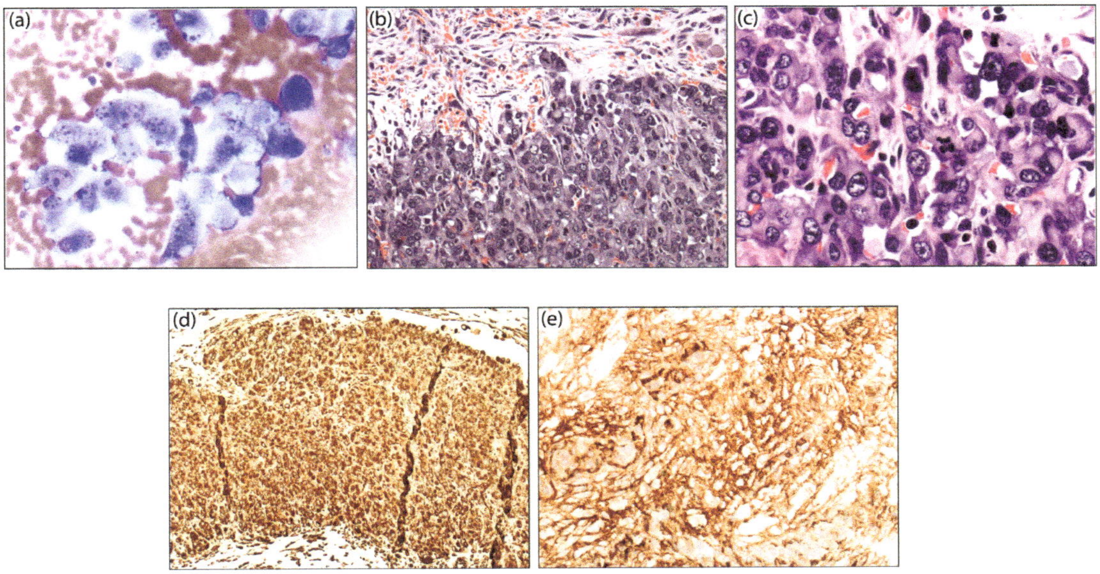

Figures 7.63a–e Mass associated with the intestine of a dog. Disseminated neoplasia was identified post-mortem and definitively diagnosed as hemangiosarcoma by immunohistochemical evaluation. (a) Cytology of a large intestinal lesion showing markedly atypical spindle cells (Wright–Giemsa, 200× magnification). (b) Histology of the intestinal mass, which has effaced the submucosa at this location (H&E, 100× magnification). (c) Higher magnification of the mass demonstrates the anaplastic appearance of the neoplastic cells (H&E, 500× magnification). (d, e) Tumor cells are positive for vimentin (d) and von Willebrand expression (e).

al., 2007; Gillespie *et al.*, 2011; Hayes *et al.*, 2013). Only a few cases of large intestinal spindle cell tumors in cats are found in the veterinary literature (Rissetto *et al.*, 2011; Kehl *et al.*, 2022). As stated previously, differentiation between GISTs and smooth muscle tumors requires biopsy and immunohistochemical characterization. GISTs are positive for vimentin and KIT (Figures 7.61a, b) but negative for desmin, whereas smooth muscle tumors (Figures 7.62a–d) are KIT negative but more consistently positive for SMA and desmin (Frost *et al.*, 2003).

Other sarcomas may arise *de novo* in the colon or metastasize from other locations, although these appear to be uncommon in the literature. Rare cases of histiocytic sarcomas, hemangiosarcomas, and fibrosarcomas have been described in the large intestine of both dogs and cats (Bonfanti *et al.*, 2006; Shor *et al.*, 2009; Rissetto *et al.*, 2011; Kehl *et al.*, 2022). The cytology of spindle cell tumors is described above. As they often appear both cytologically and histologically similar, special staining is usually necessary for definitive identification of the tissue of origin (Figures 7.63a–e).

Round cell tumors

Lymphoma

Lymphoma is considered the second most common tumor in the colon of cats (Rissetto *et al.*, 2011) but appears to occur infrequently in the large intestine of dogs (Frank *et al.*, 2007). In both species, colonic lymphomas are more often of B-cell lineage. In cats, B-cell large intestinal lymphoma is associated with a poorer long-term prognosis (Lingard *et al.*, 2009; Moore *et al.*, 2012). Contrary to cats, longer survival times are reported in dogs with colorectal lymphomas than

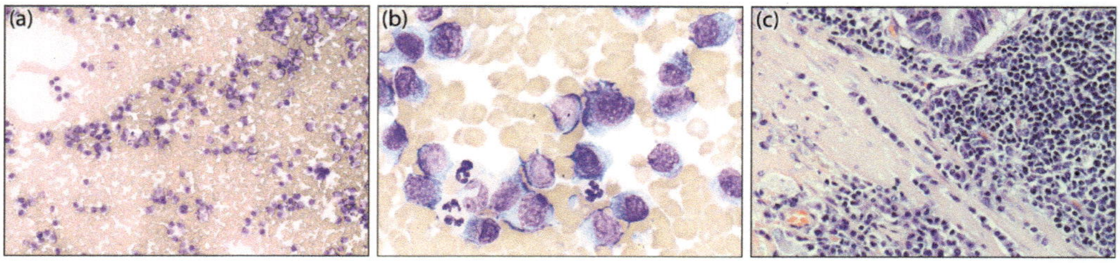

Figures 7.64a–c Dog with multiple colonic plasma cell tumors and progression to myeloma syndrome. (a) FNA of one of the masses shows a relatively monomorphic population of round cells, among a background of erythrocytes (Wright–Giemsa, 200× magnification). (b) At higher magnification cells are discrete in appearance and characteristic for atypical plasma cells (Wright–Giemsa, 1000× magnification). (c) Histology of the mass shows expansion of the mucosa and submucosa by infiltrating plasma cells (H&E 400× magnification).

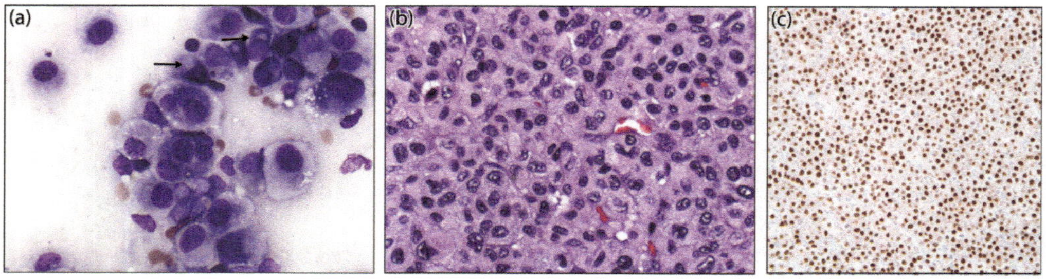

Figures 7.65a–c Plasma cell tumor in the distal rectum of a dog. (a) FNA of the mass shows a more pleomorphic population of round cells in this lesion. Golgi bodies (arrows) can still be discerned in several cells. Multinucleated cells are frequent (Wright–Giemsa, 500× magnification). (b) Histology of the same mass. Similar cellular atypia, including multinucleation, is noted in the biopsy sample (H&E, 500× magnification). (c) Neoplastic cells are positive for MUM1, a marker expressed by plasma cells (H&E, 500× magnification).

in dogs with either gastric or small intestinal lymphoma (Frank *et al.*, 2007; Van den Steen *et al.*, 2012).

Similar to lymphoma in other sites, diagnosis is made by identifying a predominance of lymphoid cells, typically large lymphocytes, often with increased mitotic activity.

Plasma cell tumors

Extramedullary plasmacytomas are relatively common in dogs and may be associated with mucocutaneous junctions; however, only a few cases of intestinal localization (mainly colorectal) have been reported in dogs or cats (Ramos-Vara *et al.*, 1998; Zikes *et al.*, 1998; Danova *et al.*, 2006; Kupanoff *et al.*, 2006). The mucosa overlying the mass is often eroded or ulcerated and may be covered by fibrinonecrotic exudate. Although neoplastic plasma cells may be confined to the submucosa, infiltration into the lamina propria and muscle layers may also occur. Cytologically, the tumor cells are typical for plasma cell tumors at other sites and are often solitary; however, multifocal masses can occur (Figures 7.64a–c). Cells may be pleomorphic and binucleate and multinucleate cells are commonly noted, thus immunochemical staining may be necessary for full differentiation from other round cell tumor types (Figures 7.65a–c) (Kupanoff *et al.*, 2006; Munday *et al.*, 2017). Most studies indicate that these tumors are not aggressive and metastasis or progression to myeloma is rare.

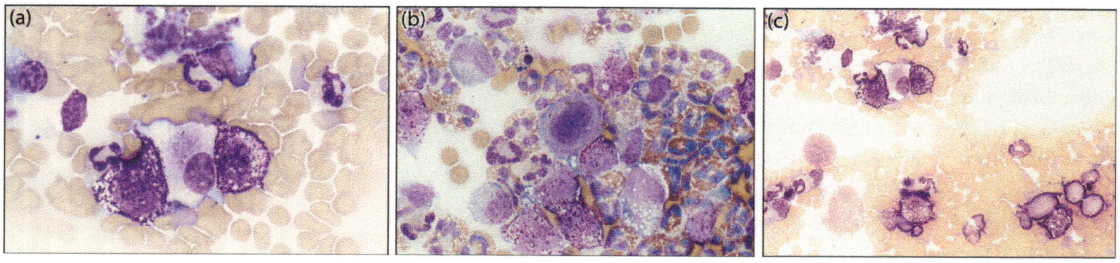

Figures 7.66a–c Colonic mast cell tumor in a dog with multifocal disease. (a) Cytology of the colonic mass is hemodilute with small clusters of well-granulated mast cells (Wright–Giemsa, 1000× magnification). (b) Abdominal fluid from the same patient. Large numbers of eosinophils are found among frequent atypical mast cells. (c) Splenic metastasis (Wright–Giemsa, 400× magnification).

Mast cell tumors

Mast cell tumors are often localized to the large intestines of cats, but are rarely diagnosed in dogs (Ozaki *et al.*, 2002; Rissetto *et al.*, 2011; Sabattini *et al.*, 2016). Similar to that noted in the small intestine above, these may occur as solitary mass lesions, but are often multifocal. Metastasis and paraneoplastic syndromes may be present at diagnosis in both species (Figure 7.66a–c).

CASES

CASE 1

Signalment/history

A 9-year-old, spayed female Siamese cat presented for progressive weight loss and diarrhea, with recent onset of anorexia and occasional vomiting.

Physical examination

Thin cat with diffuse muscle atrophy. A large mid-abdominal mass was palpated.

Ultrasound

Loss of the normal definition of the wall layers was present. The intestinal wall was hypoechoic with variable luminal width in the area of the diseased intestine. An ovoid mass was noted at the cranial border of this intestinal mass, which likely represented enlarged lymph nodes involved in the mass. A small amount of peritoneal fluid was also noted at this time.

Cytology

FNA of the mass was performed utilizing a 22-gauge needle attached to a 12 ml syringe. Mild suction was successful in acquiring a diagnostic sample. Wright–Giemsa staining of several slides revealed several aggregates of cohesive-appearing cells (Figures 7.67a, b). Individual cells were ovoid to slightly polygonal in shape. They were often poorly preserved and displayed moderate to marked criteria for malignancy including anisocytosis and increased cytoplasmic basophilia. Many also contained prominent and often multiple nucleoli, and cell borders were occasionally less distinct (Figure 7.67b). Cytoplasmic vacuolation was consistent among the cells, suggesting glandular origin. The cytologic findings were consistent with adenocarcinoma. Similar neoplastic cells were found in an aspirate of an abdominal lymph node, confirming the suspicion of metastasis. Due to a poor prognosis, the cat was humanely euthanized and necropsy was performed.

Diagnosis

Intestinal adenocarcinoma.

Necropsy

Gross necropsy revealed the mass to be associated with the mid-intestine (Figures 7.68a, b). Dilatation of the adjacent bowel was found due

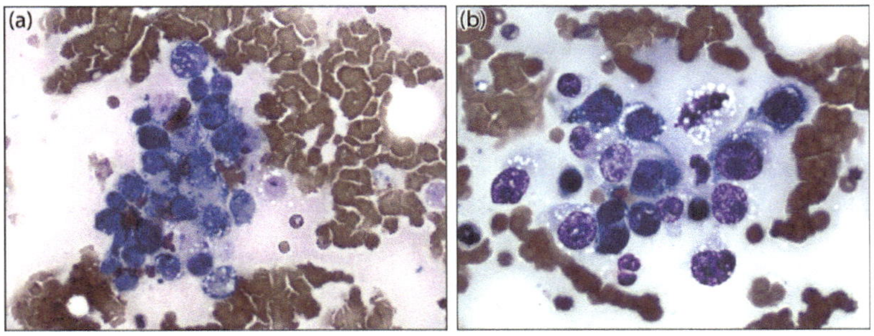

Figures 7.67a, b Intestinal mass from Case 1, feline. (a) Cohesive aggregate of neoplastic cells with moderate to marked criteria for malignancy is present. (b) Pleomorphism and cell disruption are present among the aggregates (Wright–Giemsa, 500× magnification).

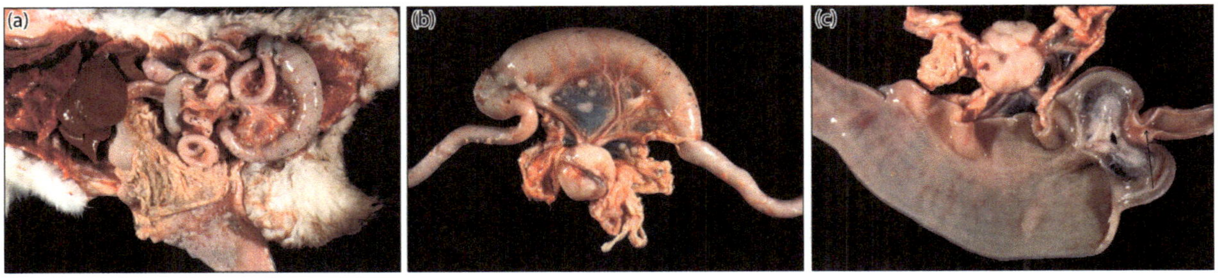

Figures 7.68a–c Intestinal mass from Case 1, feline. (a) Lesion *in situ*. (b) Mesenteric and lymph node metastases are present. (c) Annular constriction and dilatation are noted on longitudinal sectioning of the intestine. (Courtesy Barry Cooper.)

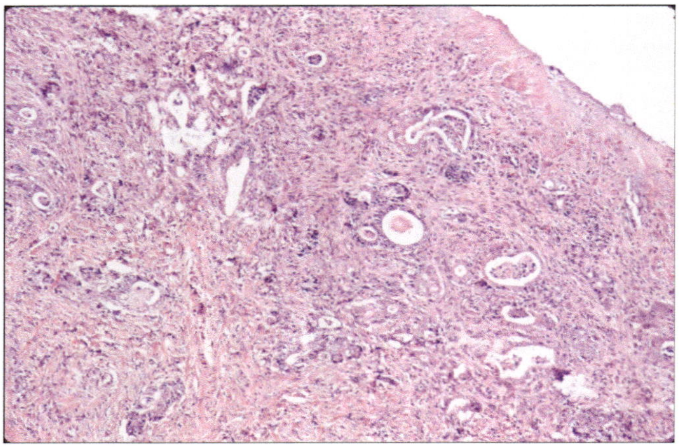

Figure 7.69 **Histology of the mass from Case 1, feline. Note the presence of glandular structures (H&E, 40× magnification). (Courtesy Barry Cooper.)**

to annular sclerosis (Figure 7.68c). Metastasis to adjacent structures, including mesentery, omentum, and lymph nodes, was present.

Histology

Histopathology from the lesion showed invasion of the intestinal wall approaching the serosa. Glandular structures were clearly visible within dense collagenous tissue, confirming the cytologic diagnosis of adenocarcinoma (Figure 7.69).

CASE 2

Signalment/history

An 8-year-old, neutered male mixed-breed dog was presented because of recent onset of exercise intolerance and inappetence. Serum biochemistry revealed hypoalbuminemia of 2.1 g/dl (21 g/l) (RI = 2.7–3.9 [27–39]) and an elevated canine-specific pancreatic lipase of >1,000 µg/l (RI = 0–200), prompting an initial, presumptive diagnosis of pancreatitis.

Physical examination

Good body condition and unremarkable findings.

Ultrasound

Mild dilation of the intestines and loss of wall layering were noted. There was also irregular folding of the jejunum at other sites (suggestive of possible irritation). In some regions of the intestine, the adjacent mesentery was hyperechoic.

Cytology

FNA of the irregular region of intestine was attempted utilizing a 22-gauge needle attached to a 12 ml syringe. Wright–Giemsa-stained slides revealed the presence of a mixed lymphoid population, which included several intermediate-sized lymphocytes (Figure 7.70). The cytology was interpreted as consistent with either atypical lymphoid hyperplasia or possible lymphoma. Biopsy of the lesion was recommended.

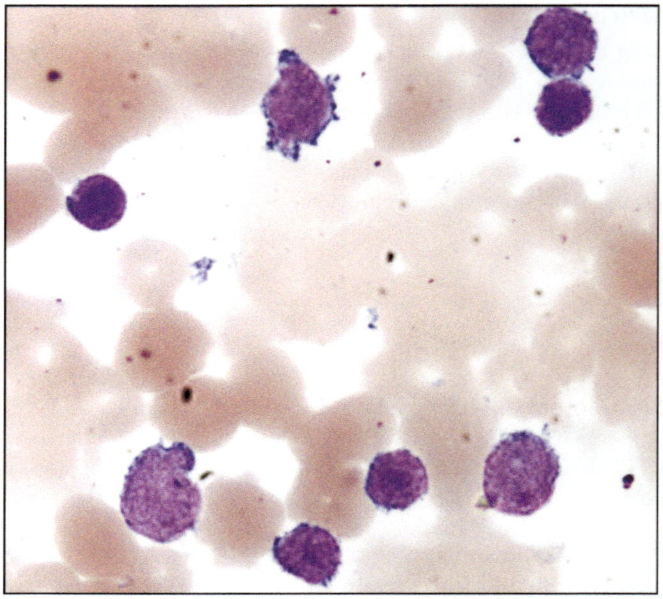

Figure 7.70 **Cytology from an aspirate of thickened intestine. Mixed lymphoid cells are present including several intermediate-sized lymphocytes. The sample was interpreted as either lymphoid hyperplasia or lymphoma (Wright–Giemsa, 1,000× magnification).**

Surgical findings

An 8 cm section of jejunum containing a circumferential, firm, yellowish 2.5 cm thickened region with omental adhesions was identified and resected (Figures 7.71a, b). Numerous plaque-like and pedunculated additional lesions in the adjacent jejunum, proximal duodenum, and omentum were also present and biopsied. Mildly enlarged mesenteric lymph nodes were appreciated and biopsied. The spleen was also mildly enlarged and therefore resected and submitted for histopathology.

A peripheral blood sample was obtained at the time of surgery. The dog had a mild anemia and mild leukocytosis due to a left shift neutrophilia. Additionally, a population of atypical intermediate-sized lymphocytes comprising approximately 11% of the nucleated cell population was identified (Figure 7.72). These cells were approximately 50% larger than neutrophils and contained oval, occasionally clefted or scalloped nuclei with smooth chromatin and indistinct nuclei. They were surrounded by small amounts of basophilic cytoplasm which, on close examination, contained fine eosinophilic granules consistent with granular lymphocytes.

Diagnosis

Lymphoma – intermediate, granular type.

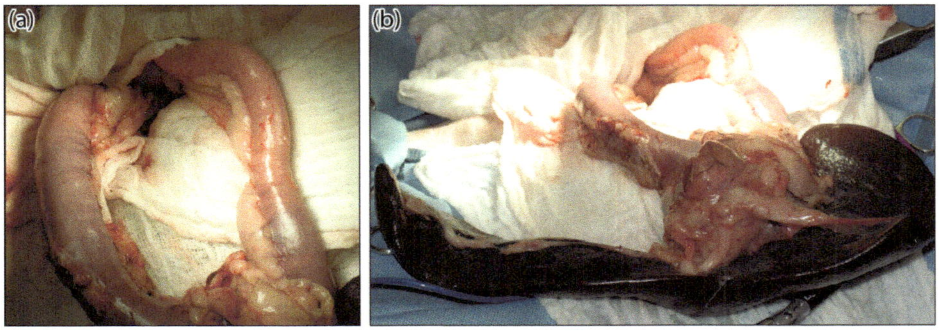

Figures 7.71a, b Intestinal mass and splenomegaly in the dog in Case 2. (a) The small intestine contains multifocal regions of thickening. (b) A larger pedunculated mass of the jejunum is present and adherent to the spleen, which is mildly enlarged.

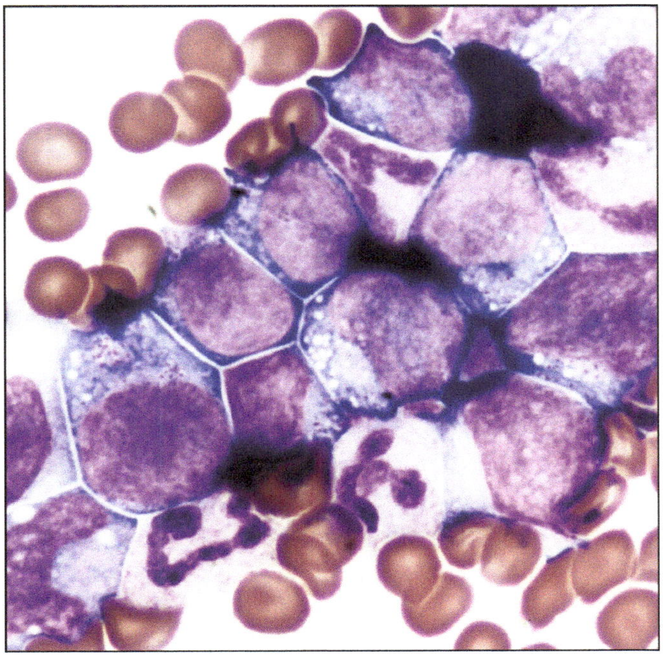

Figure 7.72 Peripheral blood smear from the dog in Case 2. Note the population of intermediate-sized atypical lymphoid cells. Cells typically contain fine eosinophilic granules consistent with granular lymphocytes (Wright–Giemsa, 1,000× magnification).

Histology

Histopathology of the intestine showed diffuse mucosal infiltration by a homogeneous population of small to intermediate-sized lymphocytes with condensed chromatin and a thin rim of indistinct cytoplasm (Figure 7.73). The cells were prominent within the superficial epithelium but not obviously epitheliotropic within the gastric glands. Neoplastic cells infiltrated the submucosa and, to a lesser degree, the muscularis. Mitotic activity was generally low. Similar lymphoid cells were found disrupting and effacing normal splenic and lymph node architecture, confirming visceral spread.

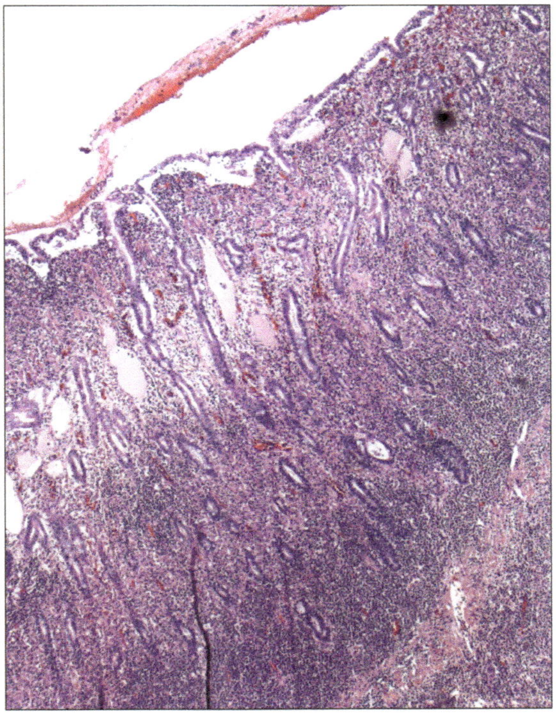

Figure 7.73 Histology of intestine from the dog in Case 2. The normal epithelial architecture is effaced by a population of small to intermediate-sized lymphoid cells. Neoplastic cells infiltrate the submucosa and the muscularis (H&E, 40× magnification).

Based on the cytologic morphology and the likelihood of a T-cell phenotype (likely CD8+, granular form), additional immunostaining for CD3 and CD79 was not pursued.

CASE 3

Signalment/history

A 3-year-old, spayed female Border Collie was presented for evaluation of chronic diarrhea, decreased appetite, and vomiting. Diarrhea

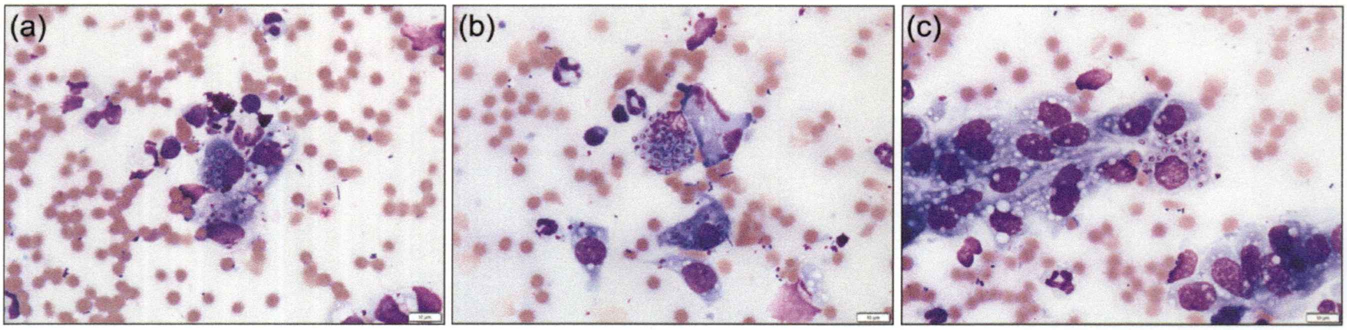

Figures 7.74a–c Cytology from a rectal scraping from a dog with chronic small bowel diarrhea and lymphadenopathy (Wright–Giemsa, 1,000× magnification). (a) Macrophages contain small, intracellular yeast-consistent organisms. Several lymphocytes are also identified. (b) Large numbers of small, circular yeast are found among disrupted cells. (c) A small raft of vacuolated colonic epithelial cells is found. Increased cytoplasmic basophilic along with several multinucleated cells are consistent with reactivity secondary to fungal colitis.

was unresponsive to a diet trial, antibiotics, steroids, or probiotics. Defecation was progressively frequent with small volume bouts of liquid stool production upwards of 14 times per day. Serum biochemistry revealed increased hepatic enzyme and total bilirubin values.

Physical examination

Severely thickened and irregular rectal mucosa and painful upon rectal exam. She was febrile (104.6F/40.3C). Generalized, peripheral lymphadenomegaly was also noted.

A rectal scraping was performed during rectal examination and direct smears of the material were made.

Cytology

Frequent mixed inflammatory cells including macrophages, lymphocytes, and occasional neutrophils were identified among a few small aggregates of colonic epithelium. Numerous small, round yeast organisms were identified among the inflammatory cells with frequent phagocytic activity noted by macrophages (Figure 7.74a–c). Erythrocytes and mixed bacteria were present consistent with hemorrhage and fecal material, respectively.

Diagnosis

Pyogranulomatous colitis secondary to *Histoplasma capsulatum* infection.

The patient was euthanized with no additional staging or treatment (case history and images courtesy of Angela Royal).

REFERENCES

Avery A.C. (2009) Molecular diagnostics of hematologic malignancies. *Top Companion Anim Med 24(3)*:144–150.

Bacha W.J., Bacha L.M. (2012) Digestive system. In: *Color Atlas of Veterinary Histology*, 3rd edn. (eds. W.J. Bacha, L.M. Bacha) Wiley-Blackwell, Ames, pp. 139–182.

Ballegeer E.A., Forrest L.J., Dickinson R.M. et al. (2007) Correlation of ultrasonographic appearance of lesions and cytologic and histologic diagnoses in splenic aspirates of dogs and cats: 32 cases (2002–2005). *J Am Vet Med Assoc 230*:690–696.

Barrand K.R., Scudamore C.L. (1999) Intestinal leiomyosarcoma in a cat. *J Small Anim Pract 40(5)*:216–219.

Barrett L.E., Skorupski K., Brown D.C. et al. (2018) Outcome following treatment of feline gastrointestinal mast cell tumours. *Vet Comp Oncol 16(2)*:188–193.

Barrs V.R., Beatty J.A. (2012) Feline alimentary lymphoma: 2. Further diagnostics, therapy and prognosis. *J Feline Med Surg 14(3)*:191–201.

Berryessa N.A., Marks S.L., Pesavento P.A. et al. (2008) Gastrointestinal pythiosis in 10 dogs from California. *J Vet Intern Med 22(4)*:1065–1069.

Berset-Istratescu C.M., Glardon O.J., Magouras I. et al. (2014) Follow-up of 100 dogs with acute diarrhoea in a primary care practice. *Vet J 199(1)*:188–190.

Bonfanti U., Bertazzolo W., Bottero E. et al. (2006) Diagnostic value of cytologic examination of gastrointestinal tract tumors in dogs and cats: 83 cases (2001–2004). *J Am Vet Med Assoc 229(7)*:1130–1133.

Bradford K., Meinkoth J., McKeirnen K. et al. (2013) Candida peritonitis in dogs: Report of 5 cases. *Vet Clin Pathol 42(2)*:227–233.

Bridgeford E.C., Marini R.P., Feng Y. et al. (2008) Gastric *Helicobacter* species as a cause of feline gastric lymphoma: A viable hypothesis. *Vet Immunol Immunopathol 123(1–2)*:106–113.

Briscoe K.A., Krockenberger M.B., Beatty J.A. et al. (2011) Histopathological and immunohistochemical evaluation of 53 cases of feline lymphoplasmacytic enteritis and low-grade alimentary lymphoma. *J Comp Pathol 145(2–3)*:187–198.

Brömel C., Sykes J.E. (2005) Histoplasmosis in dogs and cats. *Clin Tech Small Anim Pract 20(4)*:227–232.

Caniatti M., Roccabianca P., Scanziani E. et al. (1996) Canine lymphoma: Immunocytochemical analysis of fine-needle aspiration biopsy. *Vet Pathol 33(2)*:204–212.

Cave N.J. (2003) Chronic inflammatory bowel disorders of the gastrointestinal tract of companion animals. *N Z Vet J 51(6)*:262–274.

Couto K.M., Moore P.F., Zwingenberger A.L., Willcox J.L., Skorupski K.A. (2018) Clinical characteristics and outcome in dogs with small cell T-cell intestinal lymphoma. *Vet Comp Oncol 16(3)*:337–343.

Craig L.E., Hardam E.E., Hertzke D.M. et al. (2009) Feline gastrointestinal eosinophilic sclerosing fibroplasia. *Vet Pathol 46(1)*:63–70.

Cruz-Arámbulo R., Wrigley R., Powers B. (2004) Sonographic features of histiocytic neoplasms in the canine abdomen. *Vet Radiol Ultrasound 45*(6):554–558.

Dandrieux J.R.S., Mansfield C.S. (2019) Chronic enteropathy in canines: Prevalence, impact and management strategies. *Vet Med (Auckl) 10*:203–214.

Danova N.A., Robles-Emanuelli J.C., Bjorling D.E. (2006) Surgical excision of primary canine rectal tumors by an anal approach in twenty-three dogs. *Vet Surg 35(4)*:337–340.

Del Alcazar C.M., Mahoney J.A., Dittrich K. et al. (2021) Outcome, prognostic factors and histological characterization of canine gastrointestinal sarcomas. *Vet Comp Oncol 19(3)*:578–586.

Dell'Orco M., Bertazzolo W., Vergine M. et al. (2005) Gastric mucinous adenocarcinoma with cutaneous metastases in a dog: Diagnosis by fine-needle aspiration cytology. *J Small Anim Pract 46*(9):449–453.

Dennis J.S., Kruger J.M., Mullaney T.P. (1992) Lymphocytic/plasmacytic gastroenteritis in cats: 14 cases (1985–1990). *J Am Vet Med Assoc 200*(*11*):1712–1718.

Dennis M.M., Bennett N., Ehrhart E.J. (2006) Gastric adenocarcinoma and chronic gastritis in two related Persian cats. *Vet Pathol 43(3)*:358–362.

Frank J.D., Reimer S.B., Kass P.H. et al. (2007) Clinical outcomes of 30 cases of canine gastrointestinal lymphoma. *J Am Anim Hosp Assoc 43*(6):313–321.

Freiche V., Fages J., Paulin M.V. et al. (2021) Clinical, laboratory and ultrasonographic findings differentiating low-grade intestinal T-cell lymphoma from lymphoplasmacytic enteritis in cats. *J Vet Intern Med 35*(6):2685–2696.

Frost D., Lasota J. Miettinen M. (2003) Gastrointestinal stromal tumors and leiomyomas in the dog: A histopathologic, immunohistochemical, and molecular genetic study of 50 cases. *Vet Pathol 40*(*1*):42–54.

Gaastra W., Lipman L.J., De Cock A.W. et al. (2010) *Pythium insidiosum*: An overview. *Vet Microbiol 146*(*1–2*):1–16.

Gabor L.J., Canfield P.J., Malik R. (1999) Immunophenotypic and histological characterisation of 109 cases of feline lymphosarcoma. *Aust Vet J 77*(*7*):436–441.

Gabor L.J., Malik R., Canfield P.J. (1998) Clinical and anatomical features of lymphosarcoma in 118 cats. *Aust Vet J 76*(*11*):725–732.

German A.J., Hall E.J., Day M.J. (2001) Immune cell populations within the duodenal mucosa of dogs with enteropathies. *J Vet Intern Med 15*(*1*):14–25.

German A.J., Hall E.J., Day M.J. (2003) Chronic intestinal inflammation and intestinal disease in dogs. *J Vet Intern Med 17*(*1*):8–20.

German A.J., Holden D.J., Hall E.J. et al. (2002) Eosinophilic diseases in two Cavalier King Charles spaniels. *J Small Anim Pract 43*(*12*):533–538.

Gibson D., Aubert I., Woods J.P. et al. (2004) Flow cytometric immunophenotype of canine lymph node aspirates. *J Vet Intern Med 18*(*5*):710–717.

Gillespie V., Baer K., Farrelly J. et al. (2011) Canine gastrointestinal stromal tumors: Immunohistochemical expression of CD34 and examination of prognostic indicators including proliferation markers Ki67 and AgNOR. *Vet Pathol 48*(*1*):283–291.

Giordano A., Paltrinieri S., Bertazzolo W. et al. (2005) Sensitivity of Tru-cut and fine needle aspiration biopsies of liver and kidney for diagnosis of feline infectious peritonitis. *Vet Clin Pathol 34*(*4*):368–374.

Glanemann B., Schönenbrücher H., Bridger N. et al. (2008) Detection of *Mycobacterium avium* subspecies paratuberculosis-specific DNA by PCR in intestinal biopsies of dogs. *J Vet Intern Med 22*(*5*):1090–1094.

Graves T.K., Barger A.M., Adams B. et al. (2005) Diagnosis of systemic cryptococcosis by fecal cytology in a dog. *Vet Clin Pathol 34*(*4*):409–412.

Grooters A.M. (2003) Pythiosis, lagenidiosis, and zygomycosis in small animals. *Vet Clin North Am Small Anim Pract 33*(*4*):695–720.

Gualtieri M., Monzeglio M.G., Scanziani E. (1999) Gastric neoplasia. *Vet Clin North Am Small Anim Pract 29*(*2*):415–440.

Guilford W.G., Jones B.R., Markwell P.J. et al. (2001) Food sensitivity in cats with chronic idiopathic gastrointestinal problems. *J Vet Intern Med 15*(*1*):7–13.

Hall E.J. (2011) Antibiotic-responsive diarrhea in small animals. *Vet Clin North Am Small Anim Pract 41*(*2*):273–286.

Halsey C.H.C., Powers B.E., Kamstock D.A. (2010) Feline intestinal sclerosing mast cell tumor: 50 cases (1997–2008). *Vet Comp Oncol 8*(*1*):72–79.

Hart J.R., Shaker E., Patnaik A.K. et al. (1994) Lymphocytic-plasmacytic enterocolitis in cats: 60 cases (1988–1990). *J Am Anim Hosp Assoc 30*(*5*):505–514.

Hartmann K. (2011) Clinical aspects of feline immunodeficiency and feline leukemia virus infection. *Vet Immunol Immunopathol 143*(*3–4*):190–201.

Hayes S., Yuzbasiyan-Gurkan V., Gregory-Bryson E. et al. (2013) Classification of canine nonangiogenic, nonlymphogenic, gastrointestinal sarcomas based on microscopic, immunohistochemical and molecular characteristics. *Vet Pathol 50*(*5*):779–788.

Howl J.H., Petersen M.G. (1995) Intestinal mast cell tumor in a cat: Presentation as eosinophilic enteritis. *J Am Anim Hosp Assoc 31*(*6*):457–461.

Jacobs G., Collins-Kelly L., Lappin M.R. et al. (1990) Lymphocytic-plasmacytic enteritis in 24 dogs. *J Vet Intern Med 4*(*2*):45–53.

Jergens A.E. (1999) Inflammatory bowel disease. Current perspectives. *Vet Clin North Am Small Anim Pract 29*:501–521.

Jergens A.E., Andreasen C.B., Hagemoser W.A. et al. (1998) Cytologic examination of exfoliative specimens obtained during endoscopy for diagnosis of gastrointestinal tract disease in dogs and cats. *J Am Vet Med Assoc 213*(*12*):1755–1759.

Jergens A.E., Heilmann R.M. (2022) Canine chronic enteropathy-current state-of-the-art and emerging concepts. *Front Vet Sci 9*:923013.

Jergens A.E., Moore F.M., Haynes J.S. et al. (1992) Idiopathic inflammatory bowel disease in dogs and cats: 84 cases (1987–1990). *J Am Vet Med Assoc 201*(*10*):1603–1608.

Jergens A.E., Pressel M., Crandell J. et al. (2009) Fluorescence in-situ hybridization confirms clearance of visible *Helicobacter* spp. associated with gastritis in dogs and cats. *J Vet Intern Med 23*(*1*):16–23.

Johnson S.E. (1992) Canine eosinophilic gastroenterocolitis. *Sem Vet Med Surg Small Animal 7*(*2*):145–152.

Johnston L., Mackay B., King T. et al. (2021) Abdominal cryptococcosis in dogs and cats: 38 cases (2000–2018). *J Small Anim Pract 62*(*1*):19–27.

Karadsheh Z., Al-Haddad M. (2014) Endoscopic, ultrasound guided fine needle tissue acquisition: Where we stand in 2013. *World J Gastroenterol 20*(*9*):2179–2185.

Kehl A., Törner K., Jordan A., Lorenz M. et al. (2022) Pathological findings in gastrointestinal neoplasms and polyps in 860 cats and a pilot study on miRNA analyses. *Vet Sci 9*(*9*):477.

Keller R.L., Avery A.C., Burnett R.C. et al. (2004) Detection of neoplastic lymphocytes in peripheral blood of dogs with lymphoma by polymerase chain reaction for antigen receptor gene rearrangement. *Vet Clin Pathol 33*(*3*):145–149.

Kiupel M., Smedley R.C., Pfent C. et al. (2011) Diagnostic algorithm to differentiate lymphoma from inflammation in feline small intestinal biopsy samples. *Vet Pathol 48*(*1*):212–222.

Kleinschmidt S., Harder J., Nolte I. et al. (2009) Chronic inflammatory and noninflammatory diseases of the gastrointestinal tract in cats: Diagnostic advantages of full-thickness intestinal and extraintestinal lesions. *J Feline Med Surg 12*(*2*):97–103.

Kobayashi M., Sugisaki O., Ishii N. et al. (2012) Canine intestinal mast cell tumor with c-kit exon 8 mutation responsive to imatinib therapy. *Vet J 193*(*1*):264–267.

Koterbay A.M., Muthupalani S., Fox J.G., McNiel E.A. (2020) Risk and characteristics of gastric carcinoma in the chow chow dog. *Can Vet J 61*(*4*):396–400.

Krick E., Little L., Patel R. et al. (2008) Description of clinical and pathological findings, treatment and outcome of feline large granular lymphocyte lymphoma (1996–2004). *Vet Comp Oncol 6(2)*:102–110.

Kuan S., Hoffmann K., Tisdall P. (2009) Ultrasonographic and surgical findings of a gastric hyperplastic polyp resulting in pyloric obstruction in an 11-week-old French Bulldog. *Aust Vet J 87(6)*:253–255.

Kukanich K.S., Vinasco J., Scott H.M. (2013) Detection of *Mycobacterium avium* subspecies *paratuberculosis* from intestinal and nodal tissue of dogs and cats. *ISRN Vet Sci* 323–671.

Kupanoff P.A., Popovitch C.A., Goldschmidt M.H. (2006) Colorectal plasmacytomas: A retrospective study of nine dogs. *J Am Anim Hosp Assoc 42(1)*:37–43.

Lana S.E., Jackson T.L., Burnett R.C. et al. (2006) Utility of polymerase chain reaction for analysis of antigen receptor rearrangement in staging and predicting prognosis in dogs with lymphoma. *J Vet Intern Med 20(2)*:329–334.

Lane J., Price J., Moore A. et al. (2018) Low-grade gastrointestinal lymphoma in dogs: 20 cases (2010 to 2016). *J Small Anim Pract 59(3)*:147–153.

LaRock R.G., Ginn P.E. (1997) Immunohistochemical staining characteristics of canine gastrointestinal stromal tumors. *Vet Pathol 34(4)*:303–311.

Laurenson M.P., Skorupski K.A., Moore P.F. et al. (2011) Ultrasonography of intestinal mast cell tumors in the cat. *Vet Radiol Ultrasound 52(3)*:330–334.

Lingard A.E., Briscoe K., Beatty J.A. et al. (2009) Low-grade alimentary lymphoma: Clinicopathological findings and response to treatment in 17 cases. *J Feline Med Surg 11(8)*:692–700.

Linton M., Nimmo J.S., Norris J.M. et al. (2015) Feline gastrointestinal eosinophilic sclerosing fibroplasia: 13 cases and review of an emerging clinical entity. *J Feline Med Surg 17(5)*:392–404.

London C.A., Thamm D.H. (2020) Mast cell tumors. In: *Withrow and MacEwen's Small Animal Clinical Oncology*, 6th edn. (eds. D.M. Vail, D.H. Thamm, J.M. Liptak) Elsevier, St Louis, pp. 382–403.

Louwerens M., London C.A., Pedersen N.C. et al. (2005) Feline lymphoma in the post-feline leukemia virus era. *J Vet Intern Med 19(3)*:329–335.

Lubbes D., Mandigers P.J., Heuven H.C. et al. (2009) Incidence of gastric carcinoma in Dutch Tervueren shepherd dogs born between 1991 and 2002. *Tijdschr Diergeneeskd 134(14–15)*:606–610.

Lurie D.M., Milner R.J., Suter S.E. et al. (2008) Immunophenotypic and cytomorphologic subclassification of T-cell lymphoma in the boxer breed. *Vet Immunol Immunopathol 125(1–2)*:102–110.

Lyles S.E., Panciera D.L., Saunders G.K. et al. (2009) Idiopathic eosinophilic masses of the gastrointestinal tract in dogs. *J Vet Intern Med 23(4)*:818–823.

Maas C.P., ter Haar G., van der Gaag I. et al. (2007) Reclassification of small intestinal and cecal smooth muscle tumors in 72 dogs: Clinical, histological, and immunohistochemical evaluation. *Vet Surg 36(4)*:302–313.

Maeda S., Tsuboi M., Sakai K. et al. (2017) Endoscopic cytology for the diagnosis of chronic enteritis and intestinal lymphoma in dogs. *Vet Pathol 54(4)*:595–604.

Makielski K., Cullen J., O'Connor A., Jergens A.E. (2019) Narrative review of therapies for chronic enteropathies in dogs and cats. *J Vet Intern Med 33(1)*:11–22.

Manchester A.C., Hill S., Sabatino B. et al. (2013) Association between granulomatous colitis in French Bulldogs and invasive *Escherichia coli* and response to fluoroquinolone antimicrobials. *J Vet Intern Med 27(1)*:56–61.

Masuda M., Jagielski T., Danesi P. et al. (2021) Protothecosis in dogs and cats-new research directions. *Mycopathologia 186(1)*:143–152.

Moore P.F., Rodriguez-Bertos A., Kass P.H. (2012) Feline gastrointestinal lymphoma: Mucosal architecture, immunophenotype, and molecular clonality. *Vet Pathol 49(4)*:658–668.

Morini M., Gentilini F., Pietra M. et al. (2011) Cytological, immunohistochemical and mutational analysis of a gastric gastrointestinal stromal tumour in a cat. *J Comp Pathol 145(2–3)*:152–157.

Munday J.S., Löhr C.V., Kiupel M. (2017) Tumors of the alimentary tract. In: *Tumors in Domestic Animals*, 5th edn. (ed. D.J. Meuten) Wiley Blackwell Publishing, Ames, pp. 499–601.

Neiger R., Simpson K.W. (2000) *Helicobacter* infection in dogs and cats: Facts and fiction. *J Vet Intern Med 14(2)*:125–133.

Olsson M., Frankowiack M., Tengvall K. et al. (2014) The dog as a genetic model for immunoglobulin A (IgA) deficiency: Identification of several breeds with low serum IgA concentrations. *Vet Immunol Immunopathol 160(3–4)*:255–259.

Ozaki K., Yamagami T., Nomura K., Narama I. (2002) Mast cell tumors of the gastrointestinal Tract in 39 Dogs. *Vet Pathol 39(5)*:557–564.

Pastor M., Chalvet-Monfray K., Marchal T. et al. (2009) Genetic and environmental risk indicators in canine non-Hodgkin's lymphomas: Breed associations and geographic distribution of 608 cases diagnosed throughout France over 1 year. *J Vet Intern Med 23(2)*:301–310.

Patnaik A.K. (1990) Canine extraskeletal osteosarcoma and chondrosarcoma: A clinicopathologic study of 14 cases. *Vet Pathol 27(1)*:46–55.

Peaston A.E., Griffey S.M. (1994) Visceral mast cell tumour with eosinophilia and eosinophilic peritoneal and pleural effusions in a cat. *Aust Vet J 71(7)*:215–217.

Pesciaroli M., Alvarez J., Boniotti M.B. et al. (2014) Tuberculosis in domestic animal species. *Res Vet Sci 97*:S78–S85.

Porras-Silesky C., Mejías-Alpízar M.J., Mora J. et al. (2021) *Spirocerca lupi* proteomics and its role in cancer development: An overview of spirocercosis-induced sarcomas and revision of helminth-induced carcinomas. *Pathogens 10(2)*:124.

Ramos-Vara J.A., Miller M.A., Pace L.W. et al. (1998) Intestinal multinodular A lambda-amyloid deposition associated with extramedullary plasmacytoma in three dogs: Clinicopathological and immunohistochemical studies. *J Comp Pathol 119(3)*:239–249.

Rassnick K.M., Moore A.S., Collister K.E. et al. (2009) Efficacy of combination chemotherapy for treatment of gastrointestinal lymphoma in dogs. *J Vet Intern Med 23(2)*:317–322.

Richter K.P. (2003) Feline gastrointestinal lymphoma. *Vet Clin North Am Small Anim Pract 33*:1083–1098.

Rimpo K., Hirabayashi M., Tanaka A. (2022) Lymphoma in Miniature Dachshunds: A retrospective multicenter study of 108 cases (2006–2018) in Japan. *J Vet Intern Med 36(4)*:1390–1397.

Rissetto K., Villamil J.A., Selting K.A. et al. (2011) Recent trends in feline intestinal neoplasia: An epidemiologic study of 1,129 cases in the veterinary medical database from 1964–2004. *J Am Anim Hosp Assoc 47(1)*:28–36.

Rivers B.J., Walter P.A., Johnston G.R. et al. (1997) Canine gastric neoplasia: Utility of ultrasonography in diagnosis. *J Am Anim Hosp Assoc 33(2)*:144–155.

Roccabianca P., Vernau W., Caniatti M. et al. (2006) Feline large granular lymphocyte (LGL) lymphoma with secondary leukemia: Primary intestinal origin with predominance of a CD3/CD8 alpha alpha phenotype. *Vet Pathol 43(1)*:15–28.

Rossi M., Hänninen M.L., Revez J. et al. (2008) Occurrence and species level diagnostics of *Campylobacter* spp., enteric *Helicobacter* spp. and *Anaerobiospirillum* spp. in healthy and diarrheic dogs and cats. *Vet Microbiol 129(3–4)*:304–314.

Russell K.N., Mehler S.J., Skorupski K.A. et al. (2007) Clinical and immunohistochemical differentiation of gastrointestinal stromal tumors from leiomyosarcomas in dogs: 42 cases (1990–2003). *J Am Vet Med Assoc 230(9)*:1329–1333.

Sabattini S., Giantin M., Barbanera A. et al. (2016) Feline intestinal mast cell tumours: Clinicopathological characterisation and KIT mutation analysis. *J Feline Med Surg 18(4)*:280–289.

Saito T., Chambers J.K., Nakashima K. et al. (2018) Histopathologic features of colorectal adenoma and adenocarcinoma developing within inflammatory polyps in Miniature Dachshunds. *Vet Pathol 55(5)*:654–662.

Sapierzyński R., Malicka E., Zmudzka M. et al. (2006) The diagnosis of gastritis and helicobacter-like organisms infection in endoscopic biopsies of the canine gastric mucosa. *Pol J Vet Sci 9(1)*:17–21.

Sato H., Fujino Y., Uchida K. et al. (2011) Comparison between immunohistochemistry and genetic clonality analysis for cellular lineage determination in feline lymphomas. *J Vet Med Sci 73(7)*:945–947.

Schultz R.M., Johnson E.G., Wisner E.R. et al. (2008) Clinicopathologic and diagnostic imaging characteristics of systemic aspergillosis in 30 dogs. *J Vet Intern Med 22(4)*:851–859.

Seim-Wikse T., Jörundsson E., Nødtvedt A. et al. (2013) Breed predisposition to canine gastric carcinoma: A study based on the Norwegian canine cancer register. *Acta Vet Scand 55(1)*:25.

Sellon R.K., Willard M.D. (2003) Esophagitis and esophageal strictures. *Vet Clin North Am Small Anim Pract 33(5)*:945–967.

Shor S., Helfand S.C., Gorman E. et al. (2009) Diagnostic exercise: Epithelioid hemangiosarcoma mimicking metastatic prostatic neoplasia in a dog. *Vet Pathol 46(3)*:548–552.

Sims C.S., Nagle J., Tolbert K.M. et al. (2022) Correlation of cytology to histology in a case of canine granulomatous colitis in a Boxer dog. *Vet Clin Pathol 50*:83–87.

Slawienski M.J., Mauldin G.E., Mauldin G.N. et al. (1997) Malignant colonic neoplasia in cats: 46 cases (1990–1996). *J Am Vet Med Assoc 211(7)*:878–881.

Sözmen M., Tasca S., Carli E. et al. (2005) Use of fine needle aspirates and flow cytometry for the diagnosis, classification, and immunophenotyping of canine lymphomas. *J Vet Diagn Invest 17(4)*:323–330.

Stefanello D., Valenti P., Faverzani S. et al. (2009) Ultrasound-guided cytology of spleen and liver: A prognostic tool in canine cutaneous mast cell tumor. *J Vet Intern Med 23(5)*:1051–1057.

Suchodolski J.S. (2022) Analysis of the gut microbiome in dogs and cats: Review Article. *Vet Clin Pathol 50*:6–17.

Suchodolski J.S., Morris E.K., Allenspach K. et al. (2008) Prevalence and identification of fungal DNA in the small intestine of healthy dogs and dogs with chronic enteropathies. *Vet Microbiol 132*(3–4):379–388.

Suwa A., Shimoda T. (2017) Intestinal gastrointestinal stromal tumor in a cat. *J Vet Med Sci 79(3)*:562–566.

Taillieu E., Chiers K., Amorim I. et al. (2022) Gastric Helicobacter species associated with dogs, cats and pigs: Significance for public and animal health. *Vet Res 53(1)*:42.

Takahashi T., Kadosawa T., Nagase M. et al. (2000) Visceral mast cell tumors in dogs: 10 cases (1982–1997). *J Am Vet Med Assoc 216(2)*:222–226.

Tucker S., Penninck D.G., Keating J.H. et al. (2014) The clinicopathological and ultrasonographic features of cats with eosinophilic enteritis. *J Feline Med Surg 16(12)*:950–956.

Uchida E., Chambers J.K., Nakashima K. et al. (2016) Pathologic features of colorectal inflammatory polyps in miniature dachshunds. *Vet Pathol 53(4)*:833–839.

Uchiumi K., Stowe D.M., DeVanna J.C. et al. (2014) Pathology in practice. *Cryptococcus* sp. in a dog. *J Am Vet Med Assoc 245(8)*:893–895.

Valerius K.D., Powers B.E., McPherron M.A. et al. (1997) Adenomatous polyps and carcinoma in situ of the canine colon and rectum: 34 cases (1982–1994). *J Am Vet Med Assoc 33(2)*:156–160.

Van den Steen N., Berlato D., Polton G. et al. (2012) Rectal lymphoma in 11 dogs: A retrospective study. *J Small Anim Pract 53(10)*:586–591.

Vezzali E., Parodi A.L., Marcato P.S. et al. (2010) Histopathologic classification of 171 cases of canine and feline non-Hodgkin lymphoma according to the WHO. *Vet Comp Oncol 8(1)*:38–49.

von Babo V., Eberle N., Mischke R. et al. (2012) Canine non-hematopoietic gastric neoplasia. Epidemiologic and diagnostic characteristics in 38 dogs with post-surgical outcome of five cases. *Tierärztl Prax Ausg K Kleintiere Heimtiere 40(4)*:243–249.

Weese J.S. (2011) Bacterial enteritis in dogs and cats: Diagnosis, therapy, and zoonotic potential. *Vet Clin North Am Small Anim Pract 41(2)*:287–309.

Weiss A.T.A., Klopfleisch R., Gruber A.D. (2011) T-cell receptor γ chain variable and joining region genes of subgroup 1 are clonally rearranged in feline B- and T-cell lymphoma. *J Comp Pathol 144(2–3)*:123–134.

Weissman A., Penninck D., Webster C. et al. (2013) Ultrasonographic and clinicopathological features of feline gastrointestinal eosinophilic sclerosing fibroplasia in four cats. *J Feline Med Surg 15(2)*:148–154.

Willard M.D. (2012) Alimentary neoplasia in geriatric dogs and cats. *Vet Clin North Am Small Anim Pract 42(4)*:693–706.

Zikes C.D., Spielman B., Shapiro W. et al. (1998) Gastric extramedullary plasmacytoma in a cat. *J Vet Intern Med 12(5)*:381–383.

CHAPTER 8

CYTOLOGY OF THE PANCREAS

Catherine Trumel, Marie-Noëlle Lucas, Catherine Layssol, Fanny Granat, and Nathalie Bourgès-Abella

INTRODUCTION

Investigation of canine and feline pancreatic disease remains a real challenge for veterinary practitioners. The diagnostic approach usually requires several investigative tools such as CBC, biochemistry profile, diagnostic imaging, cytology, and histology.

In human medicine, for about 20 years, fine needle aspiration has been considered the standard pancreatic biopsy technique, supported by the accuracy of cytologic diagnosis and the safety of the technique (Smith et al., 1985). In the 1990s, pancreas endoscopic ultrasound-guided biopsy emerged and progressively replaced other sampling modalities, becoming the technique of choice for the detection (allowing the placement of the transducer close to the organ, providing high-quality images) and the cytologic biopsy of pancreatic lesions. Fine needle aspiration of the pancreas guided by endoscopic ultrasound (EUS FNA) is now currently used to obtain cytological and/or histological samples of solid pancreatic lesions with high diagnostic performance and a low rate of complications. Many publications (original articles and reviews) about EUS FNA performance, efficacy, technique, and complications are available, in which pancreatic EUS FNA is particularly described and debated (Siddiqui *et al.*, 2009; Dumonceau *et al.*, 2011; Baghbanian *et al.*, 2012; Eisendrath *et al.*, 2014; Fujii *et al.*, 2014; Iglesias-Garcia *et al.*, 2014; Petrone *et al.*, 2014). A recent study reported EUS FNA sensitivity, specificity, and accuracy of 88%, 100%, and 90%, respectively, for diagnosis of pancreatic adenocarcinoma (Baghbanian *et al.*, 2012). A review article described potential EUS FNA adverse effects; some are related to the endoscopic ultrasound route such as perforation or infections; other complications such as peritonitis, bleeding, or tumor seeding along the needle tract are mainly related to fine needle aspiration (Fujii & Levy, 2014). The complication rate of EUS FNA is approximately 1% (Iglesias-Garcia *et al.*, 2014). Acute pancreatitis has been reported in up to 2% of pancreatic EUS FNA, which is less than previously reported with percutaneous pancreatic FNA (Iglesias-Garcia *et al.*, 2014).

In veterinary medicine, EUS is not yet currently available and only one recent study described the feasibility and safety of EUS FNA of the pancreas in healthy Beagle dogs. It is therefore far too early to draw conclusions on EUS FNA diagnostic yield in veterinary medicine; more studies about EUS FNA in pancreatic disease are necessary. Currently, ultrasound-guided transabdominal fine needle aspiration (US FNA) remains the simplest way to obtain pancreatic cytology. The systematic use of a surgical procedure, including general anesthesia and laparotomy, is not reasonable in daily practice (Watson, 2012). The veterinary literature on canine and feline pancreatic FNA is poor but has grown somewhat in the last decade; obtaining pancreatic cytology is still probably judged as a difficult, unsafe, and irrelevant procedure by many institutions (Cordner *et al.*, 2015; Rudinsky, 2023). However, pancreatic fine needle aspiration has a good diagnostic yield and a low rate of clinical complications according to the most recent study on this topic (Cordner *et al.*, 2015; Rudinsky, 2023).

NORMAL PANCREAS STRUCTURE

Anatomy

Canine and feline pancreas have the same gross anatomic organization: the organ is divided into three linked parts or into two parts (right and left lobes) united at the body of the pancreas. In dogs, the right lobe of the pancreas lies dorsomedial to the descending duodenum, approximately from the middle of the ninth intercostal space to the fourth lumbar vertebra (Evans *et al.*, 2013). The body of the pancreas unites the right and the left lobes at an angle of about 45 degrees and is closely linked to the caudal portion of the pyloric region. The left lobe runs from the body of the pancreas to the left of the abdomen, caudo-dorsally to the stomach and craniodorsally to the transverse colon, ending at the level of the cranial pole of the left kidney. As in the dog, feline pancreas follows the descending part of the duodenum but its distal extremity curves cranially in a hook-shaped manner (Barone, 1997). Moreover, following the pyloroduodenal angle, the feline body of the pancreas is more centrally located in the abdomen than it is in the dog. Unlike the dog, the main pancreatic duct and the common bile duct share the same entry into the feline duodenum, which may explain some pathologic relations between the duodenum, the gall bladder (and its bile duct), and the pancreas in cats (Forman *et al.*, 2021).

Histology

The pancreas is a lobulated, compound, tubuloacinar gland. It is surrounded by a thin collagenous capsule that gives rise to fine connective tissue septa dividing the gland into distinct lobules. Each lobule contains both exocrine and endocrine parts (Figure 8.1). The exocrine glandular component, which constitutes 80% to 85% of the organ, is responsible for the secretion of the pancreatic juice. The

DOI: 10.1201/9781003258551-8

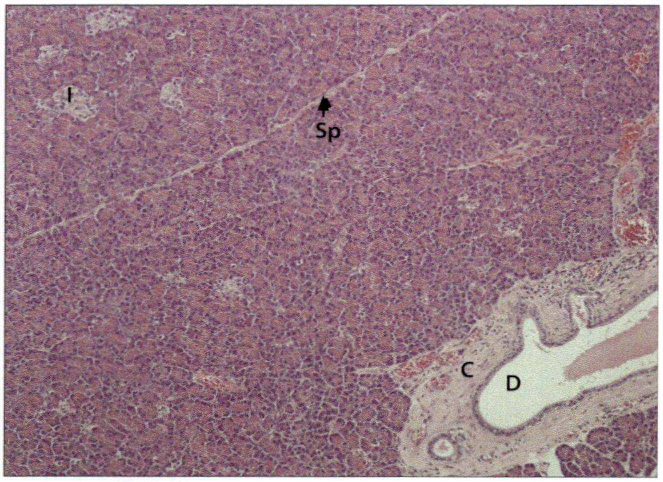

Figure 8.1 Feline pancreas. The mostly represented exocrine component consists of numerous contiguous acini and interlobular duct (D) surrounded by connective tissue (C). Delicate collagenous septa (Sp) are observed between lobules. The endocrine part is composed of clearer clusters of cells, the islets of Langerhans (I), randomly scattered throughout the exocrine part. Hematoxylin and eosin (×40).

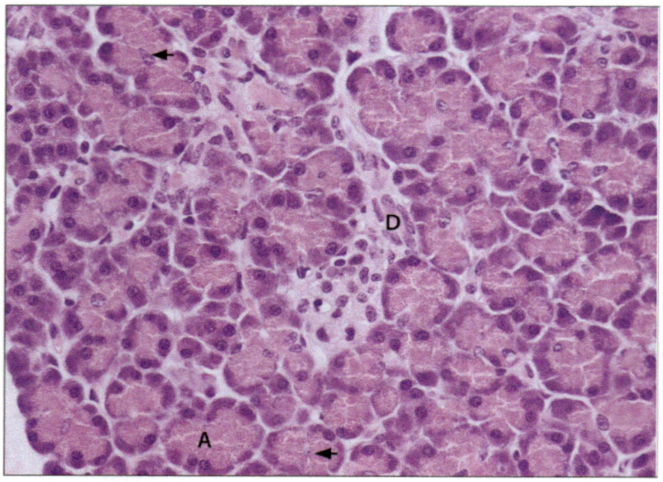

Figure 8.2 Feline pancreas. Exocrine pancreatic acini (A) consist of typical two-colored spherical clusters of cells with a very small central lumen. Pyramid-shaped acinar cells have a basal deep basophilia and an apical granular acidophilia; the spherical nucleus is basal to parabasal. The centers of the acini often contain nuclei of centroacinar cells (arrow). Intercalated duct (D) is lined by a simple low cuboidal epithelium; the small central lumen is filled with eosinophilic pancreatic juice. Hematoxylin and eosin (×400).

exocrine secretory pancreatic acini consist of typical two-colored spherical clusters of cells with a small central lumen, often difficult to see (Figure 8.2). The acinar cells are pyramidal oriented cells with a spherical basal to parabasal nucleus and prominent nucleoli. They have a basal area of the cytoplasm that is deeply basophilic resulting from the accumulation of ribosomes and rough endoplasmic reticulum and an apical granular acidophilic cytoplasmic region due to zymogen granules (Banks, 1993; Eurell & Frappier, 2006). Nuclear and cytoplasmic features are both characteristic of cells highly active in protein synthesis (Figure 8.3). The acini open into a continuous short, narrow, intercalated duct, which begins with squamous to cuboidal epithelial centroacinar cells (Eurell & Frappier, 2006; Kierszenbaum *et al.*, 2019). The latter cells extend into the lumen of the acinus and can be regarded as the intra-acinar part of the intercalated duct; their pale nuclei and sparse pale-stained cytoplasm frequently appear in the center of the acini (Figure 8.3). Weak staining of centroacinar cells and intercalated ducts is due to the secretion of water and bicarbonate ions. The intercalated ducts with narrow lumens drain then into larger intralobular ducts that present a central lumen and a cuboidal epithelium in transversal section. Intralobular ducts communicate with interlobular ducts, and progressively ductal epithelium changes from cuboidal to columnar. As the ductal system becomes confluent, the fine connective tissue associated with the acini and smaller ducts becomes thicker. Goblet cells may be observed among the epithelial cells of the larger ducts (Banks, 1993; Eurell & Frappier, 2006). The endocrine glandular component, the islets of Langerhans, produces mainly insulin and glucagon. Pancreatic islets are randomly scattered throughout the exocrine parenchyma and vary in size (Figure 8.1) (Eurell & Frappier, 2006; Young *et al.*, 2006). They are composed of clusters of pale-staining cells supported by a fine collagenous network containing blood capillaries. The endocrine pale cells appear small compared to the large surrounding exocrine acinar cells (Figure 8.3). Lamellated or Pacini's corpuscles can be observed in the connective tissue of the feline pancreas (Banks, 1993; Eurell & Frappier, 2006). Note that there are differences between histological and cytological

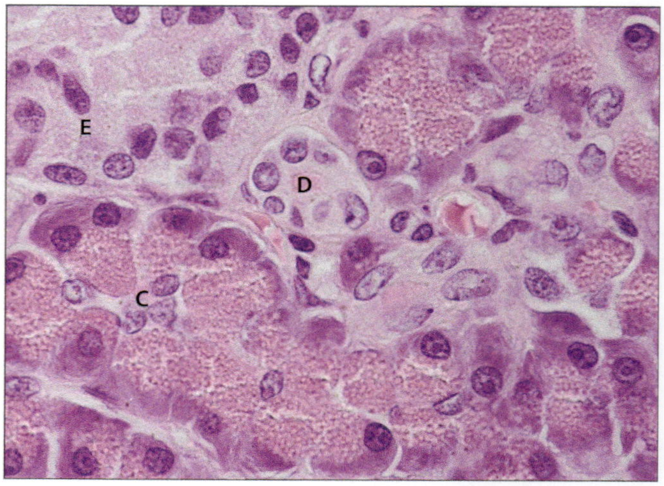

Figure 8.3 Feline pancreas. The polarity of the pyramid-shaped acinar cells can be seen easily at a higher magnification with the basal marked basophilia and the apical granular eosinophilia due to zymogen granules; their round nuclei located basally have prominent nucleoli. The pale nuclei and sparse pale-stained cytoplasm of centroacinar cells (C) appear in the lumen of an acinus. Centroacinar cells represent the intra-acinar part of the intercalated ducts (D) lined by a simple low cuboidal epithelium; the lumen is filled with eosinophilic pancreatic juice. Endocrine secretory cells (E) constitutive of an islet of Langerhans appear as small pale stained cells in contrast to the acinar cells. Hematoxylin and eosin (×1,000).

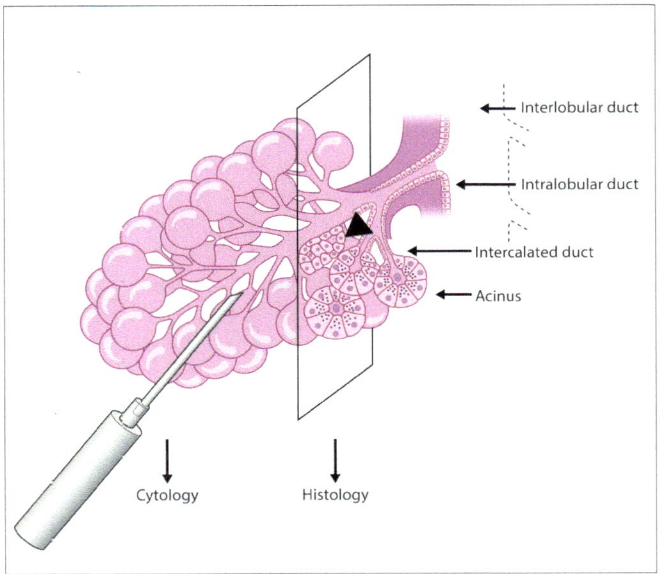

Figure 8.4 **Glandular tubuloacinar organization of a pancreatic lobule with differences between histological and cytological observations consecutive to the different sampling methods. Islet of Langerhans (arrowhead)..**

observations due to the different areas of the pancreas that samples are collected and prepared from (Figure 8.4).

Ultrasound

In dogs, the right lobe of the pancreas is more easily seen than the body and the left lobe. In cats, the left lobe which is larger than the right lobe and the body are more easily identified than the right lobe (Etue *et al.*, 2001; Hecht *et al.*, 2007; Larson, 2016; Griffin, 2020); however, in both species, the pancreas is of relatively small size (thickness ranges from 3.5 to 16 mm in clinically normal dogs and from 2.8 to 9.5 mm in healthy cats) (Etue *et al.*, 2001; Penninck *et al.*, 2013). Also, the pancreas is intimately linked to the digestive tract, which is expected to create numerous artifacts. In healthy dogs, the pancreas usually has poorly distinct margins (Larson, 2016) whereas the feline pancreas is a well-defined organ (Griffin, 2020). In both species, the pancreatic parenchyma is isoechoic to slightly hypoechoic to surrounding mesenteric fat (Hecht & Henry, 2007) even if hyperechoic pancreas has been reported in a small population of healthy dogs, suggesting pancreatic hyperechogenicity could be a rare normal variant in the dog (Granger *et al.*, 2015). The regions dorsal and dorsomedial to the descending duodenum, immediately ventral to the right kidney, are scanned for the right pancreatic lobe. The region ventral to the portal vein is scanned for the pancreatic body. Finally, the region caudal to the greater curvature of the stomach and cranial to the transverse colon is scanned for the left pancreatic lobe, extending toward the spleen and the left kidney in the cat (Robben *et al.*, 2005; Larson, 2016; Griffin, 2020).

Ultrasound-guided fine needle aspiration (US FNA)

Self-evidently, the first step in performing pancreatic US FNA is to visualize the pancreas, which may be difficult, as discussed above. Cordner *et al.* studied pancreatic cytologic FNA yield and secondary effects in 27 healthy dogs. No acute complication or significant increase in serum canine pancreatic lipase immunoreactivity (cPLI) and trypsine-like immunoreactivity (TLI) values after pancreas US FNA were noted, suggesting that the trauma to the pancreas during this procedure is minimal. However, no aspirate was of sufficient quality to be diagnostic. The authors concluded that US FNA of the normal pancreas is unlikely to provide adequate cytologic sample, incriminating the particular tightly associated fibrovascular network of the normal pancreatic tissue and the limited experience of the operator in pancreas US FNA (Cordner *et al.*, 2010). Crain *et al.* reported no increase in complication or mortality rates in cats after pancreatic aspiration, concluding feline US FNA was a safe procedure (Crain *et al.*, 2015). In dogs and cats, transabdominal US FNA feasibility is highly dependent on numerous factors such as patient conformation (deep chest, obesity), ultrasound machine performance, and experience of the radiologist (Robben *et al.*, 2005). Fortunately, pancreatic lesions usually facilitate visualization of the pancreas by significantly changing its echogenicity and its size. However, ultrasonographic findings in various pancreatic diseases overlap, usually preventing the radiologist from establishing a definitive diagnosis, and US FNA is needed to obtain additional diagnostic information (Hecht & Henry, 2007; Vanderperren *et al.*, 2014). When fluid is present in the abdomen, cytopathology of the fluid can be diagnostic in the case of exocrine carcinoma, but it has been shown to have a lower success rate than tissue aspiration (Bennett *et al.*, 2001; Armstrong *et al.*, 2012). To increase the success of pancreatic aspiration, the shortest distance as well as the safest route between the skin and the target must be chosen.

Clean, dry, and grease-free glass slides are set out before the procedure and close to the working area in order to shorten the time between the end of aspiration and the expelling of the sample onto the slide (Bjorneby *et al.*, 2002). The needles most currently mentioned in the literature are 22-gauge single-use disposable spinal or cystocentesis needles (VanEnkevort *et al.*, 1999; Bjorneby & Kari, 2002; Cordner *et al.*, 2010). However, one author suggests that a 25-gauge needle would be effective for cytologic evaluation and less traumatic than larger-gauge needles (Mansfield, 2013). This observation is in accordance with recently published 25-gauge EUS FNA needle performance on solid human pancreatic lesions (Anderson *et al.*, 2008; Siddiqui *et al.*, 2009; Varadarajulu *et al.*, 2014) but has yet to be thoroughly studied in veterinary practice in randomized studies. Crain *et al.* safely aspirated 73 feline pancreas using 20- or 22-gauge hypodermic needles (Crain *et al.*, 2015), and Kook *et al.* used 19-gauge needles for pancreas EUS FNA on 12 dogs with no reported adverse effects (Kook *et al.*, 2012). However, in human medicine, 19-gauge needles are rarely used because they are considered too rigid to pass through the echoendoscope and because of an increased risk of bleeding (Siddiqui *et al.*, 2009).

Three techniques are mentioned in the literature to guide the needle: indirect guidance, needle guidance system, and freehand guidance. Indirect guidance, which refers to the removal of the transducer before inserting the needle, is, in our opinion, highly risky and should not be considered acceptable, particularly for pancreas FNA. The needle guidance system, which uses a biopsy guide attached to the transducer, is described as the easiest biopsy method, allowing the operator to visualize the theoretical needle path by means of dots or lines superimposed on the screen. The third technique, known as freehand guidance, might sound risky but is, with a little practice, far more satisfying than the systematic use of the needle guidance system because of the movement freedom it allows. Once the needle is inserted in the pancreas, aspiration or fenestration techniques are possible as described in Chapter 1.

The smears must be prepared quickly to avoid clotting (Bjorneby & Kari, 2002); the plunger of the syringe is gently pressed to expel the needle content onto the slide. Several slides might be necessary depending on the specimen amount: indeed, a small drop is enough to avoid artifacts. The sample is then smeared using a blood smear technique, taking care not to crush the cellular material. The smears are immediately air dried and labeled before submission (Bjorneby & Kari, 2002).

Cytology

FNA smears from a normal pancreas are often bloody and of poor quality (Cordner *et al.*, 2010; Borjesson, 2014). The main cell population observed is acinar cells from the exocrine portion of the pancreas as it constitutes 98% of the pancreatic mass (Bjorneby & Kari, 2002; Borjesson, 2014). They are often present in clusters organized in a round acinar pattern, but they can also be isolated and disrupted (Figure 8.5). When samples are very cellular, larger lobules can be observed and are quite similar to other lobulated structures such as those in salivary gland cytology (Figures 8.6a and 8.6b). These cells are small to medium (their nucleus is about 10 μm in diameter), with poorly defined cytoplasmic edges, a polygonal or pyramidal form with a round and uniform basal nucleus, a medium to low nuclear to cytoplasmic (N:C) ratio, and granular cytoplasm (Figure 8.5). The cytoplasm is relatively abundant, basophilic, and contains a large quantity of very small eosinophilic granules, the zymogen granules (Borjesson, 2014). Disrupted cells are often observed and the noncellular background is often basophilic and granular (Borjesson, 2014). The nuclei contain heterogeneous chromatin (clumped and granular) with small, occasionally prominent nucleoli (Borjesson, 2014).

Ductal cells can sometimes be seen (Figures 8.7a and 8.7b). These cells are often organized into a typical tubular pattern or in a honeycomb pattern if the ductus is disrupted. The cells are

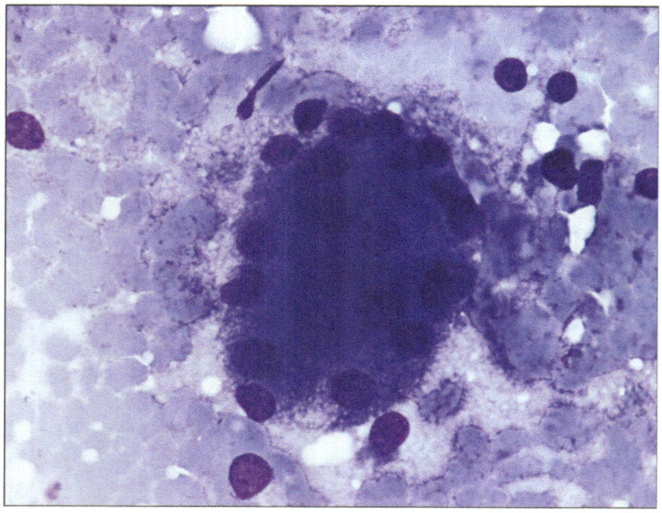

Figure 8.5 Aspirate of a normal pancreas from a dog. Acinar cells. Bloody and granular basophilic background associated with acinar cells. Medium-sized cells with a medium nuclear to cytoplasmic ratio have a pyramidal outline with indistinct cell borders. Their nuclei are eccentric, round with granular and clumped chromatin and a distinct nucleolus. Their cytoplasm is basophilic and characterized by a prominent, coarse cytoplasmic granularity due to zymogen granules. May–Grünwald–Giemsa (×1,000).

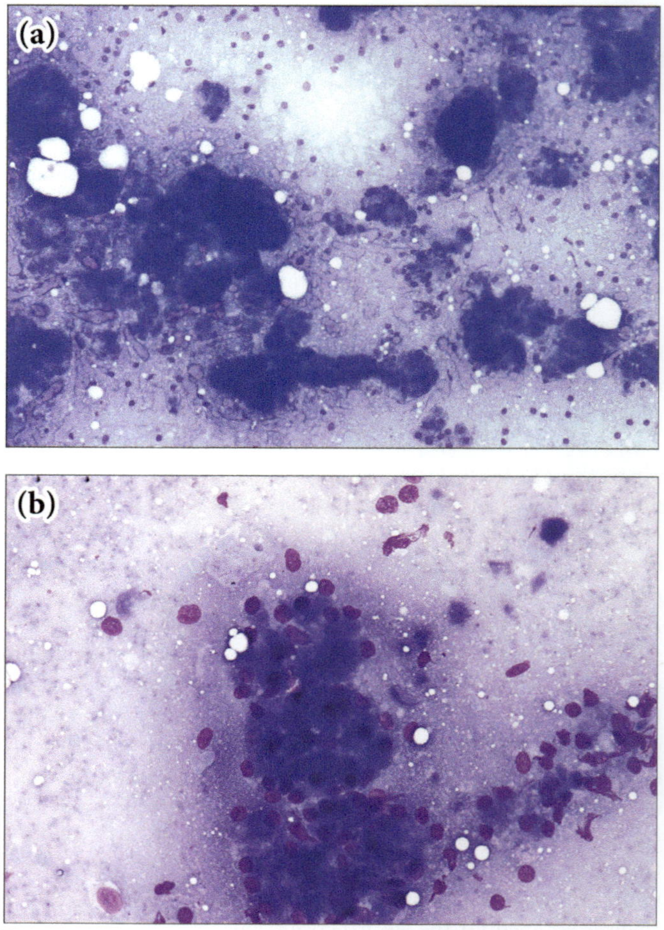

Figure 8.6 a,b Aspirate of a normal pancreas from a cat. Acinar cells. Acinar cells. Bloody and granular basophilic background associated with 2-dimensional microacinar structures and 3-dimensional grape-like clusters and collecting ductal system very similar to salivary gland. May-Grünwald Giemsa (6a: x200; 6b: x400).

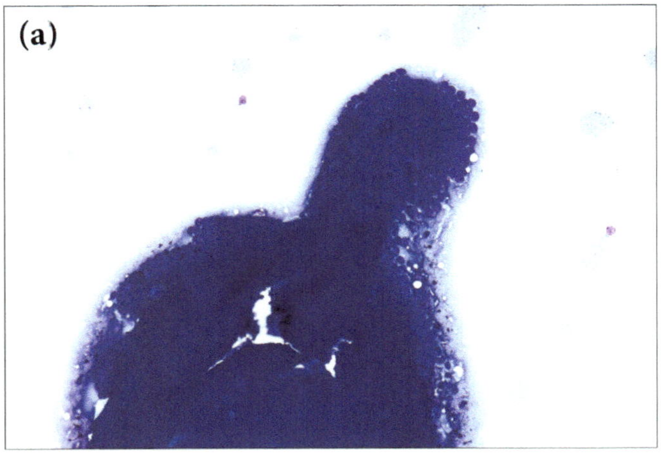

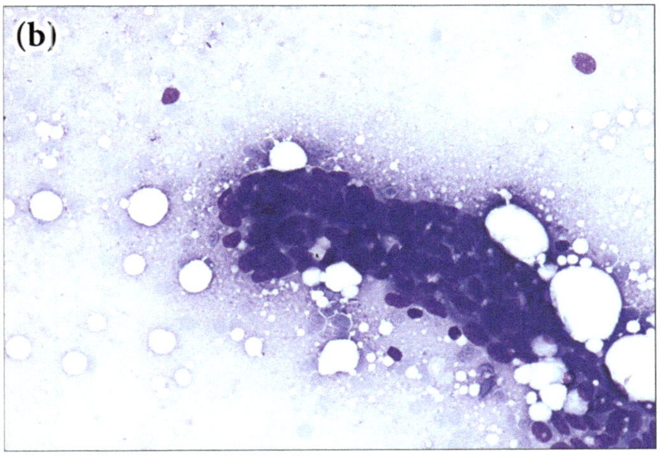

Figures 8.7a, b **Aspirate of a normal pancreas from a cat. Ductal cells. (a) Large and smaller ducts connected. May–Grünwald–Giemsa (×100). (b)Cohesive epithelial cells organized in a tubular pattern. Ductal cells are medium sized with a high nuclear to cytoplasmic ratio and a cuboidal shape. Nuclei are ovoid with a stippled chromatin. Cytoplasm is pale and scant. May-Grünwald Giemsa (x400).**

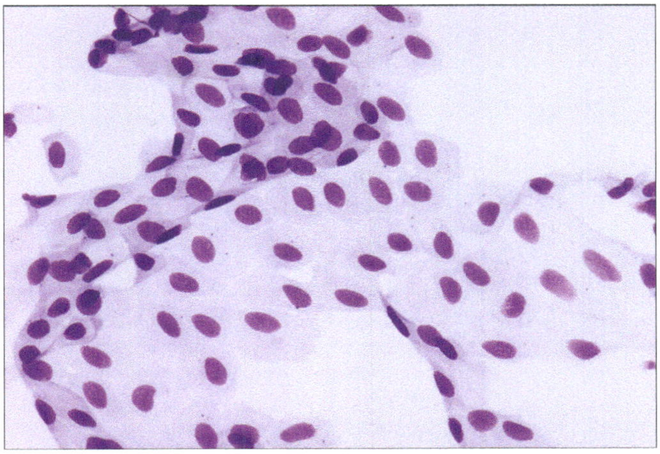

Figure 8.8 **Aspirate of a normal pancreas from a cat. Mesothelial cells. Flat sheet of cohesive uniform cells. These medium-sized cells with a medium nuclear to cytoplasmic ratio are polygonal with well-defined cell borders. Their cytoplasm is delicate, and their ovoid nucleus is finely reticulated. May–Grünwald–Giemsa (×400).**

intermediate-sized with a very high nuclear to cytoplasmic (N:C) ratio, a well-defined light basophilic cytoplasm, and an ovoid nucleus with stippled chromatin. Cells are cuboidal in the small ductus and columnar, sometimes ciliated, in the larger ductal structures (Bjorneby & Kari, 2002).

Mesothelial cells can also be seen (Figure 8.8) (Yang *et al.*, 2008). These medium to large cells are cohesive and organized in thin sheets occasionally with a cobblestone appearance. They are polyhedral, with a light blue well-defined cytoplasm and a central round to ovoid nucleus composed of finely reticular chromatin. Some inflammatory cells can be seen and should be evaluated in light of the blood contamination and leukocyte count. Because of its anatomic relationship with the stomach, intestine, spleen, and kidney, and depending on the sampling procedure, other organs may be sampled inadvertently in addition to the pancreas (Yang & Tao, 2008).

PANCREATIC CYSTIC LESIONS

Pathogenesis and description

Cystic lesions are uncommon in veterinary medicine. Although rare, cystic pancreatic neoplasia should be included as a differential diagnosis of cystic intra-abdominal and pancreatic masses (Yoshimura *et al.*, 2013; Torner *et al.*, 2020). The majority of cystic structures are pseudocysts (VanEnkevort *et al.*, 1999; Charles, 2007). Pseudocysts can be defined as intra- or peripancreatic, fluctuant pockets of pancreatic enzyme secretions, necrotic debris formed by destruction and necrosis of pancreatic tissue, usually caused by pancreatitis or pancreatic trauma. Pseudocysts lack the epithelial lining characteristic of true cysts (Branter *et al.*, 2010). Instead, the wall of a pseudocyst is composed of granulation tissue that can mature into fibrous scar tissue. The lumen contains cellular debris and pancreatic enzymes (Meuten, 2002; Head, 2003; Charles, 2007; Zachary *et al.*, 2013). Pseudocysts are filled with often turbid, sometimes blood-tinged fluid. When a cystic lesion is visualized by ultrasound, the steps necessary to confirm a pseudocyst include a high cystic fluid amylase and/or lipase activity, the exclusion of an abscess by FNA, and histology of both the pancreas and the wall of the lesion. However, no information is available on pseudocystic fluid canine pancreatic lipase (cPL) and feline pancreatic lipase (fPL) concentrations.

Additional non-neoplastic cavitary lesions of the pancreas include abscesses, congenital cysts, and retention cysts (Table 8.1) (Coleman *et al.*, 2005; Anderson *et al.*, 2008; Branter & Viviano, 2010). True cysts, like pseudocysts, are variably sized, fluid-filled lesions demarcated by a wall and located in or close to the pancreatic parenchyma (Coleman *et al.*, 2005; Charles, 2007; Branter & Viviano, 2010; Zachary & McGavin, 2013). True cysts can be unilocular or multilocular thin-walled sacs that range from millimeters to several centimeters in diameter and often contain a clear and translucent serous fluid (Bergin *et al.*, 2002; Meuten, 2002; Head, 2003; Coleman *et al.*, 2005). Histologically, pancreatic cysts are lined by a single layer of

Table 8.1 **Non-neoplastic and neoplastic lesions of the pancreas**

	Exocrine (acinar and ductular parenchyma)	Endocrine (islets of Langerhans)
Incidental findings	Pacini corpuscules (cat); stromal fat cell infiltration/lipomatosis; intrapancreatic hepatocytes; heterotopic pancreas; pancreatolithiasis	
Developmental abnormalities	Aplasia/hypoplasia; congenital ductal stenosis; congenital ductal cysts Intra-hepatic ectopic splenic tissue	Aplasia/hypoplasia
Regressive lesions	Canine juvenile acinar atrophy; primary (starvation…) or secondary atrophy (inflammation, neoplasia…); multifocal degeneration/necrosis (viruses, toxics, ductal obstruction...); lipofuscinosis; vacuolation (lysosomal storage diseases); acquired retention cyst (due to obstruction of ductular lumen)	Hydropic degeneration; amyloidosis; necrosis (selective or by extension of acute pancreatic necrosis/pancreatitis); sclerosis
Inflammatory lesions	Atrophic lymphocytic pancreatitis (first stage of canine juvenile acinar atrophy); acute lesions: acute suppurative pancreatitis/acute pancreatic necrosis/acute necrotizing pancreatitis; chronic lesions: chronic nonsuppurative pancreatitis/pancreatic fibrosis; sequelae: pseudocyst/abscess/phlegmon; ductular inflammation (parasitism, lithiasis)	
Hyperplastic lesions	Ductal hyperplasia; nodular acinar hyperplasia	Islet hyperplasia; nesidioblastosis (combined ductular and islet cells hyperplasia)
Neoplastic lesions	Epithelial: exocrine adenoma/adenocarcinoma; non-epithelial: fibroma/sarcoma, hemangiosarcoma, liposarcoma, nerve sheath tumors, lymphoma; secondary tumors (metastasis or direct extension)	Islet cell adenoma/carcinoma (insulinoma, gastrinoma, glucagonoma, pancreatic polypetide-secreting tumor)

(1–5)

1. Meuten DJ. Tumors in domestic animals. Ames, IA: Iowa State Press; 2002.
2. Zachary JF, McGavin D. Pathologic Basis of Veterinary Disease: Elsevier Health Sciences; 2013.
3. Head KW. Histological classification of tumors of the alimentary system of domestic animals: Published by the Armed Forces Institute of Pathology in cooperation with the American Registry of Pathology and the World Health Organization Collaborating Center for Worldwide Reference on Comparative Oncology; 2003.
4. Charles JA. Pancreas. In: M.; GM, editor. Jubb, Kennedy, and Palmer's Pathology of Domestic Animals, Fifth edition. Philadelphia: Elsevier Saunders; 2007.
5. Ramirez et al, JCP, 2013 "Intrapancreatic ectopic splenic tissue in dogs and cats".

low cuboidal to flattened well-differentiated ductal epithelial cells (Head, 2003; Coleman *et al.*, 2005; Charles, 2007). True cysts can be the result of congenital ductular malformations (cystic dilation of pancreatic ducts often in association with polycystic kidney and/or liver diseases) (Meuten, 2002; Head, 2003; Charles, 2007; Zachary & McGavin, 2013) or can be acquired due to obstruction of the duct system and retention of pancreatic secretion (Meuten, 2002; Head, 2003). True congenital pancreatic cysts are extremely rare. Few cases have been reported in cats, and only one in a dog (Healy *et al.*, 2022) They can be defined as a fluid-filled cyst lined with cuboidal-to-columnar epithelium and a cystic amylase concentration of <5,000 U/L (Healy *et al.*, 2022). Grossly, it can be difficult to distinguish cystic structures from abscesses, which are pockets of sterile or septic purulent exudate and necrotic debris (Head, 2003; Charles, 2007).

Ultrasound

True cysts, pseudocysts, abscesses, and cystic neoplasia may be difficult to differentiate on the sole basis of sonographic appearance (Larson, 2016; Griffin, 2020). Round to oval shape, thin and sharply demarcated wall, anechoic content, and strong distal acoustic enhancement are the usual and classical descriptions of cystic sonographic images. However, in the particular case of pancreatic pseudocysts, irregular margins, thick wall, and echoic content with slight acoustic enhancement (fluid rich in enzymes and debris) are possible findings. Obtaining a sample of cyst content under ultrasound guidance can help rule out abscess or cystic neoplasia. Aspiration and drainage of pseudocysts are reported to be safe and should be considered for the evaluation of cystic pancreatic lesions (VanEnkevort *et al.*, 1999).

Cytology

As for any cyst or pseudocyst from any organ or structure, cytology is often of low cellularity, and a clear to slightly hazy fluid is obtained, suggestive of a modified transudate. In contrast with abscesses, cystic samples are composed of an abundant amorphous background and few inflammatory cells, such as few non-degenerated neutrophils and reactive macrophages (VanEnkevort *et al.*, 1999; Bjorneby & Kari, 2002; Borjesson, 2014). One description of a congenital cyst in a dog reports a similar composition with a proteinaceous fluid associated with necrotic cellular material and mild non-septic neutrophilic inflammation with moderate to marked accumulation of uniformly blue-black pigment (Healy *et al.*, 2022). Cytology should be considered as an exclusionary diagnostic tool for abscess.

HYPERPLASIA OF THE PANCREAS

Description

Nodular hyperplasia of the exocrine parenchyma is a common incidental finding in old dogs and cats; its presence and severity are correlated with increasing age (Table 8.1) (Meuten, 2002; Newman *et al.*, 2005; Charles, 2007; Zachary & McGavin, 2013). Hyperplastic nodules should neither be considered as preneoplastic, nor reflect a response to previous pancreatic injury (Meuten, 2002; Newman *et al.*, 2005; Charles, 2007).

Pancreatic hyperplastic nodules are typically multiple, raised, smooth, firm, gray or white on cut surface, and of variable size, sometimes larger than normal lobules (Figure 8.9) (Meuten, 2002; Head, 2003; Newman *et al.*, 2005; Charles, 2007). Solitary nodular lesions are unusual and must be differentiated from pancreatic exocrine adenomas, even if the distinction between pancreatic exocrine hyperplasia and adenoma is poorly defined in domestic animals (Meuten, 2002; Newman *et al.*, 2005; Charles, 2007).

Histopathology

Due to their multiplicity, hyperplastic nodules alternate with normal lobules creating a mosaic of normal and affected lobules (Figure 8.10) (Meuten, 2002; Newman *et al.*, 2005; Charles, 2007).

Hyperplastic nodules consist of unencapsulated and minimally or non-compressive small clusters, sheets, or acini of recognizable exocrine pancreatic epithelial cells, with cytoplasmic zymogen granules, and nuclei maintained in a basal location (Figure 8.11) (Head, 2003; Newman *et al.*, 2005; Charles, 2007; Zachary & McGavin, 2013). Affected lobules may be composed of cells larger than normal pancreatic acinar cells, with an abundant brightly acidophilic cytoplasm, rich in zymogen granules, or smaller than normal cells, with a high nuclear-cytoplasmic ratio forming low cuboidal acini and a reduced cytoplasmic content of zymogen granules (Figure 8.12). The cytoplasm may be vacuolated. Mitoses are very rare (Newman *et al.*, 2005; Charles, 2007; Zachary & McGavin, 2013).

Ultrasound

Well-defined hypoechoic nodules of various sizes are described in the case of pancreatic nodular hyperplasia (Hecht & Henry, 2007).

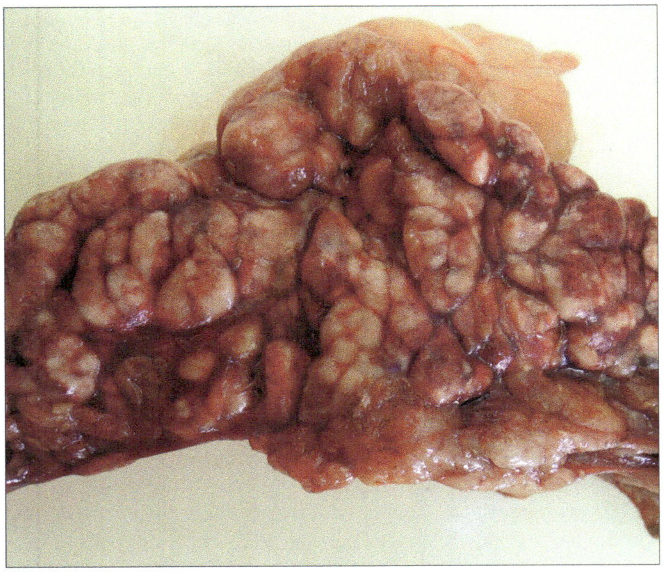

Figure 8.9 Pancreatic exocrine nodular hyperplasia from a dog. Hyperplastic nodules are multiple, smooth, well-circumscribed, pale, and raised on the pancreatic surface.

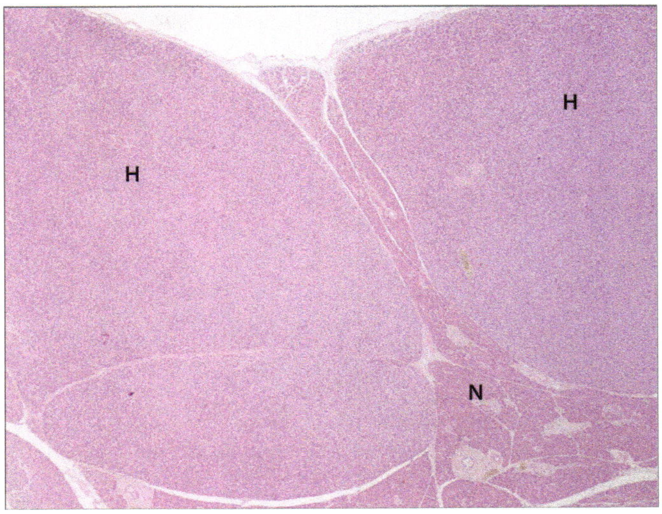

Figure 8.10 Pancreatic exocrine nodular hyperplasia from a cat. Hyperplastic lobules (H) are multiple and larger than adjacent unaffected lobules (N), creating a mosaic. They are slightly compressive and unencapsulated, only delineated by the delicate collagenous septa. Hematoxylin and eosin (×40).

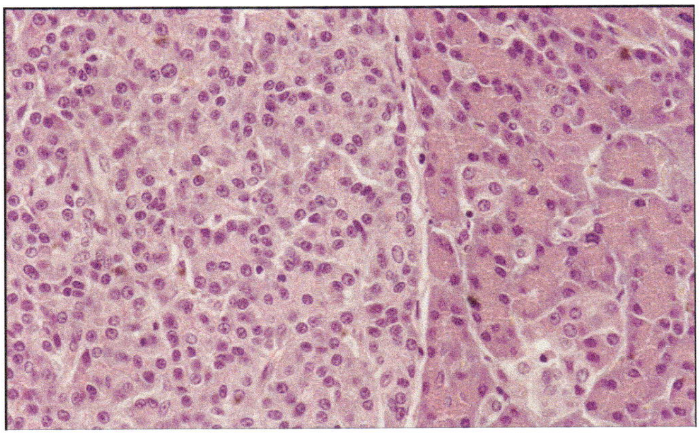

Figure 8.11 Pancreatic exocrine nodular hyperplasia from a cat. In the left part of the micrograph, the hyperplastic nodule is characterized by tightly packed aggregates of recognizable exocrine pancreatic epithelial cells, organized in acini without an obvious lumen: it closely resembles normal counterparts (right of the picture) except for cytoplasmic staining and cell size. Cells are pale, cuboid to pyramidal, with nuclei maintained in a basal location. Hematoxylin and eosin (×400).

Their sonographic appearance can be related to pancreatic endocrine neoplasia (insulinoma), pseudocysts (Penninck *et al.*, 2013), and true cysts, even if the latter are expected to produce posterior enhancement due to their fluid content.

Cytology

Cytology of nodular hyperplasia is similar to cytology of adenoma and well-differentiated carcinoma and should always be considered with the ultrasonographic findings and the observation of multiple lesions even if an overlap with neoplastic lesion could exist.

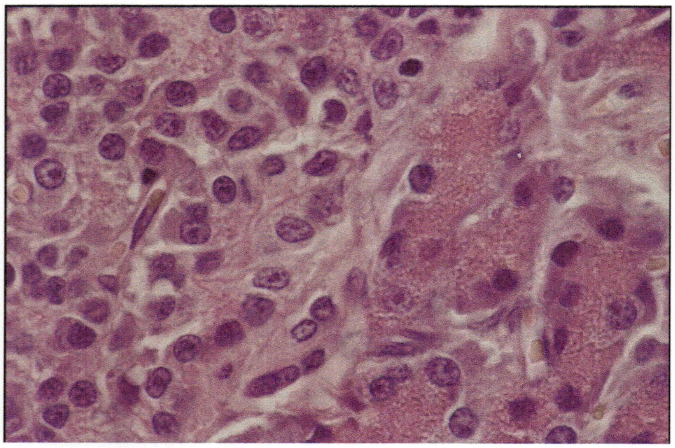

Figure 8.12 Pancreatic exocrine nodular hyperplasia from a cat. At higher magnification, epithelial cells of hyperplastic nodules (left of the picture) are smaller and paler than normal acinar cells (right of the picture), with a higher nuclear to cytoplasmic ratio. The cellular content of zymogen granules is reduced compared to those of adjacent normal exocrine parenchyma. Nuclear alterations are minimal. Hematoxylin and eosin (×1,000).

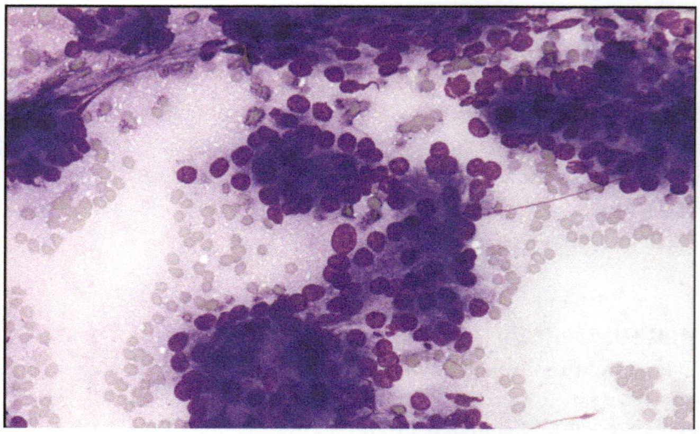

Figure 8.13 Aspirate of a nodular hyperplasia from a cat. Bloody and granular basophilic background associated with numerous cohesive cells organized in acinar and papillary structures. May–Grünwald–Giemsa (×400).

FNA are highly cellular (Figure 8.13) and characterized by numerous cohesive cells organized in papillary to acinar structures. Cells appear similar to normal pancreatic epithelial cells with some hyperplastic characteristics such as bigger cells, less granular and more basophilic cytoplasm, higher N:C ratio, bigger and more prominent nucleoli, some anisokaryosis and anisocytosis, and more noticeable binucleations (Figure 8.14) (Bjorneby & Kari, 2002; Andreasen *et al.*, 2010; Borjesson, 2014).

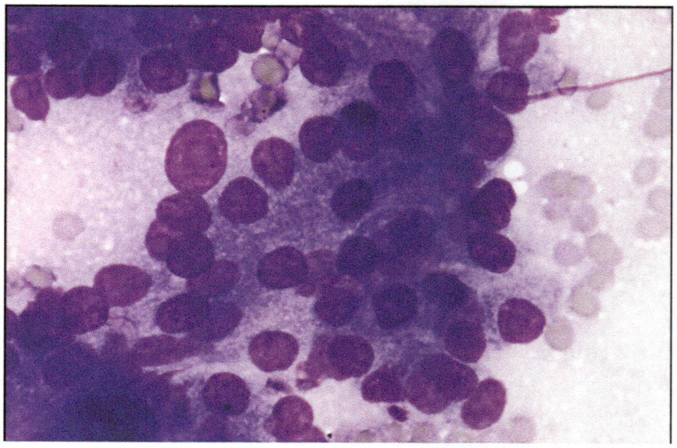

Figure 8.14 Aspirate of a nodular hyperplasia from a cat. Bloody and granular basophilic background associated with acinar cells. The medium- to large-sized cells with a medium to high nuclear to cytoplasmic ratio have a cuboidal to pyramidal outline with indistinct cell borders. Their nuclei are eccentric, round with granular and clumped chromatin and a large prominent nucleolus. Their cytoplasm is basophilic and heterogeneous and characterized by a mild eosinophilic granularity. Anisokaryosis is secondary to an isolated large naked nucleus among a homogeneously sized nucleus population. May–Grünwald–Giemsa (×1,000).

PANCREATITIS

Pancreatitis is the most common disorder of the exocrine pancreas in both dogs and cats (Washabau *et al.*, 2012). Histopathology remains the gold standard for the diagnosis of acute and chronic pancreatitis, and differentiation between pancreatitis and neoplasia (Kalli *et al.*, 2009; Washabau & Day, 2012). Acute pancreatitis is an acute and possibly reversible inflammatory process, whereas chronic pancreatitis leads to irreversible lesions such as atrophy and fibrosis (Steiner, 2010; Washabau, 2010; Washabau & Day, 2012; Watson, 2012; Borjesson, 2014). Lack of pancreatic gross lesions does not exclude the presence of pancreatitis, and a single biopsy sample is frequently insufficient to exclude pancreatitis on histology owing to the multifocal distribution of inflammation within the pancreas (Newman *et al.*, 2004). The situation is of course the same for cytology. Histopathologic grading systems for canine and feline inflammatory conditions of the pancreas have been proposed; however, there is a lack of standardization between dogs and cats and between authors (Table) (Newman *et al.*, 2004; Newman *et al.*, 2006; De Cock *et al.*, 2007; Watson *et al.*, 2007). Clinical presentations of acute and chronic pancreatitis may significantly overlap. Classification of pancreatitis can be confusing as some clinicians are inclined to differentiate acute and chronic pancreatitis based on the clinical manifestations of the disease (Charles, 2007; Steiner, 2010; Washabau, 2010; Watson, 2012). Most of the time it is very difficult to cytologically differentiate acute from chronic pancreatitis.

ACUTE PANCREATITIS

Definition

Canine and feline acute pancreatitis is characterized by variable degrees of parenchymal pancreatic necrosis often with peripancreatic fat necrosis, in association with neutrophilic inflammation, but without underlying permanent changes such as fibrosis (Watson *et al.*, 2007; Zachary & McGavin, 2013). Uncommon pancreatic complications of acute pancreatitis are abscesses, pseudocysts, and phlegmon (Charles, 2007; Washabau & Day, 2012).

Prevalence and gross anatomy

Prevalence of acute pancreatitis differs according to the authors, depending on different classification systems and inclusion criteria. In a study on 101 dogs randomly selected at necropsy (Newman *et al.*, 2006), neutrophilic inflammation was identified in 32 dogs (32%). In cats, it is uncommon to diagnose lesions of acute pancreatitis alone; however lesions of acute and chronic pancreatitis frequently occur concurrently, with a prevalence ranging from 9.6% (De Cock *et al.*, 2007) to 44% (Forman *et al.*, 2004).

The distribution of lesions of acute pancreatitis can be focal (contained in a localized area), multifocal, or diffuse. Hallmarks of acute inflammatory pancreatic lesions include swelling of the organ due to interstitial or interlobular edema; vascular lesions from hyperemia to petechiae, ecchymosis, or extensive hemorrhages; soft, gray-yellow areas of parenchymal necrosis; white chalky areas of peripancreatic fat necrosis (Figure 8.15) with hyperemic borders; and fibrin exudates on serosa (exudative peritonitis) with loose adhesions between affected portions of the pancreas and adjacent tissues (omentum, mesentery, liver…) (Charles, 2007; Zachary & McGavin, 2013).

Histopathology

Acute elementary inflammatory lesions in the pancreas are consistent with acinar cell necrosis in randomly scattered foci or involving entire lobules, often delineated by a rim of degenerate neutrophils; peripancreatic fat necrosis often with dystrophic mineralization (saponification) (Figure 8.16); interlobular septal neutrophilic infiltrate, edema, and/or fibrin exudates (Figure 8.17); and, most frequently observed in dogs, interstitial hemorrhages (Charles, 2007; De Cock *et al.*, 2007; Zachary & McGavin, 2013). These lesions can occur in variable intensity from case to case.

In cats, two distinct acute entities are recognized: acute pancreatic necrosis (or acute necrotizing pancreatitis), in which parenchymal and fat necrosis are the major components with varying amounts of inflammation, hemorrhage, and mineralization, and acute suppurative pancreatitis that differs from the former by the intensity of neutrophilic inflammation which is the predominant feature, and less parenchymal necrosis (Hill *et al.*, 1993; Charles, 2007; Washabau & Day, 2012).

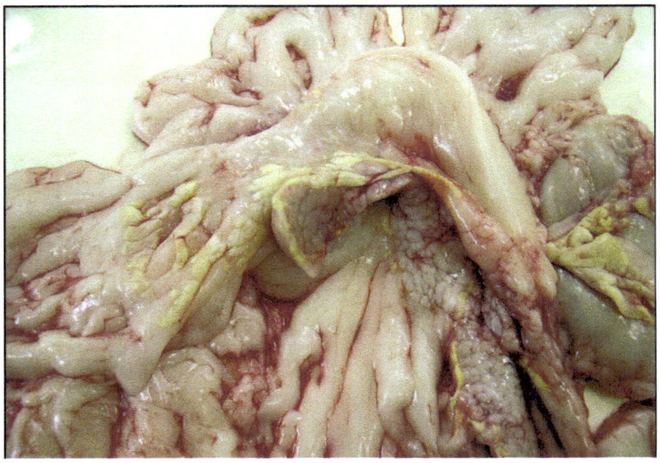

Figure 8.15 Pancreas and omentum from a cat infected by a hypervirulent calicivirus. The pancreas is moderately hyperemic and the pancreatic lobulation is exaggerated by interlobular edema. Multiple white chalky areas of fat necrosis are seen on the surface of the pancreas and in the omentum mainly close to the pancreas.

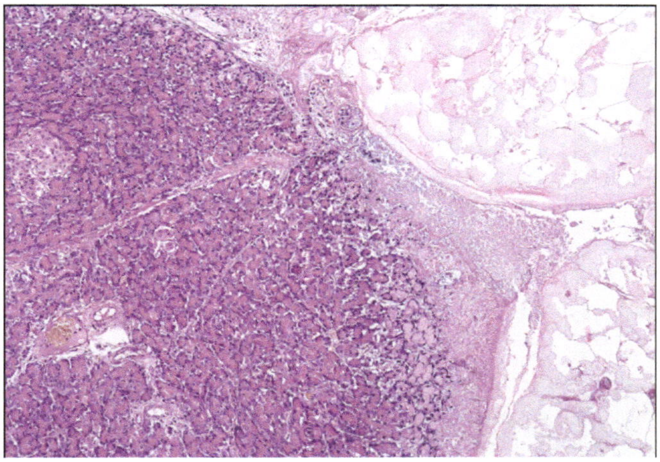

Figure 8.16 Same case as Figure 8.15: pancreas and omentum from a cat infected by a hypervirulent calicivirus. Hypervirulent caliciviruses induce subcapsular coagulative necrosis of the pancreatic exocrine parenchyma with cytoplasmic pallor and nuclear pyknosis. The peripancreatic fat (on the right of the picture) is also necrotic with dystrophic mineralization. There is fibrin exudation between necrotic omental fat and pancreatic parenchyma. Hematoxylin and eosin (×100).

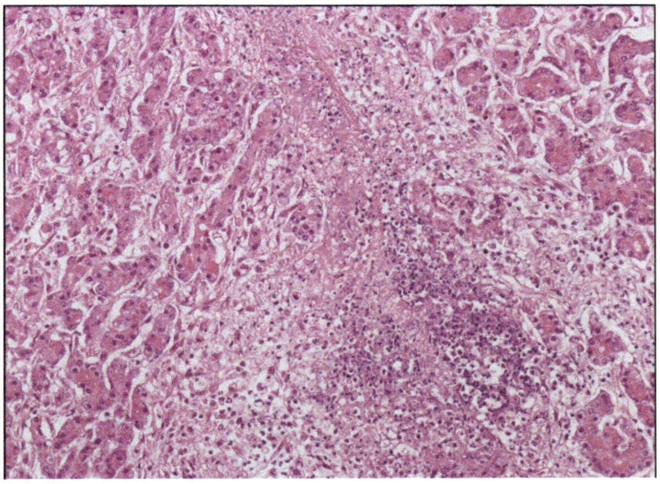

Figure 8.17 Acute suppurative pancreatitis from a cat. Pancreatic lobules are separated by interlobular collection of degenerated neutrophils (suppuration) with fibrin exudates. Pancreatic exocrine acini are separated by intralobular edema. Hematoxylin and eosin (×200).

Ultrasound

Changes observed in cases of acute pancreatitis are related to pancreatic edema, hemorrhage, and necrosis as well as focal peritonitis and fat saponification (Figure 8.18) (Nyland *et al.*, 2002; Larson,

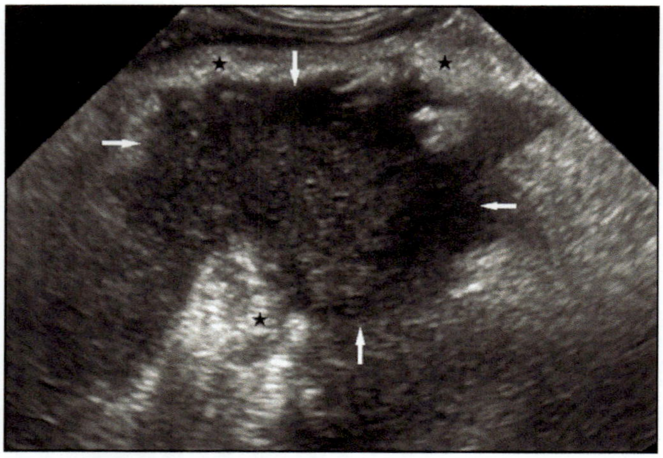

Figure 8.18 Sagittal view of the right cranial abdomen of a dog with acute pancreatitis. An enlarged hypoechoic pancreas (white arrows) surrounded by hyperechoic and bright mesenteric fat (black stars) can be seen dorsally to the descending duodenum.

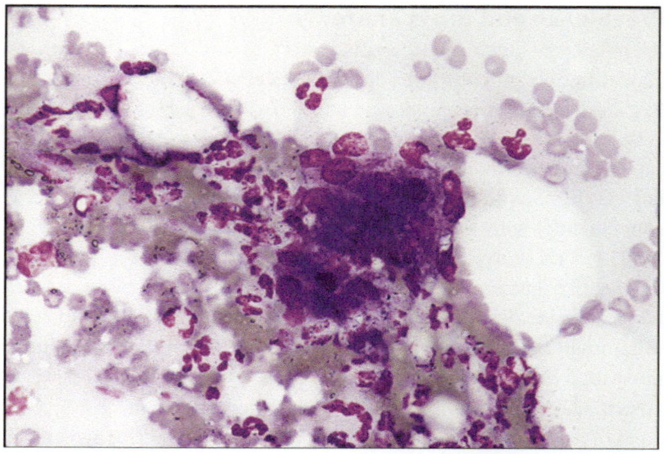

Figure 8.19 Aspirate of acute pancreatitis from a dog. The specimen is characterized by a hemorrhagic background, many nondegenerate neutrophils, and a cluster of exocrine pancreatic epithelial cells showing moderate anisokaryosis. May–Grünwald–Giemsa (×400).

2016). Sonographic appearance is variable based on the severity and the duration of the inflammation (Penninck and d'Anjou, 2013). An enlarged, ill-defined, irregularly shaped, and strongly hypoechoic organ is usually observed. However, severe pain, free abdominal fluid, excessive gas within the gastrointestinal tract, and abnormal peristalsis can make it difficult to perform the examination. In dogs, the right lobe tends to be more commonly affected, whereas in cats, the body and the left lobe are more often involved. Ultrasonographic changes in cats are often more subtle and of later onset than in dogs (Hecht & Henry, 2007; Penninck & d'Anjou, 2013; Penninck *et al.*, 2013).

Cytology

The cellularity associated with acute pancreatitis is higher than in chronic pancreatitis. Aspirates reveal a neutrophilic infiltrate with intact and degenerating neutrophils (Figure 8.19). Exocrine pancreatic epithelial cells may be present and show some degree of hyperplastic change (Figures 8.20 and 8.21); rare ductal epithelial cells may also be observed (Bjorneby & Kari, 2002; Cordner *et al.*, 2015). Necrotic background is often present (Figure 8.22). Calcified debris may also be found (Figure 8.23) (Bjorneby & Kari, 2002; Cordner *et al.*, 2015). Mixed inflammatory cells can sometimes be noted with large foamy or phagocytic macrophages in addition to the neutrophils. Note that foamy macrophages can be observed in acute or chronic pancreatitis aspirates. In some cases, only necrotic material can be found without any exocrine pancreatic epithelial cells or intact inflammatory cells.

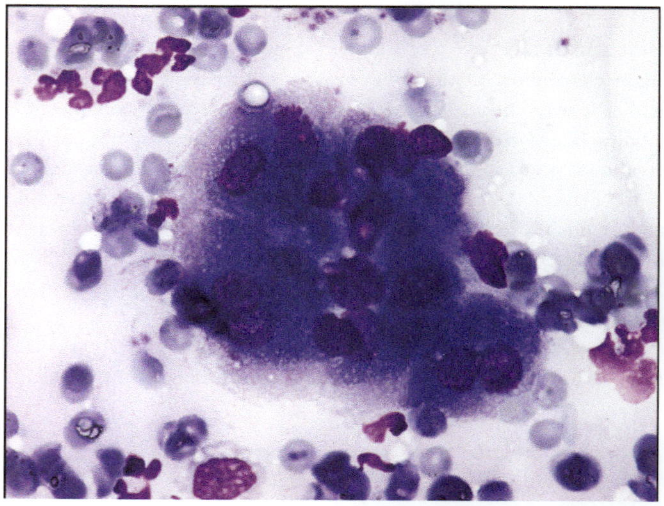

Figure 8.20 Aspirate of acute pancreatitis from a dog. Nondegenerate neutrophils surround two acini of exocrine pancreatic epithelial cells showing moderate anisokaryosis and prominent basophilic nucleoli. May–Grünwald–Giemsa (×1,000).

CHRONIC PANCREATITIS

Definition

Chronic pancreatitis is the result of progressive destruction of the pancreas by repeated mild episodes of acute pancreatic necrosis and inflammation (Bostrom *et al.*, 2013; Zachary & McGavin, 2013). Owing to modest regenerative capacity, the destruction of pancreatic parenchyma causes progressive loss of glandular tissue and its replacement by fibrosis. The hallmarks of chronic inflammation in the pancreas are fibrosis and exocrine parenchymal atrophy, which are considered permanent changes (Washabau & Day, 2012; Zachary & McGavin, 2013).

Prevalence and gross anatomy

As for acute pancreatitis, the published prevalence of chronic pancreatitis differs according to different authors but remains high. In a study based on 151 unselected canine post-mortem examinations without pancreatic autolysis, chronic pancreatitis was identified in

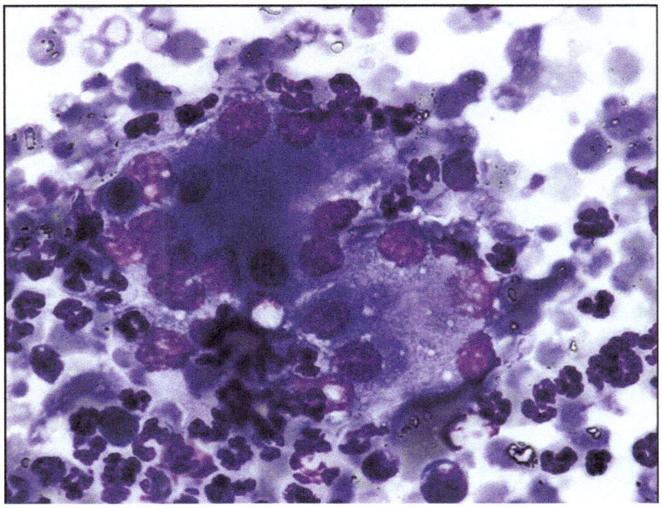

Figure 8.21 Aspirate of acute pancreatitis from a dog. The exocrine pancreatic epithelial cells show a highly basophilic cytoplasm and some binucleations. The neutrophils are mostly nondegenerate. May–Grünwald–Giemsa (×1,000).

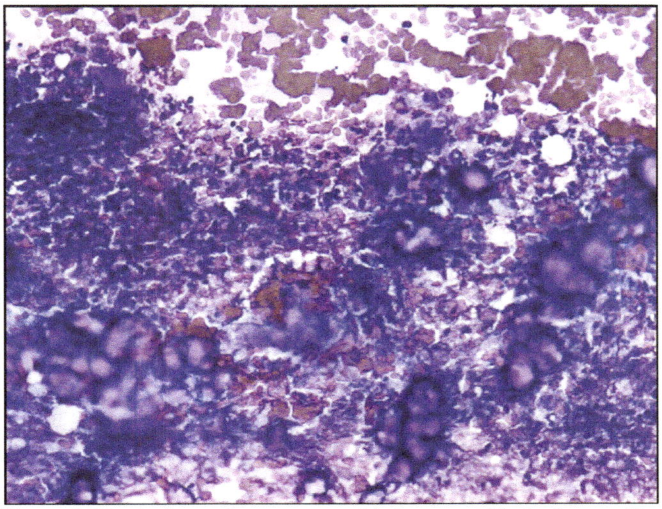

Figure 8.23 Aspirate of acute pancreatitis from a cat. The background is highly hemorrhagic and necrotic, containing many degenerate neutrophils. Calcific debris appear as tridimensional amorphous refractile material. May–Grünwald–Giemsa (×200).

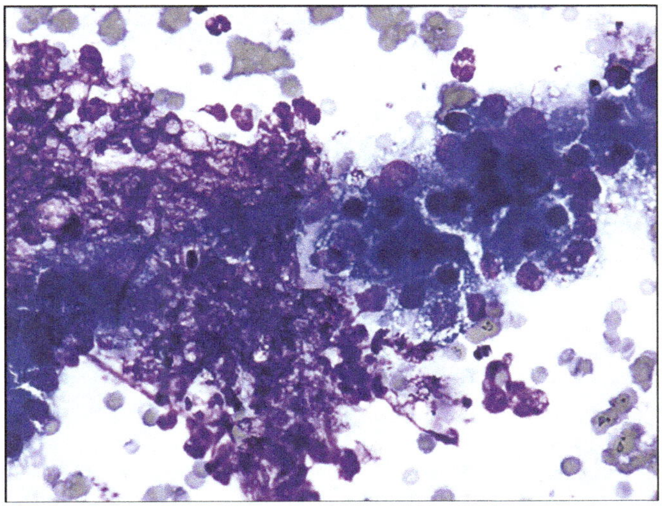

Figure 8.22 Aspirate of acute pancreatitis from a cat. The specimen is characterized by a hemorrhagic background and necrotic debris. Many degenerate neutrophils surround exocrine pancreatic epithelial cells showing marked anisocytosis and anisokaryosis. The cytoplasm of the epithelial cells shows decreased granularity and many small clear vacuoles consistent with cellular degeneration. May–Grünwald–Giemsa (×400).

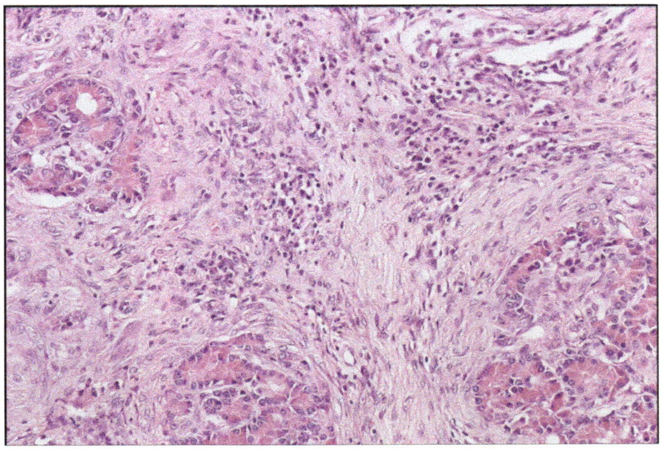

Figure 8.24 Chronic pancreatitis from a dog. Pancreatic microscopic structure is severely modified by interlobular fibrosis which extends into lobules, separating and replacing exocrine acini, associated with a sparse infiltrate of small lymphocytes. Residual exocrine pancreatic acini are well-differentiated with bright eosinophilic zymogen granules. Hematoxylin and eosin (×200).

34% of dogs (Watson *et al.*, 2007). In another study on 101 dogs randomly selected at necropsy (Newman *et al.*, 2006), lymphocytic infiltration was identified in 53 dogs (52%). In cats, an overall prevalence of 67% was identified in a group of 115 unselected feline post-mortem examinations and a prevalence as high as 45% of apparently healthy animals (De Cock *et al.*, 2007).

Chronic pancreatitis is macroscopically characterized by distortion and shrinkage of a part or the whole organ, with often exaggerated lobulation, a gray to whitish color, firm consistency, and fibrous adhesions to adjacent tissues (Charles, 2007; Zachary & McGavin, 2013).

Histopathology

The microscopic appearance of chronic pancreatitis is characterized by disruption of the normal pancreatic architecture due to variable amounts of fibrosis (Figure 8.24) in association with lymphocyte and plasma cell infiltrates, parenchymal atrophy (Figure 8.25), and occasional ductal cystic dilation in cats (Charles, 2007; De Cock *et al.*, 2007; Watson *et al.*, 2007; Zachary & McGavin, 2013).

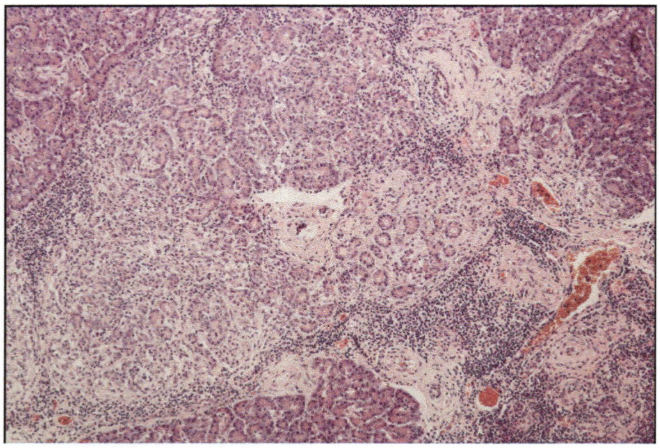

Figure 8.25 Chronic lymphocytic and atrophic pancreatitis from a cat. There is marked exocrine pancreatic lobular atrophy associated with perilobular and intralobular, dissecting, fibrosis, and lymphocytic infiltrate. Atrophic acini exhibit pale cytoplasm with severe depletion in zymogen granules. Some well-developed lobules are observed in the periphery of the atrophic one. Hematoxylin and eosin (×100).

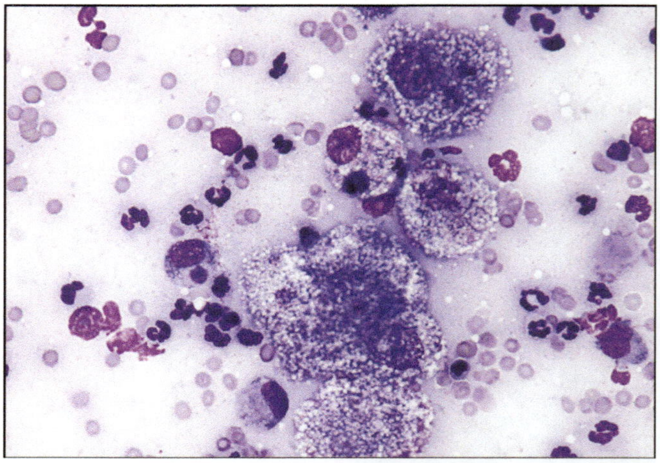

Figure 8.26 Aspirate of chronic pancreatitis from a cat. A small cluster of non-reactive exocrine pancreatic epithelial cells is surrounded by mixed inflammatory cells: many non-degenerate neutrophils and some large foamy macrophages. May–Grünwald–Giemsa (×400).

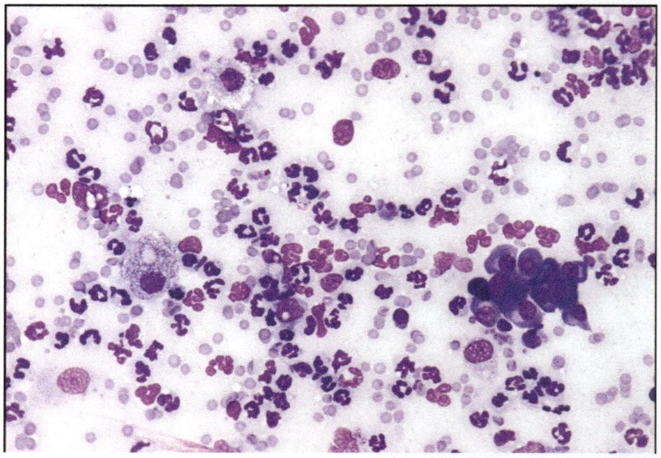

Figure 8.27 Aspirate of a chronic pancreatitis from a cat. Same case as Figure 8.26. Abundant inflammatory cells are present: mainly neutrophils but also some foamy macrophages and a small cluster of plasma cells. Some small lymphocytes are present but it is difficult to know their origin (inflammation or iatrogenic blood contamination). May-Grünwald Giemsa (x400).

Some authors have highlighted differences in histological appearance and distribution of fibrosis in different breeds of dogs and have described a periductular, interlobular pattern of fibrosis and inflammation in Cocker Spaniels compared to an acinar, dissecting intralobular pattern in other breeds (Watson *et al.*, 2007).

Acute-on-chronic pancreatitis can be observed and is characterized by edema, necrosis, neutrophils (hallmarks of acute pancreatitis) admixed with lymphocytes and plasma cells, and underlying fibrosis (hallmarks of chronic pancreatitis). These observations corroborate the theory that irreversible damage to the pancreas may be caused by repeated incidents of acute pancreatitis (Watson *et al.*, 2007; Bostrom *et al.*, 2013).

Ultrasound

In case of chronic pancreatitis, the changes may be nonexistent or very subtle (Penninck *et al.*, 2013); the pancreas usually remains a well-defined hypoechoic structure that contrasts with the slightly hyperechoic peripancreatic mesentery (Penninck and d'Anjou, 2013). Irregular margins, mild hyper/hypotrophy, heterogeneous parenchyma, calcification, and scarring can be encountered (Nyland *et al.*, 2002). Some cases of chronic pancreatitis appear as a mass-lesion on ultrasound and must not be mistaken for pancreatic neoplasia (Watson *et al.*, 2007). Ultrasonography has low sensitivity in case of chronic pancreatitis.

Cytology

Cytological specimens in cases of chronic pancreatitis are typically less cellular than in acute pancreatitis and often yield peripheral blood. Calcified debris and clusters of pancreatic acinar cells and ductal epithelial cells can be seen with hyperplastic changes sometimes mistaken for neoplasia (Bjorneby & Kari, 2002). Mixed inflammatory cells are found and include neutrophils, foamy or phagocytic macrophages, lymphocytes, and plasma cells (Figures 8.26 and 8.27) (Bjorneby & Kari, 2002; Cordner *et al.*, 2015). In our experience, fibrosis is never seen in aspirates, and the distinction between acute and chronic pancreatitis is usually not possible with cytology alone.

PANCREATIC TUMORS

Exocrine pancreatic tumors

Exocrine pancreatic adenoma

Definition and prevalence

Adenoma is a rare, incidental lesion, and less frequent than its malignant counterpart (Meuten, 2002; Head, 2003; Charles, 2007). No evidence of a transformation of a pancreatic hyperplasia through adenoma into adenocarcinoma has been demonstrated (Meuten, 2002). Distinction between pancreatic exocrine adenoma and nodular hyperplasia may be difficult, and is poorly defined in domestic animals (Zachary & McGavin, 2013).

Gross anatomy

Grossly, adenomas are solitary, small (rarely more than 5 mm in diameter), beige to fawn, compressive lesions (Meuten, 2002; Head, 2003; Charles, 2007).

Histopathology

Histologically, adenomas are masses which are expansive and compressive, tubular (of ductal origin) or acinar (of acinar cell origin) structures supported by a thin collagenous stroma surrounded by a thin capsule. Cells are cuboidal to columnar, with a variable cytoplasmic content of zymogen granules, and have a regular and round nucleus. Mitoses are rare (Meuten, 2002; Head, 2003; Charles, 2007). Metastasis does not occur, but local compressive growth patterns can result in atrophy of adjacent acini (Meuten, 2002).

Cytology

A cytological diagnosis of pancreatic adenoma is very difficult, since normal and hyperplastic pancreatic tissues are cytologically very similar (Meuten, 2002). The cytologic appearance can also be similar to some well-differentiated adenocarcinomas (Allen, 2021). Cytologic findings should be interpreted along with the ultrasonographic findings (Bjorneby & Kari, 2002). Cytological samples of a pancreatic adenoma are mainly associated with the presence of uniform and non-atypical acinar cells arranged in clusters, which can occasionally display mild anisocytosis and an increase in cytoplasmic basophilia (Bjorneby & Kari, 2002).

Exocrine pancreatic carcinoma

Definition and prevalence

Exocrine pancreatic carcinoma is the most common tumor of the exocrine pancreas (Meuten, 2002), but it remains an uncommon lesion in all species (Priester, 1974; Meuten, 2002; Charles, 2007; Zachary & McGavin, 2013). The incidence of pancreatic adenocarcinoma increases with age of animals, but it has been described in a 3-year-old dog (Priester, 1974). No sex predisposition has been described in cats; this is probably similar in dogs but needs to be confirmed because of some contradictory studies (Priester, 1974; Head, 2003; Pinard *et al.*, 2021). No clear breed predilection has been reported. Airedale terriers may be at higher risk according to one study, but this observation was not confirmed in a more recent study on a series of 23 dogs with exocrine pancreatic carcinoma (Priester, 1974; Pinard *et al.*, 2021). Comorbidities (e.g., diabetes mellitus) are frequent in cats, but they are not so obvious in dogs (Pinard *et al.*, 2021).

Gross anatomy

Carcinomas may consist of a single and discrete or more often multiple, irregular, gray to yellow nodules of variable size with a firm-to-hard consistency. The neoplastic mass can be diffuse or localized in the midportion of the pancreas in dogs, whereas the neoplastic lesion is associated with a more diffuse pattern in cats (Meuten, 2002; Pinard *et al.*, 2021). Lesions with a diffuse pattern lead to consideration of chronic pancreatitis or nodular hyperplasia in the list of differential diagnoses. The cut surface of the tumor is frequently heterogeneous with areas of softening and necrosis, mineralization, or hemorrhage. Invasion of adjacent tissues (e.g., common bile duct and duodenum) and serosal seeding with multiple transcoelomic metastases are common. The most frequent sites of metastasis are mesentery, peritoneum, adjacent gastrointestinal tract, liver, local lymph nodes, and lung, and less frequently spleen, kidney, diaphragm, and skin (Meuten, 2002; Charles, 2007). Fat necrosis of adjacent omentum or mesentery and adhesions between the pancreas and adjacent tissues are frequently observed (Meuten, 2002; Head, 2003; Charles, 2007; Zachary & McGavin, 2013).

Histopathology

Microscopic features of pancreatic carcinoma range from well-differentiated adenocarcinomas, with tubular or acinar patterns (Figure 8.28), to undifferentiated solid carcinomas. In the tubular pattern, glandular structures can be formed by cuboidal or columnar cells, presumed to originate from ducts, with occasional mucus secretion. Persistence of eosinophilic zymogen granules is only observed in well-differentiated tumors (Figure 8.29). Atypia and mitotic index are often correlated to the level of differentiation, with uniformity, regular cellular polarity, low nuclear to cytoplasmic ratio, and a low number of mitoses in well-differentiated carcinomas; and indistinct cellular borders with a high nuclear to cytoplasmic ratio, anisocytosis, anisokaryosis, and a higher number of mitoses in poorly differentiated carcinomas. The amount of supporting stroma is variable, usually greatest and scirrhous in poorly differentiated tumors. Metastatic

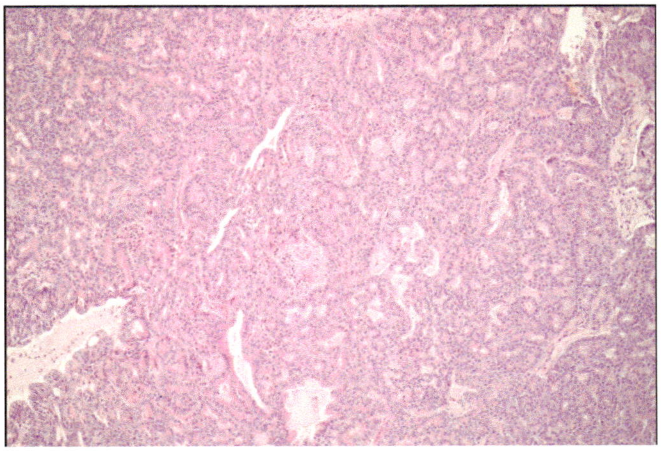

Figure 8.28 Histopathology of a pancreatic exocrine well-differentiated adenocarcinoma from a cat. Neoplastic tissue consists of relatively uniform small acinar to tubular structures with some larger ones, which appear more dilated with an eosinophilic luminal material admixed with cellular debris. Supporting stroma is sparse in this case but can be dense and desmoplastic in poorly differentiated carcinoma. Hematoxylin and eosin (×100).

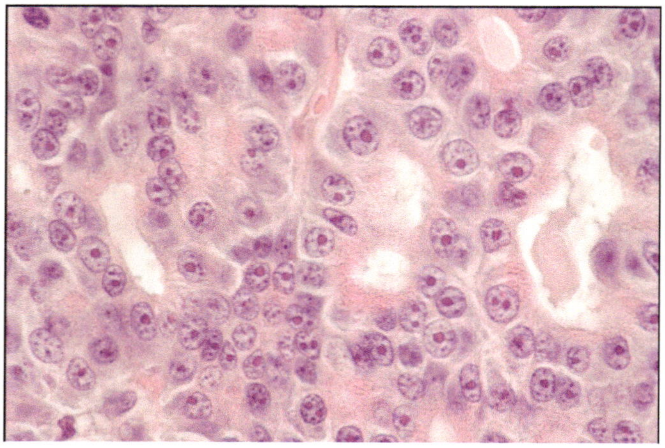

Figure 8.29 Histopathology of a pancreatic exocrine well-differentiated adenocarcinoma from a cat. Higher magnification from Figure 8.28. Neoplastic cells are cuboidal, forming acini or tubules with a small lumen. Nuclei are uniform, round to oval, with sparse chromatin and bright eosinophilic nucleoli, and are still located basally. Eosinophilic small zymogen granules are recognizable in the apical region of the cytoplasm. Despite the relative uniformity of neoplastic cells, atypical cells are noticed with anisocytosis, anisokaryosis, and multiple nucleoli. Hematoxylin and eosin (×1,000).

behavior cannot be predicted by histological morphology as well-differentiated carcinomas can metastasize widely (Meuten, 2002; Head, 2003; Charles, 2007; Zachary & McGavin, 2013).

Ultrasound

Pancreatic adenocarcinomas are described as hypoechoic nodules or masses with a tendency to develop in the central portion of the gland and invade the adjacent structures and organs (Figures 8.30a and 8.30b) (Penninck and d'Anjou, 2013). Pancreatic enlargement, abdominal effusion, and extra-hepatic biliary obstruction are also common findings with pancreatic adenocarcinomas (Hecht & Henry, 2007). Therefore, it remains challenging to differentiate pancreatic adenocarcinomas from pancreatitis or nodular hyperplasia solely on the basis of the ultrasound findings (Griffin, 2020).

Cytology

Fine needle aspirates can be useful in the diagnosis of exocrine pancreatic carcinoma (Bennett *et al.*, 2001). It has been reported as a safe procedure even if one suspected case of needle tract seeding has been reported in a cat (Jegatheeson *et al.*, 2020) In human medicine, different studies have investigated the diagnostic performance of pancreatic tissue FNA in cases of well-differentiated pancreatic adenocarcinoma. These studies have established many cytological criteria such as anisonucleosis, nuclear enlargement, nuclear crowding and overlapping, and nuclear membrane irregularity, in order to optimize the diagnostic performance of the cytology when compared to histology (with 98% sensitivity and 100% specificity) (Lin *et al.*, 2003). Other cytological criteria such as necrosis, hyperchromasia, macronucleoli, chromatin clearing, and mitosis were of more limited diagnostic significance according to this study (Lin & Staerkel, 2003). Unfortunately, no similar study has yet been performed in veterinary medicine. In general, the cytological diagnosis of exocrine pancreatic neoplasia is easier in cases of poorly differentiated neoplasms because of the presence of many anaplastic features. If the pancreatic adenocarcinoma is very well-differentiated and/or associated with an inflammatory context, the cytological diagnosis can be difficult and histopathology is needed to make a definitive diagnosis and to exclude a nodular hyperplasia, adenoma, or a reactive hyperplasia secondary to an inflammatory background (Figures 8.31–8.33) (Jegatheeson *et al.*, 2020). Furthermore, the yield of cytological sample can be dependent on the size and the degree of fibrosis of the neoplastic mass (Bjorneby & Kari, 2002).

The background of a pancreatic adenocarcinoma cytological sample is not specific and can be inflammatory, hemorrhagic, and/or necrotic (Borjesson, 2014). The cellularity is commonly high, and the cytological samples reveal many clusters of pancreatic cells organized in an acinar and/or tubular pattern, which can loose their polarity

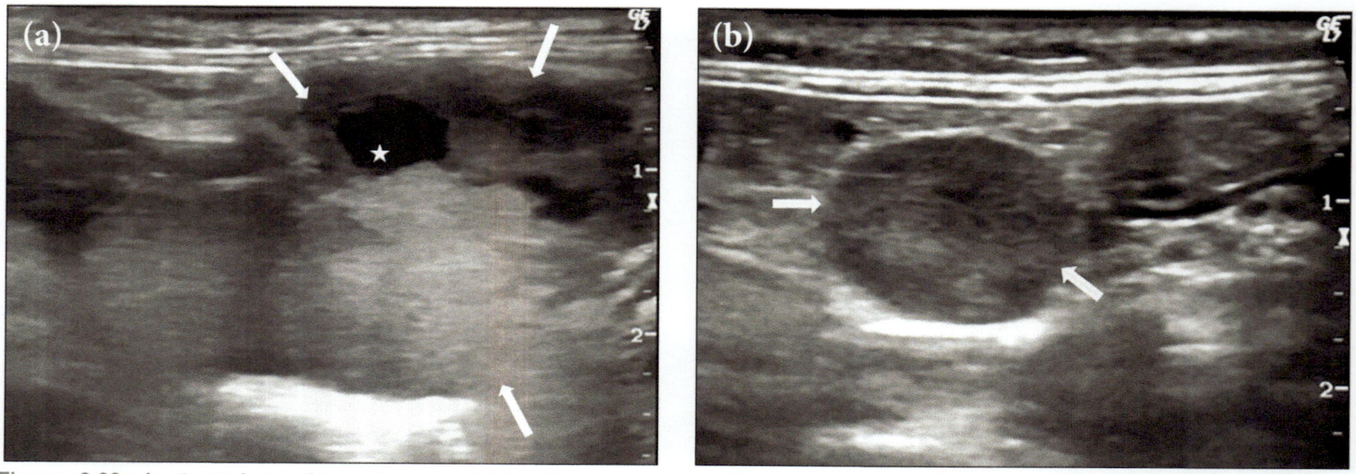

Figures 8.30a, b Sagittal view of the right pancreatic lobe of a 13-year-old cat with pancreatic adenocarcinoma. A voluminous mass (white arrows) is adjacent to the descending duodenum in an overall enlarged hypoechoic and heterogeneous pancreas. Cyst-like lesions (white star) are noted in the pancreatic parenchyma identified as necrotic centers. Enlarged mesenteric lymph node (white arrows) in the same cat.

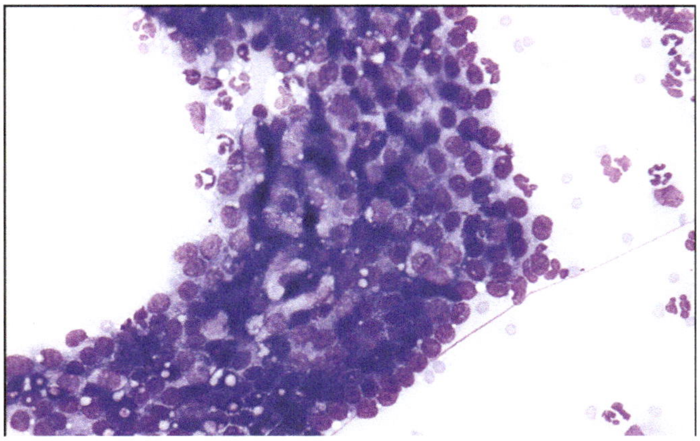

Figure 8.31 Aspirate of a well-differentiated pancreatic adenocarcinoma from a cat (same case as in Figures 8.28 and 8.29). Presence of a large pseudo-tubular structure composed of neoplastic pancreatic cells associated with an inflammatory background. The pancreatic cells are medium-sized with an increased nuclear to cytoplasmic ratio and a cuboidal shape; their cytoplasm is sometimes vacuolated (small clear and discrete vacuoles). Anisokaryosis is mild. May–Grünwald–Giemsa (×400).

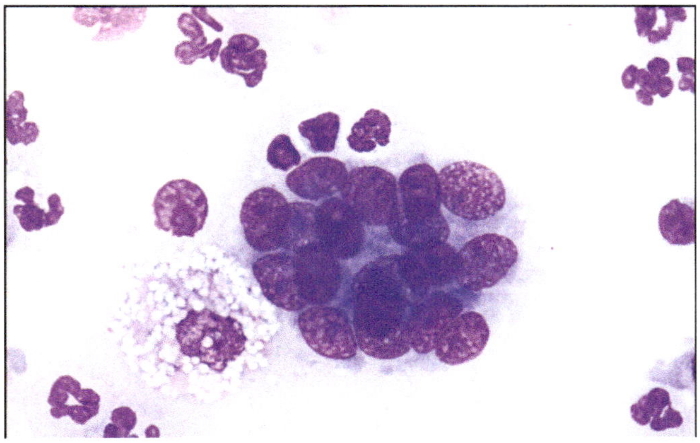

Figure 8.32 Aspirate of a well-differentiated pancreatic adenocarcinoma from a cat (same case as in Figures 8.28 and 8.29). Higher magnification from Figure 8.31. Inflammatory background composed of many neutrophils and a few foamy macrophages associated with the presence of a small acinar structure composed of acinar pancreatic neoplastic cells. The neoplastic cells are medium-sized and are characterized by a polygonal to cuboidal shape associated with a high nuclear to cytoplasmic ratio. The cytoplasm of these cells is basophilic and slightly granular, and the nuclei are round to ovoid and associated with a reticular to coarse chromatin pattern and one small to medium and round to angular nucleolus. Anisokaryosis is mild to moderate, and nuclei are overlapped. The presence of the inflammatory background can make the cytological diagnosis of exocrine pancreatic adenocarcinoma difficult in this case. May–Grünwald–Giemsa (×1,000).

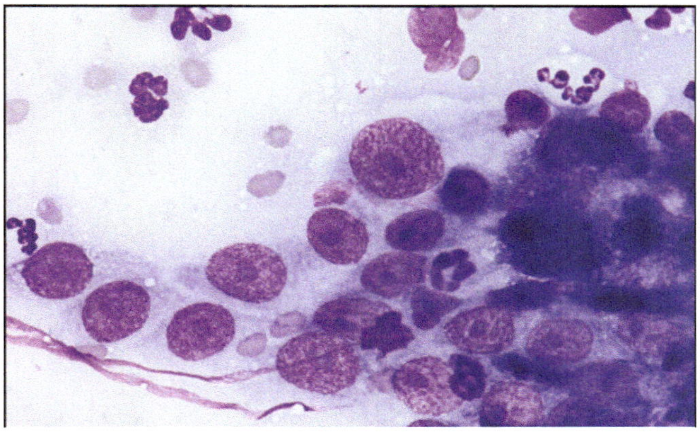

Figure 8.33 Aspirate of a well-differentiated pancreatic adenocarcinoma from a cat (same case as in Figures 8.28 and 8.29). Higher magnification from Figure 8.31 and 8.32. Inflammatory background composed of many neutrophils associated with the presence of some atypical and loosely cohesive acinar pancreatic cells. The neoplastic cells are medium- to large-sized and are characterized by a polygonal to cuboidal shape associated with a high nuclear to cytoplasmic ratio. The cytoplasm of these cells is slightly basophilic and poorly granular, and the nuclei are round to ovoid and associated with a reticular to coarse chromatin pattern and one medium to large and prominent nucleolus. Anisokaryosis and anisocytosis are marked. These more atypical pancreatic cells facilitate the cytological diagnosis of adenocarcinoma in this case associated with a marked inflammatory context. May–Grünwald–Giemsa (×1,000).

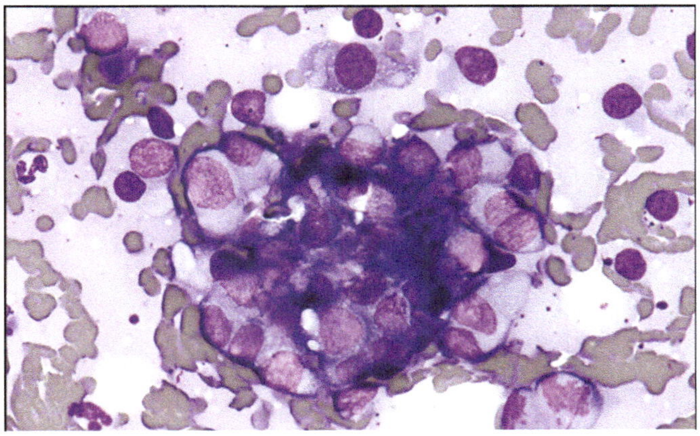

Figure 8.34 Aspirate of an anaplastic pancreatic adenocarcinoma from a cat. Bloody background associated with some naked nuclei, some inflammatory cells consisting of neutrophils and fewer lymphocytes, macrophages and mast cells, and some solid clusters of medium to large atypical and anaplastic acinar pancreatic cells organized in a pseudo-acinar pattern. These atypical cells are characterized by a round, cuboidal to polygonal shape and a high to medium nuclear to cytoplasmic ratio and disclose some criteria of malignancy, with a marked anisokaryosis, some binucleations, and an abnormal mitotic figure. May–Grünwald–Giemsa (×400).

(Figure 8.31) (Bjorneby & Kari, 2002). The cells are often associated with an increased (N:C) ratio, and their cytoplasm can be hyperbasophilic, display vacuolization (also observed in pancreatitis), and be more or less granular according to the degree of differentiation of the tumor (pale pink round granules corresponding to zymogen granules) (Figure 8.32) (Bjorneby & Kari, 2002; Borjesson, 2014). The nucleus is often enlarged with a coarse or reticular chromatin pattern and often contains one or multiple more or less prominent nucleoli (Figure 8.33) (Bjorneby & Kari, 2002; Borjesson, 2014). Nuclear molding and irregularities can also be visualized (Borjesson, 2014). Finally, the anaplastic features are variable. Moderate to marked anisokaryosis can be observed, but other anaplastic features are possible, especially in cases of poorly differentiated neoplasms (Figures 8.34

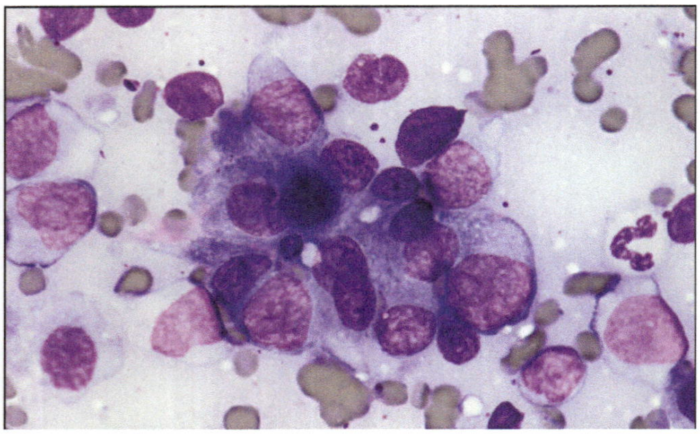

Figure 8.35 **Aspirate of an anaplastic pancreatic adenocarcinoma from a cat. Higher magnification from Figure 8.34. Bloody background associated with a large acinar structure composed of very atypical and poorly differentiated acinar pancreatic cells. The neoplastic cells are medium- to large-sized and are characterized by a round to cuboidal outline with clear to indistinct cell borders, a high to medium nuclear to cytoplasmic ratio, and a basophilic and slightly granular cytoplasm. The nuclei are round to ovoid, and associated with a finely stippled to lacy chromatin pattern and the presence of one or numerous small to large, and sometimes prominent, nucleoli. May–Grünwald–Giemsa (×1,000).**

and 8.35). Immunocytochemistry and other diagnostic testing may be necessary to differentiate poorly differentiated exocrine pancreatic adenocarcinoma and other neoplasms such as endocrine pancreatic tumor or secondary metastatic carcinoma.

Endocrine pancreatic tumors

Definition and prevalence

Pancreatic islet cell tumors are rare in domestic animals (Charles, 2007). The neoplasms most frequently related in pancreatic islets are those derived from β islet cells, named insulinoma. They are often endocrinologically active, resulting in hyperinsulinism and related hypoglycemia, regardless of the neoplasm malignancy (Charles, 2007). Non-β islet cell neoplasms, mainly secreting gastrin, glucagon, somatostatin, or pancreatic polypeptide (Meuten, 2002; Charles, 2007; Cruz Cardona *et al.*, 2010), have been reported very infrequently in dogs and cats. The macroscopic pathology as well as histopathology of these different tumors is quite similar, characteristic of an endocrine origin. Only immunohistochemistry permits the differentiation of the exact cellular lineage by identifying the hormone synthesized, even if one or more pancreatic hormones can be secreted by the tumor (Minkus *et al.*, 1997; Meuten, 2002; Head, 2003; Charles, 2007; Zachary & McGavin, 2013). Multihormonality of a tumor is not correlated with its biological behavior. The median reported age is 9 to 10 years for canine insulinoma. Medium to large breed are overrepresented, and no sex predilection has been reported (Minkus *et al.*, 1997; Bailey, 2007; Goutal *et al.*, 2012). Insulinoma is less commonly described in cats, but the prevalence also increases in older cats (Bailey, 2007). Siamese may be overrepresented, but the few reported cases in cats do not allow us to establish a breed predilection (Bailey, 2007).

Islet cell adenomas (benign insulinoma) and carcinomas (malignant insulinoma) are both encountered in domestic animals, with malignant tumors being more frequent than benign ones (Head, 2003; Charles, 2007; Zachary & McGavin, 2013). The behavior and metastatic potential of insulinoma cannot generally be reliably foretold by histological and particularly cytological features, since anaplastic features are frequently mild and inconsistent (Bjorneby & Kari, 2002; Andreasen *et al.*, 2010). Metastases are frequent, involving especially regional lymph nodes and the liver, and are reported in approximately half of cases of canine insulinoma (Caywood *et al.*, 1979; Bailey, 2007; Madarame *et al.*, 2009).

Gross anatomy and histopathology

Table 8.2 summarizes similarities and differences between islet cell adenomas and carcinomas (Charles, 2007) (Meuten, 2002; Head, 2003; Zachary & McGavin, 2013).

Ultrasound

Ultrasonography has low sensitivity to detect canine insulinoma (Robben *et al.*, 2005; Polton *et al.*, 2007) and depends on numerous factors such as the size and the distribution of the lesions, the operator's experience, equipment quality, animal conformation, and intestinal content (Penninck and d'Anjou, 2013). Insulinoma are usually nodular, lobular, or spherical and hypoechoic compared with the surrounding tissues (Goutal *et al.*, 2012; Vanderperren *et al.*, 2014) but as expected, ultrasonographic findings are non-specific (Figure 8.38).

Cytology

Insulinoma has similar cytological features as other endocrine tumors. The cellularity of malignant insulinoma is commonly higher than its benign counterpart and islet cell hyperplasia (Bjorneby & Kari, 2002). Cytological samples are mainly characterized by abundant naked nuclei on a slightly basophilic background corresponding to the cytoplasm of damaged neoplastic cells. The monomorphic cells are incohesive, individually or loosely clustered (sometimes associated with a pseudo-acinar pattern) (Figure 8.39). The neoplastic cells are of small to medium size and frequently display indistinct cytoplasmic borders, but can be round, ovoid to polygonal shaped (Figures 8.40a and 8.40b). The cytoplasm is slightly basophilic and can be associated with many small punctuate and clear vacuoles (Andreasen *et al.*, 2010; Borjesson, 2014). The nucleus is sometimes eccentrically placed, leading to a plasmacytic appearance of neoplastic cells, and can be associated with one small and indistinct to prominent nucleolus (Bjorneby Kari, 2002; Andreasen *et al.*, 2010; Borjesson, 2014). The chromatin pattern is reticular, coarse to finely clumped. Minimal cellular atypia is commonly observed, such as mild to moderate anisokaryosis and binucleation. The minimal cellular atypia cannot allow one to determine the malignancy of the tumor, in other words, its biologic behavior, and histopathology is commonly necessary. Furthermore, immunohistochemistry can be necessary to differentiate endocrine and exocrine tumors in some cases and to determine the subtype of the endocrine tumor and

Table 8.2 **Gross morphology and histopathology characteristics of islet cell neoplasia**

		Islet cell adenoma	Islet cell carcinoma
Gross morphology	Similarities	Usually single but sometimes multiple, sharply demarcated from surrounding tissues, firm, yellow-gray to purple nodular tumors	
	Differences	Small (1 to 3 cm in diameter), spherical, and homogeneous nodules	Larger than adenomas Multilobular appearance +/– extensive invasion into adjacent parenchyma Necrosis and hemorrhage Metastasis in lymph nodes, liver, omentum, and mesentery
Histopathology	Similarities	Cords, nests, trabeculae, pseudoacinar pattern Delicate fibrovascular stroma with numerous small capillaries Cells are cuboidal to polyhedral, or columnar, with an abundant, finely granular, pale eosinophilic cytoplasm Mitoses infrequent	
	Differences	Thin fibrous capsule Irregularly shaped ducts and small nests of exocrine pancreatic acinar cells, particularly towards the periphery	Infiltration through the capsule and into adjacent parenchyma by neoplastic cells = the most important feature of malignancy Cells are less uniform in size and shape (anisocytosis, anisokaryosis)

(1–4)

1. Charles JA. Pancreas. In: M.; GM, editor. Jubb, Kennedy, and Palmer's Pathology of Domestic Animals, Fifth edition. Philadelphia: Elsevier Saunders; 2007.
2. Zachary JF, McGavin D. Pathologic Basis of Veterinary Disease: Elsevier Health Sciences; 2013.
3. Meuten DJ. Tumors in domestic animals. Ames, IA: Iowa State Press; 2002.
4. Head KW. Histological classification of tumors of the alimentary system of domestic animals: Published by the Armed Forces Institute of Pathology in cooperation with the American Registry of Pathology and the World Health Organization Collaborating Center for Worldwide Reference on Comparative Oncology; 2003.

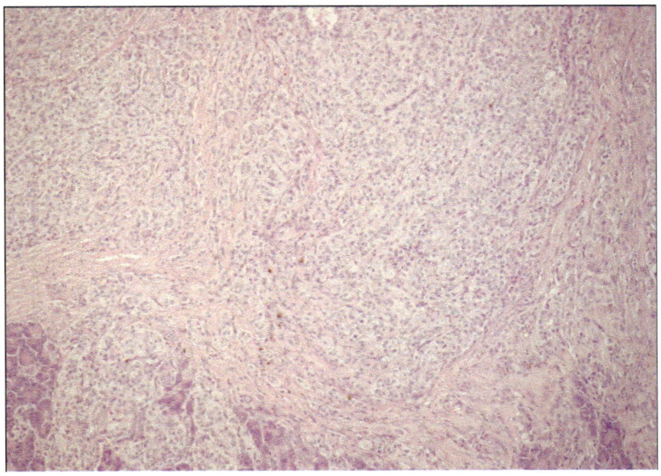

Figure 8.36 **Histopathology of a malignant insulinoma (islet cell carcinoma) from a dog. Low-power view of a pancreatic islet cell tumor infiltrating the surrounding exocrine parenchyma through a dense band of fibrous tissue (capsule). Neoplastic cells are arranged in small cords and nests supported by a thin fibrovascular stroma. Hematoxylin and eosin (×100).**

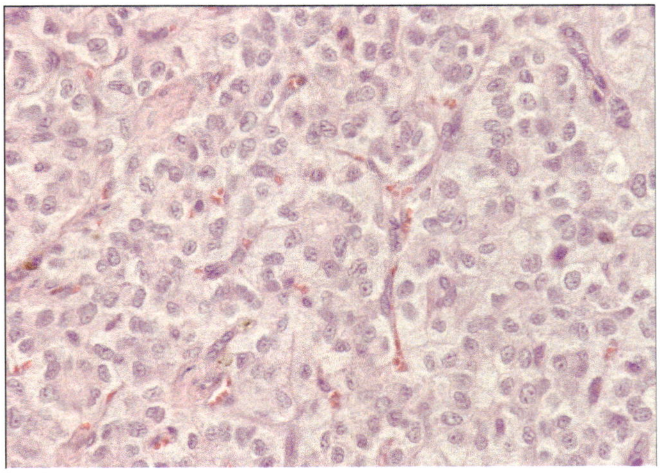

Figure 8.37 **Histopathology of a malignant insulinoma (islet cell carcinoma) from a dog. Higher magnification from Figure 8.36. Neoplastic cells are uniform, arranged in small nests supported by fine connective tissue septa containing numerous small capillaries. These cells are cuboidal to polyhedral, with an abundant, pale eosinophilic, finely granular cytoplasm, characteristic of neuroendocrine cells. Nuclei are ovoid, frequently indented, with a stippled chromatin. Hematoxylin and eosin (×400).**

so distinguish the β- and non-β islet cell neoplasms. In the case of insulinoma, the neoplastic cells predominantly secrete insulin, but other pancreatic hormones can also be secreted in lesser amounts (somatostatin, gastrin) (Madarame *et al*., 2009). Osseous metaplasia has been described in one case of canine insulinoma (Pieczarka *et al*., 2014).

Non-epithelial tumors

Primary nonepithelial tumors originating in the pancreas are rare and include fibroma, fibrosarcoma, hemangiosarcoma, liposarcoma, and nerve sheath tumors (Meuten, 2002; Head, 2003; Charles, 2007).

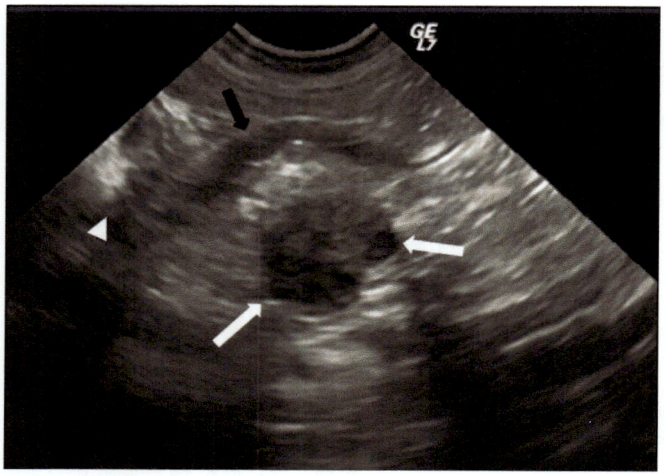

Figure 8.38 Sagittal view of the area of the left lobe of the pancreas in a 12-year-old dog. A solitary homogeneous mass of 2 cm in diameter (white arrows) was noted next to the great curvature of the stomach (arrow-head) and adjacent to the splenic vein (black arrow). Pancreatic endocrine tumor was identified histopathologically.

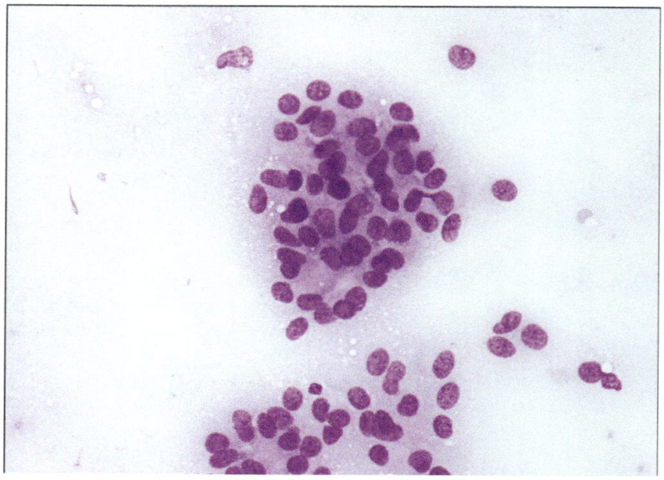

Figure 8.39 Aspirate of a malignant insulinoma (islet cell carcinoma) from a dog. Medium-power view of a pancreatic islet cell tumor characterized by some naked nuclei and loosely cohesive monomorphic medium-sized cells, organized in a pseudo-acinar pattern. Their cytoplasmic borders are very indistinct, and the rare intact cells have a cuboidal to polygonal shape. The cells display a moderate to high nuclear to cytoplasmic ratio, and minimal cellular atypia are observed. May-Grünwald–Giemsa (×400).

Secondary tumors

The pancreas may be invaded by direct extension from neoplastic diseases originating in contiguous organs such as alimentary lymphoma (Figure 8.41) and digestive (gastric or intestinal) carcinoma or may be involved in multicentric systemic disease (e.g., lymphoma, malignant histiocytosis) and disseminated malignancies through metastasis (Hayden *et al.*, 1993; Meuten, 2002; Swann *et al.*, 2002; Head, 2003; Charles, 2007). Distinguishing primitive pancreatic carcinoma from metastases of cholangiocellular or gastrointestinal carcinoma should be challenging on cytology and even on biopsies (34).

CASES

CASE 1

Signalment

A 15-year-old neutered male Domestic Shorthair cat was presented for a history of dysorexia, weakness, and weight loss for several weeks.

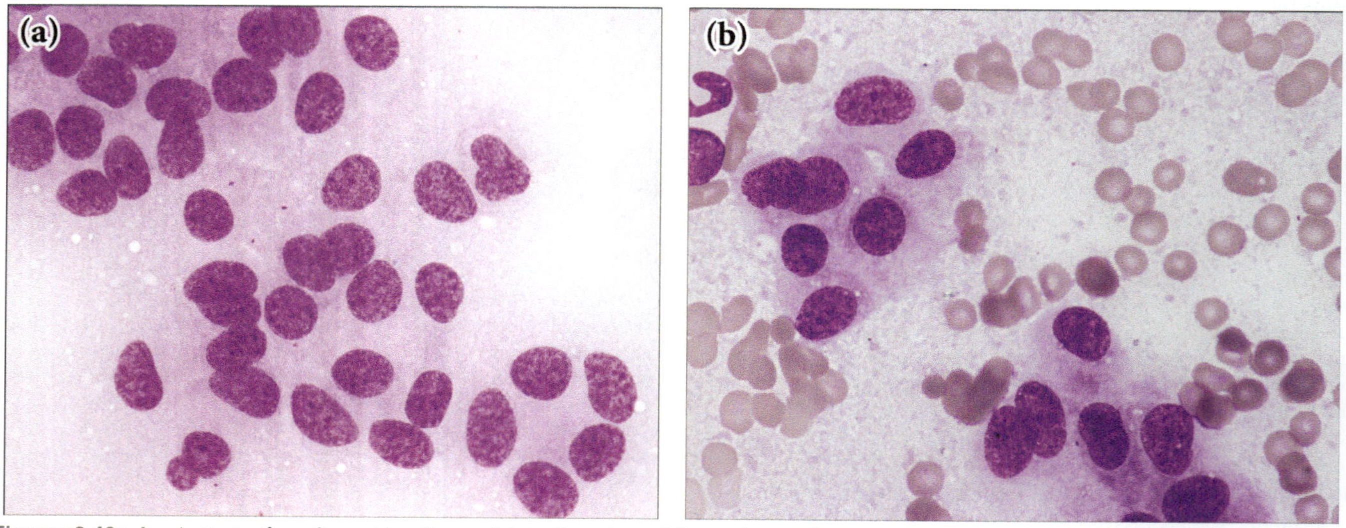

Figures 8.40a, b Aspirate of a malignant insulinoma (islet cell carcinoma) from a dog. Higher magnification from Figure 8.39. The monomorphic neoplastic cells are medium sized with a medium to high nuclear to cytoplasmic ratio, sometimes delimited by very indistinct cytoplasmic borders (8.40a) and characterized by a polygonal shape (8.40b). Cytoplasm is slightly basophilic, and nuclei are round to ovoid, sometimes eccentrically placed, with reticular to finely clumped chromatin. The main minimal cellular atypias observed are mild to moderate anisokaryosis and some binucleations. May-Grünwald Giemsa (x1000).

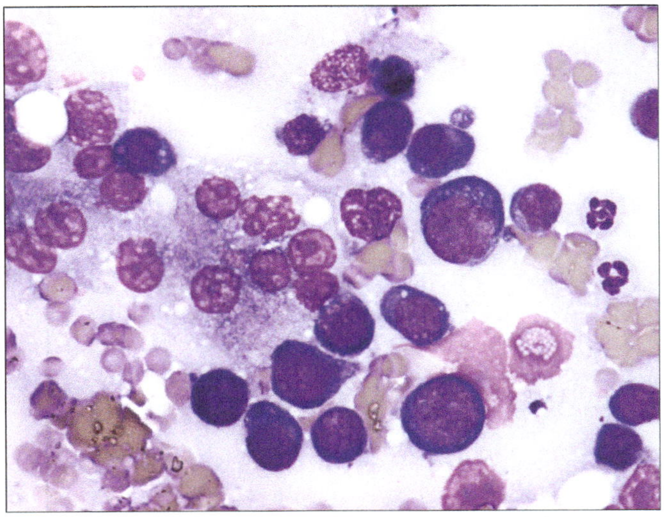

Figure 8.41 Aspirate of a pancreatic lymphoma. Presence of some hyperplastic acinar pancreatic cells associated with many round blastic cells. These blastic cells are large-sized and present a high nuclear to cytoplasmic ratio, a deeply basophilic cytoplasm, and a round to irregular nucleus associated with a finely reticulated chromatin pattern with one or numerous small to large nucleoli. These cells are highly suggestive of a high-grade lymphoma. May–Grünwald–Giemsa (×1,000).

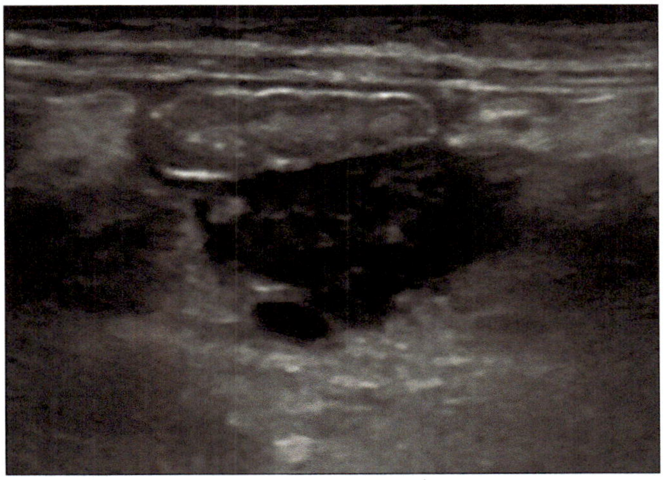

Figure 8.42 Ultrasonography of the pancreas. Pancreatic enlargement associated with diffuse hypoechogenicity and a distinct margin. The duodenum is seen in the near field, and the mesenteric fat appears hyperechoic.

Physical examination

At physical examination, the cat presented poor body condition and generalized amyotrophy. The main clinical finding was the presence of a spherical large abdominal mass (diameter: 3–4 cm). No particular abnormality was noticed at the heart and respiratory tract auscultation.

Investigation

The complete blood count was characterized by a mild leukocytosis (16.1 10^9/L, RI: 4.0–15.2 10^9/L) associated with a moderate neutrophilia (14.3 10^9/L, RI: 1.7–8.8 10^9/L), lymphopenia (0.7 10^9/L, RI: 1.2–10.2 10^9/L), and monocytosis with the presence of reactive monocytes on the blood smear (1.0 10^9/L, RI: 0.1–0.6 10^9/L), consistent with an inflammatory process and possible concurrent corticoid stress.

The biochemistry profile was dominated by a mild decrease in total proteins (51 g/L, RI: 55–71 g/L) with a mild decrease in albumin (22 g/L, RI: 27–39 g/L) which could both be more likely due to malnutrition, cachexia, malabsorption, protein loss enteropathy, and/or an inflammatory process; a mild increase in AST (72 U/L, RI: 6–44 U/L) which could be insignificant or due to hepatocellular or muscle damage; and an abnormal level of fPL with a rapid assay suggestive of a probable context of pancreatitis (IDEXX SNAP fPL Test). Electrolytes, ALP, ALT, GGT, and total bilirubin were within the reference interval, and no abnormality was noticed for the urinalysis.

A medical imaging investigation was performed to investigate a possible context of pancreatitis: the abdominal ultrasound revealed a pancreatic enlargement associated with strong and diffuse hypoechogenicity (Figure 8.42). The surrounding mesenteric fat was hyperechoic, and free fluid was noted around the pancreas. These findings were consistent with acute pancreatic inflammation or diffuse neoplasia. Thoracic radiography revealed a slight thoracic effusion.

Fine needle aspirates of the pancreas and the abdominal effusion were performed, and slides were stained with a modified May–Grünwald–Giemsa staining. Cytological evaluation of the pancreas revealed a mixed inflammation associated with secondary hyperplasia of acinar pancreatic cells, and at least a marked infiltration by an abnormal and monomorphic population of blastic cells (Figure 8.43). These blastic cells were large in size and

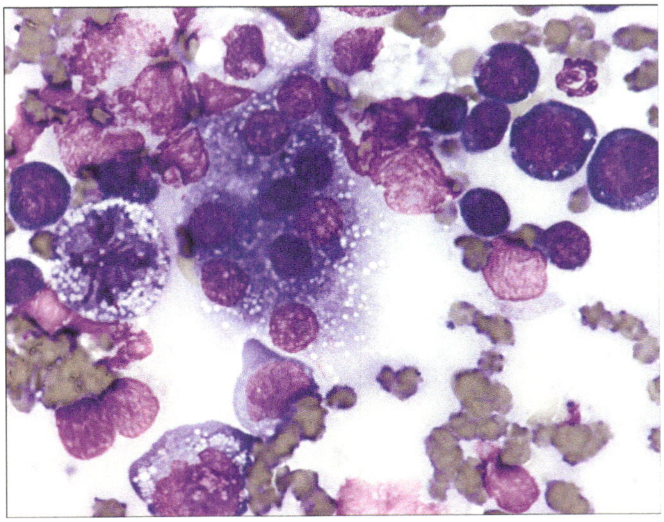

Figure 8.43 Cytology of the pancreas. Mixed inflammation characterized by macrophages and neutrophils and associated with a hyperplasia of acinar pancreatic cells characterized by the presence of a medium to large nucleoli, a moderate anisokaryosis and anisocytosis, and some binucleation of the acinar cells, and the presence of an abnormal population of blastic cells. May–Grünwald–Giemsa (×1,000).

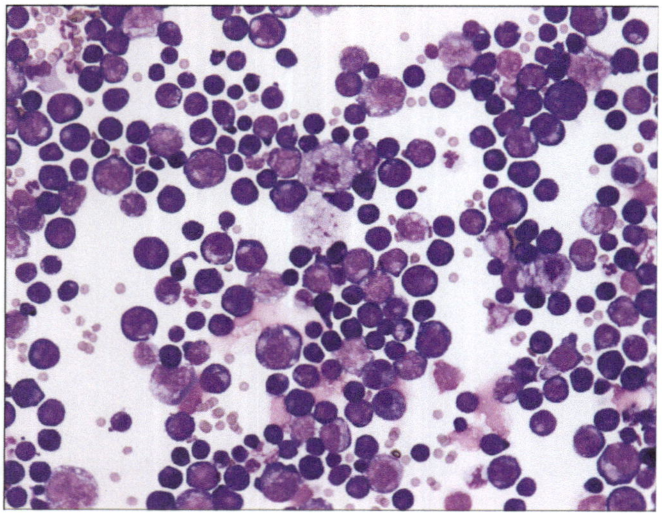

Figure 8.44 Cytology of the abdominal effusion. Presence of numerous and predominant monomorphic blastic cells cytologically similar to the neoplastic cells observed in the pancreas. May–Grünwald–Giemsa (×400).

presented a high nuclear to cytoplasmic ratio, a deeply basophilic cytoplasm sometimes finely and discretely vacuolated and/or disclosing a pseudo-arcoplasm, and a round and less frequently irregular nucleus associated with a finely reticulated chromatin pattern (Figures 8.43). One or numerous small to large nucleoli, sometimes prominent, were also observed. All these cytological features were consistent with an infiltration by blastic lymphoid cells, and the cytological diagnosis was a high-grade lymphoma. The nucleated cell count of the peritoneal fluid was 4,760 cells/µL and the protein

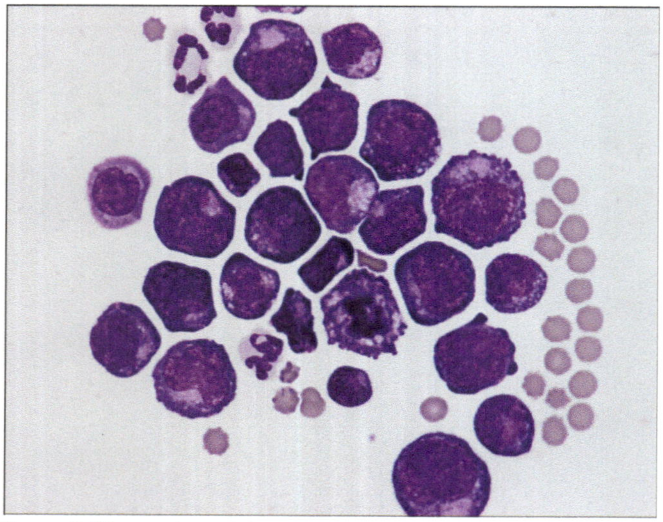

Figure 8.45 Cytology of the abdominal effusion. Presence of predominant round blastic cells consistent with the neoplastic cells observed in the pancreas. These cells are large in size and have a high nucleo-cytoplasmic ratio, a deeply basophilic cytoplasm sometimes disclosing a pseudo-arcoplasm, and a round to irregular nucleus associated with a finely reticulated chromatin pattern with one or numerous small to large nucleoli. May–Grünwald–Giemsa (×1,000).

concentration was 16 g/L. The cytological evaluation of the abdominal effusion was characterized by 87% of atypical blastic lymphoid cells, 9% neutrophils, 3% lymphocytes, and 1% macrophages (Figures 8.44 and 8.45). Immunocytochemistry was performed on the abdominal effusion to phenotype the neoplastic cells. The neoplastic population was strongly reactive for BLA36 and negative for CD3, CD79a, and a pancytokeratine (Figures 8.46a, 8.46b and 8.46c).

Based on all of these clinico-pathological findings, a final diagnosis of a B-cell high-grade lymphoma involving the pancreas was made, associated with secondary pancreatitis, even if a histiocytic neoplasm could not be excluded. The pancreatic origin of this lymphoma was suspected since no other solid organ seemed to be involved on medical imaging, but it could not be confirmed as the cat was discharged, and no outcome was available.

This clinical case stresses the fact that cytology is useful and safe to make the distinction between a pure inflammatory process such as pancreatitis and a diffuse neoplastic pancreatic infiltration such as high-grade lymphoma.

CASE 2

Signalment

A 10-year-old neutered female mixed breed dog was presented for a history of weakness, shivering for 3 days, and vomiting and diarrhea for 12 hours after dietary indiscretion. Two years ago, the dog was presented for acute blindness diagnosed as sudden acquired retinal degeneration associated with idiopathic hypertriglyceridemia.

Physical examination

At physical examination, the dog presented good body condition and abdominal distension. The main clinical finding was abdominal pain elicited by abdominal palpation. No particular abnormality was noticed at the heart and respiratory tract auscultation, but mild tachypnea was observed.

Investigation

The complete blood count was characterized by a mild neutrophilia (12.3 10^9/L, RI: 1.7–8.8 10^9/L) with a left shift and the presence of reactive monocytes and toxic neutrophils on the blood smear, consistent with an inflammatory process.

The biochemistry profile was dominated by a mild increase in total proteins (71.6 g/L, RI: 48–66 g/L), which could be due to dehydration or an inflammatory process; a mild increase in ALT (80 U/L, RI: 3–50 U/L) and ALP (331 U/L, RI: 22–155 U/L), which could be insignificant or due to hepatocellular damage and cholestasis; an abnormal level of cPL with a rapid assay suggestive of pancreatitis (IDEXX SNAP cPL Test); and an increase in creatinine, which could be suggestive of renal failure. Albumin and total bilirubin were within the reference range. The urinalysis was characterized by a low normal urinary specific gravity (1.024, RI: 1.015–1.050).

A medical imaging investigation was performed to investigate a possible context of hepatic, renal diseases, and pancreatitis: the

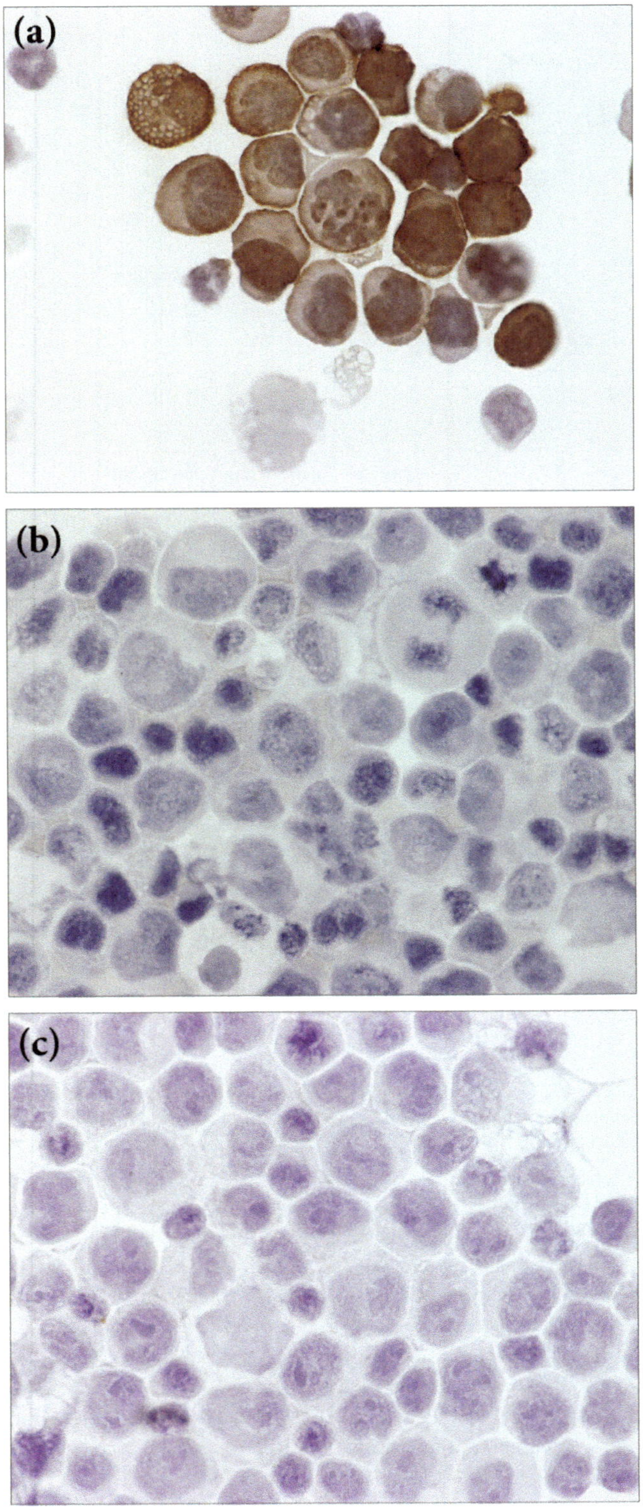

Figure 8.46a–c Immunocytochemistry of the abdominal effusion. The neoplastic cells are strongly positive with BLA36 (a) and negative for CD3 (b) and pancytokeratin (c) and are consistent with a B-cell high-grade lymphoma even if a histiocytic neoplasm could not be excluded (×1,000).

abdominal ultrasound revealed a pancreatic enlargement associated with strong and diffuse hypoechogenicity. The surrounding mesenteric fat was hyperechoic. These findings were consistent with acute pancreatic inflammation. The abdominal ultrasound also revealed a homogeneous enlarged liver and hyperechoic kidneys suggestive of diffuse vacuolar hepatopathy in the context of idiopathic hypertriglyceridemia and chronic renal failure, respectively.

Fine needle aspirates of the pancreas were performed, and slides were stained with a modified May–Grünwald–Giemsa staining. Cytological evaluation of the pancreas revealed a neutrophilic inflammation associated with a severe hyperplasia of acinar pancreatic cells (Figure 8.47). Neutrophils were sometimes degenerated and a few spumous macrophages were also observed. Based on all of these clinico-pathological findings, a final diagnosis of acute pancreatitis was made. After 3 days of supportive care, the dog improved and was discharged. The follow-up performed 1 month later showed an alert dog with stability of the chronic renal disease.

CASE 3

Signalment/history

A 5-year-old, female, Jack Russell dog was presented for a history of acute vomiting, diarrhea, and hematochezia. One month ago, the dog presented an event of acute vomiting and diarrhea simply resolved with symptomatic treatment.

Physical examination

The dog was presented in moderate body condition. The main clinical findings were marked icterus, a left apexial systolic murmur of grade I/V, and abdominal pain elicited by abdominal palpation.

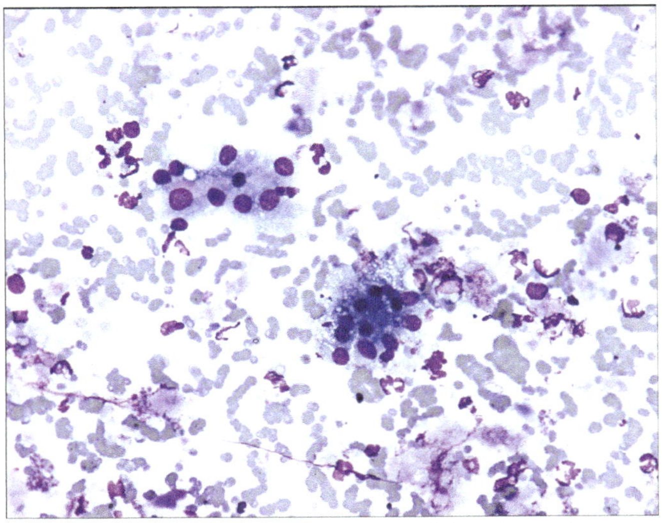

Figure 8.47 Cytology of the pancreas. Neutrophilic inflammation characterized by neutrophils associated with a hyperplasia of acinar pancreatic cells characterized by the presence of anisokaryosis and anisocytosis of the acinar cells. May–Grünwald–Giemsa (×400).

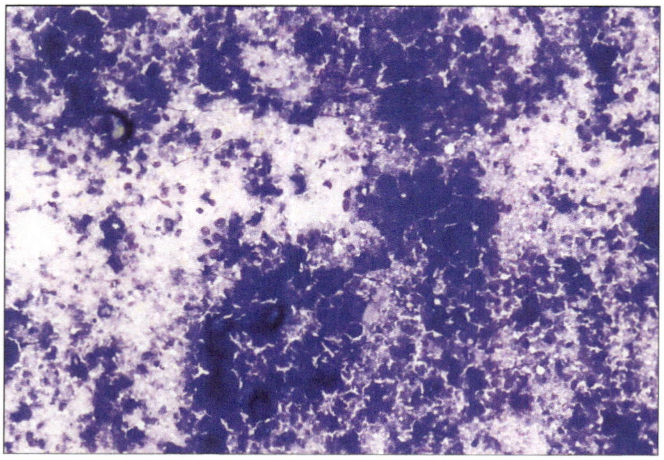

Figure 8.48 Cytology of pancreas. Necrotic background mainly associated with coagulation necrosis, damaged cells in cohesive clusters, and some calcified debris appearing as three-dimensional refractile material (May–Grünwald–Giemsa, 200× magnification).

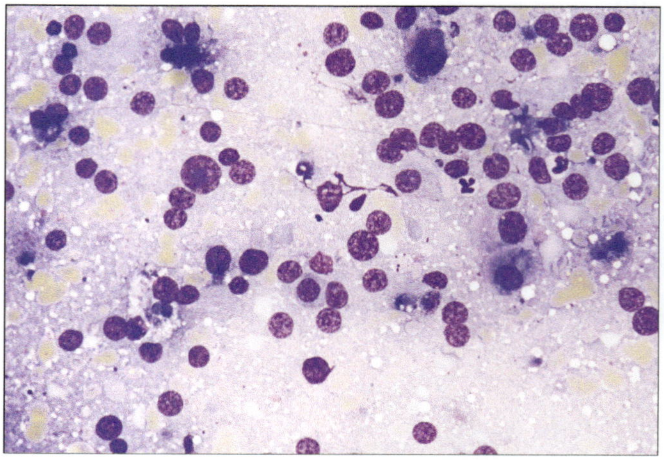

Figure 8.49 Cytology of pancreas. Hemorrhagic and necrotic background with many naked nuclei. Naked nuclei showed sometimes atypical features: gigantism, macronucleoli, and multiple nucleoli (May–Grünwald–Giemsa, 500× magnification).

Investigation

The complete blood cell count was characterized by a moderate leucocytosis (22.51.10^9/L; RI: 5.05–16.76) related to a neutrophilia (18.4.10^9/L; RI: 2.95–11.64), a monocytosis (1.32.10^9/L; RI: 0.16–1.23), and an eosinophilia (1.60.10^9/L; RI: 0.06–1.23).

The biochemistry profile was dominated by a severe increase in ALT (4062 U/L; RI: 8–60), AST (>1083 U/L; RI: 0–50), ALP (19329 U/L; RI: 30–230), and GGT (97 U/L; RI: 0–11) activities, and a marked increase in total bilirubin (38.5 mg/L; RI: 0.0–9.0), which were suggestive of hepatocellular damage and cholestasis. Urea, creatinine, glucose, and a panel of electrolytes were within reference intervals. Urinalysis was characterized by a low normal urinary specific gravity (1.015; RI: 1.015–1.050), pH equal to 8, and significant bilirubinuria (« +++ ») and possible proteinuria (« ++ ») according to dipstick analysis. Proteinuria had not been confirmed by a urinary protein to creatinine ratio.

An abdominal ultrasound mainly revealed a dilatation of the gallbladder, choledocal channel, and the rest of the biliary tract associated with the presence of a stone, many changes in the right lobe of the pancreas associated with a mass in relation to the duodenal papilla, and then a moderate pancreatic adenopathy. These findings were consistent with post-hepatic cholestasis and a possible neoplasia of the pancreas probably extended to the nearby lymph node.

A laparotomy was performed to explore the biliary tract and pancreatic anomalies, and to try to investigate more accurately the pancreatic mass. It confirmed all previously noticed changes in the biliary tract and the presence of an infiltrating and diffuse mass (size: 2 × 1 × 1 cm), in the area of the duodenal papilla but for which the origin was finally macroscopically uncertain, pancreatic, or duodenal. Surgical removal of this mass was impossible, and so FNA and biopsy of the mass and a biopsy of the enlarged pancreatic lymph node were performed to make a diagnosis.

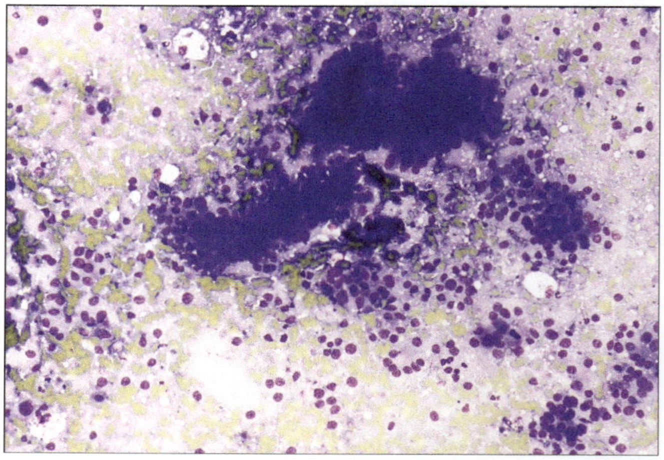

Figure 8.50 Cytology of pancreas. Abundant population of cohesive cells mainly organized in clusters with tubular, papillary, and acinar patterns. The epithelial cells were medium to large size, and round to polygonal, with a medium to high N:C ratio (May–Grünwald–Giemsa, 200× magnification).

Cytologic evaluation

There was a hemorrhagic, markedly necrotic, and slightly inflammatory background (Figure 8.48). The cellularity was high and the cells of interest were fragile; many naked nuclei (sometimes atypical) were also observed (Figure 8.49). The sample mainly revealed an abundant and predominant population of atypical cohesive cells, which were organized in many clusters with tubular, papillary, and acinar patterns (Figures 8.50 and 8.51). These epithelial cells were of medium-large size to giant, often associated with a moderate to high N:C ratio. Their cytoplasm was mainly polarized, granular (pale pink round granules suggestive of zymogen granules), and hyperbasophilic and so suggestive of acinar pancreatic cells, and their nucleus was round to oval, often polarized, and with a coarse to reticular chromatin pattern and one or two small to large nucleoli (Figures 8.51 and 8.52). These

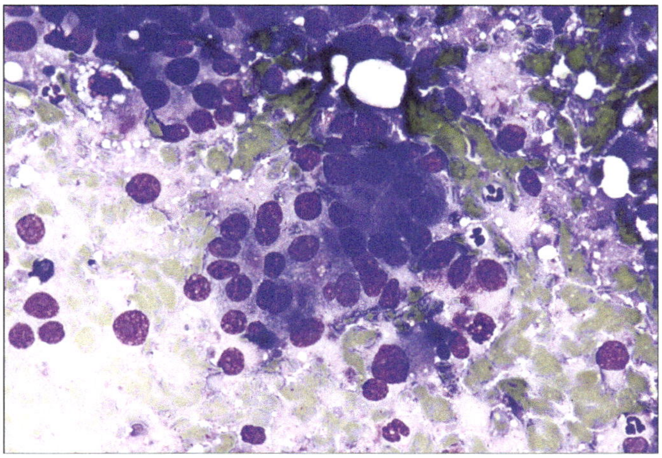

Figure 8.51 Cytology of pancreas. Epithelial cells of interest organized in clusters with acinar patterns. These cells were medium to large size, with a round to polygonal shape, and with a clearly polarized nucleus, and displayed a medium to high N:C ratio. Their cytoplasm was granular (pink round granules suggestive of zymogen granules) and hyperbasophilic and so suggestive of acinar pancreatic cells, and their nucleus was round to oval, and with a coarse to reticular chromatin pattern and one or two small to large nucleoli (May-Grünwald-Giemsa, 500× magnification).

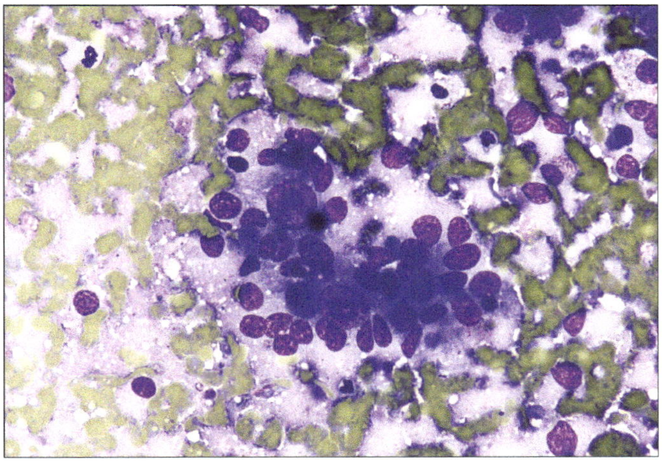

Figure 8.52 Cytology of pancreas. Acinar pancreatic cells organized in clusters with acinar patterns. These cells were medium to very large in size, with a round to polygonal shape, and with a polarized nucleus, and displayed a medium to high N:C ratio. Their cytoplasm was moderately granular and hyperbasophilic. Their nucleus was round to oval, and with a coarse to reticular chromatin pattern and one or two small to giant nucleoli. The cells showed marked atypical features: marked anisokaryosis and anisocytosis, and macronucleolation (May-Grünwald-Giemsa, 500× magnification).

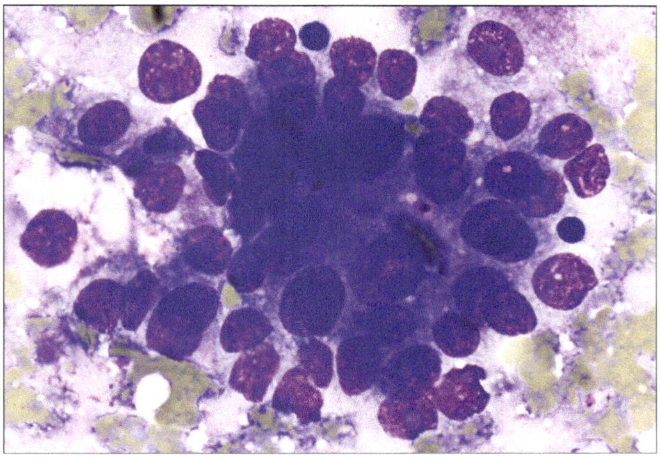

Figure 8.53 Cytology of pancreas. Acinar pancreatic cells organized in clusters with acinar patterns. These cells were medium to very large in size, with a round to polygonal shape, and with a polarized nucleus, and displayed a medium to high N:C ratio. Their cytoplasm was granular (pink granules) and hyperbasophilic. Their nucleus was round to oval, and with a coarse to reticular chromatin pattern and one or two small to large nucleoli. The cells showed marked atypical features: marked anisokaryosis and anisocytosis, some binucleation and macronucleolation (May-Grünwald-Giemsa, 1,000× magnification).

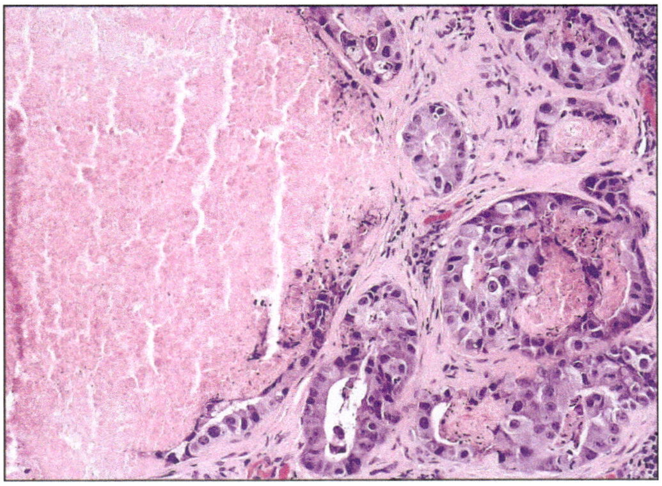

Figure 8.54 Biopsy of pancreas. The pancreatic mass consisted of anastomosed tubulo-acinar structures with variable distended lumens, supported by an abundant fibrous stroma, infiltrated by some lymphocytes, plasma cells, and neutrophils. An eosinophilic, granular necrotic material was frequently observed within neoplastic distended lumens. Tubules and acini were lined by a cuboidal to pyramidal, unicellular to multifocally stratified, severely atypical, neoplastic epithelium (Hemalun-Eosin, 200× magnification).

cells were also occasionally microvacuolated. Anaplastic features were frequently observed: marked anisocytosis and anisokaryosis, binucleation, macronucleolation, giant cells, and some mitotic figures (Figures 8.52 and 8.53). All these cytological features were highly suggestive of pancreatic adenocarcinoma. The histopathological examination of the mass and the enlarged lymph node confirmed a pancreatic adenocarcinoma with extension to the pancreatic lymph node (Figures 8.54 and 8.55). The same neoplastic tissue compatible with a pancreatic carcinoma was also observed replacing the lymphoid pulp in the nodal biopsy.

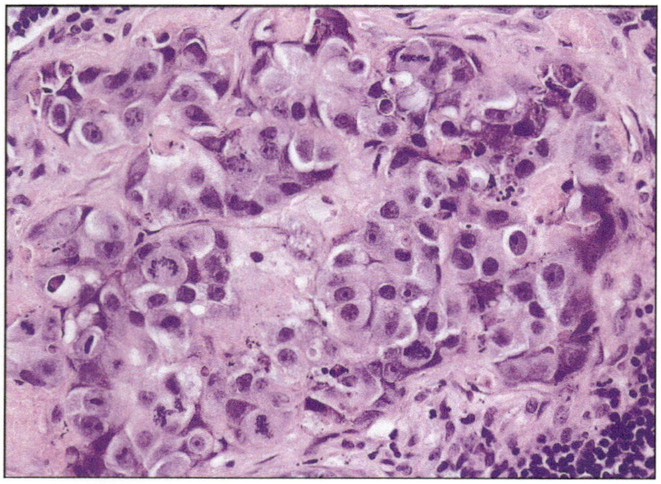

Figure 8.55 Biopsy of pancreas. Neoplastic cells, arranged in tubules or acini with a small central lumen containing necrotic hypereosinophilic debris, were large, cuboid to pyramidal, with a parabasal to basal nucleus and an abundant finely granular to rarely microvacuolated, amphophilic cytoplasm. Nuclei were round to oval, with a variably condensed chromatin, one large to several small basophilic nucleoli. Anisocytosis and anisokaryosis were marked to severe, and mitoses were numerous, and often atypical (Hemalun-Eosin, 400× magnification).

Diagnosis

Based on clinico- and histopathologic findings, a final diagnosis of pancreatic adenocarcinoma disseminated at least to the pancreatico-duodenal lymph node was made.

Outcome

Given the poor prognosis, a symptomatic and palliative treatment was decided by the owners. The dog was finally humanely euthanized 2 months later.

REFERENCES

Allen J. (2021) Pancreas (exocrine and endocrine). In: *Canine and Feline Cytopathology*, 4th edn. (ed. R.E. Raskin, D.J. Meyer, K.M. Boes) Elsevier, pp. 321–337.

Anderson J.R., Cornell K.K., Parnell N.K., Salisbury S.K. (2008) Pancreatic abscess in 36 dogs: A retrospective analysis of prognostic indicators. *J Am Anim Hosp Assoc 44(4)*:171–179.

Andreasen C.B., Jergens A.E., Meyer D.J. (2010) Oral cavity, gastrointestinal tract, and associated structures. In: *Canine and Feline Cytology* (eds. R.E. Raskin, J. Meyer) W.B. Saunders, Saint Louis, pp. 192–214.

Armstrong P.J., Williams D.A. (2012) Pancreatitis in cats. *Top Companion Anim Med 27(3)*:140–147.

Baghbanian M., Shabazkhani B., Ghofrani H., Forutan H., Dariani N., Farahvash M., Aletaha N. (2012) Efficacy of endoscopic ultrasound guided fine needle aspiration in patients with solid pancreatic neoplasms. *Saudi J Gastroenterol 18(6)*:358–363.

Bailey D. (2007) Tumors of the endocrine system. In: *Withrow & MacEwen's Small Animal Clinical Oncology* (eds. S.J. Withrow, M. Vail) W.B. Saunders, Saint Louis, pp. 583–609.

Banks W.J. (1993) *Applied Veterinary Histology. Third Edition*. Mosby Year Book, St Louis, Missouri.

Barone R. (1997) *Anatomie comparée des mammifères domestiques. Tome 3. Splanchnologie I. Appareil digestif. Appareil respiratoire*. Vigot, Paris, France.

Bennett P.F., Hahn K.A., Toal R.L., Legendre A.M. (2001) Ultrasonographic and cytopathological diagnosis of exocrine pancreatic carcinoma in the dog and cat. *J Am Anim Hosp Assoc 37(5)*:466–473.

Bergin D., Ho L.M., Jowell P.S., Pappas T.N., Paulson E.K. (2002) Simple pancreatic cysts: CT and endosonographic appearances. *AJR Am J Roentgenol 178(4)*:837–840.

Bjorneby J.M., Kari S. (2002) Cytology of the pancreas. *Vet Clin North Am Small Anim Pract 32(6)*:1293–1312, vi.

Borjesson D.L. (2014) The pancreas. In: *Cowell and Tyler's Diagnostic Cytology and Hematology of the Dog and Cat* (eds. A.C. Valenciano, R.L. Cowell) Elsevier Health Sciences, St. Louis, MO, pp. 341–353.

Bostrom B.M., Xenoulis P.G., Newman S.J., Pool R.R., Fosgate G.T., Steiner J.M. (2013) Chronic pancreatitis in dogs: A retrospective study of clinical, clinicopathological, and histopathological findings in 61 cases. *Vet J 195(1)*:73–79.

Branter E.M., Viviano K.R. (2010) Multiple recurrent pancreatic cysts with associated pancreatic inflammation and atrophy in a cat. *J Feline Med Surg 12(10)*:822–827.

Caywood D.D., Wilson J.W., Hardy R.M., Shull R.M. (1979) Pancreatic islet cell adenocarcinoma: Clinical and diagnostic features of six cases. *J Am Vet Med Assoc 174(7)*:714–717.

Charles J.A. (2007) Pancreas. In: *Jubb, Kennedy, and Palmer's Pathology of Domestic Animals*, 5th edn. (ed. M.M. Grant). Elsevier Saunders, Philadelphia.

Coleman M.G., Robson M.C., Harvey C. (2005) Pancreatic cyst in a cat. *N Z Vet J 53(2)*:157–159.

Cordner A.P., Armstrong P.J., Newman S.J., Novo R., Sharkey L.C., Jessen Emeritus C. (2010) Effect of pancreatic tissue sampling on serum pancreatic enzyme levels in clinically healthy dogs. *J Vet Diagn Invest 22(5)*:702–707.

Cordner A.P., Sharkey L.C., Armstrong P.J., McAteer K.D. (2015) Cytologic findings and diagnostic yield in 92 dogs undergoing fine-needle aspiration of the pancreas. *J Vet Diagn Invest 27(2)*:236–240.

Crain S.K., Sharkey L.C., Cordner A.P., Knudson C., Armstrong P.J. (2015) Safety of ultrasound-guided fine-needle aspiration of the feline pancreas: A case-control study. *J Feline Med Surg 17(10)*:858–863.

Cruz Cardona J.A., Wamsley H.L., Farina L.L., Kiupel M. (2010) Metastatic pancreatic polypeptide-secreting islet cell tumor in a dog. *Vet Clin Pathol 39(3)*:371–376.

De Cock H.E., Forman M.A., Farver T.B., Marks S.L. (2007) Prevalence and histopathologic characteristics of pancreatitis in cats. *Vet Pathol 44(1)*:39–49.

Dumonceau J.M., Polkowski M., Larghi A., Vilmann P., Giovannini M., Frossard J.L., Heresbach D., Pujol B., Fernandez-Esparrach G., Vazquez-Sequeiros E., Gines A., E. European Society of Gastrointestinal. (2011) Indications, results, and clinical impact of endoscopic ultrasound (EUS)-guided sampling in gastroenterology: European Society of Gastrointestinal Endoscopy (ESGE) Clinical Guideline. *Endoscopy 43(10)*:897–912.

Eisendrath P., Ibrahim M. (2014) How good is fine needle aspiration? What results should you expect? *Endosc Ultrasound 3(1)*:3–11.

Etue S.M., Penninck D.G., Labato M.A., Pearson S., Tidwell A. (2001) Ultrasonography of the normal feline pancreas and associated anatomic landmarks: A prospective study of 20 cats. *Vet Radiol Ultrasound 42(4)*:330–336.

Eurell J.A., Frappier B.L. (2006) *Dellmann's Textbook of Veterinary Histology. Sixth Edition*. Blackwell Publishing, Victoria.

Evans H.E., De Lahunta A. (2013) *Miller's Anatomy of the Dog, 4th Edition*. Saunders/Elsevier, St. Louis, Missouri.

Forman M.A., Marks S.L., De Cock H.E., Hergesell E.J., Wisner E.R., Baker T.W., Kass P.H., Steiner J.M., Williams D.A. (2004) Evaluation of serum feline pancreatic lipase immunoreactivity and helical computed tomography versus conventional testing for the diagnosis of feline pancreatitis. *J Vet Intern Med 18(6)*:807–815.

Forman M.A., Steiner J.M., Armstrong P.J., Camus M.S., Gaschen L., Hill S.L., Mansfield C.S., Steiger K. (2021) ACVIM consensus statement on pancreatitis in cats. *J Vet Intern Med 35(2)*:703–723.

Fujii L.L., Levy M.J. (2014) Basic techniques in endoscopic ultrasound-guided fine needle aspiration for solid lesions: Adverse events and avoiding them. *Endosc Ultrasound 3(1)*:35–45.

Goutal C.M., Brugmann B.L., Ryan K.A. (2012) Insulinoma in dogs: A review. *J Am Anim Hosp Assoc 48(3)*:151–163.

Granger L.A., Hilferty M., Francis T., Steiner J.M., Gaschen L. (2015) Variability in the ultrasonographic appearance of the pancreas in healthy dogs compared to dogs with hyperadrenocorticism. *Vet Radiol Ultrasound 56(5)*:540–548.

Griffin S. (2020) Feline abdominal ultrasonography: What's normal? What's abnormal? The pancreas. *J Feline Med Surg 22(3)*:241–259.

Hayden D.W., Waters D.J., Burke B.A., Manivel J.C. (1993) Disseminated malignant histiocytosis in a golden retriever: Clinicopathologic, ultrastructural, and immunohistochemical findings. *Vet Pathol 30(3)*:256–264.

Head K.W. (2003) *Histological Classification of Tumors of the Alimentary System of Domestic Animals*. Published by the Armed Forces Institute of Pathology in cooperation with the American Registry of Pathology and the World Health Organization Collaborating Center for Worldwide Reference on Comparative Oncology.

Healy D.M., Cassidy J.P., Martin S.A. (2022) A true congenital pancreatic cyst in a dog. *BMC Vet Res 18(1)*:304.

Hecht S., Henry G. (2007) Sonographic evaluation of the normal and abnormal pancreas. *Clin Tech Small Anim Pract 22(3)*:115–121.

Hill R.C., Van Winkle T.J. (1993) Acute necrotizing pancreatitis and acute suppurative pancreatitis in the cat. A retrospective study of 40 cases (1976–1989). *J Vet Intern Med 7(1)*:25–33.

Iglesias-Garcia J., Larino-Noia J., Dominguez-Munoz J.E. (2014) When to puncture, when not to puncture: Pancreatic masses. *Endosc Ultrasound 3(2)*:91–97.

Jegatheeson S., Dandrieux J.R., Cannon C.M. (2020) Suspected pancreatic carcinoma needle tract seeding in a cat. *JFMS Open Rep 6(1)*:2055116920918161.

Kalli I., Adamama-Moraitou K., Rallis T.S. (2009) Acute pancreatitis in dogs: A review article. *European Journal of Companion Animal Practice 19(2)*:147–155.

Kierszenbaum A.L., Tres L.L. (2019) *Histology and Cell Biology. An Introduction to Pathology. 5th Edition*. Elsevier.

Kook P.H., Baloi P., Ruetten M., Pantchev N., Reusch C.E., Kircher P. (2012) Feasibility and safety of endoscopic ultrasound-guided fine needle aspiration of the pancreas in dogs. *J Vet Intern Med 26(3)*:513–517.

Larson M.M. (2016) Ultrasound imaging of the hepatobiliary system and pancreas. *Vet Clin North Am Small Anim Pract 46(3)*:453–480, v–vi.

Lin F., Staerkel G. (2003) Cytologic criteria for well differentiated adenocarcinoma of the pancreas in fine-needle aspiration biopsy specimens. *Cancer 99(1)*:44–50.

Madarame H., Kayanuma H., Shida T., Tsuchiya R. (2009) Retrospective study of canine insulinomas: Eight cases (2005–2008). *J Vet Med Sci 71(7)*:905–911.

Mansfield C. (2013) Practical interpretation and application of exocrine pancreatic testing in small animals. *Vet Clin North Am Small Anim Pract 43(6)*:1241–1260, v–vi.

Meuten D.J. (2002) *Tumors in Domestic Animals*. Iowa State Press, Ames, IA.

Minkus G., Jutting U., Aubele M., Rodenacker K., Gais P., Breuer W., Hermanns W. (1997) Canine neuroendocrine tumors of the pancreas: A study using image analysis techniques for the discrimination of metastatic versus non-metastatic tumors. *Vet Pathol 34(2)*:138–145.

Newman S., Steiner J., Woosley K., Barton L., Ruaux C., Williams D. (2004) Localization of pancreatic inflammation and necrosis in dogs. *J Vet Intern Med 18(4)*:488–493.

Newman S.J., Steiner J.M., Woosley K., Barton L., Williams D.A. (2005) Correlation of age and incidence of pancreatic exocrine nodular hyperplasia in the dog. *Vet Pathol 42(4)*:510–513.

Newman S.J., Steiner J.M., Woosley K., Williams D.A., Barton L. (2006) Histologic assessment and grading of the exocrine pancreas in the dog. *J Vet Diagn Invest 18(1)*:115–118.

Nyland T.G., Wallack S.T., Wisner E.R. (2002) Needle-tract implantation following us-guided fine-needle aspiration biopsy of transitional cell carcinoma of the bladder, urethra, and prostate. *Vet Radiol Ultrasound 43(1)*:50–53.

Penninck D., d'Anjou M.-A. (2013) *Atlas of Small Animal Ultrasonography*. John Wiley & Sons.

Penninck D.G., Zeyen U., Taeymans O.N., Webster C.R. (2013) Ultrasonographic measurement of the pancreas and pancreatic duct in clinically normal dogs. *Am J Vet Res 74(3)*:433–437.

Petrone M.C., Arcidiacono P.G. (2014) Basic technique in endoscopic ultrasound-guided fine needle aspiration for solid lesions: How many passes? *Endosc Ultrasound 3(1)*:22–27.

Pieczarka E.M., Russell D.S., Santangelo K.S., Aeffner F., Burkhard M.J. (2014) Osseous metaplasia within a canine insulinoma. *Vet Clin Pathol 43(1)*:89–93.

Pinard C.J., Hocker S.E., Weishaar K.M. (2021) Clinical outcome in 23 dogs with exocrine pancreatic carcinoma. *Vet Comp Oncol 19(1)*:109–114.

Polton G.A., White R.N., Brearley M.J., Eastwood J.M. (2007) Improved survival in a retrospective cohort of 28 dogs with insulinoma. *J Small Anim Pract 48(3)*:151–156.

Priester W.A. (1974) Data from eleven United States and Canadian colleges of veterinary medicine on pancreatic carcinoma in domestic animals. *Cancer Res 34(6)*:1372–1375.

Ramírez G.A., Altimira J., García-González B., & Vilafranca M. (2013) Intrapancreatic ectopic splenic tissue in dogs and cats. *J Comp Pathol 148(4)*:361–364.

Robben J.H., Pollak Y.W., Kirpensteijn J., Boroffka S.A., van den Ingh T.S., Teske E., Voorhout G. (2005) Comparison of ultrasonography, computed tomography, and single-photon emission computed tomography for the detection and localization of canine insulinoma. *J Vet Intern Med 19(1)*:15–22.

Rudinsky A.J. (2023) Laboratory diagnosis of pancreatitis. *Vet Clin North Am Small Anim Pract 53(1)*:225–240.

Siddiqui U.D., Rossi F., Rosenthal L.S., Padda M.S., Murali-Dharan V., Aslanian H.R. (2009) EUS-guided FNA of solid pancreatic masses: A prospective, randomized trial comparing 22-gauge and 25-gauge needles. *Gastrointest Endosc 70(6)*:1093–1097.

Smith S.J., Vogelzang R.L., Donovan J., Atlas S.W., Gore R.M., Neiman H.L. (1985) Intraoperative sonography of the pancreas. *AJR Am J Roentgenol 144(3)*:557–562.

Steiner J.M. (2010) Canine pancreatic disease. In: *Textbook of Veterinary Internal Medicine: Diseases of the Dog and the Cat* (eds. S.J. Ettinger, E.C. Feldman) Elsevier Saunders, Volume 2, pp. 1695–1703.

Swann H.M., Holt D.E. (2002) Canine gastric adenocarcinoma and leiomyosarcoma: A retrospective study of 21 cases (1986–1999) and literature review. *J Am Anim Hosp Assoc 38(2)*:157–164.

Torner K., Staudacher M., Tress U., Weber C.N., Stadler C., Grassinger J.M., Muller E., Aupperle-Lellbach H. (2020) Histopathology and feline pancreatic lipase immunoreactivity in inflammatory, hyperplastic and neoplastic pancreatic diseases in cats. *J Comp Pathol 174*:63–72.

Vanderperren K., Haers H., Van der Vekens E., Stock E., Paepe D., Daminet S., Saunders J.H. (2014) Description of the use of contrast-enhanced ultrasonography in four dogs with pancreatic tumours. *J Small Anim Pract 55*(*3*):164–169.

VanEnkevort B.A., O'Brien R.T. and Young K.M. (1999) Pancreatic pseudocysts in 4 dogs and 2 cats: Ultrasonographic and clinicopathologic findings. *J Vet Intern Med 13*(*4*):309–313.

Varadarajulu S., Bang J.Y., Holt B.A., Hasan M.K., Logue A., Hawes R.H., Hebert-Magee S. (2014) The 25-gauge EUS-FNA needle: Good for on-site but poor for off-site evaluation? Results of a randomized trial. *Gastrointest Endosc 80*(*6*):1056–1063.

Washabau R.J. (2010) Feline pancreatic disease. In: *Textbook of Veterinary Internal Medicine: Diseases of the Dog and the Cat* (eds. S.J. Ettinger, E.C. Feldman) Elsevier Saunders, Volume 2, pp. 1704–1709.

Washabau R.J., Day M.J. (2012) *Canine and Feline Gastroenterology*. Elsevier Saunders.

Watson P. (2012) Chronic pancreatitis in dogs. *Top Companion Anim Med 27*(*3*):133–139.

Watson P.J., Roulois A.J., Scase T., Johnston P.E., Thompson H., Herrtage M.E. (2007) Prevalence and breed distribution of chronic pancreatitis at post-mortem examination in first-opinion dogs. *J Small Anim Pract 48*(*11*):609–618.

Yang G.C.H., Tao L.-C. (2008) Liver and pancreas. In: *Comprehensive Cytopathology* (ed. M.B. Wilbur). W.B. Saunders, Edinburgh, pp. 873–913.

Yoshimura H., Matsuda Y., Kawamoto Y., Michishita M., Ohkusu-Tsukada K., Takahashi K., Naito Z., Ishiwata T. (2013) Acinar cell cystadenoma of the pancreas in a cat. *J Comp Pathol 149*(*2–3*):225–228.

Young B., Lowe J.S., Stevens A., Heath J.W. (2006) *Wheater's Functional Histology. A Text and Colour Atlas, Fifth Edition*. Churchill Livingstone Elsevier.

Zachary J.F., McGavin D. (2013) *Pathologic Basis of Veterinary Disease*. Elsevier Health Sciences.

CHAPTER 9

LIVER CYTOLOGY

A Russell Moore

SAMPLING

Indications and contraindications

Cytologic evaluation of the liver and gallbladder contents is generally pursued to confirm and define suspected hepatobiliary disease or screen for hepatic metastasis during staging of cancer. Hepatic cytology should be considered a valued part of the diagnostic toolkit.

The liver produces most of the plasma coagulation factors; this has led some to avoid aspiration when liver failure is suspected. Several studies suggest that altered coagulation times (prothrombin time [PT], activated partial thromboplastin time [aPTT], and buccal mucosal bleeding time) are not associated with significant post-collection complications (Moritz *et al.*, 2018; Vasanjee *et al.*, 2006). However, thrombocytopenia has been strongly correlated with post-procedural bleeding (Bigge *et al.*, 2001). When hemorrhage was noted after hepatic aspiration, the clinical effects were minimal (Reece *et al.*, 2020). As a general rule, therefore, evaluation of at least PT, aPTT, and platelet count is commonly advised for most patients prior to biopsy techniques. Mildly to moderately elongated coagulation results with normal platelet counts should not be viewed as a contraindication for hepatic sampling, but instead should indicate that there is an increased likelihood of post-sampling complications and additional monitoring may be advantageous. If clinically apparent bleeding diathesis, thrombocytopenia, or severely aberrant results are found, the potential risks of post-aspiration bleeding should be weighed against the potential information gained from the procedure.

Another potential contraindication is the possibility of iatrogenic metastasis. Very few studies have evaluated the potential to disseminate cancer during biopsy in veterinary medicine; those that have been published deal with urinary tract and pulmonary cancers (Nyland *et al.*, 2002; Vignoli *et al.*, 2007). Extrapolating from human cases and animal models of human cancer, hepatocellular and biliary carcinomas are not likely to seed along the needle tract but subcutaneous implantation of hepatocellular carcinoma has been reported in dogs and humans (Peterson *et al.*, 2022). The result of one meta-analysis on the tumor metastatic effect of biopsy retrieval concluded that more was gained from sampling and identifying a lesion than was risked in the collection of the sample (Klopfleisch *et al.*, 2011). This does not mean that the risk should be ignored. Sample collection should be planned to avoid as many vital structures as possible and make resection as minimally destructive as possible.

Technique

Fine needle aspiration (FNA) of the liver can usually be performed without sedation or local or general anesthesia. For larger, palpable masses or suspected diffuse disease (lymphoma), a blind technique can be used. Ultrasound guidance is usually advantageous for most cases, especially those with nonpalpable focal lesions. Ultrasound findings should guide the choice of approach. As a general rule, approaching along the costal arch or on the right thorax at the level of the 10th intercostal space will usually allow access to the liver. Fasting the patient is not required but may ensure that the stomach is not along the path of sampling. If a focal lesion is present, aspirates of the center of the mass as well as the margin of the lesion should be taken as both sites will provide different, yet complementary findings. Aspiration of the center of a large mass often shows necrosis and an inflammatory response, while aspiration of the margin contains an obviously neoplastic population. Studies have shown that sampling of multiple sites increases the probability of obtaining a representative sample (Kemp *et al.*, 2015; Chaivoravitsakul *et al.*, 2021).

Ultrasound gel must be meticulously removed prior to aspiration. Ultrasound gel preferentially attracts most stains and can prevent full cytologic evaluation of any obtained cells (Figure 9.1). Intraoperative

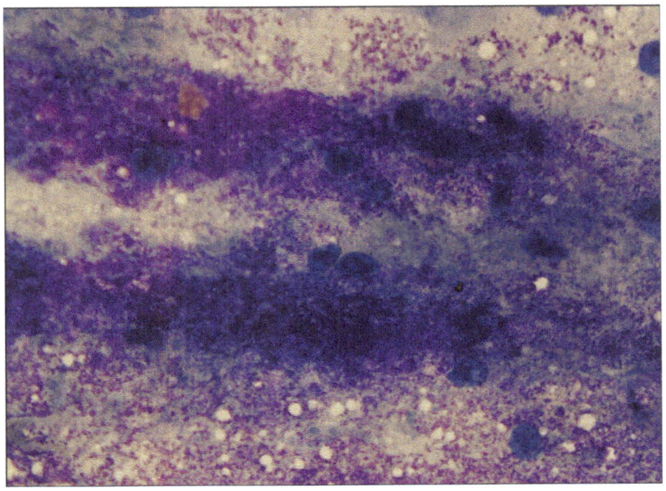

Figure 9.1 **The copious amount of purple granular material that obscures cytologic features of the underlying hepatocytes is consistent with ultrasound gel. For cytologic evaluation, it is imperative that gel be removed from the site of needle insertion prior to collection of aspirates (Wright–Giemsa, 400× magnification).**

DOI: 10.1201/9781003258551-9

evaluation of lesions and rapid evaluation can aid the surgeon in making decisions on resection and closure techniques.

A 20–22-gauge needle up to 3 inches (7.5 cm) long will allow penetration to the level of the liver in most patients. A 3 ml disposable syringe is ideal as it minimizes the amount of suction that can be applied while collecting the sample and can be either directly connected to the needle or to a segment of extension tubing. The needle should be placed at the site of the lesion and then advanced and retracted 5–10 mm multiple times along a single track (a sewing machine type action) to pack hepatocytes into the needle (Rothuizen & Twedt, 2009). Aspiration with application of negative pressure has also been described but is not recommended owing to the highly vascular nature of the liver (Rothuizen *et al.*, 2006; Rothuizen & Twedt, 2009). The application of negative pressure will frequently cause excessive blood collection. If suction is applied, it should be completely released prior to withdrawal of the needle from the sample site; this is especially important in patients with ascites to prevent contamination of the sample with ascitic fluid. After withdrawal, disconnect the syringe, fill it with air, reattach it to the needle, and gently expel the contents of the needle onto a clean, labeled glass slide. An additional slide is then used to gently make squash preparations of the sample. Biopsy samples taken for histopathology can be rolled (tru-cut type biopsies) or imprinted (wedge biopsies) on a clean glass slide to provide a quick cytologic evaluation (Chapter 1).

After the sample is air-dried, a Romanowsky stain (e.g. Wright–Giemsa, Diff-Quik®) will provide excellent staining for routine cytologic evaluation. Alternatively, special stains can be applied to unstained samples to highlight or identify pigments and structures on the slide (Table 9.1).

Efficacy

Hepatic FNA, with or without ultrasound guidance, is most accurate at detecting hepatocellular and biliary neoplasia, less accurate at detecting vacuolar change, and has only poor sensitivity and accuracy for necrosis, hyperplasia, and cystic lesions (Roth, 2001; Bahr *et al.*, 2013, Masserdotti, 2020). There are contradicting reports on the accuracy of hepatic FNA for inflammatory processes (Weiss *et al.*, 2001; Bahr *et al.*, 2013, Gardner *et al.*, 2022). As with most cytologic samples, detection of an abnormal finding is more meaningful than a lack of abnormal findings. A recent retrospective study concluded that agreement with histopathology had low sensitivity and specificity (60% and 68.6% respectively) in the diagnosis of a single mass (Cray *et al.*, 2023). If clinical suspicion is high for a disease process that is not detected on an initial sampling, repeat aspiration is recommended (Cohen *et al.*, 2003).

Ultrasound is sometimes used to identify the affected area. However, it has been shown that ultrasonographic appearance was insufficient to detect various types of canine and feline diffuse infiltrative liver disease (Feeney *et al.*, 2008). This study found that ultrasound diagnosis of liver imaged as normal had an accuracy of as low as 60%. In a similar study of canine patients known to have mast cell tumors elsewhere in the body, ultrasound failed to identify any cases of mast cell metastasis to the liver and had a reported sensitivity of 0% (Book *et al.*, 2011). Irrespective of ultrasound findings, it is of diagnostic value to sample the 'normal' appearing tissue when hepatopathy is suspected.

Table 9.1 **Selected special stains that can be applied to liver aspirates and their most common use**

Special stain	Use	Used on Romanowsky-stained slides
Rubeanic acid	Copper	Unknown
Rhodanine	Copper	Yes
Oil red O	Lipid	No
Sudan black	Lipid	No
Periodic acid–Schiff	Glycogen, fungal hyphae	Yes
Prussian blue	Iron, hemosiderin	Yes
Modified Ziehl–Neelsen	Lipofuscin, ceroid	Yes
Luxol fast blue	Lipofuscin, ceroid	Unknown
Hall's	Bilirubin	Yes – frozen or nonstained tissue preferred
Schmorl reaction	Lipofuscin	Unknown

FUNCTION AND ORGAN ARCHITECTURE

The liver plays a vital role in many catabolic and anabolic processes. Individual hepatocytes can be viewed as factory workers standing at a blood-based conveyor belt, busily picking up components and altering them either for further manufacturing work at distant sites (other body systems) or disposal (excretion, usually through the biliary or urinary system). As a result of this role, the liver has developed as a highly vascularized system with hepatocytes arranged as plates of cells, two layers thick, sandwiched between a fenestrated vascular capillary network (Figures 9.2a, b). Located within the hepatocyte bilayer is an interconnecting biliary network of fine canaliculi combining into large epithelium-lined ducts that lead to the gallbladder. This biliary network serves both as a pathway for excreta and as a method for the modification and recycling of metabolites.

NORMAL CYTOLOGIC FINDINGS

Hepatocytes

Cytologically, hepatocytes are generally found in cohesive clusters and are the predominant cell type other than red blood cells (RBCs) in a liver aspirate. They are moderately sized, polygonal cells with abundant amounts of basophilic to pink granular cytoplasm, a centrally located round nucleus with finely stippled chromatin, and a single prominent nucleolus (Figures 9.3, 9.4a). In health, there is typically minimal variability between hepatocytes. In the diseased liver, there can be hepatocytes with minimal cytologic changes juxtaposed with hepatocytes with marked pathologic changes.

Biliary epithelial cells

Biliary epithelium is usually encountered in smaller amounts as cohesive epithelium in tubular and papillary formations (Figure 9.4b). In a

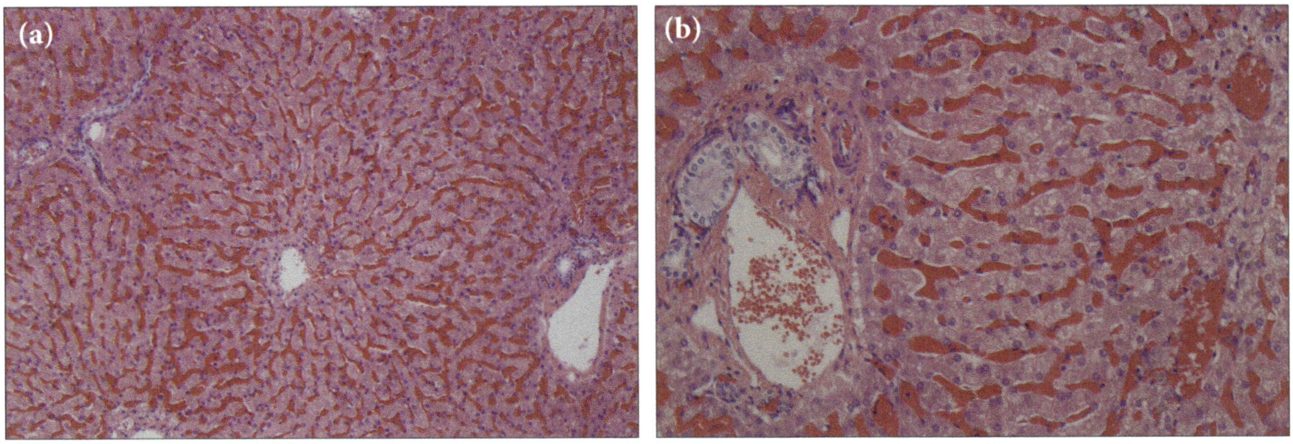

Figures 9.2a, b Histologic section of a canine liver. (a) The central vein is in the center of the image with plates of hepatocytes radiating to the portal triads along the periphery of the image. The hepatic sinusoids in this sample are filled with red blood cells (H&E, 100× magnification) (b) A closer image provides better detail of the hepatocytes and contents of the portal triad. Note the columnar epithelial cells within the bile duct, the hepatic artery surrounded by smooth muscle, and the large and open hepatic vein along the left of the image. A central vein filled with red blood cells is visible in the upper right corner of the image (H&E, 200× magnification).

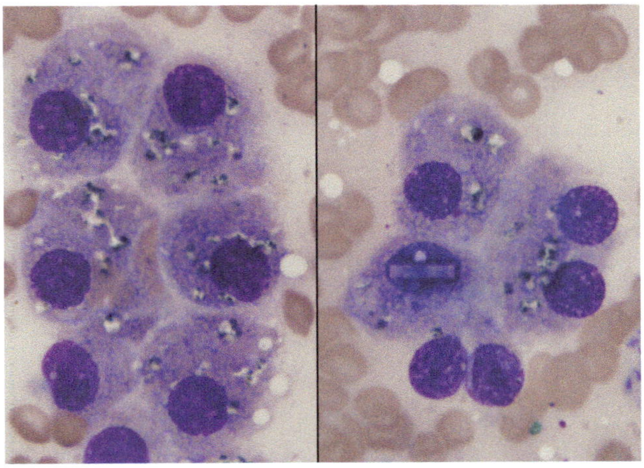

Figure 9.3 These polygonal cells are characteristic of hepatocytes. They have basophilic to pink granular cytoplasm, a centrally located nucleus with finely stippled chromatin, and a single nucleolus. Minimal pigment consistent with lipofuscin or other pigment (blue-black granular cytoplasmic material. An intranuclear brick inclusion is present (right panel) (Wright-Giemsa, 1,000× magnification).

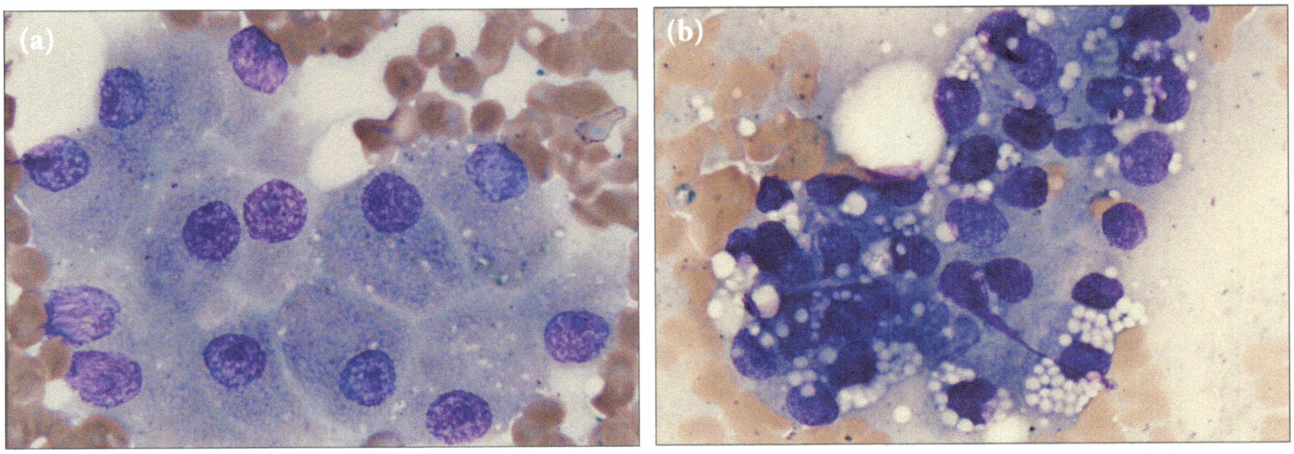

Figures 9.4a, b This canine liver aspirate has two populations of normal cells present. (a) The predominant cell population is morphologically normal hepatocytes. (b) There are also two clusters of biliary epithelial cells, which, compared with the hepatocytes, have less cytoplasm and distinct clear vacuolation (Wright-Giemsa, 1,000× magnification).

review of healthy dogs, an average of three biliary cells per two slides was observed (Stockhaus *et al.*, 2002). However, this study also found that thicker samples had relatively more biliary epithelium present. Biliary epithelium of smaller bile ducts are low columnar to cuboidal cells with minimal to moderate amounts of cytoplasm, which is lightly to deeply basophilic and filled with distinct clear vacuoles and which are smaller than hepatocytes. The nuclei are commonly basally located and more condensed. Biliary epithelium from larger ducts is columnar and can be ciliated (Masserdotti, 2020).

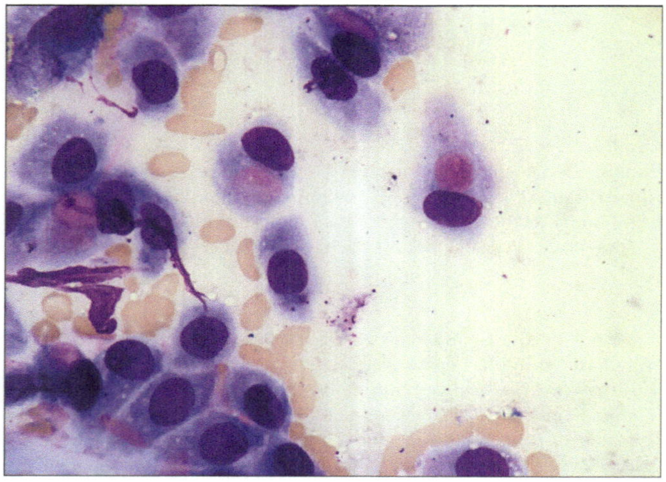

Figure 9.5 Five-year-old, male Coton de Tolear. Note the cohesive sheet of mesothelium in the lower left corner; these cells have a characteristic cobblestone appearance. The centrally located, pink cytoplasmic material noted in several of the mesothelial cells can occasionally be observed. (Courtesy Dr. Francesco Cian.)

Other cells

Few small lymphocytes, neutrophils, mature adipocytes, and mast cells are encountered during evaluation of a healthy liver. Each of these cell types makes up less than 1% of cells counted in one canine study (Stockhaus *et al.*, 2002). Mast cells can be found in higher numbers in normal canine hepatic aspirates when stained with Toluidine blue compared with May–Grünwald–Giemsa; however, even with better detection, they still total less than 1% of nucleated cells (Masserdotti, 2013). Additionally, samples of a healthy liver will typically have less than 0.1% of resident pigment-laden macrophages (Kupffer cells), mesothelium, eosinophils, and fibrocytes. When mesothelial cells are found, they will frequently be round individualized cells with basophilic to pink cytoplasm and prominent cytoplasmic blebs or will be present in cohesive sheets which have a cobblestone appearance (Figures 9.5–9.7). Due to its highly vascularized nature, hepatic aspirates often contain moderate to abundant amounts of peripheral blood elements, including RBCs, leukocytes, and platelet clumps. If peripheral blood elements are present solely as a result of the procedure, the relative numbers of cells will be similar to peripheral blood.

ABNORMAL CYTOLOGIC FINDINGS

Nuclear changes

Brick inclusions

These large blue crystalline rectangular inclusions are commonly noted in hepatocytes and are more common in older dogs (Figures 9.3, 9.8). Brick inclusions have no known pathologic

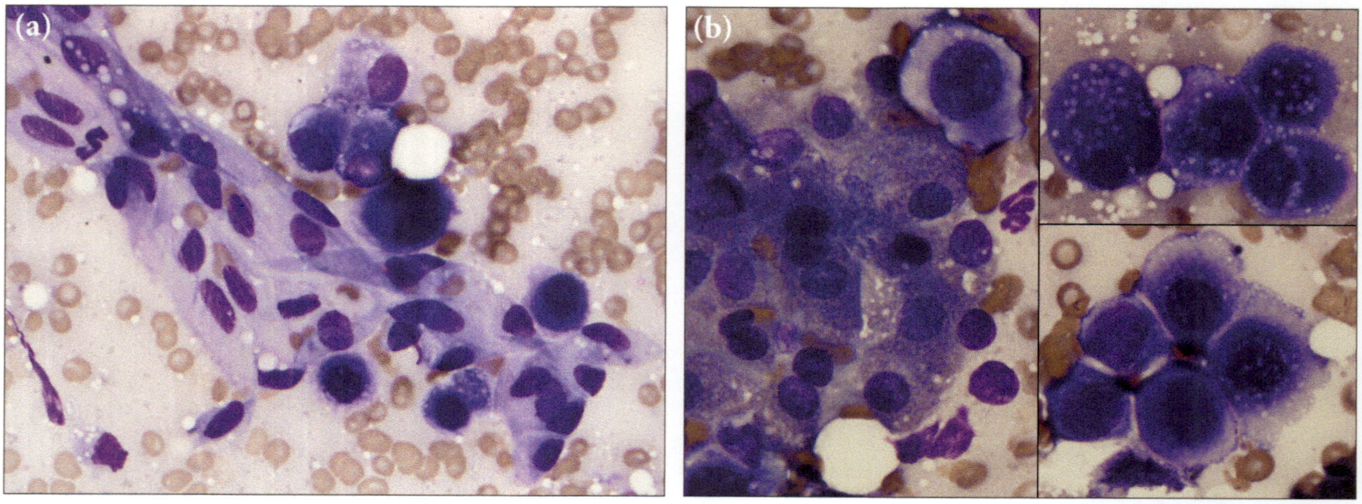

Figures 9.6a, b Liver aspirate from an Australian Shepherd Dog that had metastatic mammary carcinoma. (a) Sheets of normal mesothelium are present as an incidental finding. Note how these thin sheets can easily fold and wrinkle during slide preparation (Wright–Giemsa, 500× magnification). (b) Multiple neoplastic cells are also present (right panels), including a single macrocytic neoplastic cell with high N:C ratio (left panel), when compared with normal hepatocytes. Prominent cell–cell junctions (lower right panel) and multiple criteria of malignancy, including anisokaryosis, anisocytosis, anisonucleoliosis, and variable N:C ratio, are noted in the neoplastic population (all panels) (Wright–Giemsa, 1,000× magnification).

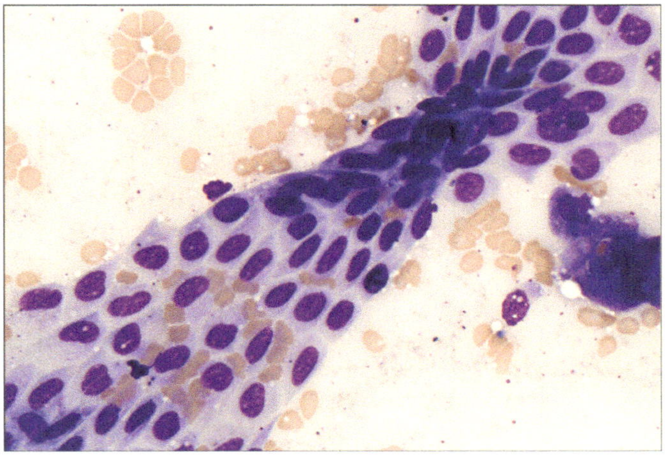

Figure 9.7 **Note the distinct cobblestone appearance of the single layer of mesothelial cells that has folded over on itself (Wright–Giemsa, 500× magnification). (Same dog as in Figure 9.20.)**

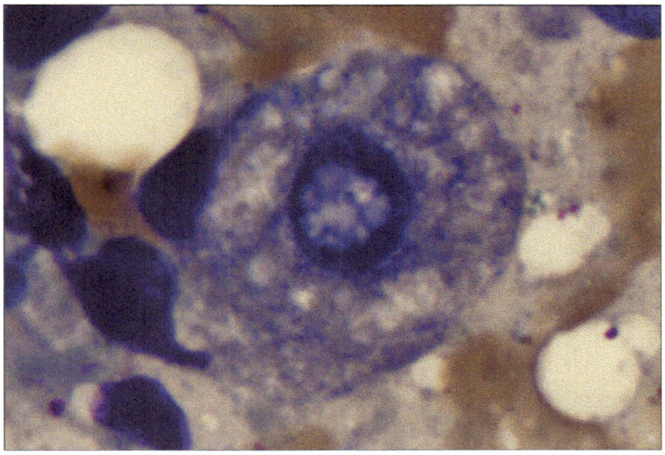

Figure 9.9 **A hepatocyte with an intranuclear cytoplasmic inclusion is noted in this image. This finding is of unknown significance. The cytoplasm is also rarefied, consistent with glycogen or hydropic degeneration (Wright–Giemsa, 1,000× magnification). (Same animal as Figure 9.12.)**

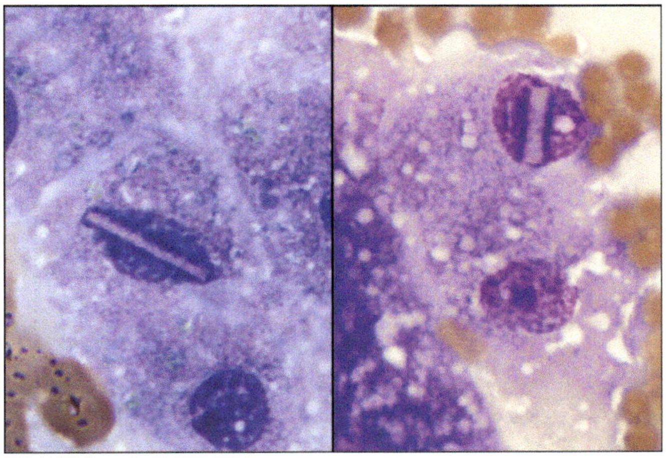

Figure 9.8 **Brick inclusions are occasionally seen in hepatocyte nuclei; they have no known significance (Wright–Giemsa, 1,000× magnification).**

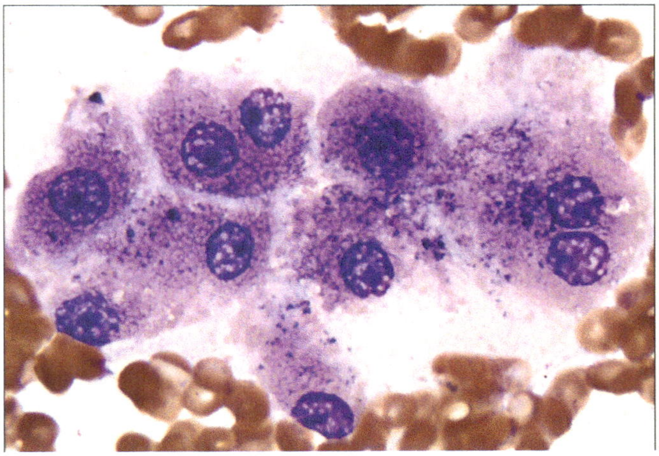

Figure 9.10 **Many binucleate hepatocytes are found. This patient also had a mild suppurative and histiocytic inflammation (not shown) (Wright–Giemsa, 1,000× magnification).**

significance, do not contain heavy metals, and are acid-fast negative, in contrast to lead inclusions, which are positive with acid-fast staining (Richter *et al.*, 1965; Reimer *et al.*, 1973).

Intranuclear cytoplasmic inclusions

Intranuclear cytoplasmic inclusions are, as the name implies, blebs of cytoplasm that appear to be within the nucleus (Figure 9.9). They are usually round, can vary in size, and are commonly thought of as a sample preparation artifact. They can be found in many cell types, including hepatocytes.

Intranuclear lead inclusions are observed infrequently, even after intentional dosing of dogs with lead (Hamir *et al.*, 1983). On electron microscopy (EM) evaluation, these acid-fast inclusions are dense with irregular borders and are surrounded by a clear zone (Hegazy & Fouad, 2014).

Binucleation

Some binucleation is seen on most, if not all, canine liver aspirates. Rarely, trinucleate cells can be observed. Increased amounts of bi- and trinucleation are most commonly associated with increased mitotic activity, as occurs with a regenerative effort (Figure 9.10). In one study, the number of binucleate and trinucleate hepatocytes in apparently healthy patients was correlated with age; this may be associated with an increased incidence of nodular regeneration in older individuals (Stockhaus *et al.*, 2002).

Anisokaryosis

Often concurrent with binucleation, mild to moderate anisokaryosis, or variably sized nuclei, will be noted in mitotically active hepatocytes.

Additionally, benign and malignant hepatic and biliary tumors can display cellular atypia, including anisokaryosis. Therefore, although nuclear size changes are more commonly found cytologically in regenerative lesions, they are not pathognomonic for hepatocellular regeneration.

Cytoplasmic changes

As a consequence of their multiple roles and varied metabolic processes, atypical hepatocytes can accumulate a wide variety of cytoplasmic inclusions, including pigments and vacuoles. Routine cytologic preparations are not the most sensitive at distinguishing these inclusions, but additional staining procedures can be used to completely identify cytoplasmic inclusions when a definitive diagnosis is required. There are several cytoplasmic changes easily noted with Romanowsky stains, as described below.

LIPID

Hepatic intracytoplasmic lipid accumulation appears as clear cytoplasmic vacuoles with a distinct margin or punched out appearance (Figures 9.11a, b). The lack of staining is due to solubilized lipid being washed away during Romanowsky staining protocols. This clear vacuolar material can often be seen in the background adjacent to ruptured hepatocytes. Oil red O or Sudan black stains can be used to confirm the presence of lipid, if needed.

Although hepatocyte lipid vacuolation is easily identified with cytologic preparations, vacuolar lipid hepatopathy is not synonymous with hepatic lipidosis. The disease entity hepatic lipidosis is a set of systemic pathologic metabolic changes and not solely lipid accumulation. Lipid vacuolation is a common secondary change associated with many different pathologic processes. A case series of four cats with cytologically diagnosed vacuolar hepatopathy had a different diagnosis which eclipsed the lipid accumulation made by subsequent histology (lymphoma, inflammation, or cholestasis) (Willard *et al.*, 1999). Ingestion of aflatoxin-contaminated commercial feed can cause hepatic failure and has been confirmed to cause lipid accumulation by histopathology and EM (Newman *et al.*, 2007). When hepatic lipid vacuolation is encountered, any pathologic process that leads to lipid accumulation, including hepatic lipidosis, must remain on the differential list until excluded.

Glycogen/hydropic degeneration

Glycogen accumulation and hydropic degeneration associated with loss of water regulation are two vastly different processes. Cytologically, however, both are noted as a fine, often foamy and indistinct cytoplasmic rarefaction (Figures 9.12, 9.13). Although glycogen accumulation is commonly referred to as a vacuolar hepatopathy, because glycogen is free in the cytosol and not within a limiting membrane it is not technically within a vacuole. The presence of glycogen can be confirmed with periodic acid–Schiff (PAS) staining which is abrogated by diastase digestion. Hepatocyte size is often markedly increased with a more rounded rather than polygonal shape. The background of the slide does not reveal the vacuolar material seen with lipid. Glycogen accumulation is more commonly seen in dogs than cats and is a fairly nondescript change. It is associated with altered glucose/glycogen metabolism, which is commonly caused by naturally occurring hyperadrenocorticism and iatrogenic glucocorticoid administration. Less frequently, insulinoma or other hormonal dysregulation can lead to hepatic glycogen accumulation (Goutal *et al.*, 2012). Most liver aspirates from aged dogs will contain a minimal amount of glycogen accumulation, a finding that has an unknown significance.

Hydropic degeneration is the result of loss of cellular control of free water, which leads to organelle swelling. Toxic injury, hypoxia, and metabolic or other insults have been associated with this ballooning degenerative process.

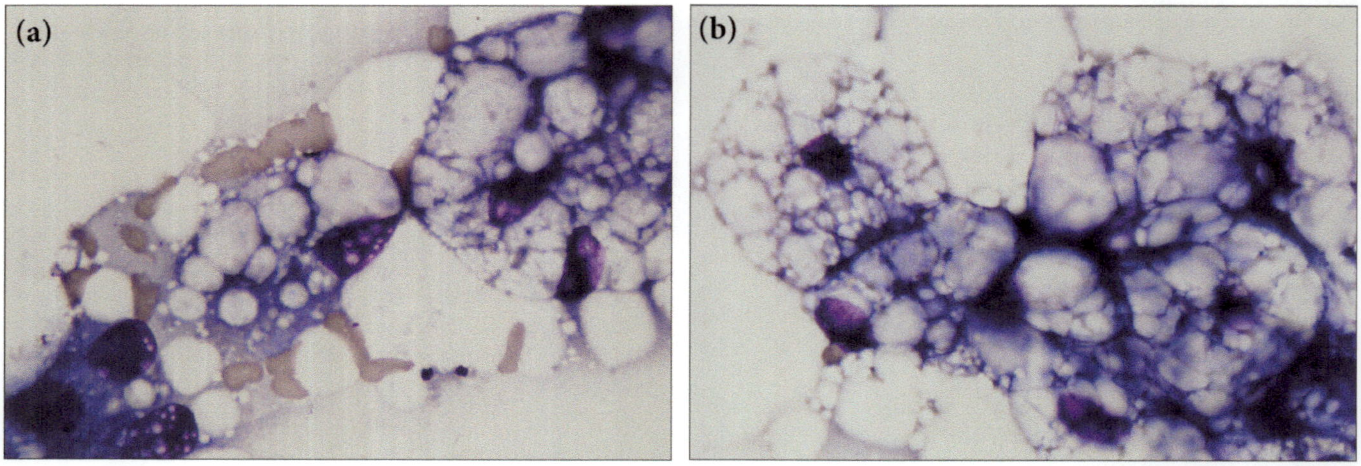

Figures 9.11a, b **Domestic shorthair cat with lipid-laden hepatocytes. (a) Note the morphologically more normal hepatocytes on the lower left of the image, progressing to cells filled with distinct lipid vacuolation in the upper right corner of the image. The origin of the highly vacuolated cells would be challenging to determine if viewed alone. (b) This cluster of hepatocytes is heavily lipid-laden and can be confused with adipocytes. Abundant free lipid is also noted as clear defects in the normally lightly blue extracellular fluid background of the images (Wright–Giemsa, 1,000× magnification).**

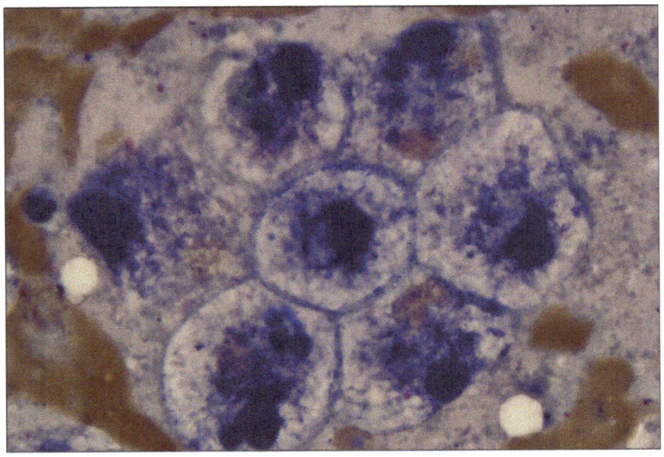

Figure 9.12 **Hepatic FNA from a 16-year-old Yorkshire Terrier. Note how the cytoplasm of these hepatocytes is rarefied by foamy cytoplasmic clearing, consistent with glycogen or hydropic degeneration. Cytologically, this type of change contrasts with the distinct lipid vacuolation seen in Figures 9.11a, b (Wright–Giemsa, 1,000× magnification).**

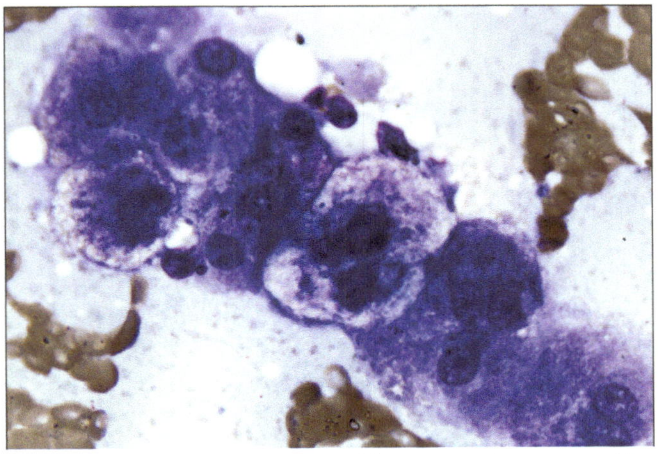

Figure 9.13 **Contrast the cytoplasm of the center two hepatocytes with those flanking them. The center hepatocytes have foamy cytoplasmic rarefaction, consistent with glycogen or hydropic degeneration (Wright–Giemsa, 1,000× magnification).**

PIGMENTARY CHANGES

Bile pigment

This green to blue to black coarse granular pigment is a normal product of the liver; however, visible quantities of bile pigment are suggestive of cholestasis. Bile pigment may be observed as a fine cytoplasmic dusting or as smaller aggregates inside the hepatocytes with intrahepatic cholestasis. With extrahepatic cholestasis, bile pigment will be in larger aggregates and forming tubular casts within the biliary canaliculi (Figures 9.14, 9.15). Occasionally, bile pigment can be present in lamellated light-brown to amber globular crystals. Hall's stain can be used to confirm the presence of bile (Figures 9.16a–d).

LIPOFUSCIN

Lipofuscin is a blue to black granular cytoplasmic material noted in many organs (Figures 9.3, 9.17a, b). It is the result of incomplete digestion of lipids and lipoproteins. In rats, chemical inhibition of lysosomal proteases will increase lipofuscin deposition in the liver; in other species it is thought to have minimal pathologic significance and increases are noted with age (Kitani *et al.*, 1989; Scott, 2006). Lipofuscin is acid-fast and will stain positive with the Schmorl reaction. In addition, lipofuscin will autofluoresce.

CEROID

Ceroid pigment is the result of peroxidation of lipids and has been correlated to age in healthy canine liver aspirates (Stockhaus *et al.*,

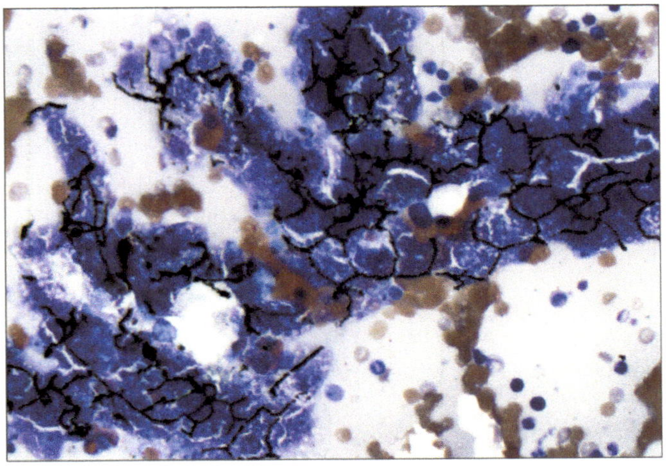

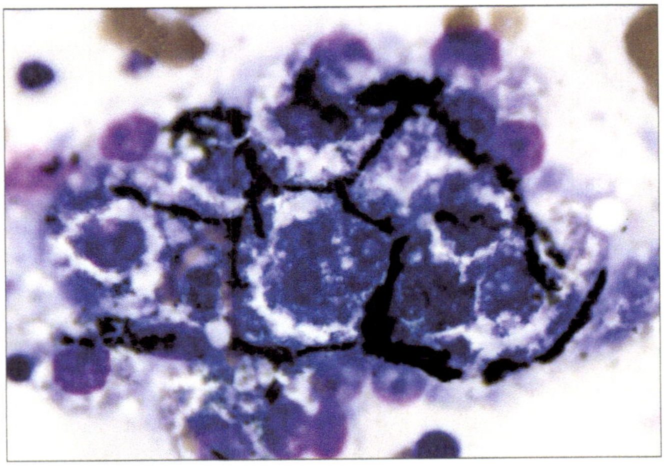

Marked cholestasis, noted as tubular accumulations of coarse green–black granular pigment, highlights the canalicular system normally present between hepatocytes

Figure 9.14 **Wright–Giemsa, 500× magnification.**

Figure 9.15 **Wright–Giemsa, 1,000× magnification.**

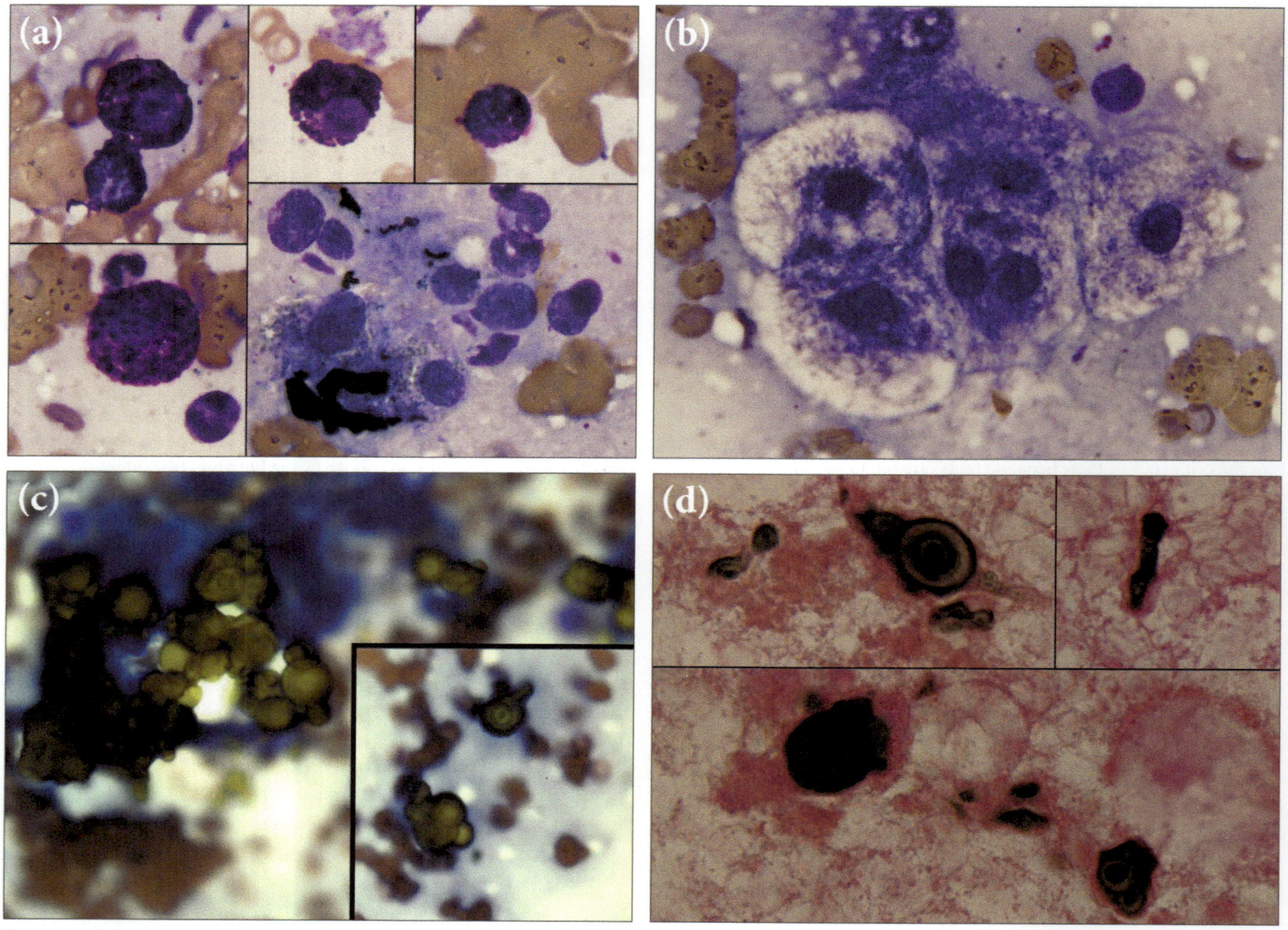

Figures 9.16a–d **Liver aspirate from a dog with cutaneous mast cell tumors that had metastasized to multiple organs. (a) Dark green–black tubular structures (lower right panel), consistent with the more commonly seen form of bile casts are very rarely seen. Well-granulated mast cells make up just over 1% of the cellular population. Multiple individualized mast cells were imaged and included along the left and upper edge of the image to display the minimal to moderate anisocytosis and anisokaryosis in this population. With knowledge of the clinical history and multiple metastatic foci, this is consistent with mast cell tumor metastasis to the liver. (b) Most hepatocytes display moderate to marked cytoplasmic rarefaction, consistent with glycogen or hydropic degeneration. (c) Globular light brown to amber round, layered crystals are found. These are occasionally present within hepatocyte clusters (not shown). (d) The globular crystals displayed in 9.16c were positive with Hall's stain, demonstrating that they are a rarely seen form of bile crystals and supporting the diagnosis of cholestasis (a–c, Wright–Giemsa, 1,000× magnification; d, Hall's bilirubin stain).**

2002). On Romanowsky-stained samples, it appears as a gold to brown granular material. Unlike lipofuscin, ceroid does not stain with the Schmorl reaction.

COPPER

Copper accumulation can be detected in Romanowsky-stained cytologic preparations as a blue–green to gray cytoplasmic crystalline material (Figure 9.18a). Copper content is not always readily apparent by Romanowsky staining but can be highlighted using rubeanic acid or rhodanine stains (Moore *et al.*, 2016; Figures 9.18b, c). Based on the low incidence of pathologically significant amounts of copper in the typical cytologic case stream, copper staining is recommended when there is a clinical concern for copper hepatopathy or an unknown pigment is found (Moore *et al.*, 2019). Often increases in liver enzyme activity are the only sign of copper accumulation (Rodrigues *et al.*, 2020). A copper grading system has been proposed which showed good correlation with quantitative hepatic copper content but does not allow distinction of where the copper is deposited within the hepatic lobule.

Hepatic copper accumulation has been associated with chronic hepatitis and altered excretion during cholestasis in both canine and feline patients (Whittemore *et al.*, 2012; Hurwitz *et al.*, 2014; Cedeño *et al.*, 2016; Eulenberg *et al.*, 2018). Data also suggest that copper may induce chronic hepatitis and contribute to the development of

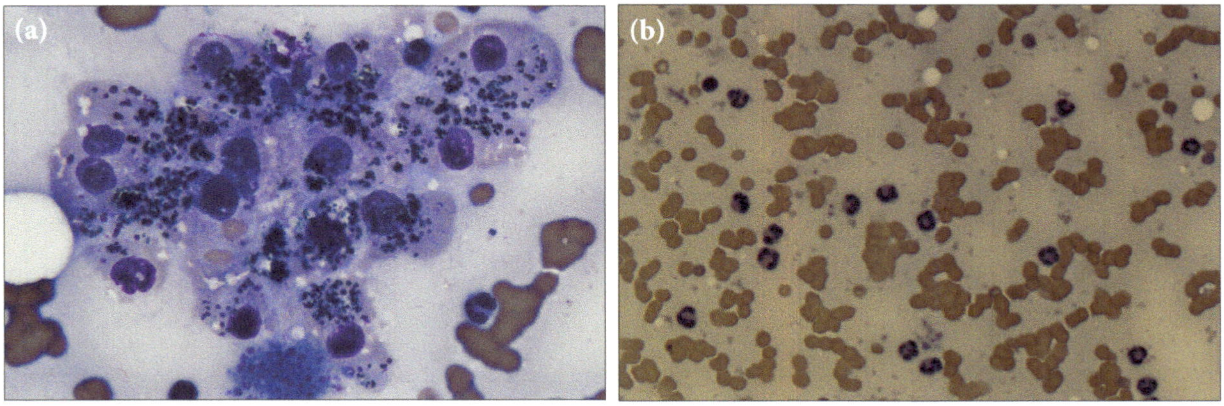

Figures 9.17a,b Canine liver sample. (a) The hepatocytes from this dog have blue to blue-green cytoplasmic material, most consistent with lipofuscin. A platelet clump is also noted in the lower center of the image (Wright–Giemsa, 1,000× magnification). (b) Neutrophils within the hepatocyte clumps, a feature commonly used to aid the diagnosis of suppurative hepatitis, are not found. The neutrophil count in this liver aspirate is higher than that of peripheral blood and myeloid precursors are not found (helping to exclude peripheral blood contamination and extramedullary hematopoiesis, respectively) (Wright–Giemsa, 500× magnification). This patient was given a diagnosis of mild suppurative hepatitis.

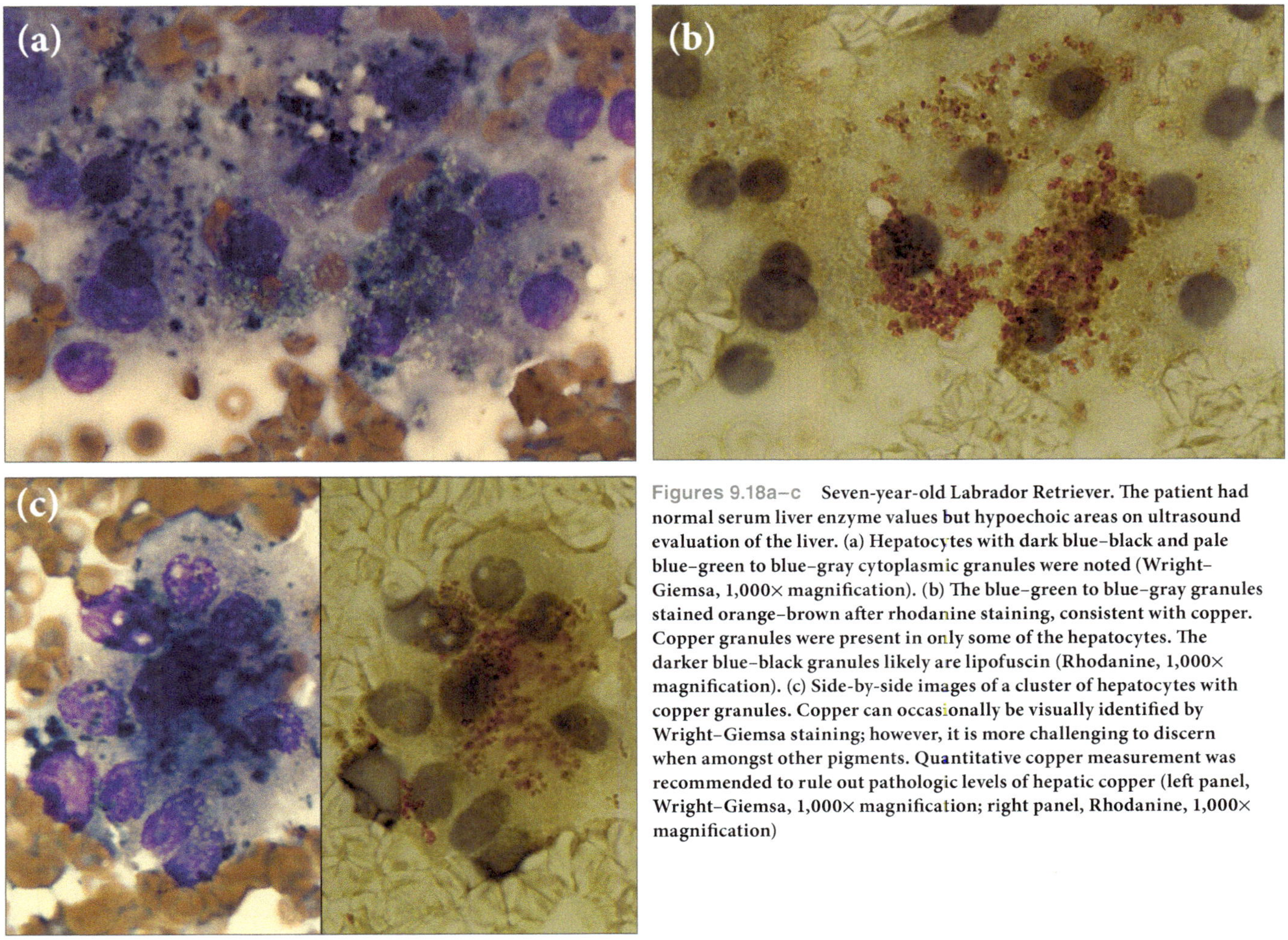

Figures 9.18a–c Seven-year-old Labrador Retriever. The patient had normal serum liver enzyme values but hypoechoic areas on ultrasound evaluation of the liver. (a) Hepatocytes with dark blue–black and pale blue-green to blue-gray cytoplasmic granules were noted (Wright–Giemsa, 1,000× magnification). (b) The blue-green to blue-gray granules stained orange-brown after rhodanine staining, consistent with copper. Copper granules were present in only some of the hepatocytes. The darker blue-black granules likely are lipofuscin (Rhodanine, 1,000× magnification). (c) Side-by-side images of a cluster of hepatocytes with copper granules. Copper can occasionally be visually identified by Wright–Giemsa staining; however, it is more challenging to discern when amongst other pigments. Quantitative copper measurement was recommended to rule out pathologic levels of hepatic copper (left panel, Wright–Giemsa, 1,000× magnification; right panel, Rhodanine, 1,000× magnification)

hepatocellular carcinoma (Harro *et al.*, 2019). A genetic copper hepatopathy has been demonstrated in Bedlington Terriers, Labrador Retrievers, and other dogs (Hoffmann, 2009). The amount of copper accumulated in the liver of Labrador Retrievers with primary copper hepatopathy is correlated with dietary copper content (Fieten *et al.*, 2012). Primary copper-associated hepatopathy was seen in young cats without cholestasis, suggesting genetic or environmental causes in the cat (Hurwitz *et al.*, 2014).

Hemosiderin/hematoidin

Hemosiderin and its iron-free homologue, hematoidin, are present in patients with increased erythrocyte turnover (hemolytic anemia or recent transfusion) and portosystemic shunts. Hemosiderin-laden macrophages are noted with copper toxicity (Smedley *et al.*, 2009). With Romanowsky staining, hemosiderin is a brown to blue–black coarse pigment. Hematoidin appears as orange rhomboid, refractile crystals. One relatively easy confirmation of hemosiderin presence is to observe the material within erythrophagocytic cells (Figure 9.19a). Because hemosiderin contains iron, it will stain strongly positive with the Prussian blue reaction (Figure 9.19b). Hematoidin is distinctive enough that it does not need a confirmatory stain. Since hematoidin is iron-free, hematoidin will not stain with the Prussian blue reaction.

HYPERPLASIA

Hepatocellular hyperplasia/nodular regeneration

The liver is capable of significant regenerative effort. In the canine liver, nodular regeneration and hyperplasia are commonly observed in older patients. Nodular hyperplasia is uncommonly encountered in the cat (Cullen & Popp, 2002). Cytologically, hyperplasia/regeneration is noted as mild to moderate hepatocellular atypia including increased cell size, altered nuclear to cytoplasmic (N:C) ratio, and bi- and trinucleation (Stockhaus *et al.*, 2002). In extreme cases, atypia can be marked, and differentiation of hyperplastic from neoplastic processes may be challenging (Figures 9.20a–c). Finding atypical hepatocytes juxtaposed with cytologically normal hepatocytes in hyperplastic cases is more consistent with hyperplasia than neoplasia (Stockhaus *et al.*, 2002). Often, distinction of hyperplasia from neoplasia is dependent on evaluation of lobular architecture, requiring a biopsy specimen and histopathology. Hyperplasia will arrange into normal bilayer plates while neoplastic liver nodules will display a more disorganized architecture disrupting the typical lobular organization (Figures 9.21a–c).

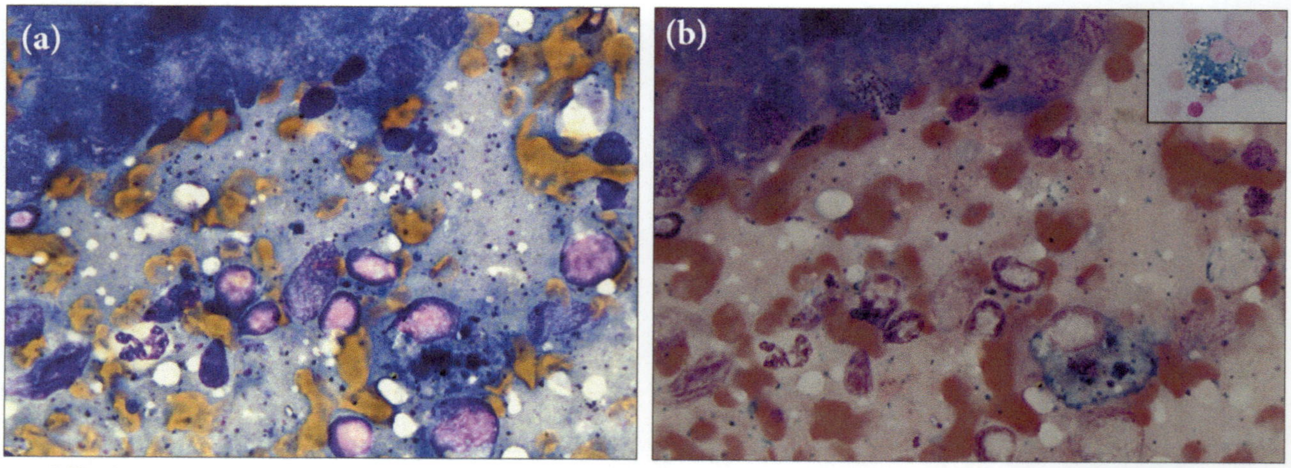

Figures 9.19a, b **Nine-year-old Terrier-cross dog with a 6-month history of weight loss and recently elevated liver enzymes. (a) Clusters of hepatocytes are present in the upper left corner. There is a mixed lymphoid population with small lymphocytes predominant, suggestive of lymphocytic inflammation. The blue–black granules are suggestive of hemosiderin. A pigment-laden macrophage is present in the lower right corner (Wright–Giemsa, 500× magnification). (b) Prussian blue stain confirms the presence of iron and helps demonstrate the amount of hemosiderin that can be present in liver samples. Hemosiderin likely accumulated secondary to inflammation. Inset image is from the control slide; note the blue-staining iron within this macrophage (Wright–Giemsa, 500× magnification). (Same dog as in Figure 9.28.)**

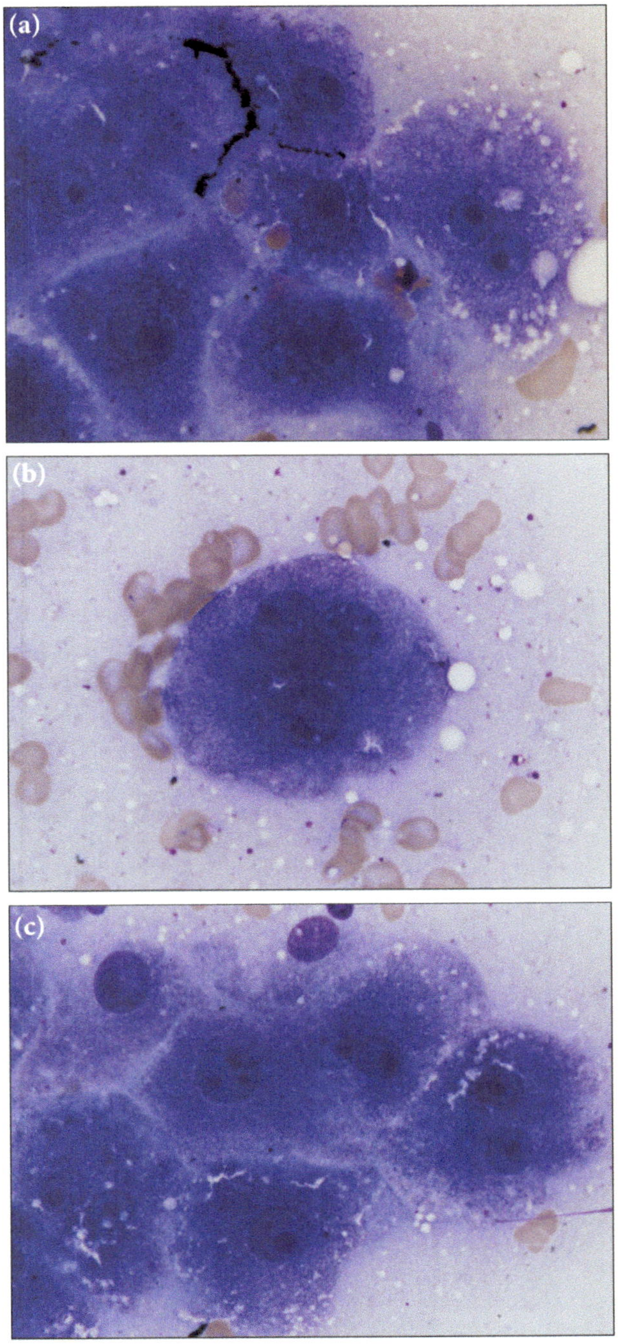

Figures 9.20a–c Liver aspirate from a Siberian Husky who was undergoing chemotherapy (CCNU). Ultrasonographic evaluation found nodules in the liver. (a) Bile is present as coarse green-black granular pigmented material in the cytoplasm and canalicular spaces. The hepatocytes frequently are binucleate with variably-sized nucleoli. (b) Rarely, large trinucleate hepatocytes with anisonucleoliosis are found. (c) Considerable size and shape variability in both nuclei and nucleoli are present. The cellular atypia is likely associated with the toxic effects of the therapeutic regimen (Wright-Giemsa, 1,000× magnification).

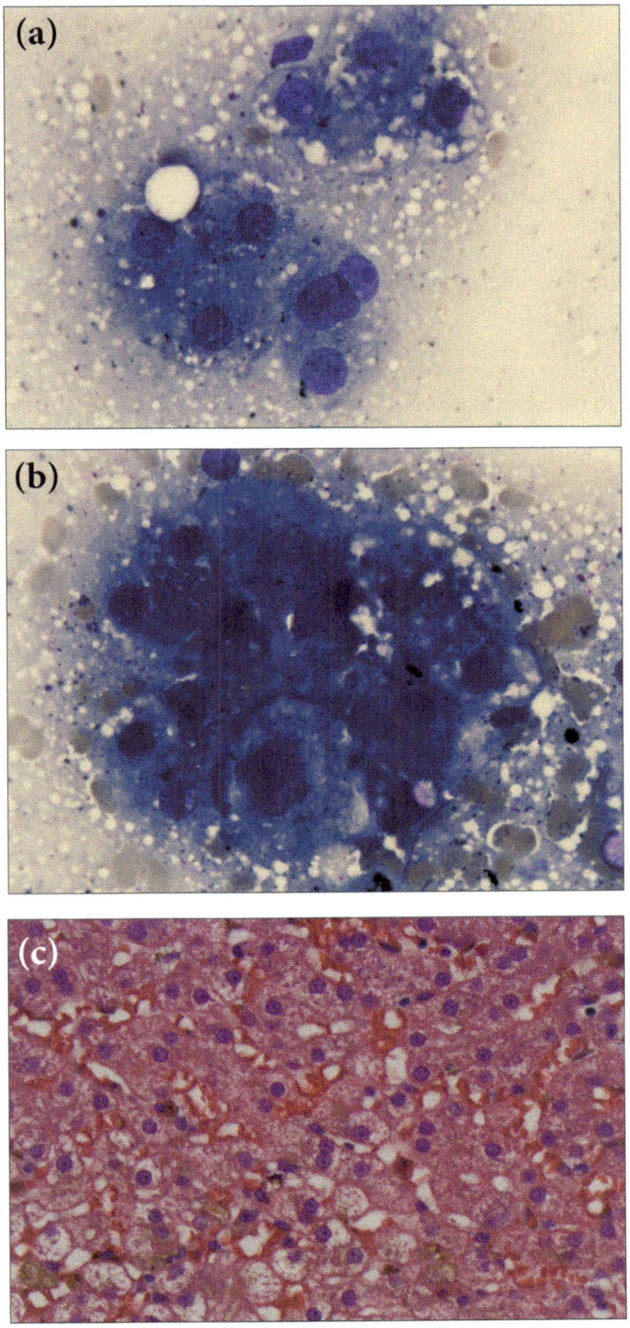

Figures 9.21a–c (a, b) Frequent binucleation, mild to moderate anisocytosis, and anisokaryosis with few hepatocytes containing multiple nucleoli are present. The black granular material in 9.21b is consistent with bile (Wright-Giemsa, 1,000× magnification). (c) Histologic evaluation of this patient's liver confirmed the frequent binucleation, anisocytosis, and anisokaryosis. Although these changes are present, hepatic plates are organized. The histologic diagnosis is nodular hyperplasia. The pale brown material present between the hepatocytes is largely cell associated and consistent with bile. A few bile casts located between hepatocytes were noted (not imaged) (Wright-Giemsa, 500× magnification).

CYSTIC HYPERPLASIA OF THE BILIARY SYSTEM

Increased numbers of cytologically normal biliary epithelial cells suggest cholestasis and biliary hyperplasia (Stockhaus *et al.*, 2004). Additionally, cirrhosis results in a relative decrease in hepatocytes which produces the appearance of increased numbers of biliary epithelium and can have concurrent biliary hyperplasia (Stockhaus *et al.*, 2004).

The hyperplastic progress can advance to a more easily diagnosed cystic hyperplasia of the biliary system. This is seen as larger accumulations of biliary epithelium, bile pigment, and aggregates of blue to blue–gray mucoid material (so-called white bile [Figures 9.22a–g]; Stalker & Hayes, 2007). Experimental studies demonstrate an association between exposure to bile salts and hyperplastic and secretory activity of biliary epithelium, implicating cholestasis as a potential initiating cause of cystic hyperplasia (Klinkspoor *et al.*, 1995; Lamote Willems, 1997). Additionally, genetic causes may play a factor; Cocker Spaniels, Shetland Sheepdogs, and Miniature Schnauzers are more predisposed to biliary mucoceles (Pike *et al.*, 2004).

Amyloid

Under certain conditions, proteins that are normally expressed in the body (e.g. serum amyloid A, immunoglobulin light chain, prion protein, and atrial natriuretic peptide, among others) can form characteristic beta pleated sheets, bind serum amyloid P, and be deposited on basement membranes. Although the substrate proteins are vastly different, at a microscopic level this material is visually indistinguishable and is collectively called amyloid. With Romanowsky staining, hepatic amyloid appears as pink fibrillar extracellular material closely

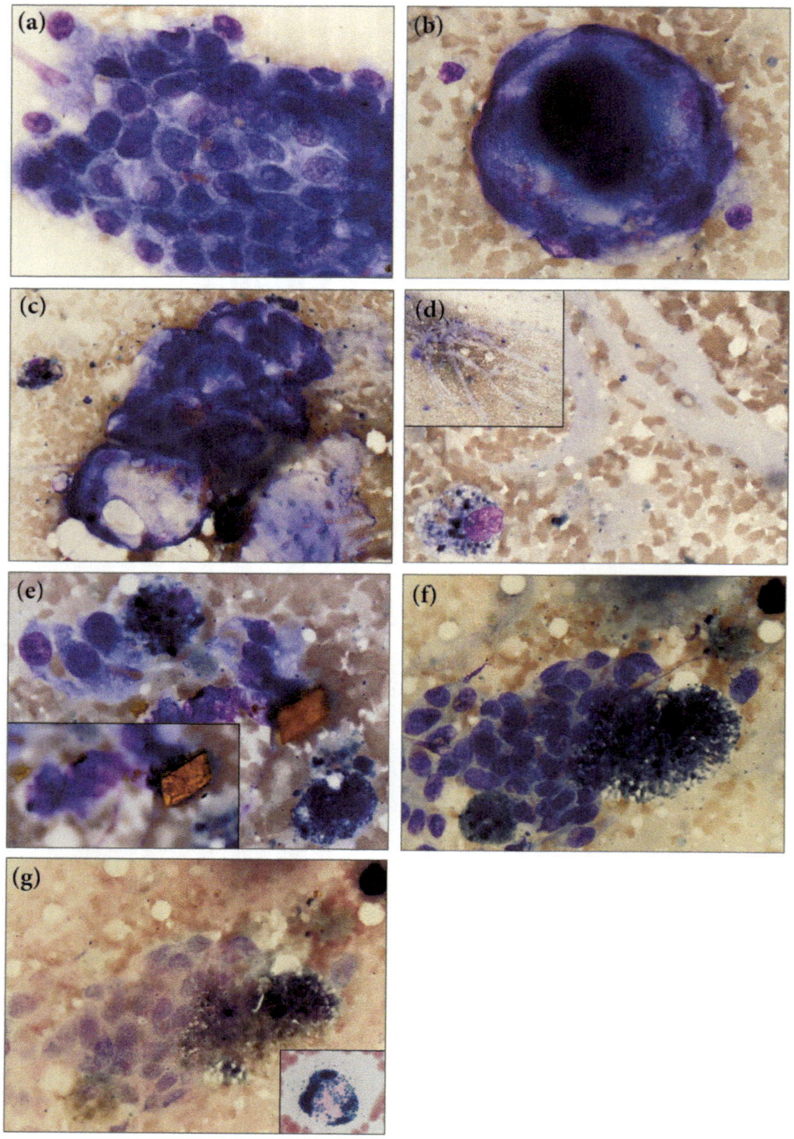

Figures 9.22a–g **Domestic shorthair cat with benign biliary hyperplasia confirmed by clinical progression and histology. (a) Rafts of biliary epithelium, which are columnar to cuboidal with basophilic to pink granular cytoplasm and mild dysplastic changes, including mild anisocytosis and variable N:C ratio, are present (Wright–Giemsa, 1,000× magnification). (b) Occasionally, these cells are found in balls and acinar-like structures around a center of blue secretory material (Wright–Giemsa, 1,000× magnification). (c) Lightly basophilic to gray extracellular material, white bile, is often found within some of these cell clusters and free in the background (Wright–Giemsa, 500× magnification). (d) White bile can cause the red blood cells to line up in linear arrangements, called windrowing. Dark blue–black material is found within cells and extracellularly. A few macrophages also display erythrophagocytosis (lower left corner) (main image, Wright–Giemsa, 1,000× magnification; inset, Wright–Giemsa, 200× magnification). (e) Columnar biliary epithelium, pigment-laden macrophages, and a single bright orange rhomboidal hematoidin crystal are present. Large hematoidin crystals are three-dimensional structures and therefore can lie in a different plane of focus from the surrounding cells (inset). Hematoidin usually suggests chronic hemorrhage but can be part of normal bile fluid (Wright–Giemsa, 1,000× magnification). (f, g) Interestingly, most of the material in this sample is Prussian blue negative, demonstrating that the blue–black material seen here is predominantly bile with minimal hemosiderin (f, Wright–Giemsa, 1,000× magnification; g, Prussian blue, 1,000× magnification; inset is from the control sample, iron forms a blue pigment with this reaction).**

associated with hepatocyte clusters. The beta pleated sheet arrangement of amyloid produces characteristic birefringence after staining with Congo red and visualization with polarized light (Beatty *et al.*, 2002). Amyloid deposition is not limited solely to the liver, but commonly involves the kidney, central nervous system, spleen, lung, pancreas, and several other organs (Segev *et al.*, 2012).

Amyloidosis has been classified as immunoglobulin-related (primary), reactive (secondary), and familial. Siamese and related breeds, Abyssinian cats, and Chinese Shar-Pei dogs have confirmed familial forms of amyloidosis (AA type amyloidosis), each with a specific amino acid substitution (Niewold *et al.*, 1999; Segev *et al.*, 2012). Half of dogs with amyloidosis had a history of infectious disease, and another quarter of the patients had a noninfectious, inflammatory disease, demonstrating the multifactorial nature of this disease (Segev *et al.*, 2012).

Insufficient data are available to characterize the accuracy of cytology at identifying hepatic amyloidosis, as the cytologically described cases are presented as single case studies in the literature and not as a case series (Roth, 2001; Meyer, 2010). Suffice it to say that amyloid can be observed cytologically, but a lack of amyloid does not rule out amyloidosis.

Extramedullary hematopoiesis

Embryologic hepatoblast cytokine production induces the niche necessary to make the liver the first site of hematopoietic production (Sugiyama *et al.*, 2011). Under conditions of increased hematopoietic need in the adult, this capacity is revived and manifests as the development of both erythroid, myeloid, and/or megakaryocytic cell proliferation associated with resident Kupffer cells (Figures 9.23a–c; Otsuka *et al.*, 2011). Although the cytologic diagnosis of extramedullary hematopoiesis (EMH) can be made based on the presence of any one hematopoietic cell line with complete maturation outside the bone marrow, EMH of multiple cell lines is commonly seen. EMH, like lipid and glycogen accumulation, is a fairly nonspecific finding. It should be considered a secondary change and an aid to help define the nature of the primary problem. Care should be taken to ensure that the sample is truly representative of the liver, as incidental aspiration of the spleen during hepatic FNA is common (colloquially termed a 'spliver' sample by the author) and the spleen is a more common site of EMH. Hepatic EMH produces a multifocal to diffuse ultrasonographic lesion, and therefore a higher cytologic accuracy for this entity could be predicted; however, data hint at poor diagnostic

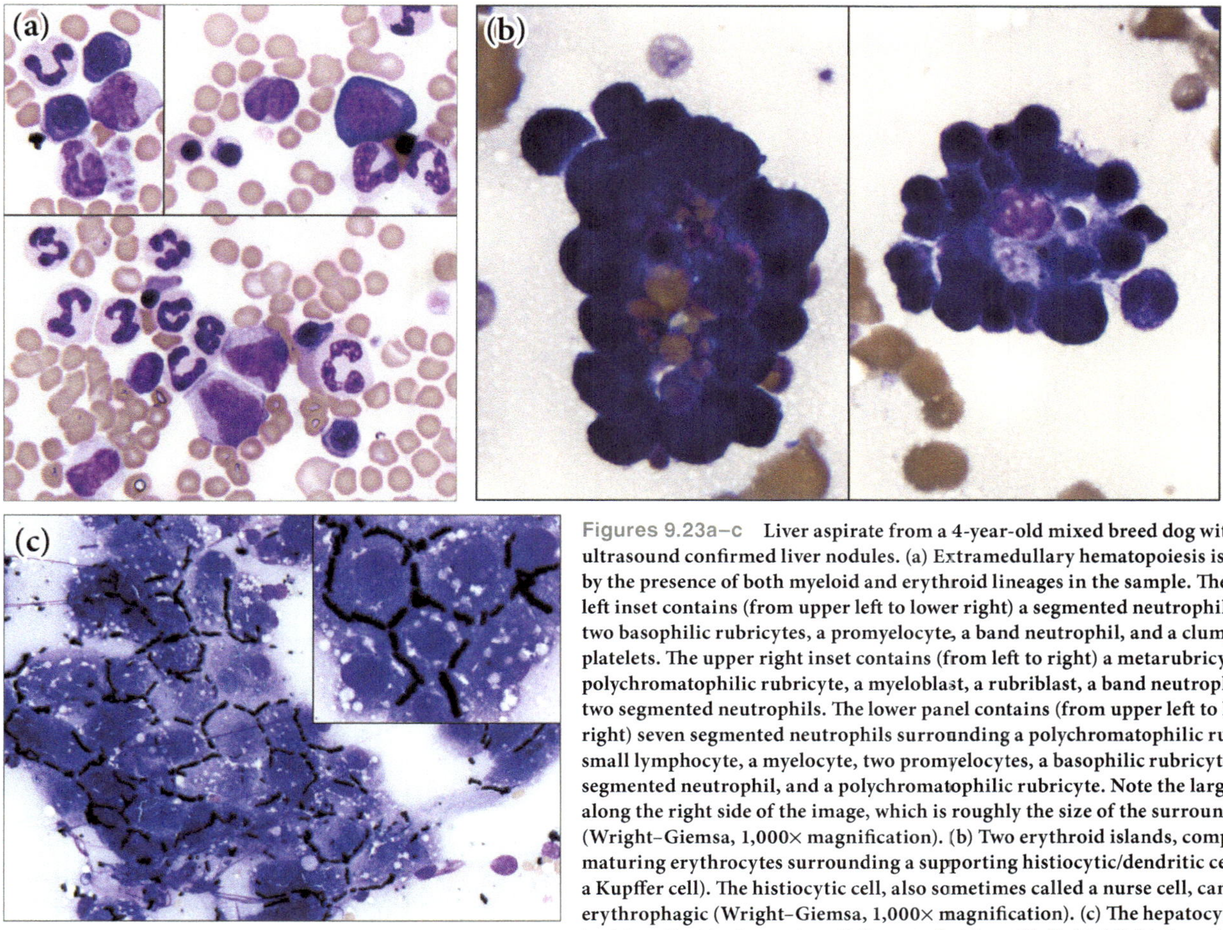

Figures 9.23a–c **Liver aspirate from a 4-year-old mixed breed dog with ultrasound confirmed liver nodules. (a) Extramedullary hematopoiesis is noted by the presence of both myeloid and erythroid lineages in the sample. The upper left inset contains (from upper left to lower right) a segmented neutrophil, two basophilic rubricytes, a promyelocyte, a band neutrophil, and a clump of platelets. The upper right inset contains (from left to right) a metarubricyte, a polychromatophilic rubricyte, a myeloblast, a rubriblast, a band neutrophil, and two segmented neutrophils. The lower panel contains (from upper left to lower right) seven segmented neutrophils surrounding a polychromatophilic rubricyte, a small lymphocyte, a myelocyte, two promyelocytes, a basophilic rubricyte, a large segmented neutrophil, and a polychromatophilic rubricyte. Note the large platelet along the right side of the image, which is roughly the size of the surrounding RBCs (Wright–Giemsa, 1,000× magnification). (b) Two erythroid islands, composed of maturing erythrocytes surrounding a supporting histiocytic/dendritic cell (likely a Kupffer cell). The histiocytic cell, also sometimes called a nurse cell, can be erythrophagic (Wright–Giemsa, 1,000× magnification). (c) The hepatocyte clusters in this patient had prominent bile casts that beautifully highlight the polygonal nature of the hepatocytes (Wright–Giemsa, 500× magnification; inset, 1,000× magnification).**

performance in small study populations (Warren-Smith *et al.*, 2012; Bahr *et al.*, 2013). Myelolipoma is an uncommon benign tumor, which presents as a nodular lesion with bone marrow elements and adipocytes cytologically. Myelolipoma can be challenging to distinguish from EMH by aspiration alone.

Necrosis

When a pathologic process pushes the microenvironment sufficiently away from homeostasis, necrosis will ensue. Necrotic but still intact cells will have a lack of cytoplasmic detail and condensed or karyorrhectic nuclei (Figure 9.24). This is apparent on cytology as basophilic amorphous to granular acellular debris (Figure 9.25). Necrotic material can be seen with infectious etiologies and within the poorly vascularized center of mass lesions. Often, re-aspiration of the margin of a lesion that previously produced necrotic debris will help identify the pathologic process leading to the necrosis.

Fibroplasia

Hepatic fibrosis results from chronic inflammation within the liver (Eulenberg *et al.,* 2018). Histologically, there is an expansion of the number of spindled mesenchymal cells, mast cells, and collagenous extracellular matrix. Several clinically different histologic patterns of fibrosis can occur (portal-portal, portal-centrilobular, centrilobular-centrilobular, dissecting fibrosis). The degree of fibrosis is clinically relevant. Importantly, fibrosis is a component of chronic hepatopathy and is a sequelae of extrahepatic bile duct obstruction, cholangitis, increased central venous pressure due to right-sided heart failure, or other causes (Eulenberg *et al.,* 2018). Congenital abnormalities, including polycystic kidney disease in cats, can induce hepatic fibrosis (Bosje *et al.*, 1998). Hepatic fibrosis is an important event in the progression to cirrhosis and is associated with prognosis (Sevelius *et al.*, 1995).

Cytologic evidence for hepatic fibroplasia is the presence of increased numbers of spindled cells associated with pink fibrillar extracellular material that often trails out of the hepatocyte cluster (Figure 9.26). Cytologic preparations from hepatic fibrosis are

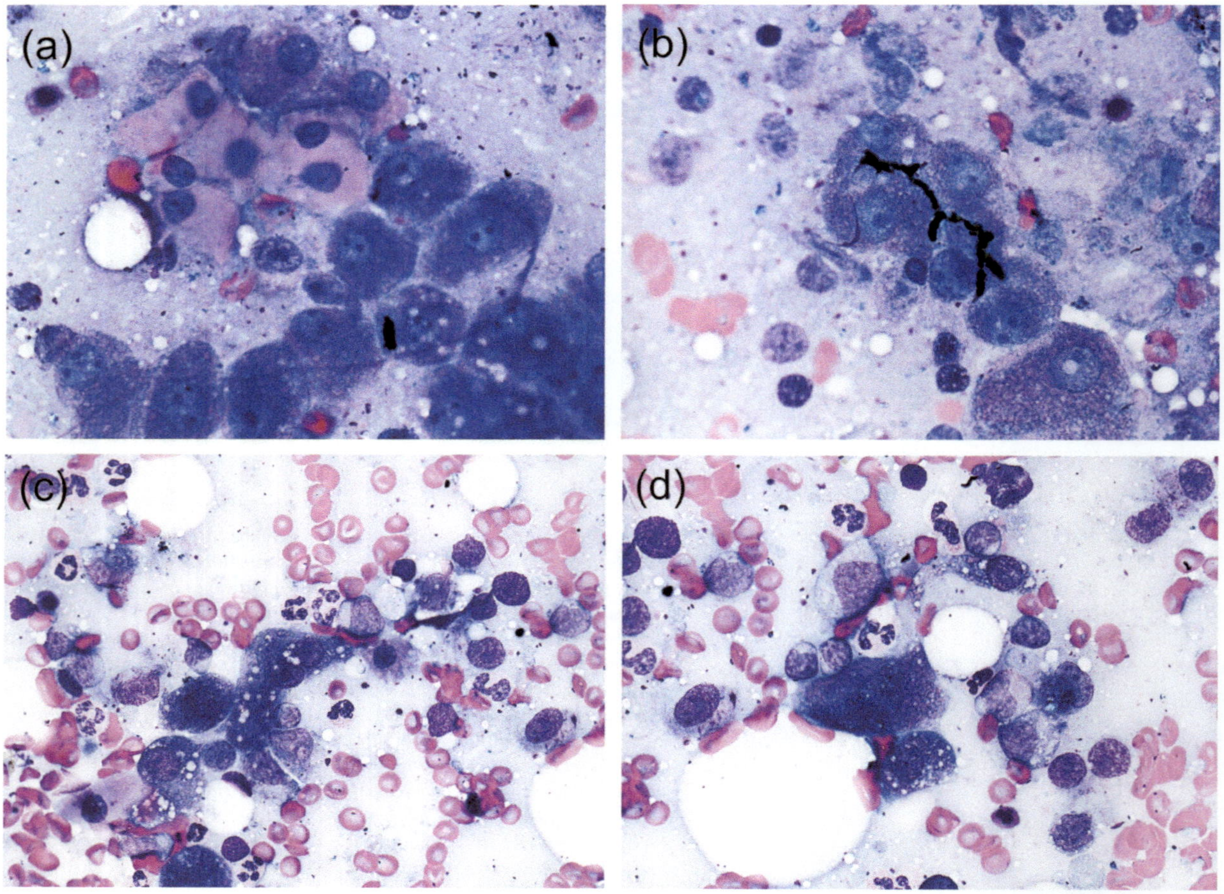

Figures 9.24a–d **Liver aspirates from a 7-year-old neutered male Golden Retriever dog with an acute history of inappetence, lethargy, and depression. (a) Individualized cells with smooth pink cytoplasm and a slightly condensed nucleus suggest single cell necrosis. Note the continuum between these cells and the hepatocytes, helping to confirm the origin of the cell population. (b) Bile casts are present and indicate cholestasis. (c&d) A mixed population of neutrophils, macrophages, and lymphocytes surround hepatocytes and a fusiform fibroblast (d) is present (Wright–Giemsa, 1,000× magnification).**

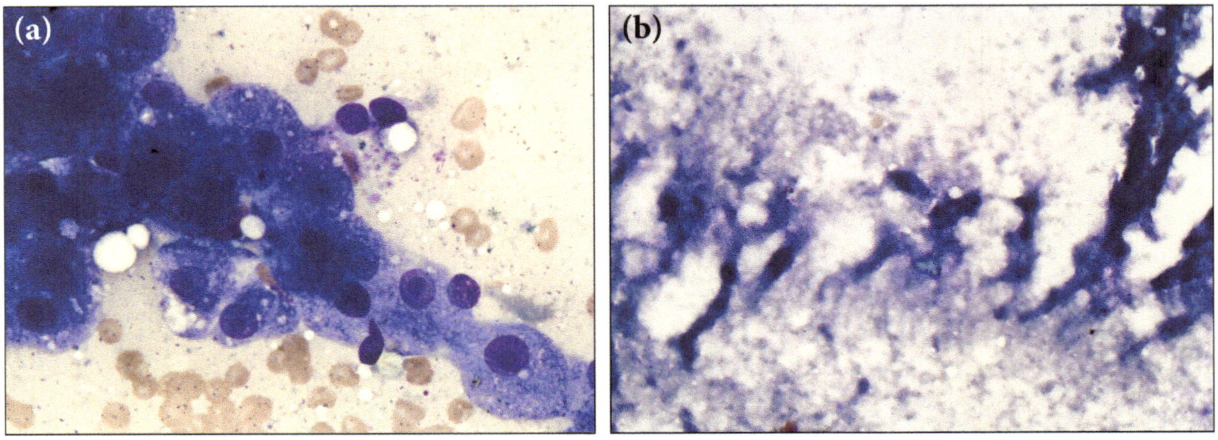

Figures 9.25a, b (a) A few clusters of intact and fairly normal hepatocytes are present from this dog (Wright–Giemsa, 1,000× magnification). (b) However, several slides contain abundant blue–gray acellular granular necrotic material. Note the ovoid structures, which may once have been nuclei. Mononuclear inflammation was present in the sample (not shown) and may have been responding to the necrosis or the process that instigated the necrosis (Wright–Giemsa, 500× magnification).

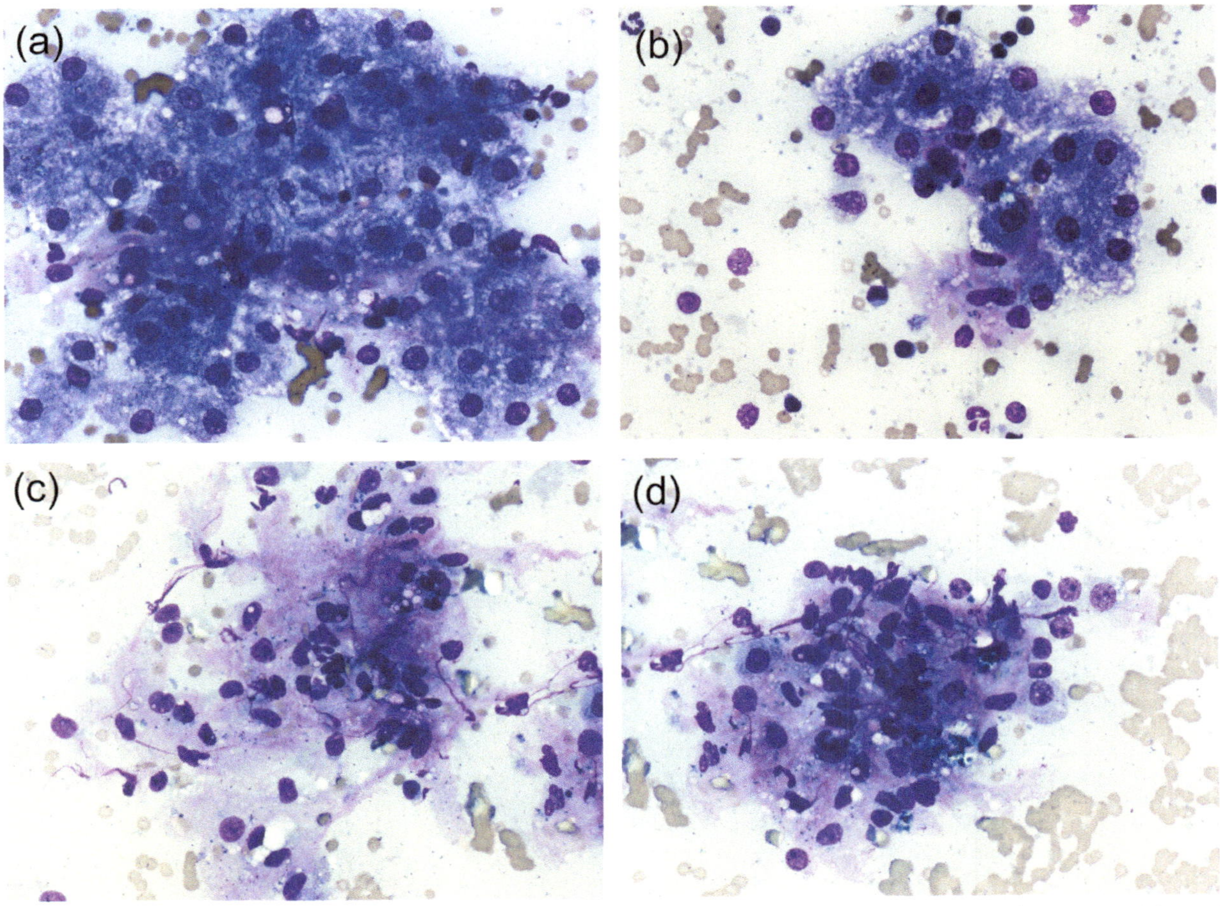

Figures 9.26a–d Liver aspirate from a 15-year-old domestic medium-haired cat. (a) Clusters of minimally pleomorphic hepatocytes with cytoplasmic rarefaction are present. Strands of pink fibrillar material are present within the clusters. (b) Cells with longer and slightly more condensed nuclei are more apparent within this cluster. (c) Larger aggregates of the extracellular material and spindled mesenchymal cells are present and few neutrophils are found within this aggregate. (d) Additionally, areas with macrophages are found within the mesenchymal component of this sample. Flow cytometry and PARR analysis (PCR for antigen receptor rearrangement) suggested a clonal CD21+ lymphocytosis from the concurrently submitted mesenteric lymph node aspirate. The neoplastic population was not apparent by cytology and the evidence of fibroplasia was considered an incidental finding (Wright–Giemsa, 500× magnification).

expected to have increased numbers of individualized and minimally pleomorphic mast cells. One study found that cytologic smears from cases with hepatic fibrosis had >10% spindled cells and >4% mast cells across 10 high-powered fields (Masserdotti *et al.*, 2016). Because of the limitations of fine needle aspiration, the pattern and degree of fibrosis cannot be determined from cytologic evaluation, but there has been suggestion that evaluation of serum biomarkers, including a proprietary algorithm of markers commonly included in serum biochemistry profiles, can provide information on the stage of fibrosis (Eulenberg *et al.*, 2018; Menard *et al.*, 2019).

Inflammatory processes

Given the bloody background of many hepatic biopsy samples, merely observing leukocytes in liver cytology is insufficient evidence of inflammation. Cytologic diagnosis of inflammation in the liver should be based on the presence of increased numbers of leukocytes relative to peripheral blood or consistent observation of inflammatory cells within or associated with clusters of hepatocytes. Different pathologic processes are more commonly associated with inflammation in specific regions of the liver, but this information is not available from cytology. Notwithstanding, significant information can be

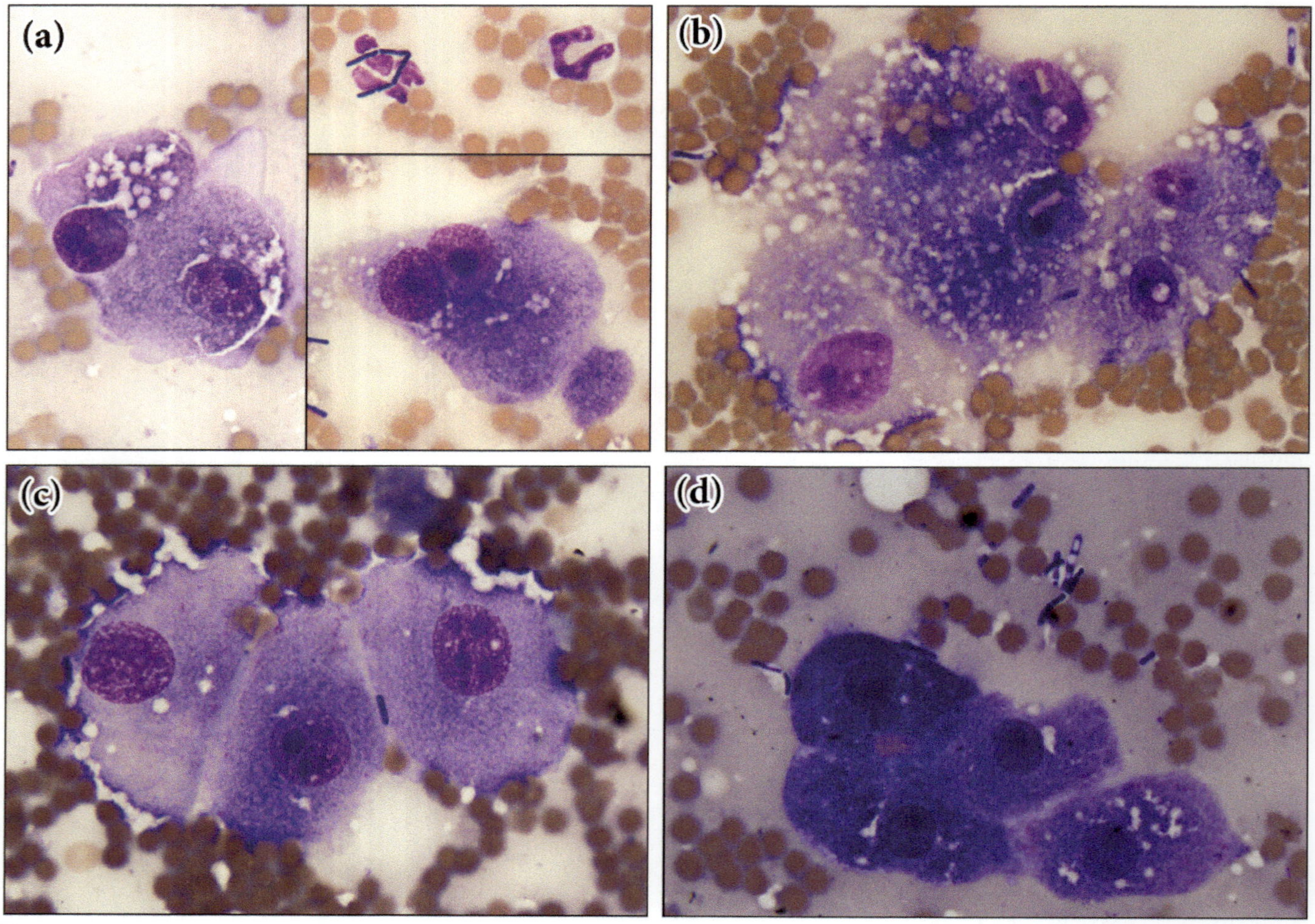

Figures 9.27a–d This dog had a remarkable septic suppurative hepatitis concurrent with hepatocellular carcinoma. (a) Degenerate neutrophils, which contain plump rod-shaped bacteria, are present (upper right panel). Cell-free bacteria are also seen (lower right panel). The hepatocytes display discrete clear vacuoles, suggestive of lipid, and dysplasia including anisocytosis, anisokaryosis, multiple nuclei, and multiple nucleoli (left and lower right panels). (b) Two brick inclusions and two intranuclear cytoplasmic inclusions are noted in this cluster of hepatocytes. Note the prominent subterminal spore found in the bacteria in the upper right-hand corner; bacterial culture determined these to be *Clostridium* species. (c) The hepatocytes have variable numbers of nucleoli and distinct cell–cell junctions. Histologic evaluation diagnosed hepatocellular carcinoma. (d) Clusters of more morphologically normal hepatocytes are also present in the slide (Wright–Giemsa, 1,000× magnification).

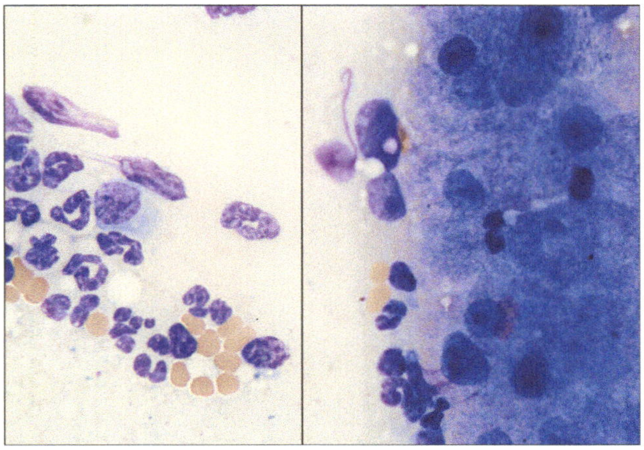

Figure 9.28 **This hepatic cytology sample is from a domestic longhair cat who was sampled after poor clinical and biochemical recovery from an episode of hepatic lipidosis. The cytology has many neutrophils interspersed around the hepatic clusters (left panel). Single neutrophils are consistently observed within the hepatocyte clusters. The hepatocytes do not have lipid-type vacuolar changes (right panel). There is a suppurative process evident (Wright–Giemsa, 1,000× magnification).**

gained cytologically, which can aid in the determination of subsequent diagnostic steps to fully understand the cause of inflammation.

SUPPURATIVE INFLAMMATION

A threshold of >7 neutrophils in close approximation with 200 hepatocytes found in clusters (i.e. 3.5% neutrophils) has been suggested for diagnosis of suppurative inflammation (Gardner *et al.*, 2022). This threshold agrees with the finding that >5% neutrophils was observed with destructive cholangitis, acute hepatitis, abscessation, and cholangiohepatitis (Figures 9.17a, b, 9.27a–d, 9.28; Weiss *et al.*, 2001; Stockhaus *et al.*, 2004). Inflammation can often be associated with hepatocellular atypia including variation in hepatocyte nuclear size, N:C ratio, and nucleoli (Stockhaus *et al.*, 2004). Both infectious and noninfectious causes of suppurative inflammation have been documented. Infectious causes include viruses such as canine adenovirus-1, canine and feline herpes viruses, and feline infectious peritonitis (corona)virus; bacterial agents including *Leptospira* spp., *Escherichia coli*, *Staphylococcus* spp., *Clostridium* spp., and *Brucella* spp.; and protozoans, including *Toxoplasma* sp. (van den Ingh *et al.*, 2006a, b). Noninfectious causes include pancreatitis and drug or toxin-induced hepatopathy and necrosis, among others (van den Ingh *et al.*, 2006a, b). Often the underlying cause of inflammation is not found. The unifying characteristic of these is the relatively acute and active nature of the disease process.

MIXED INFLAMMATION

An inflammatory population of lymphocytes, neutrophils, and macrophages is associated with both an active (represented by suppurative inflammation) and chronic (represented by macrophages and lymphocytes) disease course. Mixed inflammation is usually associated with chronic active hepatitis, destructive cholangiolitis, and metastatic neoplasms (Weiss *et al.*, 2001; Stockhaus *et al.*, 2004). As with suppurative inflammation, both infectious and noninfectious etiologies are possible. Fungi (e.g. *Histoplasma* spp., *Blastomyces* spp., *Coccidioides* spp.), atypical bacteria (e.g. *Nocardia* spp., *Mycobacteria* spp., *Rhodococcus* spp.), and parasites (e.g. *Hepatozoon* spp., *Heterobilharzia* spp.) are infectious causes, while noninfectious causes include copper-associated hepatopathy (Figures 9.29a–e; van den Ingh *et al.*, 2006a, b).

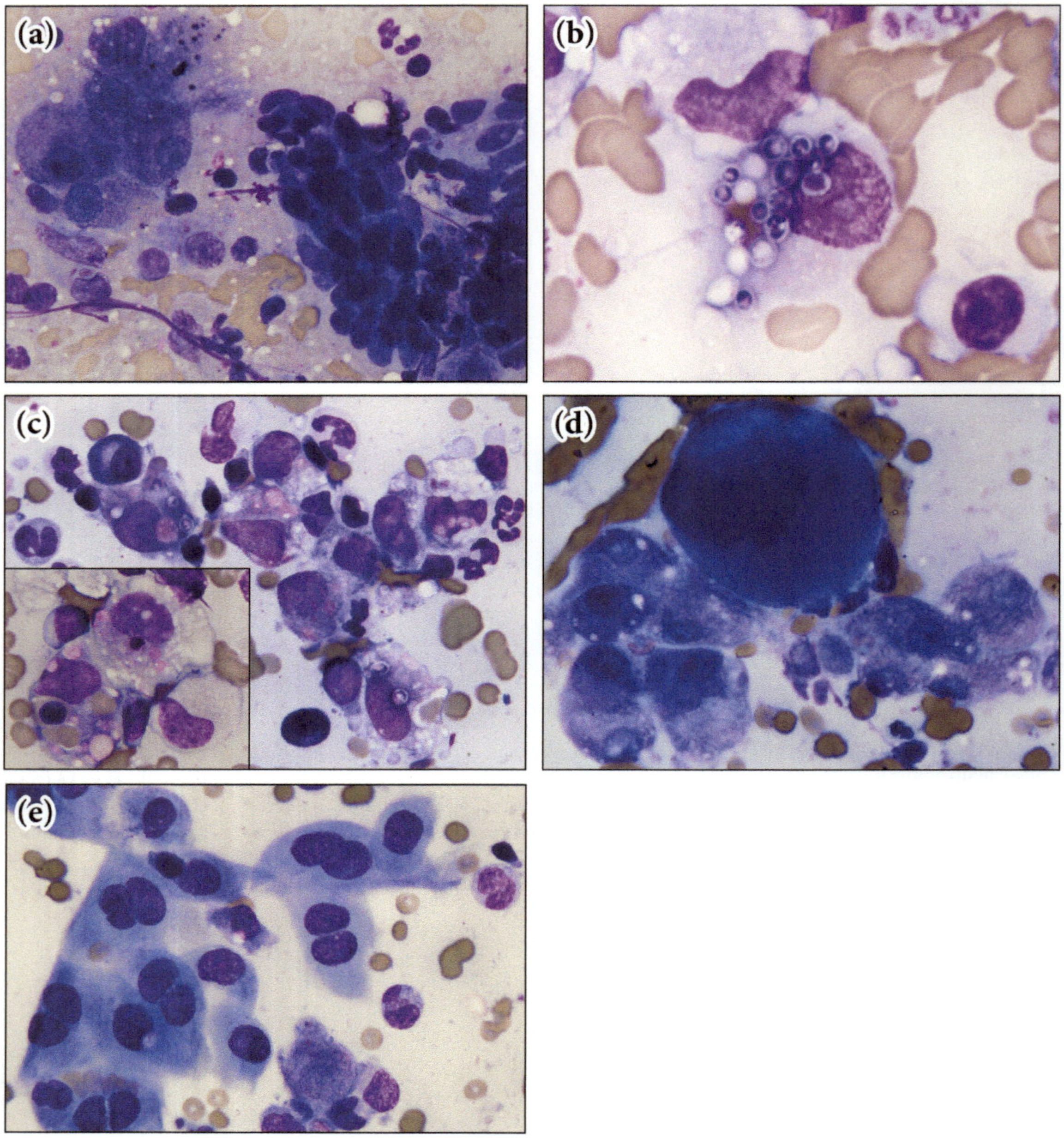

Figures 9.29a–e **Feline hepatic sample. (a) Hepatocytes (left side of image) and clusters of biliary epithelial cells (right side of image) are prevalent in some areas of the slide. (b) Highly phagocytic macrophages are also present in the sample. They contain intracellular yeast that have a distinct cell wall and crescentic nuclear basophilic material within the protoplasm, consistent with *Histoplasma* spp. yeast. (c) Macrophages, neutrophils, lymphocytes, and plasma cells are displayed. Yeasts are found in several of these macrophages as well. The inset shows erythrophagocytic macrophages, which were a common finding. (d) Rare multinucleate giant cells are present. The deeply basophilic cytoplasm and tightly aggregated nuclei mark this cell as a megakaryocyte and denote extramedullary hematopoiesis; nRBCs and fewer myeloid precursors were also present but were not imaged. (e) Few sheets of binucleated mesothelial cells are seen and suggest reactive mesothelium (Wright-Giemsa, 1,000× magnification). The cytologic diagnosis is mixed inflammation with yeast consistent with *Histoplasma* spp. and extramedullary hematopoiesis.**

LYMPHOCYTIC AND LYMPHOPLASMACYTIC INFLAMMATION

Often, lymphocytic inflammation is more regional and patchy within the liver; this has a negative effect on the sensitivity of FNA for lymphocytic inflammation. As in other locations, lymphocytic and lymphoplasmacytic inflammation is usually associated with an adaptive immune response and a more chronic duration (Figures 9.30a–c). When chronic active hepatitis progresses to cirrhosis in the dog, FNA samples have decreasing amounts of lymphocytes and increasing

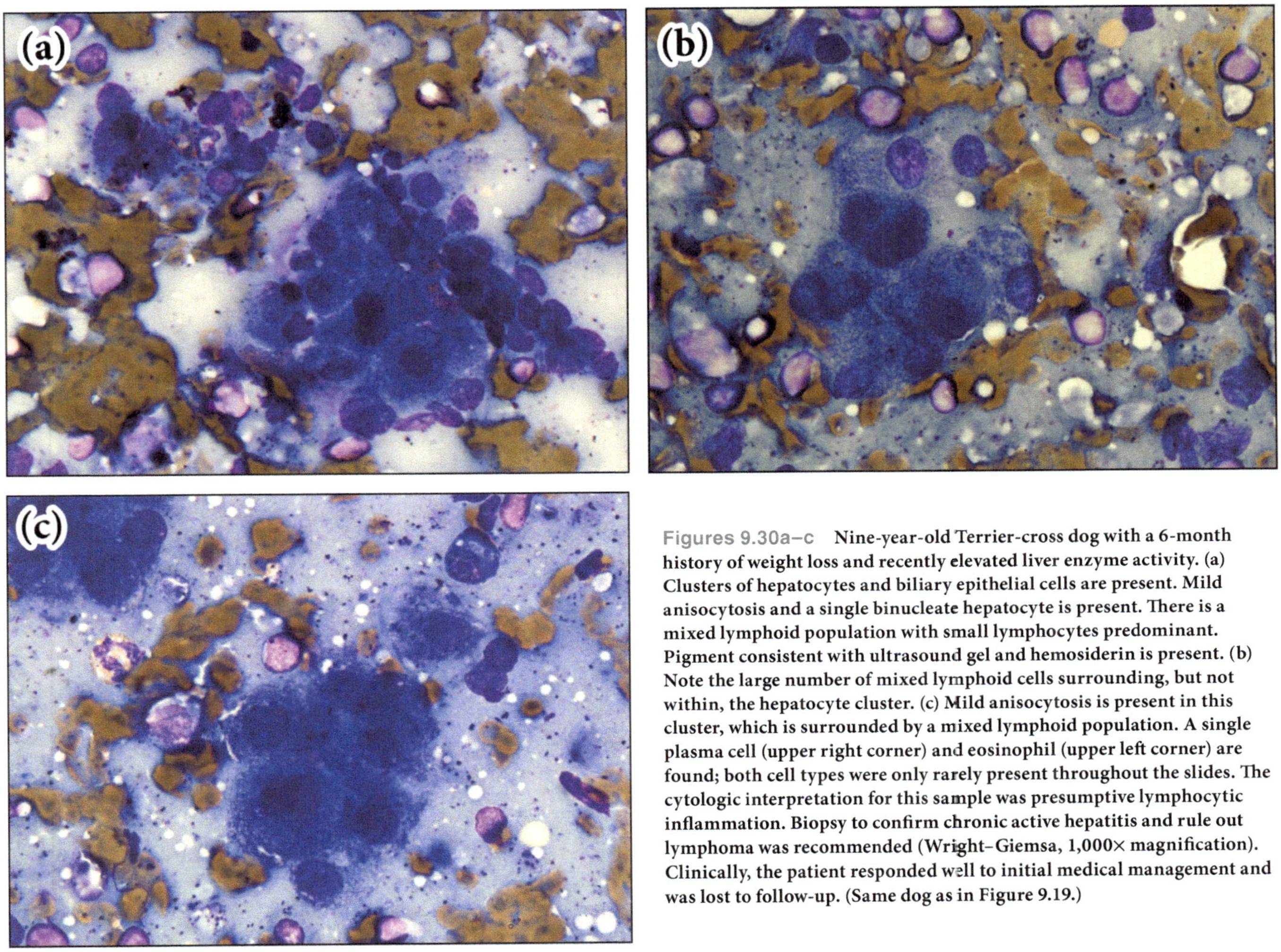

Figures 9.30a–c Nine-year-old Terrier-cross dog with a 6-month history of weight loss and recently elevated liver enzyme activity. (a) Clusters of hepatocytes and biliary epithelial cells are present. Mild anisocytosis and a single binucleate hepatocyte is present. There is a mixed lymphoid population with small lymphocytes predominant. Pigment consistent with ultrasound gel and hemosiderin is present. (b) Note the large number of mixed lymphoid cells surrounding, but not within, the hepatocyte cluster. (c) Mild anisocytosis is present in this cluster, which is surrounded by a mixed lymphoid population. A single plasma cell (upper right corner) and eosinophil (upper left corner) are found; both cell types were only rarely present throughout the slides. The cytologic interpretation for this sample was presumptive lymphocytic inflammation. Biopsy to confirm chronic active hepatitis and rule out lymphoma was recommended (Wright–Giemsa, 1,000× magnification). Clinically, the patient responded well to initial medical management and was lost to follow-up. (Same dog as in Figure 9.19.)

amounts of biliary epithelial cells (Stockhaus *et al.*, 2004). This finding fits with the expected resolution of inflammation and progression to fibrosis and hepatocyte drop-out. Care should be taken to avoid misdiagnosing lymphocytic inflammation with lymphoma (Otte *et al.*, 2017).

EOSINOPHILIC INFLAMMATION

Eosinophilic inflammation has been reported, either solely within the liver or associated with hypereosinophilic syndrome (Brellou *et al.*, 2006). Typical causes of peripheral eosinophilia (parasitic, allergic, and atypical processes such as paraneoplastic reactions or endocrinopathies) are thought to play a similar role in the liver (Figures 9.31, 9.32).

Parasitic infections

Parasites are infrequently observed in hepatic samples in the dog and cat. Cestode infection has been documented in canine liver cytology (Brosinski *et al.*, 2012; Patten *et al.*, 2013). *Toxoplasma gondii* and other Sarcocystids have been reported in hepatic cytologies as have *Echinococcus* spp., *Heterobilharzia* spp., *Hepatozoon* spp., Platynosomum spp., and *Cytauxzoon* spp., among others (van den Ingh *et al.*, 2006a, b; Aschenbroich *et al.*, 2012; Köster *et al.*, 2016). Dogs with heavy heartworm burdens can have microfilaria on hepatic

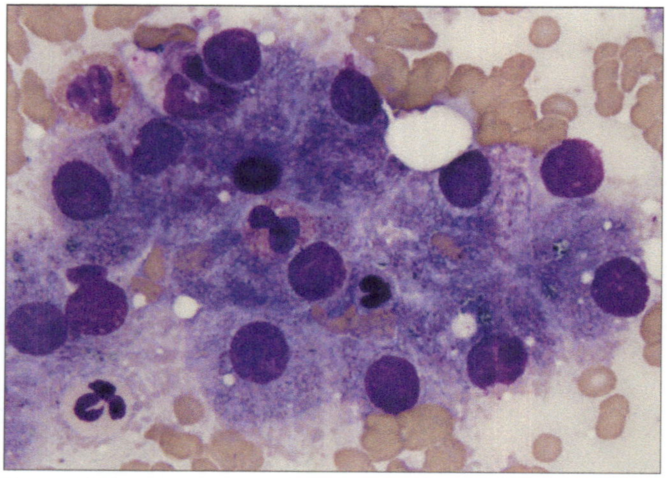

Figure 9.31 Hepatic aspirate from a domestic shorthair cat with eosinophilic inflammation in the spleen, duodenal wall, and jejunal lymph node. Eosinophils are consistently noted within clusters of hepatocytes and free in the background. Two neutrophils are also present in this image. A peripheral blood eosinophilia was not present in this patient, an important confirmation as peripheral eosinophilia can cause intrusion of eosinophils into the sinusoidal spaces (Wright–Giemsa, 1,000× magnification).

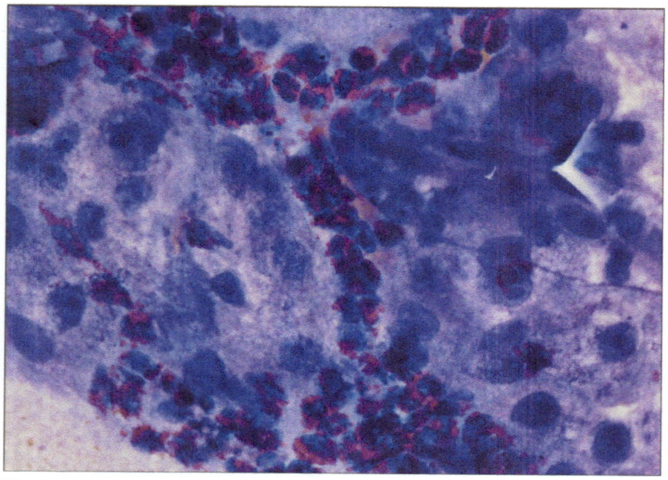

Figure 9.32 Hepatic sinuses are clogged with eosinophils in this canine patient with a marked eosinophilic hepatitis (Wright–Giemsa, 1,000× magnification).

cytology; this is an indication of blood contamination, not the true presence of the parasite specifically in the liver (Figure 9.33).

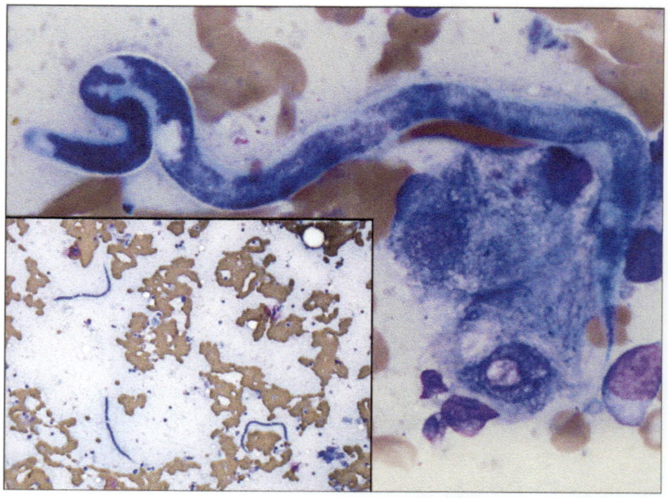

Figure 9.33 A microfilaria's tail appears to wind between hepatocytes. Two small lymphocytes are also noted. Inset shows a 200× field with multiple microfilaria (Wright–Giemsa, 1,000× magnification).

NEOPLASTIC DISEASES

Hepatic epithelial cell origin tumors

Hepatoma/hepatocellular adenoma/ hepatocellular carcinoma

Although the diagnosis of primary hepatic neoplasia can be cytologically challenging, the use of a complex logistic regression model has shown that cytologic findings can be used to diagnose hepatocellular carcinoma (Stockhaus *et al.*, 2004). This study found that hepatocytes with a high N:C ratio, larger cell diameters, increased numbers of nucleoli per nucleus, small numbers of cytoplasmic vacuoles, and small numbers of lymphocytes intermixed with hepatocytes were associated with hepatocellular carcinoma. Additionally, primary hepatic tumors will commonly display a more uniform population of abnormal hepatocytes in contrast to the mixture of dysplastic hepatocytes and cytologically unremarkable cells seen with other pathologic processes. Another canine study found that dissociated hepatocytes, acinar or palisading arrangements of neoplastic cells, and the presence of naked nuclei and capillaries, when seen with mild anisocytosis, anisokaryosis, multinucleation, and increased N:C ratio, were useful for diagnosing well-differentiated hepatocellular carcinoma (Figures 9.27, 9.34–9.36, Masserdotti Drigo, 2012).

Hepatocellular adenomas and carcinomas have been described in both dogs and cats (Trigo *et al.*, 1982; Balkman, 2009). In the dog, hepatocellular carcinoma is the most common primary liver tumor. The metastatic rate has been reported to be as high as 60% with common sites of metastasis being the lung, local lymph node, and peritoneum. Even with common metastasis, treatment has been associated with survival times of approximately 4 years (Balkman, 2009). In the cat, hepatocellular adenoma is more common.

HEPATOBLASTOMA

Hepatoblastoma has been diagnosed histologically in both the dog and the cat. It is a neoplastic proliferation of pluripotent hepatic stem cells (Shiga *et al.*, 1997; Ano *et al.*, 2011). Histologically, this cancer

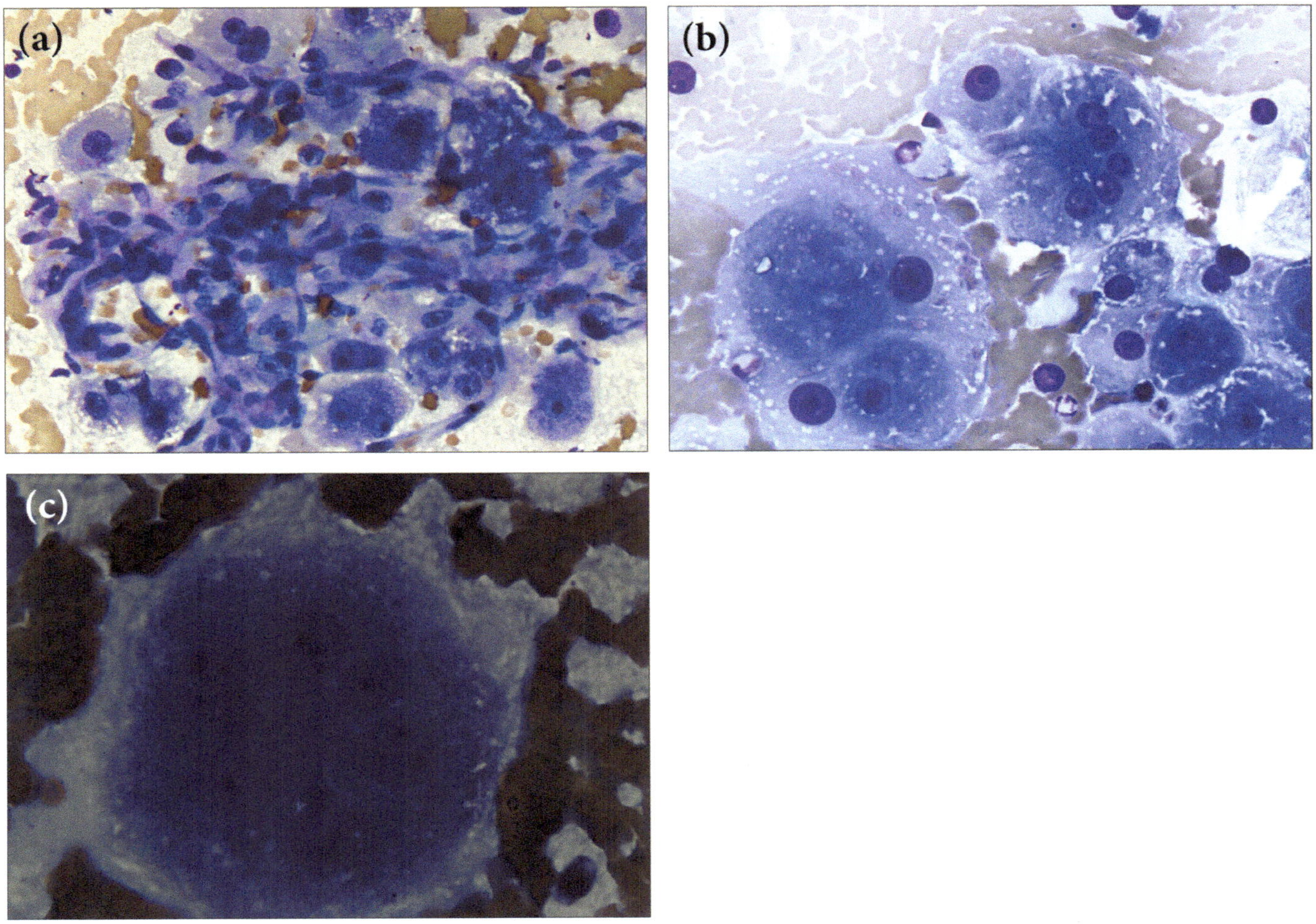

Figures 9.34a–c **Liver aspirate from a Labrador Retriever with multiple hepatic masses. (a) This slide contains a few more normal looking hepatocytes, often enmeshed in a network of capillaries. (b) Cytologically, there was a continuum of cell morphology from large cohesively clustered cells, which have pink granular to basophilic cytoplasm, to those with more basophilic cytoplasm and poorly distinct cell borders (giving a naked nuclei appearance). Marked nuclear pleomorphism was also noted. (c) Rarely, very large multinucleate cells with marked nuclear and nucleolar variability are also seen. These features have been associated with hepatocellular carcinoma. In conjunction with a history of a hepatic mass noted on ultrasound, the slides are suggestive of hepatocellular carcinoma (a and b Wright–Giemsa, 500× magnification; c, 1,000× magnification).**

presents as ovoid hepatocytes with a combination of both embryonic hepatocyte and biliary epithelial immunological markers present (Shiga *et al.*, 1997).

COMBINED HEPATOCELLULAR-CHOLANGIOCARCINOMA

Combined hepatocellular-cholangiocarcinoma is very infrequently encountered. It makes up 2–5% of primary canine liver tumors. Some of the neoplastic cells have a hepatocellular morphology while others have a distinctly biliary morphology (Terai *et al.*, 2022). Grossly, the lesions are typically large and have cystic regions. The reported prognosis after surgical excision is good.

Biliary epithelium origin tumors

Benign bile duct tumors have variably been called biliary adenoma, biliary cystadenoma, cholangiocellular adenoma, and cholangioma histologically, while the malignant form has been called biliary carcinoma, cholangiocarcinoma, and cystadenocarcinoma depending on their architectural morphology and an uncertain understanding of

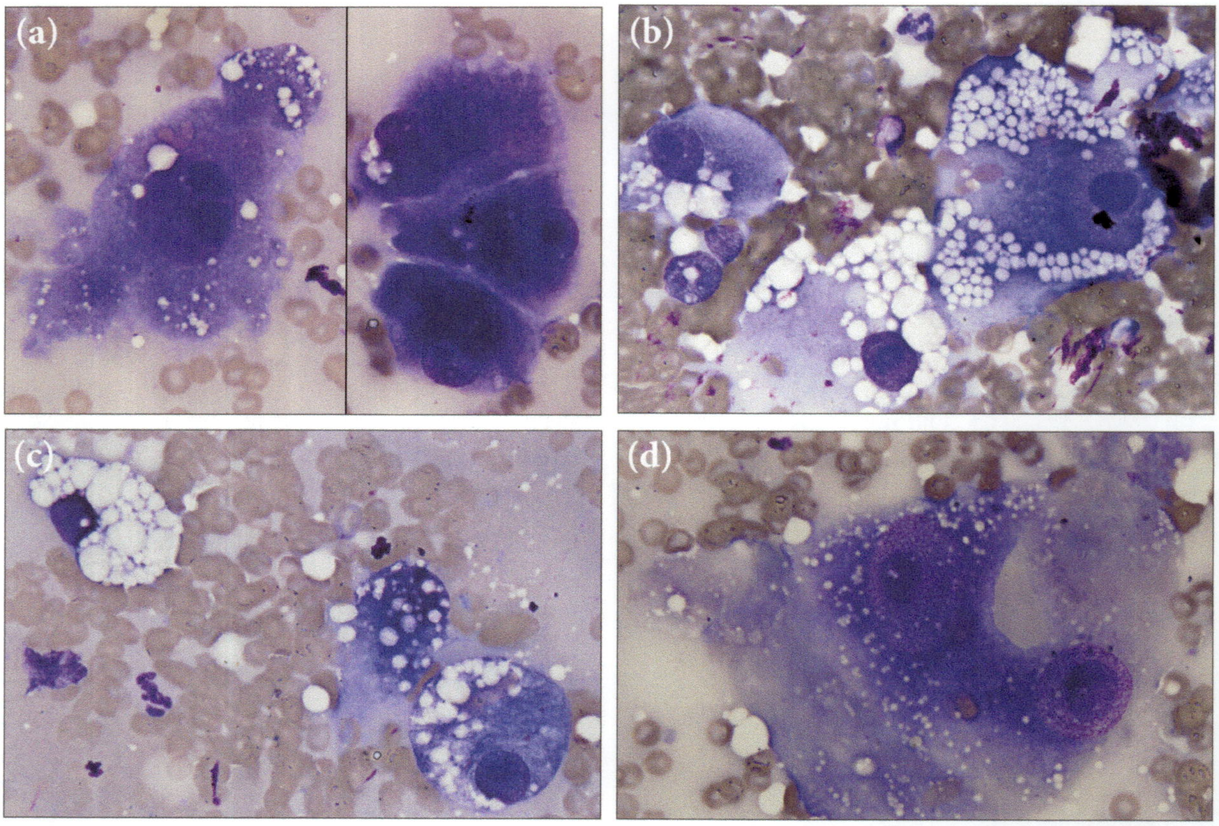

Figures 9.35a–d Liver aspirate from a Cocker Spaniel with multiple hepatic masses. Cytologically, many features suggesting hepatocellular carcinoma are present. (a) Anisocytosis, anisokaryosis, binucleation, and multiple nucleoli are present. (b) The neoplastic cell in the upper right corner has a nucleolus approximately the size of the nuclei in the other two intact hepatocytes. Most of the hepatocytes also contain abundant clear cytoplasmic vacuolation, consistent with lipid. The fuchsia material noted in the image is consistent with ultrasound gel. (c) Note the highly variable amount of clear distinct vacuolation. Without a progression of cells from minimally vacuolated to highly vacuolated, the cell in the upper left corner would be challenging to recognize as a hepatocyte. (d) Markedly cytomegalic cells are present. Again, nuclei are large and contain impressively large dark nucleoli (Wright–Giemsa, 1,000× magnification).

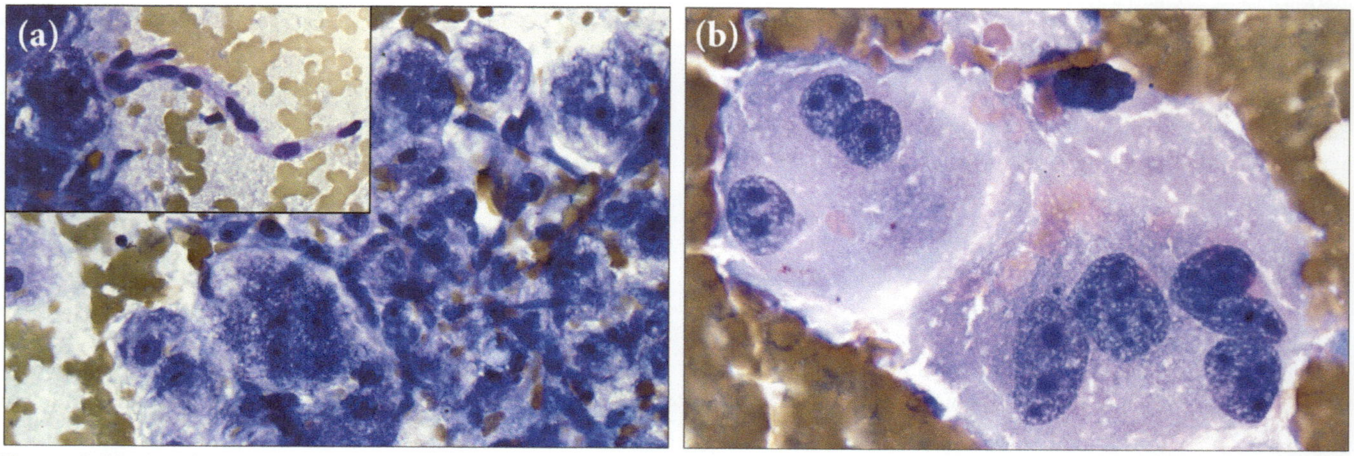

Figures 9.36a, b This dog had multiple liver nodules on ultrasound and several features suggestive of hepatocellular carcinoma on liver cytology. (a) Capillaries are commonly seen within hepatocyte clusters. (b) Many multinucleated cells with three to seven nuclei are present. Cell borders of many hepatocytes are also poorly distinct, suggesting a fragile population of cells. Note the multiple and variable size of nucleoli (Wright–Giemsa, 1,000× magnification).

the cell of origin. These distinctions cannot usually be made on cytologic evaluation.

Cytologically, neoplastic biliary epithelium commonly looks benign, irrespective of its actual clinical course. Cohesive structures that represent all morphologic features of the biliary tree can be observed, including clusters, tubules, sheets, and acinar arrangements (Figures 9.37a–c, 9.38a, b). The individual cells will frequently have less cytoplasm than a hepatocyte, making the cells appear more densely packed together. Depending on secretory function, there may be minimal to prominent vacuolation within the basophilic cytoplasm. Neoplasms that are cystic or highly secretory can be associated with either bile fluid or mucinous material, and aspiration of significant amounts of fluid can be achieved.

Benign biliary neoplasia is rarely observed in dogs, but is the most common primary hepatic tumor in the cat (Trigo *et al.*, 1982). Large fluid-filled cystadenomas have measured up to 8 cm. Many incidental cystadenomas have been reported; clinical signs, when present, are often caused by the mass acting as a space-occupying lesion (Nyland *et al.*, 1999). Malignant biliary neoplasia is more commonly observed in the dog and less commonly observed in the cat. This tumor tends to behave aggressively with 60–80% metastatic rates and spread to the local lymph node, lung, abdominal organs, and bone (Balkman, 2009).

STROMAL CELL ORIGIN TUMORS

Mesenchymal tumors

Primary mesenchymal tumors of the liver are rarely observed in both the dog and cat. As a group they tend to behave aggressively and carry a poor prognosis. Hemangiosarcoma, leiomyosarcoma, fibrosarcoma, osteosarcoma, chondrosarcoma, and liposarcoma have been reported in the dog (Galofaro *et al.*, 2008; Balkman, 2009). Hemangiosarcoma, leiomyosarcoma, rhabdomyosarcoma, and osteosarcoma have been reported in the cat (Balkman, 2009). Cytologically, these tumors tend to share many characteristics, making differentiation based on cytology alone challenging. Close

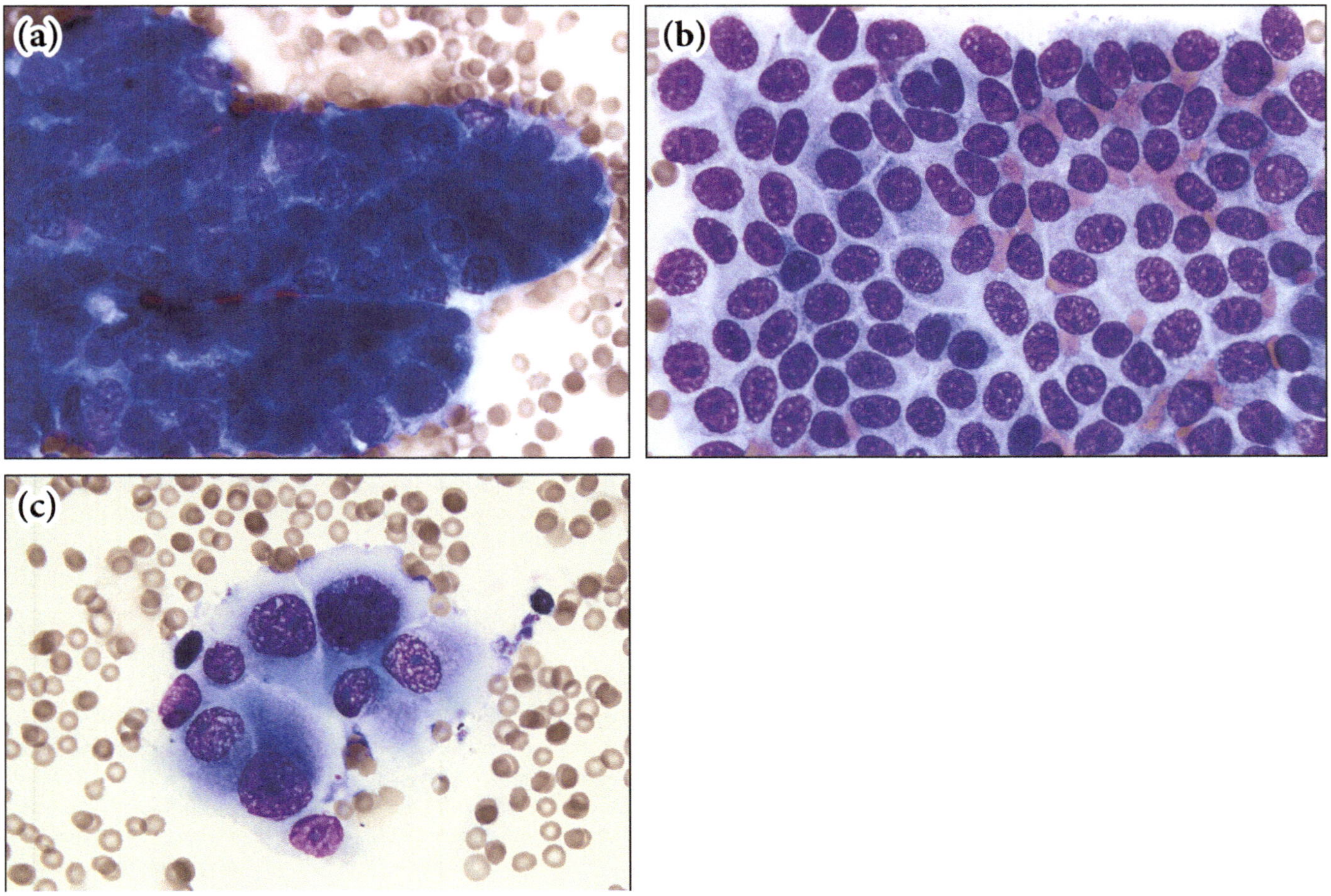

Figures 9.37a–c **(a) Large papillary structures are evident in this aspirate from a domestic shorthair cat with ultrasonographically confirmed hepatic nodules. (b) Sheets of cells help confirm that the population is predominantly cuboidal with minimal to moderate amounts of cytoplasm. (c) Cells with moderate anisocytosis and anisokaryosis are abundant. The cell morphology is most consistent with biliary origin. Although cats most commonly have benign biliary neoplasms, the criteria of malignancy noted here lead to the concern that this is a carcinoma. Biopsy and histopathology should be performed to make this distinction (Wright–Giemsa, 1,000× magnification).**

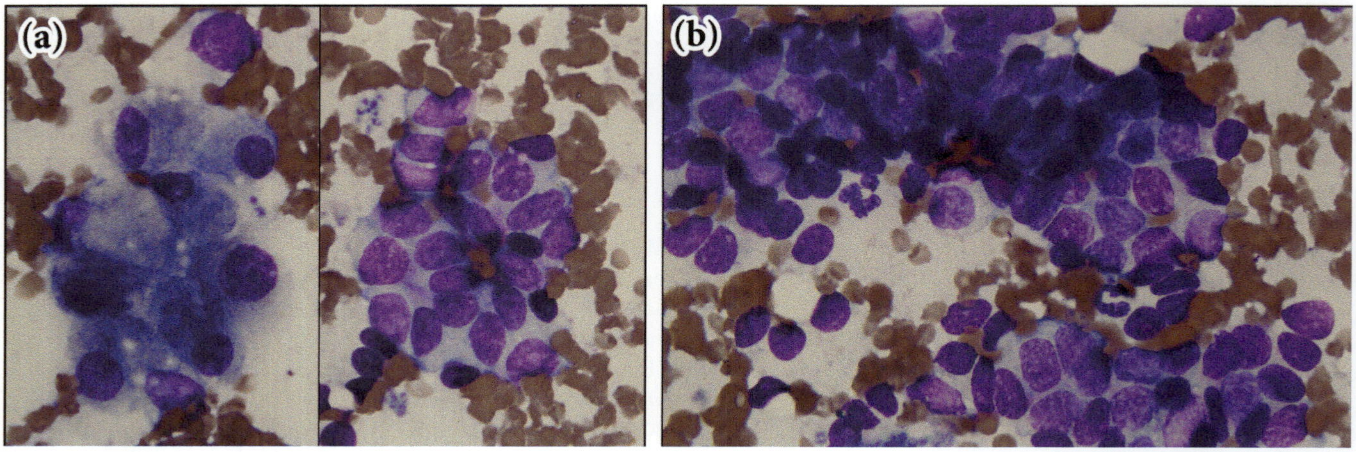

Figures 9.38a, b **(a) Contrast the hepatocytes on the left with the cuboidal epithelial cells on the right in this feline sample. The cuboidal cells are most consistent with biliary epithelium. (b) Many cells are ruptured but where intact they were found in large clusters. The pleomorphism noted suggests a biliary neoplasm, which is most likely a benign neoplastic process (Wright–Giemsa, 1,000× magnification).**

examination of slides can occasionally provide one or two characteristics that raise the index of suspicion for a specific sarcoma. For example, many large spindloid to polygonal cells with small, clear punctate vacuoles and evidence of erythrophagia are suggestive of, but not definitive for, hemangiosarcoma or histiocytic sarcoma (Barger *et al.*, 2012). Elongate spindloid cells associated with extracellular pink fibrillar matrix (collagen) can suggest fibrosarcoma among others. An abundance of large plasmacytoid cells evokes an osteosarcoma, chondrosarcoma, or plasma cell tumor. Strap-cells (large elongate cells with a row of multiple nuclei and faint to prominent cytoplasmic striations) raise suspicion for rhabdomyosarcoma. Even with recognition of one or more of these characteristics, the only accurate cytologic diagnosis is sarcoma, followed by a list of potential differentials.

MYELOLIPOMA

This rare neoplasm has been described in both the dog and cat, but reported involvement of the liver is limited to the cat (McCaw *et al.*, 1990; Kamiie *et al.*, 2009). Myelolipomas form as a nodular mass composed of islands of hematopoietic precursors and adipocytes. Cytologically, large amounts of morphologically unremarkable adipocytes and a population of erythroid, myeloid, and megakaryocytic precursors are present. Distinction of myelolipoma from EMH can be challenging. Extramedullary hematopoiesis is frequently seen as a diffuse lesion with abundant amounts of hepatocytes also present on the slides, while myelolipoma is commonly diagnosed from a nodular mass with abundant immature and mature hematopoietic cells and minimal liver tissue.

NEUROENDOCRINE TUMORS

Carcinoids, the primary neuroendocrine tumor of the liver, are uncommon but have been reported in both the dog and the cat. Cytologically, they display the classic neuroendocrine morphology of a naked-nuclei appearance; intact nuclei are observed in a mass of cytoplasm with poorly distinct cytoplasmic junctions (see Chapter 18). Occasionally, rosette and acinar structures are observed. The secretory granules characteristic of neuroendocrine tissue can be challenging to visualize with Romanowsky stains but can be enhanced with a Churukian–Schenck or other silver stain (Smith & Haggitt, 1983). Additionally, carcinoids should stain positive for common immunologic neuroendocrine markers (e.g. chromogranin-A, synaptophysin, neuron-specific enolase; Patnaik *et al.*, 2005). Carcinoids can infiltrate diffusely throughout the liver. When present as a localized mass, they are commonly associated with the bile duct or gallbladder. These tumors are highly aggressive and have been observed to metastasize to lymph node and peritoneum (Stalker & Hayes, 2007a,b).

ROUND CELL ORIGIN TUMORS

Lymphoma/leukemia

Lymphoma is the most commonly observed neoplasm in the liver and can be found as a primary hepatic lymphoma or as part of a multicentric process (e.g. stage III–V lymphoma or leukemia [Figures 9.39–9.43a, b]; Trigo *et al.*, 1982; Roth, 2001). Although most hepatic lymphoma cases will contain approximately 50% large lymphocytes, the presence of >5% large lymphocytes found in multiple

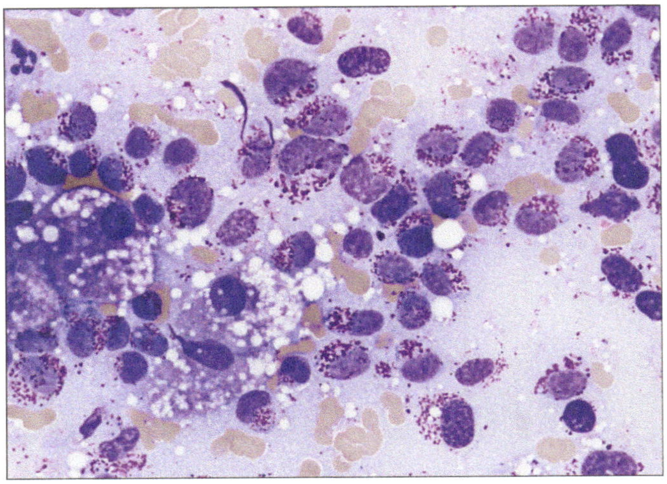

Figure 9.39 An infiltrative population of large round cells, which contain coarse fuchsia granules, are noted in this feline hepatic sample. The presumptive diagnosis is large granular lymphoma (Wright–Giemsa, 1,000× magnification). (Courtesy Dr. Amy Schnelle.)

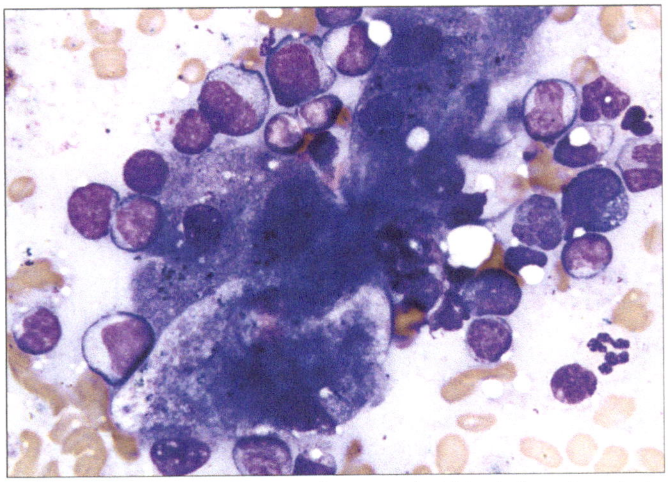

Figure 9.40 Neoplastic round cells are noted within the hepatic aspirate and were also found in samples from the spleen and peripheral blood of this Golden Retriever. Most of the round cells have scant amounts of basophilic cytoplasm and round nuclei, which are the same size or larger than the neutrophil present in the lower right corner of the image. Few neoplastic cells contain small pink cytoplasmic granules. The sample is most consistent with acute leukemia/lymphoma (Wright–Giemsa, 1,000× magnification).

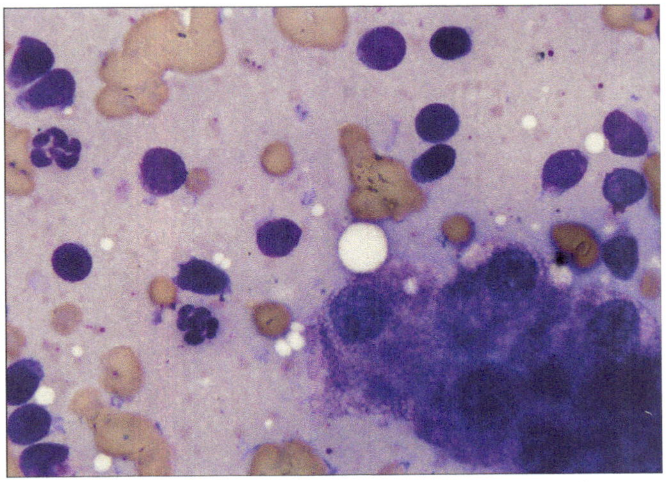

Figure 9.41 The liver aspirate from this domestic shorthair cat has very few clusters of hepatocytes and abundant lymphocytes, most of which are small cells (i.e. scant rim of cytoplasm around a nucleus smaller than a neutrophil and condensed chromatin). Very few blast cells are noted. Histologically, this was confirmed as a small-cell lymphoma (Wright–Giemsa, 1,000× magnification).

sites has been used as a criterion for diagnosing hepatic lymphoma (Stockhaus *et al.*, 2004). These cells cytologically look similar to lymphoma in other tissues (see Chapter 8). History will commonly describe hepatomegaly with a diffuse lesion or multiple target lesions noted on echography. Addition of hepatic cytology to the lymphoma staging protocols affects the perceived stage; oddly, one study found that it migrated from stage III to stage IV, but this change did not predict a change in survival (Nerschbach *et al.*, 2016).

Lymphoma is not a single disease entity but a heterogeneous group of neoplasms, all of lymphocyte origin. Distinction of B- or T-cell origin can be determined with immunocytochemical, polymerase chain reaction (PCR), or flow-cytometric techniques (Figures 9.42a, b, 9.43a, b). Subclassification into one of the several lymphoid classification systems often requires either multiple aspirations to obtain sufficient numbers of cells for immunologic testing or biopsy to evaluate the architecture of the node. The diagnosis of large granular lymphocyte lymphoma can occasionally be made by cytology on liver samples (Figure 9.39). Diagnosis of small-cell lymphoma can be difficult, especially since a small lymphocyte inflammatory population can be present in lymphocytic cholangitis and hepatitis (Otte *et al.*, 2017). The observation of a pure population of lymphocytes from several locations, potentially in conjunction with immunophenotyping or clonality testing, can help bolster a diagnosis of lymphoma or chronic lymphocytic leukemia (Figure 9.39; van den Ingh *et al.*, 2006a, b).

NONLYMPHOID LEUKEMIA

Nonlymphoid hematopoietic leukemia has been reported in small animals as both the chronic and acute forms with granulocytic, dendritic, erythroid, and megakaryocytic lineages represented

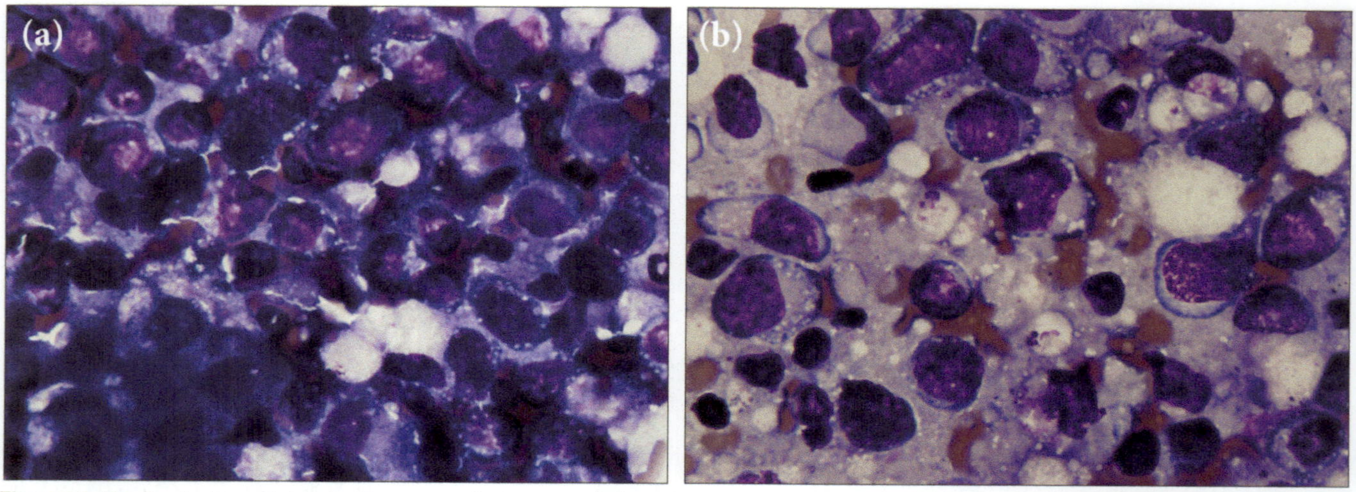

Figures 9.42a, b (a) A small cluster of hepatocytes is present in the lower left corner of the field; however, the predominant cell type in the image (and on the slide) is large lymphocytes, consistent with lymphoma. (b)A thinner area of the slide helps display the morphology of the large lymphoid cells. They are 2–3 times larger than a red blood cell, with increased amounts of basophilic cytoplasm, open chromatin, and one to several poorly distinct nucleoli. These cells were CD3 positive by immunocytochemistry, suggesting a T-cell lymphoma (Wright–Giemsa, 1,000× magnification).

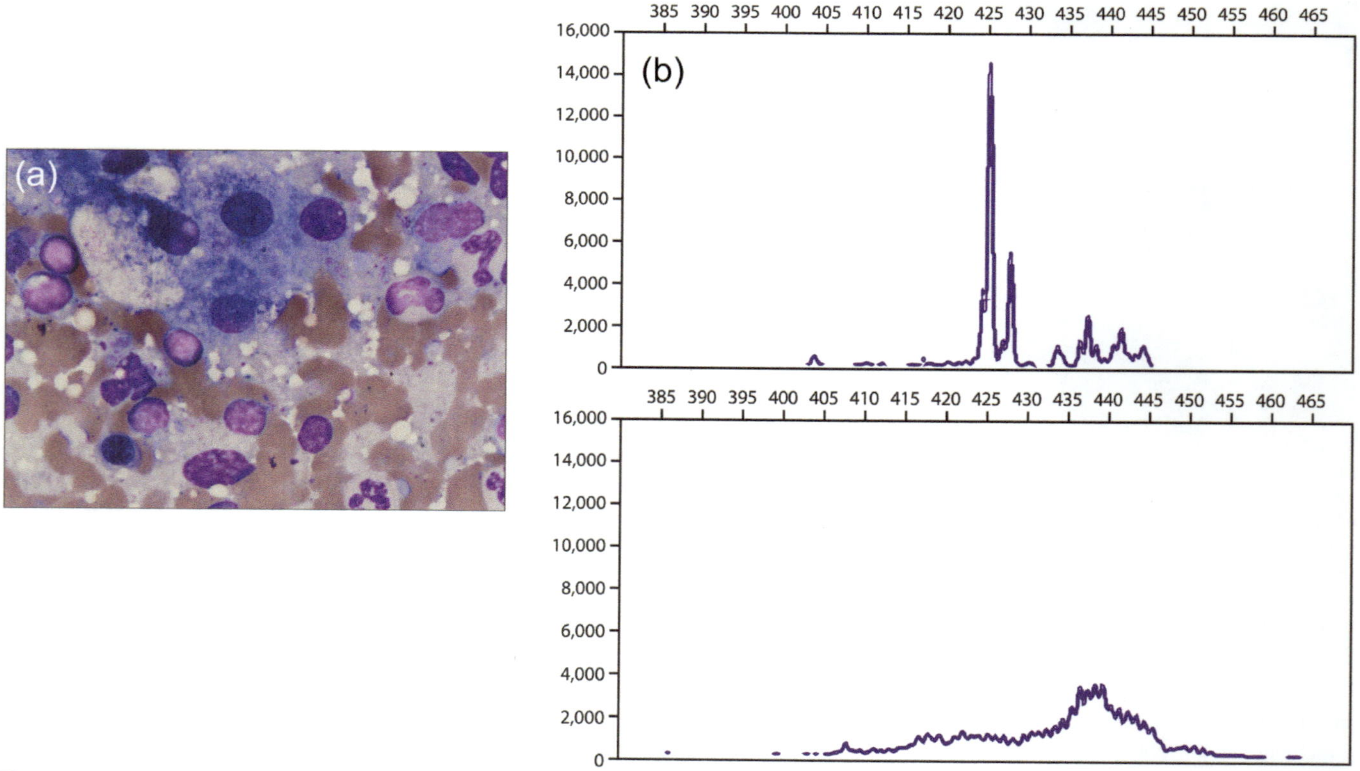

Figures 9.43a, b (a) An increased number of intermediate-sized lymphocytes with lower numbers of small and large lymphocytes is consistently found in multiple fields of this liver sample. This could suggest either lymphoid hyperplasia or lymphoma. Hepatocytes with foamy cytoplasmic rarefaction (suggesting glycogen or hydropic degeneration) and red and white blood cell precursors (suggesting extramedullary hematopoiesis) are also found (Wright–Giemsa, 1,000× magnification). (b) PARR analysis (PCR for antigen receptor rearrangement) on this sample confirmed a clonal expansion of lymphocytes and provided the diagnosis of T-cell lymphoma. The top graph depicts the patient's T-cell receptor PARR results; note the narrow, tall peak, which indicates a clonal expansion of the T-cell receptor. Compare the patient's results with the lower image from a reactive lymph node, which depicts a polyclonal T-cell receptor rearrangement. The x-axis indicates the size of the PCR product; y-axis indicates the level of fluorescence (an indication of the quantity of the PCR product). (PARR image courtesy Dr. Anne Avery.)

(Figures 9.44a–c; Fine & Tvedten, 1999; Allison *et al.*, 2008; Ameri *et al.*, 2010; Fischer *et al.*, 2012). As is typical of leukemia, a fairly monomorphic population of hematopoietic cells is observed. If immature forms (blasts) are present, an acute leukemia is diagnosed. Often, bizarre blast cells are present, which prevent determination of the cell line of origin based on Romanowsky stains alone and immunophenotyping is required. With chronic leukemia, a more mature population is present and the cell line of origin is more apparent.

MAST CELL TUMOR

Mast cells are present in low numbers in most hepatic aspirates and numbers can increase with inflammation and fibrosis; therefore, care should be used when diagnosing a hepatic mast cell tumor (Stockhaus *et al.*, 2004; Masserdotti, 2016). Mast cells are individualized round cells with distinct metachromatic purple granules, which commonly obscure nuclear morphology when stained with typical Romanowsky stains (Figures 9.16, 9.45a, b). They can occasionally appear agranular if granule content is washed away during processing. High numbers of mast cells, mast cells in clusters, or mast cells with variable granulation within the same sample have been criteria used to diagnose mast cell tumors (Stockhaus *et al.*, 2004). Most hepatic mast cell tumors are associated with disseminated disease; however, primary hepatic mast cell tumors have been diagnosed (Takahashi *et al.*, 2000).

HISTIOCYTIC SARCOMA

Histiocytic sarcoma has been described in the liver of dogs, most commonly as part of disseminated histiocytic sarcoma. However, histiocytic sarcoma rarely presents as a localized tumor found in the limbs or visceral organs, including the liver (Constantino-Casas *et al.*, 2011). The cells in histiocytic sarcoma have a marked amount of cellular atypia and mitotic activity (Figures 9.46a–d). Most cells have lightly to moderately basophilic and often faintly

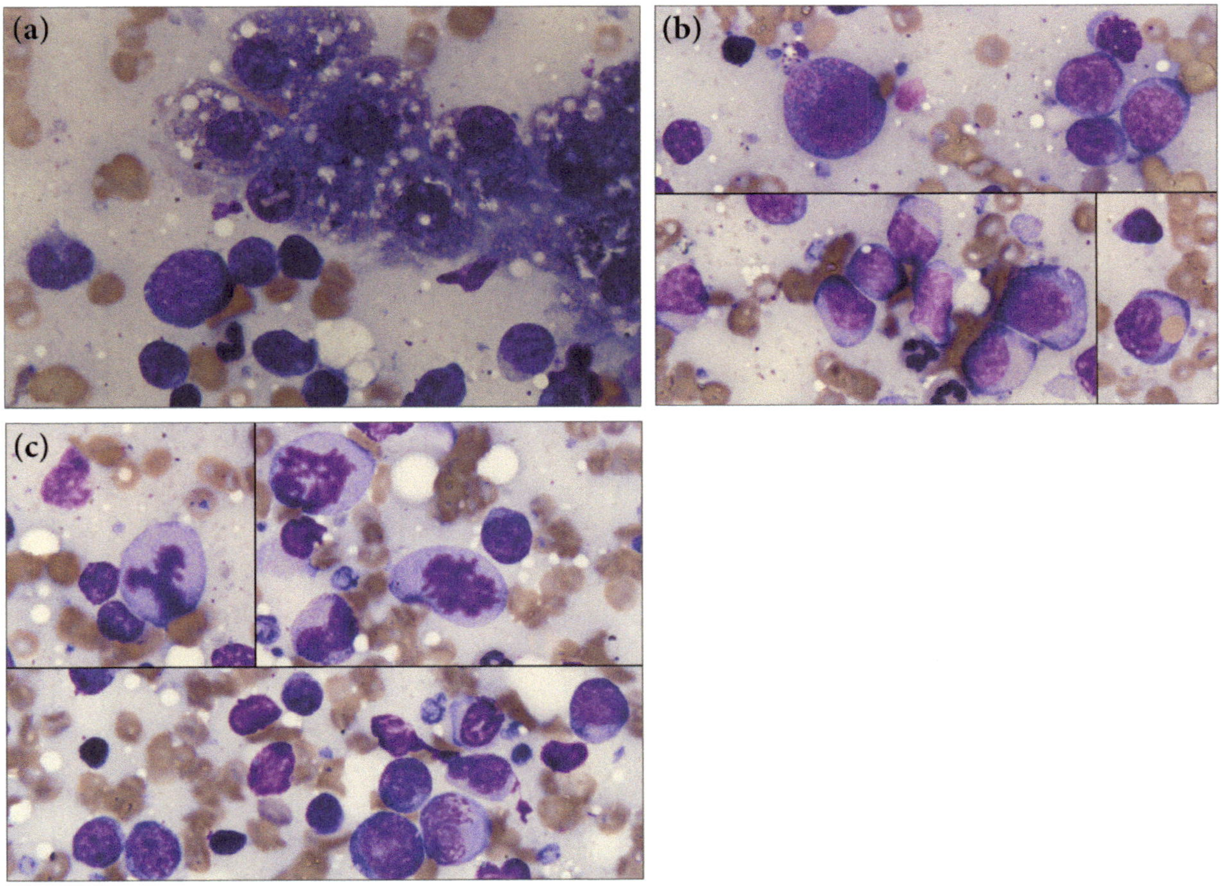

Figures 9.44a–c **Liver FNA from an 11-year-old Rottweiler. (a) Very few clusters of hepatocytes are present in this aspirate; however, there are many individualized round cells. (b) These cells have a minimal amount of deeply basophilic cytoplasm and single round nucleus, which occasionally is indented. Most cells have few to many pink to azurophilic granules. Note the erythrophagic cell in the lower right corner. (c) Mitotic figures are easily found. A bizarre mitotic figure is in the upper left corner. The large cell size, granulation, and nuclear morphology are consistent with a hematopoietic neoplasm and suggestive of a myeloid lineage; however, histopathology on the liver failed to confirm a neoplastic presence (Wright-Giemsa, 1,000× magnification).**

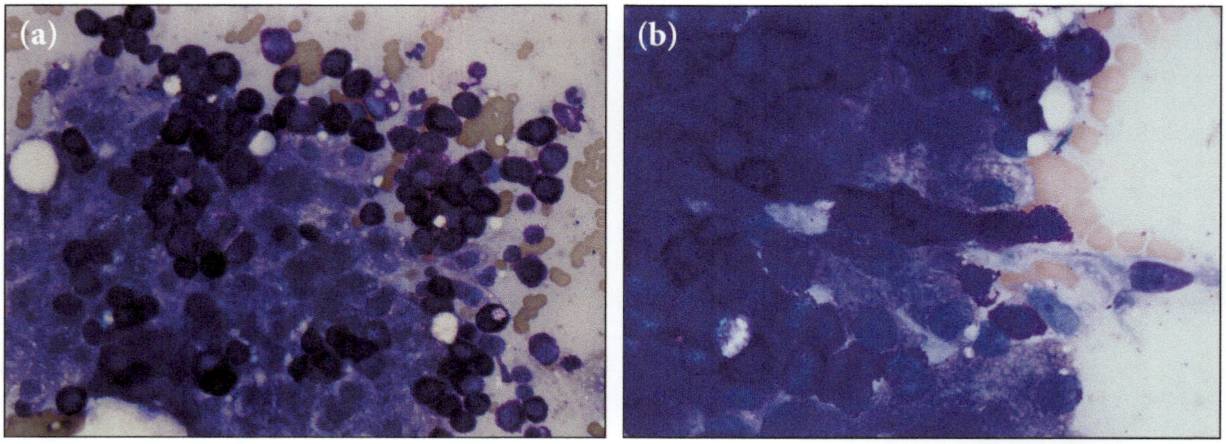

Figures 9.45a, b Liver aspirate from a domestic shorthair cat with mast cell tumors near the anus and within the spleen. (a) Copious mast cells are present throughout the entirety of this sample. Note the pleomorphism and aggregates of mast cells within the hepatic cluster (Wright–Giemsa, 500× magnification). (b) Large aggregates of mast cells with minimal atypia are wedged into the sinusoids between plates of hepatocytes (Wright–Giemsa, 1,000× magnification).

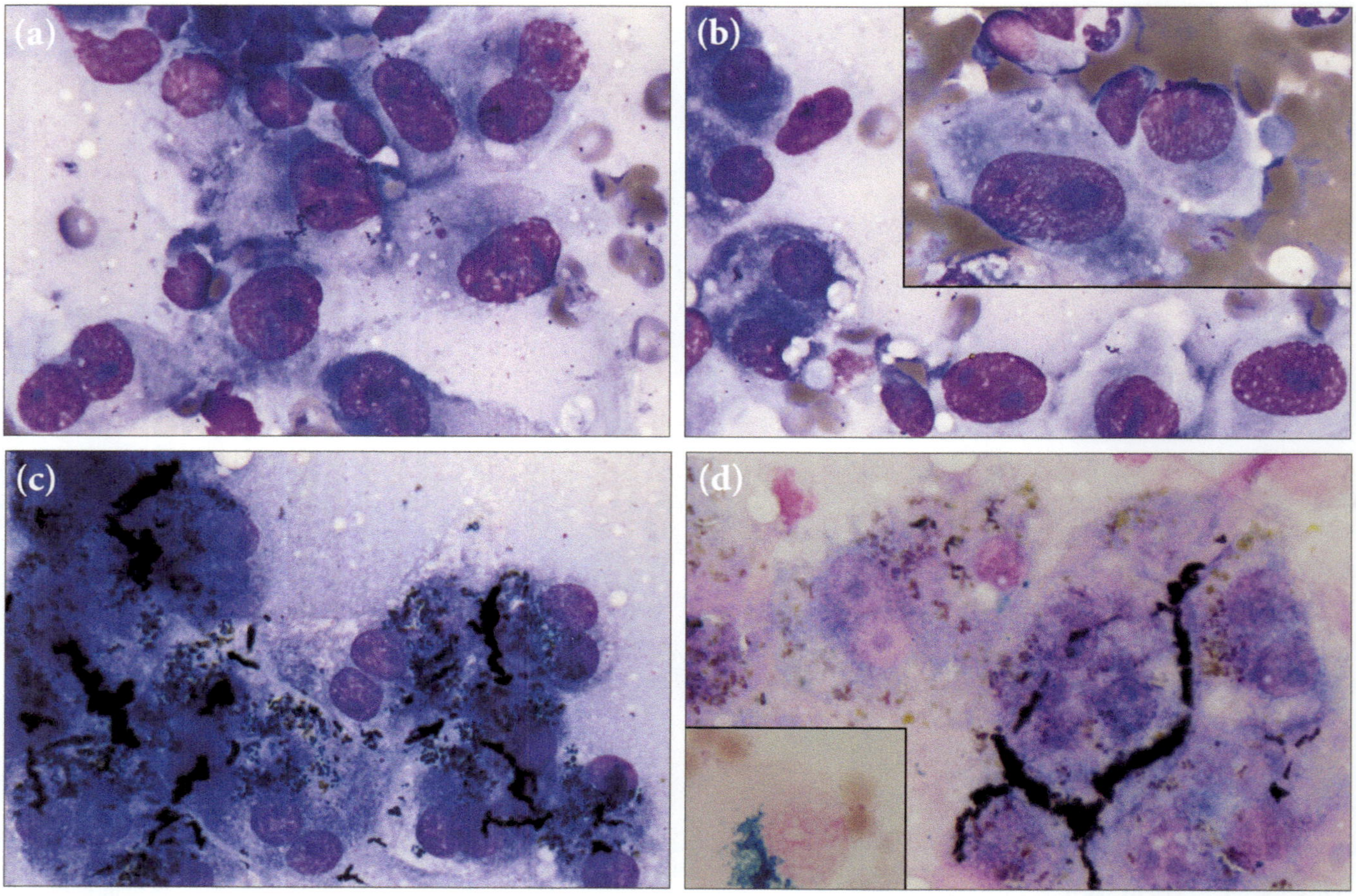

Figures 9.46a–d Histiocytic sarcoma in a Bernese Mountain Dog. (a, b) Many large spindloid to ovoid cells with multiple nucleoli, anisocytosis, and anisokaryosis are found. The overtly neoplastic mesenchymal cells and breed predilection suggest histiocytic sarcoma. (c) Hepatocytes in this sample had both coarse blue-black intracellular bile casts and cytoplasmic blue-green and pale brown granulation consistent with lipofuscin and bile. (d) Neither the blue-green material nor the brown pigment is positive for iron by the Prussian blue reaction. Inset image is from the control slide; note the blue-staining iron within this macrophage (a–c, Wright–Giemsa, 1,000× magnification; d, Prussian blue, 1,000× magnification).

granular cytoplasm, which contains fine to small punctate vacuoles. The nuclei are round to ovoid to reniform and indented with one to several prominent nucleoli. Marked variation in N:C ratio, anisocytosis, anisokaryosis, bi-, tri-, and multinucleated cells, and many exceptionally large cells are observed. Erythrophagia is another common feature; many patients with histiocytic sarcoma will present with a prominent anemia (Constantino-Casas *et al.*, 2011). Together, these criteria can give the suggestive diagnosis of histiocytic sarcoma; the addition of immunocytochemical staining has been used to confirm the diagnosis (Sapierzyński *et al.*, 2012). Histiocytic sarcoma is a malignant transformation of either dendritic cell lines (Langerhans or interstitial lineages) or macrophages. Therefore, histiocytic sarcoma should be positive for CD1, MHC-II, CD18, and vimentin; negative for CD3, CD79a, PAX5, CD20 and cytokeratin; and may display lineage-dependent markers such as CD11c, CD11d, or E-cadherin (Moore *et al.*, 2006; Constantino-Casas *et al.*, 2011; Moore, 2014).

Disseminated histiocytic sarcoma is found most commonly in Bernese Mountain Dogs, where it has a polygenic mode of inheritance. It is also common in Rottweiler and Retriever breeds and has been diagnosed in multiple other canine breeds (Padgett *et al.*, 1995; Abadie *et al.*, 2009). Flat-coated Retrievers have an increased predilection for the localized form of histiocytic sarcoma (Constantino-Casas *et al.*, 2011).

Histiocytic sarcoma is less commonly observed in cats. Both of the feline-specific histiocytic mass lesions, feline pulmonary Langerhans cell histiocytosis and feline progressive histiocytosis, have been reported to have hepatic involvement. There are very few published reports of these entities, making the description of their epidemiology, clinical progression, and morphologic characteristics uncertain; however, data suggest a poor long-term prognosis (Busch *et al.*, 2008; Moore, 2014).

PLASMACYTOMA/MULTIPLE MYELOMA

Neoplastic populations of plasma cells have been observed in the liver of both dogs and cats, either as a primary mass or as a metastatic lesion. Multiple myeloma and other myeloma-related disorders more in cats often involve the liver and spleen without bone marrow involvement (Mellor *et al.*, 2008). Cytologically, well-differentiated plasma cells have a moderate amount of basophilic to lightly basophilic cytoplasm, which frequently contains a paranuclear clearing and an eccentrically located nucleus with clumped to smooth chromatin (Figures 9.47a, b). Binucleation and atypia are common features of neoplastic plasma cells. Neoplastic plasma cell morphology can be highly atypical and not look like typical plasma cells, especially in aggressive tumors. (Mellor et al., 2008; Wachowiak *et al.*, 2022).

The distinction between solitary plasma cell tumor, multiple myeloma, and other myeloma-related disorders cannot be made solely by cytology; however, cytologic findings in conjunction with radiographic or advanced imaging, serum or urine protein electrophoresis, and immunofixation can provide enough evidence to reach an antemortem diagnosis.

Metastatic neoplasms

The liver is a highly vascularized organ, which receives the first pass at nutrients arriving from the gastrointestinal tract and is the source of much anabolic activity; therefore, it is the ideal metastasis site for

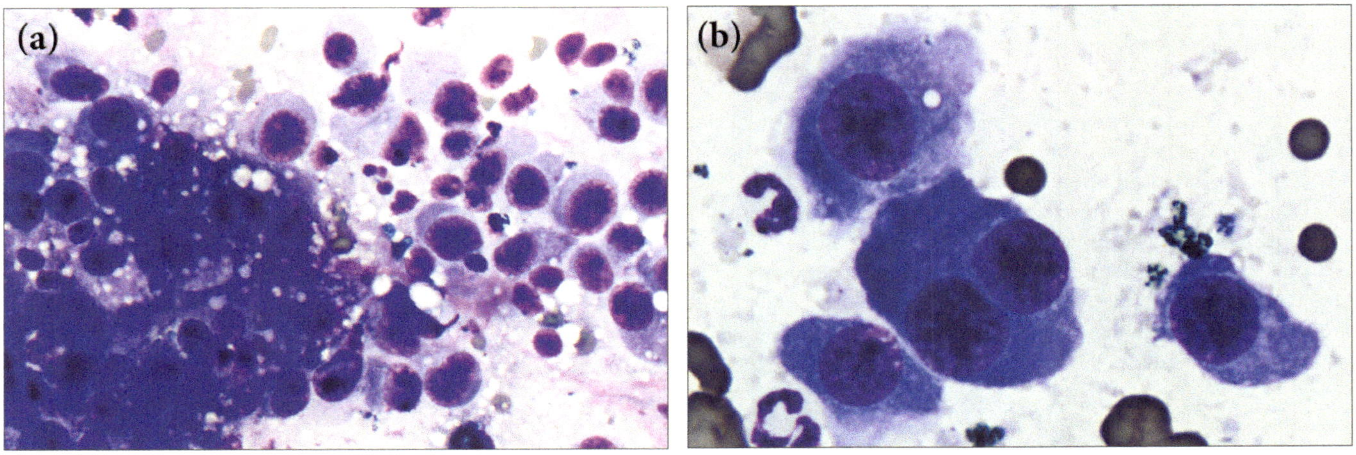

Figures 9.47a, b **(a) Large round cells with eccentric nuclei and smooth moderately basophilic cytoplasm are present within this feline hepatic aspirate. Note that many of the neoplastic cells are as large as, or larger than, surrounding hepatocytes and display marked anisocytosis and anisokaryosis (Diff-Quik®, 500× magnification). (b) Occasionally, the neoplastic cells are binucleate. Contrast the size of the neoplastic cells with the size of the neutrophils in the image (Diff-Quik®, 1,000× magnification). This cat had a plasma cell tumor.**

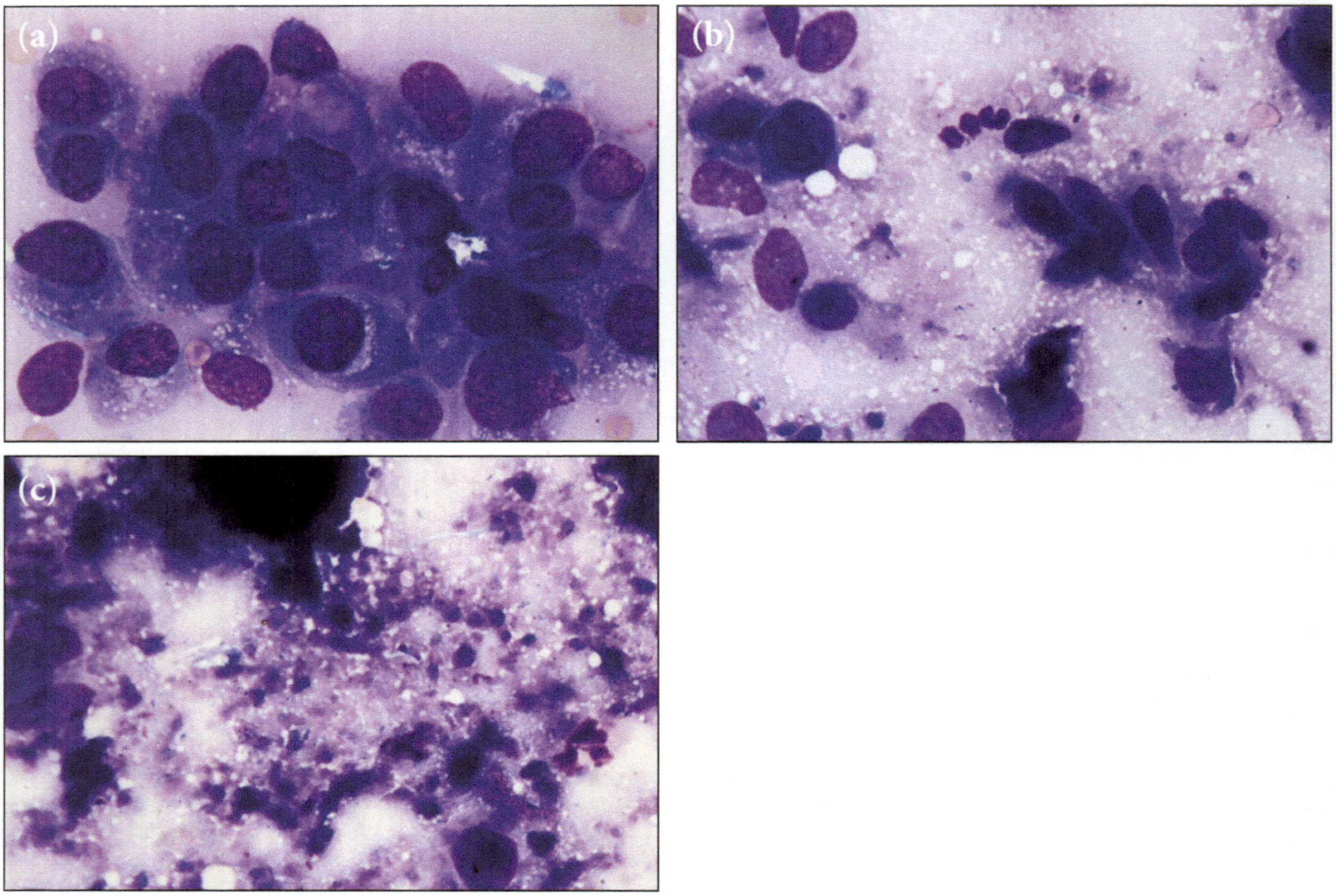

Figures 9.48a–c (a, b) Very few hepatocytes are found in this sample. Instead, abundant anaplastic neoplastic cells, which are found in both cohesive clusters and looser aggregates of spindloid cells, occasionally associated with pink extracellular material, are present. The conflicting cell morphologies prevent cytologic determination of tissue origin. If sufficient tissue architecture is present, the histogenesis of anaplastic tumors may be determined by biopsy and histopathology. (c) Several areas of blue–gray material, consistent with necrosis, are also present (Wright–Giemsa, 1,000× magnification).

many neoplasms. As a general rule, metastatic neoplasms can, but do not necessarily, retain some of the characteristic features of the tissue of origin. Often, close scrutiny will allow diagnosis of a specific metastatic tumor, sometimes diagnosis only to the cell line (epithelial versus mesenchymal) can be achieved, and other times the neoplasm is anaplastic enough that the only accurate cytologic diagnosis available is 'metastatic neoplasm' (Figures 9.48a–c). With the increased availability of immunodiagnostics, identification of specific cellular markers should be able to help differentiate more challenging tumors.

EPITHELIAL TUMORS

The presence of nonhepatocellular, distinctly malignant epithelial cells interspersed with normal hepatocytes is evidence of metastatic carcinoma or cholangiocellular carcinoma (Figures 9.6, 9.49a–c, 9.50a–c; Stockhaus *et al.*, 2004). The most common metastatic carcinomas in the liver include pancreatic, gastric/colonic, renal, mammary, ovarian, and squamous cell carcinomas (Trigo *et al.*, 1982; Stalker & Hayes, 2007a, b).

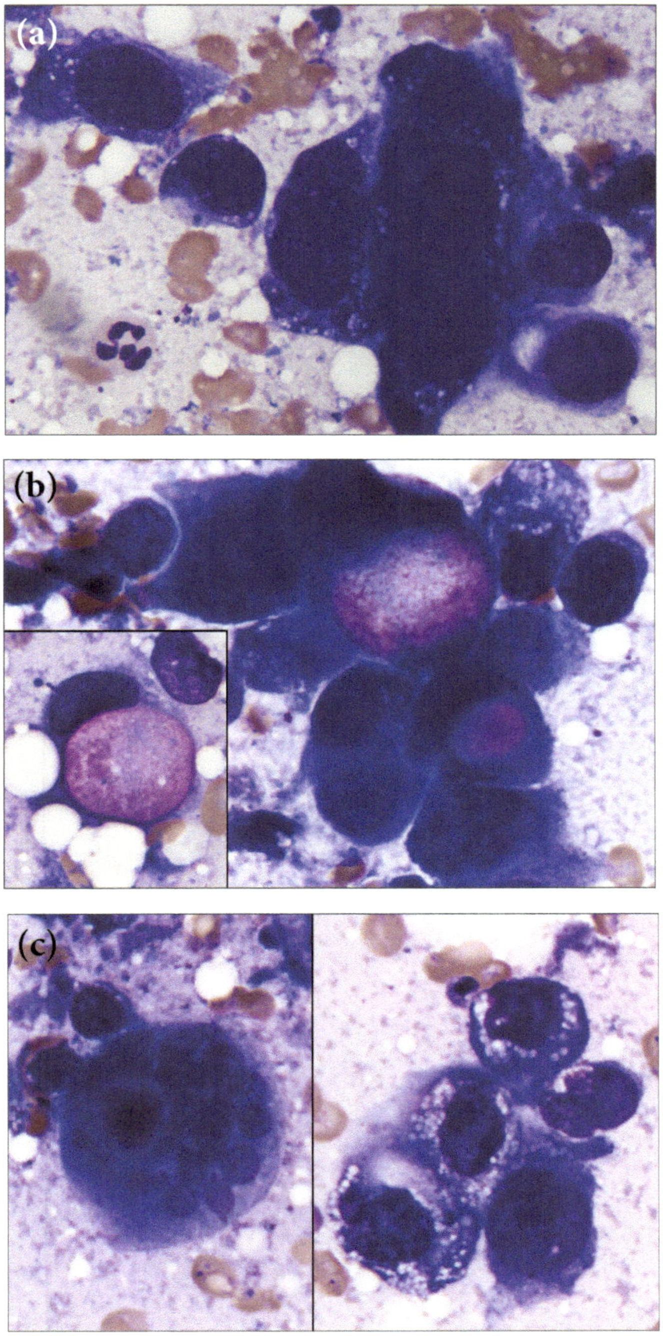

Figures 9.49a–c **Liver aspirate from a Beagle. (a) Prominent criteria of malignancy, including anisocytosis, anisokaryosis, a variable N:C ratio, and macro- and micronuclei, are noted. (b) Note the pink cytoplasmic vacuole, which displaces the nucleus, producing a signet ring appearance, in several cells in this image. The inset shows a single intact signet ring cell with a pink cytoplasmic vacuole and ovoid nucleus. Cell-free lipid is also noted as discrete clear spaces in the background outside of the cell. (c) Perinuclear clear vacuolation and micronuclei are present. Similar cells were noted in the sublumbar lymph node of this patient and were interpreted as transitional cell carcinoma or, less likely, squamous cell carcinoma (Wright–Giemsa, 1,000× magnification).**

MESENCHYMAL TUMORS

The most commonly reported metastatic mesenchymal tumors include hemangiosarcoma, fibrosarcoma, melanosarcoma, osteosarcoma, and leiomyosarcoma (Figures 9.51a–c; Trigo *et al.*, 1982; Stalker & Hayes, 2007a, b). Of significant challenge is the fact that, with the exception of melanosarcoma, these tumors can also be primary hepatic mesenchymal tumors.

NAKED NUCLEI TUMORS

Insulinoma, gastrinoma, pheochromocytoma, thyroid carcinoma, and intestinal carcinoid are among the most common neuroendocrine tumors identified in the liver of dogs and cats (Stalker & Hayes, 2007a, b). These tumors typically appear as intact nuclei within cytoplasm, which only very rarely displays cytoplasmic borders (Figures 9.52a, b). This minimal number of tissue-specific cytologic criteria, in conjunction with the unavailability or inconsistent expression of immunological identifiable markers, can make differentiation of these tumors quite challenging.

SUMMARY

Particularly challenging is the presence of neoplastic cell lines, which can be primary in the liver and other locations; this situation is commonly encountered with the mesenchymal tumors listed above or the neuroendocrine tumor, carcinoid. In all cytology cases it is wise to correlate all diagnostic data, including results from physical examination, history, imaging, and clinicopathologic and histologic evaluations, to provide the most accurate diagnosis.

EVALUATION OF GALLBLADDER FLUID

Cholecystocentesis (aspiration of gallbladder content) can be performed to obtain samples for culture and cytology. Samples can be collected laparoscopically, but ultrasound guided percutaneous sampling from right-sided transhepatic or right-ventral abdominal approaches have been reported and can be performed with sedation or light anesthesia (Peters *et al.*, 2016; Webb, 2020). Retrospective review suggests infrequent self-limiting gallbladder leakage or pericystic fluid accumulation as the most common complications and that these typically have minimal distinct clinical effect, but there are infrequent reports of more significant issues such as gallbladder rupture (Peters *et al.*, 2016; Webb, 2020). It is likely that a perceived increased risk of complication prevented sampling in the more severely affected cases during the retrospective period.

Grossly, bile fluid is opaque green-brown and variably viscous or mucoid. While bile fluid should not clot, collection into EDTA has been reported and may be appropriate if there is concern for hemorrhage. Bile fluid is harsh on cellular components; rapid preparation of slides is appropriate. Cytologic preparations can be Romanowski

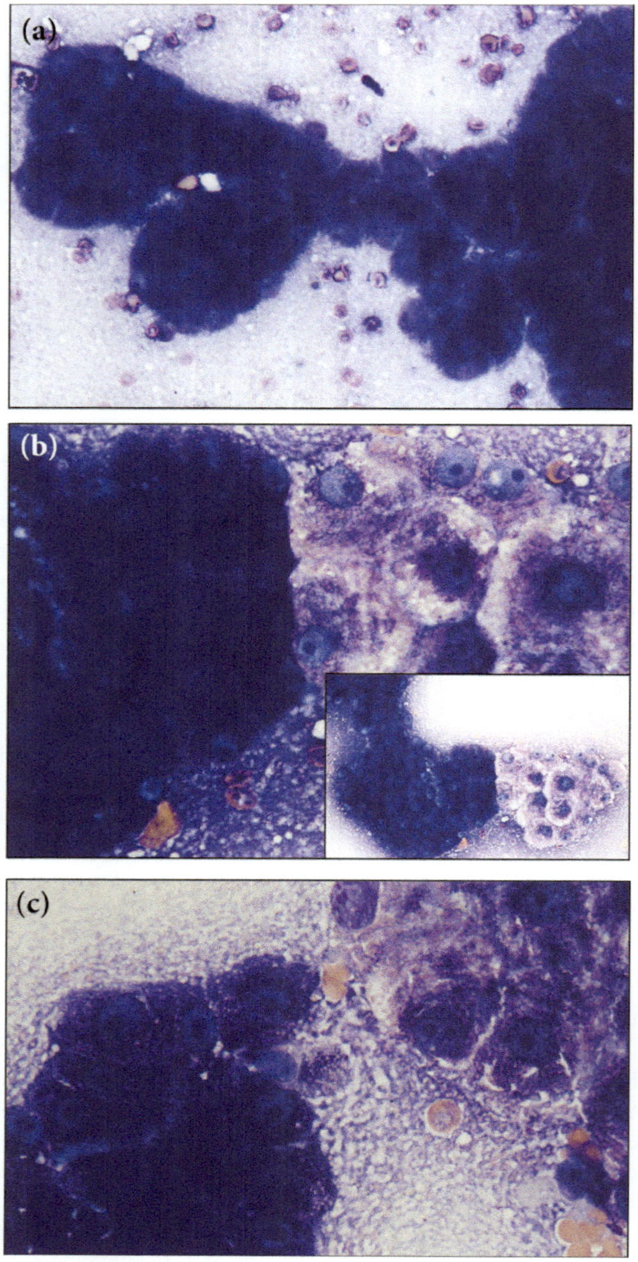

Figures 9.50a–c Canine hepatic aspirate. (a) Many distinct papillary structures are found (Wright–Giemsa, 1,000× magnification). (b) These neoplastic cells (left side of image) strikingly contrast with hepatocytes observed on the right side of the image. The hepatocytes often have cytoplasmic rarefaction consistent with glycogen or hydropic degeneration (main image, Wright–Giemsa, 1,000× magnification; inset, Wright–Giemsa, 500× magnification). (c) Where a thin enough layer of cells is present, the neoplastic cells (left side of image) have deeply basophilic cytoplasm with fine pink granules, prominent cell–cell junctions, cell crowding, multiple nucleoli, and mild anisocytosis and anisokaryosis. In combination, these findings suggest carcinoma. The background is blue-gray flecked with pink granules, similar to the cytoplasm of the neoplastic cells; this feature indicates either necrosis or fragile cells that ruptured during sample preparation. The cells in the upper right are hepatocytes (Wright–Giemsa, 1,000× magnification).

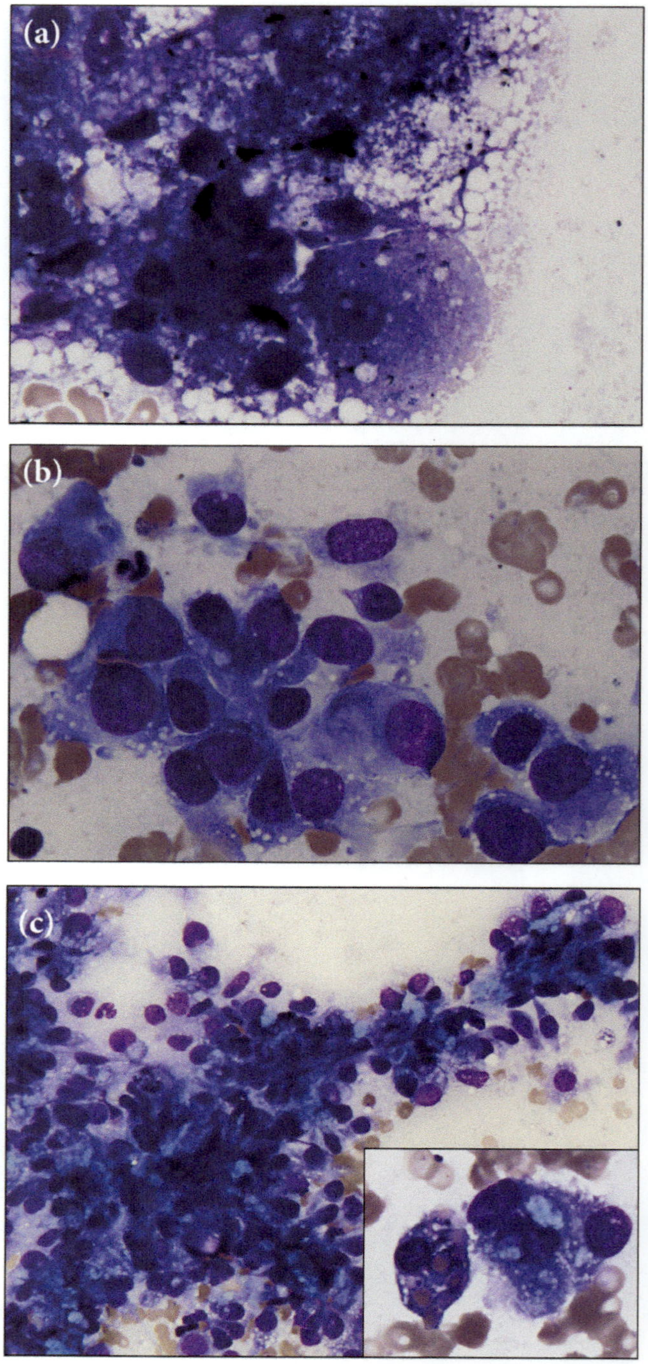

Figures 9.51a–c (a) Most hepatocytes are in poor cytologic condition in this sample. Where visible, there is distinct clear vacuolation consistent with lipid accumulation. (b) Note the spindloid nature of the cells, a cell shape seen with mesenchymal cells, while the pleomorphism suggests a neoplastic process. (c) There are also many pleomorphic mesenchymal cells with erythrophagia, or pale blue cytoplasmic material of unknown significance (a and b, Wright–Giemsa, 1,000× magnification; c, Wright–Giemsa, 500× magnification; inset, Wright–Giemsa, 1,000× magnification).

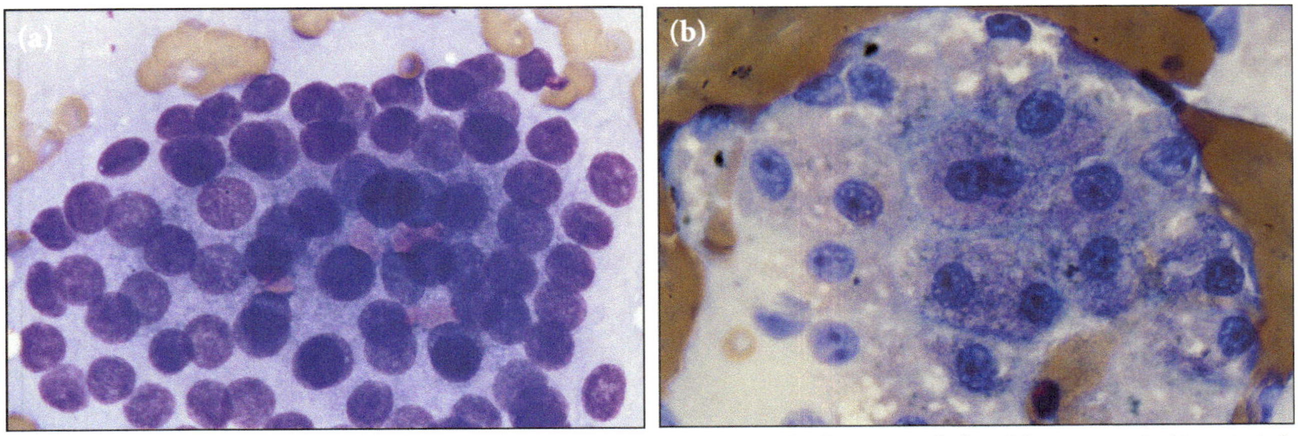

Figures 9.52a, b **Large aggregates of intact nuclei in a pool of cytoplasm without distinct borders give a naked-nuclei appearance in this aspirate from a dog. (a) This slide contains essentially only neoplastic cells. (b) A second slide contains clusters of intact hepatocytes and few neoplastic cells to help confirm that the nodule is associated with the liver. Note that several of the hepatocytes in the center of the image are binucleate. Naked nuclei tumors are most commonly of neuroendocrine histogenesis. Distinguishing the tissue of origin of naked nuclei tumors is usually not possible by cytology alone; the combination of history, clinical signs, and special stains is usually needed (Wright–Giemsa, 1,000× magnification).**

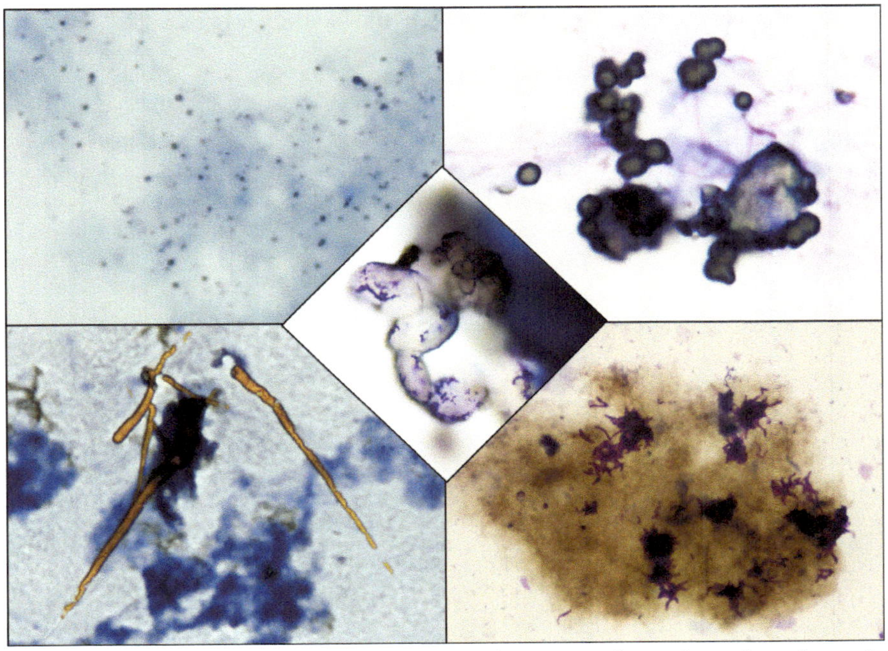

Figure 9.53 **Composite of non-cellular material encountered in bile fluid from dogs. Various forms of granular and crystal material can be found in bile fluid, including blue-black granular material (upper left), brown-green globular crystals (upper right), and orange lanceolate bile crystals (lower left), amorphous granular material (lower right) and nonstaining hemp-seed shaped crystals (center). Also note the pale basophilic mucoid material (Wright–Giemsa, 1,000× magnification).**

stained direct smears, but concentrated or cytocentrifuged preparations make evaluation of cellularity easier.

Romanowsky-stained cytologic samples of bile fluid typically have a green, blue, or gray background with variable amounts of pale basophilic mucoid material. Crystals can be found, including formed bile crystals and amorphous crystalline material (Figure 9.53).

Most often, the samples are essentially acellular. When cells are found, they often appear poorly preserved and raise concern that the cytologic preparation may not fully represent the in-vivo environment (Figure 9.54). Collection-associated peripheral blood elements can be present. Noninflammatory cellularity is most often cuboidal to columnar biliary epithelial cells and mesothelial cells but spindled mesenchymal cells and concurrently aspirated hepatocytes can be present (Figure 9.55). In a study of gallbladder cystocentesis samples from 140 dogs and cats, 70% of the cases lacked atypical

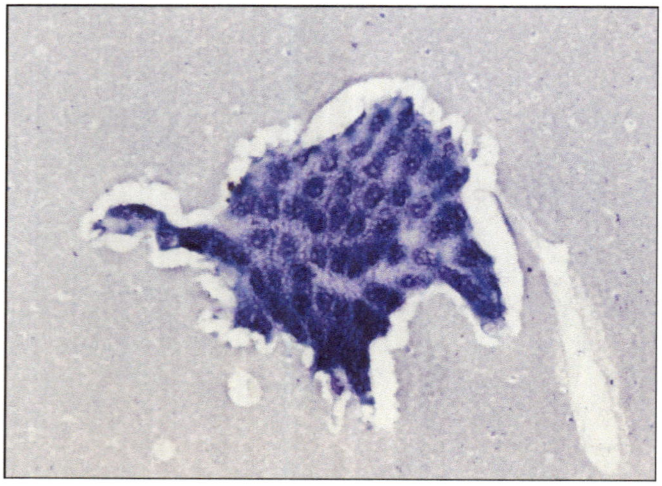

Figure 9.54 **Gallbladder aspirate from a 16-year-old castrated male domestic medium haired cat. A sheet of poorly preserved cells is present which may have been biliary epithelium.**

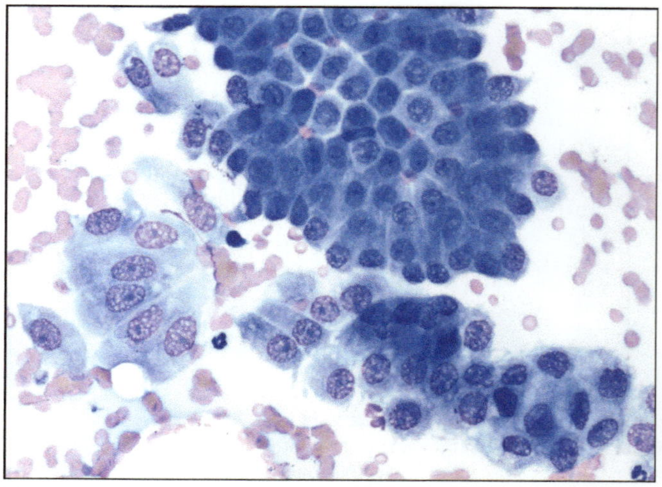

Figure 9.55 **Gallbladder aspirate from a 14-year-old castrated male Siamese cat. The sample had more red blood cells and peripheral blood elements than typically encountered in bile fluid. contained sheets of fairly unremarkable cuboidal epithelial cells and fewer columnar epithelial cells (Wright–Giemsa, 1,000× magnification).**

findings. These often receive the ontologically redundant diagnosis of bile.

When concurrent inflammation and intracellular bacteria are present, a pathologic process is easily diagnosed (Figure 9.56). When one is found without the other, interpretation is more challenging. Suppurative inflammation appears to be the most common type of inflammation but lymphoplasmacytic, eosinophilic, and other forms of inflammation can also be found (Verwey *et al.*, 2021; Peters *et al.*, 2016). Inflammation can be caused by bacteria, protozoa (*Isospora* spp., *Toxoplasma* spp., etc., Figure 9.57), liver flukes (*Platynosomum* spp.), cellular damage, and neoplasia (Palić *et al.*, 2017; Köster *et al.*, 2016).

The presence of bacteria in bile fluid is called bactibilia. Rod, cocci, and filamentous rod forms can be found on cytology (Figure 9.58). Detection of bactibilia by cytology and culture is not always correlated, and samples with both cytologic and culture confirmed bactibilia will not always have cytologic or histologic evidence of inflammation. One study found that biochemical evidence of hepatic disease or histologically confirmed cholecystitis was diagnosed at a similar frequency in apparently healthy dogs with and without bactibilia diagnosed from a bile fluid sample. This may be because enteric bacteria can transiently be present in bile fluid; advanced detection of bactibilia from healthy dogs commonly found enteric bacteria but a consistent bacterial isolate was not present between patients (Gookin *et al.*, 2023). This same study more commonly identified bacteria in the gallbladder mucus from

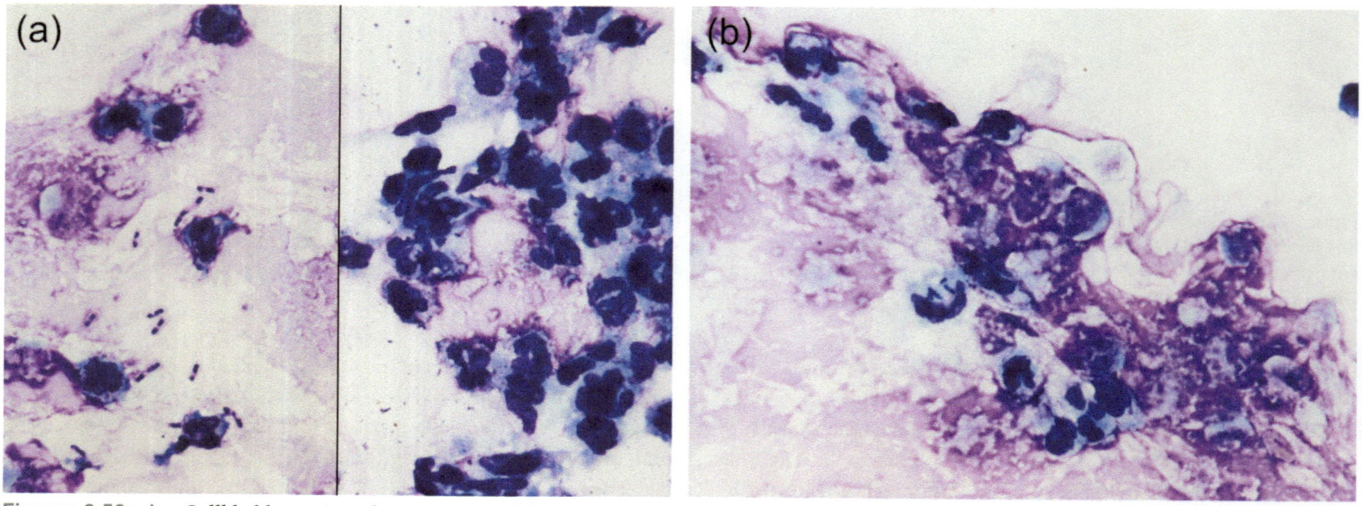

Figures 9.56a, b **Gallbladder aspirate from a 16-year-old domestic long-haired cat. (a) Many of the cells in the sample are in poor condition, but neutrophils and rod-shaped bacteria are present. (b) Rarely, phagocytized bacteria are found, helping to diagnose a septic suppurative inflammation.**

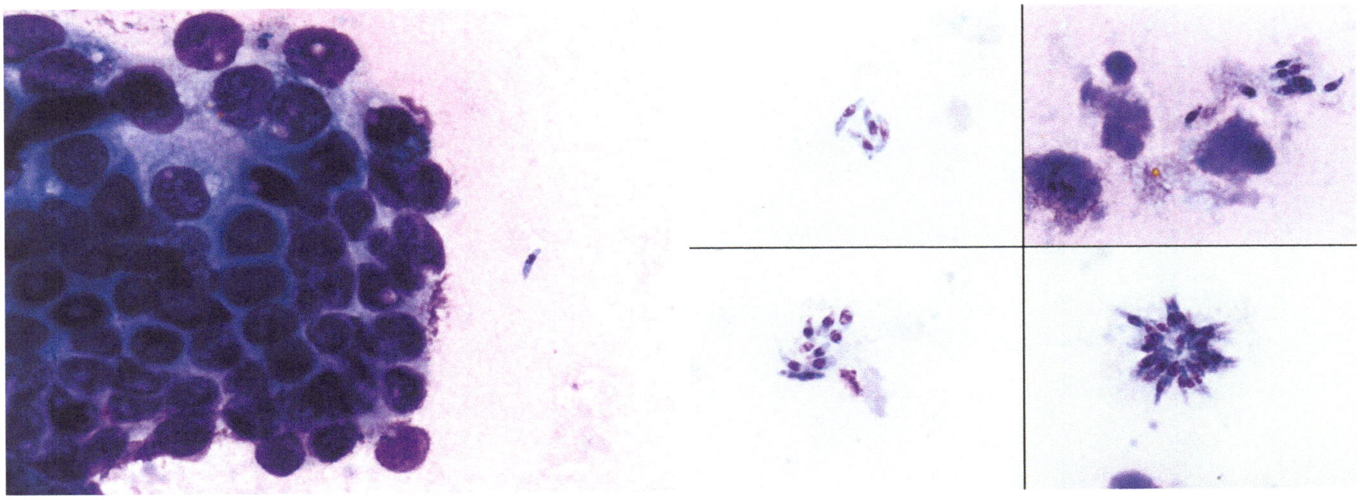

Figure 9.57 **Bile fluid aspirate from an immunosuppressed 8-year-old male intact Cocker Spaniel. Extracellular 4–5 um in length apicomplexan zoites are found. These were identified by PCR as *Hammondia* spp. (modified Wright, 1,000× magnification, images courtesy of Dr. Nora Springer).**

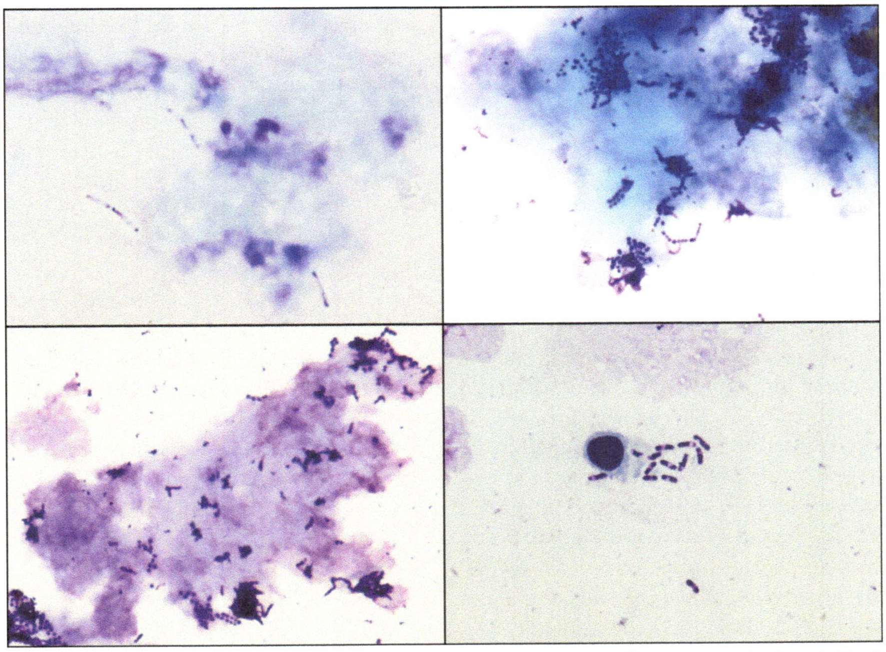

Figure 9.58 **The presence of bacteria in bile fluid is called bactibilia. Long rod, cocci, and mixed bacteria can be found. Finding bacteria alone is of unknown significance.**

dogs with a mucocele than healthy dogs but could not distinguish if the bacteria contributed to the mucocele or was a sequalae of biliary obstruction. Although the clinical significance of bactibilia without a clear inflammatory process is uncertain, some authors have argued that bactibilia is an indication for antimicrobial therapy (Palić *et al.*, 2017).

Neoplasia of the biliary tree can be diagnosed by cholecystocentesis, but the diagnostic sensitivity has not been defined in dogs and cats.

CASES

CASE 1

Signalment/history

Seven-year-old, spayed female domestic shorthair barn cat. The patient presented 2 weeks ago for significant weight loss (>50% reduction over 1 year). The owners reported normal appetite and no vomiting.

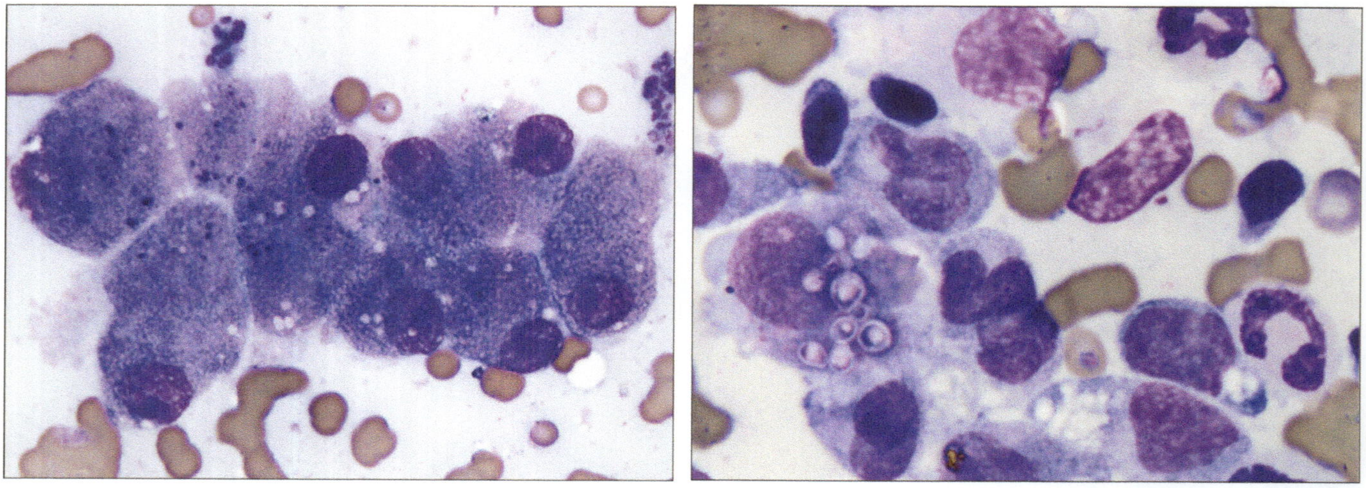

Figures 9.59 **Feline hepatic aspirate (Wright–Giemsa, 1,000× magnification).**

Diagnostics

A CBC revealed a moderate to marked normocytic normochromic anemia (Hct = 15% [0.15 l/l]; reference interval [RI] = 25–45 [0.25–0.45]), thrombocytopenia (platelets = 31 × 10^6/µl [RI = 200–500]), and normal white blood cell counts with minimal toxicity noted. A biochemistry profile showed hyperproteinemia (8.3 g/dl [83 g/l]; RI = 6.0–8.0 [60–80]), hyperglobulinemia (6.3 g/dl [63 g/l]; RI = 2.8–4.8 [28–48]), and hypoalbuminemia (2.0 g/dl [20 g/l]; RI = 2.3–2.5 [23–25]). The patient was FIV/FeLV negative and an fPLI SNAP® test was normal.

Treatment

No significant changes were reported after a 1-week course of doxycycline; however, the patient was noted to be dehydrated and had lost more weight, so was hospitalized for supportive care and additional diagnostics. Repeat blood work showed an unchanged anemia (Hct = 15% [0.15 l/l]) and mild icterus (serum bilirubin = 0.6 mg/dl [10.26 µmol/l] [RI = 0–0.3, 0–5.13]). Reticulocyte count failed to show evidence of regeneration. *Mycoplasma* PCR was negative. Abdominal radiographs were obtained and revealed decreased serosal detail; therefore an abdominal ultrasound was performed. The liver was diffusely enlarged and slightly hyperechoic, and a minimal amount of sludge was noted in the common bile duct. There was also mild splenomegaly, the duodenal and jejunal walls were slightly thickened with altered echogenicity, and a scant amount of free peritoneal fluid was noted. Aspirates of the liver, spleen, and abdominal fluid were submitted to a reference laboratory; images from the liver aspirate are shown (Figures 9.59a, b).

Cytologic description

Clusters of cohesive hepatocytes are present. These polygonal cells have an abundant amount of basophilic to pink granular cytoplasm, a single round nucleus with finely stippled chromatin, and a single prominent nucleolus. Macrophages, neutrophils, and lymphocytes are present. A macrophage contains phagocytized yeast, which are round to oval, 2–4 µm in diameter, with a thin clear capsule, narrow-based budding, and a purple crescent-shape along one end representing nuclear material. A small orange crystal is noted at the bottom center of Figure 9.59b and is consistent with hematoidin.

Cytologic interpretation

Pyogranulomatous hepatitis with *Histoplasma capsulatum.*

Outcome

The spleen had similar findings. The fluid sample was of low cellularity. The patient was started on itraconazole (10 mg/ml) and over the next week showed appropriate clinical and biochemical improvement (Hct increased to 20% [0.2 l/l], biochemical icterus resolved). The patient was discharged with instructions to follow a 4–6-month course of itraconazole and was lost to follow-up.

CASE 2

Signalment/history

Nine-year-old, spayed female Golden Retriever. The patient had a 7 cm diameter, grade II peripheral nerve sheath tumor removed from the dorsal intrascapular area 9 months ago. Adequate margins could not be confirmed and the patient was started on metronomic chemotherapy consisting of cyclophosphamide and piroxicam. The patient also suffered from arthritis, for which she was receiving carprofen. She had a history of mildly increased liver enzyme activity. She re-presented to her primary care veterinarian for vomiting and lethargy. In-house blood work revealed marked elevation of ALT, a mild anemia, and neutrophilia (Table 9.2, day 0). The chemotherapy was discontinued and antibiotic and hepatoprotectant therapies

Table 9.2 **Select values from serial evaluation of a 9-year-old, spayed female Golden Retriever dog. Results are reported as value (reference interval*). Values outside the reference interval are in bold**

	Day 0	Day 4	Day 12	Day 18	Day 47	Units
ALP	**141** (0–140)	**164** (0–140)	**156** (0–140)	**133** (7–92)	**152** (7–92)	U/l
cALP				**71** (0–40)	**101** (0–140)	U/l
ALT	**2,332** (0–120)	**906** (0–120)	**637** (0–120)	**203** (8–65)	**137** (8–65)	U/l
GGT	<10 (0–14)	<10 (0–14)	<10 (0–14)	3 (0–7)	3 (0–7)	U/l
Total bilirubin	0.1 (0–0.5)	0.1 (0–0.5)	0.1 (0–0.5)	0.2 (0.1–0.3)	0.2 (0.1–0.3)	mg/dl
RBCs	**5.04** (5.5–8.5)	6.2 (5.5–8.5)	5.77 (5.5–8.5)	5.71 (5.5–8.5)		$\times 10^6/\mu l$
Hct	33.6 (37–55)	41.5 (37–55)	38.2 (37–55)	42.2 (37–55)		%
WBCs	16.8 (6–17)	12.9 (6–17)	11.3 (6–17)	11.6 (6–17)		$\times 10^3/\mu l$
Neutrophils	**15.152** (3.0–11.5)			9.93 (3.0–11.5)		$\times 10^3/\mu l$
Band neutrophils	**0.168** (0–0.1)			0 (0–0.1)		×103/µl
Lymphocytes	0.504 (1.0–4.8)			1.08 (1.0–4.8)		×103/µl
Monocytes	0.84 (0.2–1.4)			0.559 (0.2–1.4)		×103/µl
Eosinophils	0.168 (0.1–1.0)			**0.023 (0.1–1.0)**		×103/µl
Basophils	0 (0–2)			0.048 (0–2)		×103/µl

*The analyses on days 0, 4, and 12 were performed on different analyzers from those used on days 18 and 47; therefore, there were differences in methodologies and different reference intervals are reported.

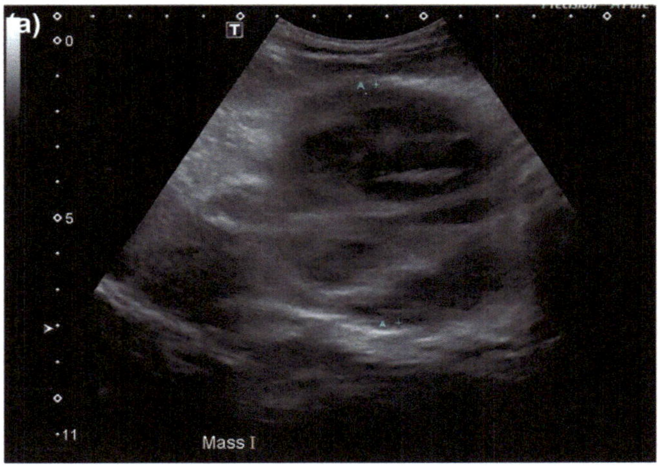

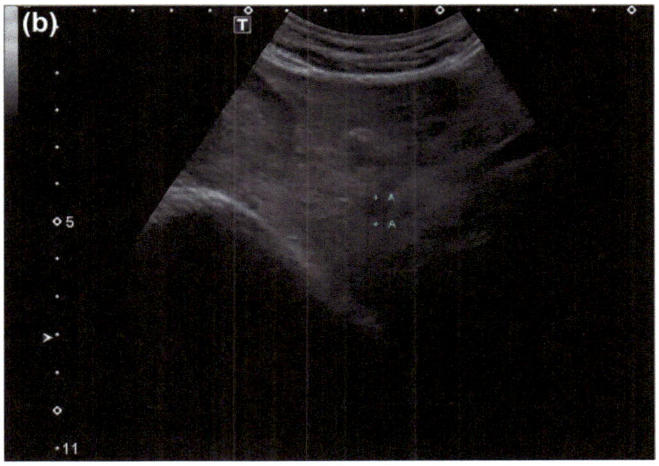

Figures 9.60a, b **Ultrasound images of abdominal masses present in a 9-year-old, spayed female Golden Retriever dog. (a) A 7.6 cm mass effect was noted in the cranial abdomen. It was challenging to determine if the mass effect was associated with the liver, spleen, or independent of these organs. (b) The liver was diffusely enlarged, and multiple small masses, some measuring up to 3.6 cm, were observed. (Courtesy Dr. Elizabeth Peters.)**

(amoxicillin/clavulanic acid and Denamarin) were started. The clinical signs quickly resolved. Over the next 3 weeks the leukocytosis, anemia, and ALT values continued to decrease while concordant mild increases in ALP were noted (Table 9.2, days 0–18).

An abdominal ultrasound was performed on day 18, which revealed an approximately 3 cm hypoechoic mass and multiple smaller hypoechoic masses in the liver and a 7 cm hyperechoic mass in the mid-abdomen, likely associated with the liver (Figures 9.60a, b). Ultrasound-guided aspirates of the liver mass and normal liver were acquired. Representative images from the liver mass cytology are shown (Figures 9.61a–c). The biochemical data are listed in Table 9.2.

Cytologic description

There are large cohesive clusters of hepatocytes present, which have an abundant amount of basophilic to pink granular cytoplasm, a centrally located round nucleus with finely stippled chromatin, and a single prominent nucleolus. These cells have a marked degree of anisocytosis, anisokaryosis, variable N:C ratio, frequent trinucleation, nuclear

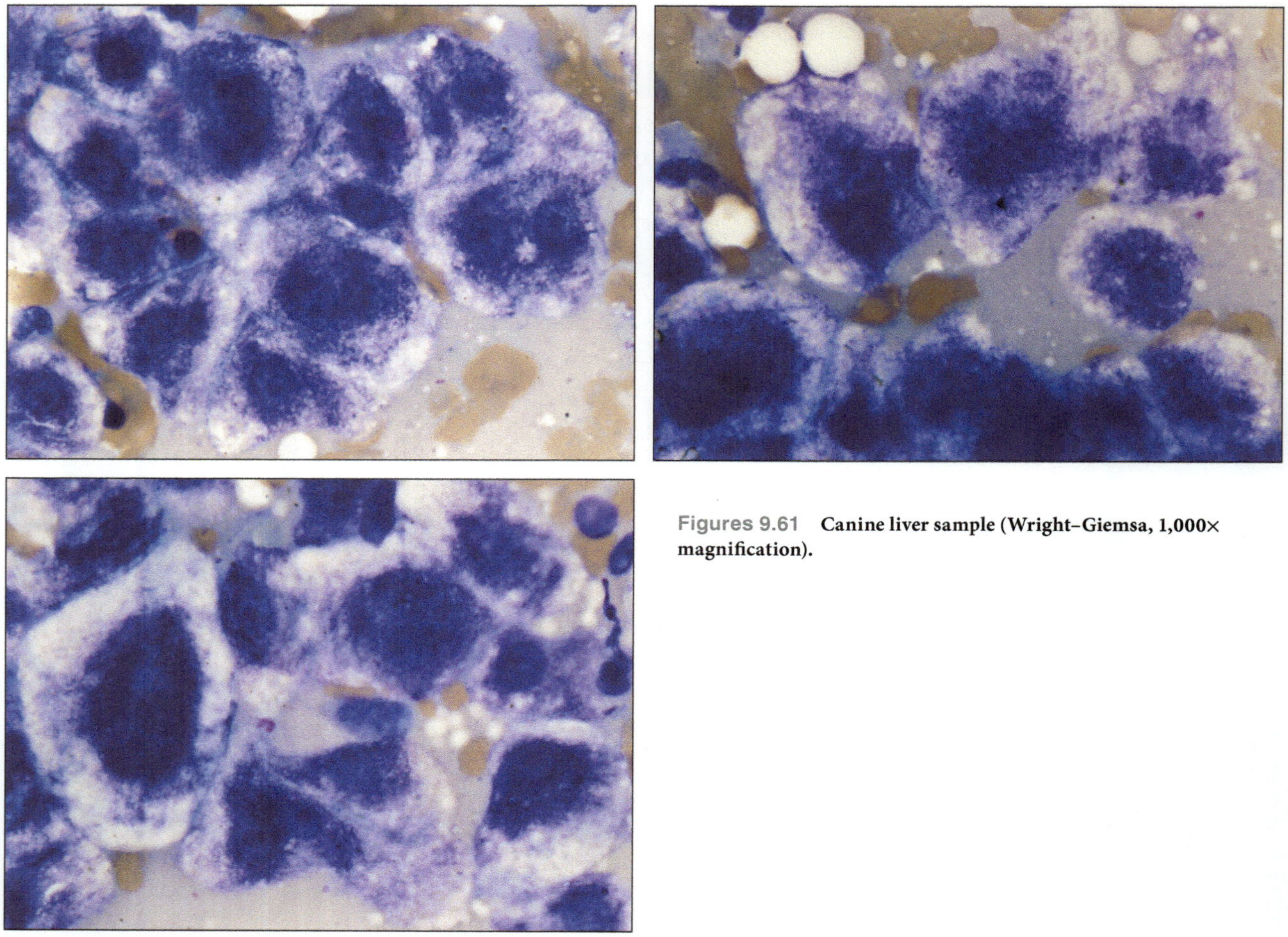

Figures 9.61 **Canine liver sample (Wright–Giemsa, 1,000× magnification).**

molding, and multiple nucleoli. These cells frequently have moderate to abundant amounts of clear foamy cytoplasmic rarefaction, consistent with glycogen or hydropic degeneration. The background consists of minimal cellular debris in a moderately proteinaceous fluid.

Cytologic interpretation

Likely regenerative nodule; rule out hepatocellular carcinoma.

Outcome

A follow-up on day 47 revealed that the biochemistry profile continued to improve but the mass was increasing in size on ultrasound. A surgical biopsy was elected.

Histology (Figure 9.62) revealed multifocal, 3 cm nodules composed of smaller nodules. The smaller nodules demonstrated a fibrous connective tissue capsule and bridging between portal triads (bridging fibrosis), atrophied hepatocytes, and serpiginous biliary ducts (biliary hyperplasia). Enlarged hepatic lobules lacked a central vein and had disorganized hepatic cords present, which were compressing adjacent parenchyma (hyperplastic nodule). Concurrently, these findings indicate hepatic cirrhosis (fibrosis and regeneration) and suggest massive hepatic necrosis. The FNA sample demonstrates the marked dysplasia that can occur with a strong regenerative effort.

CASE 3

Signalment/history

Eleven-year-old, neutered male mixed-breed dog. The patient presented with a 3-week history of sudden onset seizure activity, which was refractory to medical management.

Physical examination

At presentation the dog appeared sedated to mentally inappropriate. Examination revealed hyperthermia (102.9°F [39.4°C]), mild tachycardia (108–140 bpm), and hypertension (systolic, 140–180 mmHg). On a hand-held and bench-top glucometer, the patient was hypoglycemic, and continued to be hypoglycemic (<10–59 mg/dl [0.6–3.37

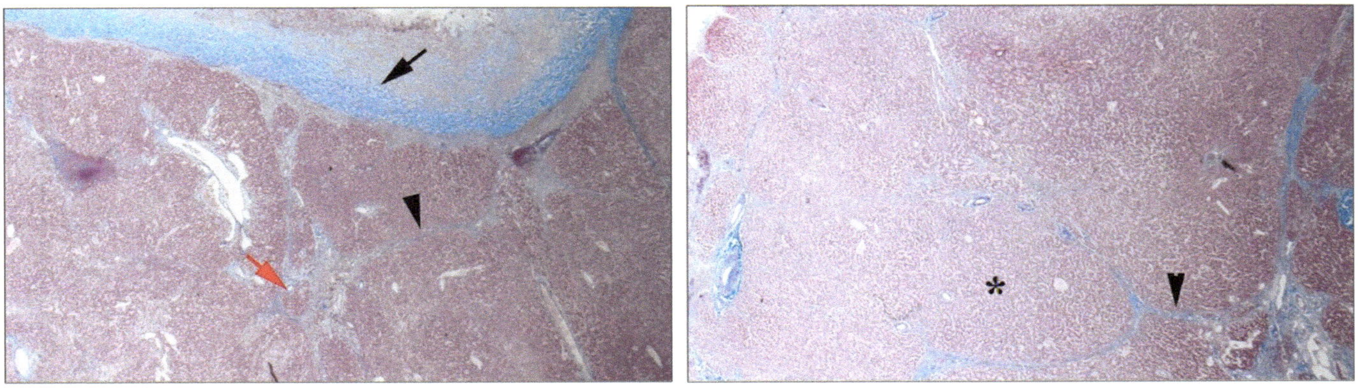

Figure 9.62 **Liver mass, histologic sections. Black arrow indicates thickened capsule. Black arrowhead indicates bridging fibrosis. Red arrow indicates lobular compression and atrophy. Asterisk indicates regenerative nodule (Mason-trichrome, 50× magnification). (Courtesy Dr. Arnon Gal.)**

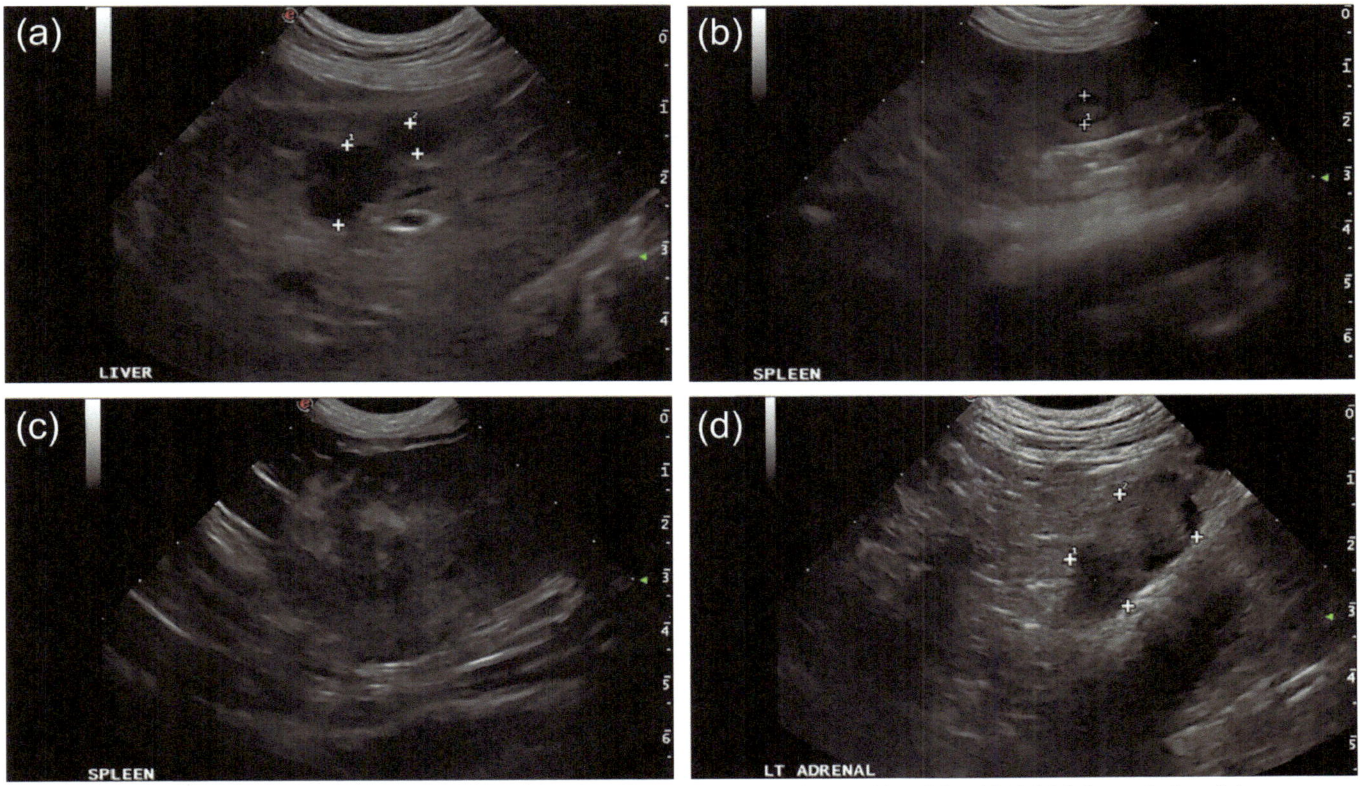

Figures 9.63a–d **Images from an abdominal ultrasound of an 11-year-old, neutered male mixed breed dog. (a) Multiple hypoechoic nodules were present in the liver, measuring between 0.44 and 1.14 cm. (b) Nodules were also present in the spleen, measuring 0.54 cm. (c) An ill-defined hypoechoic area was noted in the head of the spleen. (d) The adrenal gland was enlarged, measuring 1.25 cm at the caudal pole and 1.1 cm at the cranial pole. (Courtesy Dr. Elizabeth Peters.)**

mmol/l]) despite administration of 5% dextrose IV until a glucagon infusion was instituted. The hypertension persisted after resolution of the hypoglycemia.

An abdominal ultrasound was performed and revealed multiple hypoechoic, 0.6–1.1 cm nodules throughout the liver and spleen (Figures 9.63a, b) and an ill-defined hyperechoic area at the head of the spleen (Figure 9.63c). Additionally, the left adrenal gland was enlarged (1.25 cm caudal pole, 1.1 cm cranial pole [Figure 9.63d]; right adrenal gland: 6.9 mm caudal pole, 8.6 mm cranial pole). Ultrasound-guided FNAs of the liver and spleen were collected. Images from the liver aspirate are shown (Figures 9.64a–d).

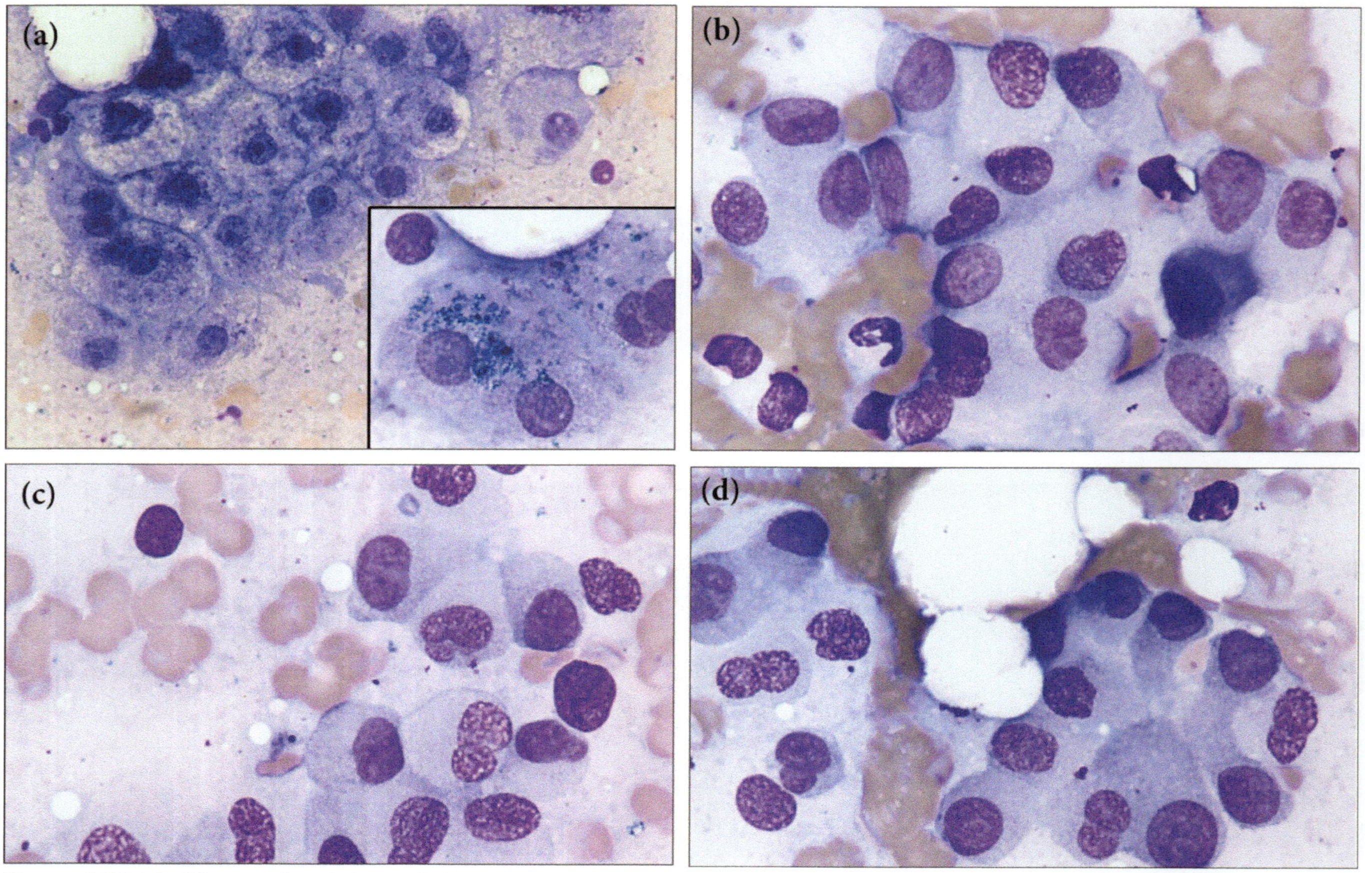

Figures 9.64a–d **Ultrasound-guided FNA of a liver mass (Wright–Giemsa: a, main image, 500× magnification, inset 1,000× magnification; b–d, 1,000× magnification).**

Cytologic description

There are many large hepatocytes with polygonal borders, basophilic to pink granular cytoplasm, a centrally located nucleus, stippled chromatin, and a prominent nucleolus (Figure 9.64a). These cells frequently are binucleate and contain blue–green, granular cytoplasmic material, consistent with lipofuscin. Moderate numbers of hepatocytes have a moderate amount of foamy cytoplasmic rarefaction, consistent with glycogen. There are also cell-free nuclei and intact, round, individualized to clustered cells (Figures 9.64b–d). These cells contain a moderate amount of lightly basophilic cytoplasm, an eccentrically located nucleus with finely stippled chromatin, and, occasionally, one to several poorly distinct nucleoli. Many of the cells have lobulated nuclei or are binucleate. Occasionally, these cells can be found in acinar-like arrangements. The background consists of minimal to moderate cellular debris in a moderately proteinaceous fluid.

Cytologic interpretation

Metastatic neoplasia versus hepatic carcinoid; suspect insulinoma given the history; hepatocellular rarefaction, consistent with glycogen or hydropic degeneration.

Outcome

Because of the worsening condition and poor prognosis the patient was euthanized and a complete necropsy was performed. Multiple pinpoint to 4 cm diameter pink to red, firm nodules were present within the liver and pancreas. These masses were neuroendocrine tumors histologically and stained positive for insulin (Figures 9.65a, b). A firm, dark red, 2 cm diameter mass was present in the left adrenal gland, which was a neuroendocrine tumor histologically. The adrenal mass was insulin negative and chromogranin-A positive. The adrenal mass was felt to be an incidental pheochromocytoma; however, a nonsecretory insulinoma metastasis could not be ruled out (Bailey Page, 2007; Gostelow et al., 2013).

The profound hypoglycemia, seizure activity, and insulin-positive pancreatic and hepatic masses suggest a primary mass with distant metastasis or stage III insulinoma (Patnaik *et al.*, 2005; Goutal *et al.*, 2012). The hepatic aspirate was of the metastatic tumor and contained the unusual finding of lobulated nuclei in neuroendocrine cells. To help confirm insulinoma antemortem, serum insulin and glucose levels should be measured concurrently to demonstrate inappropriate insulin levels (Goutal *et al.*, 2012).

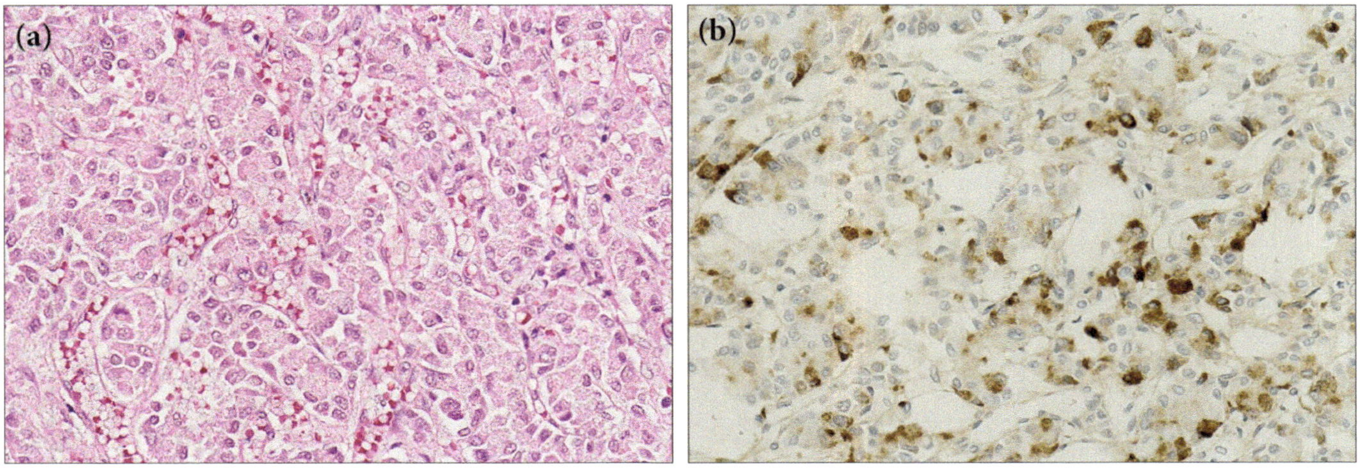

Figures 9.65a, b **Histologic sections of the liver mass. (a) Note the typical neuroendocrine appearance of round cells in nests and packets surrounded by a fine connective tissue stroma (H&E, 200× magnification). (b) The neoplastic cells stained positive for insulin (anti-insulin, diaminobenzidine, hematoxylin counterstain, 200× magnification). A histologically similar insulin-positive mass was present in the pancreas. (Courtesy Dr. Caroline Chu.)**

The atypia noted in the hepatocytes is consistent with a regenerative nodule. Insulin induces glycogen synthesis in hepatocytes, suggesting that the cytoplasmic change may be due to glycogen accumulation. Glycogen accumulation was confirmed with PAS staining, both with and without diastase digestion, of a section of liver; the hepatocytes were PAS positive before diastase and PAS negative after diastase digestion of the glycogen.

(**Note**: selected data from this case have been published previously [Moore *et al.*, 2015].)

CASE 4

Case material provided by Dr. Caitlyn Connor.

Signalment/history

Five-year-old, spayed female French bulldog. The patient was presented for a 3-week history of persistent vomiting and diarrhea, refractory to symptomatic therapy (maropitant, ondansetron, antibiotics).

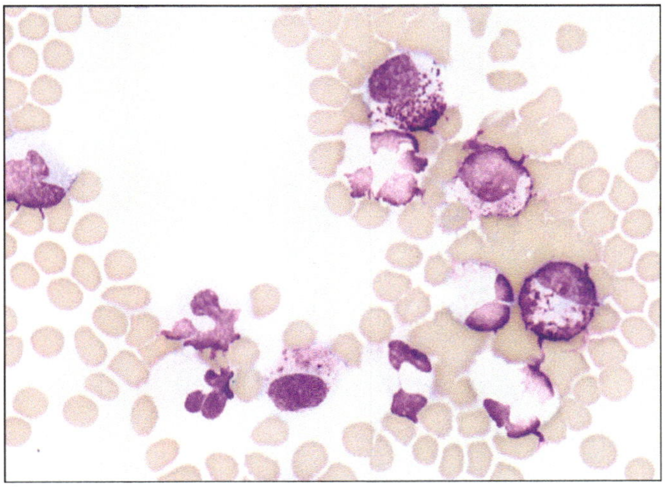

Figure 9.66 **Composite image of the nucleated cells found in the peripheral blood smear of a dog (modified Wright-Giemsa, 1,000× magnification).**

Diagnostics

A CBC revealed a moderate macrocytic, normochromic nonregenerative anemia (Hct = 28.3%; reference interval [RI] = 42–60), moderate thrombocytopenia (platelets = 95 × 10^3/µL; RI = 226–424), and a moderate leukocytosis (WBC 37.3 × 10^3/µL; RI = 4.2–12.9) characterized by a moderate neutrophilia (segmented neutrophils = 24.99 × 10^3/µL; RI = 2.70–8.50) with a minimal regenerative left shift (band neutrophils = 0.373 × 10^3/µL; RI = 0.00–0.300) with minimal signs of toxicity noted, a moderate monocytosis (monocytes = 3.357 × 10^3/µL; RI = 0.100–1.00), minimal basophilia (basophils = 0.373 × 10^3/µL; RI = 0–0), and 17% 'other cells' (Figure 9.66).

A serum biochemistry profile displayed increased liver enzyme activity (ALT = 672 U/l; RI = 12–106; ALP = 446 U/l; RI = 13–102) and cholestasis (total bilirubin = 1.20 mg/dl; RI = 0.00–0.20), a mild hypoproteinemia (5.2 g/dl; RI= 5.4–7.1) characterized by a mild hypoalbuminemia (2.8 g/dl;RI = 3.3–4.2), a mild disproportionate hypochloridemia (98 mmol/l; RI = 106–114; sodium within reference interval at 144 mmol/l; RI = 143–150), a mild to moderate hypokalemia (3.3 mmol/l; RI = 3.7–5.1), mild hypocalcemia (9.2 mg/dl; RI = 9.5–11.2), and a mild hyperphosphatemia (6.4 mg/dl; RI= 2.7–5.2).

Thoracic radiographs did not show any significant findings. Abdominal radiographs exhibited hepatosplenomegaly, and abdominal ultrasound revealed hepatosplenomegaly with multiple splenic nodules, markedly enlarged jejunal lymph nodes, abdominal effusion, and a gastro-duodenal junction ulcer. Aspirates of the liver, spleen, jejunal lymph node, and abdominal fluid were submitted to a reference laboratory. Images from the liver aspirate are shown (Figure 9.67a–d).

Cytologic description

Liver: there are many hepatocyte clusters. Hepatocytes are round to polygonal with mild to moderate amounts of deeply basophilic cytoplasm and a variable nuclear to cytoplasmic ratio. They occasionally contain blue–black granular material consistent with lipofuscin or other pigment, and many hepatocytes contain moderate amounts of distinct clear cytoplasmic vacuolization consistent with lipid. Nuclei are round to ovoid with finely reticular chromatin and one to rarely two distinct nucleoli. Anisocytosis and anisokaryosis are mild to moderate, and there are moderate numbers of binucleate cells. Few trinucleated cells are seen. There are many large discrete round cells with moderately expanded amounts of lightly basophilic cytoplasm and a round nucleus with smooth to stippled chromatin. Most of the cells have at least minimal amounts of fine to slightly coarse metachromatic cytoplasmic granulation. In most cells, this granulation is evenly distributed across the cytoplasm. In some cells, the granulation forms a small packet adjacent to the nucleus. The cells display moderate anisocytosis and anisokaryosis, with binucleation apparent and some cells having more distinct nucleoli. There are pigment-laden macrophages and few neutrophils seen in the background with cellular debris and proteinaceous fluid.

Blood smear: the leukocyte population appears moderately increased and is composed of mostly nondegenerate neutrophils with no appreciable toxic change. Monocytes appear morphologically normal and very few monocytes contain green pigment within the cytoplasm. Lymphocytes are predominantly small with a few intermediate-sized lymphocytes that are slightly smaller than the diameter of a neutrophil with deeply basophilic cytoplasm. Their nuclei are round with finely stippled chromatin and no discernible nucleoli. Eosinophils and basophils appear morphologically normal. The cells marked as 'others' are individualized mast cells. They contain moderate amounts of cytoplasm with variable numbers of fine to coarse deeply metachromatic granules distributed diffusely throughout the cytoplasm. Nuclei are centrally placed and ovoid to rarely irregular

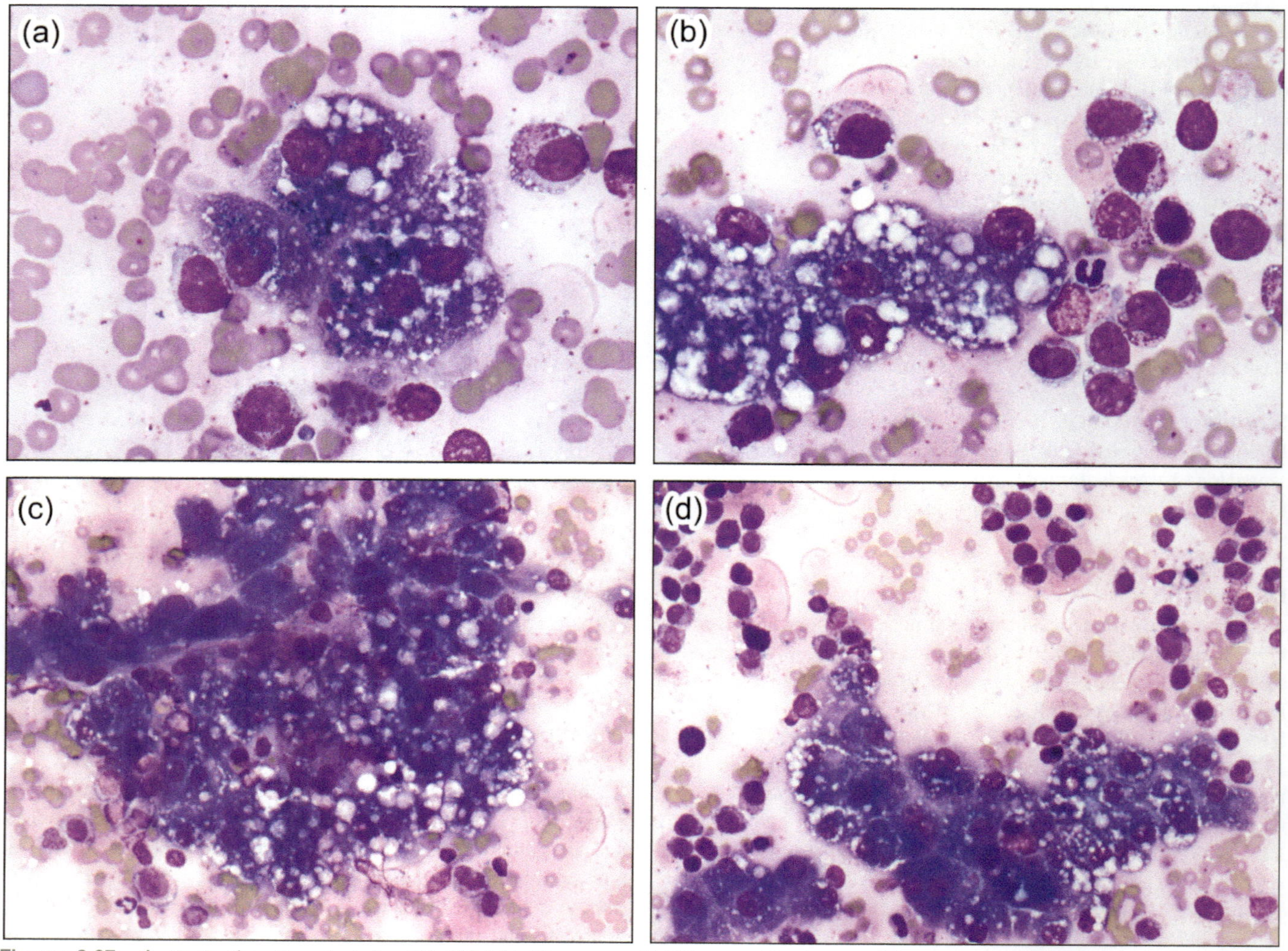

Figures 9.67a–d **Canine hepatic aspirate (modified Wright–Giemsa, a and b 500× magnification, c and d 1,000× magnification).**

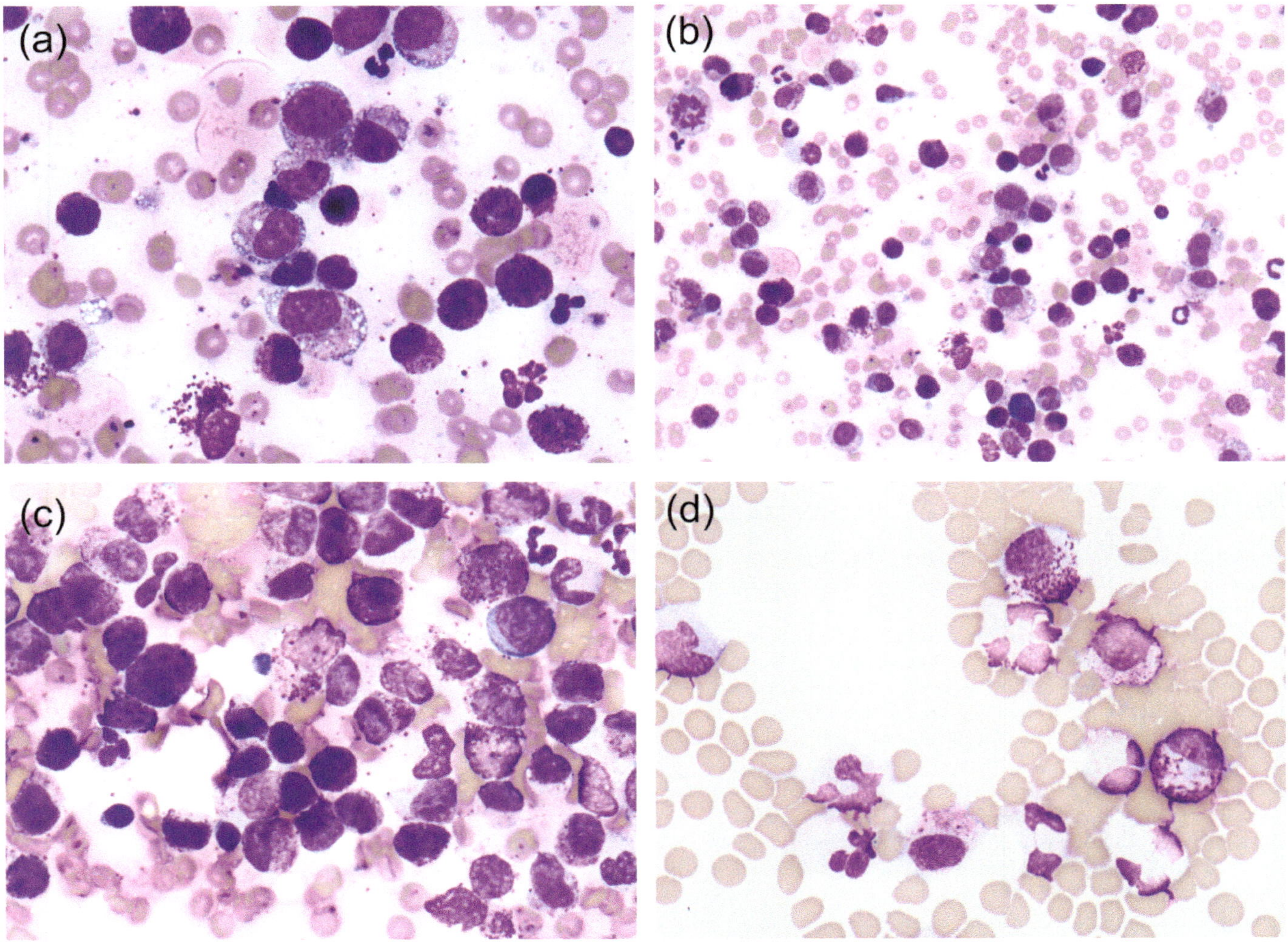

Figures 9.68a–d **Spleen, jejunal lymph node, and abdominal fluid from a 5-year-old dog with mast cell neoplasia in the liver and peripheral blood. (a) The splenic aspirate had severe infiltration of neoplastic mast cells with variable amounts of metachromatic granules. Few small lymphocytes and neutrophils are present. (b) There were only scant lymphocytes present in the jejunal lymph node, but there were abundant neoplastic mast cells with variable amounts of metachromatic granules. (c) The neoplastic mast cells found in the other organs were present in the abdominal effusion and were more prominent than could be explained by peripheral blood contribution alone (modified Wright's Giemsa, 1,000× magnification).**

with fine stippled chromatin and no discernible nucleoli. No infectious etiologic agents are seen.

Cytologic interpretation

Liver: mast cell tumor; hepatocellular vacuolization consistent with lipid.

Peripheral blood: circulating mast cells due to mast cell neoplasia; mild macrocytic, nonregenerative anemia, suspect anemia of chronic disease; mild thrombocytopenia with evidence of thrombopoiesis.

Outcome

All sampled tissue (liver, spleen, lymph node, abdominal fluid, and peripheral blood) contained the neoplastic mast cells, providing evidence of disseminated disease (Figures 9.68). A primary tumor was not evident by imaging. Because of worsening clinical condition and poor prognosis, the patient was euthanized. Necropsy was not performed.

The primary tumor site was not identified in this patient. It is possible that the tumor originated in the liver or spleen or that these sites were metastasis from another location. Very low numbers of mast cells will be seen in healthy peripheral blood. The number and morphology of the circulating mast cells, and their morphologic similarity to the cells found in the liver, spleen, and jejunal lymph node, indicate circulating neoplastic mast cells. Circulating mast cells can be seen with hematogenous spread of visceral mast cell neoplasia and can also be seen with mast cell leukemia or mast cell neoplasia originating in the bone marrow; both of these conditions have a poor prognosis (Willman *et al.*, 2021).

The hepatocellular atypia, lipid vacuolization, and the mixed hepatopathy appreciated on biochemistry were sequelae to the mast cell neoplastic infiltration of this organ rather than indicative of hepatic lipidosis. The nonregenerative anemia and thrombocytopenia are likely indirect sequelae to this disease process. The intracellular green pigment in the monocytes is nonspecific; however, it has been described in dogs with IMHA, post-blood transfusion, or even severe liver disease, which may be present in this case (Gorup *et al.*, 2017; Soos *et al.*, 2019).

ACKNOWLEDGMENTS

The author would like to thank Dr. Walter Hoffman for his assistance with this work.

REFERENCES

Abadie J., Hédan B., Cadieu E. et al. (2009) Epidemiology, pathology, and genetics of histiocytic sarcoma in the Bernese Mountain Dog breed. *J Hered 100*:S19–S27.

Allison R.W., Brunker J.D., Breshears M.A. et al. (2008) Dendritic cell leukemia in a Golden Retriever. *Vet Clin Pathol 37(2)*:190–197.

Ameri M., Wilkerson M.J., Stockham S.L. et al. (2010) Acute megakaryoblastic leukemia in a German Shepherd Dog. *Vet Clin Pathol 39(1)*:39–45.

Ano N., Ozaki K., Nomura K. et al. (2011) Hepatoblastoma in a cat. *Vet Pathol 48(5)*:1020–1023.

Aschenbroich S.A., Rech R.R., Sousa R.S. et al. (2012) Pathology in practice. *Cytauxzoon felis* infection. *J Am Vet Med Assoc 240(2)*:159–161.

Bahr K.L., Sharkey L.C., Murakami T. et al. (2013) Accuracy of US-guided FNA of focal liver lesions in dogs: 140 cases (2005–2008). *J Am Anim Hosp Assoc 49(3)*:190–196.

Bailey D.B., Page R.L. (2007) Tumors of the endocrine system. In: *Withrow & MacEwen's Small Animal Clinical Oncology* (eds. S.J. Withrow, D.M. Vail) Saunders Elsevier, St. Louis, pp. 583–609.

Balkman C. (2009) Hepatobiliary neoplasia in dogs and cats. *Vet Clin North Am Small Anim Pract 39(3)*:617–625.

Barger A.M., Skowronski M.C., MacNeill A.L. (2012) Cytologic identification of eryth-rophagocytic neoplasms in dogs. *Vet Clin Pathol 41(4)*:587–589.

Beatty J.A., Barrs V., Martin P.A. et al. (2002) Spontaneous hepatic rupture in six cats with systemic amyloidosis. *J Small Anim Pract 43(8)*:355–363.

Bigge L.A., Brown D.J., Penninck D.G. (2001) Correlation between coagulation profile findings and bleeding complications after ultrasound-guided biopsies: 434 cases (1993–1996). *J Am Anim Hosp Assoc 37(3)*:228–233.

Book A.P., Fidel J.L., Wills T.B. et al. (2011) Correlation of ultrasound findings, liver and spleen cytology, and prognosis in the clinical staging of high metastatic risk canine mast cell tumors. *Vet Radiol Ultrasound 52(5)*:548–554.

Bosje J.T., van den Ingh T.S.G.A.M., van der Linde-Sipman J.S. (1998) Polycystic kidney and liver disease in cats. *Vet Q 20(4)*:136–139.

Brellou G.D., Kleinschmidt S., Meneses F.N. et al. (2006) Eosinophilic granulomatous gastroenterocolitis and hepatitis in a 1-year-old male Siberian Husky. *Vet Pathol 43(6)*:1022–1025.

Brosinski K., Gutbrod A., Venzin C. et al. (2012) What is your diagnosis? Peritoneal fluid from a dog with abdominal pain. *Vet Clin Pathol 41(2)*:297–298.

Busch M.D.M., Reilly C.M., Luff J.A. et al. (2008) Feline pulmonary Langerhans cell histiocytosis with multiorgan involvement. *Vet Pathol 45(6)*:816–824.

Cedeño Y., López-Alonso M., Miranda M. (2016) Hepatic concentrations of copper and other metals in dogs with and without chronic hepatitis. *J Small Anim Pract 57(12)*:703–709.

Chaivoravitsakul N., Chankow K., Horoongruang K. et al. (2021) Comparison of fine-needle cytologic diagnosis between the left and right liver lobes of dogs and cats with diffuse liver disease. *Vet World 14(10)*:2670–2677.

Cohen M., Bohling M.W., Wright J.C. et al. (2003) Evaluation of sensitivity and specificity of cytologic examination: 269 cases (1999–2000). *J Am Vet Med Assoc 222(7)*:964–967.

Constantino-Casas F., Mayhew D., Hoather T.M. et al. (2011) The clinical presentation and histopathologic-immunohistochemical classification of histiocytic sarcomas in the flat-coated retriever. *Vet Pathol 48(3)*:764–771.

Cray M., Hokamp J., Abrams B. et al. (2023) Clinical utility of cytology from preoperative percutaneous fine needle aspirates of solitary liver masses in 220 dogs: A retrospective study (2009–2019). *J Am An Hosp Assoc 59*:12–19.

Cullen J.M., Popp J.A. (2002) Tumors of the liver and gall bladder. In: *Tumors in Domestic Animals* (ed. D.J. Meuten) Iowa State Press, Ames, pp. 483–508.

Eulenberg V.M., Lidbury J.A. (2018) Hepatic Fibrosis in dogs. *J Vet Intern Med 32(1)*:26–41.

Feeney D.A., Anderson K.L., Ziegler L.E. et al. (2008) Statistical relevance of ultrasonographic criteria in the assessment of diffuse liver disease in dogs and cats. *Am J Vet Res 69(2)*:212–221.

Fieten H., Hooijer-Nouwens B.D., Biourge V.C. et al. (2012) Association of dietary copper and zinc levels with hepatic copper and zinc concentration in Labrador Retrievers. *J Vet Intern Med 26(6)*:1274–1280.

Fine D.M., Tvedten H.W. (1999) Chronic granulocytic leukemia in a dog. *J Am Vet Med Assoc 214(12)*:1809–1812.

Fischer C., Tan E., Bienzle D. (2012) Erythroleukemia in a retrovirus-negative cat. *J Am Vet Med Assoc 240(3)*:294–297.

Galofaro V., Rapisarda G., Lanteri G. et al. (2008) Primary pleomorphic liposarcoma of the liver in a dog. *Pol J Vet Sci 11(4)*:385–388.

Gardner R.H., Castillo D., Constantino-Casas F. et al. (2022) Can the neutrophil count from hepatic fine-needle aspirate cytology be used to diagnose hepatitis in dogs? A pilot study. *Vet Clin Pathol 51(2)*:237–243.

Gookin J.L., Hartley A.N., Aicher K.M. et al. (2023) Gallbladder microbiota in healthy dogs and dogs with mucocele formation. *PLoS One 18*(2 February).

Gorup T., Cohen A.T., Sybenga A.B. et al. (2017) Significance of green granules in neutrophils and monocytes. *Baylor Univ Med Cent Proc 31(1)*:94–96.

Gostelow R., Bridger N., Syme H. (2013) Plasma-free metanephrine and free normetanephrine measurement for the diagnosis of pheochromocytoma in dogs. *J Vet Intern Med 27(1)*:83–90.

Goutal C.M., Brugmann B.L., Ryan K.A. (2012) Insulinoma in dogs: A review. *J Am Anim Hosp Assoc 48(3)*:151–163.

Hamir A.N., Sullivan N.D., Handson P.D. (1983) Acid fast inclusions in tissues of dogs dosed with lead. *J Comp Pathol 93(2)*:307–317.

Harrison J.L., Turek B.J., Brown D.C. et al. (2018) Cholangitis and Cholangiohepatitis in dogs: A descriptive study of 54 cases based on histopathologic diagnosis (2004–2014). *J Vet Intern Med 32(1)*:172–180.

Harro C.C., Smedley R.C., Buchweitz J.P. et al. (2019) Hepatic copper and other trace mineral concentrations in dogs with hepatocellular carcinoma. *J Vet Intern Med 33(5)*:2193–2199.

Hegazy A.M.S., Fouad U.A. (2014) Evaluation of lead hepatotoxicity: Histological, histochemical and ultrastructural study. *Forensic Med Anat Res 2*:70–79.

Hill F.I., Speelman J.P., Hui K.K.L. et al. (2022) High frequency of cholecystitis in dogs with gallbladder mucocoele in Hong Kong. *Vet J 287.*

Hoffmann G. (2009) Copper-associated liver diseases. *Vet Clin North Am Small Anim Pract 39(3)*:489–511.

Hurwitz B.M., Center S.A., Randolph J.F. et al. (2014) Presumed primary and secondary hepatic copper accumulation in cats. *J Am Vet Med Assoc 244(1)*:68–77.

Irvine K.L., Walker J.M., Friedrichs K.R. (2016) Sarcocystid organisms found in bile from a dog with acute hepatitis: A case report and review of intestinal and hepatobiliary Sarcocystidae infections in dogs and cats. *Vet Clin Pathol 45(1)*:57–65.

Kamiie J., Fueki K., Amagai H. et al. (2009) Multicentric myelolipoma in a dog. *J Vet Med Sci 71(3)*:371–373.

Kemp S.D., Zimmerman K.L., Panciera D.L. et al. (2015) Histopathologic variation between liver lobes in dogs. *J Vet Intern Med 29(1)*:58–62.

Kitani K., Ohta M., Kanai S. et al. (1989) Morphological, physiological and biochemical alterations in livers of rodents induced by protease inhibitors: A comparison with old livers. *Adv Exp Med Biol 266*:75–92.

Klinkspoor J.H., Kuver R., Savard C.E. et al. (1995) Model bile and bile salts accelerate mucin secretion by cultured dog gallbladder epithelial cells. *Gastroenterology 109(1)*:264–274.

Klopfleisch R., Sperling C., Kershaw O. et al. (2011) Does the taking of biopsies affect the metastatic potential of tumours? A systematic review of reports on veterinary and human cases and animal models. *Vet J 190(2)*:e31–42.

Köster L., Shell L., Illanes O. et al. (2016) Percutaneous ultrasound-guided Cholecystocentesis and bile analysis for the detection of Platynosomum spp.-induced Cholangitis in cats. *J Vet Intern Med 30(3)*:787–793.

Lamote J., Willems G. (1997) DNA synthesis, cell proliferation index in normal and abnormal gallbladder epithelium. *Microsc Res Techniq 38(6)*:609–615.

Masserdotti C. (2013) Proportion of mast cells in normal canine hepatic cytologic specimens: Comparison of 2 staining methods. *Vet Clin Pathol 42(4)*:522–525.

Masserdotti C. (2020) The cytologic features of biliary diseases: A retrospective study. *Vet Clin Pathol 49(3)*:440–450.

Masserdotti C., Bertazzolo W. (2016) Cytologic features of hepatic fibrosis in dogs: A retrospective study on 22 cases. *Vet Clin Pathol 45(2)*:361–367.

Masserdotti C., Drigo M. (2012) Retrospective study of cytologic features of well-differentiated hepatocellular carcinoma in dogs. *Vet Clin Pathol 41(3)*:382–390.

McCaw D.L., da Silva Curiel J.M., Shaw D.P. (1990) Hepatic myelolipomas in a cat. *J Am Vet Med Assoc 197(2)*:243–244.

Mellor P.J., Haugland S., Smith K.C. et al. (2008) Histopathologic, immunohistochemical, and cytologic analysis of feline myeloma-related disorders: Further evidence for primary extramedullary development in the cat. *Vet Pathol 173*(2008):159–173.

Menard M., Lecoindre A., Cadoré J.-L. et al. (2019) Use of serum biomarkers in staging of canine hepatic fibrosis. *J Vet Diagnostic Investig 31(5)*:665–673.

Meyer D.J. (2010) The liver. In: *Canine and Feline Cytology: A Color Atlas and Interpretation* (eds. R.E. Raskin, D.J. Meyer) Elsevier, St. Louis, pp. 226–248.

Mitsui I., Ohtsuki S., Uchida K. (2021) Chronic Cholecystitis of dogs: Clinicopathologic features and relationship with liver. *Anim 11(11)*.

Moore A.R., Chu C., Singh K. et al. (2015) What is your diagnosis? Liver aspirate from a hypoglycemic dog. *Vet Clin Pathol 44(3)*:463–464.

Moore A.R., Coffey E., Hamar D. (2016) Diagnostic accuracy of Wright-Giemsa and rhodanine stain protocols for detection and semi-quantitative grading of copper in canine liver aspirates. *Vet Clin Pathol 45(4)*:689–697.

Moore A.R., Medrano E., Coffey E. et al. (2019) Clinicopathological correlation and prevalence of increased copper in canine hepatic cytology. *J Am Anim Hosp Assoc 55(1)*:8–13.

Moore P.F. (2014) A review of histiocytic diseases of dogs and cats. *Vet Pathol 51(1)*:167–184.

Moore P.F., Affolter V.K., Vernau W. (2006) Canine hemophagocytic histiocytic sarcoma: A proliferative disorder of CD11d+ macrophages. *Vet Pathol 43(5)*:632–645.

Moritz A.K., Köhler C., Fromme V. et al. (2018) Complications of ultrasound-guided liver biopsies in dogs and cats. *Tierarztl Prax Ausg K Kleintiere Heimtiere 46(1)*:5–13.

Nerschbach V., Eberle N., Joetzke A.E. et al. (2016) Splenic and hepatic ultrasound and cytology in canine lymphoma: Effects of findings on stage migration and assessment of prognosis. *Vet Comp Oncol 14*:82–94.

Newman S.J., Smith J.R., Stenske K.A. et al. (2007) Aflatoxicosis in nine dogs after exposure to contaminated commercial dog food. *J Vet Diagn Invest 19(2)*:168–175.

Niewold T.A., van der Linde-Sipman J.S., Murphy C. et al. (1999) Familial amyloidosis in cats: Siamese and Abyssinian AA proteins differ in primary sequence and pattern of deposition. *Amyloid 6(3)*:205–209.

Nyland T.G., Koblik P.D., Tellyer S.E. (1999) Ultrasonographic evaluation of biliary cystadenomas in cats. *Vet Radiol Ultrasound 40(3)*:300–306.

Nyland T.G., Wallack S.T., Wisner E.R. (2002) Needle-tract implantation following US-guided fine-needle aspiration biopsy of transitional cell carcinoma of the bladder, urethra, and prostate. *Vet Radiol Ultrasound 43(1)*:50–53.

Otsuka H., Yagi H., Endo Y. et al. (2011) Kupffer cells support extramedullary erythropoiesis induced by nitrogen-containing bisphosphonate in splenectomized mice. *Cell Immunol 271(1)*:197–204.

Otte C.M.A., Penning L.C., Rothuizen J. (2017) Feline biliary tree and gallbladder disease: Aetiology, diagnosis and treatment. *J Feline Med Surg 19(5)*:514–528.

Padgett G.A., Madewell B.R., Keller E.T. et al. (1995) Inheritance of histiocytosis in Bernese mountain dogs. *J Small Anim Pract 36(3)*:93–98.

Palić J., Geisen V., Unterer S. et al. (2017) The beauty of bile. *Vet Clin Pathol 46(4)*:549–550.

Palić J., Unterer S., Geisen V. et al. (2022) Pathology in practice. *J Am Vet Med Assoc 259(S2)*:1–4.

Patnaik A.K., Newman S.J., Scase T. et al. (2005) Canine hepatic neuroendocrine carcinoma: An immunohistochemical and electron microscopic study. *Vet Pathol 42(2)*:140–146.

Patten P.K., Rich L.J., Zaks K. et al. (2013) Cestode infection in 2 dogs: Cytologic findings in liver and a mesenteric lymph node. *Vet Clin Pathol 42(1)*:103–108.

Peters L.M., Glanemann B., Garden O.A. et al. (2016) Cytological findings of 140 bile samples from dogs and cats and associated clinical pathological data. *J Vet Intern Med 30(1)*:123–131.

Peterson M.R., Porter B.F., Edwards E.E. et al. (2022) Subcutaneous implantation of hepatocellular carcinoma in a dog. *J Comp Pathol 199*:51–54.

Pike F.S., Berg J., King N.W. et al. (2004) Gallbladder mucocele in dogs: 30 cases (2000–2002). *J Am Vet Med Assoc 224(10)*:1615–1622.

Reece J., Pavlick M., Penninck D.G. et al. (2020) Hemorrhage and complications associated with percutaneous ultrasound guided liver biopsy in dogs. *J Vet Intern Med 34(6)*:2398–2404.

Reimer L., Roessner A., Themann H. et al. (1973) Optical diffraction on tilting series of paracrystalline intranuclear inclusions of dog liver parenchymal cells. *J Ultrastruct Res 45(5)*:356–365.

Richter W.R., Stein R.J., Rdzok E.J. et al. (1965) Ultrastructural studies of intranuclear crystalline inclusions in the liver of the dog. *Am J Pathol 47(4)*:587–599.

Rodrigues A., Leal R.O., Girod M. et al. (2020) Canine copper-associated hepatitis: A retrospective study of 17 clinical cases. *Open Vet J 10(2)*:128–134.

Roth L. (2001) Comparison of liver cytology and biopsy diagnoses in dogs and cats: 56 cases. *Vet Clin Pathol 30(1)*:35–38.

Rothuizen J., Bunch S.E., Charles J.A. et al. (2006) Sampling and handling of liver tissue. In: *WSAVA Standards for Clinical and Histological Diagnosis of Canine and Feline Liver Diseases*. Saunders, Edinburgh, pp. 5–14.

Rothuizen J., Twedt D.C. (2009) Liver biopsy techniques. *Vet Clin North Am Small Anim Pract 39(3)*:469–480.

Sapierzyński R., Jagielski D., Dolka I. et al. (2012) Cytopathological diagnosis of visceral histiocytic sarcoma in five dogs. *Pol J Vet Sci 15(4)*:751–758.

Scott M.A. (2006) Bye-Bye bile, hello Lipofuscin? Laboratory medicine: Yesterday • today • tomorrow. *Vet Clin Pathol 35(1)*:5.

Segev G., Cowgill L.D., Jessen S. et al. (2012) Renal amyloidosis in dogs: A retrospective study of 91 cases with comparison of the disease between Shar-Pei and non-Shar-Pei dogs. *J Vet Intern Med 26(2)*:259–268.

Sevelius E. (1995) Diagnosis and prognosis of chronic hepatitis and cirrhosis in dogs. *J Small Anim Pract 36(12)*:521–528.

Shiga A., Shirota K., Shida T. et al. (1997) Hepatoblastoma in a dog. *J Vet Med Sci 59(12)*:1167–1170.

Smedley R.C., Mullaney T.P., Rumbeiha W. (2009) Copper-associated hepatitis in Labrador Retrievers. *Vet Pathol 46(3)*:484–490.

Smith D.M., Haggitt R.C. (1983) A comparative study of generic stains for carcinoid secretory granules. *Am J Surg Pathol 7(1)*:61–68.

Soos M.P., Heideman C., Shumway C. et al. (2019) Blue-green neutrophilic inclusion bodies in the critically ill patient. *Clin Case Reports 7(6)*:1249–1252.

Stalker M.J., Hayes M.A. (2007a) Liver and biliary system. In: *Jubb, Kennedy & Palmer's Pathology of Domestic Animals, Vol 2*, 5th edn. (ed. M.G. Maxie) Saunders Elsevier, St. Louis, pp. 297–298.

Stalker M.J., Hayes M.A. (2007b) Hyperplastic and neoplastic lesions of the liver and bile ducts. In: *Jubb, Kennedy & Palmer's Pathology of Domestic Animals, Vol 2*, 5th edn. (ed. M.G. Maxie) Saunders Elsevier, St. Louis, pp. 382–388.

Stockhaus C., Teske E., van den Ingh T.S.G.A.M. et al. (2002) The influence of age on the cytology of the liver in healthy dogs. *Vet Pathol 39(1)*:154–158.

Stockhaus C., van den Ingh T.S.G.A.M., Rothuizen J. et al. (2004) A multistep approach in the cytologic evaluation of liver biopsy samples of dogs with hepatic diseases. *Vet Pathol 41(5)*:461–470.

Sugiyama D., Kulkeaw K., Mizuochi C. et al. (2011) Hepatoblasts comprise a niche for fetal liver erythropoiesis through cytokine production. *Biochem Biophys Res Commun 410(2)*:301–306.

Takahashi T., Kadosawa T., Nagase M. et al. (2000) Visceral mast cell tumors in dogs: 10 cases (1982–1997). *J Am Vet Med Assoc 216(2)*:222–226.

Tamborini A., Jahns H., McAllister H. et al. (2016) Bacterial Cholangitis, Cholecystitis, or both in dogs. *J Vet Intern Med 30(4)*:1046–1055.

Terai K., Ishigaki K., Kagawa Y. et al. (2022) Clinical, diagnostic, and pathologic features and surgical outcomes of combined hepatocellular-cholangiocarcinoma in dogs: 14 cases (2009–2021). *J Am Vet Med Assoc 260(13)*:1668–1674.

Trigo F.J., Thompson H., Breeze R.G. et al. (1982) The pathology of liver tumours in the dog. *J Comp Pathol 92(1)*:21–39.

van den Ingh T.S.G.A.M., Cullen J.M., Twedt D.C. et al. (2006a) Morphological classification of biliary disorders of the canine and feline liver. In: *WSAVA Standards for Clinical and Histological Diagnosis of Canine and Feline Liver Diseases*. Saunders, Edinburgh, pp. 61–76.

van den Ingh T.S.G.A.M., Van Winkle T., Cullen J.M. et al. (2006b) Hepatocellular death, hepatitis and cirrhosis. In: *WSAVA Standards for Clinical and Histological Diagnosis of Canine and Feline Liver Diseases*. Saunders, Edinburgh, pp. 85–101.

Vasanjee S.C., Bubenik L.J., Hosgood G. et al. (2006) Evaluation of hemorrhage, sample size, and collateral damage for five hepatic biopsy methods in dogs. *Vet Surg 35(1)*:86–93.

Verwey E., Gal A., Kettner F. et al. (2021) Prevalence of subclinical bactibilia in apparently healthy shelter dogs. *J Small Anim Pract 62(11)*:948–958.

Vignoli M., Rossi F., Chierici C. et al. (2007) Needle tract implantation after Fine Needle Aspiration Biopsy (FNAB) of transitional cell carcinoma of the urinary bladder and adenocarcinoma of the lung. *Schweiz Arch Tierheilkd 149(7)*:314–318.

Wachowiak I.J., Moore A.R., Avery A. et al. (2022) Atypical multiple myeloma in three young dogs. *Vet Pathol 59(5)*:787–791.

Warren-Smith C.M.R., Andrew S., Mantis P. et al. (2012) Lack of associations between ultrasonographic appearance of parenchymal lesions of the canine liver and histological diagnosis. *J Small Anim Pract 53(3)*:168–173.

Webb C.B. (2020) Evidence-based medicine: Ultrasound-guided percutaneous Cholecystocentesis in the cat. *Vet Clin North Am – Small Anim Pract 50(5)*:1123–1134.

Weiss D.J., Blauvelt M.M., Aird B. (2001) Cytologic evaluation of inflammation in canine liver aspirates. *Vet Clin Pathol 30(4)*:193–196.

Whittemore J.C., Newkirk K.M., Reel D.M. et al. (2012) Hepatic copper and iron accumulation and histologic findings in 104 feline liver biopsies. *J Vet Diagn Invest 24(4)*:656–661.

Willmann M., Yuzbasiyan-Gurkan V., Marconato L. et al. (2021) Proposed diagnostic criteria and classification of canine mast cell neoplasms: A consensus proposal. *Front Vet Sci 8(December)*:1–10.

Willard M.D., Weeks B.R., Johnson M.C. (1999) Fine-needle aspirate cytology suggesting hepatic lipidosis in four cats with infiltrative hepatic disease. *J Feline Med Surg 1(4)*:215–220.

CHAPTER 10

RENAL CYTOLOGY AND URINALYSIS

Julie L. Webb and Ashleigh W. Newman

INTRODUCTION

The urinary system includes the kidneys, ureters, urinary bladder, and urethra. Pathologic conditions can affect any segment of the urinary system, but most lesions involve the kidneys or bladder, which will be the focus of this chapter. Ureteral and urethral lesions are rare and will only be discussed briefly near the end of the chapter.

In addition to sampling renal and bladder lesions, microscopic examination of urinary sediment can provide valuable information regarding urinary tract disease. Sediment examination is one part of a complete urinalysis, which also includes gross examination, specific gravity measurement, and dipstick analysis. A description and interpretation of the complete urinalysis are beyond the scope of this text.

KIDNEYS

Sampling

The utility of renal cytology varies greatly with the underlying disease process and physical characteristics of the kidneys. In general, renal masses and diffusely enlarged kidneys are good candidates for sampling, as cytology can often classify the lesion as inflammatory, neoplastic, or cystic in nature. Small kidneys, consistent with chronic renal disease, are poor targets for sampling as they rarely contain diagnostic findings. Cytology is also not recommended when evaluating glomerulonephropathies, as such conditions require histopathologic examination of glomeruli for an accurate diagnosis.

Most renal cytologic samples are obtained via fine needle aspiration (FNA). Touch imprints can also be prepared from surgical biopsy specimens, if available. The use of ultrasound guidance is recommended to increase aspiration accuracy and reduce the risk of hemorrhage.

Normal

Kidneys contain glomeruli, tubules, a collagenous interstitium, and blood vessels. Aspirates from normal kidneys are generally poorly cellular with few tubular epithelial cells and occasional (if any) glomeruli. Blood vessels and interstitial (stromal) tissue are rarely observed. Blood contamination is frequently present in renal aspirates.

Renal tubular epithelial cells are round to polygonal cells that are often found in small clusters and, occasionally, tubular formations (Figures 10.1, 10.2). They are monomorphic in appearance with a moderate amount of lightly basophilic grainy cytoplasm. Nuclei are round and often paracentrally placed. Low numbers of small dark pigment granules may be observed. Clear, distinct, lipid vacuoles are often noted within feline renal tubular cells (Figure 10.3). Canine cells have fewer vacuoles. Glomeruli are very large multicellular structures occasionally observed in renal aspirates, comprised of a capillary tuft and supporting elements. (Figure 10.4). Some glomeruli are seen as a highly cellular capillary tuft separated from, but still attached to, poorly cellular eosinophilic stroma (potentially Bowman's capsule). Some glomeruli may be closely associated with a small cluster or long tubule of renal epithelium.

INFLAMMATION

When evaluating renal cytology samples for inflammation, the amount of blood contamination must be considered. An inflammatory process can be detected when the number or proportion of leukocytes exceeds that expected from blood contamination. Finding leukocytes in aggregates or associated with epithelium, as well as finding leukocytes that are not associated with peripheral blood (e.g. plasma cells, macrophages), provides additional support for an inflammatory process.

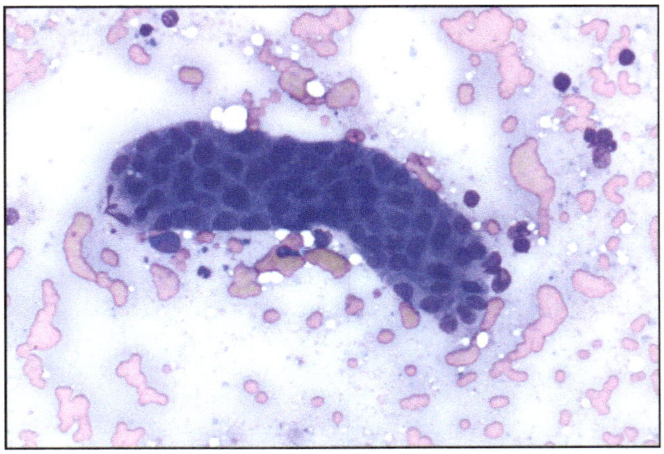

Figure 10.1 **A tubule of renal epithelium (modified Wright's, 200× magnification).**

DOI: 10.1201/9781003258551-10

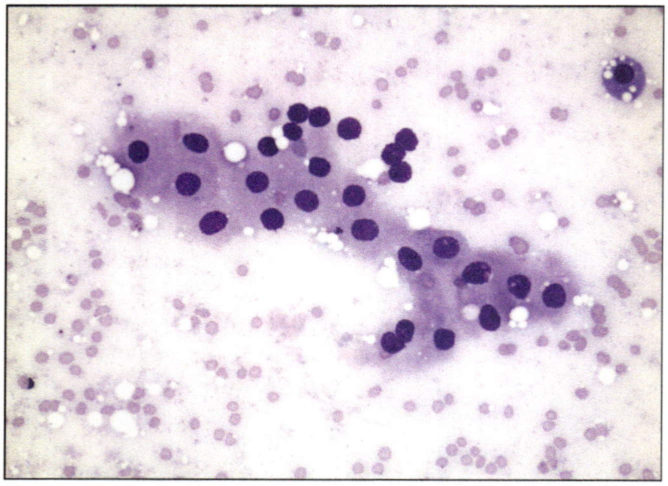

Figure 10.2 A monomorphic cluster of normal canine renal epithelium (modified Wright's, 600× magnification).

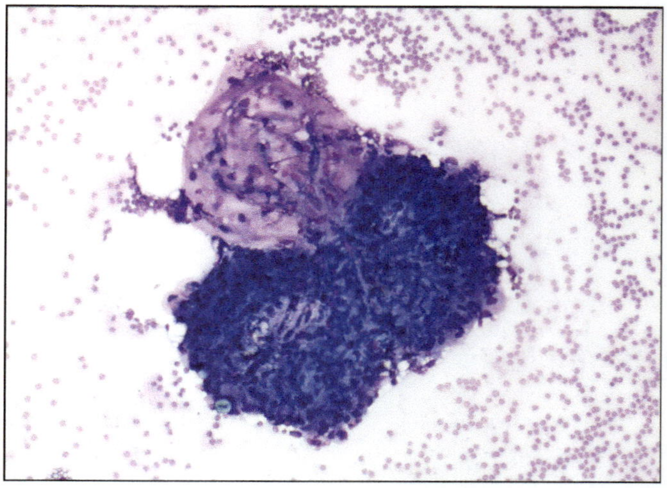

Figure 10.4 Glomerulus (modified Wright's, 200× magnification).

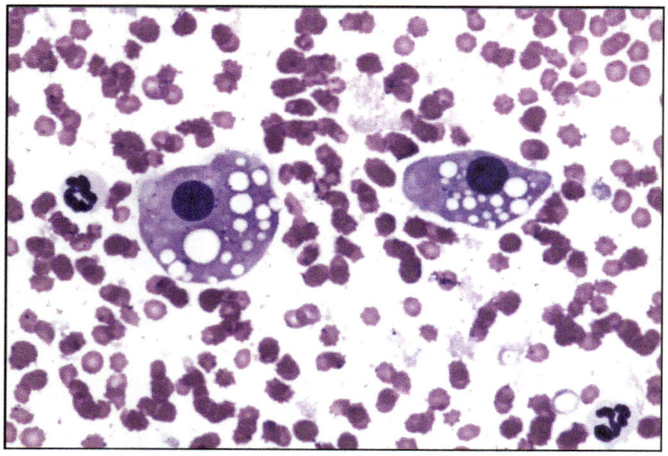

Figure 10.3 Two individualized feline renal tubular epithelial cells with many small distinct lipid droplets (modified Wright's, 1,000× magnification).

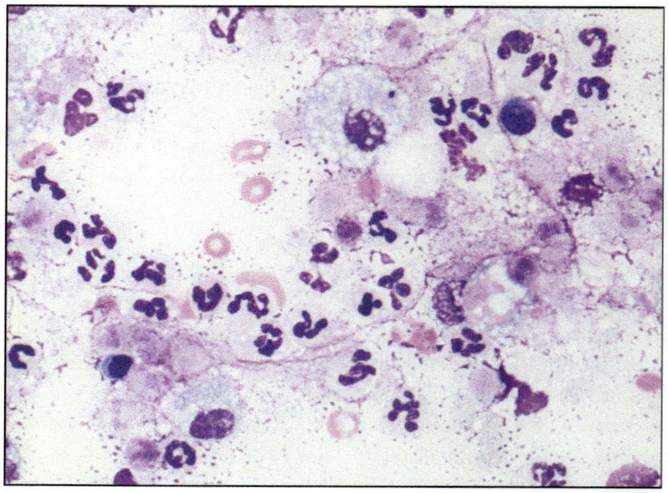

Figure 10.5 Pyelonephritis in a dog. Many neutrophils with fewer foamy macrophages. An etiology was not identified (modified Wright's, 600× magnification).

Bacterial pyelonephritis typically results from an ascending infection, although hematogenous spread is also possible. Most diagnoses are made via urinalysis and urine culture, instead of direct renal aspiration. If aspirated, samples from pyelonephritis are expected to contain increased numbers of neutrophils, potentially with a degenerate morphology (Figure 10.5). Variable numbers of bacteria may be found. A background population of renal tubular epithelial cells and a few glomeruli may also be observed.

Rarely, pyelonephritis is caused by fungal or other nonbacterial organisms and is only one symptom of systemic disease (Newman *et al.*, 2003; Pressler *et al.*, 2005). The type of inflammation varies with the causative agent but neutrophils often predominate. Macrophages, including epithelioid and multinucleated giant forms, often accompany fungal infections to produce pyogranulomatous inflammation.

Feline infectious peritonitis may be accompanied by nodular renal lesions (Giordano *et al.*, 2005). Aspirates from affected kidneys often reveal normal renal elements (tubular epithelial cells and glomeruli) with a mixed population of nondegenerate neutrophils and macrophages. Fewer lymphocytes and plasma cells may also be observed.

Lymphocytic–plasmacytic inflammation is commonly associated with interstitial nephritis and chronic kidney disease (Figure 10.6). The cause of chronic interstitial nephritis is usually not apparent (microscopically or clinically).

Neoplasia

A variety of neoplasms affect the kidneys of small animals. Renal carcinoma arises from renal tubular epithelial cells and is the most common primary renal neoplasm of both dogs and cats (Henry, 1999; Bryan *et al.*, 2006). Other carcinomas (urothelial, squamous, and metastatic) are rare (Meuten, 2002). Renal lymphoma can arise as a

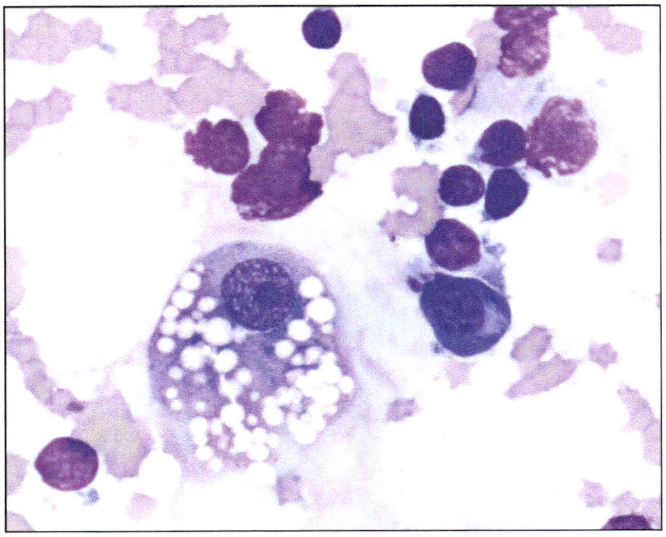

Figure 10.6 Lymphocytic–plasmacytic inflammation in a cat. Several small lymphocytes and a plasma cell associated with a lipid-laden renal tubular epithelial cell (modified Wright's, 1,000× magnification).

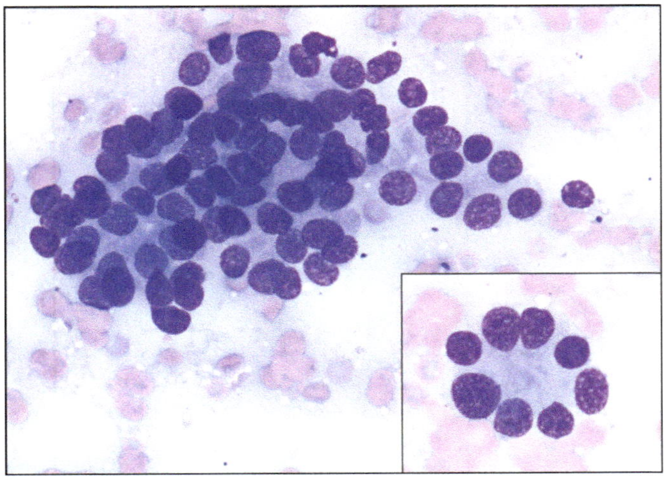

Figure 10.7 Renal carcinoma in a dog. A disorganized cluster of neoplastic epithelial cells with indistinct cell borders. Inset: acinar formation from the same tumor (modified Wright's, 600× magnification).

seemingly isolated lesion, most notably in cats, or as part of multicentric disease (Mooney *et al.*, 1987). Mesenchymal neoplasms, both primary and metastatic, can also affect the kidneys, including hemangiosarcoma, fibrosarcoma, osteosarcoma, chondrosarcoma, and histiocytic sarcoma (Hahn *et al.*, 1997; Affolter Moore, 2002; Munday et al., 2004; Bryan et al., 2006). Nephroblastoma, a mixed tumor of embryonal origin, has also been reported and may occur in very young patients (Baskin De Paoli, 1977). Most renal neoplasms are unilateral but renal carcinomas and lymphoma can be bilateral. Most renal neoplasms are malignant. Benign tumors (adenoma, papilloma, fibroma) are rare, small (2 cm), and usually an incidental finding at necropsy (pale cortical nodule in an otherwise grossly normal kidney; Baskin De Paoli, 1977).

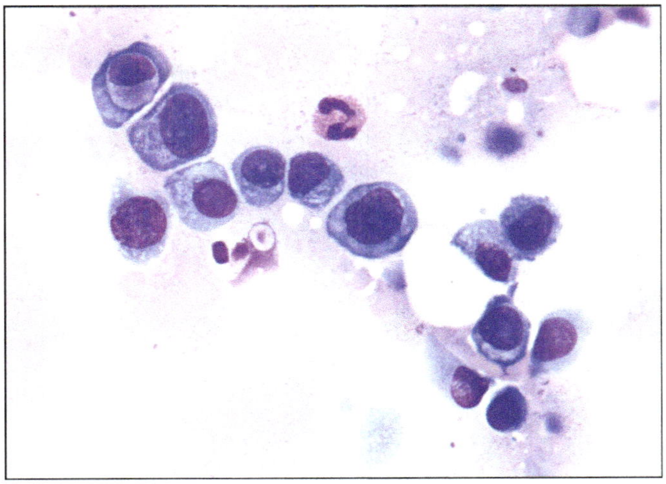

Figure 10.8 Renal carcinoma in a cat. Most of the neoplastic epithelial cells in this sample were individualized and round (modified Wright's, 600× magnification).

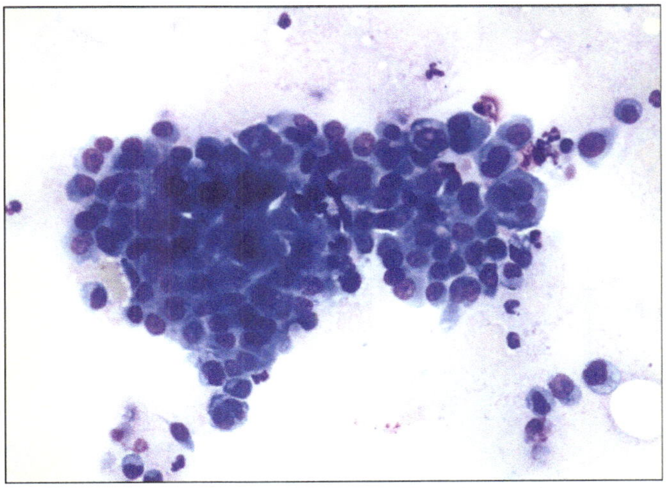

Figure 10.9 Renal carcinoma in a cat. A pleomorphic neoplastic population displaying anisocytosis, anisokaryosis, and multinucleation (modified Wright's, 400× magnification).

Aspirates from renal carcinoma are moderately to highly cellular. The epithelial cells have moderately to deeply basophilic cytoplasm and typically occur in cohesive clusters, sheets, and, rarely, acini (Figure 10.7). Cells within clusters are often tightly packed and jumbled, with irregular nuclear spacing and indistinct cell borders. In fewer tumors, the cells may be individualized and round (Figure 10.8). Nuclear to cytoplasmic (N:C) ratios are variable but are often increased above normal. Some renal carcinomas are monomorphic in appearance. Others display moderate anisocytosis and anisokaryosis with bi- and multinucleation (Figure 10.9).

Urothelial carcinomas (UCs), also known as transitional cell carcinoma (TCC), of the kidney are morphologically similar to those described later for the urinary bladder. Squamous cell carcinomas are rare and comparable to squamous cell carcinoma in cutaneous

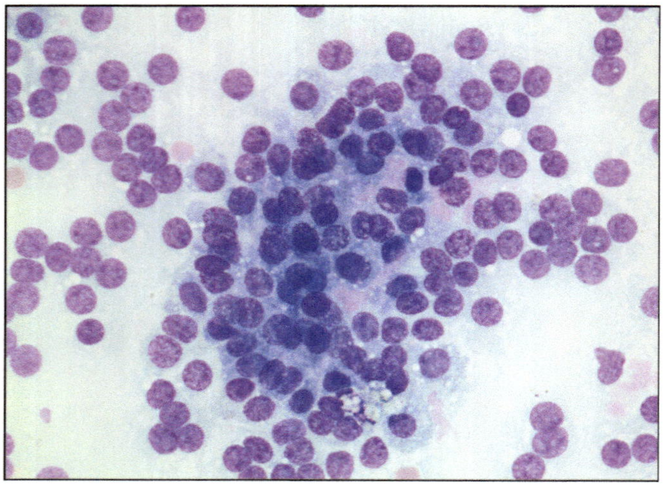

Figure 10.10 Metastatic thyroid carcinoma in a dog. A loosely cohesive epithelial population with many free nuclei suggestive of a neuroendocrine origin. A primary thyroid carcinoma with multiple metastatic lesions was identified at necropsy (modified Wright's, 600× magnification).

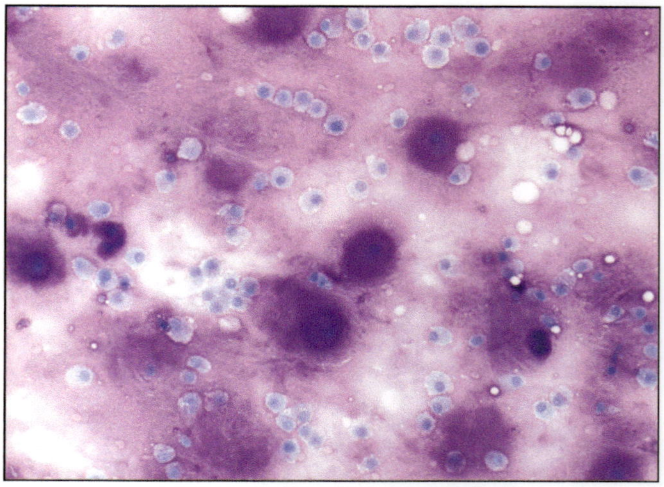

Figure 10.12 Metastatic chondrosarcoma. A large amount of extracellular matrix and cells occasionally embedded within chondroid lacunae are characteristic of this tumor (Modified Wright's, 200× magnification).

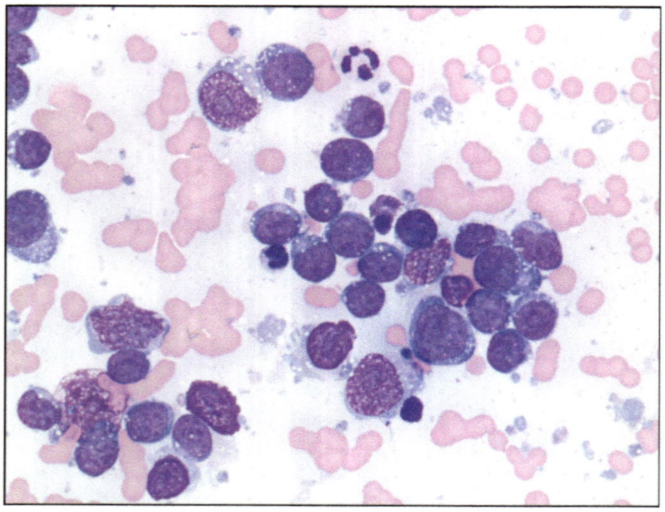

Figure 10.11 Renal lymphoma in a cat. A homogeneous population of large lymphocytes with high N:C ratios, finely stippled chromatin, and occasional nucleoli (modified Wright's, 600× magnification).

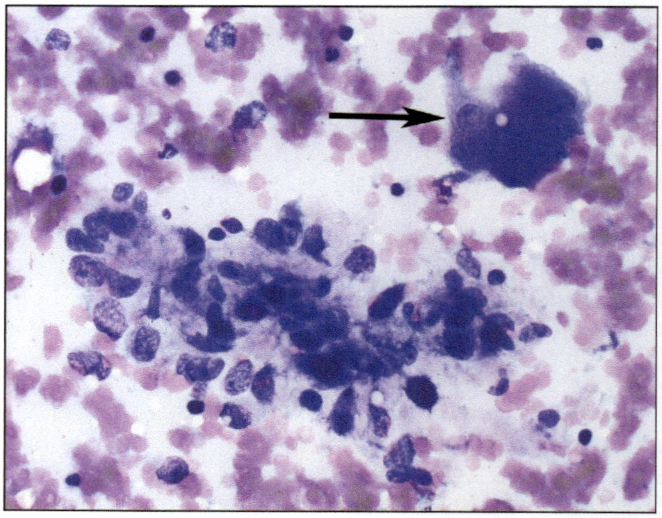

Figure 10.13 Metastatic osteosarcoma in a dog displaying an aggregate of neoplastic osteoblasts and a multinucleated osteoclast (arrow). Rare tubules of epithelium were also noted to confirm a renal origin (modified Wright's, 500× magnification).

and other locations (see Chapter 4). Metastatic carcinomas are also rare and the tissue of origin is often not obvious from cytology alone. Pertinent history and knowledge of the primary neoplasm can help identify the tumor in such cases (Figure 10.10).

Aspirates of renal lymphoma are often highly cellular and will appear cytologically like lymphoma aspirates in lymphoid and other tissues (see Chapter 5). A homogeneous population of large lymphocytes with finely stippled chromatin will be present, possibly along with a few normal renal elements (Figure 10.11). Neoplastic lymphocytes from renal lymphoma rarely exfoliate into the urine and can be noted on a urine sediment exam (Witschen *et al.*, 2020). Differentiation between neoplastic and inflammatory lymphoid populations is usually straightforward in renal aspirates. Lymphoma aspirates tend to be highly cellular with a homogeneous population of large cells. Inflammatory lymphoid populations are typically less cellular, more heterogeneous, and composed of small lymphocytes with plasma cells.

Many renal mesenchymal neoplasms aspirate poorly (fibrosarcoma) or are markedly contaminated by blood (hemangiosarcoma) and rarely provide diagnostic samples for cytology. Some sarcomas, such as chondrosarcoma and osteosarcoma, may produce more cellular aspirates, but are rare metastatic lesions (Figures 10.12, 10.13). Histiocytic sarcoma can affect the kidneys as part of disseminated

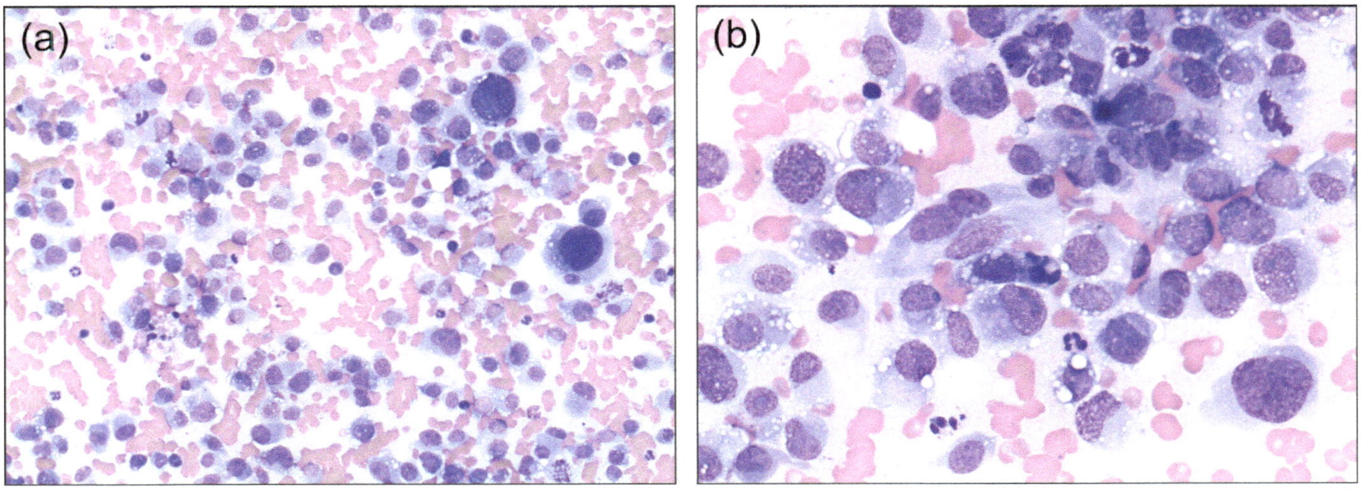

Figures 10.14a, b Histiocytic sarcoma in a dog with disseminated disease. (a) 200× magnification view displaying high cellularity and marked pleomorphism. (b) 600× magnification displaying round to spindle-shaped cells with lightly basophilic cytoplasm and small vacuoles (modified Wright's).

disease and aspirates are typically highly cellular, containing a pleomorphic population of individual round to spindle-shaped cells (Figures 10.14a, b). These cells have lightly basophilic cytoplasm and often contain a few small, distinct, clear vacuoles. Marked anisocytosis and anisokaryosis are typically evident, along with frequent bi- and multinucleation.

Nephroblastomas have a 'triphasic' pattern of epithelium, mesenchyme, and embryonic glomeruli that can be seen histologically, but all three features are rarely observed cytologically. More commonly, aspirates contain only poorly differentiated, loosely cohesive epithelial cells with lightly basophilic cytoplasm, high N:C ratios, round nuclei, and finely stippled chromatin (Neel & Dean, 2000). These poorly differentiated epithelial cells can be mistaken for large lymphocytes; however, rare cohesion, particularly rosette formation, will help suggest the true diagnosis (Figure 10.15). Small spindle cells with dark nuclei, representing the mesenchymal component of the tumor, may also be present. Glomerular structures are rare (de Lorenzi *et al.*, 2007).

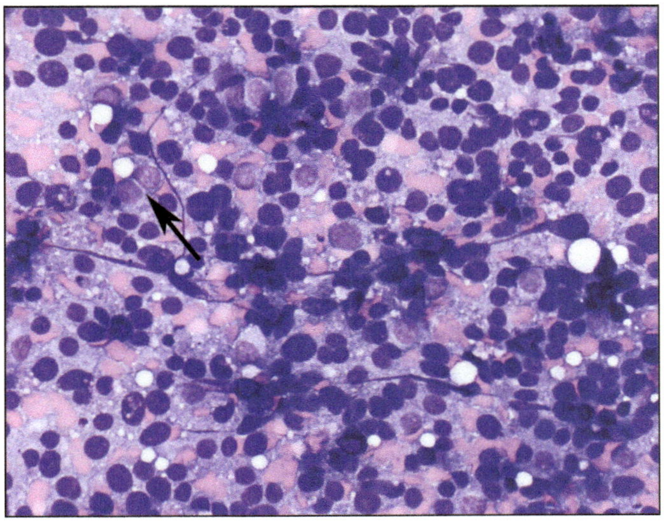

Figure 10.15 Nephroblastoma (presumed). A retroperitoneal mass in a young dog contains many free nuclei and poorly differentiated cells that could be mistaken for a lymphoid origin, but rare cohesive cells (arrow) suggest an epithelial origin. In this location, a nephroblastoma is presumed but the cytology alone is similar to other primitive neuroectodermal tumors (modified Wright's, 500× magnification).

Other renal abnormalities

Renal and perirenal cysts may be congenital or acquired and can present as single or multiple lesions. Aspirates of cysts produce a clear fluid with low cellularity. The few nucleated cells present are predominantly foamy macrophages. A few monomorphic epithelial lining cells may also be observed. Renal carcinomas can have cystic regions that mimic benign cysts. If underlying neoplasia is suspected, additional aspirates or biopsy of the suspicious tissue should be performed.

Hydronephrosis is a fluid-filled dilation of the renal pelvis due to obstructed urine flow. Diagnosis is usually made via ultrasonography. Aspirates from hydronephrotic kidneys will contain poorly cellular, watery fluid with a creatinine concentration higher than peripheral blood, consistent with urine.

BLADDER

Sampling

Cytology of urinary bladder tissue is generally reserved for investigation of masses and suspected neoplastic disease. Most inflammatory lesions affecting the bladder can be diagnosed via urine sediment examination, a minimally to non-invasive procedure for the patient.

Ultrasound-guided FNAs can be used to sample thickened bladder walls and intraluminal masses. However, the most common neoplasm of the bladder is UC and neoplastic cells from UCs can seed needle tracks after FNA attempts (Nyland *et al.*, 2002), as well as open surgical procedures (Higuchi *et al.*, 2010). Many clinicians, therefore, prefer the traumatic catheterization technique to obtain cells from intraluminal bladder masses.

Traumatic catheterizations are performed under deep sedation or a short general anesthesia, with the patient in lateral or ventral recumbency. A urinary catheter is introduced into the bladder in a sterile fashion. The bladder is emptied and the mass (usually in the trigone) is located. Rectal palpation or ultrasound guidance may be needed to localize the catheter to the mass/trigone region. If the mass is further away than the trigone, it may not be accessible via this method. Apply negative pressure to the catheter with a 10 or 20 ml syringe. While holding the negative pressure, move the catheter back and forth, rubbing against the tumor. Small pieces of tumor and blood will be seen in the catheter and syringe. Direct and sediment smears of the retrieved fluid should be prepared, but the most cellular and diagnostic samples tend to come from squash preparations of small tumor pieces. If tumor pieces are large enough, they can be placed into formalin and submitted for histopathology instead. (Procedural information contributed by Cecilia S. Robat, DVM, DACVIM [Oncology].)

Imprints of biopsied tissue may also be used for cytologic evaluation. If small samples are obtained via cystoscopy or traumatic catheterization, imprints will be difficult to make and could damage the tissue. The best option in these cases may be to leave the tissue untouched to ensure a more accurate histologic examination. Larger pieces of tissue obtained via cystotomy are better candidates for tissue imprints.

Normal

Healthy urinary bladders are typically not sampled for cytology but normal/unremarkable urothelial cells (also known as transitional epithelial cells) may be retrieved when investigating pathologic conditions. Depending on the sampling method, specimens will be poorly to moderately cellular, with catheterized samples being more cellular than aspirates or free catch methods. Urothelial cells may be found individually and in small clusters (Figure 10.16). These cells are cuboidal with a moderate amount of lightly basophilic cytoplasm. Nuclei are round to oval and often contain patchy chromatin from being exposed to urine. Mild anisocytosis is considered a normal finding in urothelial epithelium. Anisokaryosis will be minimal. A small amount of blood with associated leukocytes may also be retrieved.

Inflammation

Most cases of cystitis are diagnosed based on history, physical examination findings, and urine sediment examination. However, neutrophilic inflammation and bacterial infection can accompany neoplastic disease in the bladder. In addition, chronic infection and inflammation can result in significant, even mass-like, urothelial hyperplasia. Therefore, bacterial organisms and neutrophilic inflammation may be identified when sampling various mass lesions (Figure 10.17). This combination of factors can make interpretation of cytology difficult and is discussed further in the later hyperplasia section.

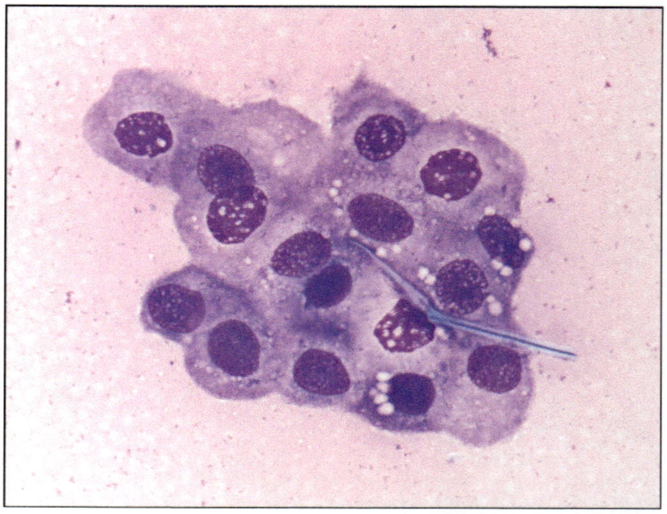

Figure 10.16 **A cluster of unremarkable urothelial epithelial cells from a catheterized routine urinalysis (modified Wright's, 600× magnification).**

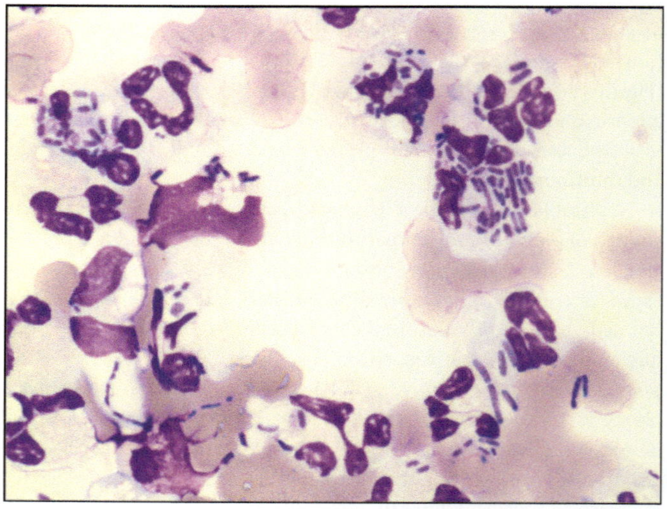

Figure 10.17 **Septic neutrophilic (suppurative) inflammation in a dog. This patient presented for a mass lesion in the bladder and was eventually diagnosed with urothelial carcinoma. Initial sampling, however, only retrieved a secondary urinary tract infection (modified Wright's, 1,000× magnification).**

Neoplasia

Urothelial carcinoma (UC) is the most common neoplasm to affect the urinary bladder in both dogs and cats, although the incidence in cats is very low compared to dogs (Griffin *et al.*, 2019). In both species, UC most commonly affects the trigone region. The gross appearance can vary in morphology from a papillary mass to a thickened bladder wall. UCs that arise in the bladder may extend into the urethra or prostate (Knapp & McMillan, 2010).

Samples from UCs, particularly squash preparations from traumatic catheterizations, can be moderately to highly cellular with urothelial cells in small clusters and large sheets (Figure 10.18). Although

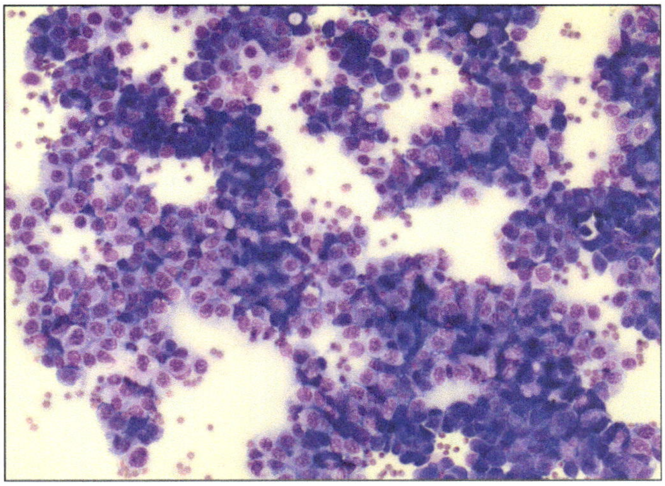

Figure 10.18 **Urothelial carcinoma. Squash preparation from traumatic catheterization procedure. Low-power view demonstrating the high cellularity that can be retrieved via this sampling method (modified Wright's, 200× magnification).**

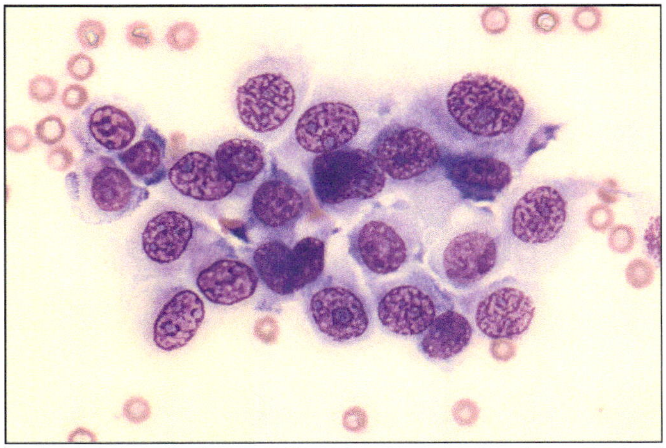

Figure 10.19 **Urothelial carcinoma. A mildly pleomorphic population of urothelial epithelial cells with increased N:C ratios. A definitive diagnosis of neoplasia could not be made from this sample. The final diagnosis was made with a surgical biopsy (modified Wright's, 600× magnification).**

typically less cellular than catheterized samples, voided urine samples may have increased urothelial cellularity to suggest neoplastic disease. Some UCs contain epithelial cells similar to normal urothelial cells (i.e. cuboidal cells with a moderate amount of basophilic cytoplasm and round central nuclei [Figure 10.19]). These cells may have an increased N:C ratio and mild pleomorphism that raises the suspicion for neoplasia, but a definitive diagnosis may not be possible by cytology alone.

When cytology is equivocal, additional testing can be recommended. Histopathologic examination is an option for these situations, but biopsy is an invasive procedure and the bladder is a difficult location to sample. Alternatively, non-invasive BRAF testing is available for suspected canine UCs with 75% of these tumors reportedly positive for the BRAF mutation (Mochizuki *et al.*, 2015). The BRAF test is currently only commercially available on urine samples so neoplastic cells must be shed in urine for testing to occur. The BRAF mutation has (thus far) not been detected in any non-neoplastic urinary or prostatic disease, so the specificity of a positive result is reportedly 100% (Mochizuki *et al.*, 2015; Grassinger *et al.*, 2019).

UCs that display significant pleomorphism can be definitively diagnosed cytologically. Cells from these tumors display marked anisocytosis, moderate anisokaryosis, frequent binucleation, rare multinucleation, multiple and prominent nucleoli, and occasional mitotic figures (Figures 10.20a, b). Large, round eosinophilic globules, known as Melamed-Wolinska bodies, are observed in the cytoplasm of some neoplastic urothelial cells (Figure 10.21). These inclusions are most associated with neoplastic urothelial cells but similar inclusions, which may have variable composition, have also been noted in other normal, degenerating, and neoplastic populations (e.g. mammary carcinoma) (Arya *et al.*, 2011; Marin *et al.*, 2023).

Other neoplastic diseases are rare in the bladder, and include SCC, lymphoma, leiomyosarcoma, and rhabdomyosarcoma (Knapp & McMillan, 2010).

Hyperplasia

Chronic irritation of the bladder wall can result in significant benign urothelial epithelial hyperplasia. The most common causes of chronic irritation are urinary tract infections and urinary calculi (Martinez *et al.*, 2003). The resulting hyperplasia can result in wall thickening and even mass-like, polypoid proliferations (polypoid cystitis).

Cytologically, hyperplastic urothelial cells may display many features suggestive of well-differentiated neoplasia. Increased basophilia, moderate anisocytosis, and binucleation are common findings (Figures 10.22a, b). Depending on the cause of the hyperplasia, concurrent inflammation or infection may also be noted.

Differentiating polypoid cystitis from UC in dogs can be a difficult process; many of the presenting signs are similar and there is cytologic overlap between the two conditions. Nuclear features of malignancy (macronuclei, abnormal nuclei, atypical mitoses, multinucleation, nuclear molding) are more suggestive of neoplastic disease and should rarely, if at all, be seen in hyperplastic lesions (Pierini *et al.*, 2022). One should be extremely cautious when attempting to diagnose UC when there is concurrent inflammation in the sample. A thorough history investigating recurrent urinary tract infections and uroliths should be taken. Abdominal ultrasound can provide relevant information; UC usually arises in the trigone region while polypoid cystitis tends to arise in the cranioventral region. Ultimately, additional testing such as histopathology and/or BRAF testing is often required to reach a diagnosis in equivocal cases.

URINARY SEDIMENT

Sampling, preparation, and evaluation

Urine sediment examination is typically part of a complete urinalysis. The basics of sediment preparation are detailed in the following

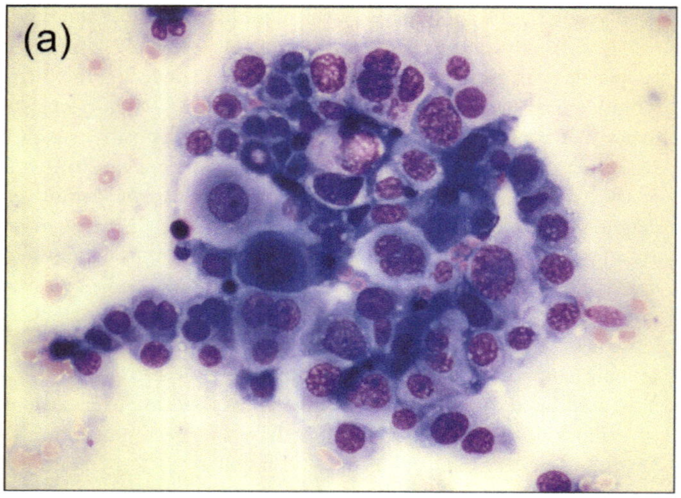

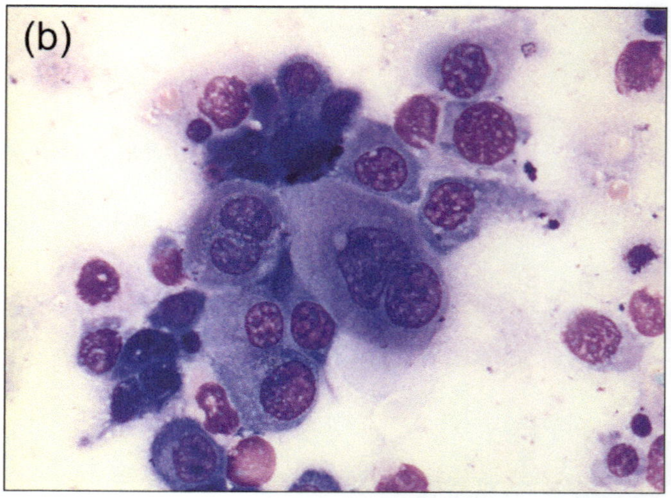

Figures 10.20a, b **Urothelial carcinoma. A pleomorphic variation of this tumor displaying marked anisocytosis, anisokaryosis, and multinucleation (modified Wright's: a, 400× magnification; b, 600× magnification).**

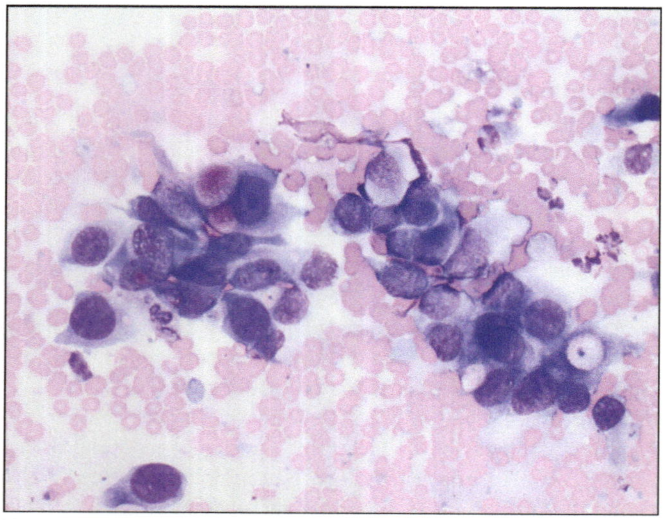

Figure 10.21 **Urothelial carcinoma. Variably sized bright eosinophilic globules (Melamed-Wolinska bodies) are found in the cytoplasm of these neoplastic urothelial cells (modified Wright's, 500× magnification).**

paragraphs (Osborne & Stevens, 1999; Gunn-Christie *et al.*, 2012). Examination of the sediment can identify various inflammatory, infectious, hemorrhagic, and metabolic processes in the patient. Neoplastic cells from prostatic and bladder tumors may also be observed in urine sediment, but this sample is not recommended for diagnosing neoplasia. Direct sampling of the suspected neoplasm, via FNA or traumatic catheterization, is recommended to obtain a higher quality sample for cytology.

Urine can be obtained via voided (free-catch), catheterization, or cystocentesis methods. Free-catch collection is a non-invasive process that is easy to perform, but these voided samples are prone to contamination with genital and skin elements. Catheterization is minimally invasive but could introduce infection and is still susceptible to external contamination. Catheterized samples often have higher numbers of urothelial cells, and these cells can be found in clusters. Cystocentesis is the most invasive method and can be complicated by iatrogenic hemorrhage or enterocentesis (Garner *et al.*, 2011). However, cystocentesis samples avoid contamination by the genital tract and are considered the best samples for urine culture.

A sterile container or plain blood collection tube is recommended for sample submission. Anticoagulants, preservatives, or clot-enhancing components can interfere with the urine dipstick reactions, sediment exam, and/or culture. To obtain the most representative results, urine should be analyzed within 30 minutes of collection. If rapid evaluation is not possible, the urine should be refrigerated. A refrigerated sample should be allowed to warm back to room temperature before being analyzed. Urine samples should ideally be analyzed within 24 hours of collection to limit in-vitro bacterial growth, crystal formation, and cast and/or cellular degradation.

To prepare a sample for microscopic examination, 5 ml of well-mixed urine is centrifuged at low speed (450 × g) for 5 minutes. The supernatant is pipetted off, leaving 0.5 ml of fluid and sediment. In healthy patients, grossly visible sediment will not be apparent. The sediment is resuspended in the remaining fluid by gentle aspiration and discharge from a pipette. A drop of the suspension is placed on a glass slide and covered with a coverslip.

The wet mount should be examined microscopically in both a low-power field (lpf, 100× magnification) and a high-power field (hpf, 400× magnification) with lighting appropriate to unstained specimens. Lighting options for most microscopes include lowering the substage condenser or closing the iris diaphragm, both of which will increase contrast and help visualize elements. Phase contrast condensers are another option for increasing contrast but are not routinely available. Cellular, crystal, and other elements are evaluated semiquantitatively at low or high power.

New methylene blue or urine stains (e.g. Sedistain) can be added to urine sediment to improve visualization of certain urine elements,

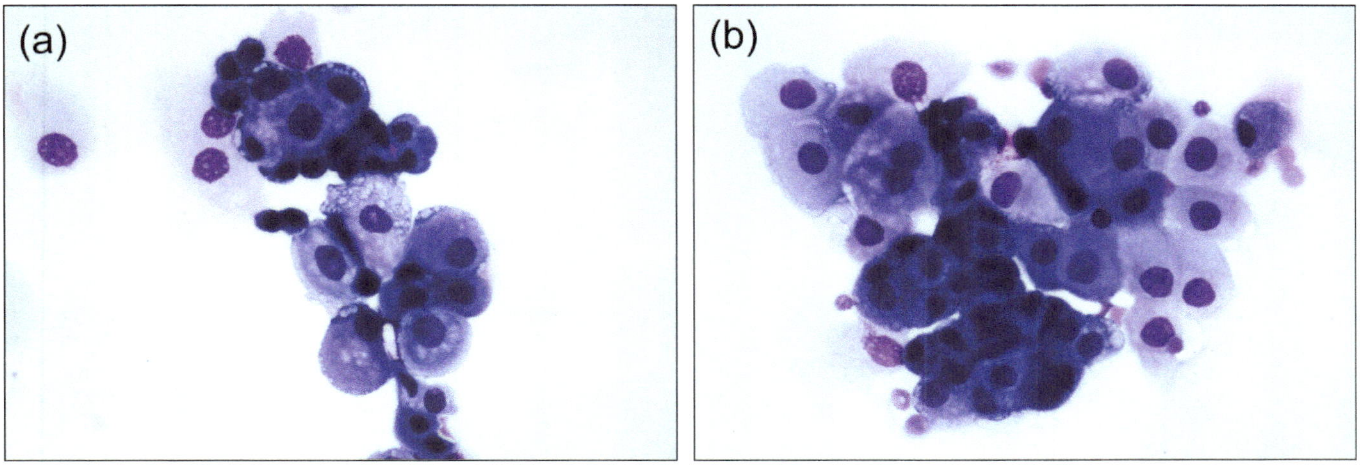

Figures 10.22a, b **Hyperplastic urothelial epithelium in a dog. This dog presented for uroliths and a thickened bladder wall. Biopsy of the bladder wall confirmed a benign hyperplastic epithelium (modified Wright's, 400× magnification).**

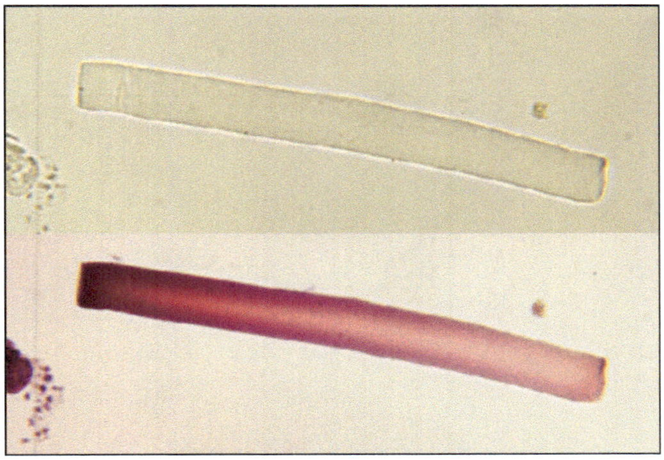

Figure 10.23 **Urine sediment unstained (top) and with Sedistain (bottom). The waxy cast is easily visualized with the addition of Sedistain (400× magnification). (Courtesy Peter S. MacWilliams.)**

most notably hyaline and waxy casts (Figure 10.23). However, they can also introduce artifactual dilution of the sample and stain debris that can be mistaken for bacteria. An alternative method to improve identification of urine elements is to prepare and stain a dry slide of the urine. A drop of resuspended urine sediment is used to make a sediment or line preparation. Once dry, the slide can be stained with Wright's, Diff-Quik, or Gram stain. Wright's- or Diff-Quik®-stained dry slides can help differentiate cellular elements (erythrocyte versus leukocyte versus epithelial cell), whereas Wright's-, Diff-Quik-, or Gram-stained slides can confirm the presence of bacteria (Swenson *et al.*, 2011).

Normal findings

Cellular elements normally found in urine include low numbers of erythrocytes, leukocytes, and epithelial cells (urothelial and/or squamous). Certain casts and crystals may also be present in low numbers, as elaborated upon in the subsequent sections. Lipid droplets are frequently encountered. Spermatozoa are expected in intact males. Abnormal findings include increased numbers of normal elements and the presence of other elements, as detailed below.

Cells

Erythrocytes are uniform in size, round or crenated in shape, and moderately refractile (shiny) in appearance (Figures 10.24a, b). They often appear colorless but may have a slight red–orange tinge (Figure 10.25). Central pallor may be visible. A few erythrocytes (0–5/hpf) are considered a normal finding. Increased numbers can be seen with uroliths, urinary tract infections, idiopathic cystitis, neoplasms, and coagulopathies. Iatrogenic hemorrhage associated with cystocentesis will also increase the number of erythrocytes.

Most leukocytes in urine are neutrophils, although they often cannot be identified as such by sediment examination. These leukocytes will be uniform in size, round in shape, and slightly granular in appearance (Figure 10.26). They are larger than erythrocytes (1.5–2 times the size) and smaller than epithelial cells. A lobulated nucleus may rarely be visible (Figure 10.27). A few leukocytes (0–5/hpf) are considered a normal finding. Increased numbers are most associated with urinary tract infections. Sterile inflammation, associated with neoplasms or uroliths, is also possible but less common.

Squamous epithelial cells in urine may originate from the skin, distal urethra, vaginal tract, or prepuce. They are large and often irregularly shaped with angular borders (Figure 10.28). They may have a small central nucleus or be anucleate. They occur singly or in sheets. Squamous cells in urine are usually the result of sample contamination and are not clinically significant. A rare exception is squamous metaplasia of the prostate (secondary to estrogen exposure) with desquamated cells found in the urine.

Urothelial cells (Figure 10.29) line the renal pelvis, ureter, bladder, and proximal urethra. They are slightly variable in size but

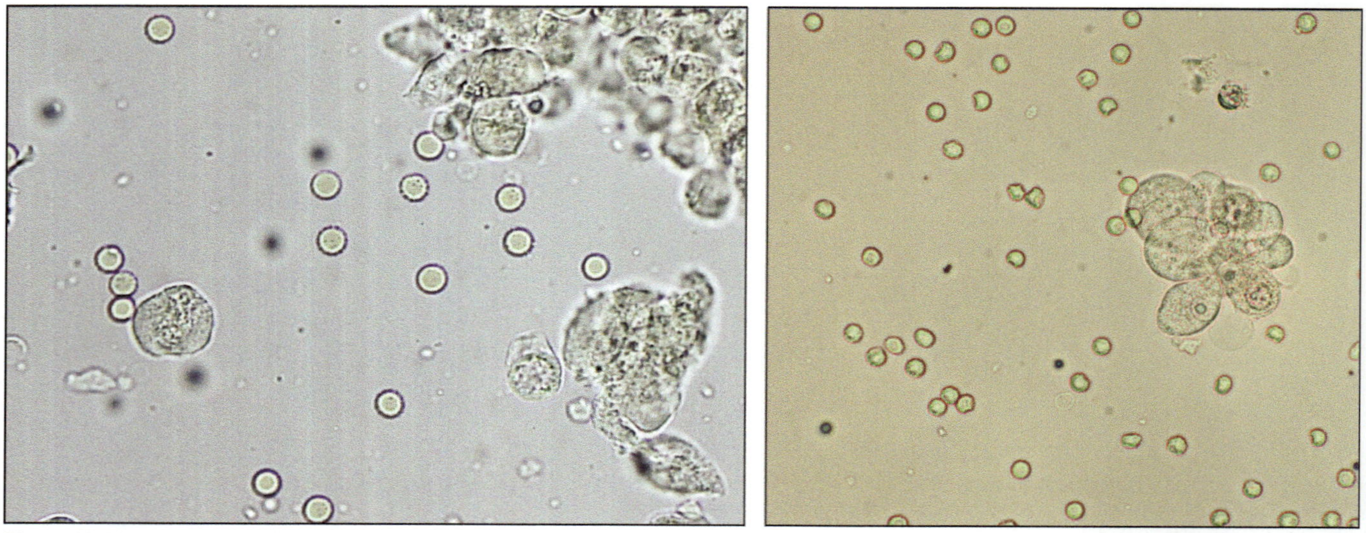

Figure 10.24a, b Many erythrocytes from a dog with hematuria secondary to urothelial carcinoma. Erythrocytes vary from round and smooth to biconcave to slightly crenated. A few larger irregular neoplastic urothelial cells are also present, found individually and in clusters (unstained, 400× magnification).

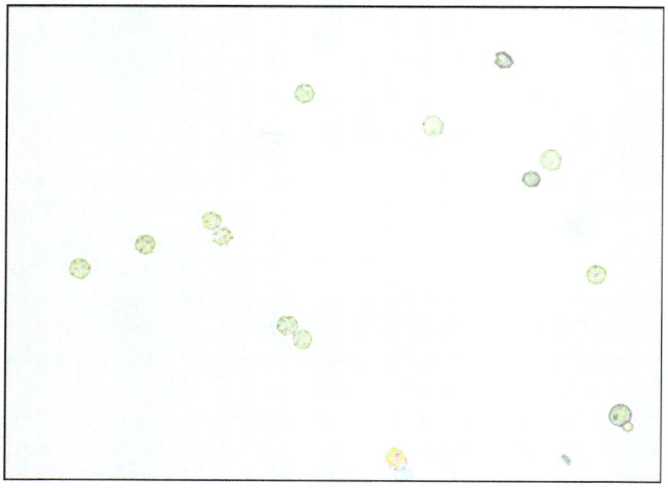

Figure 10.25 Erythrocytes with a red-orange tinge (unstained, 400× magnification).

consistently larger than leukocytes (2–4 times the size) and smaller than squamous cells (Figure 10.30). They are often round to cuboidal with a slightly granular appearance. Rarely, cells will be caudate in shape, suggestive of a renal pelvic origin. They have a round, central nucleus, although it is not always visible. Urothelial cells can be found individually or in small clusters. Low numbers of urothelial cells are considered a normal finding. Catheterized samples will have increased numbers of urothelial cells as the passage of the catheter dislodges normal cells. Increased numbers will also be seen with urinary tract infections, uroliths, and UC. The cells from UC are often pleomorphic in morphology, as described for bladder cytology (Figure 10.31). In some cases of UC, cellular details will be difficult to discern with an unstained specimen. Applying Wright's stain to a dried sediment smear may help visualize details in these cases (Figures 10.32 a, b).

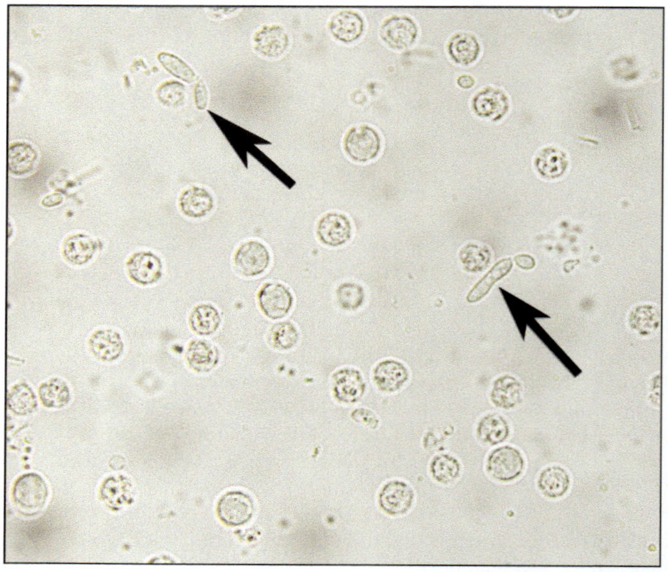

Figure 10.26 Many leukocytes (presumably neutrophils) with a diffusely granular appearance. Rare oval to elongated, budding yeast are also present (arrows) as the source of inflammation in this case (unstained, 400× magnification).

Renal epithelial cells line the renal tubules of the kidney. They are smaller than urothelial cells but slightly larger than leukocytes. Like urothelial cells, they are round to cuboidal in shape, have a round nucleus, and can be found individually or in clusters. As such, it is very difficult to accurately differentiate them from small urothelial cells. Renal epithelial cells are rarely found and definitively identified in urine. When present, they suggest renal tubular disease.

Figure 10.27 Three leukocytes with visible lobulated nuclei (neutrophils, lower right). Two red–orange erythrocytes are also present (unstained, 400× magnification).

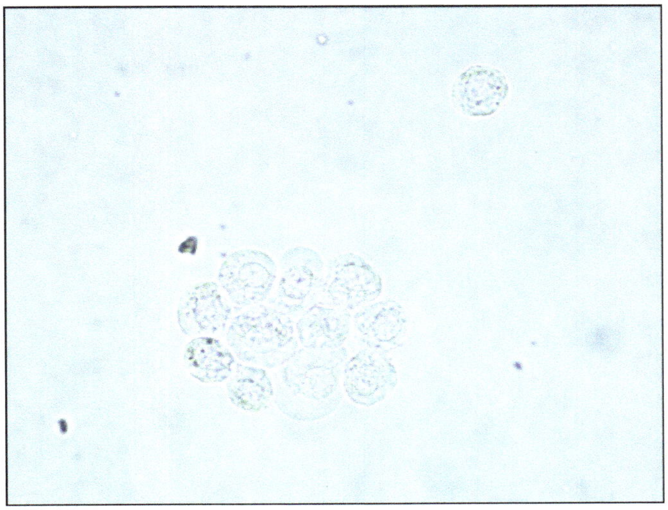

Figure 10.29 Normal urothelial cells. A small cluster and a single cell displaying mild anisocytosis. Round nuclei are occasionally visible within the cells (unstained, 400× magnification).

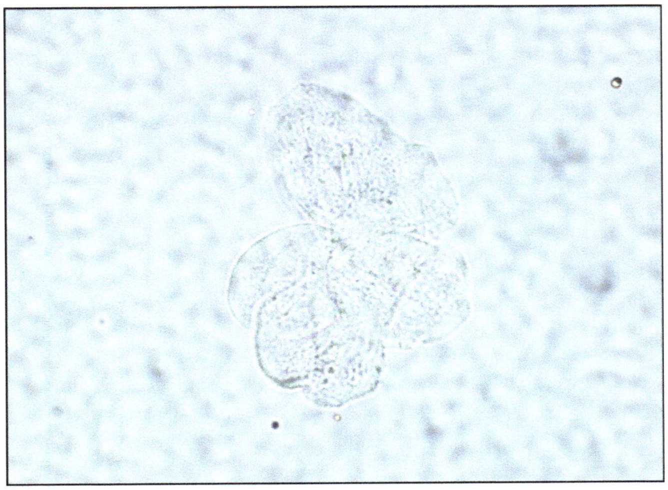

Figure 10.28 A cluster of squamous epithelial cells with irregular, angular borders (unstained, 400× magnification).

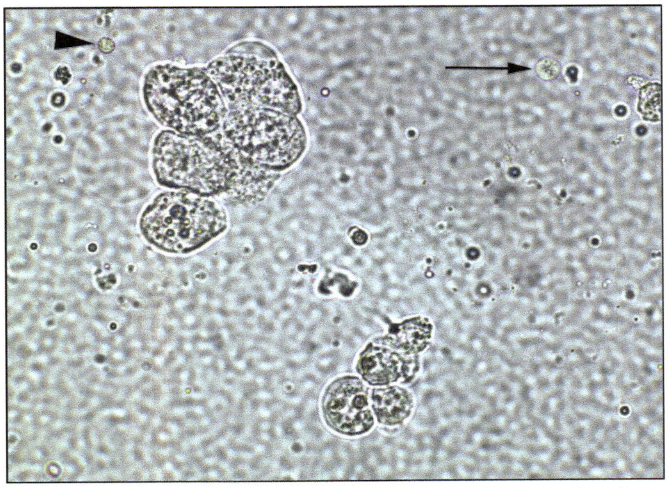

Figure 10.30 A small cluster of normal urothelial cells (bottom) with size comparisons to squamous epithelial cells (upper left), a leukocyte (arrow), and an erythrocyte (arrowhead) (unstained, 400× magnification).

Casts

Casts are cylindrical molds of renal tubules composed of mucoproteins and, often, cellular elements. Casts are variable in length but all have parallel sides and are approximately 3–4 leukocytes in width. Casts do not preserve well in urine sediment; they easily fragment into short pieces, making identification difficult. Also complicating identification is the fact that mucus strands, fibers, and aggregates of debris sometimes mimic casts.

Hyaline casts are composed of protein only. They are very faint (almost transparent) and homogeneous with rounded ends (Figure 10.33). A low number of hyaline casts is a normal finding. Increased numbers can be seen with proteinuria, glomerular disease, and renal tubular damage. Cellular casts contain intact renal tubular epithelial cells embedded within a glycoprotein matrix (Figure 10.34). Rarely, entire segments of intact tubules will slough (Figure 10.35). Both forms are an abnormal finding and indicate renal tubular damage. Granular casts may result from the breakdown of cellular casts or the precipitation of proteins. They vary from finely to coarsely granular in appearance, with no intact cells (Figure 10.36). Low numbers of granular casts are considered a normal finding. Increased numbers are associated with renal tubular damage and may accompany cellular casts and/or waxy casts. Waxy casts are the presumed final breakdown product of cellular and granular casts. They are faint, smooth, and wide with blunt ends (Figure 10.37). They are an uncommon finding and thought to indicate chronic renal tubular disease. Multiple types of casts and mixed casts can be observed in a single urine sample (Figures 10.38, 10.39).

Rarely, other cells or elements that are present in the renal tubules can become trapped within a mucoprotein matrix, creating unique casts. The significance of the cast varies with the embedded material.

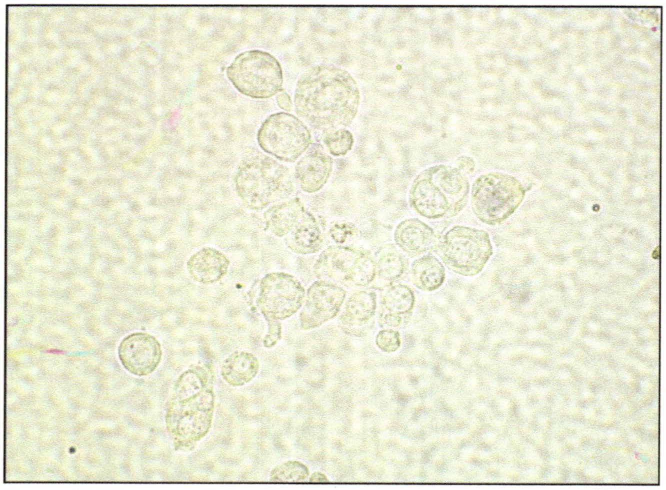

Figure 10.31 A population of neoplastic urothelial cells with moderate anisocytosis, anisokaryosis, and binucleation (unstained, 400× magnification).

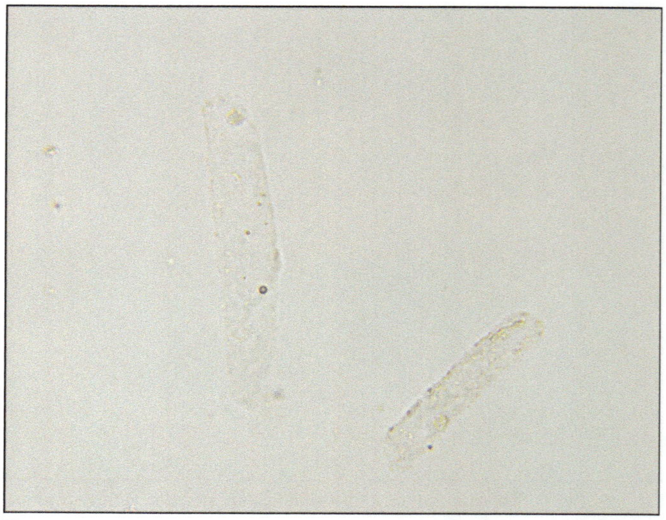

Figure 10.33 Two faint hyaline casts with parallel walls and rounded ends (unstained, 400× magnification).

Leukocyte casts indicate renal inflammation while erythrocyte casts indicate renal hemorrhage. Hemoglobin casts indicate intravascular hemolysis and subsequent hemoglobinuria (Figure 10.40). Myoglobin casts indicate severe muscle damage and subsequent myoglobinuria. Bilirubin casts could be associated with any cause of conjugated hyperbilirubinemia and bilirubinuria. Bacterial casts have been reported with bacterial pyelonephritis (Phelps *et al.*, 2022) and amorphous crystalline casts have been reported in a dog with massive uric acid crystalluria (Tvedten *et al.*, 2019).

Crystals

Some crystals are considered a normal finding in low or moderate numbers while other crystals are considered an abnormal finding at any number. Large numbers of any crystal are considered a risk for, but not definitive evidence of, urolith formation. Fresh urine is the best sample to evaluate for crystals. Refrigeration and storage can both enhance *in-vitro* crystal formation, making accurate interpretation difficult.

Magnesium ammonium phosphate (a.k.a. struvite or triple phosphate) crystals are colorless, variably sized crystals that are often rectangular in shape with a three-to-six-sided 'coffin-lid' appearance (Figure 10.41). In cats, struvite crystals may have fewer sides and lack the coffin-lid morphology (Figure 10.42). Struvite crystals are typically found in alkaline urine and can be seen in healthy animals and animals with uroliths. Struvite crystals can also form in patients with urinary tract infections if those infections raise the urine pH.

Calcium oxalate dihydrate crystals appear as colorless, variably sized squares with intersecting diagonal lines (envelope shape;

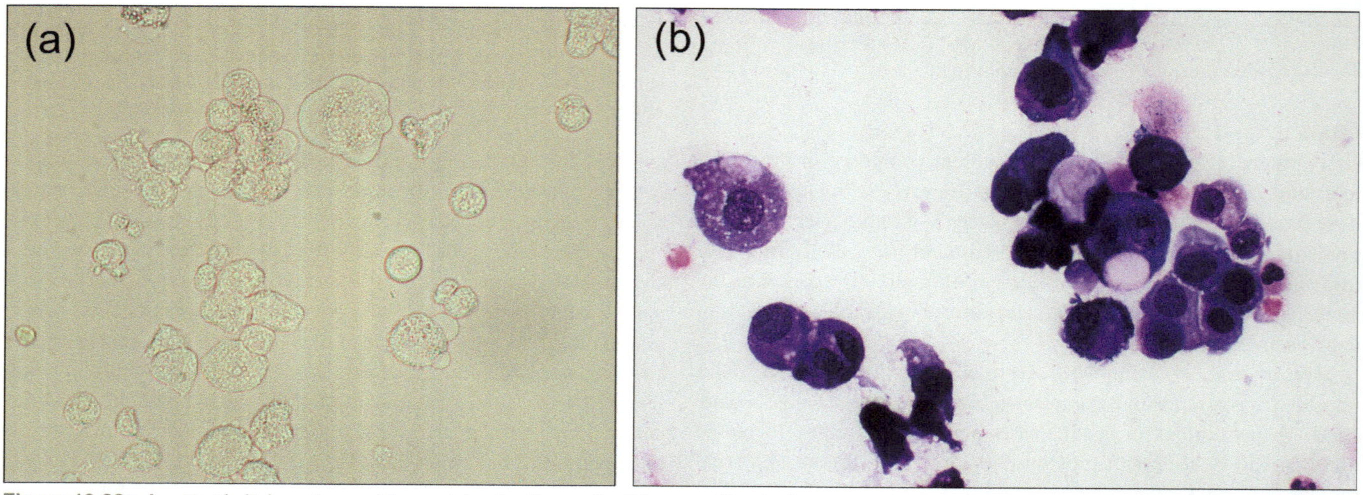

Figure 10.32a, b Urothelial carcinoma. The unstained sediment (a, 400× magnification) contains clusters of epithelial cells that vary in size and are suspicious for neoplasia, but additional cellular details are difficult to visualize. A stained specimen (b) further displays anisokaryosis and binucleation to support the diagnosis of neoplasia (modified Wright's, 500× magnification).

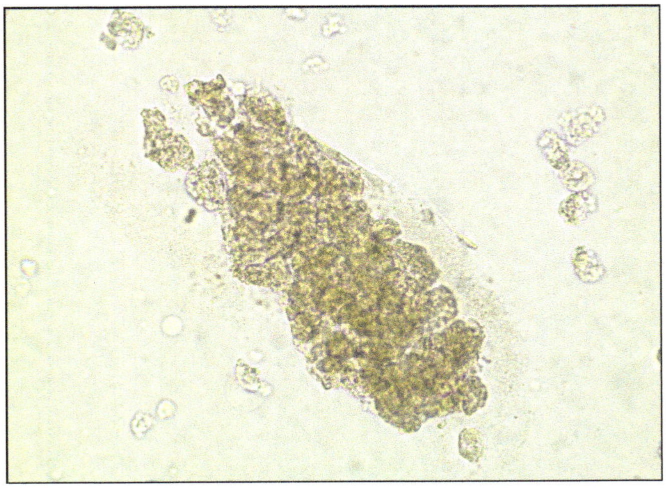

Figure 10.34 Cellular cast. Outlines of tubular epithelial cells are discernible in a cylindrical form (unstained, 400× magnification).

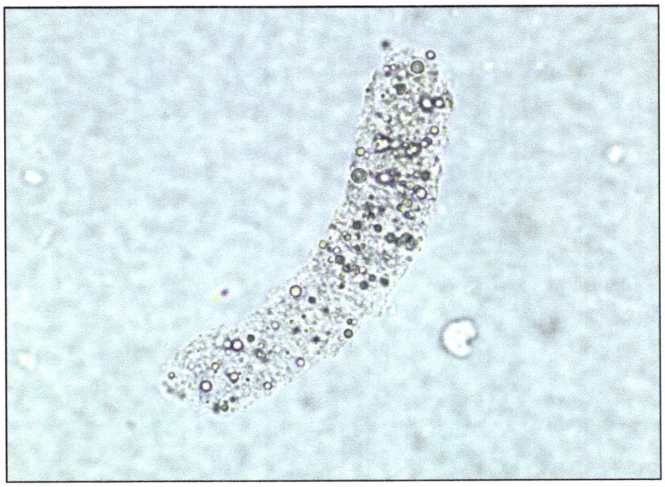

Figure 10.36 Granular cast. Variably sized fat droplets are adhered to the surface (unstained, 400× magnification).

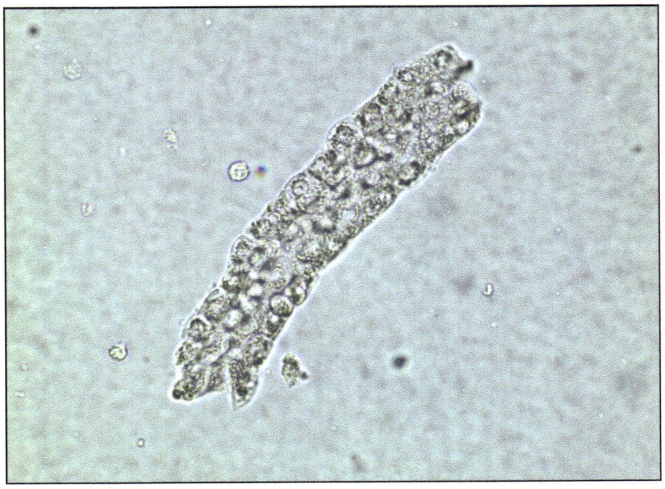

Figure 10.35 An intact fragment of renal tubule that sloughed during acute tubular injury (unstained, 400× magnification).

Figure 10.43). They are considered a normal finding in low to moderate numbers and can also form in vitro with storage. Larger numbers may be associated with uroliths.

Calcium oxalate monohydrate crystals vary in size and shape. Possible shapes include rectangles with pointed ends (picket fence), ovals (hemp seed), spindles, and dumb-bell forms (Figures 10.44, 10.45). Large numbers of these crystals are often observed with ethylene glycol toxicosis. The significance of lower numbers is uncertain; they may be a normal or non-specific finding, although even low numbers of the picket fence morphology should raise concern for ethylene glycol toxicity.

Bilirubin crystals are small golden-brown to red needles or granules that are often found in aggregates (Figure 10.46). They are occasionally associated with a fat droplet on one end, giving them a flashlight appearance. A few bilirubin crystals may be found in concentrated urine of normal dogs. Increased numbers indicate conjugated hyperbilirubinemia with subsequent bilirubinuria.

Ammonium biurate crystals are golden-brown spheres that often have irregular thorn-like protrusions (Figure 10.47). Smooth forms (lacking thorn-like protrusions) are less commonly seen (Figure 10.48). In most patients, ammonium biurate crystals are an abnormal finding indicating hepatic failure or portosystemic shunting. A few canine breeds, especially Dalmatians, form these crystals as part of a congenital defect in uric acid metabolism. These dogs may also form uric acid crystals, colorless blunted diamonds, or ovals that often aggregate into rosettes (Figure 10.49).

Cystine crystals are colorless, hexagonal crystals that often aggregate into layers (Figure 10.50). They are an abnormal finding seen in patients with acquired or congenital defects in urinary cysteine reabsorption.

Amorphous crystals are lightly colored, refractile granules that form variably sized aggregates (Figure 10.51). Such aggregates can be mistaken for colonies of cocci bacteria. Amorphous crystals will be more variable in size and more refractile than bacteria, but a stained slide of sediment should be examined if there is any doubt regarding identity. These crystals may be urates or phosphates in origin and their significance is often unclear.

Certain medications, including ampicillin, sulfadiazine, and ciprofloxacin, and radiographic contrast agents can precipitate in urine and produce variably shaped crystals (Figure 10.52). Fan-like aggregates and bundles of rectangular crystals have been reported, but the exact morphology of these crystals is hard to predict in veterinary medicine (Escobar & Grindem, 2010).

Other crystals are rarely reported in veterinary medicine and often have an uncertain significance. Calcium phosphate forms long, thin, colorless, rectangular crystals that often aggregate (Figure 10.53). Cholesterol crystals are flat, colorless rectangles (often with a notched corner). Xanthine crystals are morphologically identical to ammonium biurate crystals (Davis & Grindem, 2015). They are rarely reported and have a distinct association with allopurinol administration.

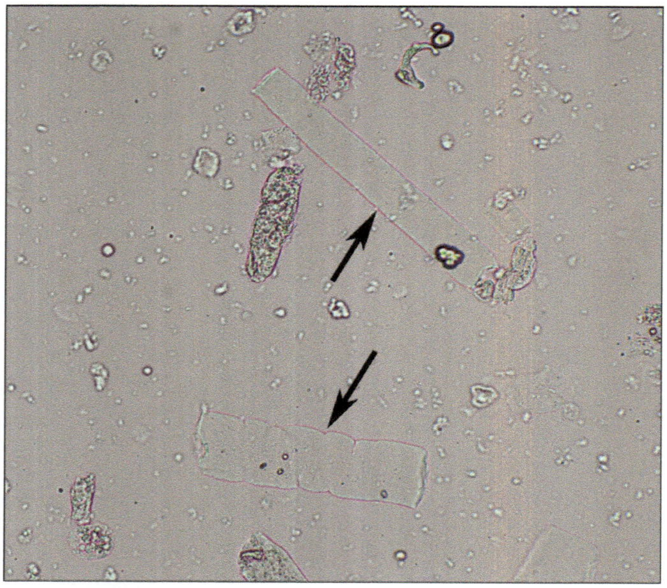

Figure 10.37 Two waxy casts (arrows) with blunt ends (unstained, 400× magnification).

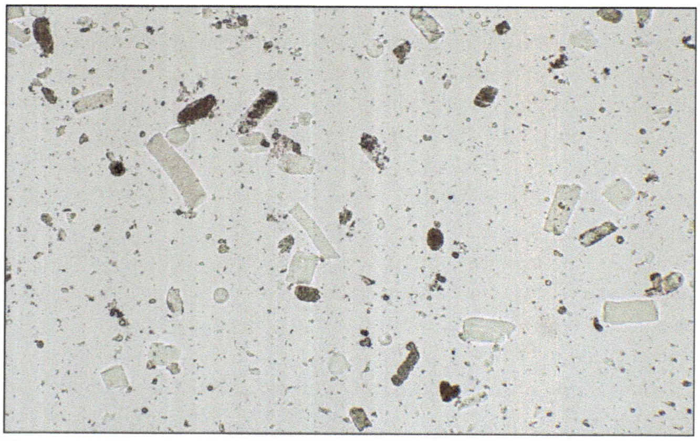

Figure 10.38 Multiple casts (granular, waxy, and mixed) in a dog with severe acute kidney injury (unstained, 100× magnification).

When crystals cannot be identified by routine sediment examination, dissolution studies may help better characterize their origin. One drop of urine sediment is mixed with one drop of a specific chemical, and the sediment is re-examined to determine whether the crystals are soluble or insoluble with that chemical. The process is repeated with additional chemicals and/or heat, and the combination of results can sometimes assist in crystal identification (Figure 10.54). However, dissolution results are only known for common crystals, and some discrepant results have been reported (Table 10.1) (Lee *et al.*, 2022; Thompson, 1981).

Organisms

Bacteria are small and refractile in appearance on wet mount preparations. Rods are the easiest form to identify, especially in large

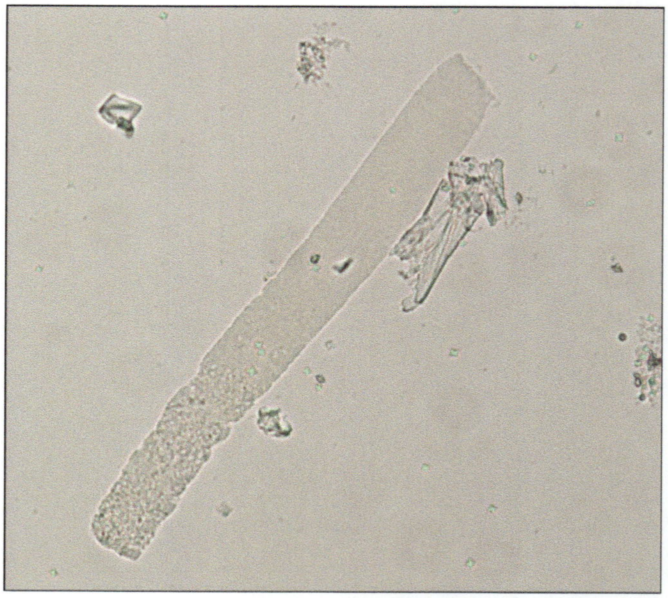

Figure 10.39 Mixed cast. Although most of the cast is homogeneous (waxy), there is some granularity visible at the lower end (unstained, 400× magnification). (Courtesy Kristen R. Friedrichs.)

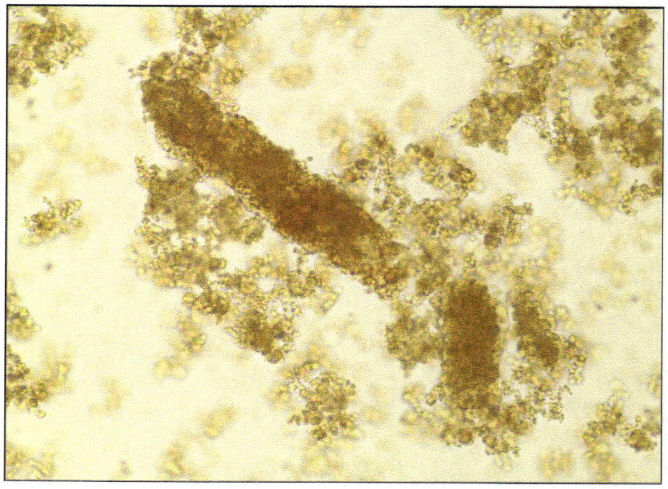

Figure 10.40 A fragmented hemoglobin cast from a dog with intravascular hemolysis (unstained, 400× magnification).

numbers, because their shape is unique (Figure 10.55). Fewer rods can be difficult to identify definitively. Cocci and small pleomorphic organisms are more difficult to identify overall and can be confused with debris or amorphous crystals (Myers *et al.*, 2022). If cocci or low numbers of rods are suspected, preparation of a dry slide stained with Gram, Wright's, or Diff-Quik stain is recommended for confirmation (Figures 10.56a, b and 10.57a, b). The significance of bacteriuria varies with the method of collection, type of bacteria, and host response. Free-catch samples are easily contaminated with a mixed population of mucocutaneous bacteria. Catheterized samples are less susceptible to contamination, but it can still occur. Bacteria in cystocentesis samples are considered pathologic unless accidental enterocentesis has

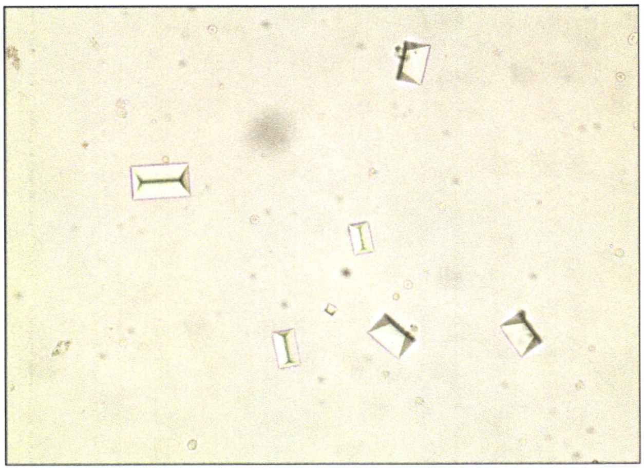

Figure 10.41 Struvite crystals in a dog with the classic 'coffin-lid' appearance (unstained, 250× magnification).

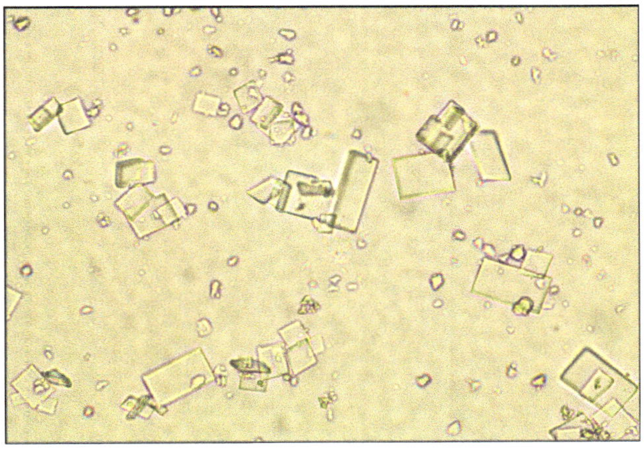

Figure 10.42 Struvite crystals in cats do not always have the classic 'coffin-lid' appearance (unstained, 400× magnification).

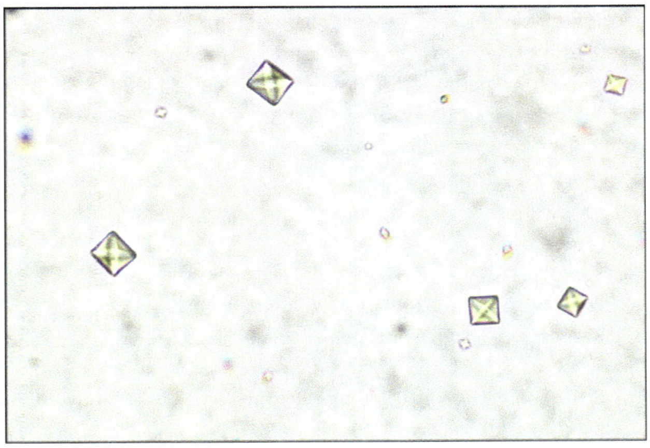

Figure 10.43 Calcium oxalate dihydrate crystals with intersecting diagonal lines (envelope shape) (unstained, 400× magnification).

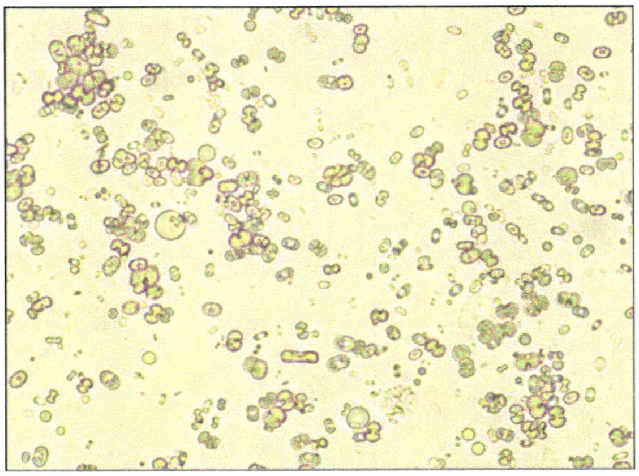

Figure 10.44 A low-power view demonstrating the pleomorphic nature of calcium oxalate monohydrate crystals (unstained, 400× magnification).

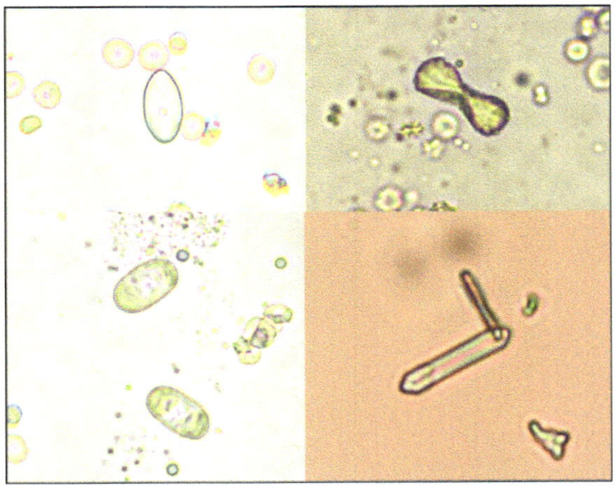

Figure 10.45 Closer view of the variable forms of calcium oxalate monohydrate crystals (unstained, 400× magnification). (Lower right courtesy Anne Barger.)

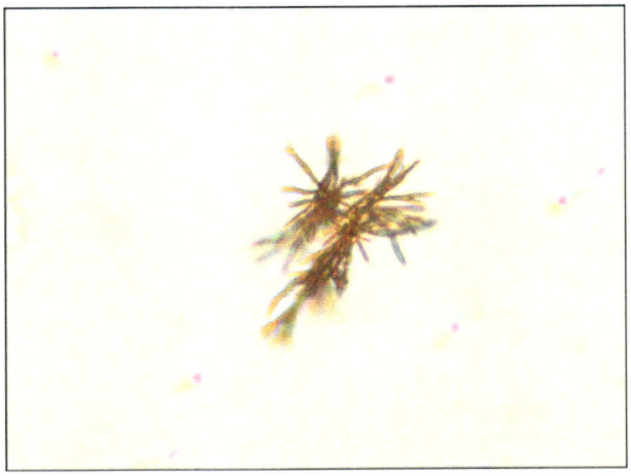

Figure 10.46 Small, red-brown, needle-shaped bilirubin crystals (unstained, 400× magnification).

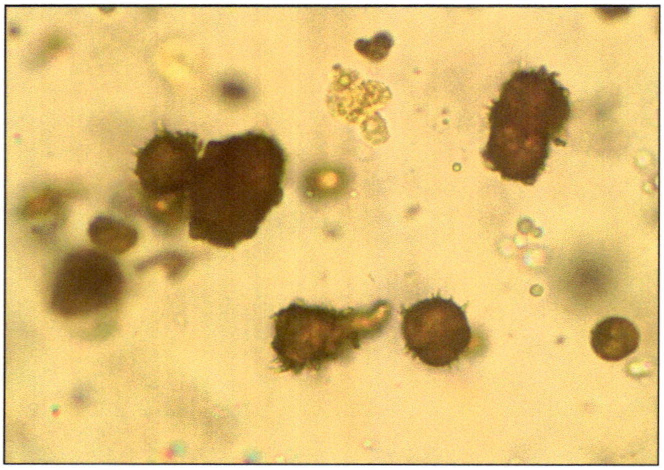

Figure 10.47 **Ammonium biurate crystals with irregular surface spicules (thorn-apple morphology) (unstained, 400× magnification).**

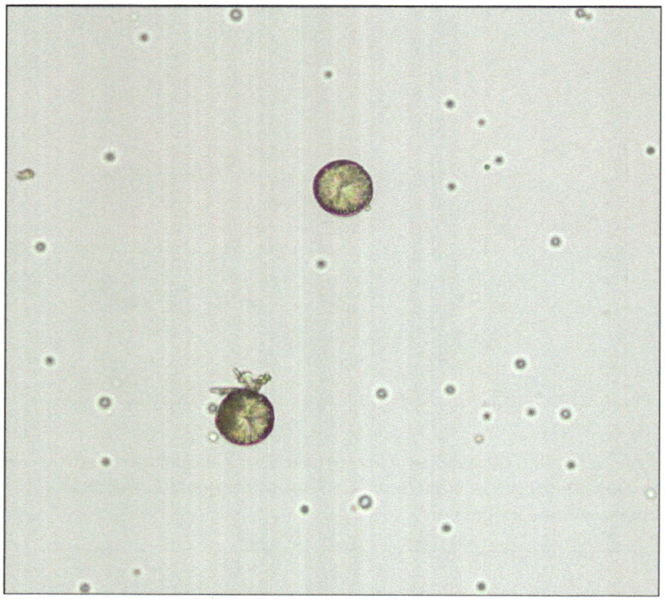

Figure 10.48 **Round ammonium biurate crystals with a predominantly smooth surface (unstained, 400× magnification).**

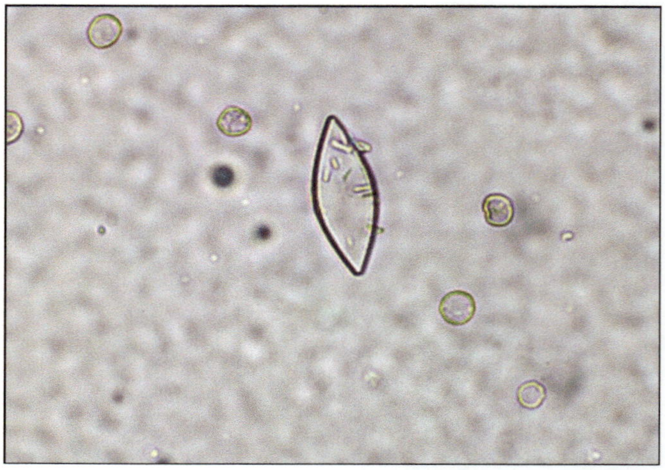

Figure 10.49 **Uric acid crystal with a pointed oval/blunted diamond shape (unstained, 400× magnification). (Courtesy Ruth A. Houseright.)**

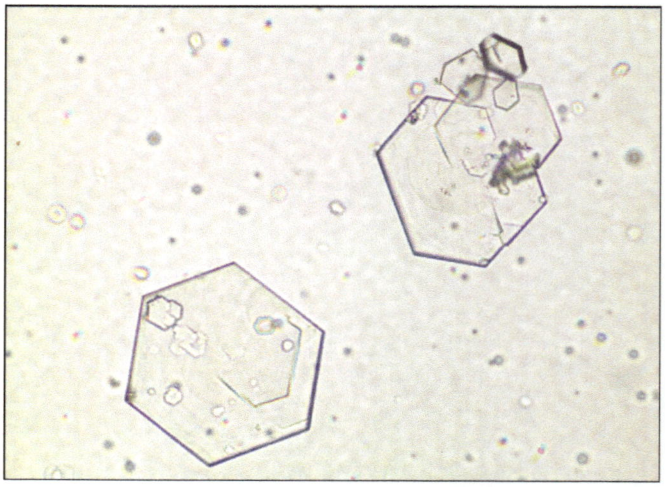

Figure 10.50 **Hexagonal cystine crystals (unstained, 400× magnification).**

occurred (Figures 10.58a, b). With all collection methods, true infection is expected to be accompanied by an inflammatory response, unless the patient is immunocompromised by neutropenia, steroids, chemotherapy, hyperadrenocorticism, or other disease.

Yeast and fungal organisms are rarely observed in urine samples. Yeast are round to oval structures that may display budding. Low numbers of certain yeasts (e.g. *Candida, Malassezia*) may be the result of contamination, especially if the sample was voided. Low numbers of other yeasts (e.g. *Blastomyces, Cryptococcus*) indicate true infection, often associated with systemic disease (Brandt & Blauvelt, 2010). High numbers of any yeast indicate true infection, which can arise as a primary disease or secondary to immunosuppression or chronic antibiotic usage, depending on the organism. Fungal hyphae are long branching structures with parallel walls and occasional septations (Figure 10.59). Any fungal hyphae in urine are presumed pathogenic, although environmental contamination should also be considered in voided samples.

Parasite eggs are rare findings in urine samples, including those from the kidney worm, *Dioctophyma renale* (Vieira *et al.*, 2011), and bladder worm, *Pearsonema plica* (Figure 10.60). Gastrointestinal parasite eggs may also be seen in urine contaminated with feces.

Other elements

Lipid droplets are small, variably sized, and highly refractile (Figure 10.61). They must be differentiated from erythrocytes, which will be uniform in size. In addition, lipid droplets float under the coverslip and will often focus on a different plane than other urine elements. Mucus often comes in a cylindrical form and can easily be mistaken for a cast. Whereas casts will be uniform in width, mucus threads will vary in width and often have an irregular shape with tapered

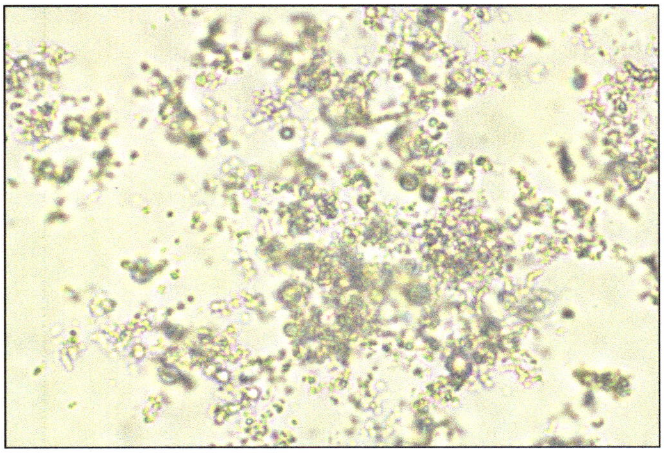

Figure 10.51 An aggregate of amorphous crystals. Their high refractility helps distinguish them from debris and bacteria (unstained, 400× magnification).

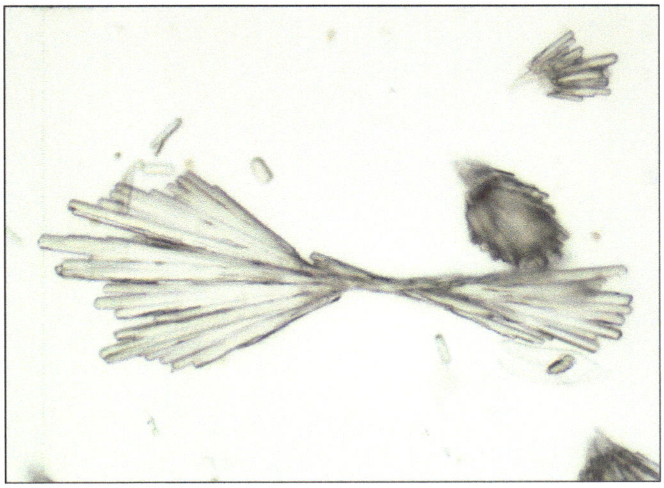

Figure 10.52 Fan-like aggregates of crystals in a dog receiving multiple antibiotics (unstained, 400× magnification).

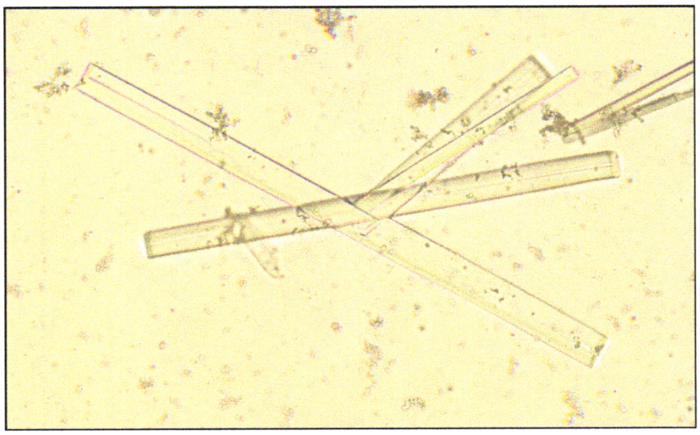

Figure 10.53 Suspect calcium phosphate crystals (unstained, 400× magnification).

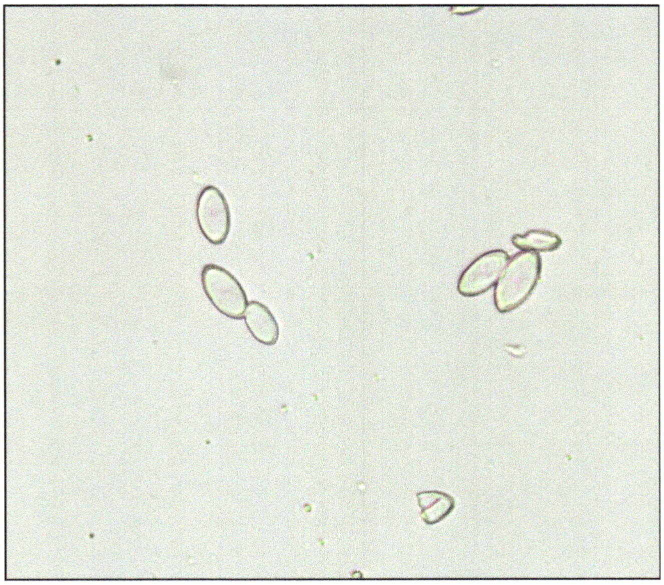

Figure 10.54 Oval (hemp seed) crystals in a cat. Morphology is suggestive of calcium oxalate monohydrate but difficult to confirm in isolation. Dissolution studies revealed the crystals to be soluble in hydrochloric acid, insoluble in acetic acid, and partially soluble in sodium hydroxide, results further consistent with a calcium oxalate origin (unstained, 400× magnification).

ends (Figure 10.62). Fibers can also be mistaken for casts but are typically larger and contain an internal structure suggesting a processed origin (Figure 10.63). Glove powder (Figure 10.64) contains corn starch, which could be mistaken for a urinary crystal. Glass shards (from slides or coverslips) are irregular refractile fragments that could also be mistaken for a crystal but are more variable in appearance (Figure 10.65). Multiple types of pollen may be encountered in urine sediment. They are variable in size and shape but typically quite large and golden-brown (Figure 10.66). Sperm are easy to identify, with a characteristic appearance including a pointed head and long tail (Figure 10.67).

URETERS AND URETHRA

The ureters are lined by urothelium, making urothelial carcinoma a possible but very rare diagnosis in this location. Ureteral fibroepithelial polyps have also rarely been reported (Etzioni *et al.*, 2020). The urethra is lined by urothelium proximally and squamous epithelium distally. Urethral UC (sometimes extending from the bladder), squamous cell carcinoma, and leiomyomas have been reported (Knapp & McMillan, 2010) with morphologies described earlier in this chapter and elsewhere in this textbook (Figure 10.68). Urethritis has also been reported, both in isolation and associated with cystitis (Hostutler *et al.*, 2004).

Table 10.1 Dissolution results for common crystals

CRYSTAL	SOLUBLE WITH	INSOLUBLE WITH	DISCREPANT RESULTS	NOTES
Calcium oxalate	HCl	AA	NaOH, heat	
Calcium carbonate	HCl, AA	NaOH, heat		CO_2 gas produced when dissolving with HCl or AA
Triple phosphate	HCl, AA	NaOH, heat		
Calcium phosphate	HCl, AA	NaOH, heat		
Amorphous phosphate	HCl, AA	NaOH, heat		
Amorphous urate	NaOH, heat		HCl, AA	May dissolve in HCl or AA to produce uric acid
Ammonium biurate	HCl, AA, NaOH, heat			Ammonia gas produced when dissolved with NaOH. HCl or AA dissolve crystals slowly to form uric acid
Uric acid	NaOH	HCl, AA	Heat	
Cystine	NaOH, HCl	AA, heat		
Bilirubin	HCl, AA, NaOH	Heat		

HCl = 30% hydrochloric acid, AA = 30% acetic acid, NaOH = 10% sodium hydroxide, heat = 60° Celsius.

Note: 10% potassium hydroxide (KOH) can be substituted for NaOH with equivalent results.

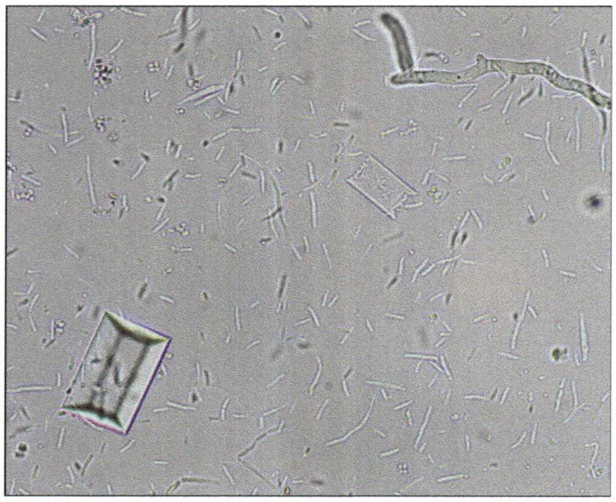

Figure 10.55 Large numbers of bacterial rods can usually be identified in wet preparations. Also present is a section of fungal hyphae (upper right) and a single struvite crystal (lower left) (unstained, 500× magnification).

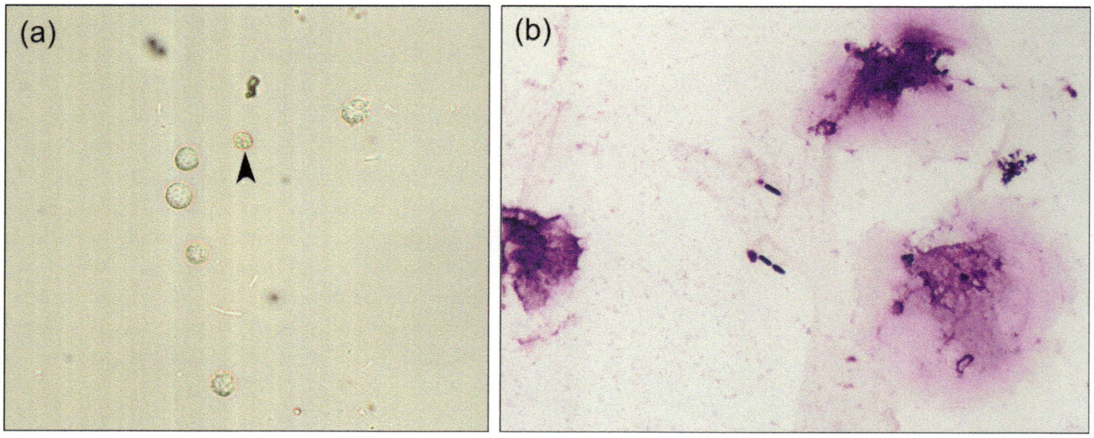

Figure 10.56a, b (a) A few leukocytes, one crenated erythrocyte (arrowhead) and low numbers of rod bacteria (unstained, 400× magnification). (b) A stained specimen confirms the rod bacteria (modified Wright's, 500× magnification).

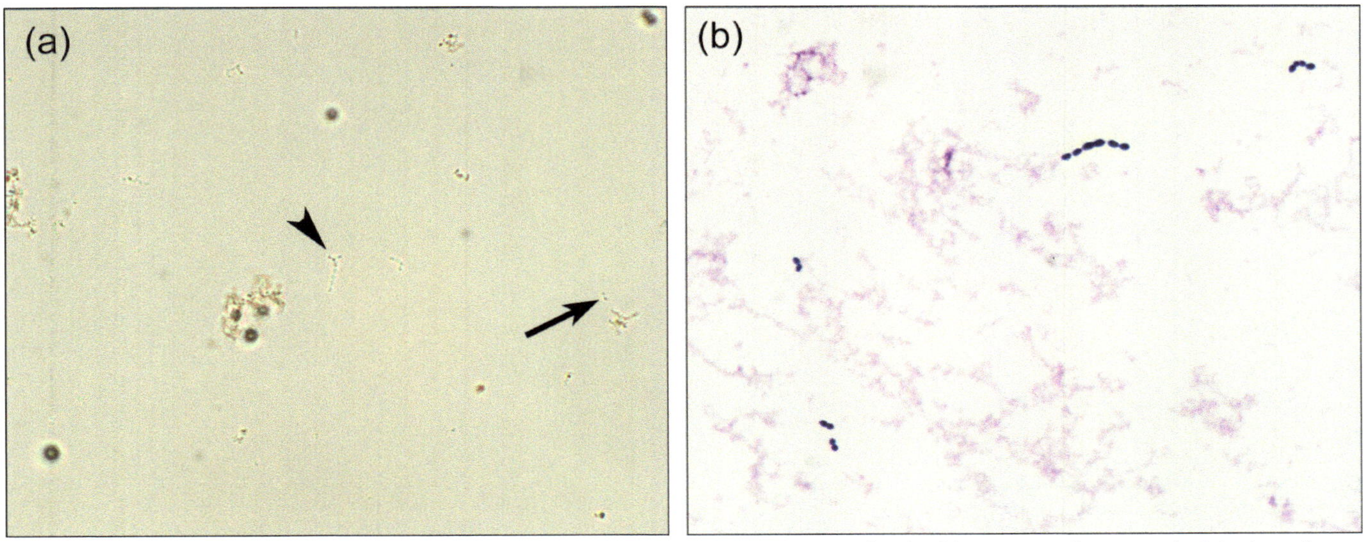

Figures 10.57a, b (a) Bacterial cocci can be difficult to identify in wet preparations, being mistaken for debris or amorphous crystals. Pairs (arrow) and chains (arrowhead) of organisms can help with identification (unstained, 400× magnification). (b) Modified Wright's stain of the same specimen, confirming the presence of cocci (1,000× magnification).

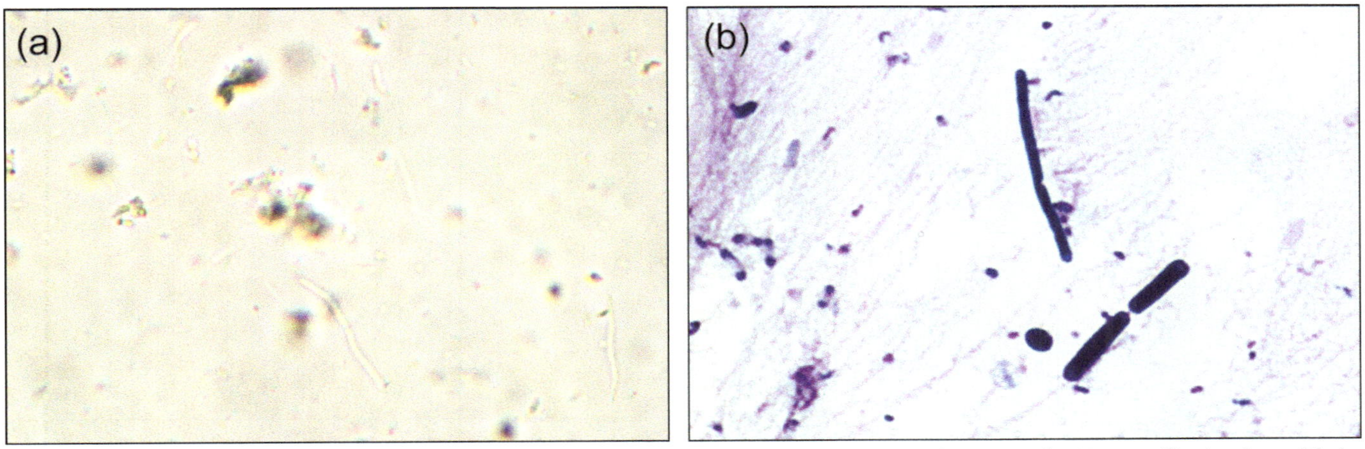

Figures 10.58a, b Fecal contamination. A mixed population of bacteria with no inflammatory reaction (a: unstained, 400× magnification; b: modified Wright's, 1,000× magnification).

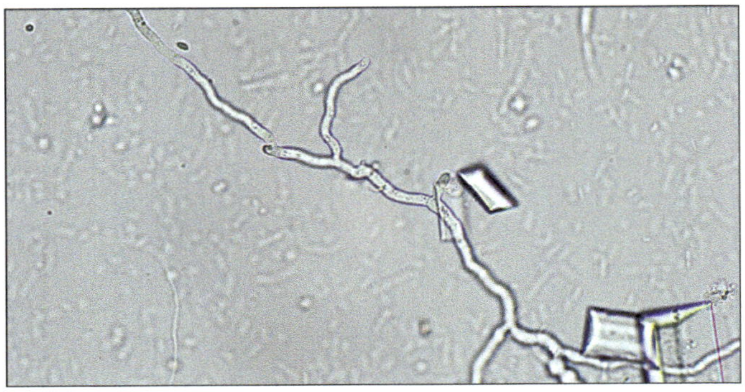

Figure 10.59 Branching fungal hyphae (unstained, 500× magnification).

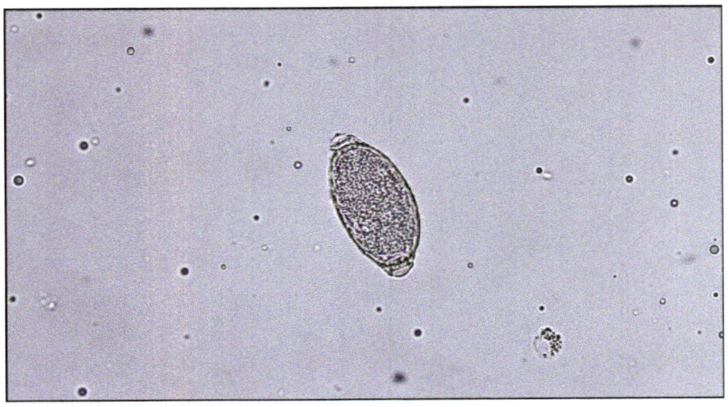

Figure 10.60 *Pearsonema plica* egg (unstained, 500× magnification).

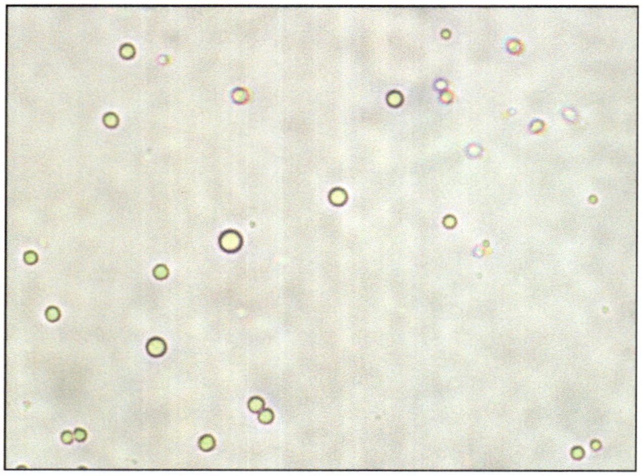

Figure 10.61 Variably sized and highly refractive lipid droplets (unstained, 400× magnification).

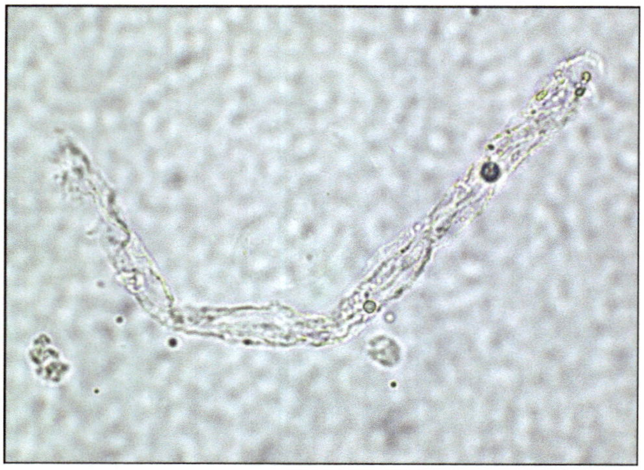

Figure 10.62 Mucus. The irregular borders help differentiate mucus threads from casts (unstained, 400× magnification).

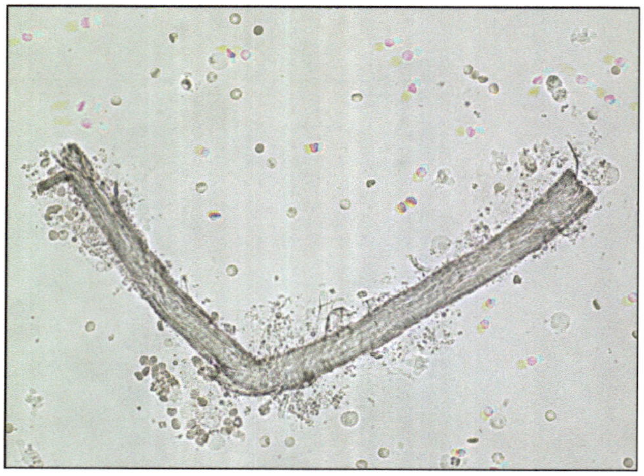

Figure 10.63 A large textile fiber (unstained, 200× magnification).

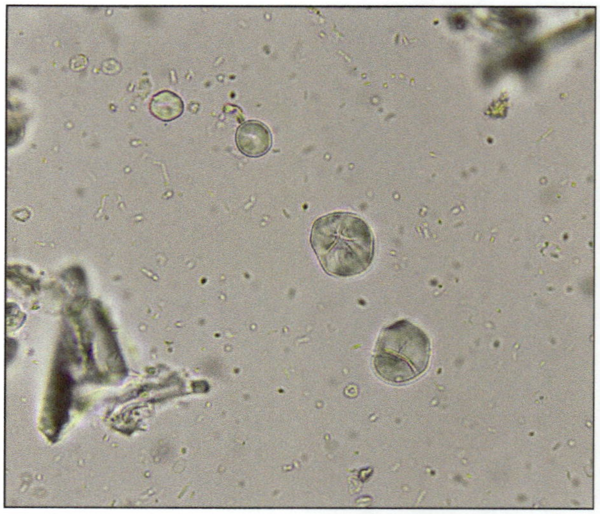

Figure 10.64 Starch (glove powder) granules (unstained, 400× magnification).

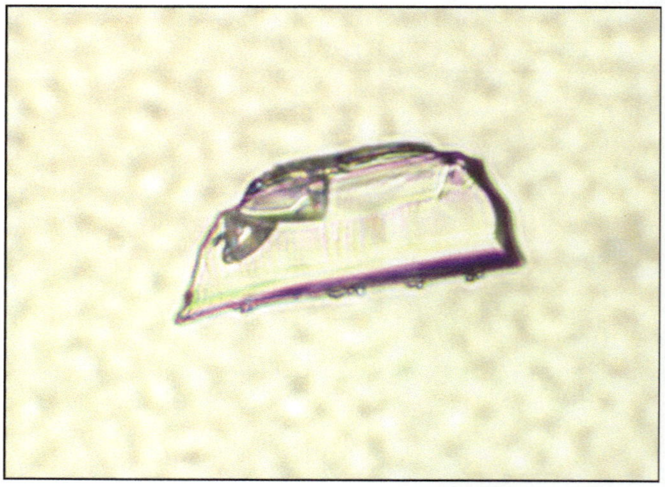

Figure 10.65 Glass shard. The irregular shape helps differentiate this from a urinary crystal (unstained, 400× magnification).

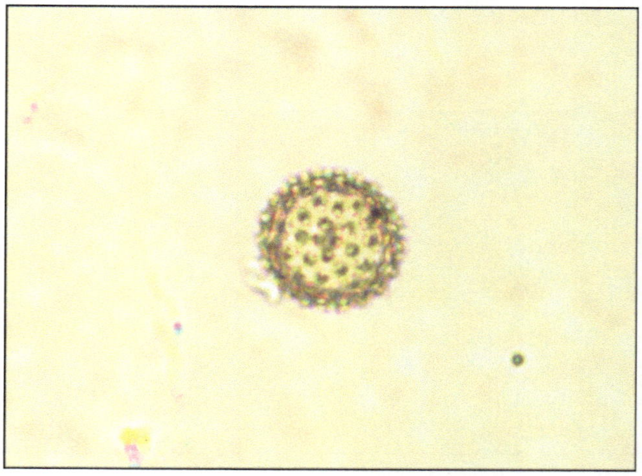

Figure 10.66 A spiculated pollen granule (unstained, 400× magnification).

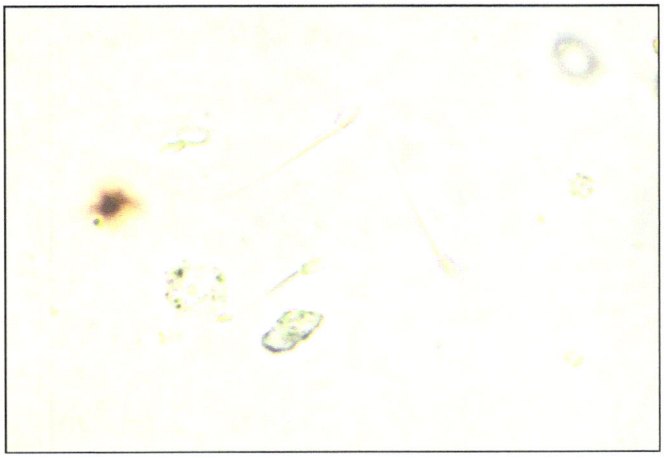

Figure 10.67 Sperm from the urinalysis of an intact male dog (unstained, 400× magnification).

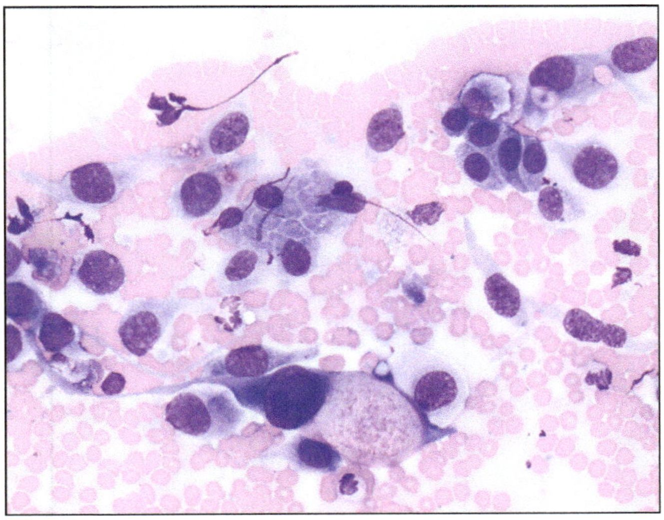

Figure 10.68 Urothelial carcinoma originating in the urethra and extending into the vagina of a female dog. A pleomorphic population of neoplastic cells varies from cuboidal to spindle in shape. Multiple eosinophilic globules (Melamed-Wolinska bodies) help suggest a urothelial origin (modified Wright's, 500× magnification).

CASES

CASE 1

Signalment/history

A 9-year-old spayed female domestic shorthair cat presents for a 1-week history of lethargy and progressive anorexia. The cat is dehydrated and has small ulcerations below her tongue. Blood work reveals azotemia with marked increases in both urea nitrogen and creatinine. An abdominal ultrasound shows bilaterally enlarged kidneys. FNAs are obtained from both kidneys (Figures 10.69a, b, representative of both aspirates).

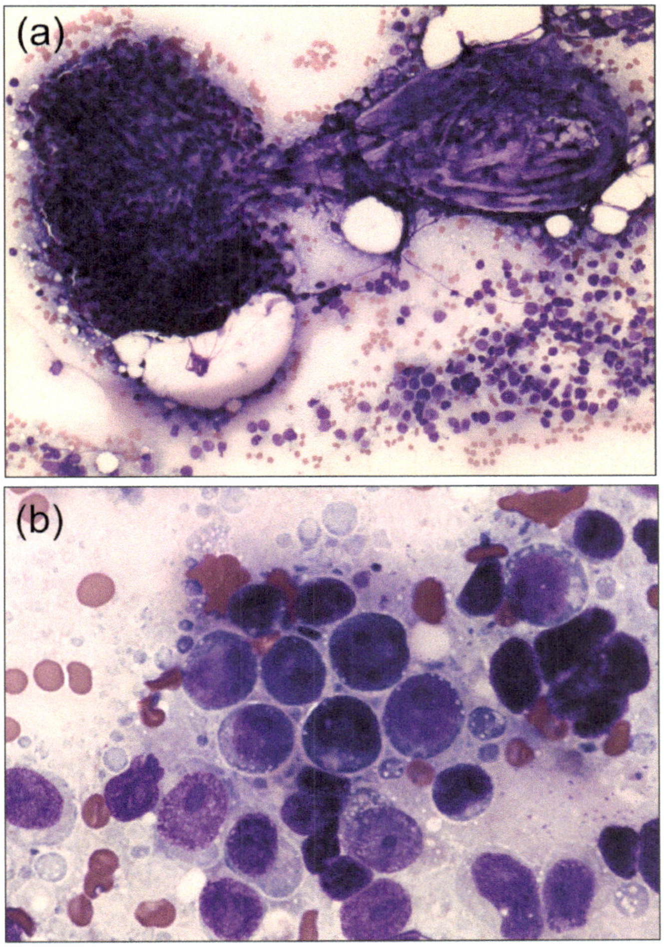

Figures 10.69a, b (a) 200× magnification view of the renal aspirate. (b) 600× magnification view of a highly cellular region (Diff-Quik®).

Cytology

A single glomerulus is present, confirming the aspirate is renal in origin. No other renal tissue is observed. Instead, the high cellularity is attributed to a proliferation of large lymphocytes with deeply basophilic cytoplasm, finely stippled chromatin, and multiple nucleoli.

Diagnosis

Bilateral renal lymphoma causing acute kidney injury.

CASES 2 AND 3 (compare and contrast)

Signalment/history

- Case 2. A 12-year-old neutered male Miniature Pinscher presents for occasional straining to urinate. An abdominal ultrasound reveals a large mass originating in the trigone region of the

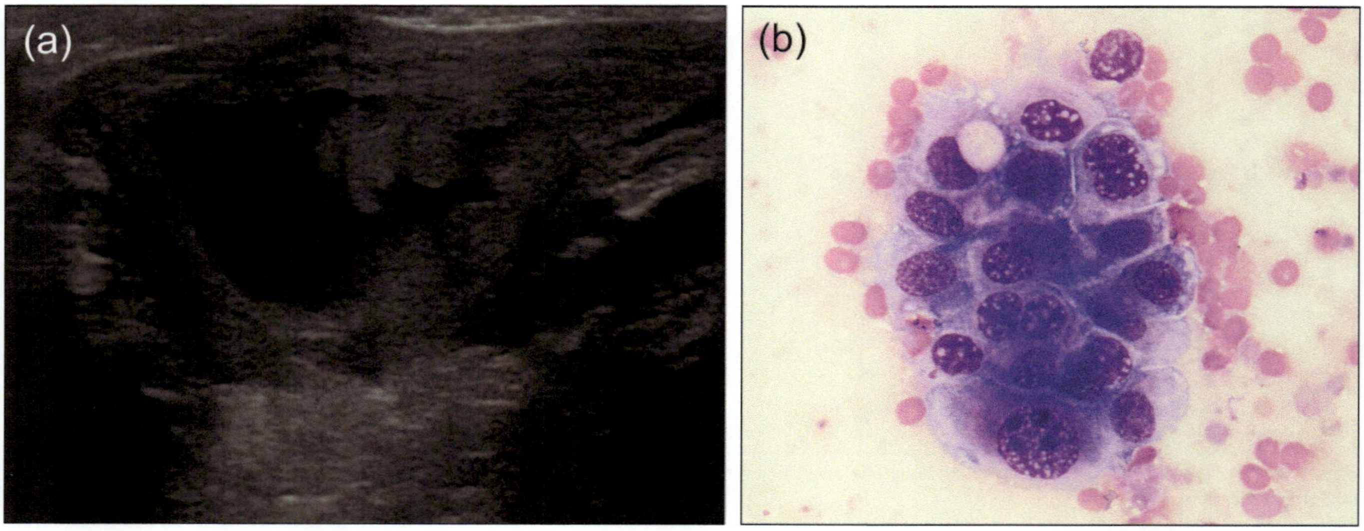

Figures 10.70a, b (a) Ultrasound of the bladder mass (trigone region). (b) A representative cluster of urothelial cells recovered via traumatic catheterization (modified Wright's, 600× magnification).

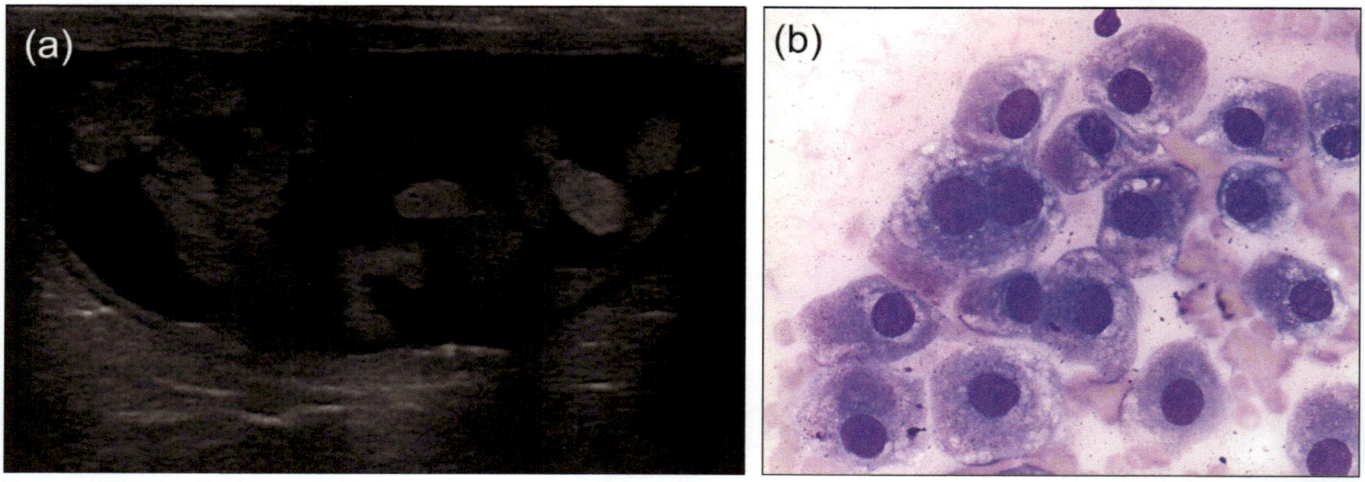

Figures 10.71a, b (a) Ultrasound of the bladder mass (cranioventral region) (b) A representative cluster of urothelial cells recovered via traumatic catheterization (modified Wright's, 600× magnification).

bladder (Figure 10.70a). A traumatic catheterization of the mass is performed (Figure 10.70b).

- Case 3. A 10-year-old neutered male Yorkshire Terrier presents for sporadically urinating blood. An abdominal ultrasound reveals a papillary mass in the cranioventral region of the bladder (Figure 10.71a). Several small bladder stones are also seen on ultrasound. A traumatic catheterization of the mass is performed (Figure 10.71b).

Cytology

- The cells from Case 2 display pleomorphism suggestive of urothelial carcinoma: moderate anisocytosis, moderate anisokaryosis, increased and variable N:C ratios, frequent binucleation, and multiple nucleoli.
- The cells from Case 3 display mild anisocytosis and occasional binucleation with monomorphic nuclei, changes suggestive of hyperplastic urothelial cells, with uroliths the presumed predisposing factor. Both cases have very suggestive ultrasonographic and cytologic findings, but histopathology and/or BRAF testing is recommended because cytology results are not definitive.

Diagnosis

- Case 2. Urothelial carcinoma (confirmed by cytoscopic biopsy).
- Case 3. Polypoid cystitis (confirmed by cystotomy, urolith removal, and excisional biopsy).

CASE 4

Signalment/history

An 8-month-old female Yorkshire Terrier is referred for surgical correction of a portosystemic shunt. The shunt was diagnosed 2 months earlier based on clinical signs and blood work abnormalities (decreased albumin and urea nitrogen, increased bile acids). At this visit, the owner reports a new problem of inappropriate urination. A urine sample is collected by cystocentesis (Figure 10.72).

Microscopy

A single intact ammonium biurate crystal is present, consistent with this patient's portosystemic shunt. In addition, there are large numbers of leukocytes and rare erythrocytes. There are many small, variably shaped structures that are difficult to identify. They may be bacteria, but they could also be fragments of crystals. A single large struvite crystal is also present.

Additional test results

Gram staining reveals low numbers of bacterial cocci, and urine culture identifies a *Staphylococcus* sp. The urine pH is high (8.0). The majority of the small, variably shaped structures from the wet mount do not stain with Wright's or Gram stain, consistent with crystal fragments.

Diagnosis

(1) Urinary tract infection with urease-producing *Staphylococcus* sp. and secondary struvite crystal formation. (2) Ammonium biurate crystals, consistent with portosystemic shunt.

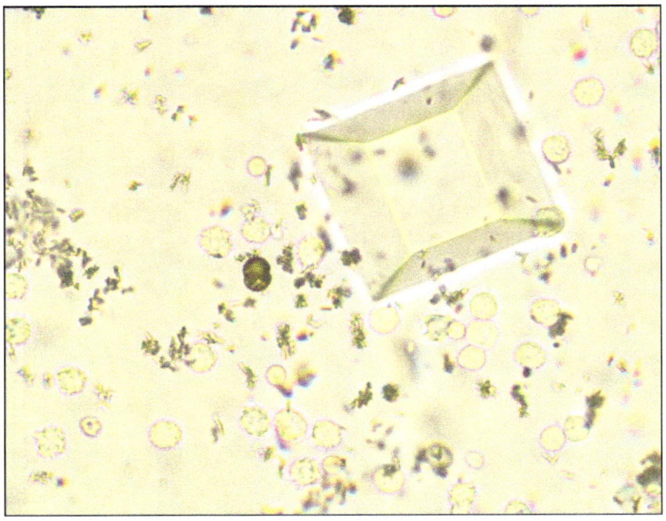

Figure 10.72 Wet-mount preparation of the urine sediment (unstained, 400× magnification).

CASE 5

Signalment/history

An 8-year-old female spayed domestic shorthair cat presents with a history of recurrent urinary tract infections, presumed the result of lifelong urinary and fecal incontinence secondary to neurologic injury. The patient has been treated with multiple courses of various antibiotics in the past. Her most recent urine culture, performed one month prior to this visit, revealed large numbers of multi-drug resistant *Enterococcus faecium*. A cytocentesis urine sample is collected as follow-up to that infection (Figure 10.73).

Microscopy

Numerous round to oval refractile structures are noted, along with rare leukocytes. Differentials for the structures include erythrocytes, fat droplets, and yeast organisms. Small narrow-based buds are occasionally noted, most consistent with yeast.

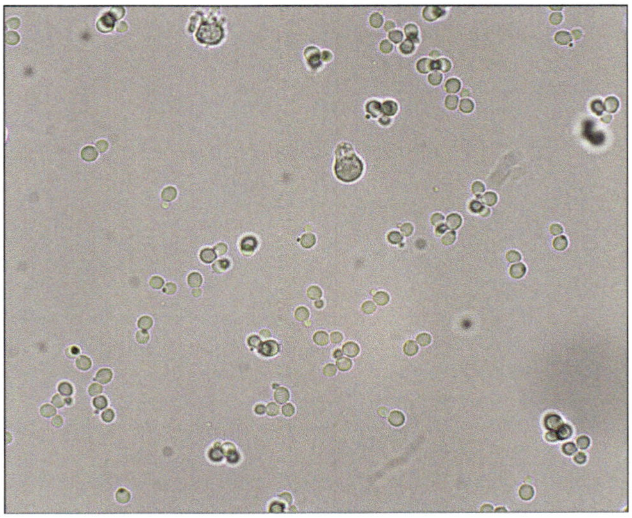

Figure 10.73 Wet-mount preparation of the urine sediment (unstained, 500× magnification).

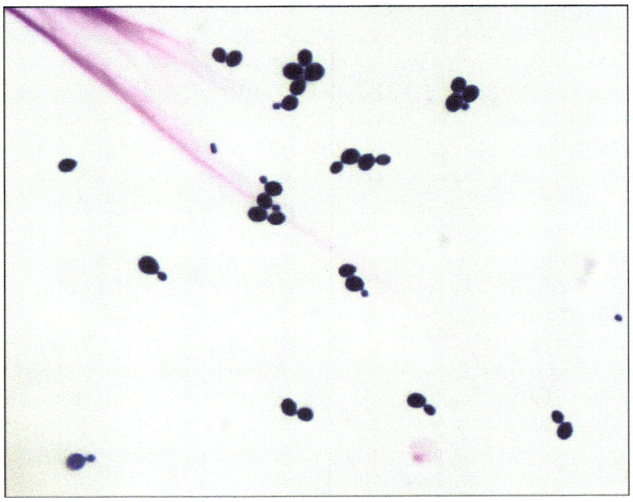

Figure 10.74 Line preparation of urine sediment. Deeply basophilic round to oval yeast organisms display occasional narrow-based budding (modified Wright's, 1,000× magnification).

Additional test results

A line preparation of urine sediment is prepared, dried, and stained with Wright's stain (Figure 10.74). The structures stain deeply basophilic, inconsistent with erythrocytes (which would stain lightly eosinophilic) or fat droplets (which would not stain). Instead, this staining is consistent with a yeast organism, confirming the initial sediment exam suspicion. Culture reveals a pure population of *Candida glabrata*.

Diagnosis

Candida infection. Very low numbers of *Candida* organisms may represent mucocutaneous contamination in voided samples, but large numbers are a pathologic finding. The yeast infection in this patient has likely arisen secondary to the chronic antibiotic usage, although the neurologic injury and incontinence may also have predisposed to this infection. The inflammatory reaction is minimal, which could indicate underlying immunosuppression.

REFERENCES

Affolter V.K., Moore P.F. (2002) Localized and disseminated histiocytic sarcoma of dendritic cell origin in dogs. *Vet Pathol 39*:74–83.

Arya P., Khalbuss W.E., Monaco S.E. (2011) Melamed-Wolinska bodies. *Diagnostic Cytopathology 40*(2):150–151.

Baskin G., de Paoli A. (1977) Primary renal neoplasms of the dog. *Vet Pathol 14*:591–605.

Brandt L.E., Blauvelt M.M. (2010) What is your diagnosis? Urine sediment from a southern California cat with weight loss. *Vet Clin Pathol 39*:517–518.

Bryan J.N., Henry C.J., Turnquist S.E. et al. (2006) Primary renal neoplasia of dogs. *J Vet Intern Med 20*:1155–1160.

Davis K.U., Grindem C.B. (2015) What is your diagnosis? Urine crystals from a dog. *Vet Clin Pathol 44*:331–332.

de Lorenzi D., Baroni M., Mandara M.T. (2007) A true "triphasic" pattern: Thoracolumbar spinal tumor in a young dog. *Vet Clin Pathol 36*:200–203.

Escobar C., Grindem C.B. (2010) What is your diagnosis? Urine crystals in a dog. *Vet Clin Pathol 39*:510–514.

Etzioni A.L., Raskin R.E., Alstine W.G., Yu J. (2020) The cytologic and histologic diagnosis of ureteral fibroepithelial polyp in a dog. *Vet Clin Pathol 49*:646–651.

Garner B., Zimmerman S., Brown H.M. (2011) Unique urinalysis. *Vet Clin Pathol 40*:279.

Giordano A., Paltrinieri S., Bertazzolo W. et al. (2005) Sensitivity of tru-cut and fine-needle aspiration biopsies of liver and kidney for diagnosis of feline infectious peritonitis. *Vet Clin Pathol 34*:368–374.

Grassinger J.M., Aupperle-Lellbach H., Erhard H. et al. (2019) Detection of BRAF mutation in canine prostatic diseases. *Tierarztl Prax Ausg K Kleintiere Heimtiere 47*:313–320.

Griffin M.A., Culp W.T., Giuffrida M.A. et al. (2019) Lower urinary tract transitional cell carcinoma in cats: Clinical findings, treatments, and outcomes in 118 cases. *J Vet Intern Med 34*:274–282.

Gunn-Christie R.G., Flatland B., Friedrichs K.R. et al. (2012) ASVCP quality assurance guidelines: Control of preanalytical, analytical, and postanalytical factors for urinalysis, cytology, and clinical chemistry in veterinary laboratories. *Vet Clin Pathol 41*:18–26.

Hahn K.A., McGavin M.D., Adams W.H. (1997) Bilateral renal metastases of nasal chondrosarcoma in a dog. *Vet Pathol 34*:352–355.

Henry C. (1999) Primary renal tumours in cats: 19 cases (1992–1998). *J Feline Med Surg 1*:165–170.

Higuchi T., Burcham G.N., Childress M.O. et al. (2010) Characterization and treatment of urothelial cell carcinoma of the abdominal wall in dogs: 24 cases (1985–2010). *J Am Vet Med Assoc 242*:499–506.

Hostutler R.A., Chew D.J., Eaton K.A. et al. (2004) Cystoscopic appearance of proliferative urethritis in 2 dogs before and after treatment. *J Vet Intern Med 18*:110–116.

Knapp D.W., McMillan S.K. (2010) Tumors of the urinary system. In: *Small Animal Clinical Oncology*, 5th edn. (eds. S.J. Withrow, D.M. Vail, R.L. Page) Elsevier, St. Louis, pp. 572–582.

Lee A-J., Yoo E.-H., Bae Y.-C. et al. (2022) Differential identification of urine crystals with morphologic characteristics and solubility test. *J Clin Lab Anal 36*:e24707.

Marin J., Ferris K., Gruber E. (2023) What is your diagnosis? Perineal swelling in a dog. *Vet Clin Pathol*:1–3.

Martinez I., Matton J.S., Eaton K.A. et al. (2003) Polypoid cystitis in 17 dogs (1978–2001). *J Vet Intern Med 17*:499–509.

Meuten D.J. (2002) Tumors of the urinary system. In: *Tumors in Domestic Animals*, 4th edn. (ed. D.J. Meuten) Iowa State Press, Ames, pp. 509–546.

Mochizuki H., Shapiro S.G., Breen M. (2015) Detection of BRAF mutation in urine DNA as a molecular diagnostic for canine urothelial and prostatic carcinoma. *PLoS ONE 10*(*12*):e0144170.

Mooney S., Hayes A., Matus R. et al. (1987) Renal lymphoma in cats: 28 cases (1977–1984). *J Am Vet Med Assoc 191*:1473–1477.

Munday J.S., Egins J., Selcer B.A. et al. (2004) Renal osteosarcoma in a dog. *J Small Anim Pract 45*:618–622.

Myers J.M., Schexnayder M.M., Mekuria Z. et al. (2022) What is your diagnosis? Urine sediment from a dog. *Vet Clin Pathol*:1–3.

Neel J., Dean G.A. (2000) A mass in the spinal column of a dog. *Vet Clin Pathol 29*:87–89.

Newman S.J., Langston C.E., Scase T.J. (2003) Cryptococcal pyelonephritis in a dog. *J Am Vet Med Assoc 222*:180–183.

Nyland T.G., Wallack S.T., Wisner E.R. (2002) Needle-track implantation following US-guided fine-needle aspiration biopsy of urothelial cell carcinoma of the bladder, urethra, and prostate. *Vet Radiol Ultrasound 43*:50–53.

Osborne C.A., Stevens J.B. (1999) Urine sediment. In: *Urinalysis: A Clinical Guide to Compassionate Patient Care* (eds. C.A. Osborne, J.B. Stevens) Bayer, Shawnee Mission, pp. 125–150.

Phelps S.M., Gorman E., Johns J. (2022) What is your diagnosis? Urinalysis from a dog. *Vet Clin Pathol 51*:595–597.

Pierini A., Criscuolo M.A., Bonfanti U. et al. (2022) Usefulness of squash preparation cytology in the diagnosis of canine urinary bladder carcinomas. *Vet Clin Pathol 51*:498–506.

Pressler B.M., Gookin J.L., Sykes J.E. et al. (2005) Urinary tract manifestations of protothecosis in dogs. *J Vet Intern Med 19*:115–119.

Swenson C.L., Boisvert A.M., Gibbons-Burgener S.N. et al. (2011) Evaluation of modified Wright-staining of dried urinary sediment as a method for accurate detection of bacteriuria in cats. *Vet Clin Pathol 40*:256–264.

Thompson A. (1981) Crystalluria. In: *Urine Sediment: A Textbook Atlas* (ed. M.H. Haber) American Society of Clinical Pathologists, Chicago, pp. 29–32.

Tvedten H., Lilliehook I., Ronnberg H. et al. (2019) Massive uric acid crystalluria and cylinduria in a dog after l-asparaginase treatment for lymphoma. *Vet Clin Pathol 48*:425–428.

Vieira A.B., Rodrigues M.D.R., de Castro T. et al. (2011) What is your diagnosis? Unexpected finding in sedimented urine from a dog. *Vet Clin Pathol 40*:403–404.

Witschen P.M., Sharkey L., Seelig D.M. et al. (2020) Diagnosis of canine renal lymphoma by cytology and flow cytometry of the urine. *Vet Clin Pathol 49*:137–142.

CHAPTER 11

CYTOLOGY OF THE REPRODUCTIVE SYSTEM

Amy L. MacNeill

INTRODUCTION

Cytologic evaluation of the female and male reproductive systems is more commonly performed in dogs than cats. Typically, vaginal cytology and semen samples are analyzed in healthy animals for breeding purposes. Cytology of other reproductive organs is more likely to occur if disease is suspected. With the exception of the prostate and penis, surgical removal of the diseased reproductive organ is almost always the treatment of choice. In these cases, analysis of impression smears from the surgically excised tissue can be very beneficial in reaching a quick, definitive diagnosis.

FEMALE REPRODUCTIVE SYSTEM

CYTOLOGY OF THE VULVA AND VAGINA

Introduction

In the dog, vaginal cytology is frequently used to optimize timing for breeding and improve pregnancy rates (England, 1992). Collection of vaginal cytology can be performed daily beginning 3–5 days after a bloody vaginal discharge is detected. When vaginal cytology is indicative of estrus, dogs are encouraged to mate within 48 hours. A recent study of the reliability of vaginal cytology results indicated some inaccuracy, even when an experienced person evaluated the samples. In this study, 4 people reviewed 32 vaginal cytology samples; their cytologic interpretations correlated with histologic changes in the uterus in 20–40% of proestrus, 25–50% of estrus, 60–100% of early diestrus, 33–67% of late diestrus, and 0–100% of anestrus samples (Moxon *et al.*, 2010). For this reason, it is common to correlate vaginal cytology results with plasma progesterone concentration (expected to be 5 ng/ml at ovulation). Collection of vaginal cytology is not critical when breeding cats because ovulation is often induced by mating in this species. However, vaginal cytology may be important to perform in previously spayed dogs and cats with suspected ovarian remnants. The method of collection and cytologic appearance of vaginal samples are similar at each stage of the estrous cycle in dogs and cats.

Sample collection

Vaginal swabs are collected from the anterior aspect of the vagina to avoid contamination with either labial or cervical epithelial cells. Clean gloves should be worn. A clean cotton swab is moistened with saline. The labia are gently separated (Figure 11.1). A sterile metal speculum can be inserted into the vagina for limited visual examination of the vagina, but this is not necessary for collection of an adequate sample (Kustritz, 2006). The moistened swab is advanced into the vagina at a 45° angle and rubbed on the vaginal surface (Figure 11.2). The swab is carefully removed, the labia are released, and the swab is gently rolled down the length of a glass slide several times (Figure 11.3). The sample is allowed to air dry and then stained with a Romanowsky-type stain (e.g. Diff-Quik®).

Estrus stages (Table 11.1)

Proestrus

Proestrus lasts 3 days to 3 weeks in dogs and typically 1–3 days in cats. The onset of proestrus correlates with the presence of a bloody vaginal discharge, but this is often not recognized in cats. Behavioral changes including vocalizing, head rubbing, and playfulness may be noted. Maturation of ovarian follicles occurs during proestrus and anechoic follicles can be seen ultrasonographically. Cytology of a vaginal swab will contain high numbers of superficial squamous epithelial cells, low to moderate numbers of anucleate squamous epithelial cells, and low numbers of neutrophils (Figures 11.4, 11.5). Both types of epithelial cells are considered cornified epithelial cells because their cytoplasm contains keratin. These cells are large and polygonal to angular with pink or light blue to aqua colored cytoplasm. Superficial squamous epithelial cells have a small round nucleus with dense chromatin, whereas (as the name implies) no nucleus is present in anucleate squamous epithelial cells.

Estrus

Estrus lasts 3 days to 3 weeks in dogs and cats. This stage is associated with receptiveness to mating. During this stage, estrogen concentration decreases, triggering a peak in luteinizing hormone (LH)

DOI: 10.1201/9781003258551-11

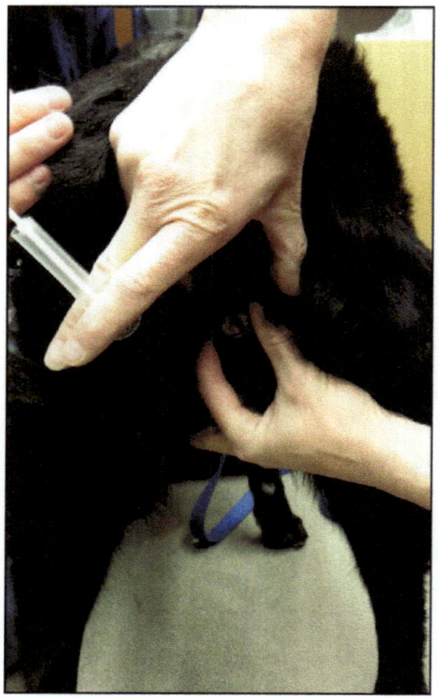

Figure 11.1 Step 1. The labia are gently separated manually to collect a vaginal swab sample.

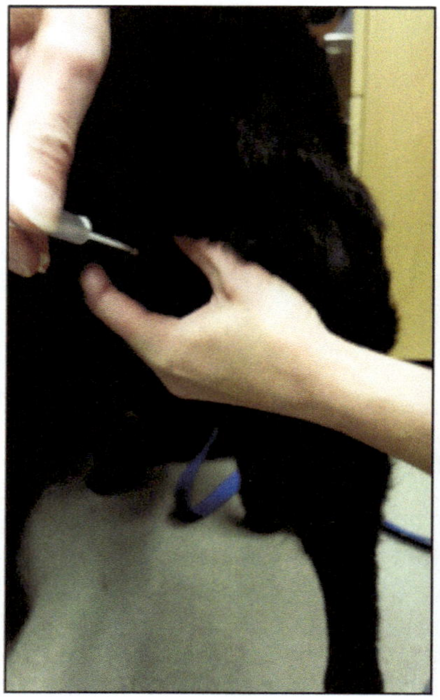

Collection of samples for vaginal cytology.

Figure 11.2 Step 2. A moistened swab is introduced into the vagina at a 45° angle and rubbed on the vaginal surface. Care should be taken to avoid the clitoris and the labia.

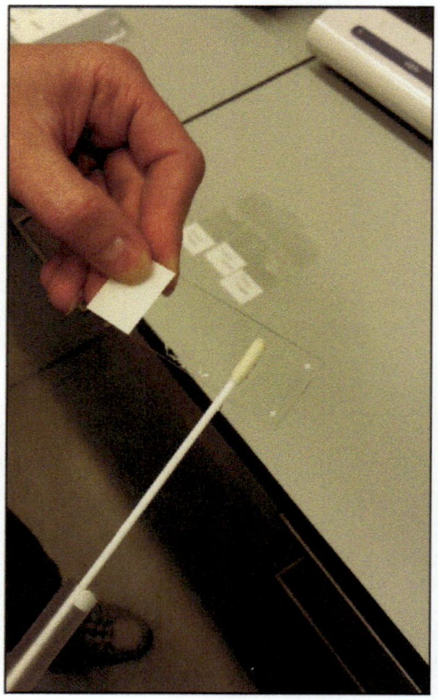

Figure 11.3 Step 3. The swab is rolled onto a clean glass slide for staining and cytologic evaluation.

Table 11.1 **List of cell types expected during different estrus stages in cytologic samples from the vagina, uterus, and ovary**

Estrus stage	Proestrus	Estrus	Early diestrus	Late diestrus	Anestrus
Vaginal cytology	Squamous epithelial cells; anucleate epithelial cells; neutrophils	Anucleate epithelial cells; squamous epithelial cells	Parabasal cells; small intermediate cells; neutrophils	Small and large intermediate cells; parabasal cells; neutrophils	Parabasal cells; small intermediate cells; neutrophils
Uterine cytology	Endometrial cells; neutrophils; lymphocytes	Endometrial cells; neutrophils; lymphocytes	Endometrial cells; neutrophils	Degenerate endometrial cells; neutrophils; macrophages	Endometrial cells; macrophages; lymphocytes
Ovarian cytology	'Round' cells; granulosa cells; mesenchymal cells	Granulosa cells; mesenchymal cells	Luteal cells; 'round' cells; granulosa cells; mesenchymal cells	Luteal cells; 'round' cells; granulosa cells; mesenchymal cells	Granulosa cells; mesenchymal cells

concentration, ovulation occurs, and progesterone concentration increases sharply. In dogs, ovulation occurs 36–50 hours after the LH peak (Kustritz, 2012). Ultrasound of the ovaries shows flattening of follicles and thickening of the corpora luteal walls. Cytologically, nearly 100% of cells from a vaginal swab are cornified epithelial cells with >50% of these cells being anucleate squamous epithelial cells. Neutrophils are notably absent (Figures 11.6, 11.7).

Diestrus

Diestrus in dogs lasts 50–80 days if not pregnant or until whelping (58–68 days) if pregnant. In cats, diestrus typically lasts 7–14 days if not pregnant or for the duration of pregnancy (63–69 days). Corpus lutea are maintained during diestrus. Decreasing LH and prolactin concentrations and an increase in prostaglandin concentration may trigger regression of the corpora lutea during the late stages of diestrus (Kustritz, 2012).

In early diestrus, vaginal cytology samples contain noncornified parabasal and small intermediate epithelial cells as well as several neutrophils (Figures 11.8, 11.9). Parabasal cells are smaller than cornified epithelial cells and are round with a moderate amount of basophilic cytoplasm and a large round nucleus with a slightly open chromatin pattern. Intermediate cells are at an intermediate stage of maturation between parabasal cells and squamous epithelial cells. During maturation of surface epithelial cells, cellular diameter increases and nuclear diameter decreases. Therefore, small intermediate cells are round to polygonal and, compared with parabasal cells, have slightly more abundant, lightly basophilic cytoplasm and a round nucleus with moderately condensed nuclear chromatin. Large intermediate cells have still more abundant polygonal, lightly basophilic cytoplasm and have a slightly smaller nucleus with denser chromatin. In late diestrus, the number of parabasal cells decreases, small and large intermediate cells are frequent, and neutrophils begin to decrease (Figures 11.10, 11.11). Rare lymphocytes and eosinophils may be present.

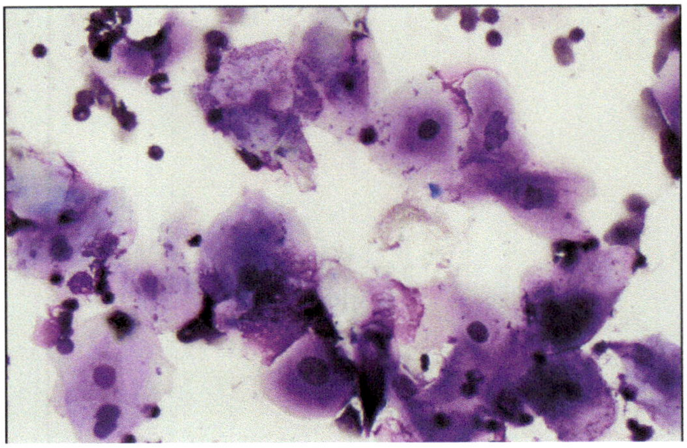
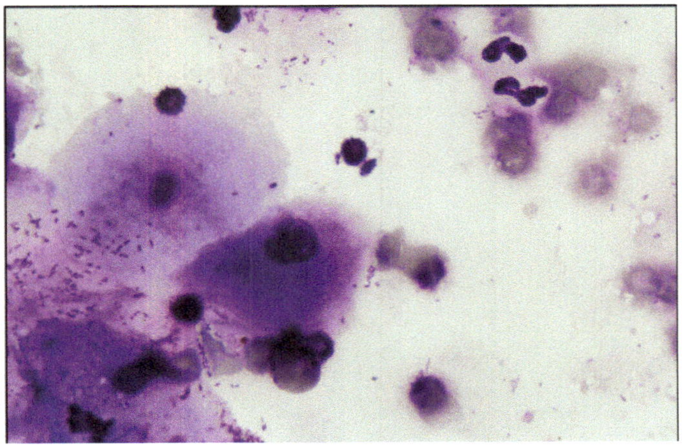

Proestrus. Vaginal swab cytology from a 2-year-old, intact female mixed-breed dog.

Figure 11.4 The majority of cells are large, cornified, nucleated squamous epithelial cells with fewer anucleate squamous epithelial cells. One, more rounded, large intermediate cell is present. Bacterial cocci and fewer rods are seen adhered to the epithelial cells. Neutrophils are expected but are not present in this image. Low numbers of erythrocytes are noted in the background (Diff-Quik®, 500× magnification).

Figure 11.5 Large, cornified, nucleated squamous epithelial cells predominate. Lower numbers of anucleate squamous epithelial cells are seen. A few nondegenerate neutrophils are present. Low numbers of erythrocytes and scattered bacterial organisms are observed in the background (Diff-Quik®, 1,000× magnification).

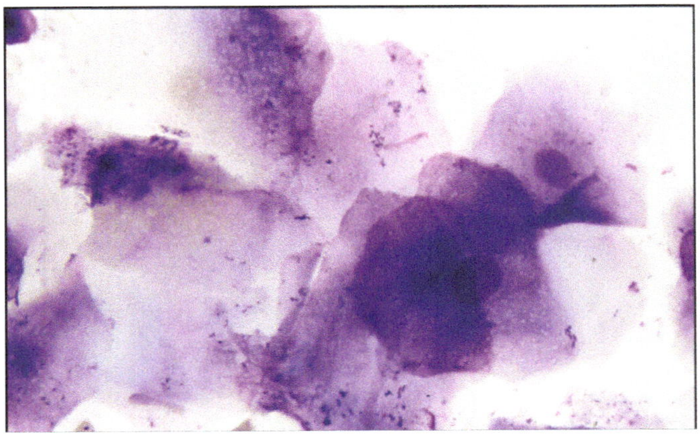
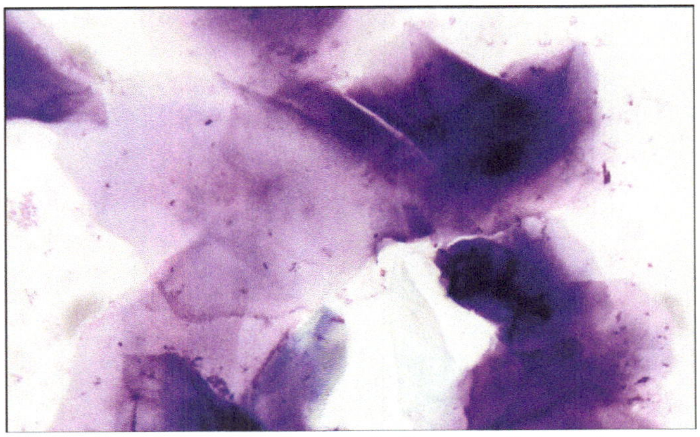

Figures 11.6, 11.7 Estrus. Vaginal swab cytology from a 3-year-old, intact female Labrador Retriever. The majority of cells are cornified, anucleate, squamous epithelial cells. Low numbers of nucleated squamous epithelial cells and bacterial organisms are seen, but neutrophils are not present (Diff-Quik®, 1,000× magnification).

Anestrus

Anestrus lasts anywhere from 30 to 240 days in dogs (Kustritz, 2012), but may not occur at all in queens. In cats, the occurrence of anestrus is dependent on photoperiod (Faya *et al.*, 2011). During this stage, involution of the uterus occurs. Estrogen concentration increases toward the end of anestrus causing the LH concentration to increase, which stimulates growth of new follicles in the ovary (Kustritz, 2012). Cytologically, vaginal samples taken during anestrus contain predominantly parabasal cells, moderate numbers of small intermediate cells, and low numbers of neutrophils (Figures 11.12, 11.13).

Inflammation

Vaginitis or vulvovaginitis may be difficult to assess cytologically because low to moderate numbers of neutrophils are a normal finding during proestrus, diestrus, and anestrus. Additionally, during proestrus and estrus, the vulva may be mildly edematous and swollen. Studies of vaginal bacterial flora in healthy dogs indicate that extracellular and phagocytized intracellular bacteria can be observed in vaginal cytology samples (Groppetti *et al.*, 2012). Bacteria commonly cultured from canine vaginal swabs include *Enterococcus faecalis*, *Streptococcus β-haemolyticus*, *Escherichia coli*, *Pasteurella multocida*, and *Staphylococcus* spp. (Groppetti *et al.*, 2012; Maksimovic *et al.*,

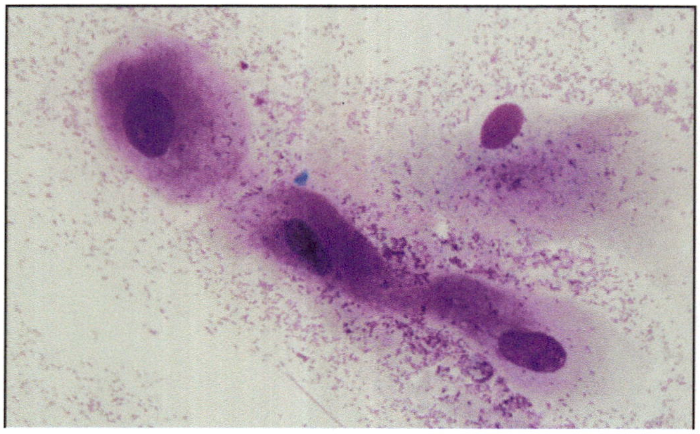
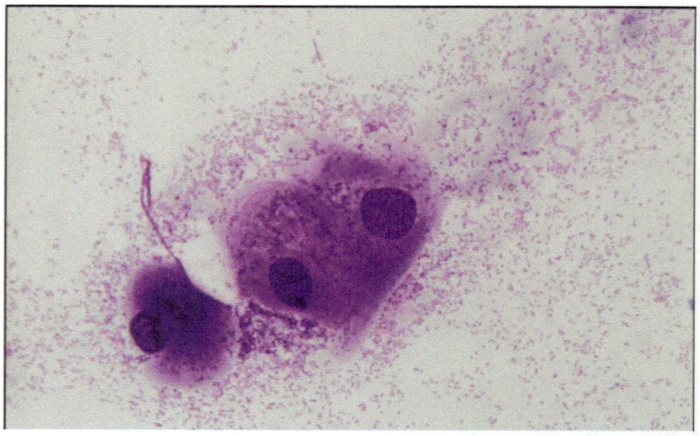

Figures 11.8, 11.9 Early diestrus. Vaginal swab cytology from a 4-year-old, intact female Collie (Diff-Quik®, 1,000× magnification). Figure 11.8: Two parabasal cells (left and center) and a cell transitioning into a small intermediate cell (lower right) are present. A partially lysed, small intermediate cell also is seen (upper right). A large number of bacterial organisms are observed. Moderate numbers of neutrophils are expected but are not present in this image. Figure 11.9: Three parabasal cells are shown. There are a large number of bacterial organisms in the background. Moderate numbers of neutrophils are expected but are not present in this image.

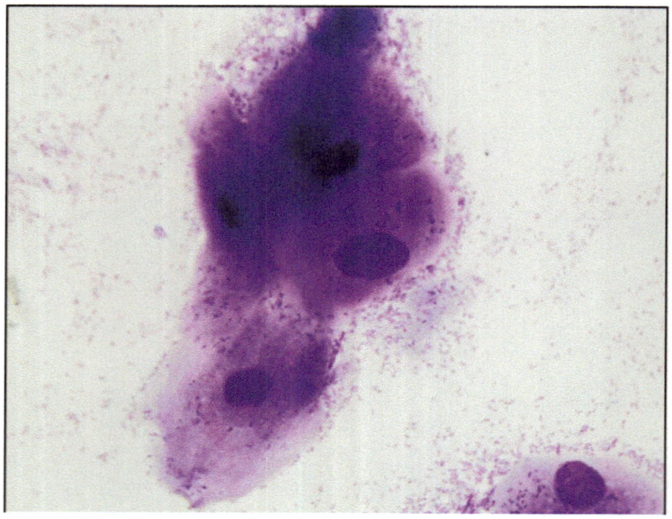
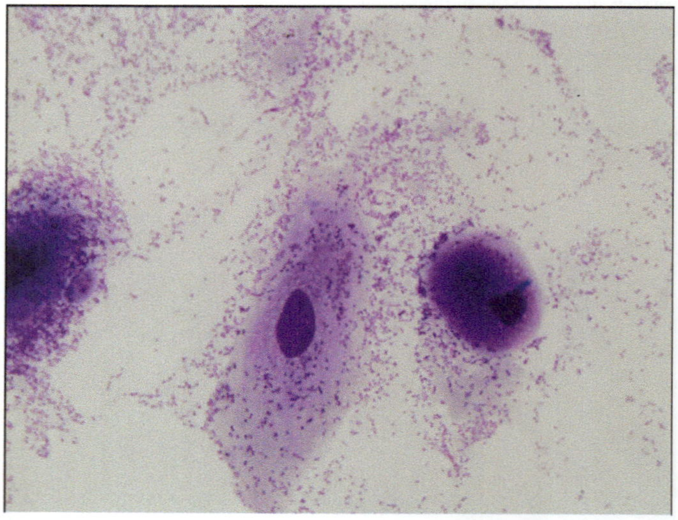

Figures 11.10, 11.11 Mid to late diestrus. Vaginal swab cytology from a 2-year-old, intact female Beagle (Diff-Quik®, 1,000× magnification). Figure 11.10: Three cells transitioning from parabasal to small intermediate cells (top) and two large intermediate cells (bottom) are shown. There are a large number of bacterial organisms in the background. Low numbers of neutrophils are expected but are not present in this image. Figure 11.11: A large intermediate cell (left) and a parabasal cell (right) are present. A large number of bacterial organisms also are observed. Note: low numbers of neutrophils are expected but are not present in this image.

2012). If clinical signs strongly support inflammation as a differential, and cytologic evaluation indicates suppurative or pyogranulomatous inflammation with or without intracellular bacteria, then a diagnosis of vaginitis or vulvovaginitis can be made (Figure 11.14).

Neoplasia

Neoplasia of the vulva must be distinguished from an enlarged clitoris (often observed in intersex animals) or from vaginal prolapse. Neoplastic conditions of the vulva and vagina account for 2.4–3% of tumors in dogs, and approximately 83% of these tumors are benign (Thacher & Bradley, 1983; Saba & Lawrence, 2013). Leiomyoma, fibroma, and fibroleiomyoma are considered more common tumors, whereas lipoma, polyps, melanoma, myxoma, myxofibroma, and adenocarcinoma are uncommon (Ortega-Pacheco *et al.*, 2012).

Leiomyoma/fibroleiomyoma

Benign mesenchymal tumors involving smooth muscle of the vulva, vestibule, and vagina have a similar cytologic appearance to leiomyomas arising from other areas of the body (Figures 11.15, 11.16). The overall cellularity of the sample may be scant. Cells tend to have thin, elongated, lightly basophilic, spindle-shaped cytoplasm and a centrally located, thin, long, oval nucleus with dense to stippled

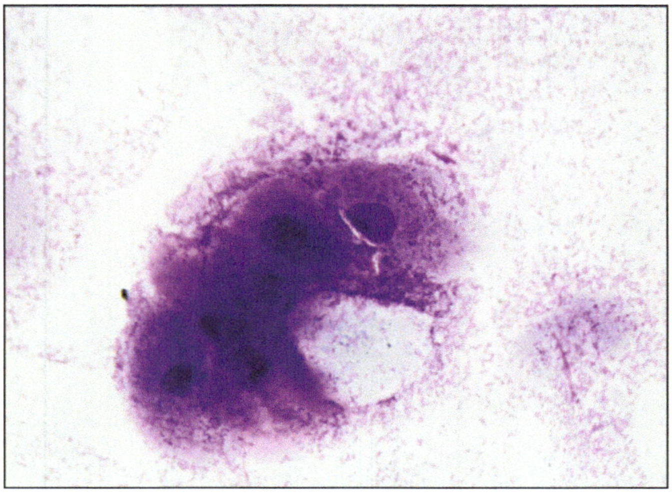

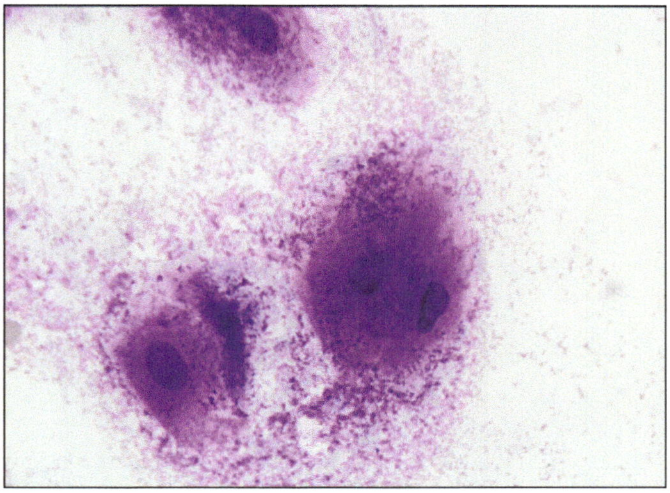

Figures 11.12, 11.13 Anestrus. Vaginal swab cytology from a 1-year-old, intact female Boxer (Diff-Quik®, 1,000× magnification). Figure 11.12: A group of parabasal cells are present. A large number of bacterial organisms are also observed. Figure 11.13: One small intermediate cell (left) and two parabasal cells (right) are present. A large number of bacterial organisms also are observed. Note: low numbers of neutrophils are expected but are not depicted in these images.

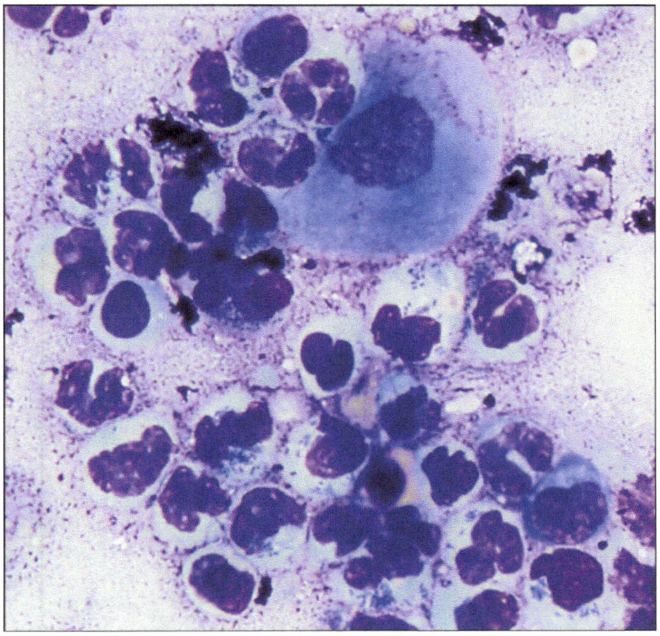

Figure 11.14 Bacterial vaginitis. Vaginal discharge cytology from a 6-year-old, spayed female Labrador Retriever mix. Clinical history included 2 years of intermittent, mucinous, bloody vaginal discharge. The cytology sample has a stippled, proteinaceous background, rare nucleated squamous epithelial cells, and large numbers of degenerate neutrophils. Many of the neutrophils contain phagocytized bacterial organisms (Wright–Giemsa, 1,500× magnification).

chromatin. Cells are generally uniform in appearance and lack overt criteria of malignancy. Histopathology is needed for a final definitive diagnosis of leiomyoma or fibroleiomyoma.

Fibroma

Fibromas tend not to exfoliate well when aspirated for collection of a cytologic sample. These tumors are derived from fibroblasts, so cells have a moderate amount of lightly basophilic, spindle-shaped cytoplasm and a centrally located, oval nucleus. The chromatin of these cells is usually stippled and there are typically two small nucleoli, located apart from each other at opposite ends of the oval nucleus (Figure 11.17).

Polyp

Vaginal polyps are commonly observed in older dogs and tend to be solitary masses located on the ventral aspect of the vagina. These lesions cannot be distinguished from leiomyoma on gross examination and are often ulcerated (Brown *et al.*, 2012; Foster, 2012a). In general, polyps are difficult to diagnose cytologically because cells are morphologically identical to hyperplastic epithelial cells, which are well-differentiated and may not to exfoliate well.

Adenocarcinoma

Adenocarcinoma is not a common tumor of the vulva, vestibule, or vagina. However, the lesion is worth mentioning here because the cytology and histology are similar to what is seen in samples from apocrine gland anal sac adenocarcinomas. Cytologically, these lesions have a neuroendocrine appearance with abundant lightly basophilic cytoplasm that has indistinct cell junctions and is associated with several small, rounded nuclei. Occasionally, nuclei may be loosely arranged in a circle around a central area of cytoplasm, forming acinar structures (Figure 11.18). Histologically, these tumors are classic adenocarcinomas with nests of neoplastic polygonal epithelial cells and frequent acini.

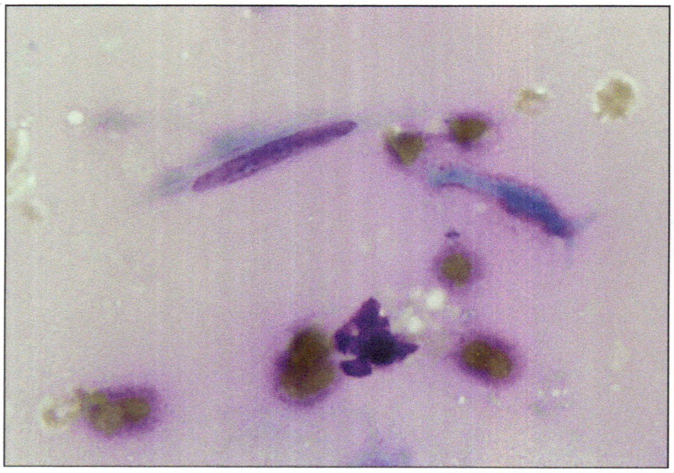

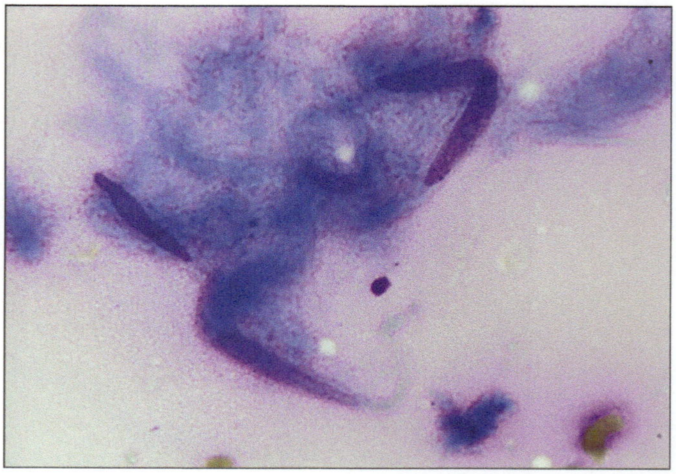

Figures 11.15, 11.16 Leiomyoma (Wright–Giemsa, 1,500× magnification). Figure 11.15: A small spindle-shaped cell with a thin, long, oval nucleus is shown. Small cytoplasmic fragments, low numbers of erythrocytes, and a partially lysed neutrophil also are present. Figure 11.16: Four intact cells have spindle-shaped to wispy basophilic cytoplasm and a thin, long, oval nucleus with finely stippled chromatin and an indistinct round nucleolus. Several cytoplasmic fragments are observed. Note: differential diagnoses include leiomyoma, leiomyosarcoma, and other soft tissue sarcomas. Histopathology is needed to confirm the cytologic diagnosis.

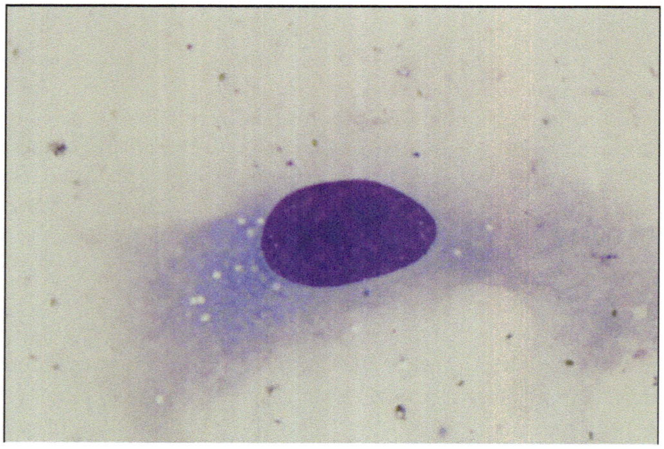

Figure 11.17 Reactive fibroblast. This cell has abundant spindloid basophilic cytoplasm and a centrally located oval nucleus with stippled chromatin and two, relatively indistinct, round nucleoli that are mildly variable in size (Wright–Giemsa, 2,000× magnification).

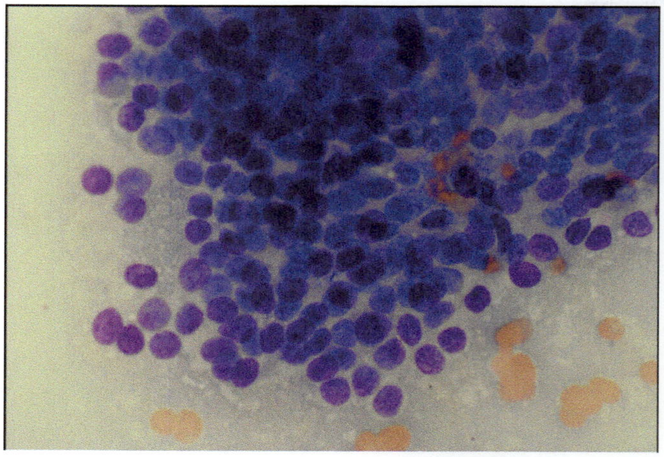

Figure 11.18 Adenocarcinoma. FNA of a clitoral mass on an 11-year-old, spayed female Basset Hound. The sample is highly cellular with several clusters of cells that have a neuroendocrine appearance. Cells have lightly basophilic cytoplasm with indistinct cytoplasmic borders and a small, round nucleus with dense chromatin. Nuclei arranged in a circular, acinar structure are observed slightly lower and to the left of the center of the image (Wright–Giemsa, 1,000× magnification).

Transmissible venereal tumor

Transmissible venereal tumors (TVTs) likely arise from canine histiocytic cells (Mozos *et al.*, 1996; Marchal *et al.*, 1997). Theoretically, this tumor line developed in a dog approximately 11,000 years ago (Murchison *et al.*, 2014). Both male and female dogs can develop TVTs. The tumors tend to be present on the preputial and vaginal areas as well as around the nose. The lesion is typically a large, multilobular, ulcerated mass that exfoliates very easily by fine needle aspiration (FNA). Cytologic samples contain large numbers of round cells with abundant lightly basophilic cytoplasm; numerous clear, distinct cytoplasmic vacuoles; and a round, centrally located nucleus with finely stippled chromatin. Mitotic figures are frequently observed cytologically (Figures 11.19, 11.20). In immunocompetent animals, TVTs may spontaneously regress and are responsive to vincristine; however, metastasis is not uncommon in unhealthy animals (Foster, 2012a).

CYTOLOGY OF THE UTERUS

Introduction

Uterine cytology is not commonly performed in dogs and cats. Touch imprints of the mucosal surface of the uterus or of uterine lesions may

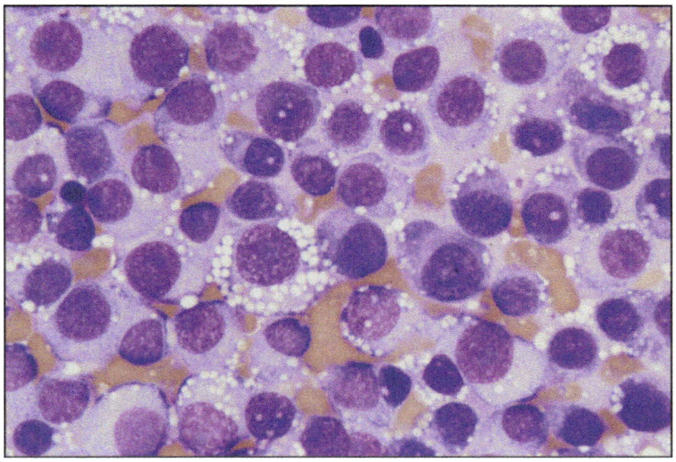

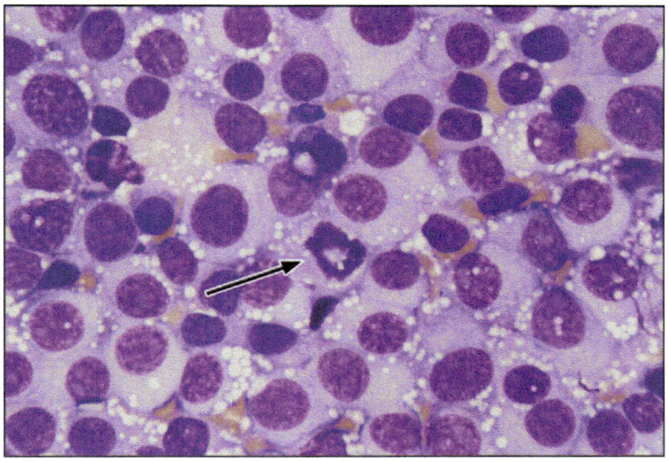

Figures 11.19, 11.20 Transmissible venereal tumor. FNA of a vaginal mass from a 4-year-old, intact female mixed-breed dog. Cells exfoliate well and are individualized and round. Most cells have abundant, lightly basophilic cytoplasm with numerous, clear, distinct, round vacuoles. Nuclei are large and round with stippled chromatin and often a prominent, large, round nucleolus. Moderate anisocytosis and anisokaryosis are noted. A mitotic figure is shown at the center of Figure 11.20 (arrow). Low numbers of erythrocytes are trapped in between the neoplastic cells (Wright–Giemsa, 1,000× magnification).

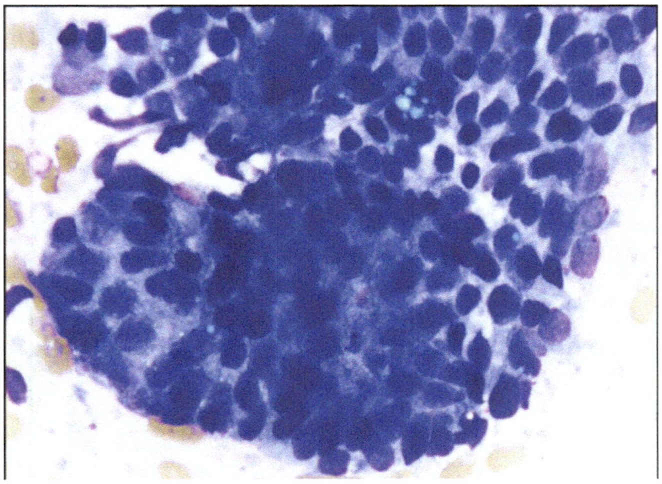

Figure 11.21 Endometrial cells. Impression smear from the uterus of an adult cat. A sheet of endometrial cells is shown. Cells have lightly basophilic, cuboidal to columnar cytoplasm and a small, round, nucleus with dense chromatin (Wright–Giemsa, 1,000× magnification).

be obtained perioperatively. Collection of cells via vaginal endoscopy with transcervical catheterization and uterine flushing has been described (Wilson, 2001). As expected, the estrous cycle greatly affects the cytologic appearance of uterine samples (Table 11.1). In dogs, during proestrus and estrus, Groppetti *et al.* (2010) reported finding clusters of endometrial cells with few neutrophils and rare lymphocytes. In early diestrus, they saw similar clusters of endometrial cells and few neutrophils, but lymphocytes were not observed (Figure 11.21). In late diestrus, endometrial cells became degenerate with evidence of cytoplasmic vacuolation and nuclear pyknosis, and inflammatory cells were not found. As dogs entered anestrus, endothelial cells became foamy and macrophages and neutrophils were observed. Finally, during late anestrus, endometrial cells appeared healthy and a mixed mononuclear inflammatory cell population was noted, including macrophages, lymphocytes, and plasma cells.

Inflammation

Metritis is uncommon in dogs and cats, but there is a moderate amount of information about endometritis in dogs. At least 70% of canine endometritis cases are caused by bacterial infection (Fontaine *et al.*, 2009). Bacteria commonly isolated from uterine samples include *Escherichia coli, Proteus* spp., *Streptococcus* spp., and *Staphylococcus* spp. (Ortega-Pacheco *et al.*, 2012). Cytologic sampling of a uterus affected by endometritis is unlikely to be rewarding, but may include endometrial cells, rare fibroblasts, and increased numbers of neutrophils.

Pyometra and uterine stump pyometra are diagnosed more commonly in dogs and cats. Cytologic samples from uterine flushing contain degenerate endothelial cells, large numbers of neutrophils, and scattered macrophages, lymphocytes, and plasma cells (Groppetti *et al.*, 2010). Additionally, necrotic material can be observed in vaginal smears from most of these patients (Figure 11.22).

Hyperplasia

Endometrial hyperplasia is uncommon in cats. In dogs, it is often cystic and has been associated with the development of pyometra (Schlafer & Gifford, 2008). In patients with cystic endometrial hyperplasia, cells collected by vaginal endoscopy with transcervical catheterization and uterine flushing included degenerate, foamy endometrial cells, and neutrophils (Groppetti *et al.*, 2010).

Neoplasia

Leiomyoma/leiomyosarcoma

Uterine neoplasms in dogs and cats are very rare. In dogs, most uterine tumors are benign leiomyomas (Saba & Lawrence, 2013). As described

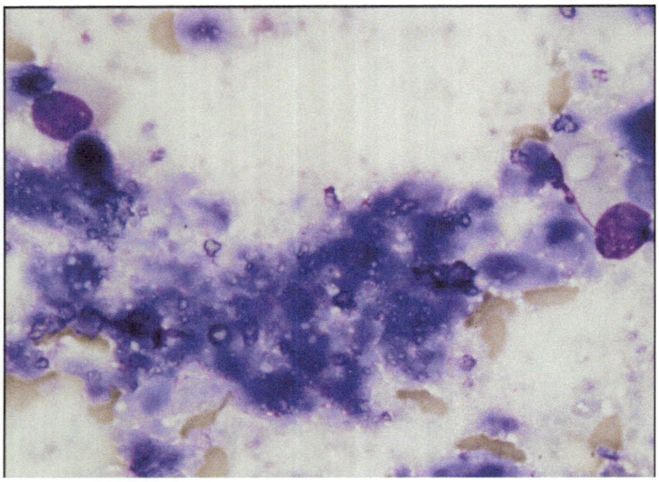

Figure 11.22 Necrosis. Blue-gray necrotic cellular debris may be observed in vaginal smears of dogs with pyometra if uterine epithelial cells are dying and sloughing off. Small, nonstaining pieces of mineralized material may be associated with the necrosis. Rare lysed nuclei are seen (Wright–Giemsa, 1,000× magnification).

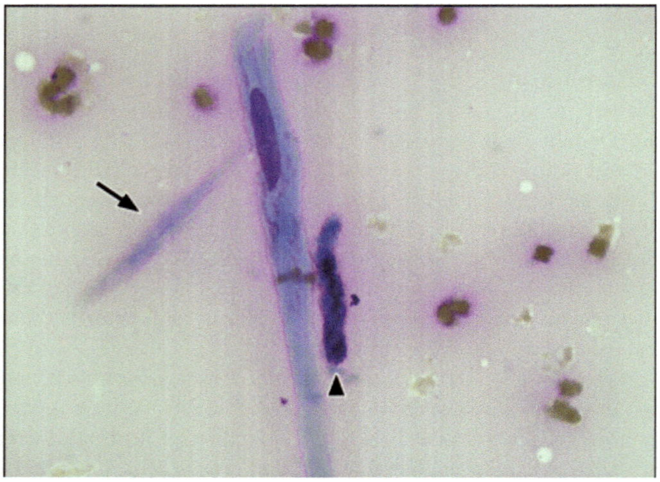

Figure 11.23 Leiomyosarcoma. The intact cell in the center of the image is strap-like with elongated rectangular basophilic cytoplasm and a thin, long, oval nucleus with finely stippled chromatin, and an indistinct round nucleolus. A cytoplasmic fragment is observed to the left of the large cells (arrow). A smaller spindle-shaped cell with a high nuclear to cytoplasmic ratio is seen at the right of the image (arrowhead). There are low numbers of erythrocytes in the background. Differential diagnoses include leiomyoma, leiomyosarcoma, and other soft tissue sarcomas. Histopathology is needed to confirm the cytologic diagnosis (Wright–Giemsa, 1,000× magnification).

for the vaginal area, the overall cellularity from a leiomyoma may be low. Smooth muscle tumor (leiomyoma and leiomyosarcoma) samples contain spindle-shaped cells with elongated, lightly basophilic cytoplasm. Benign tumors have a centrally located, thin, long, oval nucleus with dense to stippled chromatin. More malignant cells can have larger, plumper nuclei and coarse chromatin with one or more prominent nucleoli (Figure 11.23). Other characteristics of malignancy, including binucleation, anisocytosis, and anisokaryosis, are expected with leiomyosarcomas. Neoplastic smooth muscle cells can look similar to other sarcoma cells; therefore, histopathology is needed for a final definitive diagnosis of leiomyoma or leiomyomasarcoma.

Adenocarcinoma

Although rare overall, adenocarcinoma of the uterus is the most common uterine tumor in cats (Saba & Lawrence, 2013). These tumors are typically diagnosed histologically. Immunohistochemical staining indicates they are positive for cytokeratin, cyclo-oxygenase-2, E-cadherin, and β-catenin and may express progesterone receptors (Gil da Costa *et al.*, 2009).

CYTOLOGY OF OVARIAN TISSUE

Introduction

It is unusual to obtain cytology samples from ovaries of dogs and cats. Ovarian remnant syndrome is the most common complication associated with this tissue; diagnosis is typically based on the occurrence of estrous behavior in ovariectomized animals. A vaginal cytology sample containing nearly 100% cornified epithelial cells is evidence of estrus and supports the clinical suspicion of an ovarian remnant. Cytologic samples of the ovary may be collected by ultrasound-guided FNA or perioperative impression smears. Cytology of healthy ovarian tissue varies throughout the estrous cycle. Recently, Piseddu *et al.* (2012) described their cytologic findings in 16 dogs undergoing elective ovariohysterectomy (Table 11.1). Low numbers of benign mesenchymal cells were seen in ovarian aspirates at all stages of the estrous cycle. Luteal cells were only observed in dogs during diestrus. These cells are large and have abundant basophilic cytoplasm, distinct cytoplasmic vacuoles, and a rounded nucleus with finely stippled chromatin (Figure 11.24). A small amount of extracellular

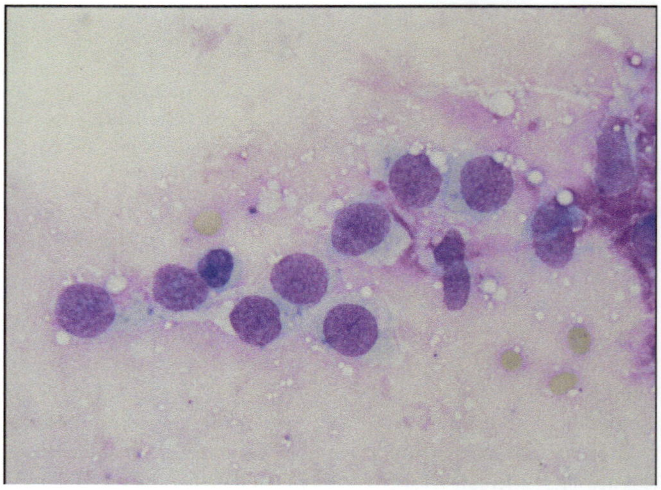

Figure 11.24 Luteal cells. FNA of an ovary from an adult cat. There are several individualized, rounded cells with lightly basophilic cytoplasm and a large, round nucleus with finely stippled chromatin. A single prominent nucleolus can be seen in some cells. One smaller granulosa cell (third cell from the left) also is present (Wright–Giemsa, 1,000× magnification).

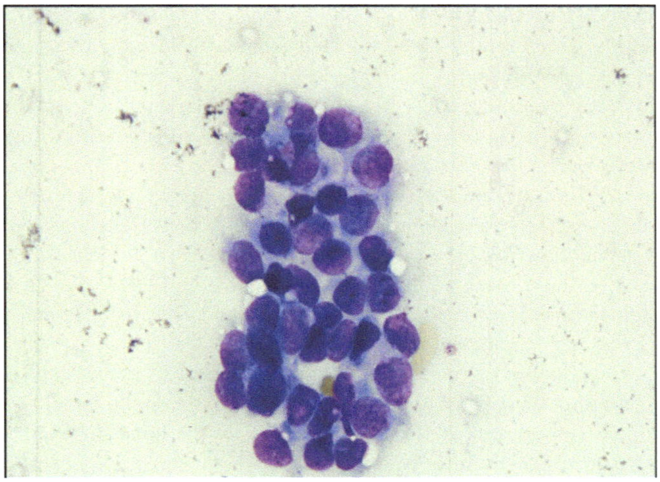

Figure 11.25 **Granulosa cells. Imprint of an ovary from an adult cat. A loose sheet of granulosa cells is shown. Cells are round and have a moderate amount of lightly basophilic cytoplasm and a round nucleus with dense chromatin (Wright–Giemsa, 1,000× magnification).**

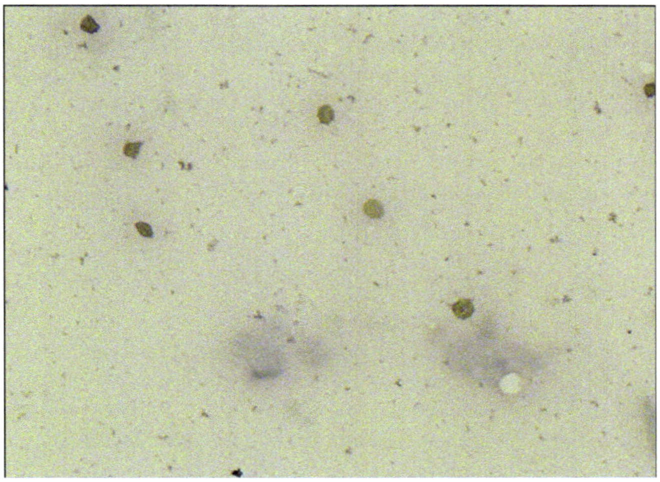

Figure 11.26 **Cystic fluid. The sample is nearly acellular with a thin layer of proteinaceous material in the background of the slide. A few erythroctyes are seen (Wright–Giemsa, 800× magnification).**

matrix was reported in some samples during proestrus and diestrus. Ovarian cytology samples from dogs in proestrus often contained 'round' cells (possibly germ cells) and a few granulosa cells. During estrus, no round cells were identified but a few granulosa cells were seen. In diestrus, luteal cells were apparent in most animals and often there were moderate numbers of round cells and many granulosa cells. Finally, during anestrus, there were no round cells and a few granulosa cells. Four of the 16 dogs were sexually immature; ovarian aspirates from these animals contained moderate numbers of granulosa cells and few round cells and mesenchymal cells. Granulosa cells often exfoliate in loose clusters and have a scant to moderate amount of basophilic cytoplasm and small, round nuclei with dense chromatin (Figure 11.25).

Inflammation

Oophoritis is extremely uncommon in dogs and cats. Bacterial oophoritis must be differentiated from granulomas caused by feline infectious peritonitis in cats. Cytologically, one would expect to see severe neutrophilic inflammation with bacterial infection.

Cystic structures

Periovarian cysts are commonly seen in dogs and cats during ovariectomy. Intraovarian cysts may also be observed and are often derived from the rete ovarii (Foster, 2012b). Classically, cytologic samples of cystic structures are acellular and have a thin basophilic proteinaceous background consistent with the fluid aspirated from the cyst (Figure 11.26).

Neoplasia

The incidence of ovarian tumors in dogs and cats is low, with higher prevalence reported in intact animals (as expected), and ranges from 0.5 to 6.25% in dogs and 0.7 to 3.6% in cats (Saba & Lawrence, 2013). There are four categories of ovarian neoplasms: epithelial tumors and sex cord stromal tumors (specifically granulosa-theca cell tumors) are the most common tumor types, whereas germ cell tumors and mesenchymal tumors are rare.

Epithelial neoplasms

Tumors of the ovarian epithelium include undifferentiated carcinomas, papillary adenomas, adenocarcinomas, and cystadenomas, among others. Adenocarcinomas are the most common ovarian tumors in the dog and often metastasize (Patnaik & Greenlee, 1987). Carcinomas are often immunoreactive for cytokeratin, desmin, vimentin, cyclo-oxygenase-2, and endothelin-1, but nearly all carcinomas are negative for inhibin-a (Pelkey *et al.*, 1998; Akihara *et al.*, 2007). Most tumors are unilateral. Cysts in the contralateral ovary and/or endometrial hyperplasia may occur concurrently. Cytologically, adenocarcinomas contain clusters of rounded epithelial cells with a variable amount of deeply basophilic cytoplasm and round nucleus. Cells occasionally may be arranged in an acinar pattern. Several characteristics of malignancy, including binucleation and prominent nucleoli, are seen.

Sex cord stromal tumors

Granulosa cell tumors are the most common ovarian sex cord stromal tumors. Most granulosa cell tumors are benign, but there is a subset (20%) that has metastatic potential (Saba & Lawrence, 2013). Immunohistochemical staining of the tumors indicates they express vimentin, S100, and often express inhibin-a and endothelin-1

(Akihara *et al.*, 2007; Borzacchiello *et al.*, 2010). They exfoliate well and are cytologically distinctive. Small clusters of granulosa cells are often found forming acinar structures. The cells are large and round with a moderate amount of lightly basophilic cytoplasm and an eccentric, round nucleus with stippled chromatin. Cells often contain distinct cytoplasmic vacuoles. Other, less common ovarian sex cord stromal tumors include Sertoli–Leydig tumors, luteomas, and thecomas.

Germ cell tumors

Dysgerminomas and teratomas are germ cell tumors of the ovary. Each tumor type accounts for approximately 10% of ovarian tumors in dogs (Greenlee & Patnaik, 1985). Concurrent cysts in the contralateral ovary, endometrial hyperplasia, and/or pyometra may be observed. Neither of these tumor types is commonly diagnosed cytologically. Dysgerminomas are reported to be immunohistochemically positive for vimentin and negative for cytokeratin, desmin, S100, and inhibin-a (Akihara *et al.*, 2007). Teratomas are comprised of at least two types of embryonic tissue (ectoderm, mesoderm, and/or endoderm). Histologically, haired skin, bone, cartilage, adipose tissue, and other tissue types are often observed together in a disorganized mass (Foster, 2012b). Cytologically, teratomas are difficult to diagnose definitively. The malignant version of this tumor (teratocarcinoma) is extremely rare.

MALE REPRODUCTIVE SYSTEM

SEMEN

Semen collection and storage

Canine semen can be collected by digital massage. Having a bitch in estrus present can be beneficial. Ideally a latex collection cone is used; however, a sterile, clear, plastic bag (e.g. a baby bottle liner) is adequate for collection of the ejaculate. Digital massage is performed by exposing the tip of the penis, placing the collection bag over the penis, and pushing the prepuce back over the bulbis glandis. Pressure is applied to the penis using a forward and backward movement. As the dog begins to thrust, the ejaculate should begin to fill the collection bag. Three fractions of ejaculate can be identified. The first fraction is clear to slightly cloudy and does not contain sperm. The second fraction should be cloudy and white and is sperm-rich. The third fraction is clear and is from the prostate. The three portions of ejaculate together have a volume of 1–30 ml (Johnston, 1991). Typically, the collection bag is removed as soon as the prostatic fraction is observed and analysis of semen is performed on the combination of the first and second fractions of the ejaculate.

Collection of semen from cats can be done using a teaser queen and artificial vagina or by electroejaculation. The first method may require some training before successful collection of fluid. The total volume of the feline ejaculate ranges from 110 to 740 μl (Zambelli & Cunto, 2006).

Analysis of semen

Canine semen samples are evaluated for fluid volume, clarity, and color; aerobic and anaerobic bacteria; pH (reference interval 6.3–6.7); alkaline phosphatase concentration; and motility, quantity, and morphology of spermatozoa (Johnston, 1991). Samples from healthy dogs should have <10,000 bacteria/ml (Johnston, 1991). There are several bacterial species associated with disease, including mycoplasmas. Alkaline phosphatase should be 5,000–40,000 U/l in healthy dogs; obstruction between the epididymis and meatus of the urethra is suspected if the concentration is decreased (Johnston, 1991). Analysis of feline samples is restricted by the volume of fluid collected; often only microscopic parameters are evaluated.

A wet mount of the ejaculate fluid is examined microscopically for motility of spermatozoa. Greater than 70% of sperm should be progressively motile in semen. To quantitate the concentration of spermatozoa, the sample is diluted 1:10^6, sperm are counted using a hemocytometer, and the number of sperm/ml is calculated. Healthy dogs produce 50–500 million spermatozoa/ml of ejaculate. Cats produce 3–600 million sperm per ejaculate sample. A cytocentrifuged sample of the fluid is stained with a Romanowsky-type stain and examined microscopically to look at the morphology of the sperm. Abnormalities in spermatozoa are described as primary or secondary defects. Fewer than 20% of sperm should have primary defects, which include proximally coiled tails, retained proximal cytoplasmic droplets, double heads, and double tails (Table 11.2). These abnormalities occur during development in the testes. Secondary defects tend to develop secondary to fever, inflammation, trauma, or infection while

Table 11.2 **Diagrams of sperm illustrating morphologic differences between normal spermatozoa and sperm with primary defects (proximally coiled tails, retained proximal cytoplasmic droplets, double heads, and double tails) and secondary defects (bent tails, hairpin tails, heads broken at the midpiece, retained distal cytoplasmic droplets, and detached acrosomes)**

Normal spermatozoon	Primary defects	Secondary defects
Acrosome, oval head and long tail 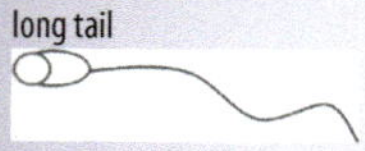	Proximally coiled tails 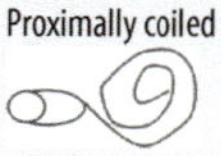	Bent tails 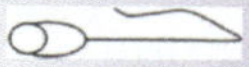
	Retained proximal cytoplasmic droplets 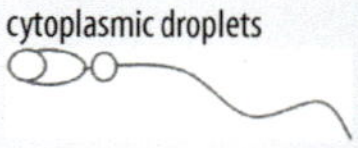	Hairpin tails 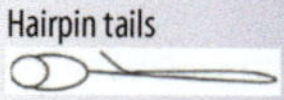
	Double heads 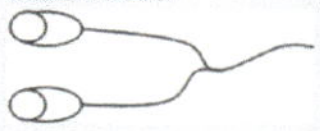	Heads broken at the midpiece 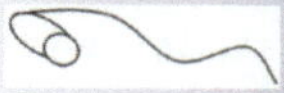
	Double tails 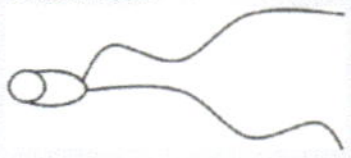	Retained distal cytoplasmic droplets 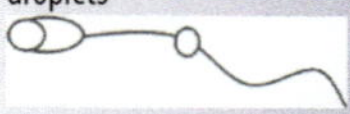
		Detached acrosome 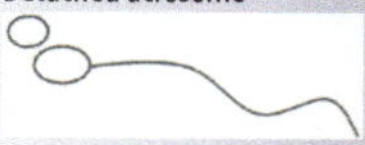

sperm are in the epididymis. Secondary defects include bent tails, hairpin tails, heads broken at the midpiece, retained distal cytoplasmic droplets, and detached acrosomes (Table 11.2). The percentage of sperm with secondary defects also should be <20%.

CYTOLOGY OF THE TESTES

Introduction

FNA of the testes is safe to perform and can yield important diagnostic information. No effect on production or quality of spermatozoa has been reported, but a small amount of hemorrhage can be detected for up to a week following the procedure (Gouletsou *et al.*, 2010, 2011, 2012). Cytologic evaluation of testicular tissue may be warranted in cases of infertility, suspected orchitis, and when masses are palpated.

The cell types observed in cytologic samples from normal canine testes were recently described in detail (Santos *et al.*, 2012) and are similar to the cell types observed histologically in cat testicles (Diagone *et al.*, 2011). As a brief review, the normal cells present in aspirates of testicles include mesenchymal cells, Leydig cells, Sertoli cells, spermatogonia, spermatocytes, spermatids, and spermatozoa. Mesenchymal cells are rare, individualized cells that appear benign with scant, spindle-shaped, lightly basophilic cytoplasm and a small, centrally located, oval nucleus with stippled chromatin. Leydig cells also are rare, but may be seen individually and in small sheets. They are round with abundant, basophilic cytoplasm that contains large, clear, distinct vacuoles. The nucleus is round to ovoid and has clumped chromatin. Sertoli cells are fragile, but when found intact, they are large, round to oval cells with abundant, poorly defined, lightly basophilic to eosinophilic cytoplasm and a large round nucleus with finely stippled chromatin and a prominent nucleolus (Figure 11.27). Development of spermatozoa should be orderly and complete, with few spermatogonia and large numbers of spermatozoa. Spermatogonia are large, round cells with pale basophilic cytoplasm and a large oval nucleus often containing a crescent-shaped section of condensed chromatin (Figure 11.28). Spermatocytes are slightly larger than spermatogonia and are round with a moderate amount of lightly basophilic cytoplasm. The nuclei of these cells are large and round with ropey chromatin resembling a mitotic figure in prophase (Figure 11.29). Spermatids are slightly smaller than spermatogonia and much smaller than spermatocytes. These cells undergo four identifiable stages of maturation: the Golgi phase, cap phase, acrosomal phase, and maturation phase. Early spermatids in the Golgi phase are round with scant, lightly basophilic cytoplasm; small, distinct, clear cytoplasmic vacuoles; and a round nucleus with coarsely stippled chromatin. These cells are often binucleate (Figure 11.30). During the

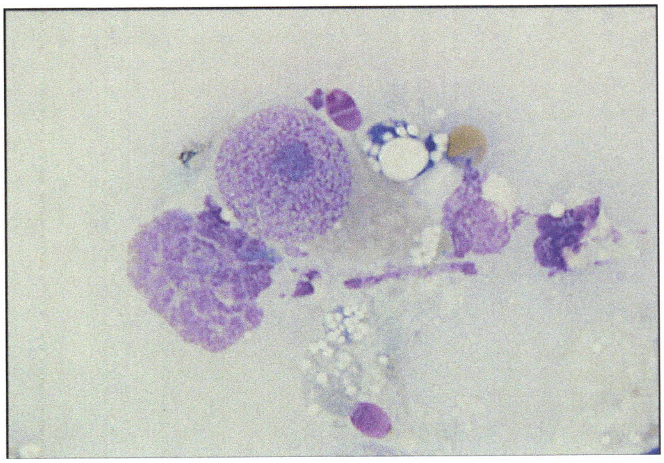

Figure 11.27 **Sertoli cell. Imprint of a testicle from an adult dog. A Sertoli cell is shown in the center of the image. The cell has abundant, pale cytoplasm and a large, round nucleus with open chromatin and a prominent, round nucleolus (Wright–Giemsa, 1,500× magnification).**

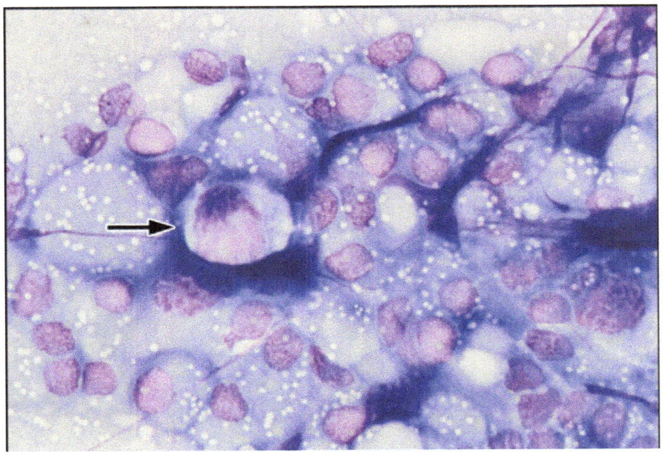

Figure 11.28 **Spermatogonium. Imprint of a testicle from an adult dog. The large cell to the left of center is a spermatogonium (arrow). The cell has abundant, lightly basophilic cytoplasm and a large nucleus with open chromatin except for a condensed, crescent-shaped area at the top of the nucleus. Large numbers of early spermatids also are present in the image (Wright–Giemsa, 1,000× magnification).**

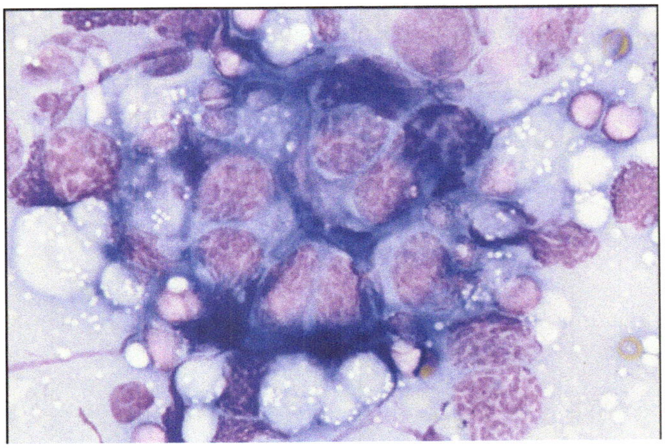

Figure 11.29 **Spermatocytes. Imprint of a testicle from an adult dog. Spermatocytes are large, round cells with basophilic cytoplasm and a round nucleus with ropey, clumped chromatin (Wright–Giemsa, 1,000× magnification).**

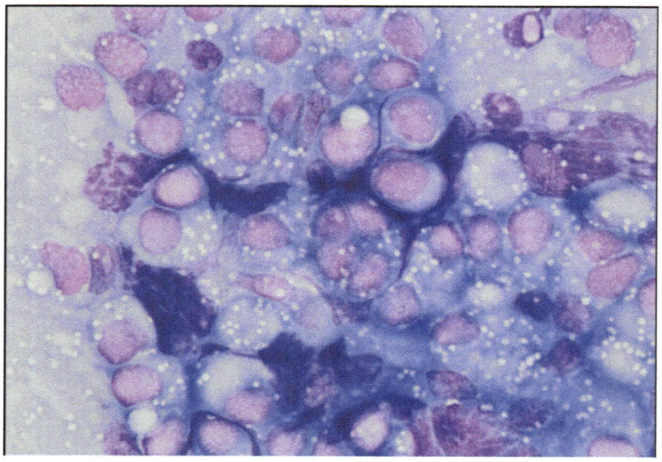

Figure 11.30 Early spermatids. Imprint of a testicle from an adult dog. Spermatids are present in large numbers. They are round cells with a moderate amount of basophilic cytoplasm that contains low to moderate numbers of distinct, clear, cytoplasmic vacuoles. The nucleus is rounded with finely stippled chromatin. Binucleated and multinucleated cells are frequently seen (Wright–Giemsa, 1,000× magnification).

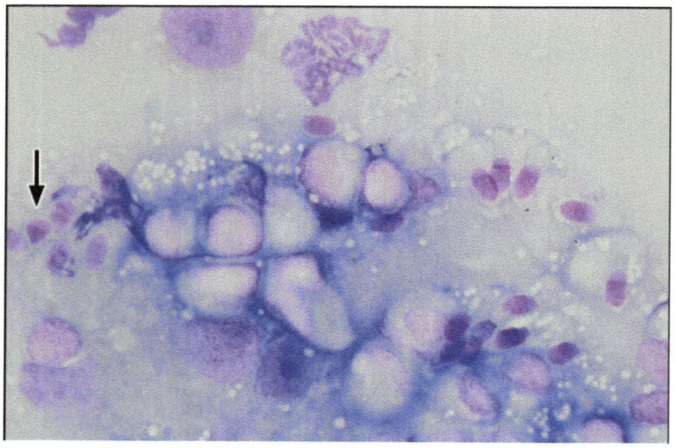

Figure 11.31 Cap phase spermatid. Imprint of a testicle from an adult dog. One cap phase spermatid is shown at the left of the image (arrow). The cell has a nucleus with a rounded edge and a pointed edge. Several early and late spermatids are observed. A few Sertoli cells and a spermatocyte also are present (Wright–Giemsa, 1,000× magnification).

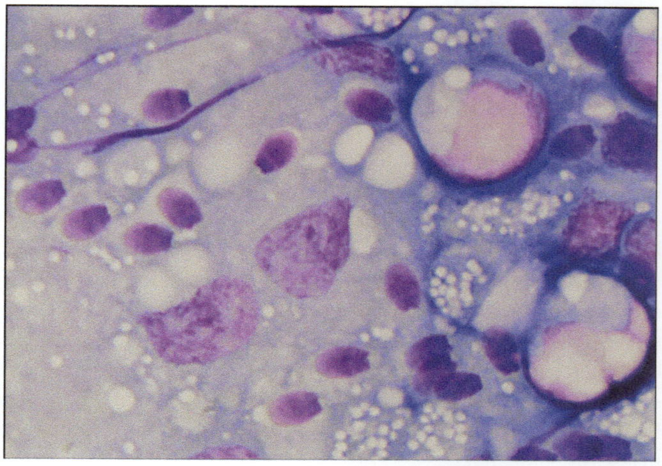

Figure 11.32 Late spermatids. Imprint of a testicle from an adult dog. Several late spermatids are present in this image. Cell cytoplasm is scant and pale. The nucleus is dense with an oval edge and a flattened edge (Wright–Giemsa, 2,000× magnification).

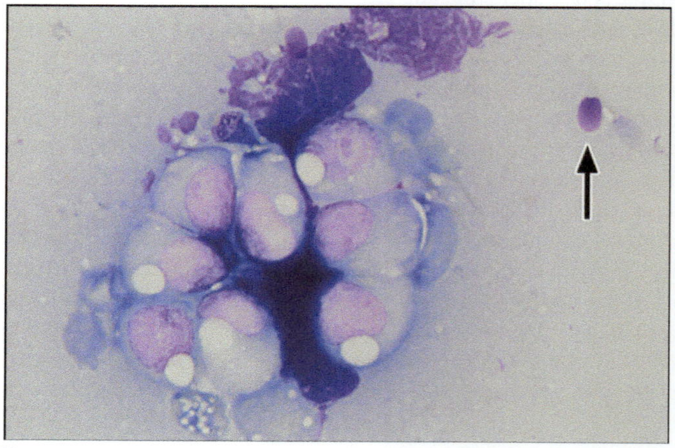

Figure 11.33 Spermatozoon. Imprint of a testicle from an adult dog. A mature spermatozoon is shown at the upper right of the image (arrow). The cell has a pale, light blue head and a long, nonstaining tail. Several early spermatids and two late spermatids also are shown (Wright–Giemsa, 1,500× magnification).

cap phase, the spermatid cytoplasm becomes paler and less distinct and the nucleus becomes bell-shaped as one end begins to elongate toward the location from which the tail forms. A thin crescent-shaped clear zone (cap) can be observed covering the rounded portion of the nucleus, opposite from where the tail is developing (Figure 11.31). Late spermatids in the acrosomal and maturation phases are morphologically similar to spermatozoa but have a very scant amount of pale basophilic cytoplasm at the base of the nucleus around the area of tail formation. During these stages the nucleus becomes progressively smaller, denser, and more oval in shape (Figure 11.32). Finally, spermatozoa are small cells that lack visible cytoplasm and have a dense, oval nucleus and a long, thin tail (Figure 11.33).

Infertility

Morphologic abnormalities observed in spermatozoa in wet mounts of semen samples can also be recognized during cytologic evaluation of testicular aspirates. These abnormalities are important findings in infertile animals.

Inflammation

Neutrophils can be seen cytologically in testicular aspirates from animals affected by orchitis, periorchitis, or epididymitis. In these cases, it is recommended that the clinician submit a sample for bacterial culture for detection of *Babesia canis*. Transient, sterile, neutrophilic inflammation is observed following chemical castration by injection of

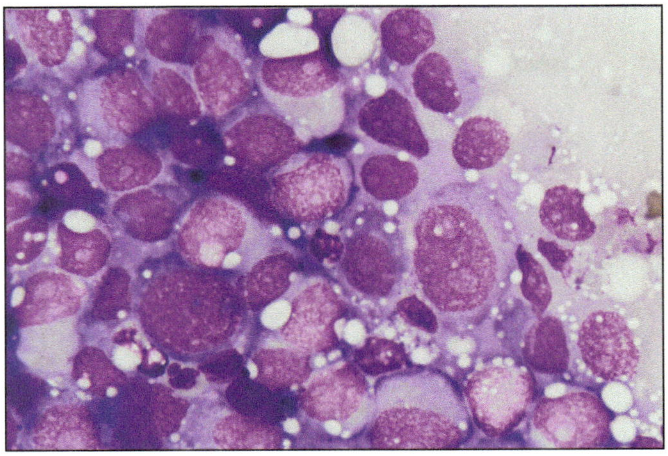

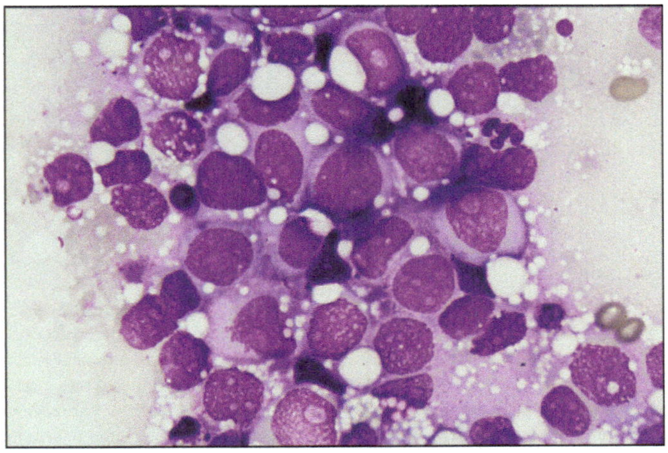

Figures 11.34, 11.35 **Sertoli cell tumor. FNA of an enlarged testicle from an adult intact male mixed-breed dog. Neoplastic cells are individualized and large with abundant, lightly basophilic cytoplasm that often contains one or more clear vacuoles. The nucleus is large and round with stippled to ropey chromatin and one to two large prominent nucleoli. Moderate anisocytosis and moderate to marked anisokaryosis are observed (Wright–Giemsa, 1,000× magnification).**

the testes with zinc compounds. Inflammation should be minimal and decreased semen volume and azoospermia are expected by 3 months following this procedure (Fahim *et al.*, 1993; Fagundes *et al.*, 2014).

Hematocele and hydrocele

Hematoceles and hydroceles are formed when blood or ascitic fluid, respectively, fills the cavity formed by the vaginal tunics. Aspiration of these lesions will yield a poorly cellular fluid sample that may contain low numbers of macrophages. If the macrophages contain phagocytized erythrocytes and black pigment (hemosiderin), a hematocele is suspected.

Neoplasia

Testicular tumors include epithelial tumors, sex cord stromal tumors, and germ cell tumors. In dogs, testicular tumors tend to be benign (metastasis occurs in <15% of canine cases) and it is common to find two types of tumors developing concurrently (Lawrence & Saba, 2013a). In cats, testicular tumors are rare, although all tumor types described in this section have been reported in both cats and dogs (Lawrence & Saba, 2013b).

Epithelial tumors

Epithelial tumors include rete adenomas and carcinomas. Both are rare compared with the other tumor types in testes.

Sex cord stromal tumors

Sertoli cell tumors and interstitial tumors are the sex cord stromal tumors that develop within testicles. Both tumor types can cause feminization due to expression of estrogens. Sertoli cell tumors are the most common type of testicular tumor and are particularly common in cryptorchid testicles. These tumors form from neoplastic sustentacular cells and are grossly firm, lobulated, and white. Sertoli cell tumors express vimentin, inhibin-a, and anti-Müllerian hormone (Banco *et al.*, 2010, 2012). Cytologically, Sertoli cell tumors comprise individualized cells with abundant, lightly basophilic cytoplasm and a large, round nucleus with stippled chromatin. A prominent, round nucleolus may be seen. Cells often contain a few large, clear, cytoplasmic vacuoles (Figures 11.34, 11.35). Interstitial tumors are derived from Leydig cells and are often an incidental finding at necropsy. Grossly, these tumors are soft, expansive, and yellow. On cytology, interstitial tumors contain aggregates of cells that may be associated with capillaries. Cellular characteristics can vary. Cells may have basophilic columnar cytoplasm with a round, relatively dense or stippled nucleus. If cells are partially ruptured, a dark, prominent nucleolus is often seen. Anisocytosis and anisokaryosis are common (Figures 11.36–11.40). Other tumors may be composed of smaller cells with scant lightly basophilic cytoplasm and a small, round nucleus with dense chromatin (Figures 11.41, 11.42).

Germ cell tumors

Seminomas are common germ cell tumors of dogs. As with Sertoli cell tumors, seminomas more often affect cryptorchid testicles. Grossly, seminomas are soft, small to lobulated, and ivory. Aspirates of seminomas contain large, individualized cells with a moderate amount of basophilic cytoplasm and a large, round nucleus that has finely stippled chromatin. A prominent nucleolus may be observed. Binucleation and mitotic figures are frequent findings (Figures 11.43, 11.44).

CYTOLOGY OF THE PROSTATE

Introduction

Cytology of prostatic tissue is performed when the gland is enlarged. Good quality samples of prostatic cells may be safely collected by

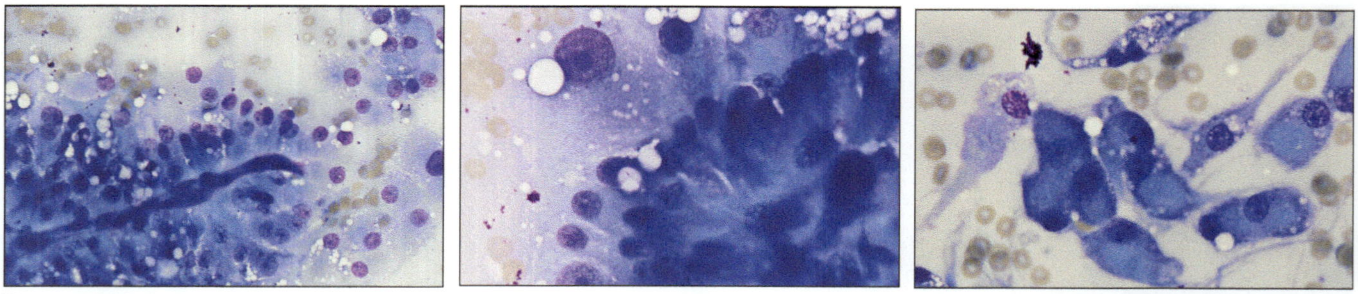

Figures 11.36–11.38 Interstitial cell tumor. FNA of an enlarged testicle from an adult intact male mixed-breed dog. Figure 11.36: Neoplastic cells are aggregated and often associated with vessels. Cells have basophilic, columnar cytoplasm and a round nucleus. Nuclei in this sample have stippled chromatin and a single, prominent nucleolus. Moderate anisocytosis and anisokaryosis are observed (Wright–Giemsa, 500× magnification). Figure 11.37: Aggregates of the neoplastic cells have basophilic, columnar cytoplasm and a round, basally located nucleus. Stippled chromatin and a single, prominent nucleolus are observed in most cells. Marked anisocytosis and anisokaryosis are shown (Wright–Giemsa, 1,000× magnification). Figure 11.38: Cells are arranged individually and in small aggregates. Cells have abundant cuboidal to columnar to spindloid basophilic cytoplasm, a round, basally located nucleus, stippled chromatin, and a single prominent nucleolus. Moderate anisocytosis was noted (Wright–Giemsa, 1,000× magnification).

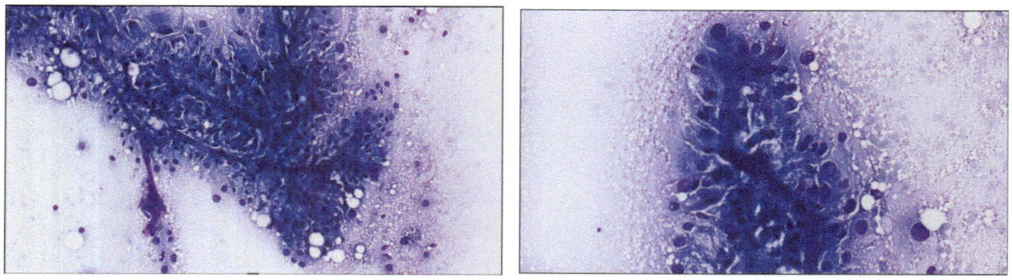

Figures 11.39, 11.40 Interstitial cell tumor. FNA of a testicular mass on a 10-year-old, male Golden Retriever. Figure 11.39: Neoplastic cells are closely associated with blood vessels and streams of brightly eosinophilic extracellular matrix. They have a moderate amount of basophilic cytoplasm and a round nucleus. Several cells contain clear cytoplasmic vacuoles. Anisocytosis and anisokaryosis are observed (Wright–Giemsa, 500× magnification). Figure 11.40: Cells are closely associated with blood vessels. They have a moderate to large amount of columnar, basophilic cytoplasm and contain small, distinct, clear cytoplasmic vacuoles. The nucleus is round with stippled chromatin. Many cells have a large, prominent, round nucleolus. Marked anisocytosis and anisokaryosis are seen (Wright–Giemsa, 1,000× magnification).

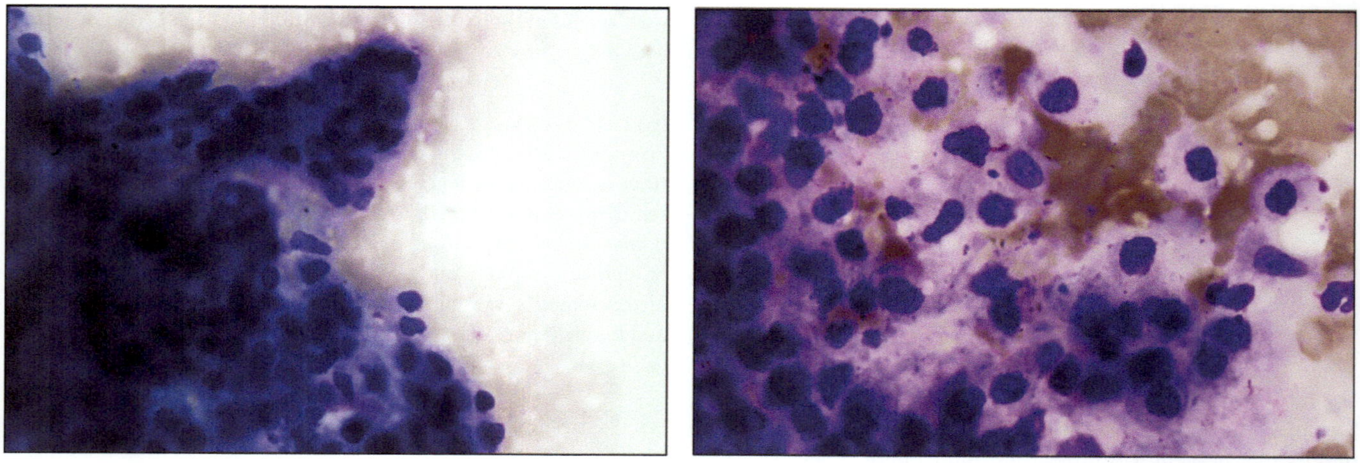

Figures 11.41, 11.42 Interstitial cell tumor. FNA of a testicular mass on an adult intact male Rottweiler. Figure 11.41: Cells are aggregated and have a small amount of lightly basophilic cytoplasm and a small, round nucleus with dense chromatin (Wright–Giemsa, 1,000× magnification). Figure 11.42: A small prominent nucleolus can be appreciated in some of the partially lysed cells in Figure 11.40 (Wright–Giemsa, 1,500× magnification).

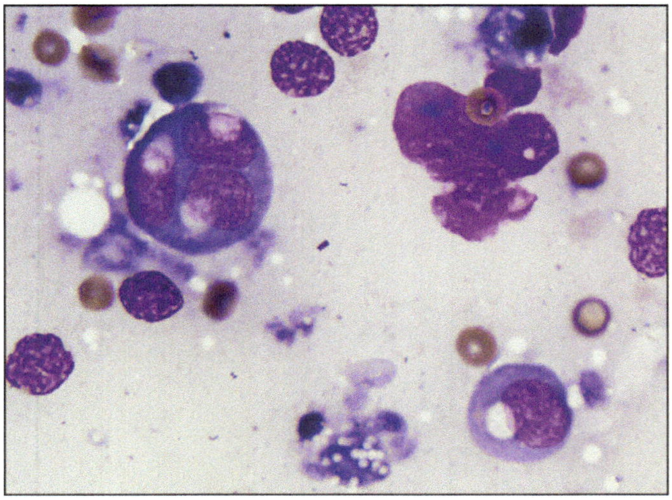

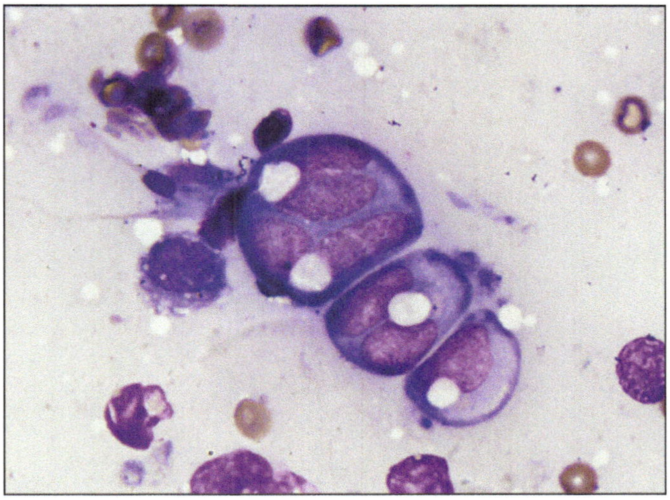

Figures 11.43, 11.44 Seminoma. FNA of a testicular mass on a 14-year-old, intact male Cocker Spaniel. Large, individualized, round cells with basophilic cytoplasm and low numbers of round, clear, distinct cytoplasmic vacuoles are observed. These cells have one or more round to oval nuclei with stippled chromatin. Several lysed cells and few erythrocytes are seen in the background (Wright–Giemsa, 1,500× magnification).

ejaculation, prostatic massage, prostatic wash, traumatic catheterization, and impression smears during surgery. Note that if manual ejaculation or prostatic massage is performed, the first and third fractions contain the prostatic epithelial cells (Kustritz, 2006). Additionally, ultrasound-guided, perirectal, or transrectal FNA can yield excellent quality samples, but these procedures have some risk for seeding the abdomen with neoplastic cells if the patient has a carcinoma. Powe *et al.* (2004) reported that cytologic interpretations of prostatic aspirates agreed with the histopathologic diagnosis 80% of the time. Only 2 of the 25 cytology samples they evaluated were nondiagnostic due to low cellularity; both of the nondiagnostic samples were collected by ultrasound-guided FNA.

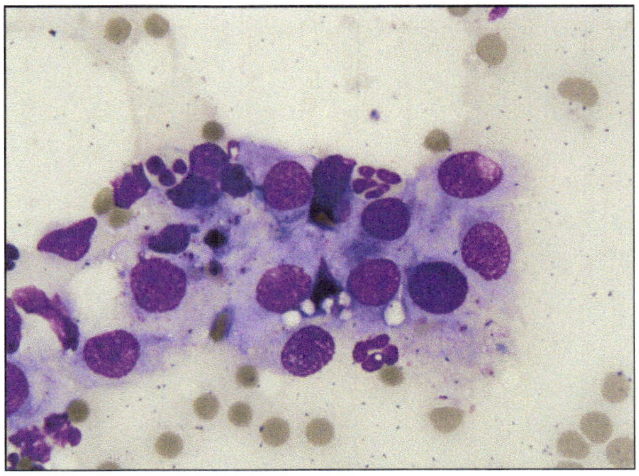

Figure 11.45 Prostatitis. Ultrasound-guided FNA of an enlarged prostate from a 12-year-old, intact male German Shepherd Dog. The image shows a slightly ruptured cluster of prostatic epithelial cells with abundant, lightly basophilic cytoplasm and a round nucleus with stippled chromatin. Closely associated with the prostatic epithelial cells are several neutrophils (Wright–Giemsa, 1,000× magnification).

Inflammation

If inflammation is present, the prostate may be uniformly enlarged or may contain soft, swollen pockets consistent with abscesses. Cytologically, the sample contains large numbers of nondegenerate to markedly degenerate neutrophils. There also should be low numbers of prostatic epithelial cells that are arranged in clusters. Prostatic epithelial cells are small and cuboidal with scant basophilic cytoplasm, distinct cell junctions, and a round nucleus with stippled chromatin (Figure 11.45). Mild anisocytosis and anisokaryosis are not commonly observed in the epithelial cell population but may be caused by dysplastic changes secondary to the inflammation. A moderate amount of blue-gray amorphous debris consistent with necrotic cellular material also may be seen. The sample should be closely examined for bacteria, especially if neutrophils appear degenerate. Infectious organisms that can cause prostatitis include bacteria (*Escherichia coli*, *Proteus vulgaris*, *Brucella canis*, among others), fungi (*Blastomyces dermatitis*, *Cryptococcus neoformans*, *Coccidioides immitis*), and parasites (*Leishmania* spp.) (Palmieri *et al.*, 2022).

Cysts

Cysts can develop in the prostate following obstruction of ducts. Clinical signs are usually associated with complications of prostatic enlargement. Fluid aspirated from prostatic cysts is typically straw-colored. Fluid cytology samples are of overall low cellularity and may contain low numbers of prostatic epithelial cells, macrophages, neutrophils, and lymphocytes (Boland *et al.*, 2003).

Hyperplasia

Hyperplasia tends to cause uniform enlargement of the prostate, but may be irregular if cysts are present. Prostatic hyperplasia is detected

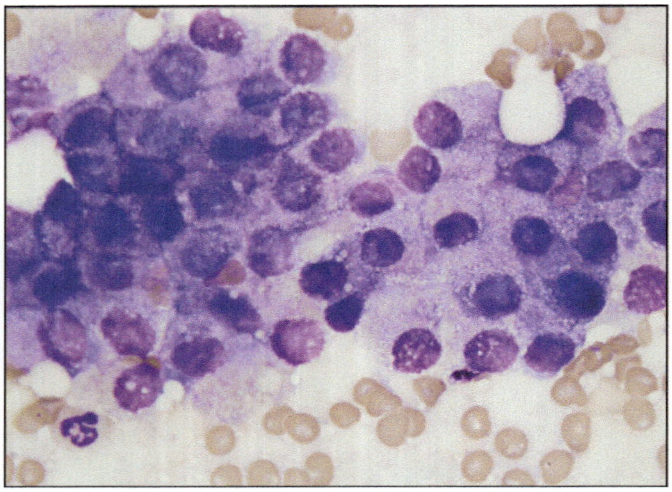
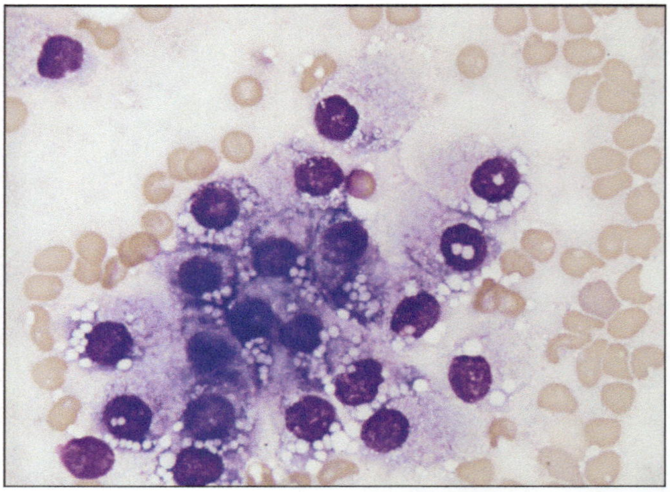

Figures 11.46, 11.47 Benign prostatic hyperplasia. Transrectal FNA of an enlarged prostate from an adult neutered male Bernese Mountain Dog. Sheets of cuboidal epithelial cells with a moderate to abundant amount of basophilic cytoplasm and a round nucleus are observed. Cells often contain numerous, clear, cytoplasmic vacuoles. The nuclei are relatively uniform in diameter and have smooth chromatin. A small, round nucleolus can be seen in low numbers of cells (Wright–Giemsa, 1,000× magnification).

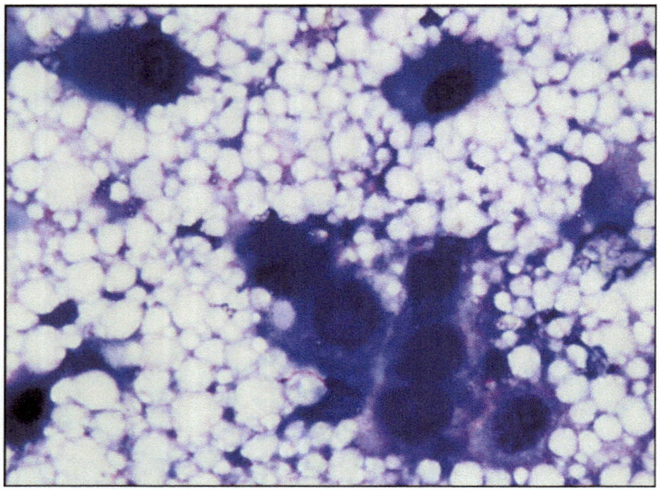

Figures 11.48 Squamous metaplasia. FNA from the enlarged prostate of a 6-year-old, neutered male Samoyed. Dysplastic prostatic epithelial cells have abundant, deeply basophilic cytoplasm and a large, round nucleus with clumped chromatin. Four individualized cells to the left and upper aspects of the image have glassier, blue, keratinized cytoplasm and a more condensed nucleus consistent with squamous metaplasia. The background is filled with basophilic proteinaceous material and lipid vacuoles (Wright–Giemsa, 1,000× magnification).

in many middle-aged to older, intact dogs. Aspiration of hyperplastic prostatic tissue yields large clusters of prostatic epithelial cells with scant to moderate amounts of deeply basophilic, sometimes vacuolated, cytoplasm and a round nucleus with stippled chromatin (Figures 11.46, 11.47). Cells have a uniform appearance and lack significant criteria of malignancy. The treatment of choice for prostatic hyperplasia is castration.

Metaplasia

Squamous metaplasia may occur in the prostate following trauma, inflammation, or exposure to an increased concentration of estrogen (which may be observed with Sertoli cell tumors and interstitial tumors of the testes). It is not considered a preneoplastic process. This condition is diagnosed when mildly dysplastic squamous epithelial cells with abundant, pale, polygonal cytoplasm and a round dense nucleus are found within or near prostatic epithelial cell clusters (Figure 11.48).

Neoplasia

Neoplastic changes in the prostate tend to form in one of the lobes of the prostate, and so the prostate palpates unevenly. The most common neoplasm of the canine prostate is prostatic carcinoma/adenocarcinoma and this can occur in intact or neutered male dogs. Transitional cell carcinomas, squamous cell carcinomas (SCCs), and mixed carcinomas are other relatively frequent neoplasms of the prostate. Less commonly, sarcomas (including fibrosarcoma, leiomyosarcoma, osteosarcoma, and hemangiosarcoma) have been reported (Foster, 2012c; Lawrence & Saba, 2013).

Prostatic/urothelial carcinoma

Cytology samples from neoplastic lesions of the prostate are often highly cellular. Morphologic differentiation between prostatic adenocarcinoma (originating from glandular prostatic epithelium) and urothelial carcinoma (originating from the prostatic urethra or periurethral ducts) is not possible without immunochemical stains. Uroplakin III and cytokeratin 7 expression by tumor cells support a diagnosis of urothelial carcinoma, but have relatively poor sensitivity and specificity (Palmieri *et al.*, 2022). Neoplastic cells tend to be grouped in clusters

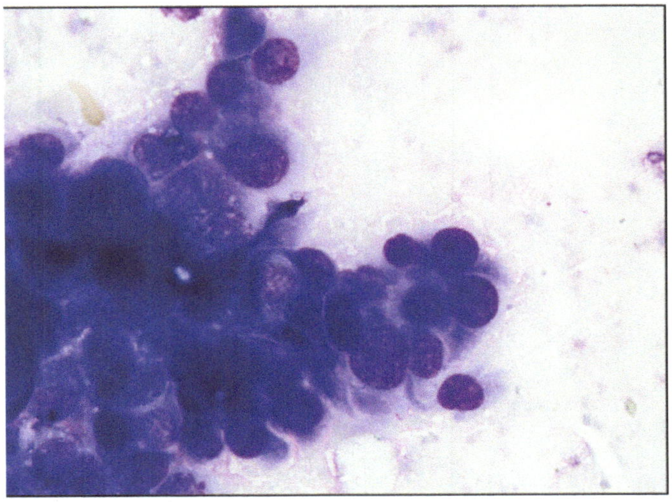

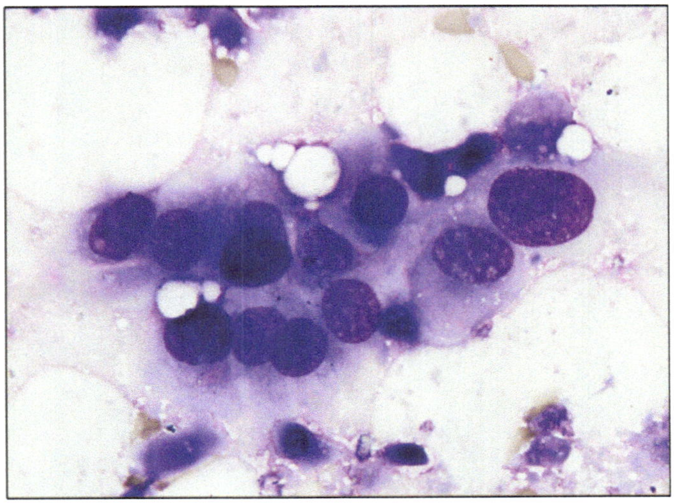

Figures 11.49, 11.50 **Prostatic adenocarcinoma. Ultrasound-guided FNA from the enlarged prostate of a 9-year-old, neutered male mixed-breed dog. The sample is highly cellular and has several crowded clusters of epithelial cells with rounded, lightly basophilic cytoplasm, a large rounded nucleus, and stippled to clumped chromatin. One or two prominent nucleoli are seen in low numbers of cells. Nuclear molding can be appreciated. Marked anisocytosis and anisokaryosis are observed (Wright–Giemsa, 1,000× magnification).**

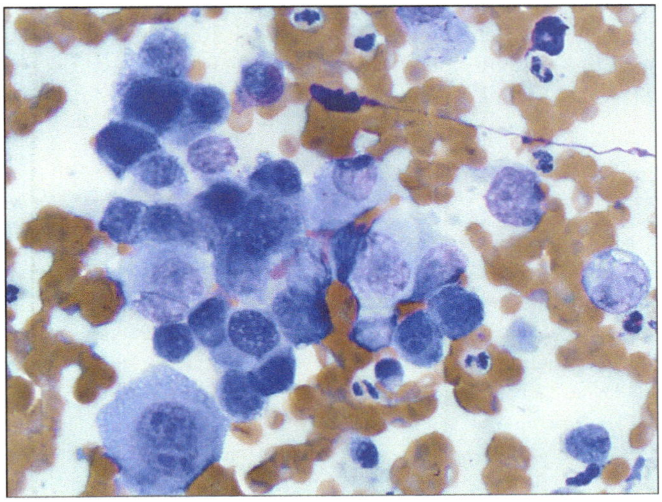

Figure 11.51 **Urothelial carcinoma (metastatic). FNA of a lytic bone lesion from a 14-year-old, spayed female dog. The sample is highly cellular and has several clusters of transitional epithelial cells with rounded, lightly basophilic cytoplasm, a large round nucleus, and stippled chromatin. One to three prominent nucleoli are seen in many cells. Binucleation and nuclear molding can be appreciated. Marked anisocytosis and anisokaryosis are observed (Wright–Giemsa, 800× magnification).**

and exhibit marked criteria of malignancy. Variable amounts of deeply basophilic cytoplasm can be seen. The cytoplasm may contain numerous small, clear vacuoles or one large, clear to eosinophilic vacuole that pushes the nucleus to the edge of the cell. Nuclei are variably sized and have coarse, clumped chromatin and one or more prominent nucleoli. Binucleation, nuclear molding, and mitotic figures often are observed (Figures 11.49–11.51). Prostatic (adeno)carcinomas tend to metastasize to regional lymph nodes, lung, and bone, particularly the lumbar vertebrae. It is a very common tumor of humans, but is less common in dogs (1% of all canine tumors) and is rare in cats (Lawrence Saba, 2013b). The median survival time of dogs with prostatic adenocarcinoma is less than 30 days and most cats die within 3 months of diagnosis (Lawrence Saba, 2013c).

CYTOLOGY OF THE PENIS AND PREPUCE

Introduction

Disease or trauma of the penis and prepuce occurs in low numbers of dogs and is even less common in cats. These lesions typically cause swelling of the region and are rarely aspirated unless a mass-effect is present. A few non-neoplastic diseases in the dog that may lead to swelling in the area include balantitis, paraphimosis, phimosis, priapism, foreign body reaction, and fracture of the os penis. In the cat, urethritis and damage secondary to urolith formation are more common (Foster, 2012c). Healthy cells of the penis are uniform, cuboidal to columnar epithelial cells (Kustritz, 2006).

Neoplasia

Several tumor types have been associated with the penis and prepuce. Any of the tumors arising from the skin and subcutis can be found in this location. In dogs, the most common tumors of the penis are TVT and SCC. Virtually no information exists about tumors that occur on the penis of cats (Foster, 2012c; Lawrence & Saba, 2013c).

Transmissible venereal tumor

TVT is the most common tumor of the penis in dogs. The behavior and appearance are identical to those described for tumors of the

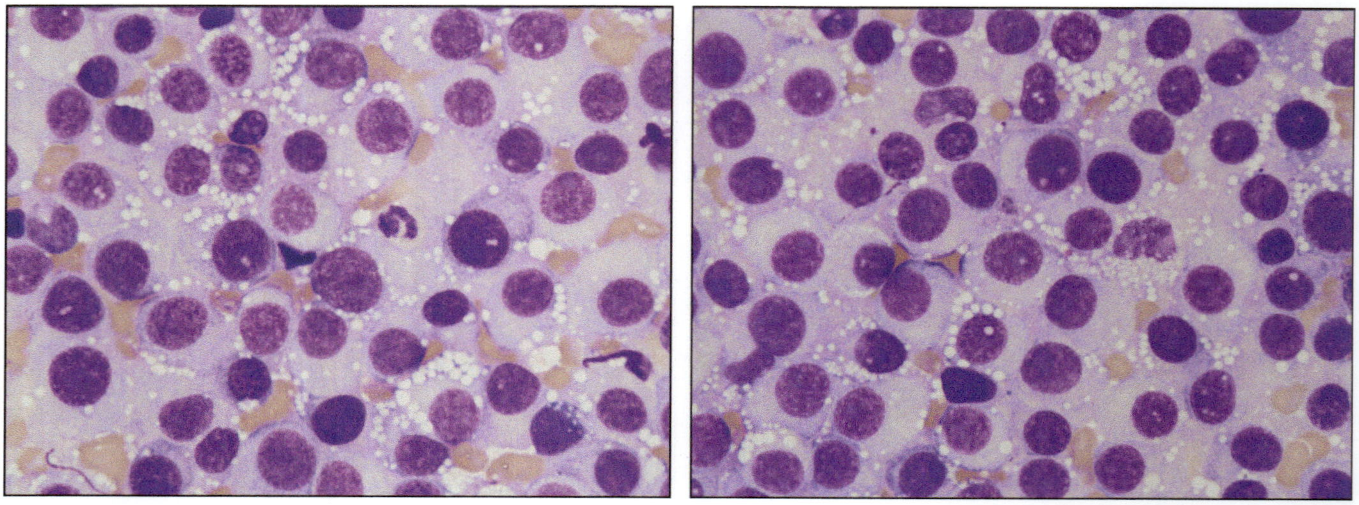

Figures 11.52, 11.53 **Transmissible venereal tumor. FNA from a penile mass on a 7-year-old, neutered male Labrador Retriever. Cells are individualized and round with abundant, lightly basophilic cytoplasm and a large, round nucleus. The nuclei have stippled chromatin and a prominent, large, round nucleolus is often seen. Clear, distinct, round, cytoplasmic vacuoles are observed in most cells. Moderate anisocytosis and anisokaryosis are noted. Low numbers of erythrocytes and rare neutrophils are present in the background (Wright–Giemsa, 1,000× magnification).**

vagina. As mentioned previously, cytologic samples are highly cellular and contain round cells with abundant lightly basophilic cytoplasm, distinct cytoplasmic vacuoles, and a round nucleus with finely stippled chromatin (Figures 11.52, 11.53).

Squamous cell carcinoma

SCCs tend to exfoliate well. Cells are primarily individualized and round to polygonal with abundant lightly basophilic to aqua cytoplasm. Nuclei are variably sized and round to irregular with coarse to clumped chromatin. Many classic characteristics of malignancy can be identified. Additionally, aberrant nuclear to cytoplasmic maturation is commonly observed, especially a large nucleus with immature chromatin within a keratinized cell. Perinuclear vacuoles indicative of aberrant keratinization also are common. Tadpole-shaped cells may be seen; these cells have a tail of lightly basophilic cytoplasm and an eccentrically located, rounded nucleus. Cells that contain a large cytoplasmic vacuole that flattens and displaces the nucleus to the side, giving them a signet ring appearance, may also be found (Figures 11.54–11.57).

CYTOLOGY OF THE SCROTUM

Introduction

Most pathology of the scrotum involves the scrotal skin. Lesions can be due to a large variety of etiologies including trauma, infection, atopy and other immune-mediated dermatopathies, endocrinopathies, toxicities, zinc deficiency, frostbite, sunburn, and neoplasia (Cerundolo & Maiolino, 2002). Scrotal necrotizing dermatitis has been associated with testicular injection of specific chemicals used for sterilization (Forazán *et al.*, 2014). Rarely, disease can occur in deeper fascial layers of the scrotal sac (Figure 11.58). The deepest facial layer is the tunica vaginalis, which communicates with the peritoneal cavity and is lined by mesothelial cells. Scrotal cestodiasis has been described in a dog with a peritoneal infestation of *Mesocestoides* sp. (Zeman *et al.*, 1988). The organisms likely migrated along the tunica vaginalis into the scrotum.

NEOPLASIA

In a study of 676 scrotal masses, 96% were neoplastic (Trappler *et al.*, 2014). The vast majority (396 of 676 cases, 58.6%) were round cell tumors; more specifically, 369 of 676 cases (54.6%) were mast cell tumors (Figure 11.59). Melanocytomas were slightly more common than malignant melanomas (7.1% and 4.7%, respectively). Other neoplasms included vascular hamartoma (6.8%), hemangiosarcoma (5.0%), hemangioma (4.6%), and histiocytoma (3.4%). Twenty-nine masses (4.3%) were epithelial in origin; of these, squamous cell carcinoma was the most common (the exact number was not indicated).

CASES

CASE 1

Signalment/history

A 7-year-old, neutered male Standard Poodle presented for a 5-day history of hematuria and dysuria.

Physical examination

Physical examination was normal except for an ulcerated hemorrhagic mass on the penis. FNAs of the mass were submitted for cytologic examination (Figures 11.60, 11.61; Bolfer *et al.*, 2015).

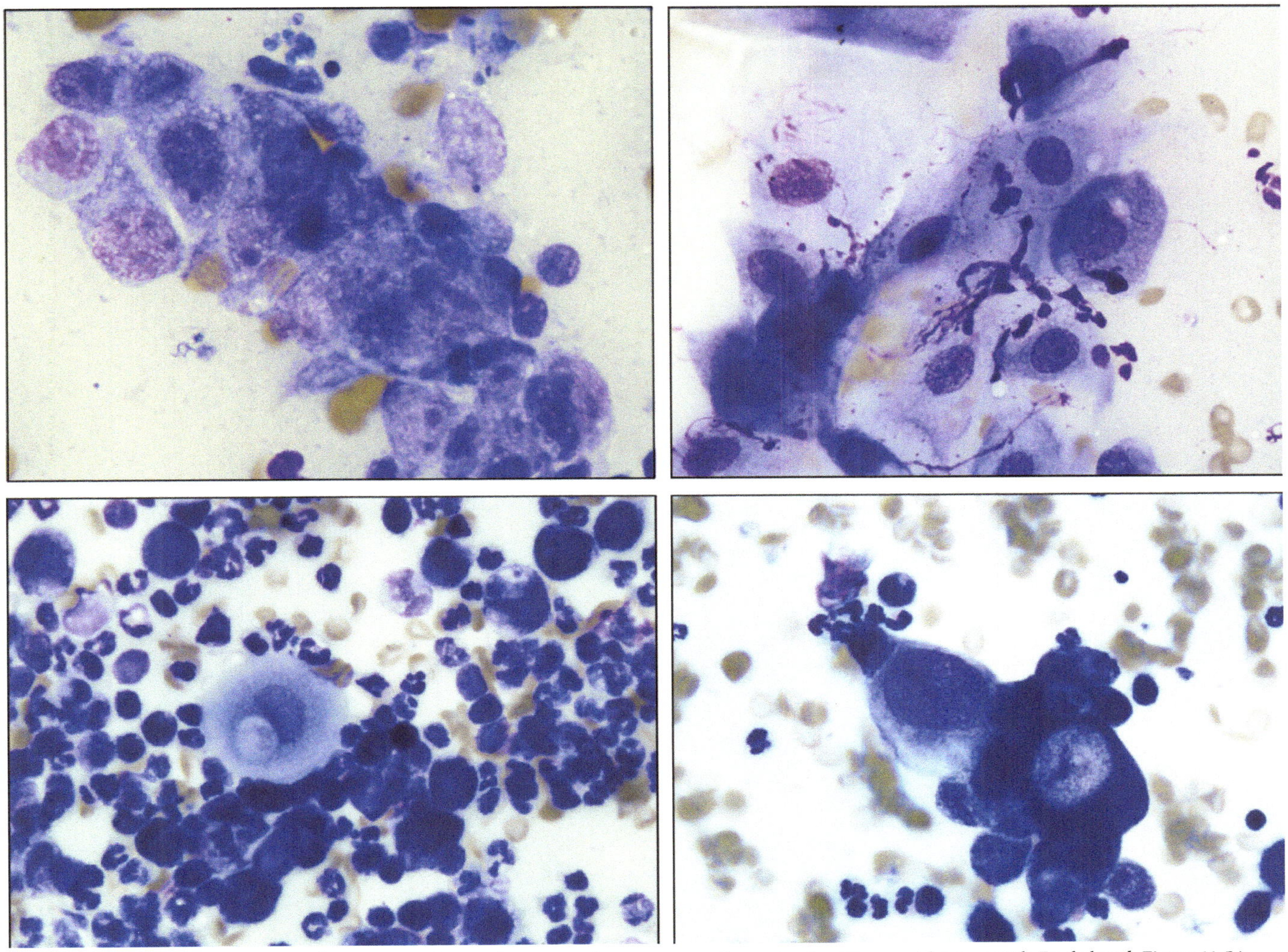

Figures 11.54–11.57 Squamous cell carcinoma. Impression smears from a mass on the penis of an 11-year-old, intact male Dachshund. Figure 11.54: Cells in this image are arranged in a cluster. Cells are large when compared with the neutrophil at the top of the image. They have scant, basophilic cytoplasm and a large, rounded nucleus with finely stippled chromatin and multiple nucleoli. Moderate anisocytosis and anisokaryosis are seen. This morphology supports a diagnosis of carcinoma (Wright–Giemsa, 1,500× magnification). Figure 11.55: Cells in this area of the slide are more individualized and some are keratinized. Cells are large and round to angular with abundant, lightly basophilic cytoplasm and a round nucleus with stippled chromatin. A prominent nucleolus can be seen in low numbers of cells. A few neutrophils also are present (Wright–Giemsa, 1,000× magnification). Figure 11.56: Large numbers of neutrophils and fewer macrophages are seen in some areas of the slide. A single, anaplastic, squamous epithelial cell with abundant light-blue-green cytoplasm, an aberrant cytoplasmic vacuole, and a distorted, rounded nucleus is present at the center of the image (Wright–Giemsa, 1,000× magnification). Figure 11.57: A large cluster of highly variably sized epithelial cells is shown. Cells have scant to abundant, lightly to deeply basophilic, rounded cytoplasm. The nucleus is round with open chromatin. A prominent, crescent-shaped nucleolus is observed in one of the larger cells. Many of the smaller cells have a high nuclear to cytoplasmic ratio. Low numbers of neutrophils are closely associated with the neoplastic cells (Wright–Giemsa, 1,000× magnification).

Cytologic description

The sample contained moderate numbers of large spindloid cells with deeply basophilic cytoplasm and an ovoid nucleus. Many cells contained punctate clear cytoplasmic vacuoles. Eosinophilic product was seen in low numbers of cells. Multinucleation, anisocytosis, anisokaryosis, and multiple prominent variably sized nucleoli were observed.

Cytologic interpretation

Sarcoma. Primary differential diagnoses are hemangiosarcoma and fibrosarcoma.

Management/outcome

Penile amputation was performed and the mass was submitted for histopathology. The histologic diagnosis was completely excised

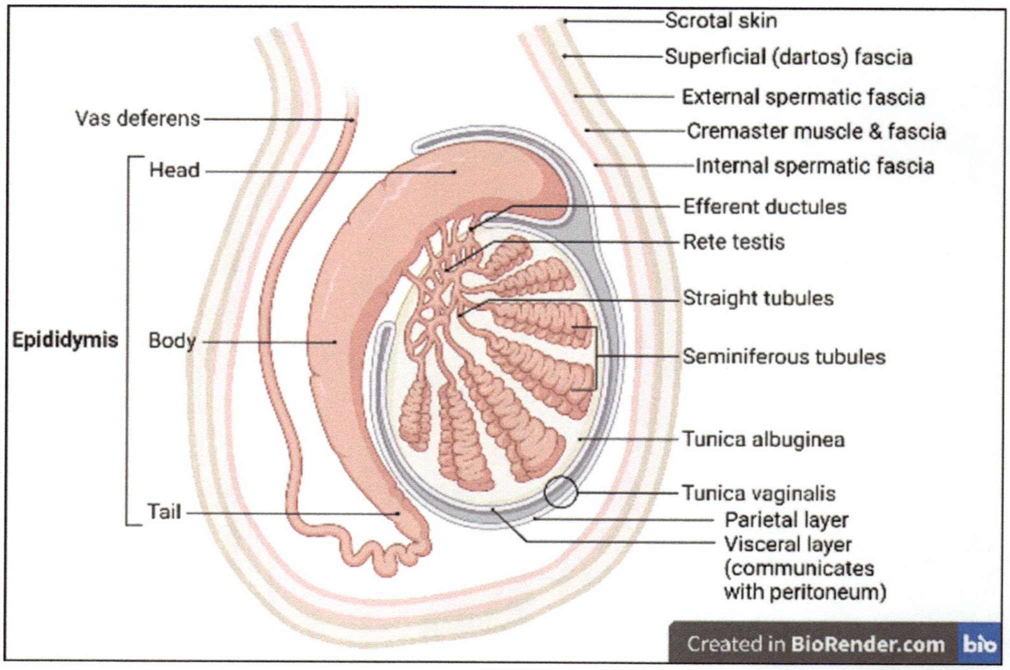

Figure 11.58 Anatomy of the scrotum. The most superficial layer of the scrotal sac is the skin. Deeper facial layers include the superficial (dartos) fascia, the external spermatic fascia, the cremaster muscle and fascia, the internal spermatic fascia, the parietal layer of the tunica vaginalis, and the visceral layer of the tunica vaginalis. Created with BioRender.com.

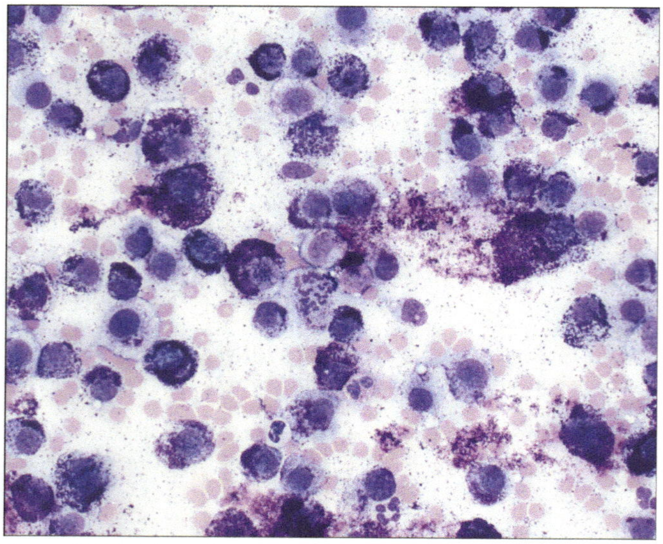

Figure 11.59 Mast cell tumor. FNA from a scrotal mass on a 9-year-old, neutered male American Bulldog. Cells are individualized and round with abundant, lightly basophilic cytoplasm and a large, round, centrally located nucleus. The nuclei have smooth to finely stippled chromatin and an indistinct nucleolus. Cells contain variable numbers of pinpoint metachromatic cytoplasmic granules. Moderate anisocytosis and anisokaryosis are noted. There are occasional mitotic figures. Low numbers of neutrophils and eosinophils, and moderate numbers of erythrocytes are present in the background. Free metachromatic granules are scattered throughout the sample (Wright–Giemsa, 500× magnification).

hemangiosarcoma. Two hundred and five days after the surgery, the patient presented to an emergency clinic with ascites and was euthanized due to presumptive disseminated hemangiosarcoma.

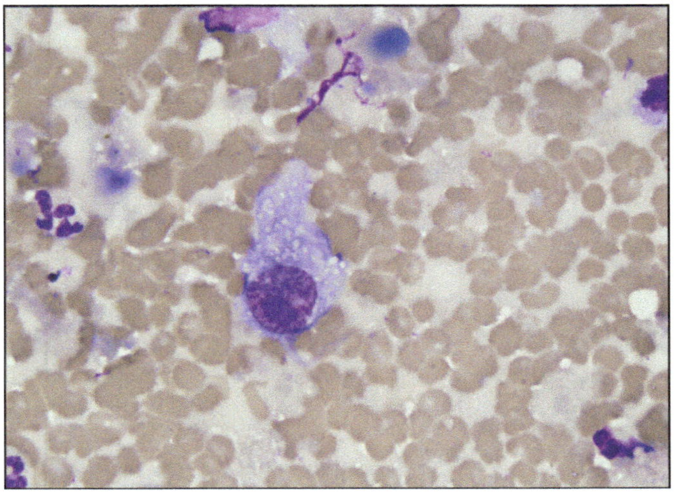

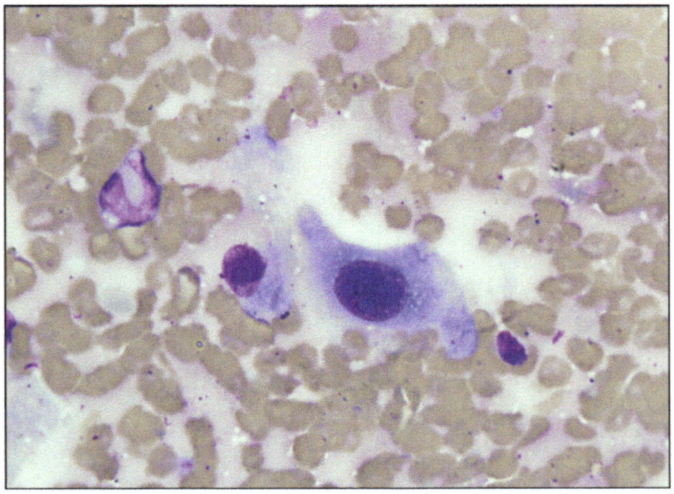

Figures 11.60, 11.61 Hemangiosarcoma. FNA from a mass on the penis of a 7-year-old, neutered male Standard Poodle. Individualized large spindle-shaped cells with abundant basophilic cytoplasm, often several cytoplasmic vacuoles, and a large ovoid nucleus are seen (Wright–Giemsa, 1,000× magnification).

CASE 2

Signalment/history

A 10-year-old, spayed female Golden Retriever presented with a 2-month history of mucinous vaginal discharge.

Physical examination

No physical abnormalities were detected. A vaginal swab was submitted for cytologic examination (Figure 11.62).

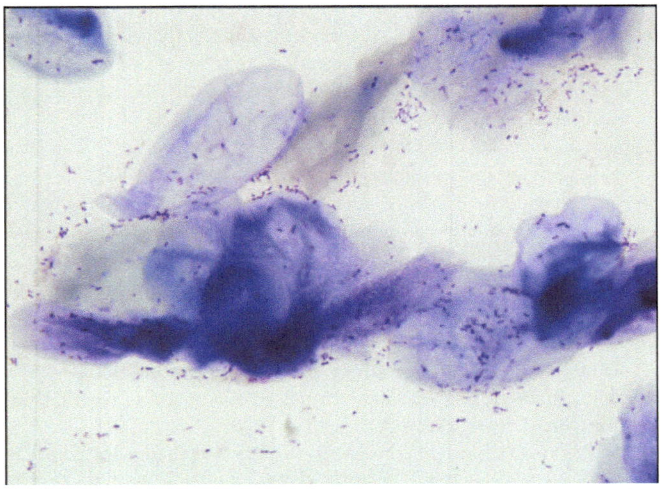

Figure 11.62 Possible estrus. Vaginal swab from a 10-year-old, spayed female Golden Retriever. The majority of cells are anucleate squamous epithelial cells. Large numbers of bacterial cocci and rods are observed in the background, but no inflammatory cells are seen (Wright–Giemsa, 1,000× magnification).

Cytologic description

The majority of cells were anucleate squamous epithelial cells with fewer nucleated squamous epithelial cells. Large numbers of bacterial cocci and rods were observed in the background. No inflammatory cells were seen.

Cytologic interpretation

Mature squamous epithelium. The bacteria are likely commensal organisms. If the sample is representative of the vaginal wall, not inadvertently sampled from the vulva or clitoris, it is consistent with estrus. In a spayed female, this is commonly associated with a retained ovarian remnant. Given the patient's age and duration of the vaginal discharge, exogenous sources of estrogen (including neoplasms) should be considered.

Management/follow-up

The patient was fully evaluated for mass lesions. None were found. The sample was suspected of being more representative of the vulva than the vaginal wall.

CASE 3

Signalment/history

A 10-year-old, male castrated American Pit Bull Terrier presented for swelling of the caudoventral abdomen and scrotum.

Physical examination

The patient was in moderate pain and was administered analgesics. He had pitting edema of the abdomen and scrotum. His popliteal lymph nodes were enlarged. Ultrasonography revealed medial iliac

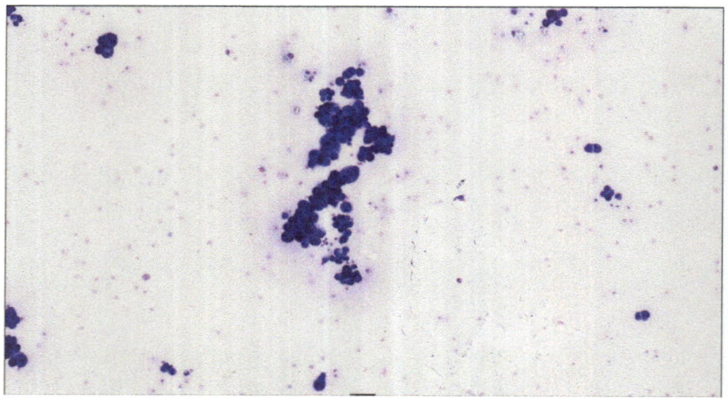

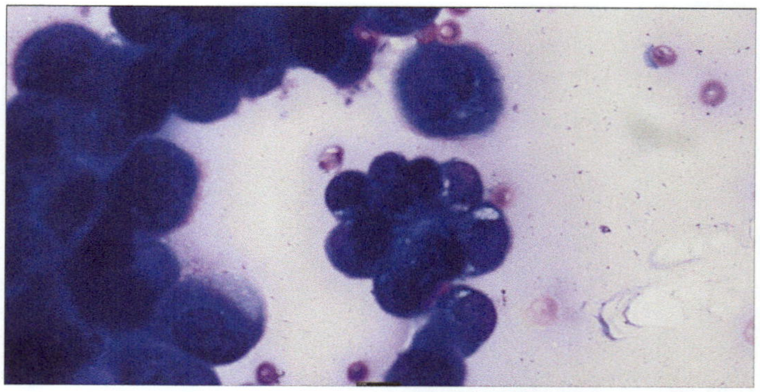

Figures 11.63, 11.64 **FNA from a scrotal swelling on a 10-year-old, male castrated Pit Bull. Figure 11.63: Clusters of mesothelial cells are observed (Wright–Giemsa, 200× magnification). Figure 11.64: Mesothelial cells are present in clusters. They have a variable amount of round, deeply basophilic cytoplasm with a thin pink fringe at the cytoplasmic border. The nucleus is round or slightly cleaved and had coarse chromatin. One to two nucleoli are often seen. Anisocytosis and anisokaryosis are marked (Wright–Giemsa, 2,000× magnification).**

and inguinal lymphadenopathy, and a prostatic cyst. FNA of the scrotum was performed (Figures 11.63, 11.64).

Cytologic description

The sample was highly cellular. The majority of cells were clustered together. Most cells had a small amount of deeply basophilic cytoplasm, while others had more expanded, moderately basophilic cytoplasm. Cells frequently had a bright pink cytoplasmic fringe. The nucleus was round to ovoid with coarsely stippled chromatin and one to multiple distinct nucleoli. There were low numbers of binucleate cells. Marked anisocytosis and anisokaryosis were observed. Low numbers of vacuolated macrophages also were seen. No infectious organisms were present.

Cytologic interpretation

Probable malignant neoplasm. Differential diagnoses include reactive mesothelial tissue, mesothelioma, or an atypical carcinoma (possibly a prostatic or urogenital carcinoma).

Management/follow-up

Enlarged lymph nodes were aspirated for cytologic evaluation. The samples contained a reactive lymphoid population and cells similar to those observed in the swollen scrotum. The top differential diagnosis was a metastatic mesothelioma. Due to the pain the patient was in and the poor disease prognosis, the dog was euthanized.

REFERENCES

Akihara Y., Shimoyama Y., Kawasako K. et al. (2007) Immunohistochemical evaluation of canine ovarian tumors. *J Vet Med Sci 69(7)*:703–708.

Banco B., Giudice C., Veronesi M.C. et al. (2010) An immunohistochemical study of normal and neoplastic canine sertoli cells. *J Comp Pathol 143*:239–247.

Banco B., Veronesi M.C., Giudice C. et al. (2012) Immunohistochemical evaluation of the expression of anti-Mullerian hormone in mature, immature and neoplastic canine sertoli cells. *J Comp Pathol 146*:18–23.

Boland L.E., Hardie R.J., Gregory S.P. et al. (2003) Ultrasound-guided percutaneous drainage as the primary treatment for prostatic abscesses and cysts in dogs. *J Am Anim Hosp Assoc 39(2)*:151–159.

Bolfer L., Schmit J.M., MacNeill A.L. et al. (2015) Penile amputation and scrotal urethrostomy followed by chemotherapy in a dog with penile hemangiosarcoma. *J Am Anim Hosp Assoc 51(1)*:25–30.

Borzacchiello G., Mogavero S., Tortorella G. et al. (2010) Expression of endothelin-1 and endothelin receptor a in canine ovarian tumours. *Reprod Domest Anim 45(6)*:465–468.

Brown P.J., Evans H.K., Deen S. et al. (2012) Fibroepithelial polyps of the vagina in bitches: A histological and immunohistochemical study. *J Comp Pathol 147(2–3)*:181–185.

Cerundolo R., Maiolino P. (2002) Review cutaneous lesions of the canine scrotum. *Veterinary Dermatology 13*:63–76.

Diagone K.V., Feliciano M.A.R., Pacheco M.R. et al. (2011) Histology and morphometry of the testes of adult domestic cats (*Felis catus*). *J Feline Med Surg 14(2)*:124–130.

England G.C.W. (1992) Vaginal cytology and cervicovaginal mucus arborisation in the breeding management of bitches. *J Small Anim Pract 33*:577–582.

Fagundes A.K.F., Oliveira E.C.S., Tenorio B.M. et al. (2014) Injection of a chemical castration agent, zinc gluconate, into the testes of cats results in the impairment of spermatogenesis: A potentially irreversible contraceptive approach for this species. *Theriogenology 81*:230–236.

Fahim M.S., Wang M., Sutcu M.F. et al. (1993) Sterilization of dogs with intra-epididymal injection of zinc arginine. *Contraception 47*:107–122.

Faya M., Carranza A., Priotto M. et al. (2011) Domestic queens under natural temperate photoperiod do not manifest seasonal anestrus. *Anim Reprod Sci 129*:78–81.

Fontaine E., Levy X., Grellet A. et al. (2009) Diagnosis of endometritis in the bitch: A new approach. *Reprod Domest Anim 44(S2)*:196–199.

Forzán M.J., Garde E., Pérez G.E., Vanderstichel R.V. (2014) Necrosuppurative orchitis and scrotal necrotizing dermatitis following intratesticular administration of zinc gluconate neutralized with arginine (EsterilSol) in 2 mixed-breed dogs. *Vet Pathol 51(4)*:820–823.

Foster R.A. (2012a) Female reproductive system and mammary gland. In: *Pathologic Basis of Veterinary Disease*, 5th edn. (eds. J.F. Zachary, M.D. McGavin) Elsevier Saunders, St. Louis, p. 1120.

Foster R.A. (2012b) Female reproductive system and mammary gland. In: *Pathologic Basis of Veterinary Disease*, 5th edn. (eds. J.F. Zachary, M.D. McGavin) Elsevier Saunders, St. Louis, pp. 1097–1098.

Foster R.A. (2012c) Common lesions in the male reproductive tract of cats and dogs. *Vet Clin North Am Small Anim Pract 42*:527–545.

Gil da Costa R.M., Santos M., Amorim I. et al. (2009) An immunohistochemical study of feline endometrial adenocarcinoma. *J Comp Pathol 140(4)*:254–259.

Gouletsou P.G., Galatos A.D., Leontides L.S. et al. (2010) Impact of fine or large needle aspiration on the dog's testis: In vitro ultrasonographic, bacteriological, gross anatomy and histological assessment. *Theriogenology 74*:1604–1614.

Gouletsou P.G., Galatos A.D., Leontides L.S. et al. (2011) Impact of fine- or large-needle aspiration on canine testes: Clinical, in vivo ultrasonographic and seminological assessment. *Reprod Domest Anim 46*:712–719.

Gouletsou P.G., Galatos A.D., Sideri A.I. et al. (2012) Impact of fine needle aspiration (FNA) and of the number of punctures on the feline testis: Clinical, gross anatomy and histological assessment. *Theriogenology 78*:172–181.

Greenlee P.G., Patnaik A.K. (1985) Canine ovarian tumors of germ cell origin. *Vet Pathol 22(2)*:117–122.

Groppetti D., Pecile A., Arrighi S. et al. (2010) Endometrial cytology and computerized morphometric analysis of epithelial nuclei: A useful tool for reproductive diagnosis in the bitch. *Theriogenology 73*:927–941.

Groppetti D., Pecile A., Barbero C. et al. (2012) Vaginal bacterial flora and cytology in proestrous bitches: Role on fertility. *Theriogenology 77*:1549–1556.

Johnston S.D. (1991) Performing a complete canine semen evaluation in a small animal hospital. *Vet Clin North Am Small Anim Pract 21(3)*:545–551.

Kustritz M.V.R. (2006) Collection of tissue and culture samples from the canine reproductive tract. *Theriogenology 66*:567–574.

Kustritz M.V.R. (2012) Managing the reproductive cycle in the bitch. *Vet Clin North Am Small Anim Pract 42*:423–437.

Lawrence J.A., Saba C.F. (2013a) Tumors of the male reproductive system. In: *Withrow & MacEwen's Small Animal Clinical Oncology*, 5th edn. (eds. S.J. Withrow, D.M. Vail) Elsevier Saunders, St. Louis, p. 558.

Lawrence J.A., Saba C.F. (2013b) Tumors of the male reproductive system. In: *Withrow & MacEwen's Small Animal Clinical Oncology*, 5th edn. (eds. S.J. Withrow, D.M. Vail) Elsevier Saunders, St. Louis, p. 561.

Lawrence J.A., Saba C.F. (2013c) Tumors of the male reproductive system. In: *Withrow & MacEwen's Small Animal Clinical Oncology*, 5th edn. (eds. S.J. Withrow, D.M. Vail) Elsevier Saunders, St. Louis, pp. 564–566.

Maksimovic A., Maksimovic Z., Filipovic S. et al. (2012) Vaginal and uterine bacteria of healthy bitches during different stages of their reproductive cycle. *Vet Rec 171(15)*:375–376.

Marchal T., Chabanne L., Kaplanski C. et al. (1997) Immunophenotype of the canine transmissible venereal tumour. *Vet Immunol Immunopathol 57(1–2)*:1–11.

Moxon R., Copley D., England G.C.W. (2010) Quality assurance of canine vaginal cytology: A preliminary study. *Theriogenology 74*:479–485.

Mozos E., Méndez A., Gómez-Villamandos J.C. et al. (1996) Immunohistochemical characterization of canine transmissible venereal tumor. *Vet Pathol 33(3)*:257–263.

Murchison E.P., Wedge D.C., Alexandrov L.B. et al. (2014) Transmissible [corrected] dog cancer genome reveals the origin and history of an ancient cell lineage. *Science 343(6169)*:437–440.

Ortega-Pacheco A., Gutiérrez-Blanco E., Jiménez-Coello M. (2012) Common lesions in the female reproductive tract of dogs and cats. *Vet Clin North Am Small Anim Pract 42*:547–559.

Palmieri C., Fonseca-Alves C.E., Laufer-Amorim R. (2022) A review on canine and feline prostate pathology. *Frontiers in Veterinary Science 26(9)*:881232.

Patnaik A.K., Greenlee P.G. (1987) Canine ovarian neoplasms: A clinicopathologic study of 71 cases, including histology of 12 granulosa cell tumors. *Vet Pathol 24(6)*:509–514.

Pelkey T.J., Frierson H.F. Jr, Mills S.E. et al. (1998) The diagnostic utility of inhibin staining in ovarian neoplasms. *Int J Gynecol Pathol 17(2)*:97–105.

Piseddu E., Masserdotti C., Milesi C. et al. (2012) Cytologic features of normal canine ovaries in different stages of estrus with histologic comparison. *Vet Clin Pathol 41(3)*:396–404.

Powe J.R., Canfield P.J., Martin P.A. (2004) Evaluation of the cytologic diagnosis of canine prostatic disorders. *Vet Clin Pathol 33(3)*:150–154.

Saba C.F., Lawrence J.A. (2013) Tumors of the female reproductive system. In: *Withrow & MacEwen's Small Animal Clinical Oncology*, 5th edn. (eds. S.J. Withrow, D.M. Vail) Elsevier Saunders, St. Louis, p. 535.

Santos M., Marcos R., Caniatti M. (2012) Cytologic study of normal canine testis. *Theriogenology 73*:208–214.

Schlafer D.H., Gifford A.T. (2008) Cystic endometrial hyperplasia, pseudo-placentational endometrial hyperplasia, and other cystic conditions of the canine and feline uterus. *Theriogenology 70*:349–358.

Thacher C., Bradley R.L. (1983) Vulvar and vaginal tumors in the dog: A retrospective study. *J Am Vet Med Assoc 183(6)*:690–692.

Trappler M.C., Popovitch C.A., Goldschmidt M.H. et al. (2014) Scrotal tumors in dogs: A retrospective study of 676 cases (1986–2010). *Canadian Veterinary Journal 55(1)*:1229–1233.

Wilson M.S. (2001) Transcervical insemination techniques in the bitch. *Vet Clin North Am Small Anim Pract 31(2)*:291–304.

Zambelli D., Cunto M. (2006) Semen collection in cats: Techniques and analysis. *Theriogenology 66(2)*:159–165.

Zeman D.H., Cheney J.M., Waldrup K.A. (1988) Scrotal cestodiasis in a dog. *Cornell Vet. 78(3)*:273–279.

CHAPTER 12

MUSCULOSKELETAL CYTOLOGY

Amy N. Schnelle

INTRODUCTION

Cytology of the musculoskeletal system can present unique challenges, in particular poor exfoliation of lesions or contamination of the sample with significant quantities of peripheral blood. However, cytology of joints, skeletal muscle, and bone can provide important diagnostic information. Even in instances in which a definitive cytologic diagnosis is not achievable, the results of cytologic evaluation may help guide selection of subsequent diagnostic steps.

SYNOVIAL FLUID

Sampling

Aspiration of synovial fluid from the joints of dogs and cats is often performed on effusive joints, although fluid may occasionally be collected from joints without obvious effusion. These joints may have accompanying masses, be associated with clinical lameness, or have previously displayed clinical or cytological abnormalities.

Collection of joint fluid requires limited supplies. Materials for aseptic preparation of the site, an appropriately sized hypodermic needle, 3 ml or 6 ml syringe, an EDTA tube, and a sterile glass tube should be gathered in preparation. The patient should be appropriately restrained, with sedation or anesthesia, as indicated. Pain control should be instituted as needed. The site should be selected by reviewing anatomic landmarks and flexing and extending the joint of interest; this allows identification of a site in which the joint space may be accessed without a high likelihood of encountering significant vessels, nerves, cartilage, or bone. Review of individual joint anatomy may be helpful, and illustrated guides are available in clinical technique textbooks and elsewhere (Johnson & Mackin, 2012a). Once selected, the site should be clipped and prepared with a sterile scrub, and the synovial fluid should be carefully collected using sterile technique (Figures 12.1a–c). This ensures that an appropriate sample

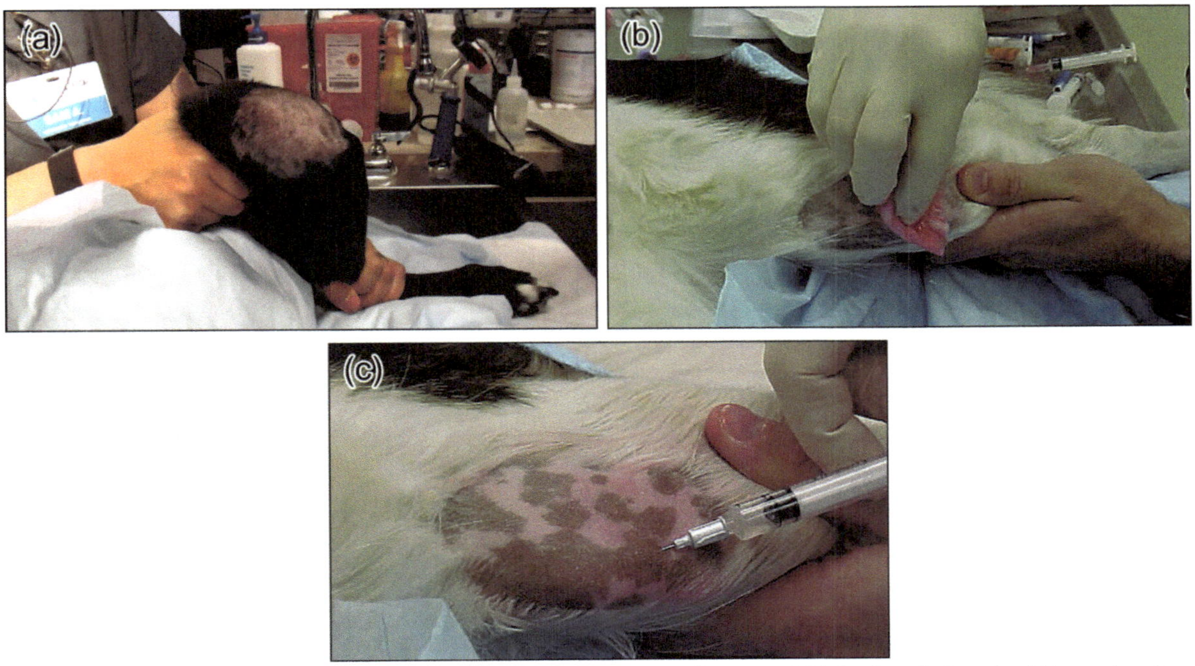

Figures 12.1a–c The site should be prepared with a surgical clip (a) and then aseptically prepared (b). Sterile technique should be employed in sample collection (c). These steps ensure that microorganisms are not introduced into the synovial space during sampling and that the sample remains free of microorganism contamination. (Courtesy Brian Husbands.)

DOI: 10.1201/9781003258551-12

for culture is available, if needed, as well as avoiding introduction of microorganisms into the synovial space. Synovial fluid can be collected using a 22- or 25-gauge hypodermic needle of length sufficient to penetrate the joint of interest. Aspiration is applied to collect the fluid; however, aspiration should be discontinued before withdrawing the needle to help reduce blood contamination. A notation should be made if obvious blood contamination occurs during collection.

Synovial fluid should be collected into an EDTA tube for cytologic analysis, a sterile glass tube for any serologic testing or culture, and/or a culturette for bacterial culture, if needed. Collection of fluid into an EDTA tube is helpful for prevention of cell clotting in samples with peripheral blood contamination. Clotting and cell aggregation can interfere with determination of accurate cell estimates. Preparation of one or more direct smears at the time of fluid collection is also beneficial. This provides a baseline for assessment of cell morphology and can help distinguish real findings from *in-vitro* artifacts. This is particularly helpful when trying to discern true hemorrhage from *in-vitro* peripheral blood contamination.

Analysis

Analysis of synovial fluid typically consists of measurement of the total protein concentration (generally estimated by a refractometer), a nucleated cell count, and cytologic assessment. It may also include assessment of mucin clot quality and viscosity if sufficient sample is available. Normal synovial fluid is typically thick in character, clear, and pale yellow or colorless.

A normal total nucleated cell count of <3,000 cells/μl is generally accepted for canine synovial fluid and <1,000 cells/μl in feline synovial fluid (Pacchiana *et al.*, 2004). Nucleated cells within synovial fluid may be counted via an automated analyzer or a hemocytometer or estimated via review of a direct smear of synovial fluid. The determination of a numerical value is affected by synovial fluid properties and some variability exists in the literature with regards to the most accurate means of counting. The viscous nature of synovial fluid can result in uneven distribution of cells within fluid, which may hamper accurate counting. The addition of a small amount of hyaluronidase to a synovial fluid sample can reduce this quality and may facilitate counting of nucleated cells (Ekmann *et al.*, 2010). Standing synovial fluid samples may develop a gelatinous nature that dissipates with agitation; this property is referred to as thixotropy. Smearing of synovial fluid in this state may contribute to uneven cell distribution. This property should not be confused with sample clotting, which occurs with peripheral blood contamination of samples and may necessitate collection of a new sample for accurate analysis. Use of automated hematology analyzers to count nucleated cells within synovial fluid has been described in human, equine, and canine samples (Salinas *et al.*, 1997; de Jonge *et al.*, 2004; Ekmann *et al.*, 2010; Dusick *et al.*, 2014; Froom *et al.*, 2013). Evaluation of the nucleated cellularity of direct smears of synovial fluid may help assess the accuracy of an automated cell count; the identification of many cellular aggregates may raise concerns for a falsely low automated cell count.

Visual estimation may be attempted in cases with limited sample volume, although this may result in a falsely elevated estimation (Gibson *et al.*, 1999). A study evaluated a detailed protocol for the estimation of a nucleated cell count by visual review of direct smears of synovial fluid and found that 78% of estimated samples were correctly categorized as within the reference interval, mildly to moderately increased, or markedly increased, relative to automated counts (for details of the protocol, refer to Dusick *et al.*, 2014). In samples with aggregates of nucleated cells and/or a high degree of viscosity, obtaining an accurate nucleated cell count or estimate may be challenging.

To evaluate the viscosity of the sample, the mucin clot test can be performed. The mucin clot test is used to assess the amount of hyaluronic acid in synovial fluid via a semiquantitative rating scheme. The test consists of the application of one part of the plain or heparinized synovial fluid sample to four parts 2.5% glacial acetic acid (MacWilliams & Friedrichs, 2003), with an assessment of the mucin clot formed thereafter. The mucin clot is assessed as 'good' for a firm, cohesive clot surrounded by clear fluid, 'fair' for a soft clot with less cohesion and cloudy surrounding fluid, and 'poor' for a friable clot in murky fluid.

Synovial fluid viscosity, another method of estimating hyaluronic acid content, is assessed by touching a wooden applicator stick to a small amount of sample at the mouth of the tube and measuring the distance the strand will stretch with applicator withdrawal before breaking (approximately 2 cm in normal fluid).

Both the mucin clot test and assessment of fluid stranding are attempts to estimate the hyaluronic acid content of the synovial fluid, with reduced viscosity raising concern for underlying disease; however, a retrospective study of dogs with polyarthritis found that fluid viscosity was decreased in only 17 of 36 joints in which it was assessed (Jacques *et al.*, 2002). In the author's experience, fluid viscosity is often normal in joints with overt clinical and microscopic abnormalities, and assessment of this characteristic of synovial fluid should be omitted if only a limited sample volume is available for diagnostic testing.

Protein concentrations of 1.5–3 g/dl (15–30 g/l) are commonly observed in healthy synovial fluid (MacWilliams & Friedrichs, 2003). Protein concentrations may be elevated with the addition of inflammatory proteins or may decrease with fluid influx associated with effusion. Protein concentrations may also be normal in samples with other evidence of joint disease.

Assessment of direct smears of synovial fluid on low power (100× magnification) typically reveals an eosinophilic, stippled background, with windrowing (linear arrangement) of cells within this material, which reflects the high viscosity of the fluid (Figures 12.2a–d). This material is often thick and prevents adequate cell spreading. Since this material obscures much of the fine cytologic detail, the nucleated cells within the sample should be evaluated in the thinnest portions of the smear for more accurate determination of cell size, cytologic and nuclear features, and presence of inclusions or infectious organisms. The amount of blood that is present should be noted, as this may influence the cells observed. Cells within normal synovial fluid samples consist primarily of large mononuclear cells, which may include macrophages, monocytes, and synovial lining cells, as well as small mononuclear cells (consistent with small lymphocytes). Macrophages and monocytes within synovial fluid are similar in appearance to those observed elsewhere within the body; macrophages may or may

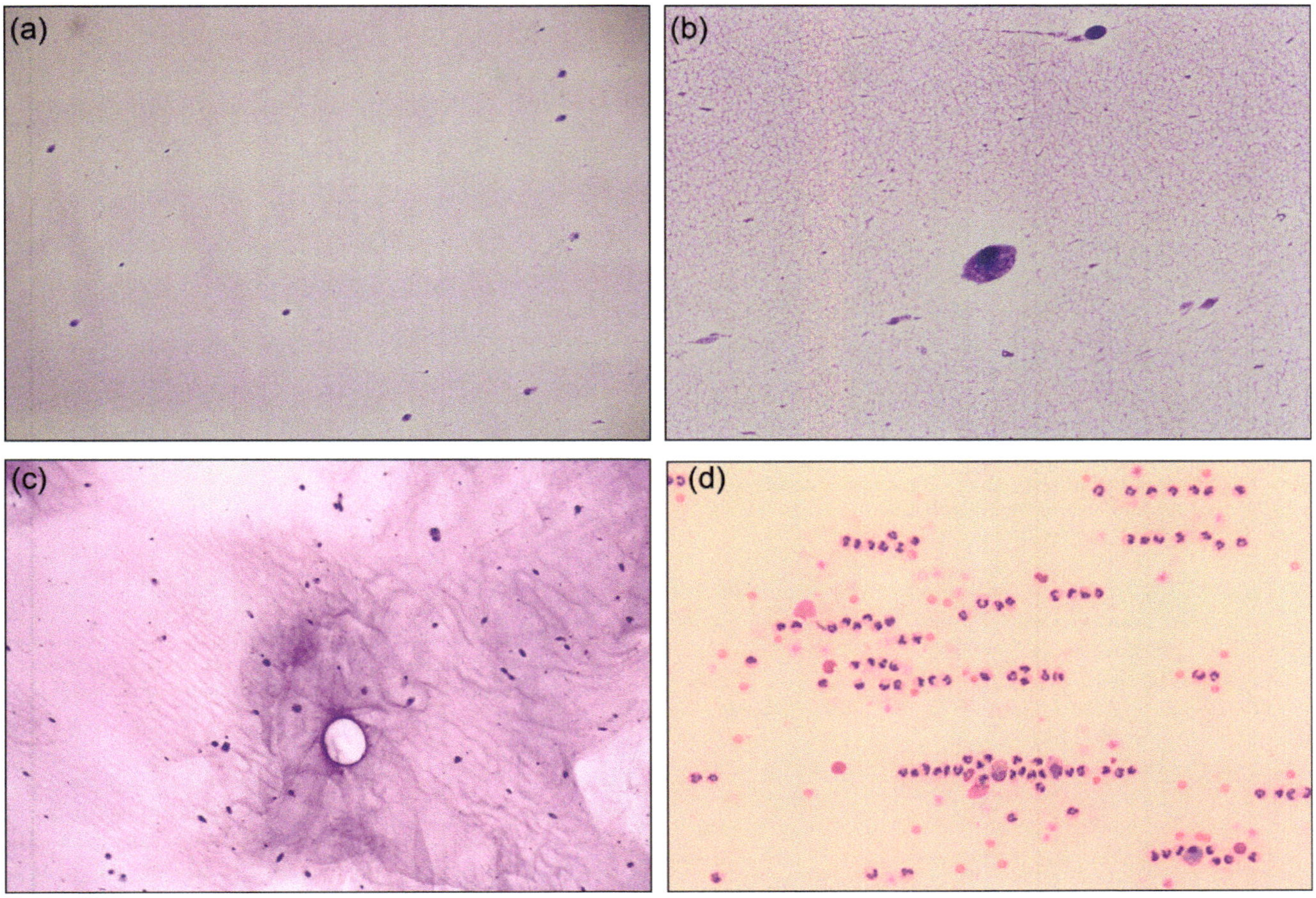

Figures 12.2a–d (a, b) Normal synovial fluid is of low nucleated cellularity with eosinophilic stippled background material (Wright–Giemsa: a, 100× magnification; b, 500× magnification). (c) The viscous nature of synovial fluid can result in uneven distribution of nucleated cells within a smear, posing a challenge in estimating cellularity (Wright–Giemsa, 100× magnification). (d) The linear arrangement (windrowing) of cells is demonstrated in this synovial fluid sample with marked suppurative inflammation. Note the stippled, eosinophilic background; this highly viscous material results in the cellular arrangement observed in the image (Wright–Giemsa, 250× magnification).

not have vacuolated cytoplasm. Synovial lining cells may be rounded to spindloid in shape, with moderate to abundant basophilic cytoplasm, rounded or ovoid nuclei, and stippled chromatin. Neutrophils are infrequently identified and should be nondegenerate if observed in otherwise normal synovial fluid. Although variable percentages of neutrophils have been reported in synovial fluid, most samples contain less than 10% neutrophils (Pacchiana *et al.*, 2004).

Inflammatory arthritides

Inflammatory joint disease of infectious and noninfectious causes often is characterized by increased numbers of nucleated cells; generally, significantly increased fractions of neutrophils are part of the process. Since infectious and noninfectious diseases may have a similar cytologic appearance, clinical impression and suspicion are often very important in the selection of subsequent diagnostic testing for further differentiation.

Suppurative inflammation

Infectious disease

A variety of organisms can result in inflammatory joint disease, including bacterial, rickettsial, spirochetal, fungal, mycoplasmal, and viral pathogens. Observation of intracellular bacteria within synovial neutrophils indicates a need for culture of synovial fluid. Unfortunately, bacteria may not be visually identified in all cases of septic arthritis; therefore, bacterial culture may have value in cases with increased clinical suspicion, such as a juvenile animal with multiple effusive joints or a patient with a previous trauma to an affected joint. Culture may be generally valuable in cases with increased fractions of neutrophils without identified organisms, particularly those samples with moderately to markedly elevated nucleated cell counts (Figure 12.3). A retrospective study of 31 cases of septic arthritis reported a range in neutrophil fractions from 25% to 99%, with a median of 90% (Clements *et al.*, 2005).

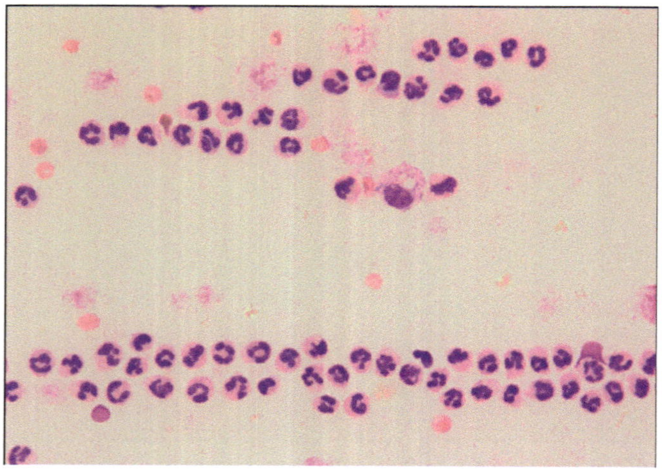

Figure 12.3 **Suppurative arthritis in a dog. The sample is cellular and consists of nondegenerate neutrophils exhibiting marked windrowing (Wright–Giemsa, 500× magnification).**

A variety of organisms can be identified. One study cultured *Staphylococcus intermedius* most frequently from ten cases of septic arthritis; *S. haemolyticus*, *Streptococcus canis*, and *Enterococcus faecalis* were among other cultured organisms (Riggio *et al.*, 2014). Another study similarly cultured *Staphylococcus* spp. most commonly, followed by *Streptococcus* spp. and others (Clements *et al.*, 2005). Using polymerase chain reaction (PCR), bacterial DNA was detected in joints with cranial cruciate rupture and medial patellar luxation, as well as normal synovial fluid, though the clinical significance is unclear (Bhandal *et al.*, 2013). *Mycoplasma gateae* induced erosive joint disease in multiple joints in a young cat; the organism was isolated via anaerobic culture (Zeugswetter *et al.*, 2007). Dogs experimentally infected with the spirochete *Borrelia burgdorferi* developed joint inflammation that was primarily suppurative during acute disease, transitioned to a mixed inflammatory population of neutrophils and mononuclear cells in intermediate stages, and was typically lymphoplasmacytic in chronic disease (Summers *et al.*, 2005). Rickettsial morulae may be observed in cells within synovial fluid and are cytologically consistent with those observed in peripheral blood leukocytes (Figures 12.4a–d). The protozoan *Leishmania donovani* can result in joint inflammation, and amastigotes have been identified within macrophages alone or within both macrophages and neutrophils in synovial fluid (McConkey *et al.*, 2002; Santos *et al.*, 2006). A retrospective study of 13 cases of dogs with *L. donovani* found that synovial fluid nucleated cell counts ranged from 34,000 to 66,000 cells/µl; neutrophils ranged from 34% to 89%, and lymphocytes ranged from 18% to 62% (Sbrana *et al.*, 2014). *Blastomyces dermatitidis* can be identified within the synovial fluid of infected dogs (Woods *et al.*, 2013). Diagnostic testing for underlying infectious disease may be useful prior to starting immunosuppressive therapy for suspected immune-mediated joint disease.

Noninfectious disease

Immune-mediated arthritides include idiopathic polyarthritis, polyarthritis secondary to drug or vaccine administration, breed-specific conditions (e.g., Akitas and Shar Peis), steroid-responsive meningitis–arteritis, systemic lupus erythematosus, and polyarthritis/polymyositis syndrome; these conditions are not typically associated with erosive lesions of articular cartilage or underlying bone (Johnson & Mackin, 2012b). They typically affect young adult dogs, although the polyarthritis that affects Akitas occurs in dogs less than 1 year of age (Johnson & Mackin, 2012b). In cats, idiopathic polyarthritis, systemic lupus erythematosus, and chronic progressive polyarthritis have been reported (Oohashi *et al.*, 2009). In animals in which other causes of cartilage and bone destruction have been ruled out, erosive polyarthritis should raise concern for rheumatoid arthritis in dogs and chronic progressive polyarthritis in cats, as these conditions are associated with radiographic changes in these species (Johnson & Mackin, 2012b). When synovial fluid is altered by suppurative inflammation and immune-mediated joint disease is a clinical concern, negative test results for likely infectious diseases (through culture, PCR, serology, etc.) and assessment of radiographic findings can help support clinical suspicion. Identification of multiple inflamed joints is an expected finding, although rare cases with single joint involvement are reported (Johnson & Mackin, 2012b). Neutrophils containing large, rounded, deeply eosinophilic inclusions (lupus erythematosus cells) and small, variably sized, rounded inclusions (ragocytes) have sometimes been associated with cases of suppurative arthritis due to an immune-mediated etiology. This material is thought to represent phagocytized nuclear material or complexes of immunoglobulin with cell or nuclear material (Figures 12.5a–c). However, these inclusions are infrequently identified, and care must be taken not to misinterpret intracellular bacteria or phagocytized cell debris. If used judiciously in patients with other strong clinical evidence, testing for rheumatoid factor and antinuclear antibodies, respectively,

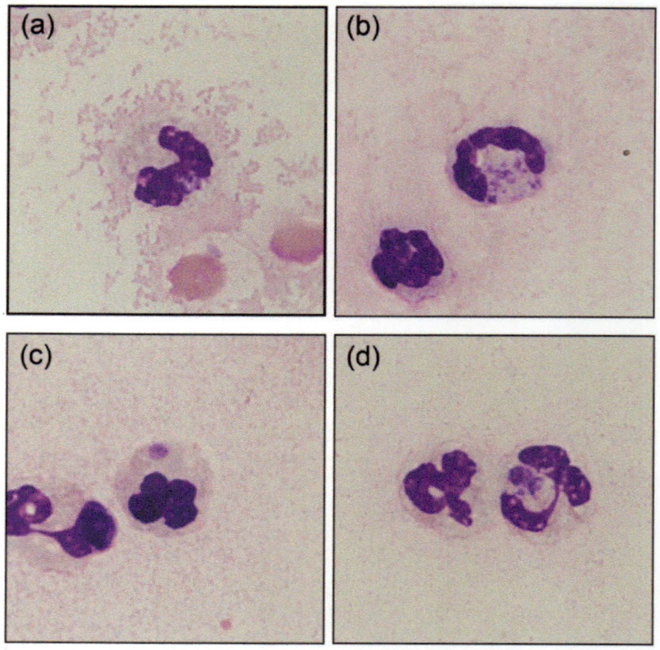

Figures 12.4a–d **Rickettsial arthritis in a dog; molecular testing was not performed to determine species. Neutrophils contain basophilic, stippled morulae (Wright–Giemsa, 1000× magnification).**

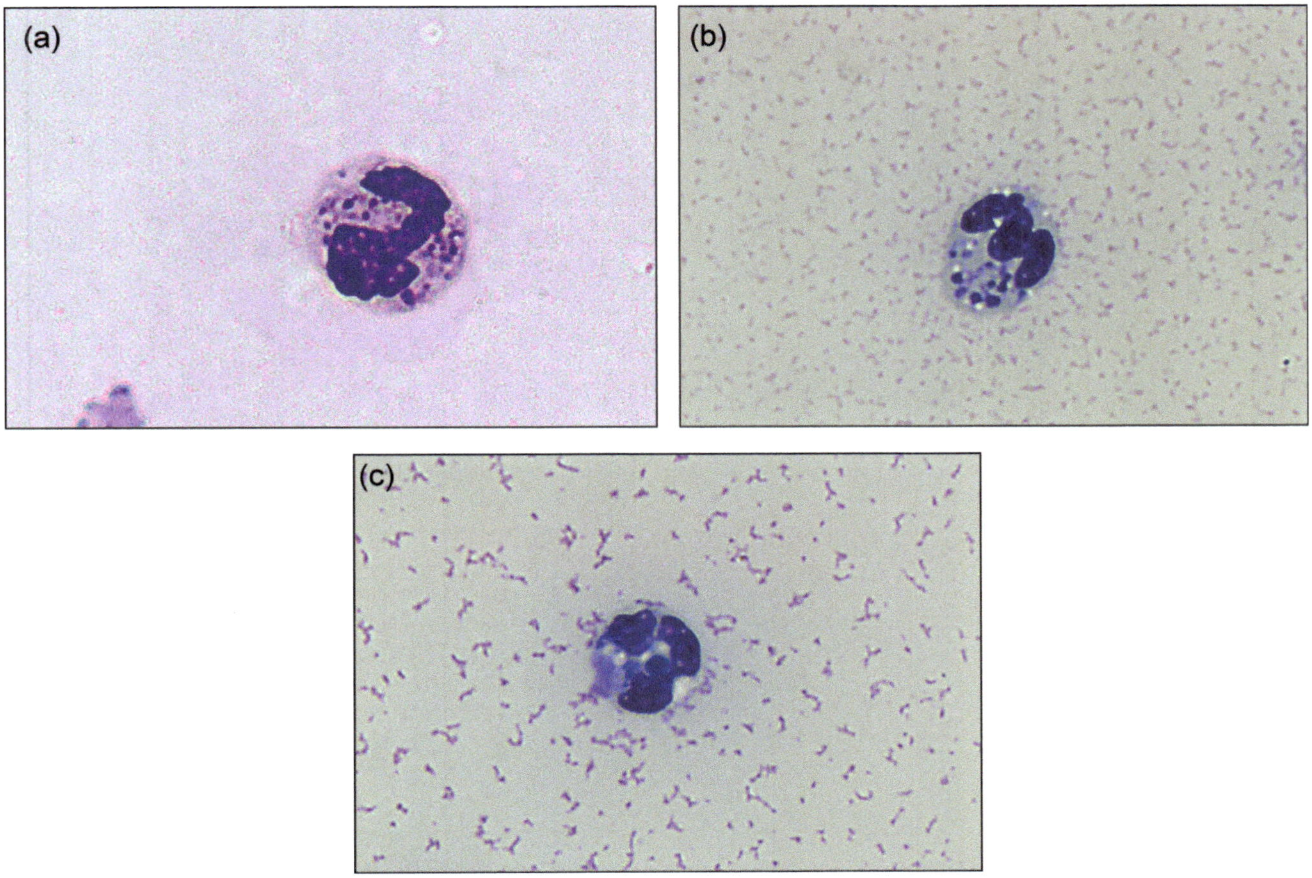

Figures 12.5a–c **Synovial fluid from a dog with immune-mediated polyarthritis. (a) A neutrophil contains many basophilic structures; this cell is consistent with a ragocyte (Wright–Giemsa, 4,000× magnification). (Courtesy Anne Barger.) (b) Synovial fluid from a different dog; a ragocyte is also pictured (Wright–Giemsa, 3,000× magnification). (c) Same dog as 14.4b. A single lupus erythematosus cell is noted with a large basophilic inclusion (Wright–Giemsa, 3,000× magnification). (Courtesy Amy MacNeill.)**

can help lend support for diagnosis of rheumatoid arthritis or systemic lupus erythematosus, respectively (Johnson & Mackin, 2012a, 2012b). Alone, positive results for either test are not pathognomonic for those conditions, and interpretation should be done with caution.

Mononuclear inflammation

Mononuclear inflammation of synovial fluid consists of increased numbers of large mononuclear cells, typically with a smaller fraction of small lymphocytes within the fluid (Figures 12.6a, b). This type of inflammation is typically mild to moderate in degree and is associated with degenerative joint disease or trauma. Radiographic evaluation can help identify evidence of osteoarthritis and may identify overt traumatic injuries.

HEMARTHROSIS

Hemarthrosis is hemorrhage within a synovial space, which may be seen secondary to trauma, anticoagulant rodenticide intoxication, hereditary coagulation abnormalities, and other bleeding diatheses. Observation of uniformly red synovial fluid during collection is supportive of hemarthrosis (as opposed to a wisp of red that may appear with peripheral blood contamination). Identification of macrophages containing phagocytized erythrocytes, as well as hemosiderin pigment (blue-black, granular material) and hematoidin crystals (orange, rhomboid, refractile, crystalline material), is indicative of joint hemorrhage in smears prepared immediately after synovial fluid collection (Figure 12.7). Care must be taken in interpreting erythrophagia in fluid samples that have been shipped or had other delays in sample processing, as *in-vitro* erythrophagia may have occurred.

Tumors of the joint

A varied population of cells makes up the synovial lining, including vascular and adipose tissue and cells of fibroblast (synoviocytes) and macrophage origin. A review of 35 synovial tumors in dogs found 18 histiocytic sarcomas diagnosed in part by positive staining for CD18, and 5 synovial cell sarcomas were identified via positive staining for cytokeratin. The other tumors were synovial myxomas and several other sarcomas, including fibrosarcoma and chondrosarcoma (Craig *et al.*, 2002).

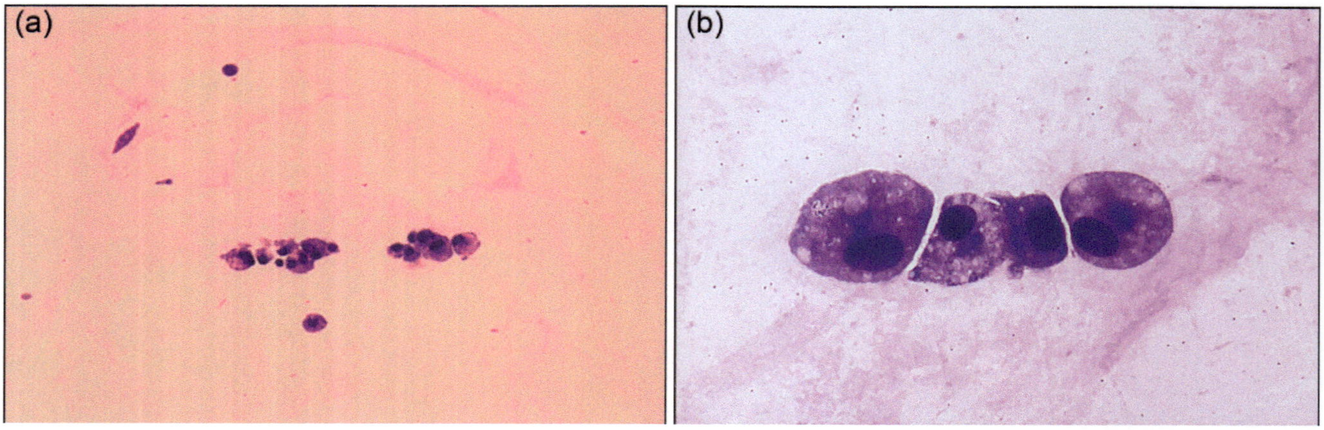

Figures 12.6a, b **Mononuclear inflammation due to osteoarthritis in a dog. This synovial fluid had a mildly increased nucleated cell count, due to increased numbers of large mononuclear cells (Wright–Giemsa: a, 250× magnification; b, 1,000× magnification).**

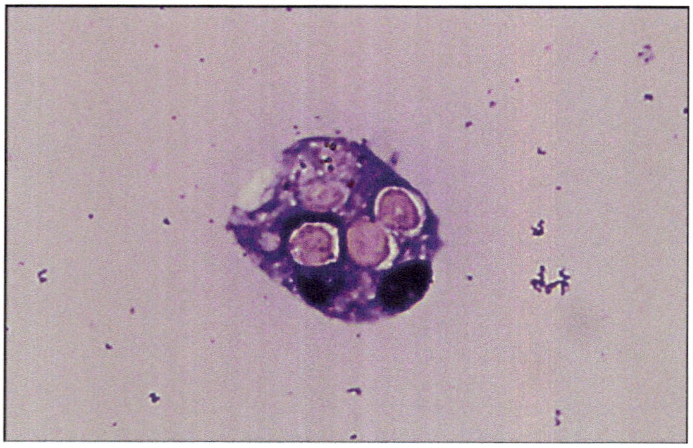

Figure 12.7 **Phagocytized erythrocytes within a degenerating synovial macrophage (Wright–Giemsa, 3,000× magnification).**

Sarcomas of multiple types can have similar cytologic features (Figures 12.8a–c). These include spindloid or stellate borders, wispy cytoplasmic projections, variable amounts of moderately basophilic cytoplasm, nuclear pleomorphism, and prominent nucleoli. The cells can display mild to marked variations in cell, nuclear, and nucleolar size, as well as increases in the nuclear to cytoplasmic (N:C) ratio. Histiocytic sarcoma may share these features, but cells with rounded borders, cytoplasmic vacuolation, multinucleation, and lobulated nuclei may be observed as more prominent features (Figures 12.9a, b). Similarly, synovial cell sarcoma has an appearance that can be difficult to differentiate from other sarcomas cytologically (Figure 12.10). Individualized and aggregated spindloid to rounded cells are observed, with moderate to marked criteria of malignancy. Special staining of histopathologic sections may be necessary for definitive diagnosis. A case report of a biphasic (spindloid and epithelioid components) synovial cell sarcoma was negative for the cytokeratin used in the immunohistochemical staining of the study, but foci of cells were positive for epithelial membrane antigen (Loukopoulos *et al.*, 2004). Tumors of other cell types that involve the joint, such as lymphoma or metastatic carcinoma, are rare (Lahmers *et al.*, 2002).

It should be noted that in human medicine, the term 'synovial sarcoma' has replaced 'synovial cell sarcoma', as research has determined that the cell of origin is a mesenchymal stem cell, rather than synoviocytes, with diagnosis made via genetic marker (Craig *et al.*, 2015). This nomenclature has been adopted by some in veterinary medicine, with one report suggesting the term 'cytokeratin-positive joint associated sarcoma' for use in tumors with appropriate IHC markers (Monti *et al.*, 2018).

Skeletal muscle

Sampling

Standard aspiration or fenestration techniques are employed in sampling skeletal muscle or tumors of skeletal muscle.

Normal cytology

In general, normal striated skeletal muscle is poorly exfoliative; however, fragments of skeletal muscle can be observed in a wide variety of samples, due to incidental aspiration (Figures 12.11a, b). The cytoplasm of the myocytes found in these fragments is deeply basophilic staining and, with adjustment of the fine focus of the microscope, the internal striation of the cells is often appreciable. Low numbers of nuclei are typically visible as small and oval-shaped with dark chromatin, although frequently a high level of detail is not appreciable. The nuclei are expected to be uniform in size and shape.

Inflammation (myositis)

Myositis is uncommonly observed on cytology. A presumptive or suspected cytologic diagnosis may be possible in samples containing significant numbers of inflammatory cells observed in close association with fragments of skeletal muscle; however, histopathology is recommended for definitive diagnosis.

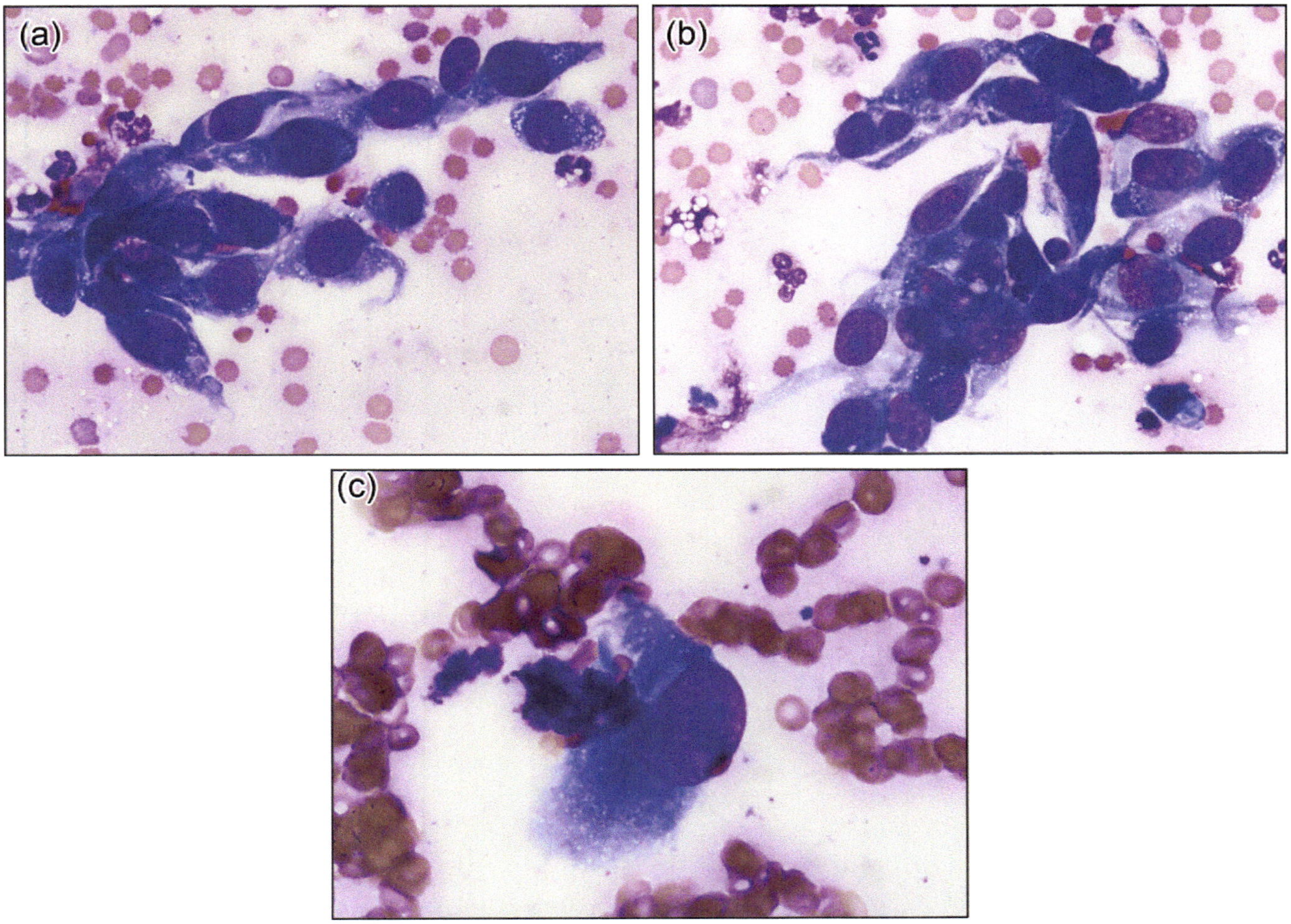

Figures 12.8a–c (a) Sarcoma cells demonstrating spindloid borders, moderately basophilic cytoplasm, rounded to ovoid nuclei, coarsely stippled chromatin, and prominent nucleoli (Wright–Giemsa, 500× magnification). (b) Criteria of malignancy observed in sarcoma: anisocytosis, anisokaryosis, anisonucleoliosis, binucleation, and anisokaryosis within a binucleated cell (Wright–Giemsa, 500× magnification). (c) Cell demonstrating nucleolar irregularity (Wright–Giemsa, 800× magnification).

TUMORS OF SKELETAL MUSCLE

Tumors arising from skeletal muscle are uncommon. Rhabdomyosarcomas reportedly make up less than 1% of tumors in domestic animals; in dogs, many of the reports involve young animals (Ginel *et al.*, 2002). Normal striated skeletal muscle does not exfoliate easily, and aspirates of tumors of musculoskeletal origin also may be contaminated with peripheral blood, of low cellularity, and nondiagnostic. The cytologic features of rhabdomyosarcoma samples are not easily distinguishable from other sarcomas (described above). The cells may have subtle striations within the cytoplasm, but these are often absent or difficult to find. 'Strap cells' or 'strap-like cells' are multinucleated cells in which the nuclei are arranged in a linear fashion within the cytoplasm. This cellular morphology is sometimes associated with rhabdomyosarcomas, but it is not a pathognomonic feature and may occur with other tumor types, as well.

BONE

Sampling

While obtaining a bone aspirate of diagnostic cellularity can be challenging, the benefits of bypassing a more involved bone biopsy are valuable if a sample of diagnostic cellularity can be obtained. Aspirates of lytic or proliferative bone lesions are less invasive than biopsy, and histopathology of bone requires additional time for the decalcification process required prior to standard processing. Poorly exfoliative lesions or those with considerable peripheral blood contamination may require biopsy for diagnosis. Aspiration or fenestration is performed with an 18–22-gauge needle. Using a smaller gauge needle risks collecting a poorly cellular, nondiagnostic sample but may be more appropriate in lesions with considerable bone lysis or smaller patients to avoid iatrogenic trauma. Sampling at the periphery of a lesion can result in high numbers of reactive osteoblasts, which

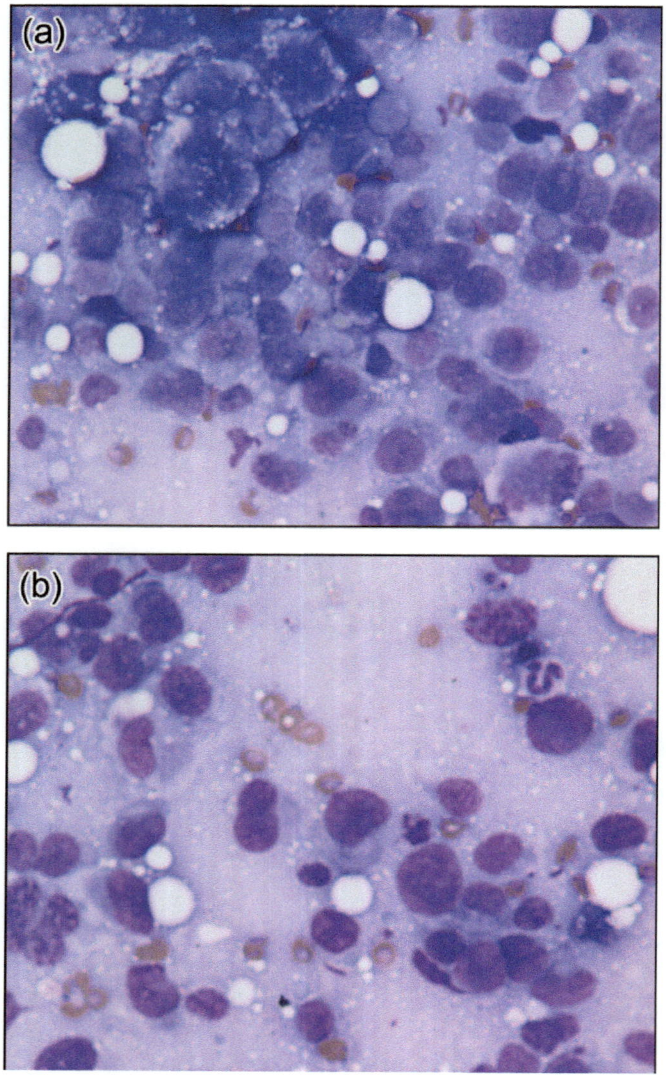
(a)
(b)

Figures 12.9a, b **Histiocytic sarcoma in a dog. Rounded, irregular, and spindloid mesenchymal cells displaying marked pleomorphism (Wright–Giemsa, 700× magnification). (Courtesy Anne Barger.)**

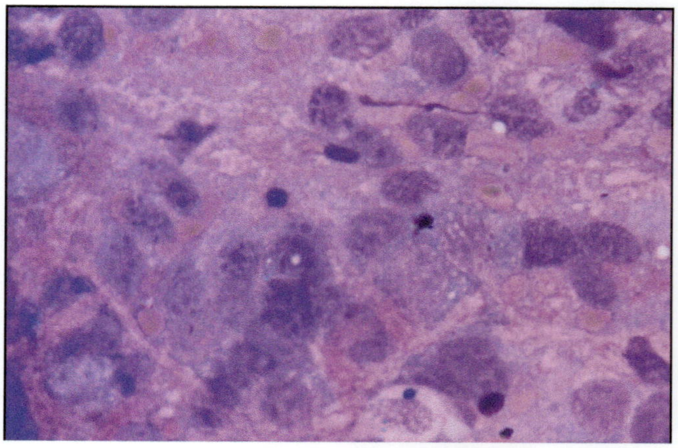

Figure 12.10 **Synovial sarcoma in a dog. Spindloid to rounded cells demonstrate several criteria of malignancy within a background of eosinophilic, granular material (Wright–Giemsa, 800× magnification). (Courtesy Anne Barger.)**

may preclude accurate diagnosis of the primary pathology. Peripheral blood contamination is a common problem, and discontinuation of negative pressure on the syringe when blood enters the needle hub may help limit the amount of background blood.

Normal cytology

Bone cytology samples are often of low cellularity and primarily consist of peripheral blood. Healthy bone is not expected to exfoliate well on cytology. Bone aspirates are typically performed on lesions observed on radiographs (lysis, proliferation) or palpable masses or abnormalities noted on physical examination. Consequently, the expectation of exfoliation on aspiration is greater than normal due to the presence of pathologic change. In a study of 36 lytic, proliferative, or lytic and proliferative bone lesions aspirated via ultrasound guidance, diagnostic samples were obtained in 32 cases (Britt *et al.*, 2007).

Reactive bone

A significant complicating feature of aspirating bone lesions is the exfoliation of nonneoplastic reactive osteoblasts into a sample, either in place of or in concert with inflammatory or neoplastic cells. Reactive osteoblasts are typically rounded or ovoid in shape and have a plasmacytoid or 'flag' appearance, with a round, eccentric nucleus and polarized cytoplasm (Figure 12.12). The cytoplasm is expected to be moderately basophilic and moderate to abundant in amount, and perinuclear clearing, consistent with a prominent Golgi apparatus, may be appreciated. The cells may contain variable numbers of fine, azurophilic granules within the cytoplasm. The chromatin pattern is generally finely to coarsely stippled, and nucleoli are often indistinct or absent; however, observation of nucleoli is not pathognomonic for neoplastic cells. Reactive osteoblasts often display mild to moderate anisocytosis and anisokaryosis and may be present in aggregates. A small amount of wispy to glassy, eosinophilic, extracellular matrix may be present, and nucleated cells may be found in close association with this matrix. Osteoclasts may be present in lesions with bone lysis or remodeling and appear as large, multinucleated cells with rounded or irregular cell borders, variable cytoplasmic projections, and basophilic cytoplasm with dark eosinophilic stippling (Figure 12.13). The nuclei are oval with reticular chromatin and a small, typically single nucleolus; the nuclei are typically fairly uniform in appearance within a cell. Osteoclasts may contain extremely variable numbers of nuclei; it is not uncommon to identify cells with more than ten nuclei and care must be taken not to confuse osteoclasts for neoplastic cells (Figures 12.13, 12.14a, b).

On occasion, hematopoietic precursors will be observed in bone aspirates, particularly when lysis allows considerable penetration of the collecting needle into the medullary cavity.

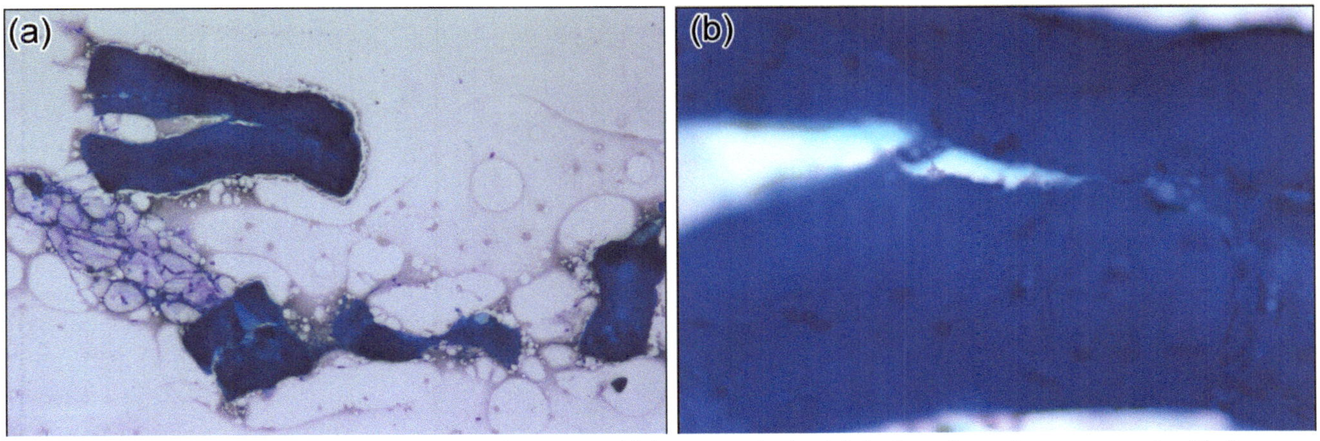

Figures 12.11a, b Striated skeletal muscle and mature adipose tissue. (a) Fragments of striated skeletal muscle may be seen on occasion. The linear arrangement of myocytes is typically preserved. (b) By adjusting the fine focus of the microscope, the cytologist can often appreciate the fine striations within the myocytes (Wright–Giemsa: a, 100× magnification; b, 500× magnification).

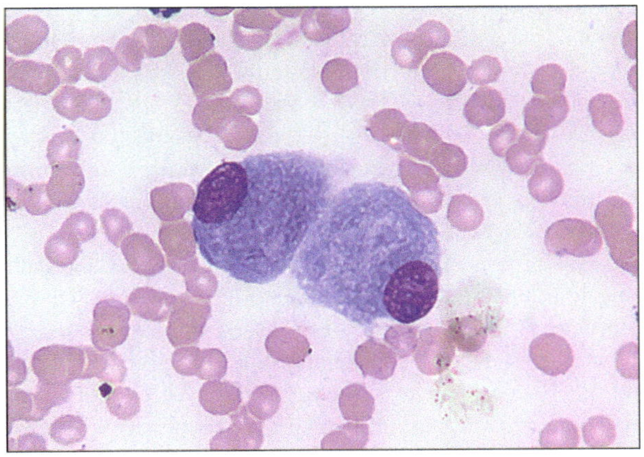

Figure 12.12 Reactive osteoblasts in a bone aspirate. The cells have a low N:C ratio, abundant basophilic cytoplasm, and a round, eccentric nucleus (Wright–Giemsa, 1,000× magnification). (Courtesy Anne Barger.)

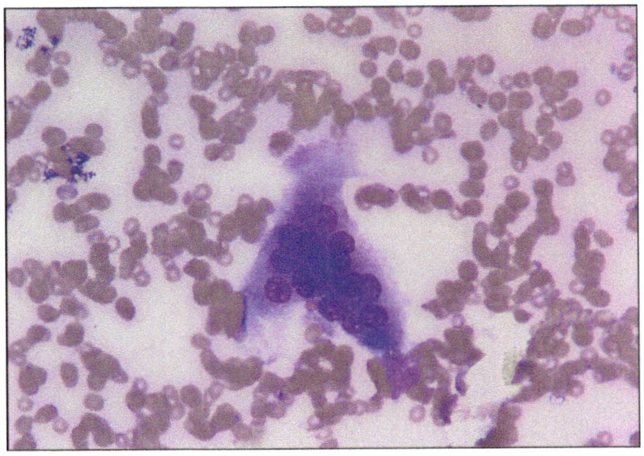

Figure 12.13 Osteoclast. Large cell with variable borders and multiple uniform nuclei (Wright–Giemsa, 1,000× magnification). (Courtesy Anne Barger.)

Inflammation

Inflammation of the bone is referred to as osteomyelitis. Inflammatory bone disease can be associated with lytic and/or proliferative lesions on radiographs, and lesions must be differentiated from similar radiographic findings that may be seen with a bone tumor. Aspirates of an inflamed bone may contain variable amounts of peripheral blood. In addition to disproportionately high numbers of leukocytes, the presence of degenerate neutrophils and phagocytic macrophages (as opposed to monocytes) can help differentiate inflammation from normal blood leukocytes. Careful review of the sample for infectious organisms should ensue. Identification of bacteria, particularly intracellular organisms, indicates the need for bacterial culture and susceptibility testing (Figure 12.15); culture of suppurative and pyogranulomatous bone lesions is also advisable when organisms cannot be identified. Several organisms have been associated with osteomyelitis, including *Streptococcus* spp., *Nocardia* spp., *Mycobacterium* spp., *Bartonella* spp., and *Leishmania* spp. (de Souza *et al.*, 2005; Varanat *et al.*, 2009; Lo *et al.*, 2012; França *et al.*, 2014; Hilligas *et al.*, 2014). Lytic and proliferative lesions due to blastomycosis, histoplasmosis, coccidioidomycosis, cryptococcosis, and aspergillosis can be seen (Figures 12.16a–c; Walker *et al.*, 2012; Block et al., 2017; Fielder et al., 2019; Shaver et al., 2022; Washington et al., 2022). Pyogranulomatous inflammation is expected more commonly with fungal disease, although suppurative or chronic suppurative inflammation may also be observed (Figure 12.17).

Tumors of bone and cartilage

Osteosarcoma

Osteosarcoma is a malignant proliferation of osteoblasts. Osteosarcomas are often associated with concurrent bone proliferation. Many samples are a mixture of neoplastic and reactive osteoblasts, and differentiation of the two can prove challenging. Additionally, reliable differentiation of osteosarcoma from other

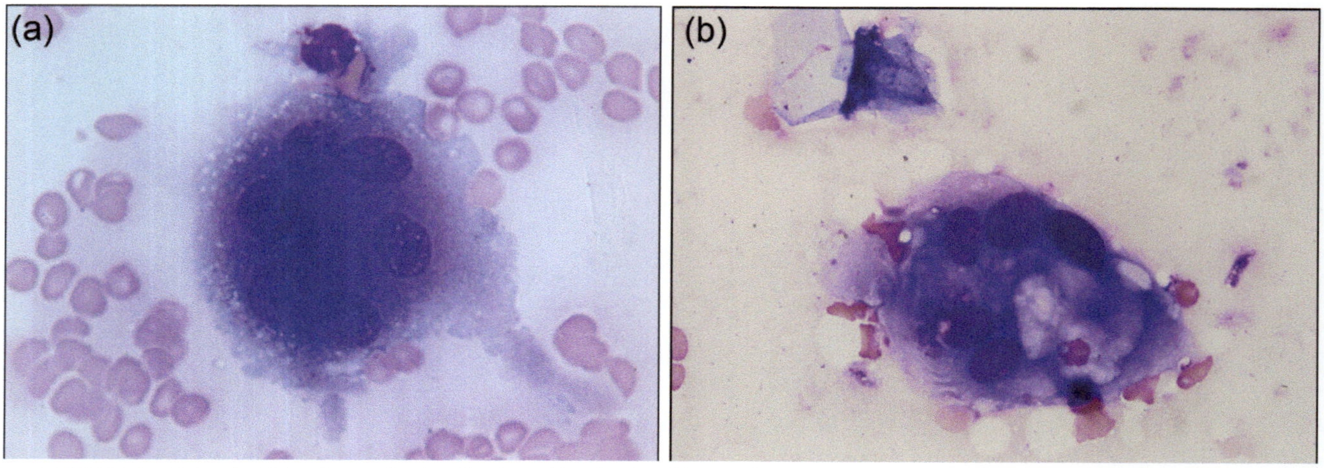

Figures 12.14a, b Osteoclast (a) and a neoplastic cell with multinucleation (b). Note the eosinophilic stippled cytoplasm and relative nuclear uniformity displayed by the osteoclast (Wright–Giemsa, both, 1,000× magnification). (12.14a courtesy Anne Barger.)

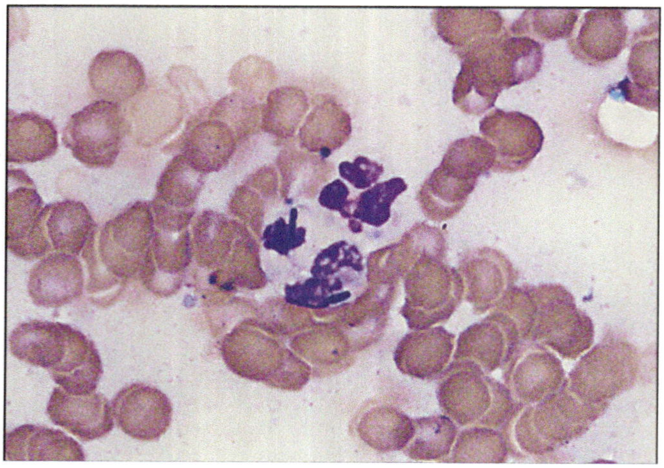

Figure 12.15 Septic osteomyelitis, with rod-shaped intracellular bacteria (Wright–Giemsa, 2,000× magnification).

sarcomas based purely on cytologic appearance is typically not possible. The features of reactive osteoblasts have been described above. Neoplastic osteoblasts can display a range of atypia (Figures 12.18a, b). The cells may be rounded or spindloid in shape, with a small to large amount of basophilic cytoplasm. The cells may contain a few small (approximately 0.5–1 µm), rounded or angular, variably sized eosinophilic granules within the cytoplasm. The cells are expected to display variable degrees of anisocytosis, anisokaryosis, and anisonucleoliosis. The cells may be associated with a variable amount of wispy to glassy eosinophilic extracellular matrix, although this is not a criterion of malignancy and may also be seen in samples of reactive bone. The nuclei are often round or oval, and the chromatin pattern may range from fine to coarse to open, even within a single sample. Nucleoli are often prominent, multiple, and may vary considerably in size and shape. Erythrophagia may be observed within the cytoplasm of osteosarcoma cells but is not specific for this tumor type (Barger *et al.*, 2012). Several subtypes of osteosarcoma exist and may influence cytologic sample features. A 2020 study that assessed 153 cases of canine osteosarcoma found osteoblastic osteosarcoma was the most common at 56.9%, followed by chondroblastic (13.7%), telangiectatic (11.8%), fibroblastic (7.8%), giant cell-rich (5.2%), and poorly differentiated neoplasms (4.6%) (Guim *et al.*, 2020). Low case numbers among several subtypes precluded accurate determination of subtype influence on prognosis in this study.

Once a diagnosis of sarcoma has been made on a bone aspirate, staining additional slides for alkaline phosphatase (ALP) activity can be helpful in differentiating between several types of sarcoma. This is evidenced by dark brown–black staining within the cytoplasm following incubation with nitroblue tetrazolium chloride/5-bromo-4-chloro-3-indolyl phosphate (NBT/BCIP) toluidine salt, which acts as a substrate for alkaline phosphatase in the cell (Barger *et al.*, 2012). Cells displaying significant criteria of malignancy, such as marked increases in the N:C ratio, multinucleation, or marked anisocytosis, must be confirmed positive to differentiate neoplastic cells from positively staining reactive osteoblasts that may also be present (Figure 12.18c). Osteoclasts are expected to be negative for alkaline phosphatase activity. Counterstaining of apparently negative slides with a Romanowsky stain is recommended to confirm that neoplastic cells are present. A study assessing the utility of ALP activity in differentiating between vimentin-positive tumors found that 33/33 osteosarcomas, 1/4 chondrosarcomas, and 1/1 multilobular tumor of bone were positive, while 3/4 chondrosarcomas, 2/2 fibrosarcomas of bone, 4/4 synovial cell sarcomas, and 2/2 plasma cell tumors were negative (Barger *et al.*, 2005). Another study determined that slides previously stained with Wright–Giemsa could also be utilized for staining for ALP activity, allowing additional diagnostic testing on samples with limited cellularity (Ryseff & Bohn, 2012). This study found that 15/17 osteosarcomas were positive for ALP activity.

A 2022 study assessing immunohistochemical staining of primary bone tumors found that sequential use of ALP, followed by the transcription factor runx2, provided 87% sensitivity and 85% specificity

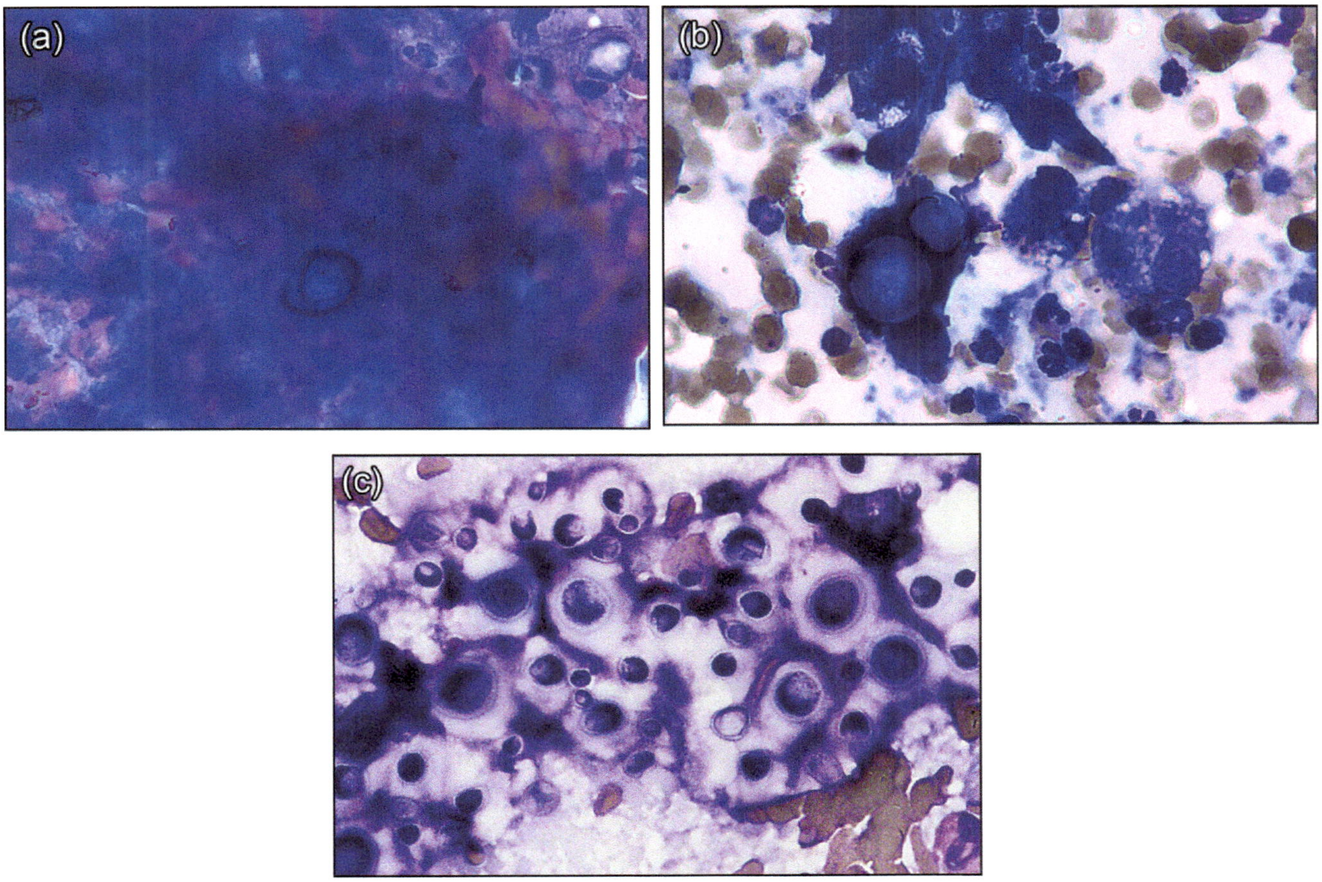

Figures 12.16a–c (a) *Blastomyces dermatitidis* (near bottom of image) with inflammatory cells. This fungal yeast is deeply basophilic staining, with a double-contoured cell wall, is typically 10–15 μm in diameter, and displays broad-based budding (not pictured). (Courtesy Anne Barger.) (b) *Coccidioides* spp. This fungus forms spherules that range in size from 10 to 200 μm in diameter. Endospores (2–4 μm) may be visible within larger forms or within the background on spherule rupture (not pictured). (Courtesy Anne Barger.) (c) *Cryptococcus* spp. The yeasts demonstrate the prominent mucoid capsule characteristic of this fungus. They typically display narrow-based budding and variable staining (Wright–Giemsa: a, 2,000× magnification; b and c, 1,000× magnification).

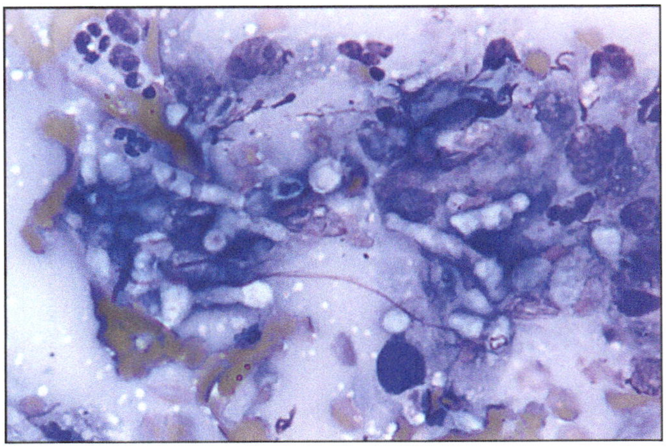

Figure 12.17 Fungal osteomyelitis in a dog. Lytic changes were noted on radiographs, and a bone neoplasm was suspected. Cytologic review of lesion aspirates revealed pyogranulomatous inflammation and fungal hyphae (Wright–Giemsa, 1,000× magnification). (Courtesy Anne Barger.)

in distinguishing osteosarcoma from chondrosarcoma, fibrosarcoma, and histiocytic sarcoma; alone, ALP was highly sensitive (100%) but poorly specific (30%), and runx2 was moderately sensitive (87%) and specific (78%) (Barger *et al.*, 2022).

Chondrosarcoma

Chondrosarcomas (malignant proliferations of chondroblasts) are cytologically similar to osteosarcomas. Chondrosarcomas are often associated with a large amount of stippled to wispy, brightly eosinophilic, extracellular matrix (chondroid) that fills the background (Figures 12.19a, b). However, osteosarcomas and fibrosarcomas may also be associated with a significant amount of pink extracellular material. Chondrosarcomas tend to arise in the nasal cavity and in flat bones; a retrospective analysis of 31 cases of non-nasal chondrosarcomas in dogs found 13 cases occurred in appendicular long bones, 12 in ribs, 4 in the mandible, and 1 each in the maxilla and scapula (Waltman *et al.*, 2007).

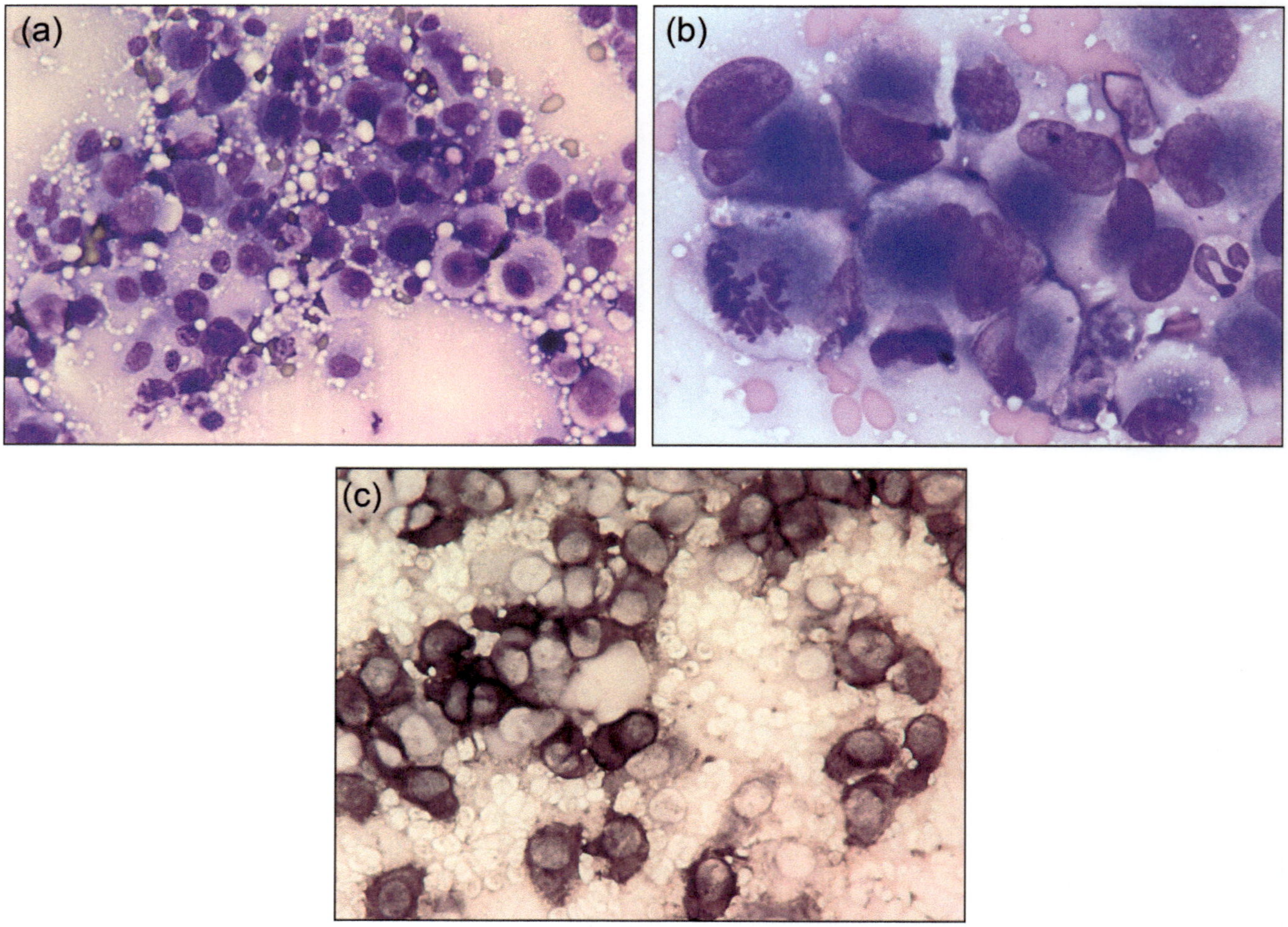

Figures 12.18a–c Osteosarcoma in a dog. (a, b) Pleomorphic rounded to spindloid cells (Wright–Giemsa: a, 500× magnification; b, 1,000× magnification). (c) Brown–black staining indicates ALP activity within the neoplastic cells. Criteria of malignancy should be identified within positive-staining cells to differentiate from reactive osteoblasts (NBT/BCIP, 500× magnification). (Courtesy Anne Barger.)

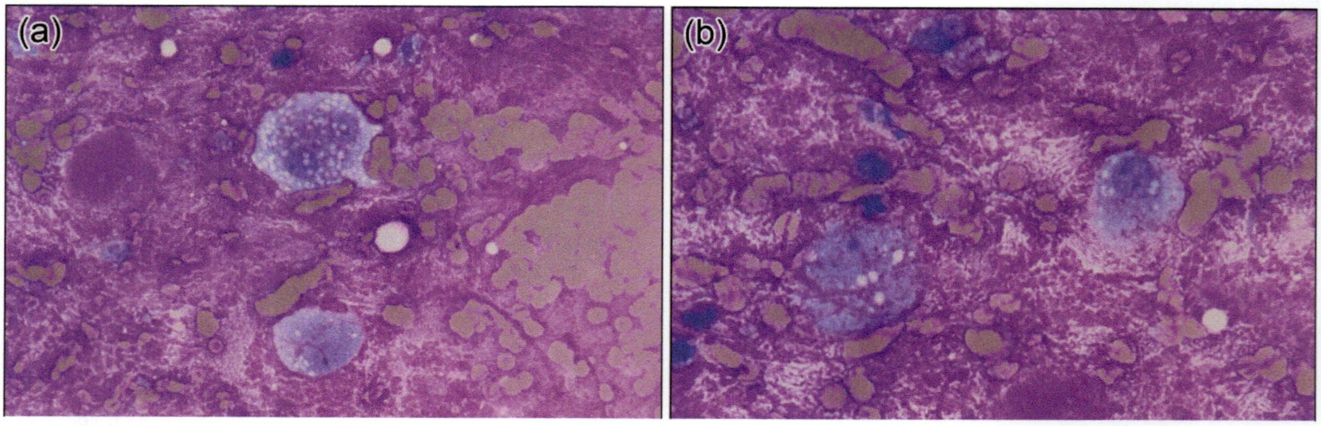

Figures 12.19a, b Chondrosarcoma in a dog. Pleomorphic mesenchymal cells within a distinctive background of thick, brightly eosinophilic, extracellular matrix (Wright–Giemsa: 1,000× magnification). (Courtesy Anne Barger.)

FIBROSARCOMA AND HEMANGIOSARCOMA

Fibrosarcoma and hemangiosarcoma are two additional types of primary bone tumor. These tumor types share cytologic features with other sarcomas (described above) and may be difficult to conclusively identify on cytology. The cells of both tumor types may be found individually and in aggregates. Fibrosarcomas may be associated with a small amount of eosinophilic extracellular matrix. Hemangiosarcoma cells may occasionally be seen in densely cellular groups that appear semicohesive. Hemangiosarcoma cells may display erythrophagia, and black granular material (hemosiderin, a hemoglobin breakdown product) may be identified within the cytoplasm of some cells. Histopathologic assessment of tissue architecture and special staining are often required for definitive diagnosis of many tumors of mesenchymal origin.

Other tumors of bone and muscle

Benign variants of bone and cartilage tumors (osteomas and chondromas) can arise, but histopathology is usually necessary to differentiate these from other mesenchymal proliferations. Other sarcomas, including hemangiosarcoma, fibrosarcoma, and histiocytic sarcoma, may occasionally affect bone or muscle, but often cannot be definitively distinguished on cytology from osteosarcoma, chondrosarcoma, and rhabdomyosarcoma. Histiocytic sarcoma may also result in bone tumors; the cytologic appearance is described above (Figures 12.9a–b). Multilobular tumor of bone is a rare tumor that has a characteristic nodular 'popcorn ball' appearance on radiographs and is often associated with the skull; it has been described in both dogs and cats (Dernell *et al.*, 1998; Yildiz *et al.*, 2003). Additionally, metastasis of other tumor types, especially carcinoma, may be identified, particularly in bone lesions (Figures 12.20a–c). Squamous cell carcinoma (SCC) may also invade adjacent bone (Figure 12.21). In cats, metastasis of pulmonary adenocarcinoma and SCC to the digits is of particular note (Helm Morris, 2012). Metastasis of pulmonary adenocarcinoma to the digit appears to be uncommon. A 2023 study that found 42 cases of pulmonary carcinoma among 1,940 cats submitted for post-mortem examination detected digital metastasis in only a single case of the 39 cases that met inclusion criteria (2.5%) (Santos *et al.*, 2023).

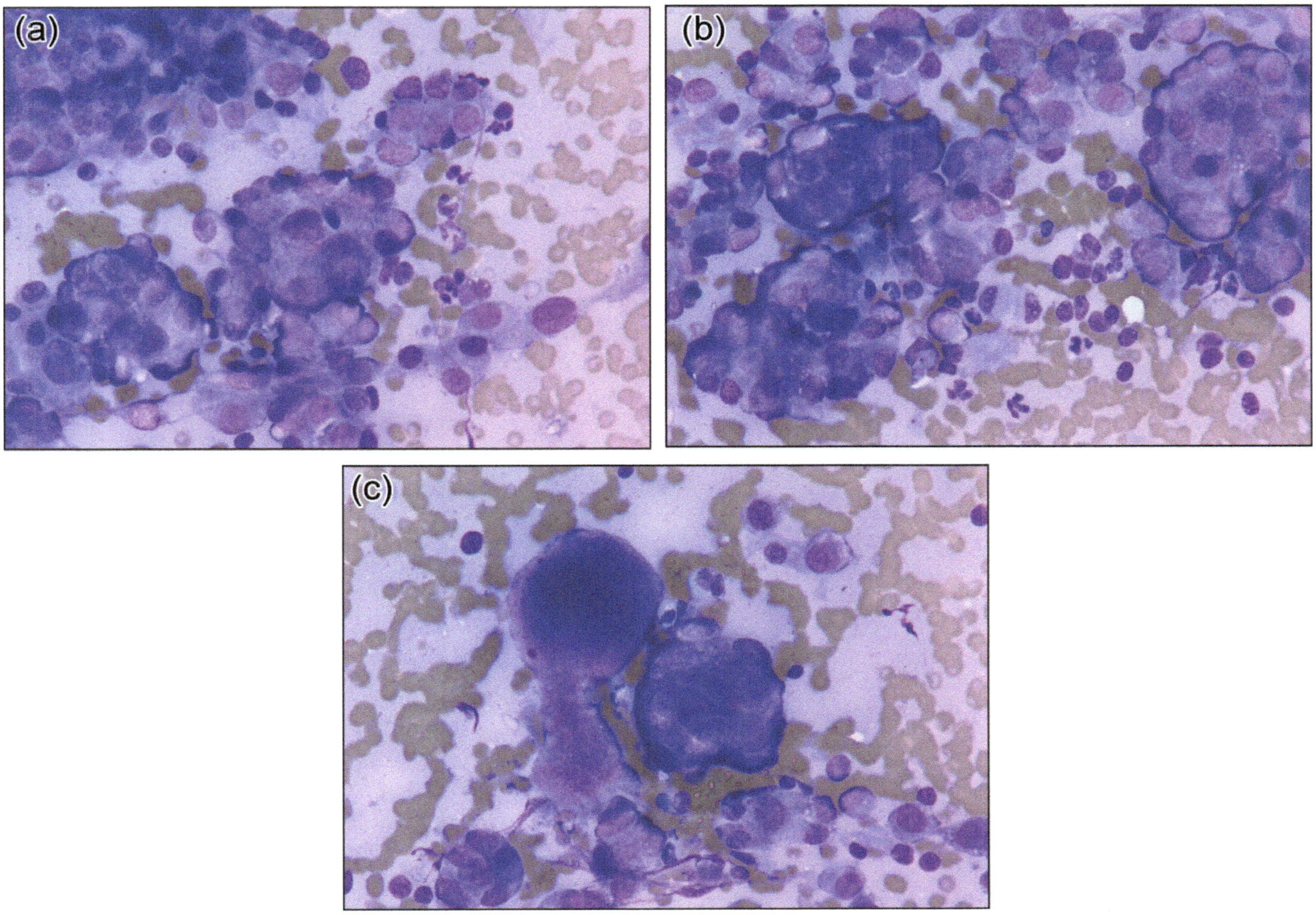

Figures 12.20a–c Metastatic carcinoma in a dog. Clusters of cohesive cells are observed in aspirates from a lytic bone lesion. Osteoclasts and reactive osteoblasts may also be present in samples from such lesions (Wright–Giemsa, 500× magnification). (Courtesy Anne Barger.)

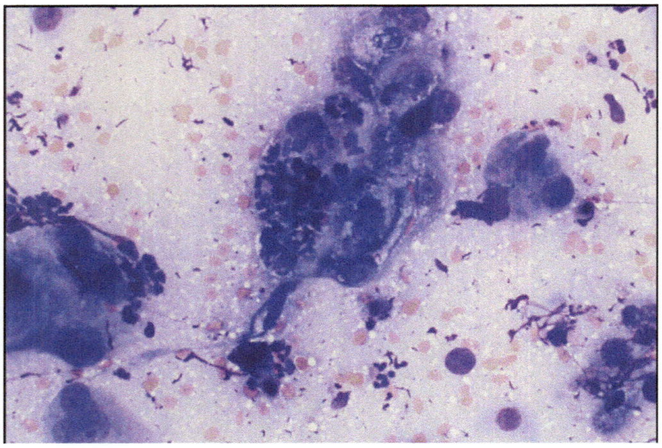

Figure 12.21 Squamous cell carcinoma in a cat. Squamous cell carcinoma, like this poorly differentiated tumor associated with the maxilla, can invade adjacent bone. Osteoclasts and reactive osteoblasts (not pictured) may be observed in conjunction with neoplastic epithelial cells (Wright–Giemsa, 700× magnification).

Plasma cell neoplasia of bone may be part of the spectrum of multiple myeloma or represent a solitary osseous plasmacytoma. The cytologic appearance of each is similar, and additional diagnostics should be performed to assess for evidence of multiple myeloma (hyperglobulinemia due to monoclonal gammopathy, Bence-Jones proteinuria, increased plasma cells within the bone marrow). Lytic bone lesions due to plasma cell neoplasia tend to exfoliate well with aspiration and contain numerous discrete round cells; these typically have recognizable plasmacytoid features that must be differentiated from reactive osteoblasts. Neoplastic plasma cells are expected to have moderate to abundant deeply basophilic cytoplasm, perinuclear clearing (prominent Golgi), a round, eccentric nucleus, and distinctly clumped chromatin (Figure 12.22). Binucleate cells are often identified, and multinucleate cells may be observed. Less differentiated tumors may display significant anisocytosis and anisokaryosis, considerable increases in the N:C ratio, and may have prominent nucleoli. Plasma cell neoplasia involving the bone was uncommon in a study of cats with myeloma-related disorder; only 1 cat of 12 that were radiographed had evidence of bone involvement (Mellor *et al.*, 2006).

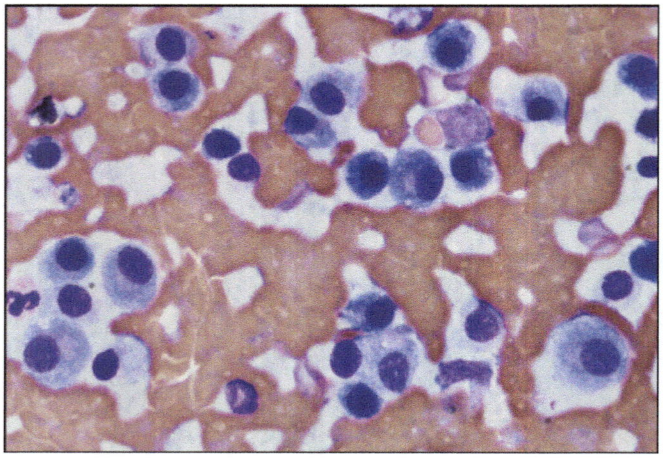

Figure 12.22 Plasma cell neoplasia in a dog. Aspirate is from lytic bone lesion. These neoplastic plasma cells display moderate pleomorphism (Wright–Giemsa, 700× magnification).

Lymphoma may rarely result in bone lysis (Brockley *et al.*, 2012). Neoplastic proliferations of other hematopoietic cells of the bone marrow are not expected to affect the cortical bone.

CASES

CASE 1

Signalment/history

A 10-year-old neutered male Labrador Retriever-mix dog was presented for forelimb lameness.

Physical examination

The patient was toe-touching lame on the right forelimb and a swelling was detected in the area of the distal radius. Radiographic imaging revealed a lytic and proliferative lesion affecting the distal radius (Figure 12.23a).

Cytology

An aspirate of the lesion was obtained using a 20-gauge needle and syringe, and smears of the sample were prepared. The slides were stained with Wright–Giemsa and examined cytologically.

A pleomorphic population of individualized cells was present. The cells varied from rounded to spindloid in shape, with a small to moderate amount of basophilic cytoplasm, a round or oval nucleus, moderate to high N:C ratio, finely to coarsely stippled chromatin, and prominent nucleoli (Figure 12.23b). The cells displayed moderate anisocytosis, anisokaryosis, and anisonucleoliosis, and occasional binucleation. Low numbers of cells contained a few fine, magenta granules within the cytoplasm.

Diagnosis

The cytologic interpretation was sarcoma, with osteosarcoma as the top differential.

Management/outcome

Because of financial limitations, the owners elected limb amputation without other therapeutic modalities. The histopathologic diagnosis was osteosarcoma (Figure 12.23c). Thoracic radiographs prior to surgery did not reveal appreciable metastatic lesions. Four months following limb amputation, the patient was presented for weight loss and lethargy. Thoracic radiographs were repeated, and several discrete nodular lesions, compatible with metastatic disease, were identified (Figure 12.23d). Due to the poor prognosis and declining patient quality of life, the owners elected humane euthanasia.

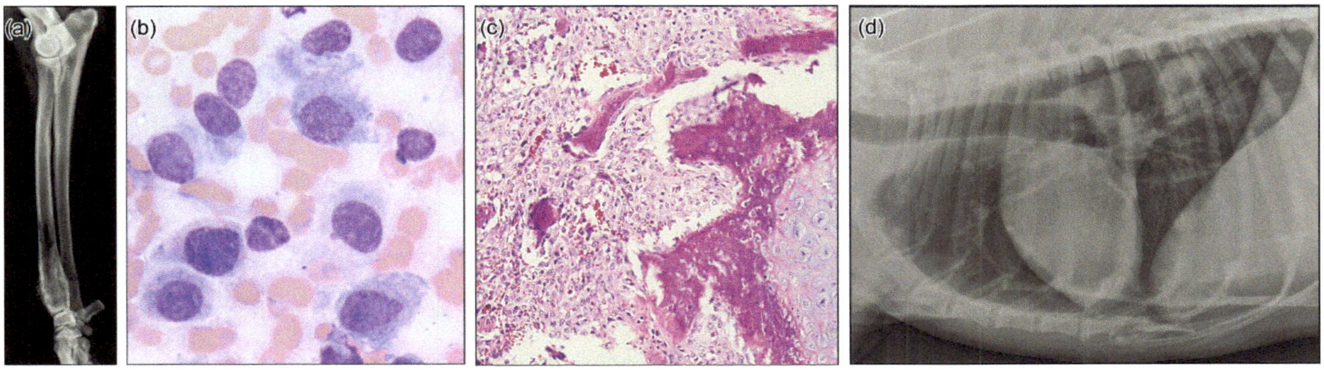

Figures 12.23a–d (a) Digital radiographic image of the lateral aspect of the right forelimb demonstrating a lytic and proliferative bone lesion affecting the distal radius. (Courtesy Laura Garrett.) (b) Cytology of the bone lesion revealed pleomorphic rounded to spindloid neoplastic cells, consistent with sarcoma (Wright–Giemsa: a and b, 1,000× magnification). (Courtesy Anne Barger.) (c) Histopathology of the bone lesion (H&E, 100× magnification). (d) Lateral thoracic radiograph with nodular pulmonary lesions, compatible with metastatic neoplasia. (Courtesy Laura Garrett.)

Discussion

Osteosarcoma is a proliferation of malignant neoplastic osteoblasts that can be identified in the axial and appendicular skeleton. Lesions often arise in the metaphyseal region of long bones. Lesions display variable radiographic changes, but many are both lytic and proliferative. Atypical, pleomorphic mesenchymal cells may be identified on cytologic examination of aspirates of bone lesions, although peripheral blood contamination is common and may limit the conclusiveness of cytology. Staining for ALP activity may be helpful in samples of appropriate cellularity, but neoplastic cells must be differentiated from reactive, non-neoplastic osteoblasts that may be present concurrently. Histopathology may be necessary to differentiate osteosarcoma from other sarcomas that may be found in bone lesions. Pulmonary metastasis is common, although other sites, including skin and organ metastasis, are also observed.

CASE 2

A young adult male neutered domestic shorthair cat was presented for evaluation due to lethargy and pain upon being picked up. The cat had an indoor/outdoor lifestyle and was up to date on vaccinations.

Physical examination

The patient demonstrated pain responses to palpation over all four limbs, and radiographs revealed multifocal lytic bone lesions, primarily affecting long bones.

Cytology

An aspirate of a lytic humeral lesion was obtained using a 20-gauge needle and syringe, and smears of the sample were prepared. The slides were stained with Wright–Giemsa and examined cytologically. An inflammatory population was present and consisted of a mix of nondegenerate and mildly degenerate neutrophils, rounded and spindloid macrophages, and occasional multinucleated giant cells. Several macrophages contained rounded or oval fungal yeast, which ranged from approximately 2 to 4 microns wide (Figure 12.24). The yeast structures were surrounded by a thin area of clearing and contained a crescent-shaped or rounded basophilic nucleus. A few organisms were also observed free in the background blood. Low numbers of hematopoietic precursors were also noted, consistent with incidental sampling of bone marrow.

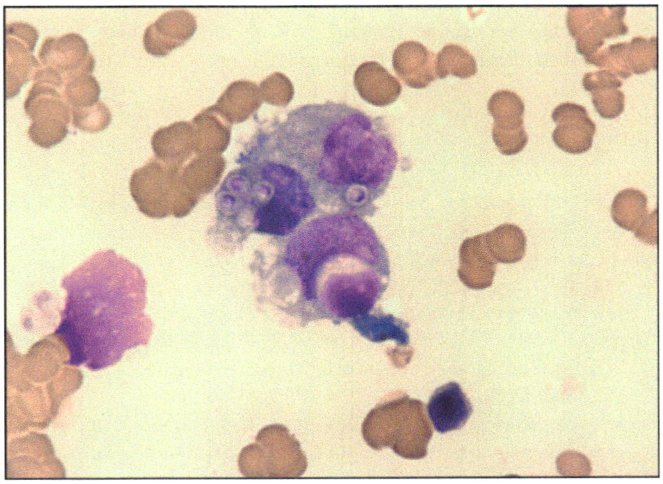

Figure 12.24 Cytology of the bone lesion revealed macrophages that contained fungal yeast (Wright–Giemsa, 1,000× magnification). (Courtesy Anne Barger.)

Diagnosis

The cytologic interpretation was pyogranulomatous inflammation with intralesional fungal yeast. The morphology was consistent with *Histoplasma capsulatum*.

Management/outcome

Due to a guarded prognosis, the owner declined further diagnostic testing (PCR) and treatment. The patient was humanely euthanized, and necropsy was not performed.

Discussion

A 2012 review of a group of 22 cats with histoplasmosis found that weakness (68%), weight loss (50%), and anorexia (45%) were the most common presenting complaints. Physical examination information was available for 20 of the cats, and only 4 had recorded lameness (Aulakh, 2012). Fielder *et al.* reviewed 25 cases of feline histoplasmosis with lameness or joint effusion and found bone lesions in 29 of 33 radiographs (88%) of carpi and tarsi. Diagnosis was made via cytology of one or more tissues in 22/25 cats (88%). Of cats for which serum ALP concentration was available (n = 18), no cat demonstrated an elevation in this value (Fielder *et al.*, 2019). The Aulakh 2012 study assessed outcome and found that 12/22 cats (55%) survived to discharge; three died during the first week of treatment, and seven died or were euthanized without treatment.

REFERENCES

Aulakh H.K., Aulakh K.S., Troy G.C. (2012) Feline histoplasmosis: A retrospective study of 22 cases (1986–2009). *J Am Anim Hosp Assoc 48*(3):182–187.

Barger A., Baker K., Driskell E. et al. (2022) The use of alkaline phosphatase and runx2 to distinguish osteosarcoma from other common malignant primary bone tumors in dogs. *Vet Pathol 59*(3):427–432.

Barger A., Graca R., Bailey K. et al. (2005) Use of alkaline phosphatase staining to differentiate canine osteosarcoma from other vimentin-positive tumors. *Vet Pathol 42*(2):161–165.

Barger A.M., Skowronski M.C., MacNeill A.L. (2012) Cytologic identification of erythrophagocytic neoplasms in dogs. *Vet Clin Pathol 41*(4):587–589.

Bhandal J., Hayashi K., Kim S.Y. et al. (2013) Detection of bacterial DNA by PCR in dogs with stifle pathology. *Vet Surg 42*(7):814–818.

Block K., Battig J. (2017) Cryptococcal maxillary osteomyelitis and osteonecrosis in an 18-month-old dog. *J Vet Dentist 34*(2):76–85.

Britt T., Clifford C., Barger A. et al. (2007) Diagnosing appendicular osteosarcoma with ultrasound-guided fine-needle aspiration: 36 cases. *J Small Anim Pract 48*(3):145–150.

Brockley L.K., Heading K.L., Jardine J.E. et al. (2012) Polyostotic lymphoma with multiple pathological fractures in a six-month-old cat. *J Feline Med Surg 14*(4):285–291.

Clements D.N., Owen M.R., Mosley J.R. et al. (2005) Retrospective study of bacterial infective arthritis in 31 dogs. *J Small Anim Pract 46*:171–176.

Craig L.E., Dittmer K.E., Thompson K.G. (2015) Tumors and tumor-like lesions of joints. In: *Jubb, Kennedy, Palmer's Pathology of Domestic Animals*, 6th edn. (ed. M. Grant Maxie) W.B. Saunders, Oxford, pp. 159–163.

Craig L.E., Julian M.E., Ferracone J.D. (2002) The diagnosis and prognosis of synovial tumors in dogs: 35 cases. *Vet Pathol 39*(1):66–73.

de Jonge R., Brouwer R., Smit M. et al. (2004) Automated counting of white blood cells in synovial fluid. *Rheumatology 43*(2):170–173.

de Souza A.I., Juliano R.S., Gomes T.S. et al. (2005) Osteolytic osteomyelitis associated with visceral leishmaniasis in a dog. *Vet Parasitol 129*(1–2):51–54.

Dernell W.S., Straw R.C., Cooper M.F. et al. (1998) Multilobular osteochondrosarcoma in 39 dogs: 1979–1993. *J Am Anim Hosp Assoc 34*(1):11–18.

Dusick A., Young K.M., Muir P. (2014) Relationship between automated total nucleated cell count and enumeration of cells on direct smears of canine synovial fluid. *Vet J 202*(3):550–554.

Ekmann A., Rigdal M.L., Gröndahl G. (2010) Automated counting of nucleated cells in equine synovial fluid without and with hyaluronidase pretreatment. *Vet Clin Pathol 39*(1):83–89.

Fielder S.E., Meinkoth J.H., Rizzi T.E. et al. (2019) Feline histoplasmosis presenting with bone and joint involvement: Clinical and diagnostic findings in 25 cats. *J Fel Med Surg 21*(10):887–892.

França S.D.A., Braga J.F.V., Moreira M.V.L. et al. (2014) Splendore-Hoeppli phenomenon in a cat with osteomyelitis caused by *Streptococcus* species. *J Feline Med Surg 16*(2):189–193.

Froom P., Diab A., Barak M. (2013) Automated evaluation of synovial and ascitic fluids with the Advia 2120 hematology analyzer. *Am J Clin Pathol 140*:828–830.

Gibson N.R., Carmichael S., Li A. et al. (1999) Value of direct smears of synovial fluid in the diagnosis of canine joint disease. *Vet Rec 144*:463–466.

Ginel P.J., Martin de las Mulas J., Lucena R. et al. (2002) Skeletal muscle rhabdomyosarcoma in a dog. *Vet Rec 151*:736–739.

Guim T.N., Bianchi M.V., De Lorenzo C. et al. (2020) Relationship between clinicopathological features and prognosis in appendicular osteosarcoma in dogs. *J Comp Path 180*:91–99.

Helm J., Morris J. (2012) Musculoskeletal neoplasia: An important differential for lumps or lameness in the cat. *J Feline Med Surg 14*(1):43–54.

Hilligas J., van Wie E., Barr J. et al. (2014) Vertebral osteomyelitis and multiple cutaneous lesions in a dog caused by *Nocardia pseudobrasiliensis*. *J Vet Intern Med 28*(5):1621–1625.

Jacques D., Cauzinille L., Bouvy B. et al. (2002) A retrospective study of 40 dogs with polyarthritis. *Vet Surg 31*(5):428–434.

Johnson K.C., Mackin A. (2012a) Canine immune-mediated polyarthritis: part 2: Diagnosis and treatment. *J Am Anim Hosp Assoc 48*(2):71–82.

Johnson K.C., Mackin A. (2012b) Canine immune-mediated polyarthritis: part 1: Pathophysiology. *J Am Anim Hosp Assoc 48*(1):12–17.

Lahmers S.M., Mealey K.L., Martinez S.A. et al. (2002) Synovial T-cell lymphoma of the stifle in a dog. *J Am Anim Hosp Assoc 38*:165–168.

Lo A.J., Goldschmidt M.H., Aronson L.R. (2012) Osteomyelitis of the coxofemoral joint due to *Mycobacterium* species in a feline renal transplant recipient. *J Feline Med Surg 14*(12):919–923.

Loukopoulos P., Heng H.G., Arshad H. (2004) Canine biphasic synovial sarcoma: Case report and immunohistochemical characterization. *J Vet Sci 5*(2):173–180.

MacWilliams P.S., Friedrichs K.R. (2003) Laboratory evaluation and interpretation of synovial fluid. *Vet Clin North Am Small Anim Pract 33*:153–178.

McConkey S.E., López A., Shaw D. et al. (2002) Leishmanial polyarthritis in a dog. *Can Vet J 43*:607–609.

Mellor P.J., Haugland A., Murphy A. et al. (2006) Myeloma-related disorders in cats commonly present as extramedullary neoplasms in contrast to myeloma in human patients: 24 cases with clinical follow-up. *J Vet Intern Med 14*:1376–1383.

Monti P., Barnes D., Adrian A.M., Rasotto R. (2018) Synovial cell sarcoma in a dog: A misnomer—Cytologic and histologic findings and review of the literature. *Vet Clin Pathol 47*:181–185.

Oohashi E., Yamada K., Oohashi M. et al. (2009) Chronic progressive polyarthritis in a female cat. *J Vet Med Sci 72*(4):511–514.

Pacchiana P.D., Gilley R.S., Wallace L.J. et al. (2004) Absolute and relative cell counts for synovial fluid from clinically normal shoulder and stifle joints in cats. *J Am Vet Med Assoc 225*(12):1866.

Riggio M.P., Lappin D.F., Bennett D. (2014) Bacteria and Toll-like receptor and cytokine mRNA expression profiles associated with canine arthritis. *Vet Immunol Immunopathol 160*(3–4):158–166.

Ryseff J.K., Bohn A.A. (2012) Detection of alkaline phosphatase in canine cells previously stained with Wright-Giemsa and its utility in differentiating osteosarcoma from other mesenchymal tumors. *Vet Clin Pathol 41(3)*:391–395.

Salinas M., Rosas J., Iborra J. et al. (1997) Comparison of manual and automated cell counts in EDTA preserved synovial fluids. Storage has little influence on the results. *Ann Rheum Dis 56(10)*:622–626.

Santos I.R., Raiter J., Lamego E.C. et al. (2022) Feline pulmonary carcinoma: Gross, histological, metastatic, and immunohistochemical aspects. *Vet Pathol 60(1)*:8–20.

Santos M., Marcos R., Assunção M. et al. (2006) Polyarthritis associated with visceral leishmaniasis in a juvenile dog. *Vet Parasitol 141*(3–4):340–344.

Sbrana S., Marchetti V., Mancianti F. et al. (2014) Retrospective study of 14 cases of canine arthritis secondary to *Leishmania* infection. *J Small Anim Pract 55(5)*:309–313.

Shaver S.L., Foy D.S., Carter T.D. (2022) Clinical features, treatment, and outcome of dogs with *Coccidioides* osteomyelitis. *J Am Vet Med Assn 260(1)*:63–70.

Summers B.A., Straubinger A.F., Jacobson R.H. et al. (2005) Histopathological studies of experimental Lyme disease in the dog. *J Comp Pathol 133(1)*:1–13.

Varanat M., Travis A., Lee W. et al. (2009) Recurrent osteomyelitis in a cat due to infection with *Bartonella vinsonii* subsp. *berkhoffii* genotype II. *J Vet Intern Med 23*:1273–1277.

Walker J.T., Frazho J.K., Randell S.C. (2012) A novel case of canine disseminated aspergillosis following mating. *Can Vet J 53*:190–192.

Waltman S.S., Seguin B., Cooper B.J. et al. (2007) Clinical outcome of non-nasal chondrosarcoma in dogs: Thirty-one cases (1986–2003). *Vet Surg 36(3)*:266–271.

Washington C., Paulman A., Stapleton B.L. (2022) Mandibular blastomycosis in a 5-year-old dog. *J Vet Dentist 39*(3):269–277.

Woods K.S., Barry M., Richardson D. (2013) Carpal intra-articular blastomycosis in a Labrador retriever. *Can Vet J 54*:167–170.

Yildiz F., Gurel A., Yesildere T. et al. (2003) Frontal chondrosarcoma in a cat. *J Vet Sci 4*(*2*):193–194.

Zeugswetter F., Hittmair K.M., de Arespacochaga A.G. et al. (2007) Erosive polyarthritis associated with *Mycoplasma gateae* in a cat. *J Feline Med Surg 9*(3):226–231.

CHAPTER 13

RESPIRATORY TRACT CYTOLOGY

Amelia Goddard and Yolandi Rautenbach

INTRODUCTION

Cytologic evaluation of a high-quality sample from the respiratory tract can, together with history, clinical data, and imaging, provide invaluable diagnostic information toward patient management. Clinical indications for cytologic evaluation of the respiratory tract in dogs and cats include sneezing, nasal discharge, epistaxis, ocular discharge, pawing at the nose, facial deformity, chronic coughing, dyspnea, and radiographic evidence of bronchial or pulmonary parenchymal disease. One of the major factors determining the diagnostic value of cytologic specimens is the quality of the sample.

NASAL CAVITY

The most common reported causes for chronic nasal disease in dogs and cats include neoplasia, followed by lymphocytic-plasmacytic rhinitis or chronic rhinitis, and fungal infection. Primary bacterial rhinitis is rare in dogs and cats and is usually secondary to foreign bodies or disorders where there is disruption of normal mucociliary mucosal integrity (Lobetti, 2009; Meler *et al.*, 2008; Cohn, 2020; Henderson *et al.*, 2004).

Collection techniques and sample preparation

A thorough visual inspection of the nasal cavity through endoscopy (rhinoscopy), as well as localization of the lesion(s), using imaging modalities such as radiography or computed tomography (CT), should be performed prior to obtaining samples for cytologic examination. It is advisable to perform a complete blood count (CBC) and hemostatic profile prior to sample collection since most sampling techniques result in significant hemorrhage due to the rich vascular supply of the nasal mucosa. Hemorrhage may obscure proper visualization of the cavity and hamper radiographic interpretation; therefore, radiography should be performed prior to rhinoscopy and sample collection. Rhinoscopic evaluation of the nasal cavity is unable to predict the presence or absence of inflammation and, therefore, it is important to obtain samples for microscopic evaluation either through nasal swabs, nasal flushing, nasal brushing, fine needle aspiration (FNA) biopsy, or pinch biopsy techniques. General anesthesia, together with a properly inflated endotracheal tube and packing of the oropharynx with gauze, is recommended during sample collection. Tilting the patient's nose downward will further prevent any aspiration during the procedure (Tasker *et al.*, 1999; Elie & Sabo, 2006; Miller, 2007).

Superficial and deep nasal swabs are easily obtained and nontraumatic but are limited to identifying superficial inflammation, secondary bacterial infection, hemorrhage, or necrosis and do not provide much information on disease processes involving the deeper lying nasal mucosa. However, some infectious diseases, such as cryptococcosis in cats, are easily diagnosed by cytologic examination of the nasal discharge. Samples obtained through nasal flushing can also be very unrewarding; therefore more invasive techniques are needed to yield diagnostic material. A traumatic nasal flush can be accomplished by nicking the catheter, creating a rough surface that will assist with dislodging material. Care must be taken not to penetrate the cribriform plate. The distance from the external nares to the medial canthus of the eye should be measured beforehand, and the catheter should be marked or cut to the appropriate length. Small amounts (5–10 ml) of nonbacteriostatic, sterile saline are flushed into the cavity via a 20–35 ml syringe with alternating positive and negative pressure. The catheter should be moved back and forth against the mucosa as the fluid enters the cavity, in an attempt to acquire deeper lying tissue cells. An alternative method involves directing the catheter into the nasopharynx via the oral cavity and retroflexing it around the soft palate. Once the bulb of the catheter is inflated, saline can be lavaged through the nasal cavity and collected at the external nares. This technique is especially useful in patients with very small nasal passages, such as cats and small dogs (Tasker *et al.*, 1999; Kuehn, 2006). Any fluid retrieved through either method should be collected in an EDTA-anticoagulated tube for microscopic examination. EDTA is considered to be bacteriostatic; therefore samples for microbiology should be collected using a sterile swab or into a sterile tube. If the fluid is very turbid, direct smears can be made of the particulate matter using the 'squash' preparation technique. Briefly, a drop of fluid is placed on a clean slide with a second slide placed on top, perpendicularly. Once the fluid has spread, the two slides are pulled apart in a horizontal fashion with minimal vertical pressure applied. If the fluid is clear, the sample can be centrifuged and smears prepared of the sediment. If available, cytocentrifugation can be used for further concentration of the sample. One study described a minimally invasive hydropulsion method of forceful nasal flushing, which was able to obtain a large sample for biopsy of nasal tumors in dogs and cats. The study reported a success rate for definitive diagnosis of 90.2%, higher than previous reports of nasal flushing and endoscopic pinch

DOI: 10.1201/9781003258551-13

biopsy techniques. This technique was successful in obtaining tissue from a variety of tumors, and the gross rhinoscopic appearance of the mass did not influence the success of the hydropulsion (Ashbaugh *et al.*, 2011).

A cytobrush or endoscopic brush can be used to collect tissue to roll on a clean glass slide for cytologic examination; however, brush cytology often misses the deeper inflammatory cells and may not correlate with histologic findings. One study reported very poor agreement between cytologic and histologic samples in cats, with only 25% of samples having the same predominant cell type (Michiels *et al.*, 2003). Brush cytology has been shown to correctly identify neoplasia of epithelial origin in 86–88% of cases, but diagnoses of mesenchymal tumors are less likely (Clercx *et al.*, 1996; Caniatti *et al.*, 2012). Brush cytology samples with high cellularity are reported to have lower sensitivity for the diagnosis of neoplasia compared with samples having low or moderate cellularity (Caniatti *et al.*, 2012). Fine needle aspiration biopsy or biopsy, using a large gauge polypropylene urinary catheter with the end cut at a 45° angle, attached to a syringe, has been shown to yield the most diagnostic material when a mass lesion is present. It is important, however, to accurately identify the location of the mass using various imaging techniques. Care should again be taken not to penetrate the cribriform plate. Alligator biopsy forceps can be used to obtain a pinch biopsy for impression cytology and histopathology (Withrow *et al.*, 1985; Tasker *et al.*, 1999).

Normal cytology of the nasal cavity

In healthy animals, samples collected from the nasal cavity contain few cells and a small amount of mucus. Large, nonkeratinized squamous epithelial cells, often associated with low numbers of mixed population extracellular bacteria (normal bacterial flora) colonizing their surface, are obtained from the oropharynx and external nares (Figure 13.1). The presence of *Conchiformibius* spp. (previously known as *Simonsiella* spp.) in the sample confirms oropharyngeal contamination. *Conchiformibius* spp. are large, rod-shaped bacteria that align in a row after division, giving them a distinctive 'bar code' appearance (Figure 13.2) (Nyby *et al.*, 1977a).

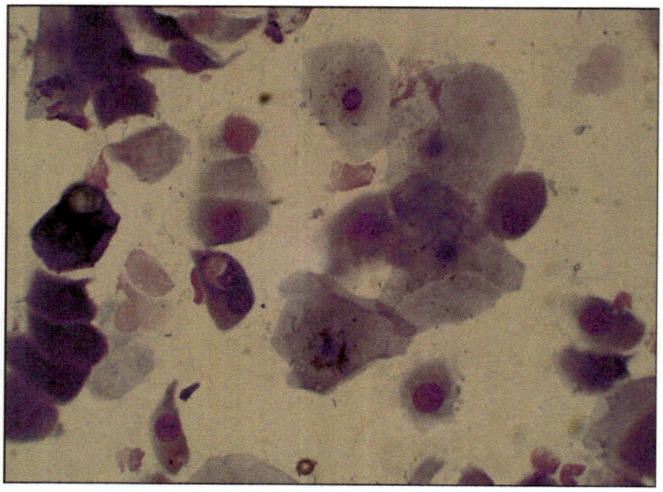

Figure 13.1 **Oropharyngeal contamination. Large, keratinized and nonkeratinized squamous epithelial cells with low numbers of mixed population extracellular bacteria (normal bacterial flora) obtained from the oropharynx and external nares (Diff-Quik, 500× magnification).**

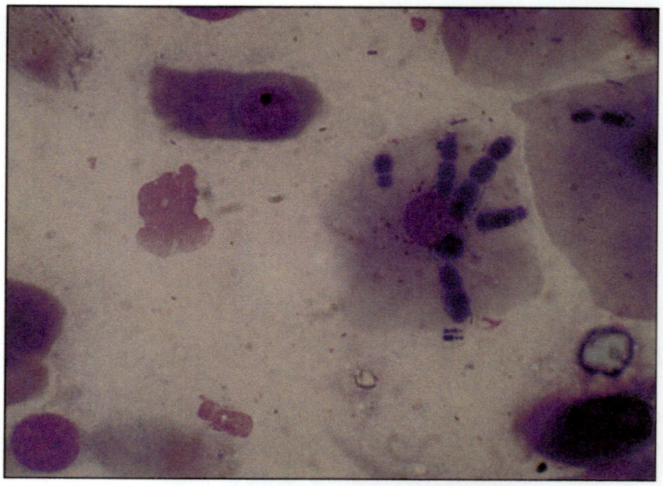

Figure 13.2 **Oropharyngeal contamination. A superficial squamous epithelial cell with several *Conchiformibius* organisms (previously *Simonsiella* spp.). *Conchiformibius* spp. are large, rod-shaped bacteria that align in a row after division and indicate that there was oropharyngeal contamination of the sample (Diff-Quik, 1,000× magnification).**

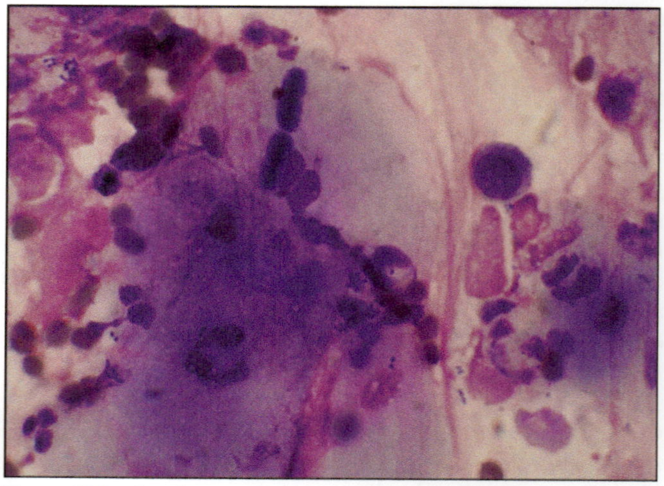

Figure 13.3 **Oropharyngeal contamination with inflammation. Neutrophilic inflammation in the presence of oropharyngeal contamination can make it difficult to determine the origin of the inflammation. Inflammatory cells, specifically neutrophils, may be seen in patients with oral inflammation or dental disease (Diff-Quik, 1,000× magnification).**

Neutrophils are usually absent with oropharyngeal contamination; however, in patients with oral inflammation or dental disease, inflammatory cells may be seen (Figure 13.3). The predominant cell type from the nasal turbinate is typically ciliated columnar respiratory epithelial cells, which appear elongated or cone shaped with eosinophilic staining cilia on their flattened apical ends and a round nucleus present in the basal end of the cell (Figure 13.4). These

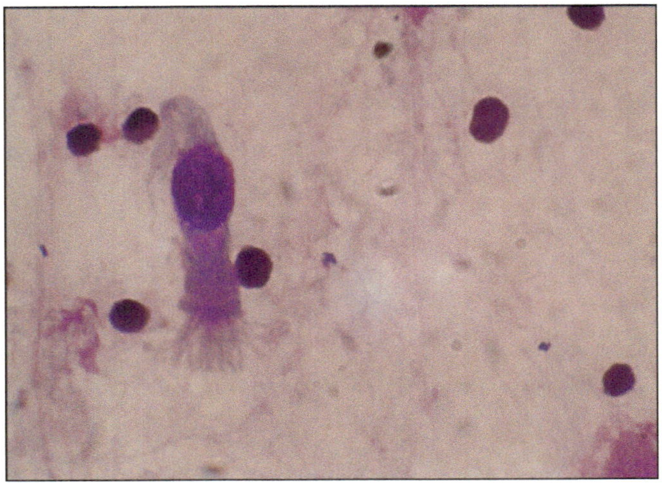

Figure 13.4 Respiratory epithelial cell. The predominant cell type from the nasal turbinates is typically ciliated columnar respiratory epithelial cells, of which one can be seen in this picture. They appear elongated or cone shaped with eosinophilic staining cilia on their flattened apical ends and a round nucleus present in the basal end of the cell (Diff-Quik, 1,000× magnification).

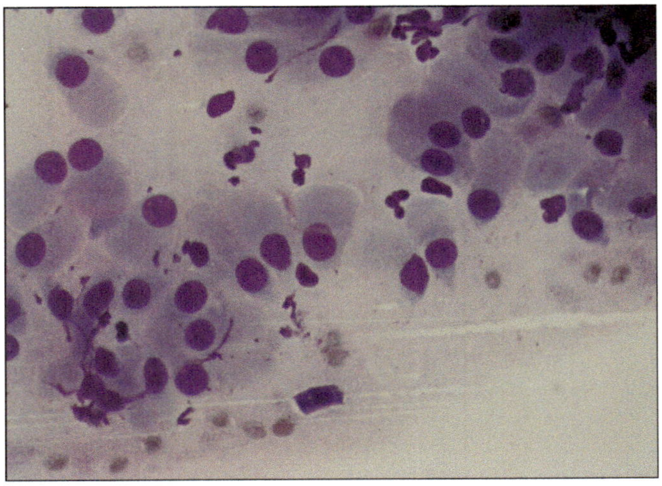

Figure 13.5 Nasal respiratory epithelial cells. Clusters of normal nonciliated respiratory epithelial cells from the nasal cavity (Diff-Quik, 500× magnification).

respiratory epithelial cells can be seen as single cells or in clusters (Figure 13.5). Occasionally, basal epithelial cells may be seen, depending on the collection method used. These cells are round to cuboidal with scant, deeply basophilic cytoplasm and a round nucleus that is centrally located (Figure 13.6). Mucus appears as eosinophilic amorphous extracellular material, often containing entrapped cells (Figure 13.7). Hemorrhage during sampling is a common occurrence and will result in the presence of red blood cells (RBCs), few white blood cells (WBCs), and sometimes platelet clumps. Iatrogenic contamination of a sample is suspected if the proportion of RBCs and WBCs is similar to that in peripheral blood (approximately 1 WBC per 500–1,000 RBCs) (Burkhard & Millward, 2010; Arndt, 2014).

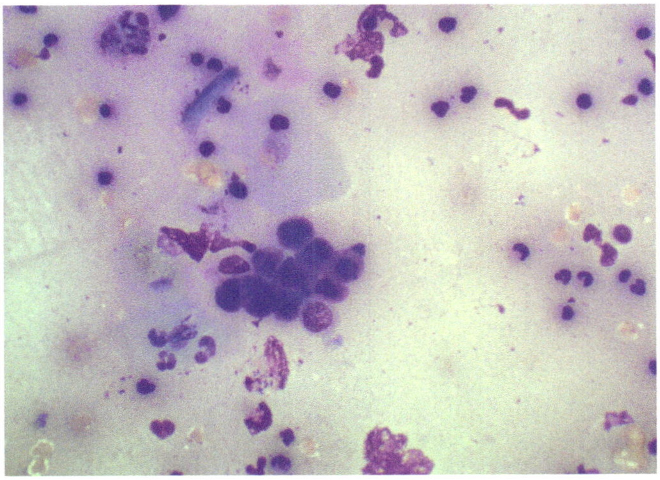

Figure 13.6 Basal epithelial cells. A group of basal epithelial cells, commonly seen as sheets of small cells with scant, round to cuboidal, deeply basophilic cytoplasm and a round nucleus that is centrally located (Diff-Quik, 500× magnification).

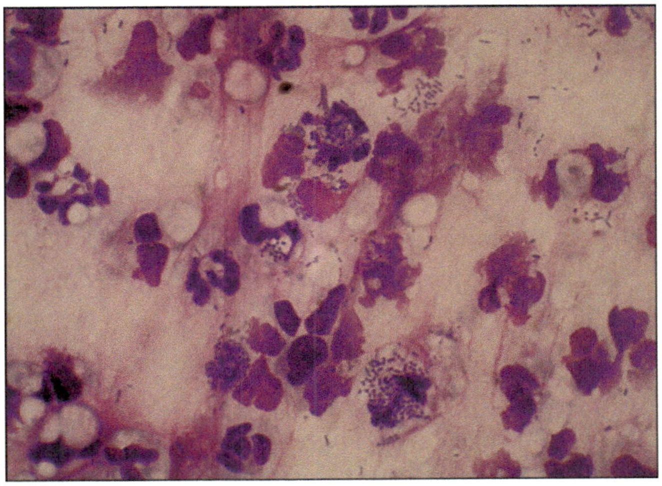

Figure 13.7 Nasal bacterial infection. Neutrophils with phagocytized bacteria indicating a bacterial nasal infection. Some mucus strands are present in the background appearing as eosinophilic amorphous extracellular material, containing entrapped cells (Diff-Quik, 1,000× magnification).

INFLAMMATION OF THE NASAL CAVITY

Infectious

Neutrophils predominate in nasal exudates associated with bacterial, viral, and some fungal infections. Other inflammatory cells, such as macrophages, lymphocytes, and plasma cells, may also be present (Figure 13.8). The normal bacterial flora in the nasal and oral cavities is generally pleomorphic; therefore a monomorphic bacterial population suggests either infection or bacterial overgrowth (Figure 13.9; French, 1987; Michiels *et al.*, 2003). Neutrophils containing phagocytized bacteria consisting of a monomorphic population strongly suggest infection (Figure 13.7). Primary bacterial infections are rare and

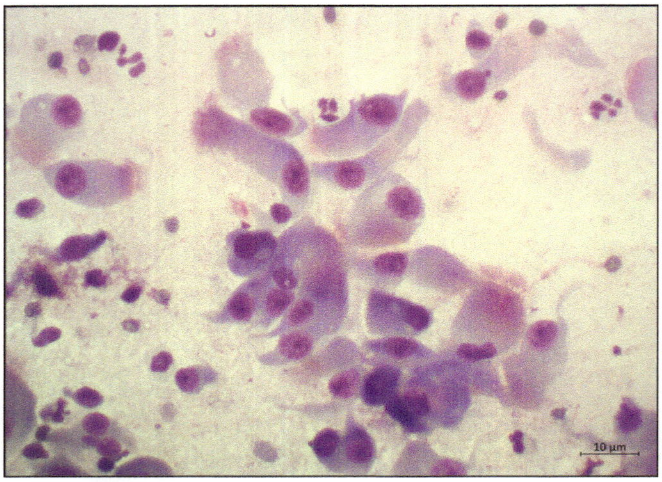

Figure 13.8 Neutrophilic inflammation. Several neutrophils and a few lymphocytes are seen amongst clusters of ciliated and nonciliated respiratory epithelial cells (Wright–Giemsa, 500× magnification).

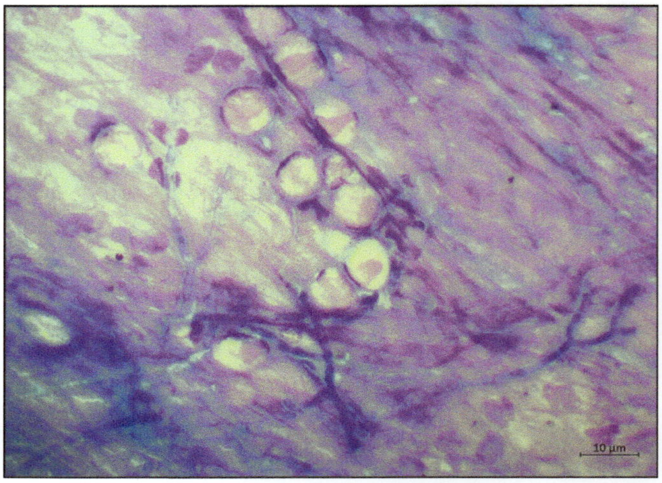

Figure 13.10 Fungal infection. Fungal hyphae – branching, septate with straight, parallel walls and globose terminal ends – arranged in mats and individually. The hyphae resembled that of *Aspergillus* or *Penicillium* spp. (Wright–Giemsa, 500× magnification).

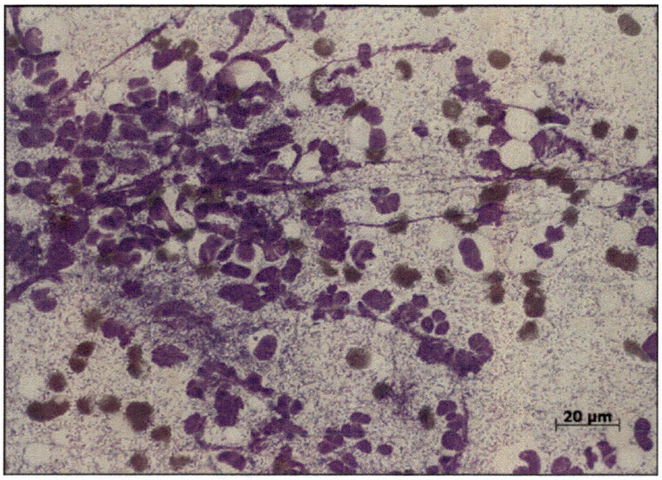

Figure 13.9 Bacterial overgrowth. An overgrowth of a monomorphic population of bacteria. The high number of neutrophils most likely indicates a bacterial infection despite the fact that all of the bacteria appear to be extracellular (Diff-Quik, 500× magnification).

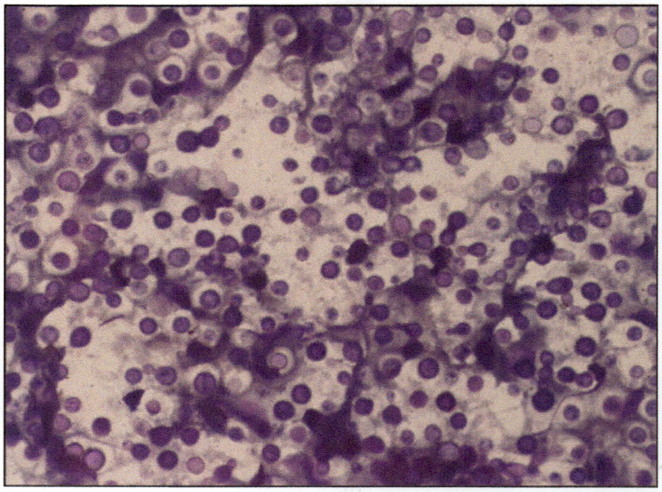

Figure 13.11 Nasal cryptococcosis. Numerous round to oval, basophilic staining yeasts surrounded by a thick nonstaining polysaccharide capsule. This is the typical presentation for *Cryptococcus neoformans*. Narrow-based budding is also often seen cytologically (Diff-Quik, 500× and 1,000× magnification, respectively).

usually secondary to mucosal injury, viral, parasitic, or fungal infections, dental disease, oronasal fistulas, idiopathic lymphoplasmacytic rhinitis, and neoplasia. These conditions should be suspected in a patient with sinusitis that is unresponsive to antimicrobial therapy. Cytologic findings with viral rhinitis are nonspecific and often only secondary bacterial infection, with the presence of various types of inflammatory cells, can be seen (Windsor & Johnson, 2006; Windsor *et al.*, 2006). With mycotic rhinitis, fungal hyphae may be difficult to identify between cells and debris because they may not stain well with Romanowsky stain and appear as clear filamentous structures. The most common fungal agents responsible for mycotic rhinitis in dogs are *Aspergillus* spp. and *Penicillium* spp. (Figure 13.10), whereas *Cryptococcus* spp. occur more frequently in cats (Figure 13.11). *Aspergillus* spp. and *Penicillium* spp. are morphologically similar and present as septate, branching hyphae (2–4.5 µm wide), associated with serosanguineous to mucopurulent nasal exudates, nasal mucosal necrosis, and turbinate destruction (Peeters & Clercx, 2007; Day, 2011). Although fungal rhinosinusitis, caused by *Aspergillus* spp., occurs less frequently in cats, two forms have been described, namely sinonasal aspergillosis and sinoorbital aspergillosis (most common). Both infections start in the nasal cavity and brachycephalic breeds of cats, especially Persian and Himalayan, are predisposed. Feline sinonasal aspergillosis is usually noninvasive with a favorable prognosis, whereas feline sinoorbital aspergillosis carries a guarded to poor prognosis (Barrs & Talbot, 2020; Barachetti *et al.*, 2009). *Cryptococcus*

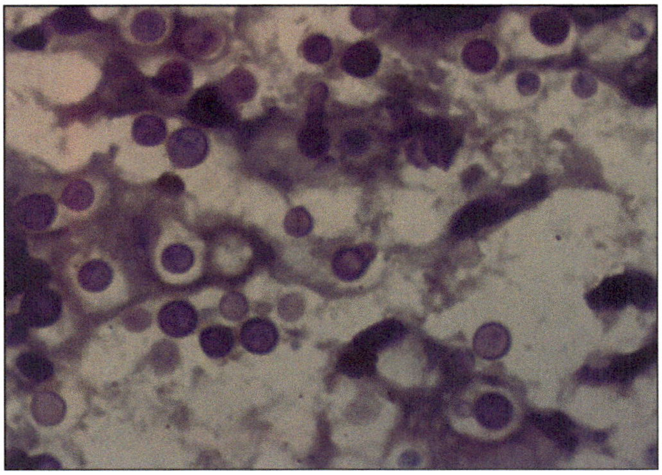

Figure 13.12 **Nasal cryptococcosis. Numerous round to oval, basophilic staining yeasts surrounded by a thick nonstaining polysaccharide capsule. This is the typical presentation for *Cryptococcus neoformans*. Narrow-based budding is also often seen cytologically (Diff-Quik, 500× and 1,000× magnification, respectively).**

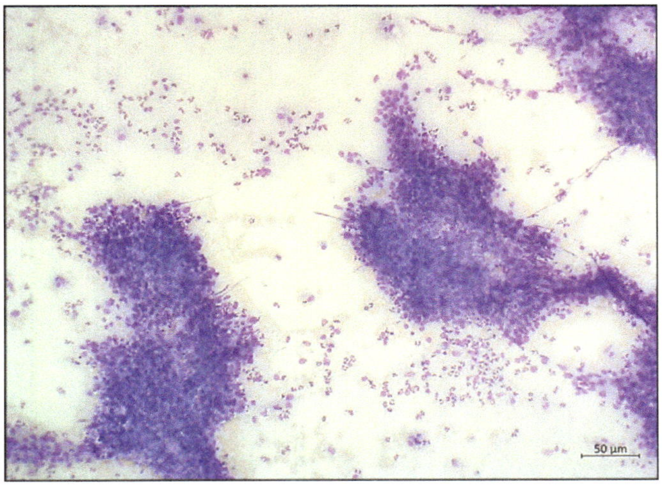

Figure 13.13 **Nasal adenocarcinoma. Several cohesive sheets of epithelial cells from a nasal mass (Wright–Giemsa, 100× magnification).**

neoformans is a saprophytic yeast that is round to oval (3.5–7.0 µm in diameter), stains basophilic, and is surrounded by a thick polysaccharide capsule (1–30 µm) that stains poorly with Wright–Giemsa or Diff-Quik® stains. Narrow-based budding is a feature of the organism (Figure 13.12). The organism is often diagnosed by examining only touch imprints of nasal lesions or exudates (Lester *et al.*, 2011; Sykes & Malik, 2012). An increase in the prevalence of subclinical cryptococcosis and asymptomatic dog and cat carriers of *Cryptococcus gattii* has been reported, which may contribute to outbreaks of clinical cryptococcosis in humans and animals (Duncan *et al.*, 2005).

Noninfectious

Foreign bodies such as plant awns or twigs are fairly common in dogs and are either directly inhaled or enter the nasal cavity traumatically through the external nares, the nasal planum, or through the palate via the oral cavity. Typically, a marked, suppurative to pyogranulomatous, inflammatory reaction is present and close attention should be paid to identifying any foreign material. Eosinophils may predominate in nasal exudates resulting from allergic rhinitis, but may also be present in response to parasites, fungi, bacteria, and neoplasia (Burkhard & Millward, 2010; Arndt, 2014).

Neoplasia of the nasal cavity

Neoplasia of the nasal cavity is uncommon in dogs and cats, but carries a poor prognosis when present because the majority of nasal tumors are malignant (80–90%). Malignant tumors, such as carcinomas, are more often seen in older animals, involve the caudal two-thirds of the nasal cavity, and result in destruction of the nasal turbinates and septum. Metastasis, however, is uncommon and may only be present in the late stages of the disease. Malignant epithelial tumors are seen more frequently and include adenocarcinoma, squamous cell carcinoma, transitional carcinoma, and undifferentiated carcinoma (Norris, 1979; Legendre, 1983).

Adenocarcinomas are cytologically characterized by the presence of small aggregates to large sheets of neoplastic epithelial cells (Figures 13.13, 13.14). Malignant cells show various anaplastic changes such as macrocytosis, mild to moderate anisocytosis and anisokaryosis, basophilic cytoplasm that may contain numerous discrete vacuoles, an increased nuclear to cytoplasm (N:C) ratio, and increased number of visible nucleoli per nucleus, some with shape variations (Figure 13.15). Adenocarcinomas may be associated with the production of mucus, which appears as extracellular, amorphous to fibrillar, eosinophilic material. Anaplastic cells may individualize and appear as discrete round cells. These neoplastic changes may be difficult to differentiate from other 'normal', adaptive changes that may be seen with chronic inflammation or irritation. Hyperplasia and/or dysplasia are mechanisms for tissue cells to undergo adaptive changes in

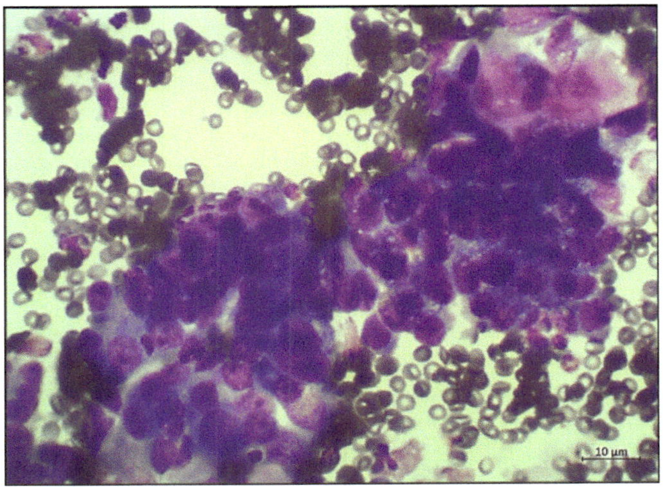

Figure 13.14 **Nasal adenocarcinoma. A sheet of pleomorphic epithelial cells showing anisocytosis, anisokaryosis, and prominent nucleoli (Wright–Giemsa, 500× magnification).**

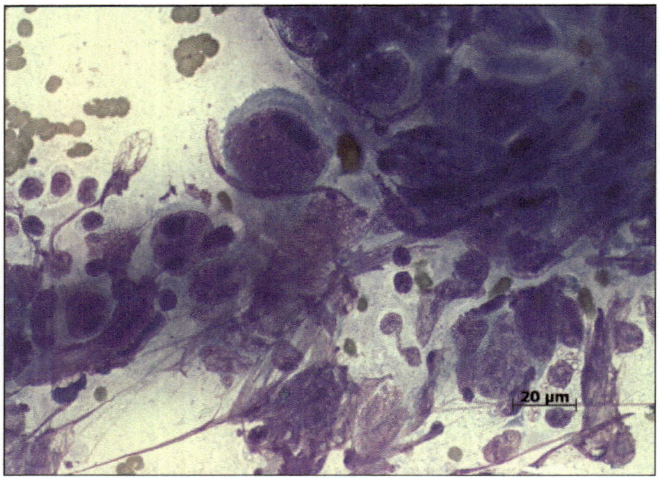

Figure 13.15 Nasal adenocarcinoma. Neoplastic epithelial cells display various cytologic signs of malignancy such as macrocytosis, marked anisocytosis and anisokaryosis, basophilic cytoplasm, an increased nuclear to cytoplasm ratio, and increased number of visible nucleoli per nucleus, some with shape variations (Diff-Quik, 500× magnification).

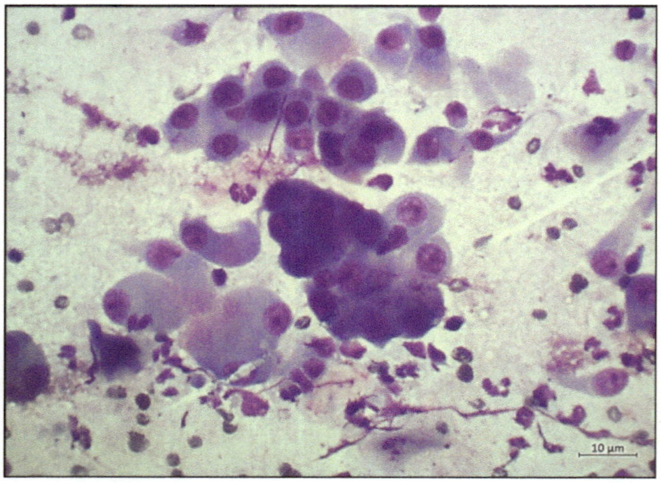

Figure 13.16 Epithelial hyperplasia and/or dysplasia. Nasal epithelium undergoes hyperplastic changes in order to survive amid a pathologic stimulus such as chronic inflammation. Hyperplasia is often accompanied by dysplasia and may present as sheets of epithelial cells with an increased nuclear to cytoplasm ratio, mild to moderate anisocytosis, and basophilic cytoplasm (Wright–Giemsa, 500× magnification).

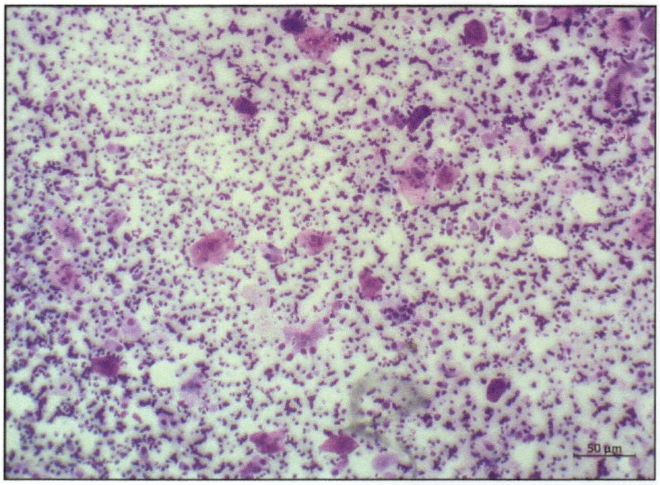

Figure 13.17 Squamous metaplasia. Chronic ongoing inflammation may result in the normal cell type changing into one that is better able to endure the environmental stress while losing specialized function (squamous cells) (Wright–Giemsa, 100× magnification).

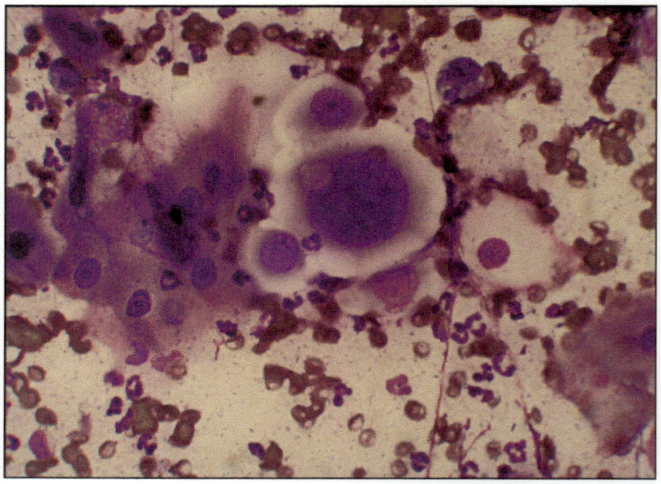

Figure 13.18 Squamous cell carcinoma. Squamous cell carcinomas present cytologically as large cells with angular borders, abundant cytoplasm, and centrally placed nuclei. The neoplastic epithelial cells can vary from immature, small, cuboidal, nucleated cells with deeply basophilic cytoplasm to large, mature, angular cells with abundant, pale cytoplasm and large nuclei. Cytologic criteria include marked anisokaryosis accompanied by a moderate to marked neutrophilic inflammatory response (Diff-Quik, 500× magnification).

order to survive amid a pathologic stimulus such as chronic inflammation. Hyperplasia (increased number of cells) is often accompanied by dysplasia (loss of architectural organization) and may present as sheets of epithelial cells with an increased N:C ratio, mild to moderate anisocytosis, basophilic cytoplasm, and the presence of mitotic figures (Figure 13.16). Chronic ongoing inflammation may result in squamous metaplasia (Figure 13.17), where the normal cell type is transformed into one that is better able to endure the environmental stress while losing specialized function (squamous cells). Both hyperplasia and metaplasia may result in neoplasia. Squamous cell carcinomas present cytologically as large cells with angular borders, abundant cytoplasm, and centrally placed nuclei (Figure 13.18). The neoplastic epithelial cells can present in various stages of maturation: from immature, small, cuboidal, nucleated cells with deeply basophilic cytoplasm to large, mature, angular cells with abundant, pale cytoplasm and large nuclei. Cytologic preparations are often associated with marked anisokaryosis accompanied by a moderate to marked neutrophilic inflammatory response. The presence of perinuclear vacuoles strongly suggests squamous cell origin (Burkhard

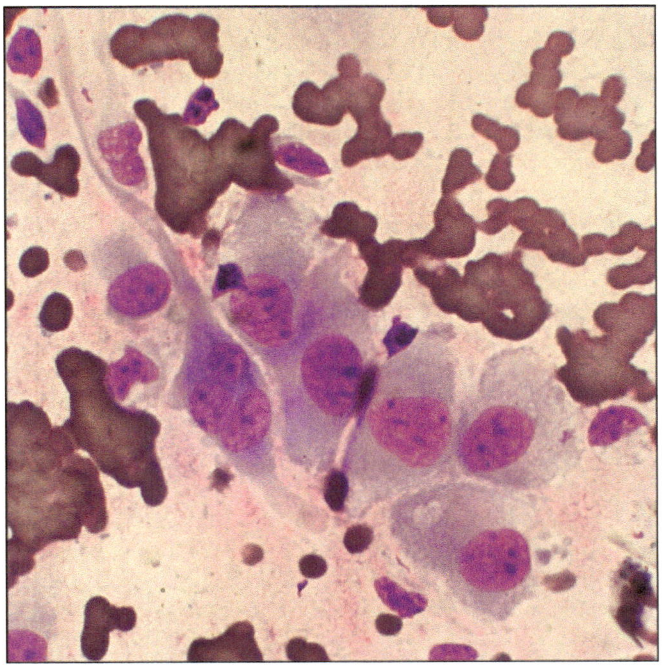

Figure 13.19 **Osteosarcoma. The presence of individual or aggregates of plump, fusiform, or spindle-shaped cells, with cytoplasm streaming away from the nuclei may indicate a mesenchymal tumor of the nasal cavity (Diff-Quik, 500× magnification).**

Millward, 2010; Arndt, 2014). Mesenchymal tumors of the nasal cavity are uncommon and normally these tumors exfoliate poorly, which complicates cytologic diagnosis. Cytologic samples typically present as low cellular samples with the occasional individual or aggregate of plump, fusiform, or spindle-shaped cells. Mesenchymal tumors most often seen include osteosarcoma (Figure 13.19), fibrosarcoma, and chondrosarcoma. Round cell (discrete cell) tumors, such as lymphoma, mast cell tumors (Khoo *et al.*, 2017), and transmissible venereal tumors, have been reported to occur in the nasal cavity of dogs and cats. Cytologic characteristics include highly cellular samples consisting of a homogeneous population of individualized, neoplastic round cells with distinct cytoplasmic borders, and morphologic characteristics resembling those seen in other sites (Arndt, 2014; Burkhard Millward, 2010).

TRANSTRACHEAL WASH AND BRONCHOALVEOLAR LAVAGE

Collection techniques and sample preparation and preservation

Transtracheal wash (TTW) and bronchoalveolar lavage (BAL), with or without bronchial brushing, are generally used to evaluate the larger airways and smaller airways, including the alveoli, respectively. The cytologic results between the two techniques can differ significantly, and should therefore be interpreted accordingly (Hawkins & DeNicola, 1989). Material is collected in a sterile manner from the tracheal lumen with tracheal washes, allowing cytological investigation for the presence of inflammation, infection, allergy, parasitic infestation, or neoplasia. Samples from a TTW can be collected either directly by entering through the cricothyroid ligament between two tracheal rings, or via an endotracheal (ET) tube. As muscle coverage increases towards the thoracic inlet, insertion of the needle between tracheal rings is easier in more anterior locations. For direct penetration of the tracheal wall, sedation is optional because it will impair the cough reflex, which is necessary for fluid retrieval. Depending on the size of the patient a 16- to 19-gauge jugular catheter is used. After numbing the area with local anesthetic, the catheter should be inserted with the bevel of the needle facing down, in a downward direction, to avoid laceration of the larynx and avoid contamination by the oropharynx. The catheter is then passed over the needle up to the level of the corina (4th intercostal space) and the needle removed. Approximately 0.1–0.2 ml/kg (maximum 10 ml) of warm, sterile, nonbacteriostatic saline is used, of which only half is initially injected using a 12 ml or larger syringe. A different syringe is used for aspiration of the fluid. Injected fluid remaining in the tracheobronchial tree will be absorbed and is not cause for concern. Although uncommon, complications may include subcutaneous emphysema, tracheal laceration, hemorrhage, cellulitis, hemoptysis, pneumomediastinum, and pneumothorax (Johnson & Vernau, 2011). A mild neutrophilic influx into the airways and transient bronchoconstriction may also occur (Kaneko *et al.*, 1996). The method using an ET tube requires general anesthesia and should be reserved for small dogs and cats. Care should be taken not to contaminate the ET tube tip in the oropharynx. Once the tube is in place, the cuff should be inflated and the patient placed in lateral recumbency. A jugular catheter or sterile polypropylene urinary catheter is then inserted into the ET tube up to the point of the carina, after which saline is instilled and collected as previously described (Creevy, 2009; Creighton, 1974; McCullough & Brinson, 1999b).

Bronchoalveolar lavage is indicated in patients with chronic coughing, bronchial or interstitial patterns on thoracic radiographs, and lung masses. Bronchoscopy is the ideal technique to obtain samples through BAL. Since BAL is used to sample the smaller airways and the alveoli, bronchoscopy will allow the operator to select specific lobes of the lung based on localization or severity of the lesion, as well as visualize masses that can be biopsied. The patient should be maintained under general anesthesia and the bronchoscope passed through an ET tube to allow visualization of the airways. Aliquots of warmed, sterile, nonbacteriostatic saline are injected through the biopsy channel. This is immediately reaspirated with a syringe or pump (Woods *et al.*, 2014a). Multiple lung lobes should be lavaged to increase the possibility of identifying an etiologic agent (Hawkins *et al.*, 1990, 1995; McCullough & Brinson, 1999b). In cats with lower respiratory disease, total and differential cell counts in BAL samples often differ significantly between lung segments and, therefore, clinicians should be cautious when using a single BAL cytology to define the inflammatory process present (Ybarra *et al.*, 2012). If a bronchoscope is unavailable or the patient is too small for a scope, the ET tube technique may be used. As with TTW, the patient should be maintained under general anesthesia, the ET tube passed, and the patient placed in lateral recumbency with the most severely affected side down. A sterile tube, long enough to reach up to the level of the 11th rib, should be inserted through the ET tube. The recommended total volume of warm, sterile saline for infusion, as previously described, is 1–3 ml/kg or 5–20 ml per site in dogs and 3–10 ml aliquots per site in cats (Hawkins *et al.*, 1990; Finke, 2013; Johnson & Drazenovich, 2007; Dehard *et al.*, 2008; Rajamäki *et al.*, 2001a). The suction pump aspiration technique has been shown to improve BAL fluid retrieval compared with manual aspiration; however, the increased fluid retrieval did not significantly improve the rate of diagnostic success in dogs with pulmonary disease (Woods *et al.*, 2014b). Preferably >50% of the infused volume should be recovered and it should have a foamy appearance which indicates the presence of surfactant and therefore adequate lavage of the lower airways (Woods *et al.*, 2014a; Finke, 2013; Andreasen, 2003; Hawkins *et al.*, 1990). The main complications associated with BAL are transient hypoxia, bronchoconstriction, and exacerbation of respiratory insufficiency (Johnson & Vernau, 2011; Johnson & Drazenovich, 2007; Allerton *et al.*, 2013). Therefore, patients should be supplied with supplemental oxygen before, during, and up to 20 minutes after the procedure.

Tracheobronchial brush samples allow cytological evaluation of visible endobronchial lesions (Rebar *et al.*, 1980; Hawkins *et al.*, 2006; Zhu *et al.*, 2015). Samples are obtained using an endoscopic brush passed through the biopsy channel of the endoscope or, alternatively, a protected sterile cytology brush or culture swab can be introduced directly through the oral cavity and larynx into the tracheal for sample collection. It is a useful adjunct but not a replacement for BAL and useful when a potentially hypocellular BAL sample is collected. The agreement of tracheobronchial brush cytology with BAL cytology is good for detecting inflammation, with the type of inflammation identified dependent on the technique used (Zhu *et al.*, 2015). Inflammation in dogs with chronic cough is more readily identified on bronchial brushing cytology compared to BAL cytology (Hawkins *et al.*, 2006). Bronchial brushings are also useful for detecting *Bordetella* organisms that are adherent to epithelial cells (Canonne *et al.*, 2016).

The processing of fluid samples should be standardized. Samples obtained through TTW or BAL should be divided into two portions: one portion should be placed into an EDTA tube to preserve cellular morphology and the other portion into a sterile container for possible microbial culture. Samples should ideally be placed on ice and processed within 30–60 minutes, since cell morphology is not well preserved in TTW/BAL samples (Andreasen, 2003; McCullough & Brinson, 1999b; Rebar *et al.*, 1980). If this is not possible, the sample should be placed on ice or stored at 4°C and processed within 4 hours. The laboratory should be contacted before sample collection; however, if the sample cannot reach the laboratory within 60 minutes, direct smears should be made of turbid samples or mucoid material present in the sample, in an attempt to avoid cellular changes due to the low-protein environment as well as enzyme release by the cells. Macrophages and neutrophils may phagocytize RBCs, bacteria, and other debris if the sample is not processed within the prescribed period of time (McCullough & Brinson, 1999b; Rakich & Latimer, 1989a). The protein concentration in BAL samples is not routinely measured as it is very low. The determination of cell counts on BAL samples is questionable due to increased mucus and lack of standardization of techniques and therefore an inconsistent degree of dilution (Creevy, 2009; Woods *et al.*, 2013). Cell counts can, however, be helpful in determining whether the BAL sample was adequate. A sample with a cell count <250 cells/μl should be repeated (Hawkins & DeNicola, 1989). The cellular component of the fluid should be concentrated either through standard centrifugation or cytocentrifugation. Squash preparations should be made of large mucus plugs observed in the sample, as cells and organisms are frequently embedded in the mucus (Andreasen, 2003; McCullough & Brinson, 1999b). If a TTW/BAL sample is deemed unacceptable for various reasons, it should be repeated either immediately or only after 48 hours. However, it has been shown that even though a sterile solution is used during the procedure, it induces a neutrophilic response that peaks 24 hours after the procedure was performed (Damiano *et al.*, 1980; Rakich & Latimer, 1989a). Differential cell counts of BAL fluid provide important information in the assessment of various bronchial and pulmonary diseases. A 500-cell differential count is required for all types of cells to be quantified with adequate reproducibility. Although neutrophils, alveolar macrophages, and eosinophils had high reproducibility by counting 200 cells, only adequate reproducibility was reached for lymphocytes and bronchial epithelial cells by counting 500 cells (De Lorenzi *et al.*, 2009). Measurement of cytokine concentrations in bronchoalveolar samples may provide a tool to more accurately define disease processes in veterinary patients (Richard *et al.*, 2014).

Normal cytologic features

Normal cytologic findings for TTW and BAL include a small amount of mucus, low numbers of columnar or cuboidal epithelial cells (<1% in BAL), goblet cells, alveolar macrophages, and neutrophils (<5%), occasional lymphocytes, and superficial squamous cells (fewer with BAL). A small amount of mucus is usually present in clinically normal dogs and cats. Mucus appears as amorphous sheets ranging from blue to pink or as homogeneous strands that are frequently twisted or whorled (Figures 13.20, 13.21). The trachea and bronchi are lined by pseudostratified ciliated and nonciliated epithelial cells, which are typically seen in washings from the trachea, large bronchi, and bronchioles, as opposed to alveolar space, from normal dogs and cats (Figure 13.22). Like those seen in the nasal cavity, ciliated columnar cells are elongated, or cone shaped with cilia on their flattened apical ends. The nucleus is present in the basal end of the cell. Ciliated cuboidal cells look similar except that these cells are as wide as they are tall (Figure 13.23) (Andreasen, 2003; Creevy, 2009). Cilia can detach if there is a delay in sample processing and care should be taken not to confuse them with bacterial rods (Andreasen, 2003; McCullough & Brinson, 1999b). Nonciliated columnar epithelial cells look the same except for the absence of cilia. These cells may be present individually or in clusters and are usually of no clinical significance. Due to the low protein content of the fluid in which the cells are collected, most columnar epithelial cells may be poorly preserved in many samples. Compared with BAL fluid, tracheal wash fluid is more hypocellular and has a different cytologic appearance. Tracheal wash fluid reflects the larger airways, which are lined with ciliated columnar epithelium and, therefore, will contain a larger population of these cells, a few goblet cells, rare macrophages, and other leukocytes. Tracheal or

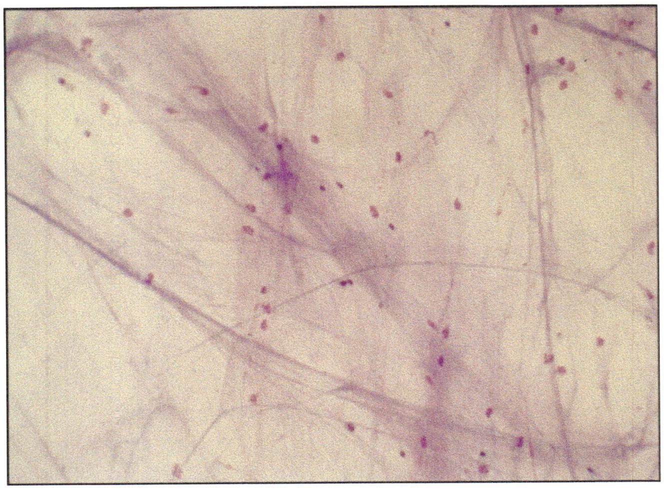

Figure 13.20 **Mucus. Mucus from a normal transtracheal wash or bronchoalveolar lavage appears as blue to pink amorphous sheets or homogeneous strands that are frequently twisted or whorled (Diff-Quik, 100× magnification).**

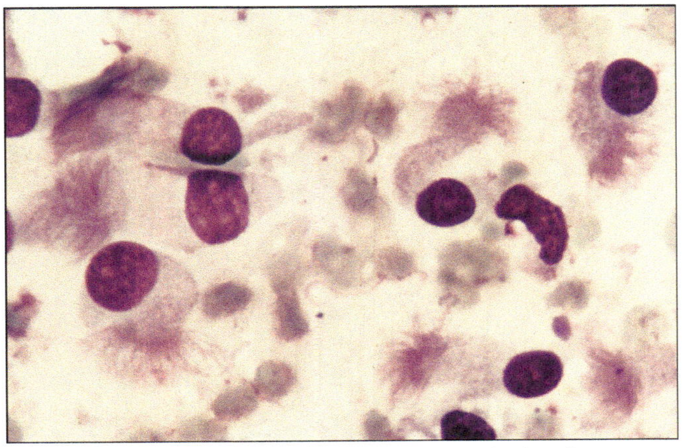

Figure 13.22 **Respiratory epithelial cell. A transtracheal wash or bronchoalveolar lavage with a cluster of normal respiratory epithelial cells (Diff-Quik, 1,000× magnification).**

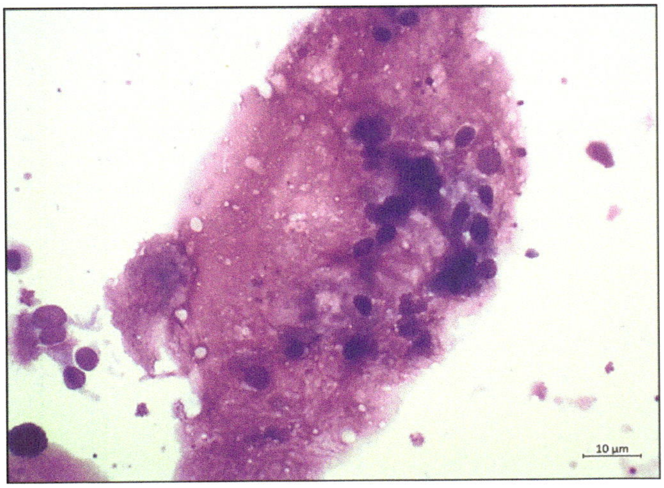

Figure 13.21 **Mucus. Amorphous and granular sheet of mucus from a bronchoalveolar lavage with alveolar macrophages, some respiratory epithelial cells and leukocytes embedded in it. A granular appearance is often associated with increased cellularity (Wright–Giemsa, 500× magnification).**

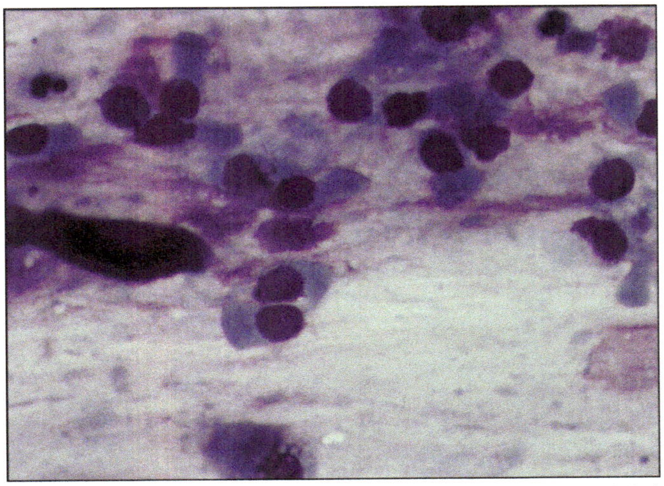

Figure 13.23 **Respiratory epithelial cells. Cuboidal respiratory epithelial cells look like columnar epithelial cells except that they are as wide as they are tall (Diff-Quik, 500× magnification).**

bronchial brushings in healthy dogs consist mainly of epithelial cells, with >7% leukocytes noted in dogs with cough (Hawkins *et al.*, 2006). On the other hand, alveolar macrophages are more commonly seen in the BALs of healthy dogs and cats (>70%) and are useful indicators of washes that have adequately washed the alveolar spaces (Figure 13.24) (Creevy, 2009; Hawkins *et al.*, 1995; McCullough & Brinson, 1999b). Alveolar macrophages have abundant blue–gray cytoplasm and an eccentrically positioned, round to bean-shaped nucleus. When activated, their cytoplasm becomes more abundant and vacuolated and may contain phagocytized material (Figures 13.25, 13.26) (Burkhard & Millward, 2010; English, 2014; Rebar *et al.*, 1980). Occasional binucleated alveolar macrophages may be an incidental finding, while multinucleated are associated with cell activation and increased phagocytosis. Leukocytes such as neutrophils and eosinophils are frequently seen in washes and look like those seen in the blood (Figure 13.27). Normal differential cell counts for BALs have been established for dogs and cats and are generally considered more important than absolute counts (Table 13.1) (Woods *et al.*, 2014a; Rajamäki *et al.*, 2001a; Rebar *et al.*, 1980). Neutrophils usually represent <5–10% of the nucleated cell count and an increase would indicate inflammation. Eosinophils, in species other than cats, should be <5% and a hypersensitivity reaction should be suspected when eosinophils are increased. In thick areas on a smear, where cells are not well spread out, careful distinction should be made between neutrophils and eosinophils, as individual granules may be hard to see (Figure 13.28). Eosinophil numbers in cats have been shown to vary markedly from those in dogs, and a range from 6% to 28% may be seen in BAL samples from healthy cats (Padrid *et al.*,

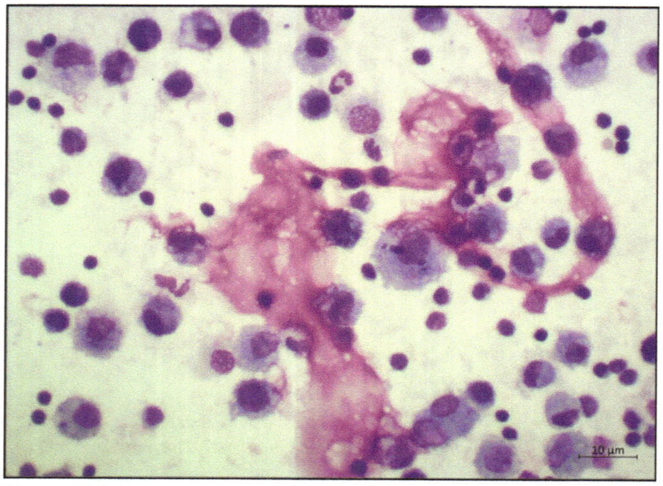

Figure 13.24 Alveolar macrophages and mucus from a bronchoalveolar lavage. Alveolar macrophages are commonly seen and are useful indicators of washes that have adequately washed the alveolar spaces. They have abundant blue–gray cytoplasm and an eccentrically positioned, round to bean-shaped nucleus (Wright–Giemsa, 500× magnification).

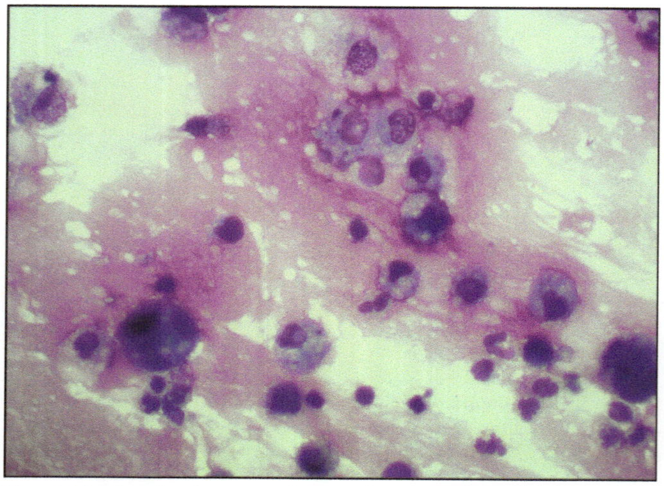

Figure 13.25 Alveolar macrophages and mucus. When activated, such as during chronic inflammation, the cytoplasm of alveolar macrophages becomes more abundant and vacuolated ('foamy'), and may contain phagocytized debris and display multinucleation (Wright–Giemsa, 500× magnification for both).

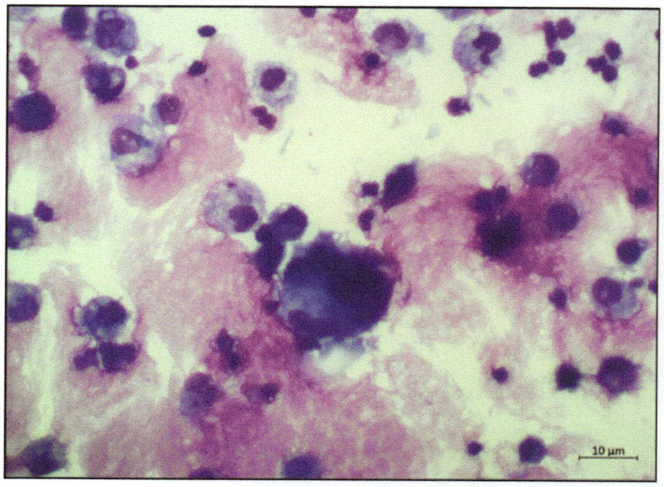

Figure 13.26 Alveolar macrophages and mucus. When activated, such as during chronic inflammation, the cytoplasm of alveolar macrophages becomes more abundant and vacuolated ('foamy'), and may contain phagocytized debris and display multinucleation (Wright–Giemsa, 500× magnification for both).

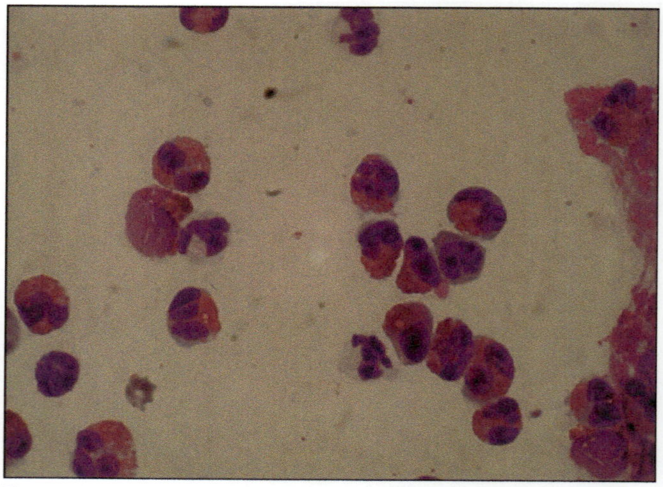

Figure 13.27 Leukocytes. Leukocytes, when present in transtracheal or bronchoalveolar lavage, look like those seen in the blood. This bronchoalveolar lavage contained high numbers of both neutrophils and eosinophils, as can be seen with hypersensitivity reactions (Diff-Quik, 1,000× magnification).

Table 13.1 Total and differential cell counts for bronchoalveolar lavage fluid from clinically healthy dogs and cats*

	Total cells/Ml	Macrophages	Lymphocytes	Eosinophils	Neutrophils	Mast cells
Dog	<400–600	70–100%	<7%	<6%	<5%	<1%
Cat	<400	70–100%	<5%	<10%	<7%	<2%

* Adapted from Alice Defarges Bichot, Dorothee Bienzle (2021) Lower Respiratory Tract of the Dog and Cat. In: *Veterinary Cytology*, 1st edn. (eds. L. C. Sharkey, M. J. Radin and D. Seelig) Wiley-Blackwell 2021, p. 287.

1991; Dehard *et al.*, 2008; Hawkins *et al.*, 1990; Kirschvink *et al.*, 2007; Norris *et al.*, 2003; Hawkins *et al.*, 1994; Dye *et al.*, 1996; Lécuyer *et al.*, 1995). The presence of eosinophils in samples from cats should therefore be interpreted carefully. A small percentage of lymphocytes may be present in the washes of normal dogs and cats and resemble those seen in the blood. Mature plasma cells may also be rarely seen (Figure 13.29). Increased numbers of lymphocytes may generally indicate nonspecific inflammation and is a common response to airway injury, independent

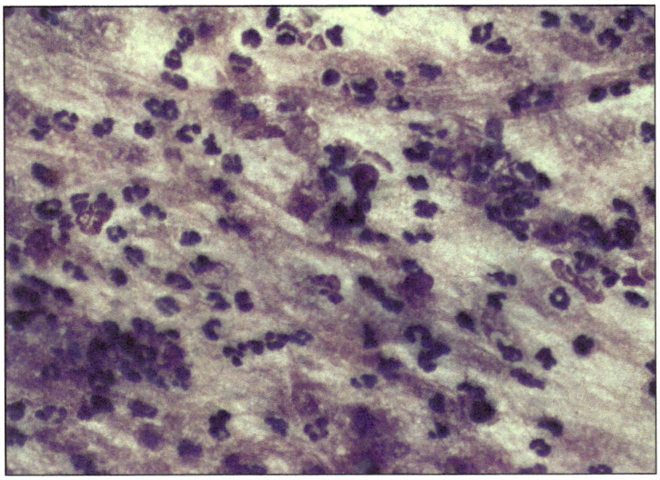

Figure 13.28 Leukocytes. Thick areas on a smear, where cells are not well spread out, should be examined with caution, especially if a lot of mucus is present. Neutrophils and eosinophils may be difficult to differentiate in these areas (Diff-Quik, 500× magnification).

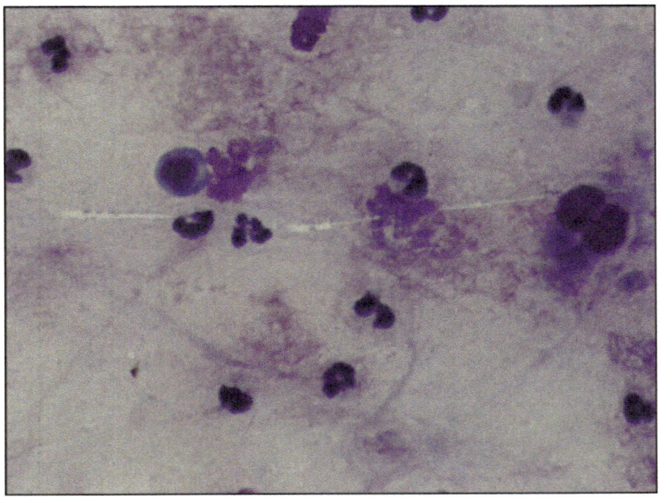

Figure 13.29 Leukocytes. Lymphocytes and plasma cells may also be present in the washes of normal dogs and cats, as well as in inflammatory conditions. This picture shows several neutrophils along with a single plasma cell, which resemble those seen in lymphoid tissue (Diff-Quik, 500× magnification).

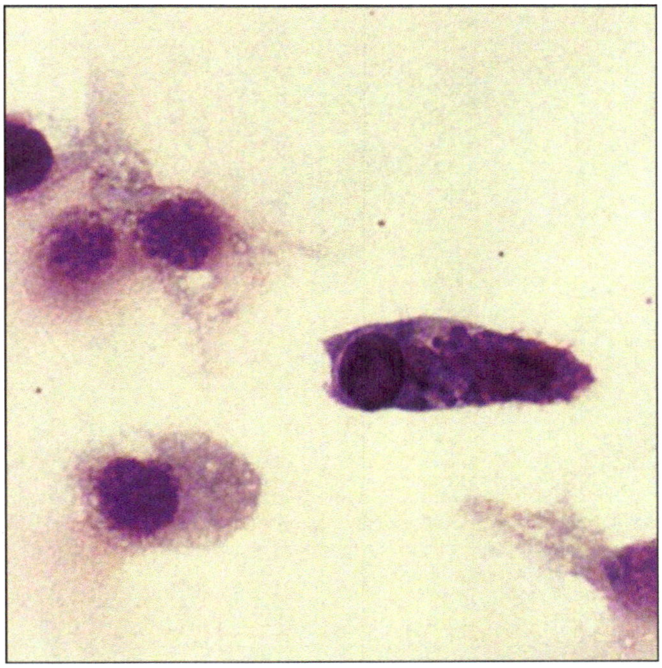

Figure 13.30 Goblet cells. Goblet cells are mucus-producing bronchial cells that are occasionally seen in normal transtracheal and bronchoalveolar washings. They are elongated cells and contain round granules of mucin that stain from red to blue to clear (Diff-Quik, 1,000× magnification).

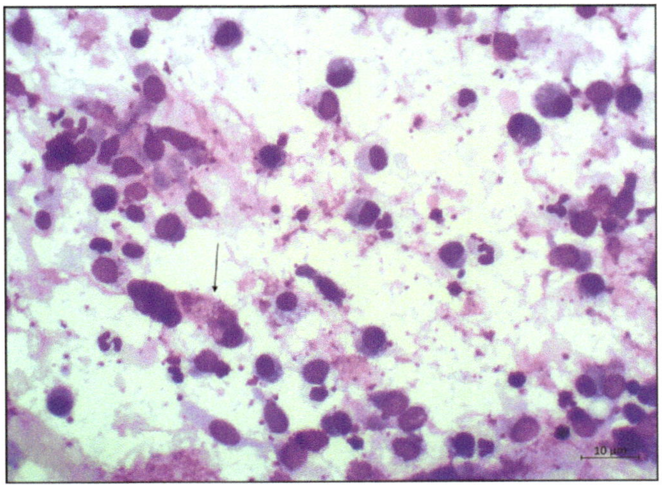

Figure 13.31 Goblet cells. Goblet cells are mucus-producing bronchial cells that are occasionally seen in normal transtracheal and bronchoalveolar washings. They are elongated cells and contain round granules of mucin that stain from red to blue to clear (Wright–Giemsa, 500× magnification).

of the type or duration of injury (Peeters *et al.*, 2000). Airway hyperreactivity, viral diseases, and chronic infections are associated with mildly increased numbers of lymphocytes (Creighton, 1974; Hirshman *et al.*, 1986). Low numbers of mast cells (<2%) are occasionally observed in samples from normal dogs and cats; however, increased numbers have been reported with many different inflammatory lung disorders, but are of little diagnostic significance (Hawkins *et al.*, 1990; Lécuyer *et al.*, 1995; Rebar *et al.*, 1980; Padrid *et al.*, 1991; Vail *et al.*, 1995). Airway hyperreactivity is associated with a mild increase in mast cell numbers (Hirshman *et al.*, 1986). Globule leukocytes are cells with eosinophilic cytoplasmic granules and round to oval eccentric nuclei. They have been observed in BAL specimens, but their cellular origin is unknown (Rebar *et al.*, 1980; Spoor *et al.*, 2011). Goblet cells are mucus-producing bronchial cells that are occasionally seen in normal washings and are not considered abnormal. Goblet cells are elongated, containing round granules of mucin that stain from red to blue to clear and often distend the cytoplasm (Figures 13.30–13.33) (Johnson *et al.*, 2013; McCullough

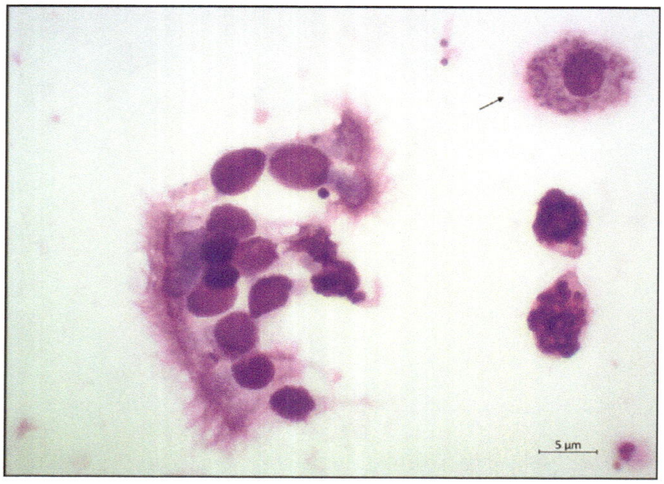

Figure 13.32 Goblet cells from a bronchoalveolar lavage. Two goblet cells with a rounded appearance, a small cluster of ciliated respiratory epithelial cells and a macrophage containing mucinous material (arrow) (Wright–Giemsa, 1,000× magnification).

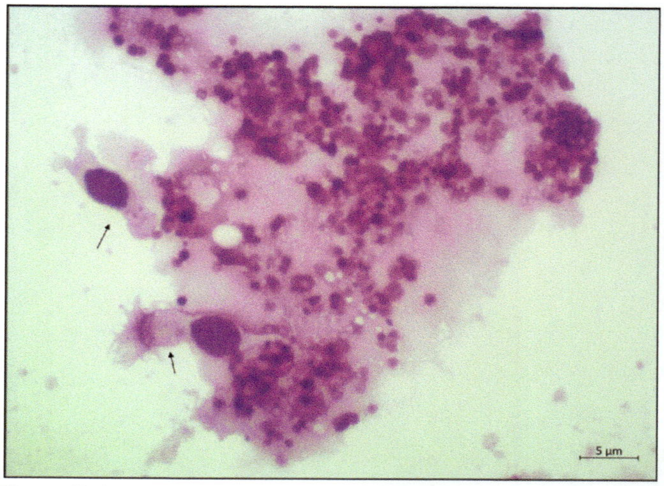

Figure 13.34 Free granules from ruptured goblet cells in bronchoalveolar lavage fluid. A goblet cell and ciliated respiratory epithelial cells indicated by arrows (Wright–Giemsa, 1,000× magnification).

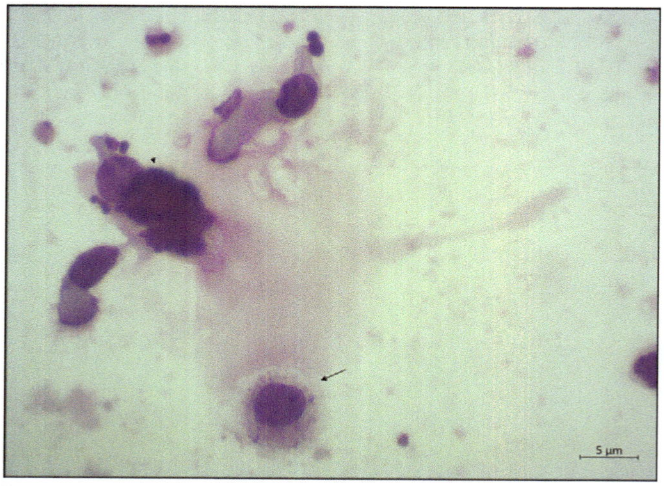

Figure 13.33 Goblet cell. Single elongated goblet cell with a cytoplasm distended by granules (arrowhead). A single macrophage (arrow) (Wright–Giemsa, 1,000× magnification).

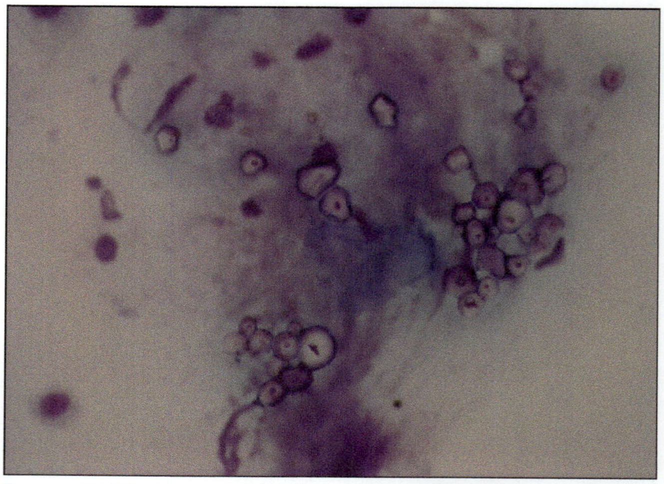

Figures 13.35 Corn starch. A transtracheal or bronchoalveolar wash from a dog containing corn starch (glove powder), which is occasionally seen in samples and is considered an incidental finding. Cytologically, corn starch appears as large, round to hexagonal structures that stain clear or blue and have a central fissure (Diff-Quick, 500× magnification).

& Brinson, 1999b). Free granules from ruptured cells may be seen on smears (Figure 13.34). Goblet cells can be differentiated from mast cells in that they have larger granules. Any chronic pulmonary irritant may result in an increased number of goblet cells (English, 2014). Corn starch or glove powder is occasionally seen in samples from TTW or BAL and is an incidental finding. Cytologically, they appear as large, round to hexagonal structures that stain clear or blue and have a central fissure (Figures 13.35). Pollen or plant cells may also occasionally be present in TTW or BAL samples (Figure 13.36).

Cytologic interpretation

Samples of TTWs and BALs are usually interpreted according to the type, quantity, and proportion of cells recovered; however, information gathered from history taking, physical examination, and radiography should be considered. The cell proportions often differ between TTW and BAL samples. In general, cellular patterns can be categorized as: (a) insufficient sample, (b) oropharyngeal contamination, (c) eosinophilic infiltrate, (d) neutrophilic infiltrate, (e) macrophage infiltrate, and (f) the presence of atypical cells.

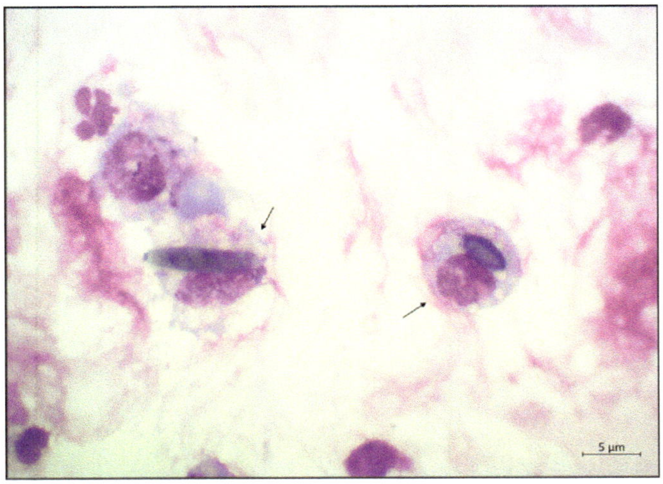

Figure 13.36 Pollen and plant material. Phagocytized pollen and plant material (arrows) in tracheal wash fluid (Wright–Giemsa, 1,000× magnification).

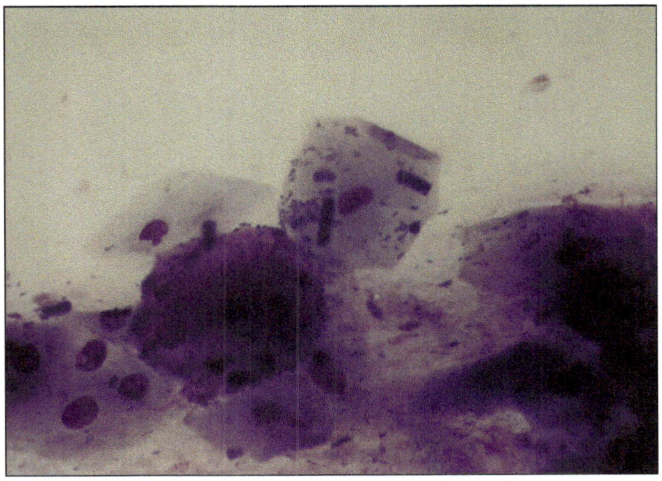

Figure 13.37 Oropharyngeal contamination. The presence of several large, superficial squamous cells associated with *Conchiformibius* spp. bacteria is a hallmark of oropharyngeal contamination (Diff-Quik, 500× magnification).

Insufficient sample

The absence of cells on a direct or concentrated preparation may indicate that the sample is not representative of the cytology of the respiratory tract. Similarly, when a predominance of only columnar respiratory epithelial cells, in the absence of alveolar macrophages, is seen in a BAL specimen, it indicates that only the airways and not the alveolar space has been effectively sampled.

Oropharyngeal contamination

Contamination is much more likely when TTWs or BALs are performed through an ET tube. Superficial squamous cells and a mixed population of bacteria (specifically *Conchiformibius* spp.) are the hallmarks for oropharyngeal contamination (Figures 13.37, 13.38) (Nyby *et al.*, 1977b). Many bacteria may be seen adhered to the surface of squamous epithelial cells and generally without the presence of neutrophils. However, neutrophils may be present in a contaminated sample if the patient has a purulent or ulcerative oropharyngeal lesion or suffers from dental disease (Figure 13.39). Oropharyngeal contamination may therefore have a significant effect on the interpretation of the cytologic evaluation and culture results.

Inflammation

Normally, neutrophils are present in very low numbers (<5%) in TTW/BAL samples of dogs and cats (Andreasen, 2003; McCullough & Brinson, 1999b; Rebar *et al.*, 1980). Neutrophil numbers are increased in nearly all conditions (infectious and noninfectious) that cause inflammation (Figures 13.40, 13.41). Neutrophils may show degenerative changes because of bacterial toxins or may be smudged (ruptured) secondary to trauma from collection and preparation

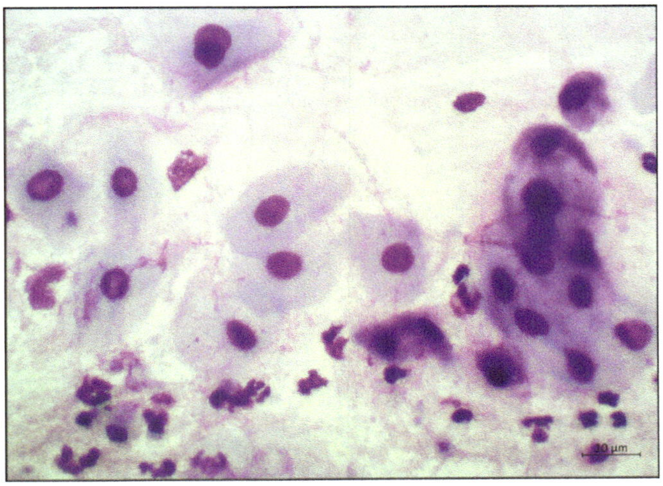

Figure 13.38 Oropharyngeal contamination. Sheet of squamous epithelial cells and some neutrophils in slightly mucinous background (Diff-Quik, 500× magnification).

(Figure 13.42) (Andreasen, 2003; Hawkins *et al.*, 1990). Degenerative changes occur when neutrophils are unable to control water homeostasis and undergo hydropic degeneration, of which the hallmark feature is nuclear swelling. Compared with non-degenerate neutrophils (Figure 13.43), the nucleus of the degenerative cell swells and appears thicker, stains a lighter eosinophilic color, and loses nuclear lobulation (karyolysis; Figure 13.44). When neutrophils are the predominant cell type, especially when the neutrophils appear degenerative, the sample should be examined closely for infectious agents, specifically bacteria (Figure 13.41). Confirmation of lower respiratory tract infection is challenging and organisms can be isolated from patients

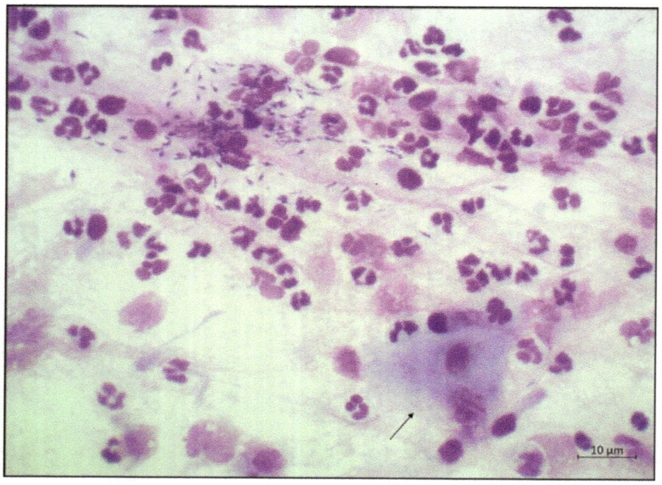

Figure 13.39 Oropharyngeal contamination. Neutrophils may be present in samples contaminated by the oropharynx, specifically when the patient suffers from oral or dental disease. Many neutrophils, a squamous epithelial cell (arrow), and extracellular bacteria are present in this bronchoalveolar lavage (Wright–Giemsa, 500× magnification).

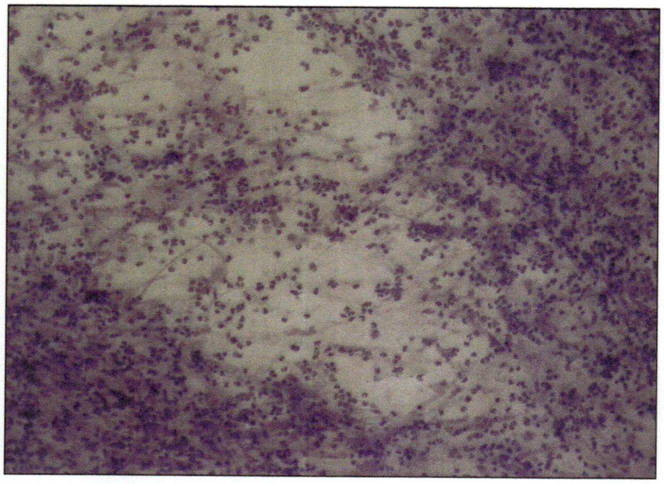

Figure 13.40 Inflammation. A bronchoalveolar lavage from a dog with inflammation of the lower respiratory tract. High numbers of neutrophils and some mucus strands are shown. When neutrophils are the predominant cell type, the sample should be closely examined for the presence of an infectious agent, such as bacteria (arrow) (Diff-Quik, 100× magnification).

in which bacteria were not detected on cytologic evaluation; therefore it is recommended to submit samples with marked neutrophilic inflammation for culture (Johnson *et al.*, 2013). The combination of BAL quantitative cultures with quantitating intracellular bacteria on Gram stain BAL cytology is useful in identifying lower respiratory tract infection in dogs (Peeters *et al.*, 2000). Other infectious disorders include mycotic, viral, or protozoal diseases (Figures 13.45, 13.46). Noninfectious disorders include tissue irritation or necrosis secondary to inhalation of a toxic substance, as well as neoplasia (Andreasen, 2003; McCullough & Brinson, 1999b). Neutrophilic inflammation can also be induced with the aspiration of water that contains diatom

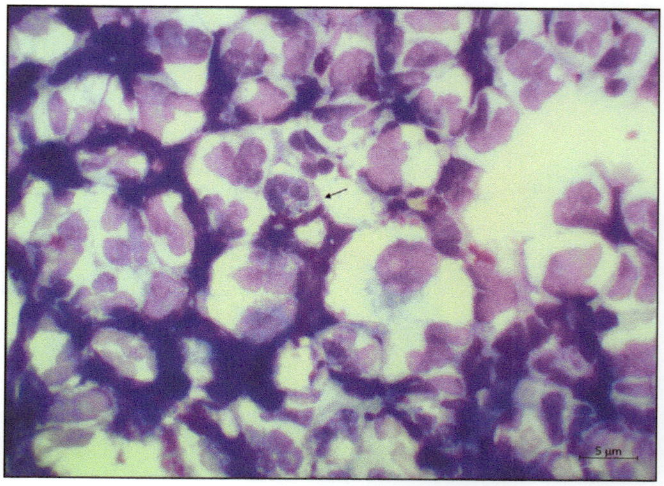

Figure 13.41 Inflammation. A bronchoalveolar lavage from a dog with inflammation of the lower respiratory tract. High numbers of neutrophils and some mucus strands are shown. When neutrophils are the predominant cell type, the sample should be closely examined for the presence of an infectious agent, such as bacteria (arrow) (Wright–Giemsa, 1,000× magnification).

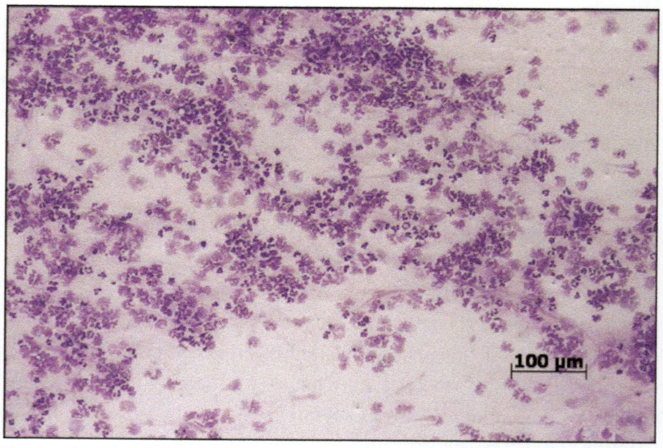

Figure 13.42 Inflammation. Neutrophils may show degenerative changes in the presence of bacterial toxins or may be smudged (ruptured) secondary to trauma from collection and preparation (Diff-Quik, 100× magnification).

algae (Benson *et al.*, 2013). The presence of neutrophils with phagocytosed nuclear material, morphologically consistent with presumed lupus erythematosus cells, has been reported in the BAL fluid from a dog with a clinical diagnosis of systemic lupus erythematosus (Black *et al.*, 2017). An increased amount of mucus can be seen with inflammation, irritation, or upper airway damage (chronic respiratory disease) due to increased numbers of goblet cells (Figure 13.47). Mucus usually stains more eosinophilic with inflammatory conditions due to the incorporation of inflammatory proteins and material from lysed cells (Figure 13.48) (Creighton, 1974). Curschmann's spirals are mucus casts of small bronchioles that appear as spiral, twisted masses of mucus that may have perpendicular radiations (bottle-brush-like appearance; Figures 13.49, 13.50, 13.51). They are seen with

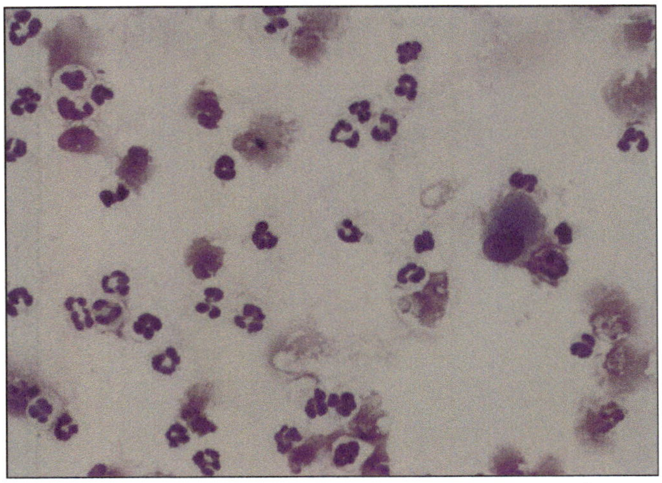

Figure 13.43 **Inflammation. Bronchoalveolar lavage with several non-degenerate neutrophils. The nuclei of the non-degenerate neutrophils are slender with clear lobulation and stain darkly (Diff-Quik, 500× magnification).**

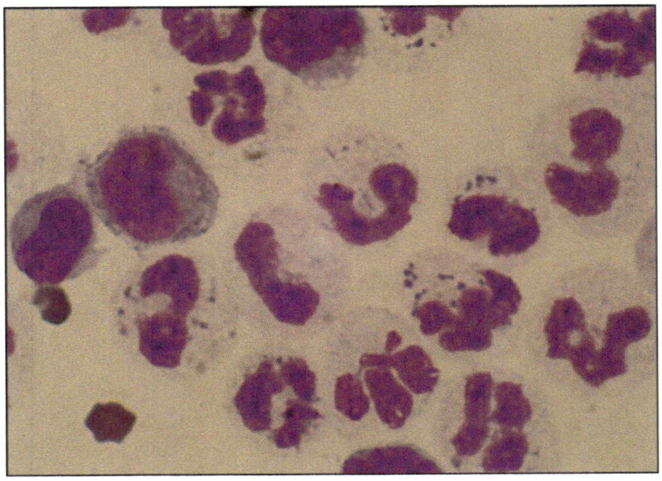

Figure 13.44 **Inflammation. Cytologic appearance of degenerative neutrophils in samples includes a thicker nucleus that stains a lighter eosinophilic color and loses nuclear lobulation (karyolysis) (Diff-Quik, 1,000× magnification).**

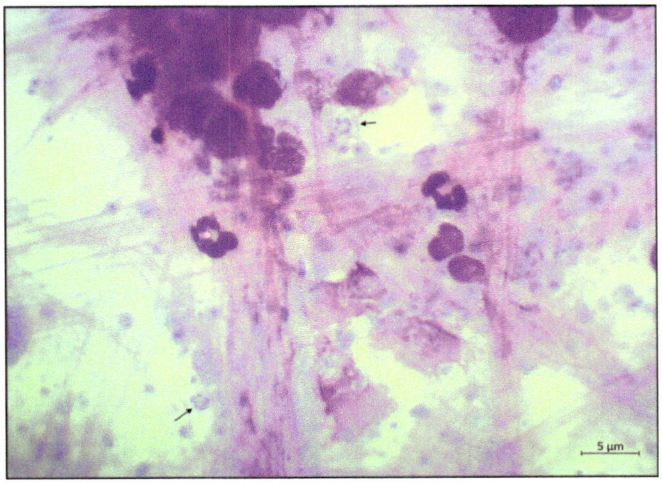

Figure 13.45 **Inflammation in a tracheal wash of a dog. Numerous small (1–2 µm) oval organisms with a clear cytoplasm and peripheral nucleus, either occurring singly or arranged in a ring formation inside a cyst (arrows), in the background. These organisms are consistent with *Pneumocystis* spp. (Wright–Giemsa, 1,000× magnification).**

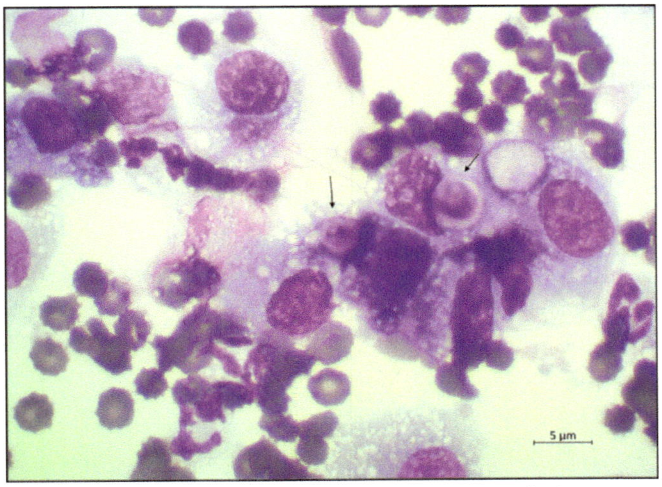

Figure 13.46 **Inflammation in a bronchoalveolar lavage of a dog. Activated alveolar macrophages displaying phagocytosis of *Cryptococcus neoformans* yeast-like organisms (arrows) (Diff-Quik, 1,000× magnification).**

disorders that result in chronic, excessive mucus production and are usually an indication of bronchiolar obstruction (Andreasen, 2003; Johnston, 1986). Increased numbers of alveolar macrophages are frequently seen with subacute and chronic pulmonary disorders, such as chronic persistent inflammation (Figure 13.52). Activated alveolar macrophages can also become bi- and multinucleated, known as giant cell macrophages (Figures 13.53, 13.54), with pulmonary disorders associated with chronic or pyogranulomatous inflammation (Andreasen, 2003). Epithelioid macrophages, characterized by granular eosinophilic cytoplasm, tend to cluster at sites of granuloma formation. Anthracotic pigment (dark or black granules) may be present within macrophages from clinically normal animals living in large cities or areas with polluted air (Roza & Viegas, 2007). Hyperplastic epithelium, together with goblet cell hyperplasia and increased mucus, is an additional change that can be seen with chronic inflammation. Cytologically, hyperplastic epithelium presents as variably sized, deeply basophilic epithelial cells (Figure 13.55).

Hypersensitivity

Healthy animals normally have a very low percentage (<5%) of eosinophils in TTW or BAL samples. In healthy dogs the proportion of eosinophils in BAL samples has been reported to be <11%; however it is mostly <5% (Clercx & Peeters, 2007b; Barçante *et al.*, 2008). Clinically healthy/asymptomatic cats may have significantly

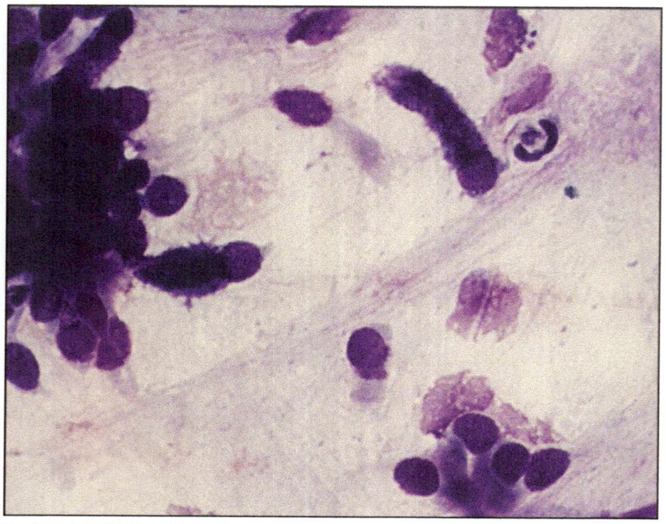

Figure 13.47 Goblet cells. An increased amount of mucus can be seen with inflammation, irritation, or upper airway damage (chronic respiratory disease) due to increased numbers of goblet cells. Goblet cells are distinguished from normal respiratory epithelial cells based on the presence of distinct large, intracytoplasmic, purple globules (Diff-Quik, 1,000× magnification).

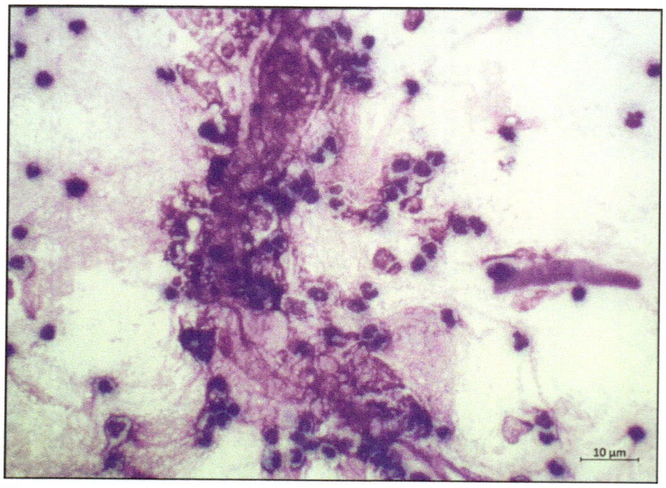

Figure 13.48 Mucus. Dark eosinophilic mucus is commonly seen with inflammatory conditions due to the incorporation of inflammatory proteins from lysed cells (Wright–Giemsa, 500× magnification).

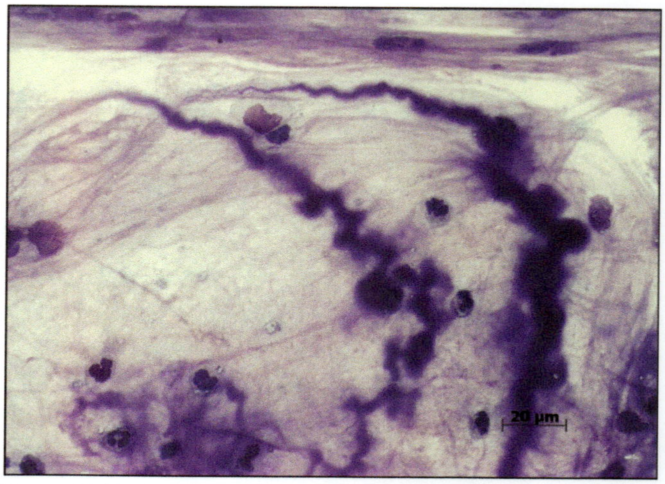

Figure 13.49 Curschmann's spirals. Curschmann's spirals are twisted mucus casts of small bronchioles that have a bottle-brush appearance due to perpendicular radiations. They are seen with disorders that result in chronic, excessive mucus production and are usually an indication of bronchiolar obstruction (Diff-Quik: both, 500× magnification).

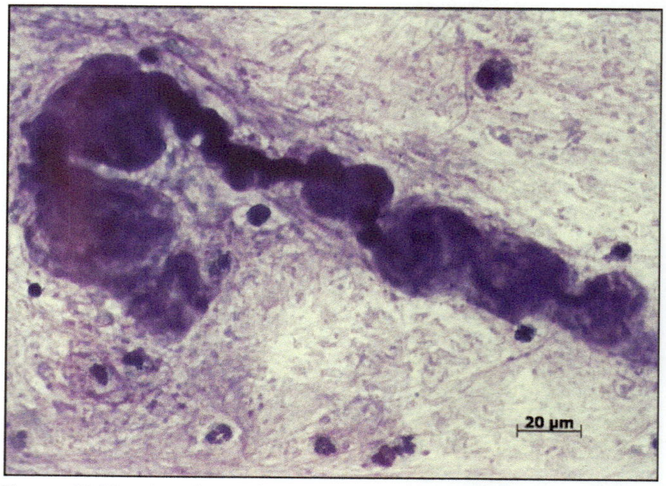

Figure 13.50 Curschmann's spirals. Curschmann's spirals are twisted mucus casts of small bronchioles that have a bottle-brush appearance due to perpendicular radiations. They are seen with disorders that result in chronic, excessive mucus production and are usually an indication of bronchiolar obstruction (Diff-Quik: both, 500× magnification).

higher numbers (up to 28%); however, >10% eosinophils in BAL from companion cats are considered abnormal (Lécuyer *et al.*, 1995; Padrid *et al.*, 1991; Rebar *et al.*, 1980; Alice Defarges Bichot, 2021; Clercx & Peeters, 2007b; Barçante *et al.*, 2008). In dogs, samples with >10% eosinophils are indicative of a significant hypersensitivity disease process (Figure 13.56) (Rajamäki *et al.*, 2001b; Hawkins *et al.*, 2006) and may be associated with increased numbers of neutrophils, macrophages, mast cells, lymphocytes, and plasma cells if tissue irritation is sufficient to induce an inflammatory response. Eosinophils are often trapped in strands of mucus and therefore may predominate in certain areas of the slide. They sometimes also do not stain completely (Figure 13.57). Rounded nuclei may be seen in dogs with allergic pneumopathy (Baldwin & Becker, 1993). Disorders associated with increased eosinophils in samples from TTW/BAL include allergic bronchitis/pneumonitis, feline asthma, lung worms, eosinophilic bronchopneumopathy, and heart worms (Clercx & Peeters, 2007b).

Hemorrhage

Erythrocytes are not commonly present in BAL. Erythrophagocytosis (consistent with acute hemorrhage) (Figure 13.58) and/or

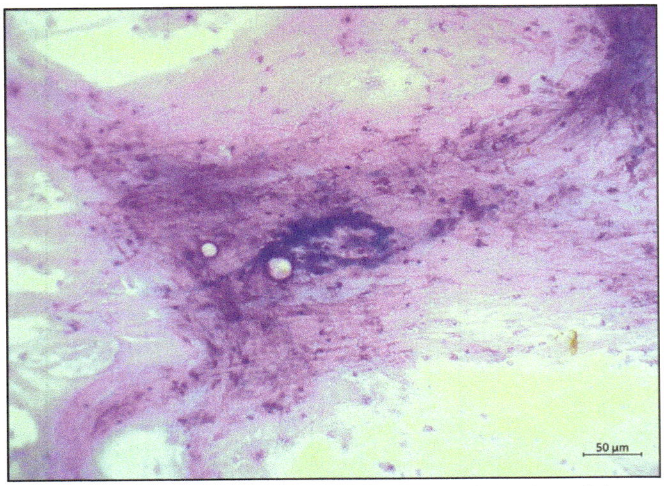

Figure 13.51 Curschmann's spirals. Densely wound, deep basophilic mucus strands in a background of streaming eosinophilic mucus and cells (Wright–Giemsa, 100× magnification).

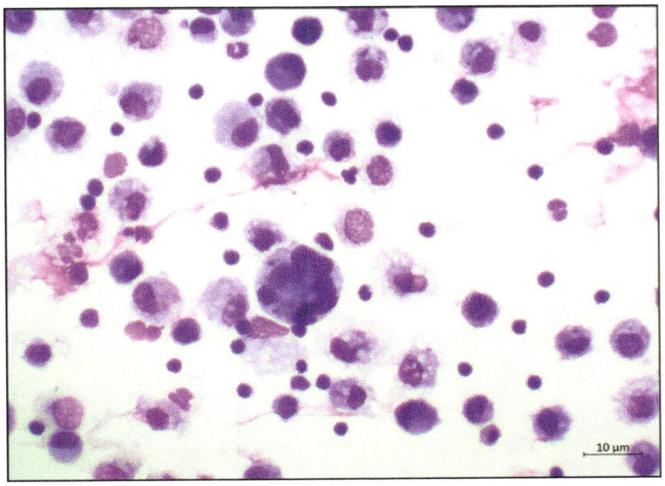

Figures 13.53 Giant cell macrophages. In chronic pulmonary inflammation, activated alveolar macrophages can become multinucleated and are then known as giant cell macrophages (Wright–Giemsa: both, 500× magnification).

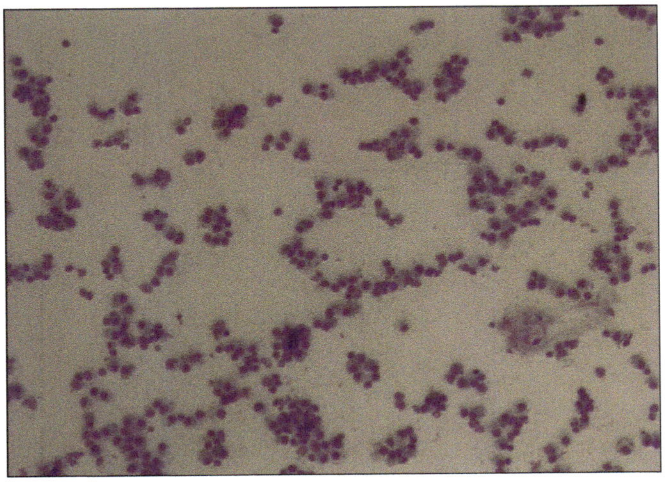

Figure 13.52 Alveolar macrophages. Increased numbers of alveolar macrophages are typically seen with subacute and chronic pulmonary disorders (Diff-Quik, 100× magnification).

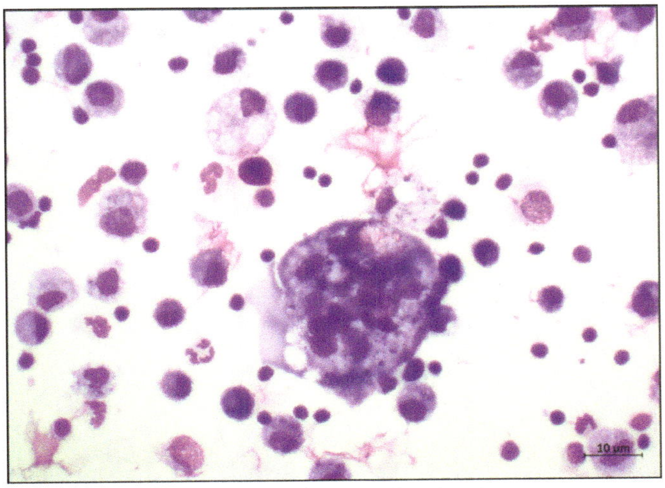

Figure 13.54 Giant cell macrophages. In chronic pulmonary inflammation, activated alveolar macrophages can become multinucleated and are then known as giant cell macrophages (Wright–Giemsa: both, 500× magnification).

macrophages containing pigmented hemoglobin breakdown products (hemosiderophages; associated with chronic hemorrhage) may be seen in conditions that cause pulmonary hemorrhage (Figures 13.59, 13.60). Hemoglobin breakdown products include hemosiderin (granular, bright blue to black pigment; Figures 13.61, 13.62) or hematoidin (small, bright yellow to orange crystals; Figure 13.63). These cytologic findings are essential for differentiating between iatrogenic hemorrhage and hemorrhage caused by pulmonary pathology such as congestive heart failure, feline asthma, neoplasia (primary and metastatic), infectious pneumonia, foreign body migration, heartworm emboli, coagulopathies, trauma, pulmonary embolism, neurological disease, tracheal collapse, and lung lobe torsion (DeHeer & McManus, 2005; McCullough & Brinson, 1999b; Pérez-Arellano *et al.*, 1992). Cats are 13 times more likely to have pulmonary hemosiderosis on BAL cytology compared with dogs (Hooi *et al.*, 2019). Although no risk factors associated with pulmonary hemosiderosis have been identified in cats, increased respiratory rates, prolonged bronchoalveolar lavage times, concurrent transthoracic FNA biopsies, and cytologic diagnoses are associated with an increased risk in dogs (Hooi *et al.*, 2019). Low to moderate numbers of hemosiderophages may be seen in tracheal wash fluid in cats with rhinitis and asthma (DeHeer & McManus, 2005).

Necrosis

Samples containing necrotic material can be seen with inflammatory or neoplastic conditions. Cytologically, necrosis is characterized by

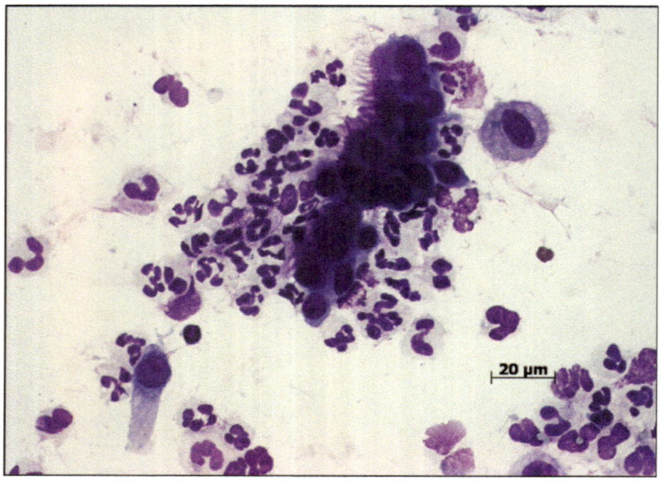

Figure 13.55 Hyperplastic respiratory epithelium. Hyperplastic respiratory epithelium is a change that can be seen with chronic inflammation. Cytologically, hyperplastic epithelium presents as variably sized, deeply basophilic epithelial cells (Diff-Quik, 500× magnification).

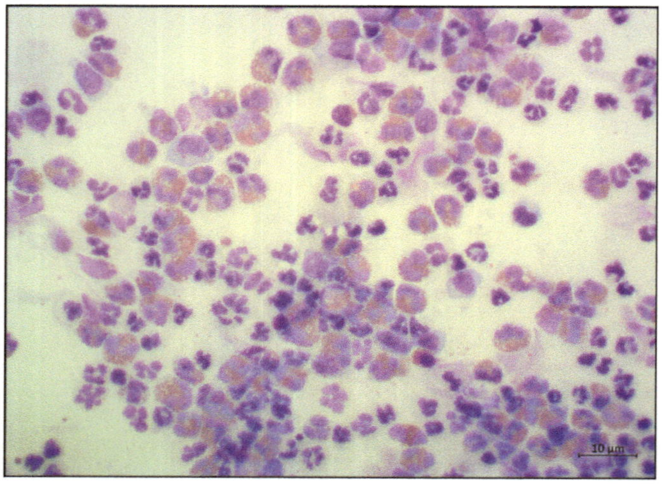

Figure 13.56 Eosinophils. In dogs, samples with >10% eosinophils are indicative of a significant hypersensitivity disease; however, clinically healthy/asymptomatic cats may have significantly higher numbers of eosinophils (up to 28%) (Wright–Giemsa, 500× magnification).

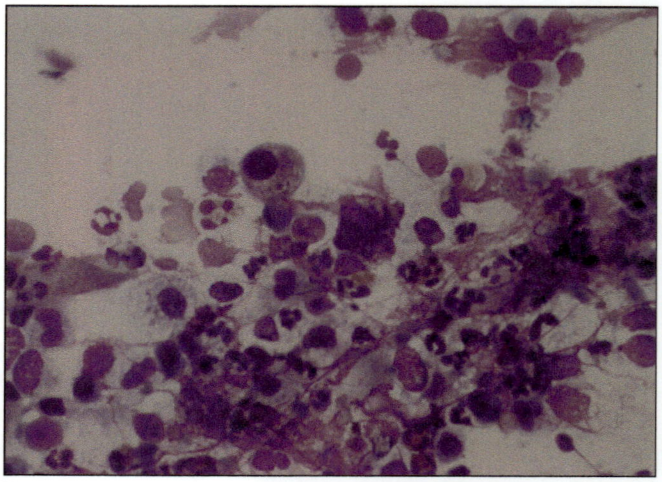

Figure 13.57 Eosinophils. When the sample contains a lot of mucus, eosinophils may become trapped and therefore predominate in certain areas of the slide. Their granules sometimes do not stain properly (Diff-Quik, 500× magnification).

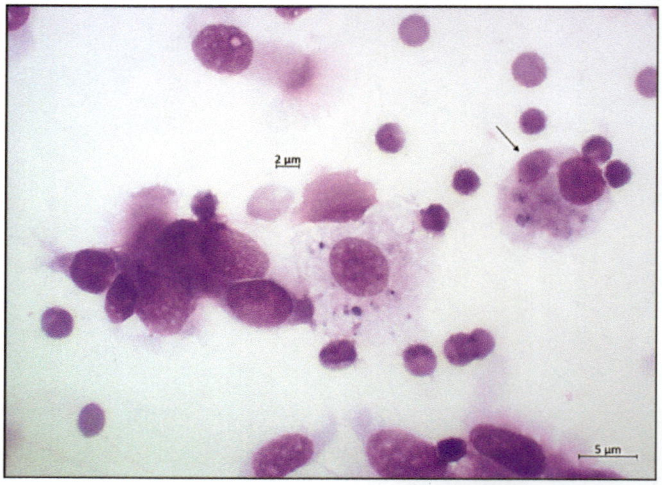

Figure 13.58 Hemorrhage. An alveolar macrophage showing erythrophagocytosis (arrow), indicating acute hemorrhage (Diff-Quik, 1,000× magnification).

the presence of basophilic granular to amorphous background material (Figures 13.64, 13.65). The material is often acellular, but inflammatory or even neoplastic cells may occasionally be imbedded in the material.

Neoplasia

Primary lung tumors or metastatic tumors are generally interstitial, and therefore neoplastic cells are rarely found in TTW/BAL samples unless the tumor has eroded into the airways or if it is a primary tumor involving the bronchial tree. Sometimes, the affected portion of the bronchial tree can be clogged with secretions and necrotic material, preventing cells from being collected via TTW/BAL. A definitive or supportive diagnosis yielded by BAL has been reported in 10 of 14 lung carcinomas (Hawkins *et al.*, 1994). In contrast, a definitive diagnosis of canine primary pulmonary tumors, by tracheal wash, was only possible in 1 of 6 cases (McNiel *et al.*, 1997). A very good agreement has been reported for the diagnosis of pulmonary carcinoma in dog and cat samples when comparing cytopathologic and histopathologic interpretation (Wood *et al.*, 1998a; DeBerry *et al.*, 2002b). Hyperplastic epithelial cells may appear as clusters with cells showing changes such as anisocytosis and, therefore, may be misinterpreted as neoplastic. Carcinomas (epithelial cell tumors) are most commonly seen (up to 80% of primary lung tumors). If clusters of cells are present, the cells should be examined for criteria of malignancy such as anisocytosis, anisokaryosis, multiple nuclei, prominent and multiple

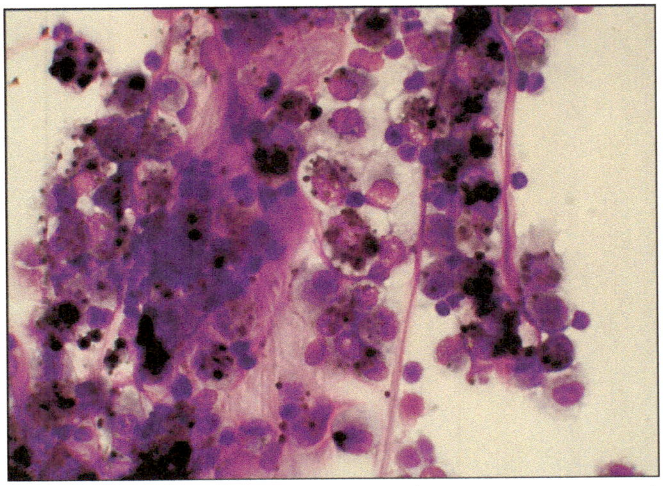

Figure 13.59 Hemorrhage. Alveolar macrophages containing pigmented hemoglobin breakdown (hemosiderophages) products are typically seen with conditions associated with chronic pulmonary hemorrhage (Diff-Quik: both, 500× magnification).

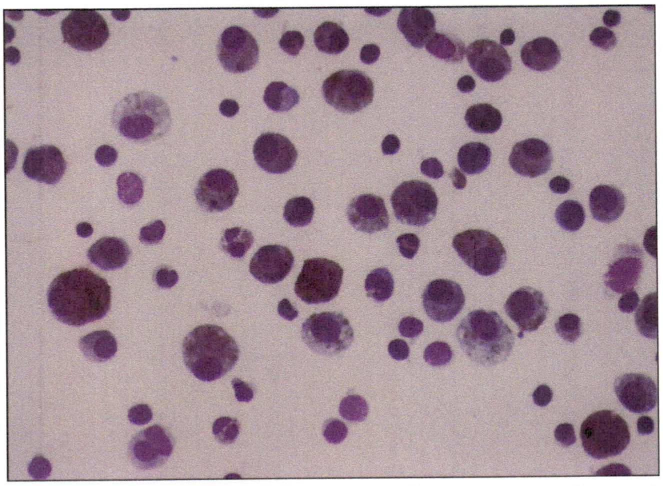

Figure 13.60 Hemorrhage. Alveolar macrophages containing pigmented hemoglobin breakdown (hemosiderophages) products are typically seen with conditions associated with chronic pulmonary hemorrhage (Diff-Quik: both, 500× magnification).

nucleoli, and nuclear molding. If there is cytologic evidence of acini formation or secretory product production (i.e., signet ring cell formation), it is classified as adenocarcinoma (Figure 13.66). In the case of lymphoma, pulmonary involvement may be determined through TTW/BAL samples (Andreasen, 2003; Hahn *et al.*, 1996; Hawkins *et al.*, 1993; McCullough & Brinson, 1999b).

LUNG PARENCHYMA

Collection techniques and sample preparation

Intrathoracic FNA biopsy of the lung parenchyma may result in the cytologic diagnosis of inflammatory conditions, neoplasia, and

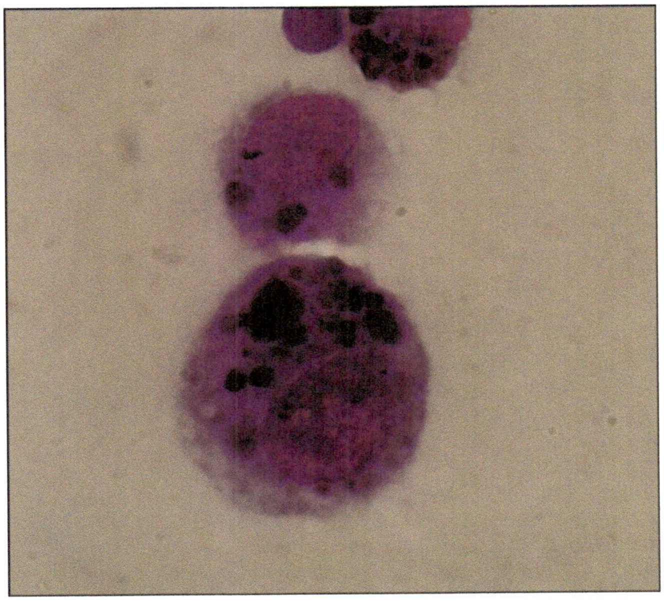

Figures 13.61 Hemorrhage. Hemosiderin, a breakdown product of hemoglobin, is often observed in macrophages of dogs and cats with chronic pulmonary hemorrhage and appears as a granular, bright blue to black pigment (Diff-Quik: both, 1,000× magnification).

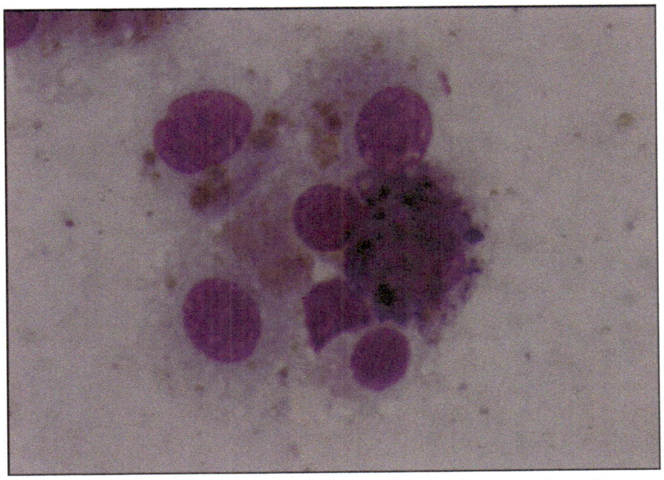

Figure 13.62 Hemorrhage. Hemosiderin, a breakdown product of hemoglobin, is often observed in macrophages of dogs and cats with chronic pulmonary hemorrhage and appears as a granular, bright blue to black pigment (Diff-Quik: both, 1,000× magnification).

infectious agents. Limitations of FNA biopsy cytopathology include poor cellular yield, especially for certain cell types (e.g. mesenchymal cells), necrosis, failure to obtain a representative sample, and its inability to provide information regarding architectural changes (DeBerry *et al.*, 2002a). Although complications may occur, it is generally considered a safe procedure. The procedure is performed using a 22-gauge needle (20–25 gauge) of variable length (depending on the depth and size of the lesion). A 5–12 ml syringe should be attached to the needle, either directly or via an extension tube. The use of an

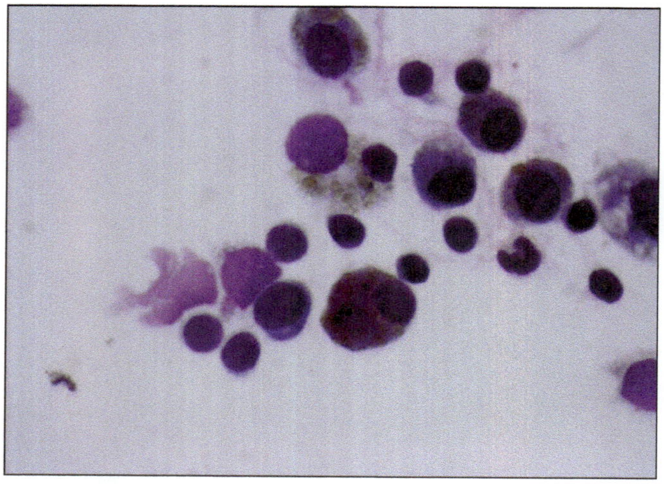

Figure 13.63 Hemorrhage. Hematoidin is also a breakdown product of hemoglobin and appears as small, bright yellow to orange crystals inside the macrophage (Diff-Quik, 1,000× magnification).

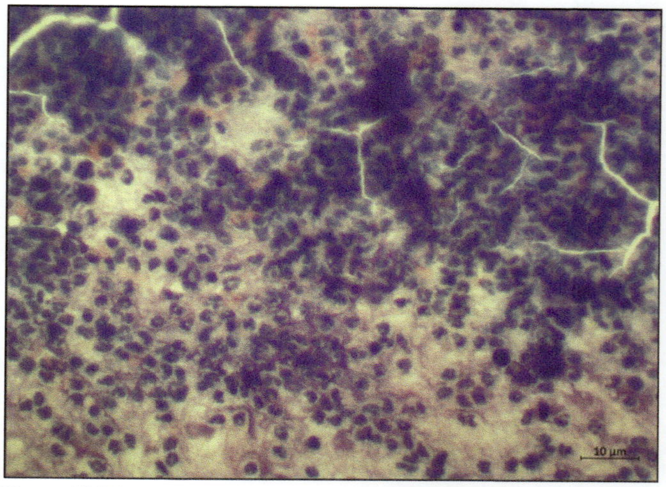

Figure 13.65 Necrosis. Necrosis can be seen with inflammatory or neoplastic conditions. Necrotic material appears cytologically as basophilic granular to amorphous background material (Wright–Giemsa, 500× magnification).

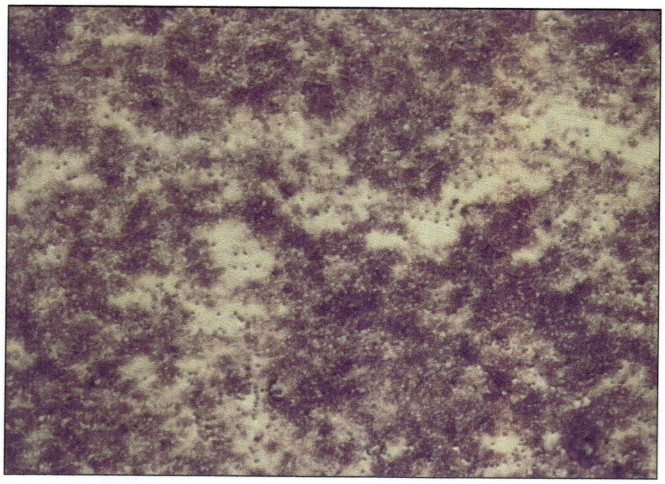

Figure 13.64 Necrosis. Necrosis can be seen with inflammatory or neoplastic conditions. Necrotic material appears cytologically as basophilic granular to amorphous background material (Diff-Quik, 100× magnification).

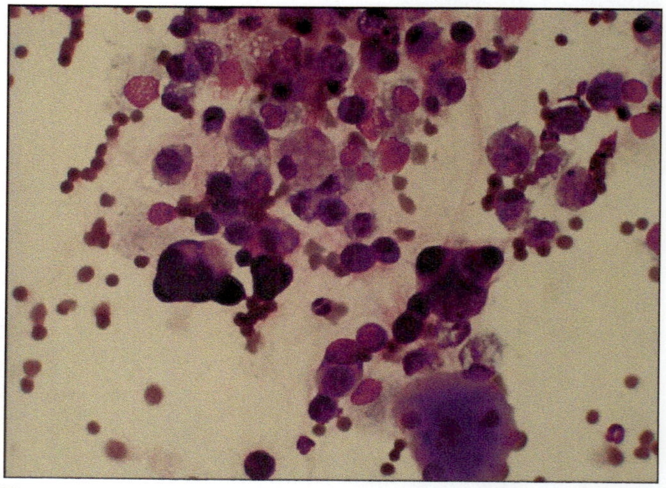

Figure 13.66 Primary lung neoplasia. Primary lung tumors or metastatic tumors are rarely found in bronchoalveolar samples. Carcinomas are most commonly seen and may show malignant criteria such as anisocytosis, anisokaryosis, very basophilic cytoplasm, multiple nuclei, and prominent and multiple nucleoli (Diff-Quik, 500× magnification).

imaging modality such as thoracic radiographs, fluoroscopy, ultrasonography, or CT is strongly advised in order to obtain a representative sample of the lesion. Blind aspiration may, however, be attempted with diffuse, infiltrative pulmonary disease. The right caudal lung lobe is usually sampled with diffuse disease and the standard sampling site is the 7th to 9th intercostal space, one-third of the distance from the spinal column to the costochondral junction. If the chest is entered too far caudally, the liver can be accidentally aspirated. Hemostatic screening should preferably be performed before the procedure and should include a platelet count and other routine hemostatic assays. The procedure can either be performed with sedation only or under general anesthesia, depending on the clinical status of the patient. The hair over the sampling site should be clipped and the area prepared aseptically. Samples can be obtained using aspiration or nonaspiration techniques. Once the sample is in the bore of the needle it should be transferred efficiently to the surface of a clean slide. To create a monolayer of cells the 'squash' preparation technique can be used (described above under 'Nasal Cavity'). If the material is very bloody, a normal blood smear preparation technique should be used. Possible complications for the procedure include pneumothorax and hemorrhage, both mild and self-limiting, and needle tract implantation, which is rare (Rakich & Latimer, 1989b; Teske *et al.*, 1991; Wood *et al.*, 1998b; Warren-Smith *et al.*, 2011). Contraindications for the procedure include bleeding disorders, bullous emphysema, uncooperative

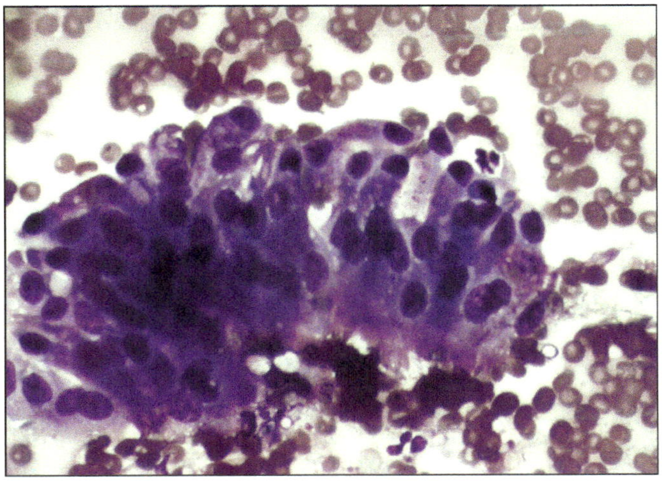

Figure 13.67 Respiratory epithelial cells. Respiratory epithelial cells may be seen with aspiration cytology of the lung. The epithelial cells can be cuboidal to columnar, are often ciliated, with a round, eccentric nucleus and lightly basophilic cytoplasm (Diff-Quik, 500× magnification).

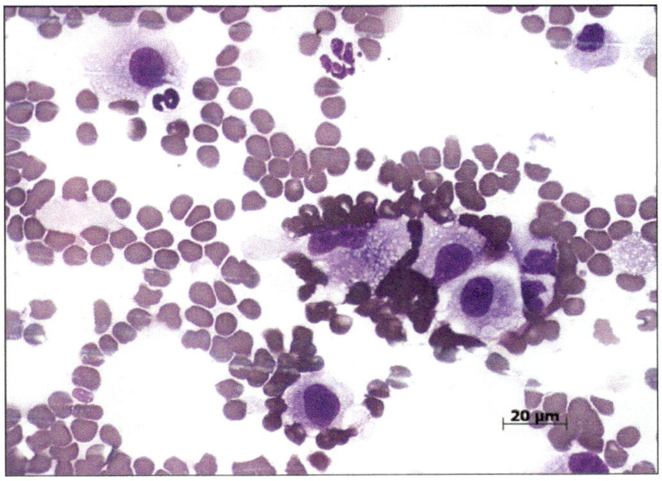

Figure 13.68 Alveolar macrophages. Low numbers of alveolar macrophages can be seen in samples obtained through aspiration of a lung lesion (Diff-Quik, 500× magnification).

patient, severe uncontrolled coughing, and pulmonary hypertension (Rakich & Latimer, 1989b; Wood *et al.*, 1998b). Agreement of 82–89% between percutaneous FNA biopsy cytopathology and histopathology has been reported for dogs and cats (DeBerry *et al.*, 2002a; Bonfanti *et al.*, 2004).

Normal cytologic features

Samples from normal lung parenchyma usually have a marked blood admixture and may contain a small amount of mucus. Typically, the nucleated cell count is low and consists mainly of respiratory epithelial cells. The epithelial cells are cuboidal to columnar, often ciliated, with a round, eccentric nucleus and lightly basophilic cytoplasm (Figure 13.67). Low numbers of alveolar macrophages are also commonly seen (Figure 13.68). Due to the blood admixture leukocytes will be present; however, their number should not exceed that which is expected in the blood. Other contaminants include ultrasound gel, corn starch (glove powder), and squamous cells from the skin. Samples may also contain mesothelial cells (Figure 13.69) and elements from an effusion (if present) due to the transthoracic technique used. If the sample is taken too far caudally, well-differentiated hepatocytes and skeletal muscle may be observed due to inadvertent aspiration of the liver or diaphragm (McCullough & Brinson, 1999a; Grimes *et al.*, 2014).

CYTOLOGIC INTERPRETATION

Inflammation

Inflammation of the lung parenchyma appears very similar to that seen in other tissue, with neutrophils being the predominant cell type. Typical causes include bacterial infection, neoplasia, necrosis, presence of foreign material, and other noninfectious causes. Necrotic

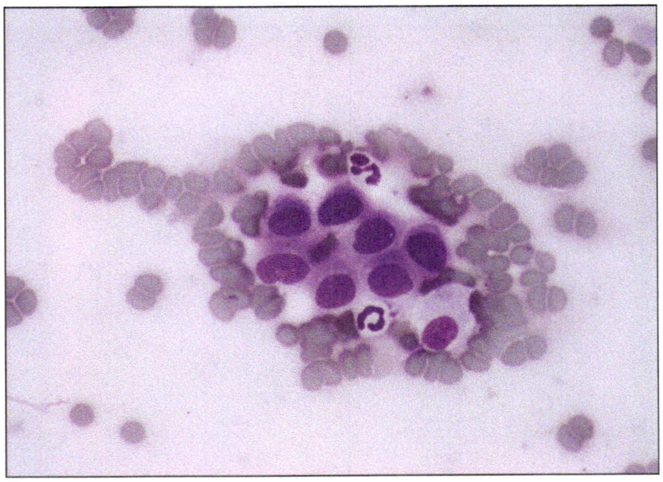

Figure 13.69 Contaminants in FNAs of lung tissue. A plaque of normal mesothelial cells can be seen due to contamination from the pleural lining during sample collection (Diff-Quik, 500× magnification).

debris is often aspirated and appears as amorphous, bluish-gray to pink material that may be scattered throughout the smear or concentrated in certain dense aggregates (Figures 13.70, 13.71). Foreign material may sometimes be observed surrounded by aggregates of inflammatory cells. Increased numbers of alveolar macrophages (Figure 13.72) may be seen with both acute and chronic inflammatory disorders such as necrosis, atelectasis, lung lobe torsion, hemorrhage, neoplasia, and pneumonia due to foreign material. An increased number of epithelioid macrophages, together with multinucleated giant cell macrophages, is termed granulomatous inflammation. Epithelioid macrophages are plump, round with well-defined cytoplasmic borders and blue-gray to pale pink cytoplasm. Granulomatous inflammation is most commonly associated with certain infectious agents, including fungi, protozoa, mycobacteria, other bacteria such as *Nocardia* spp., or foreign bodies (Grimes *et al.*, 2014).

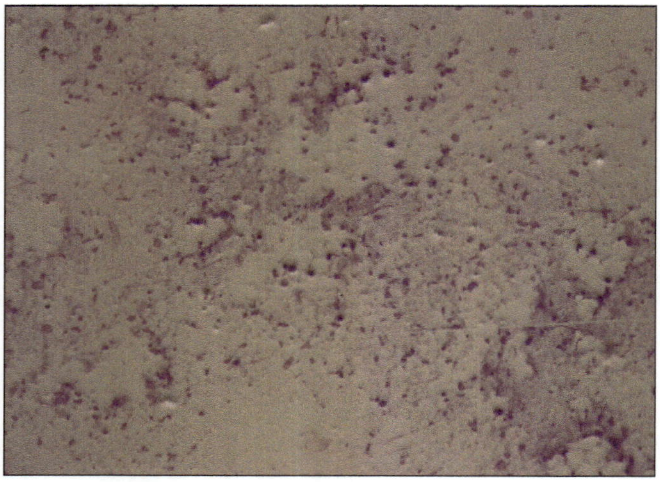

Figure 13.70 Necrosis. A sample taken from the necrotic center of a lung lesion can appear as amorphous, bluish-gray to pink material that may be scattered throughout the smear or concentrated in certain dense aggregates (Diff-Quik: 100× magnification).

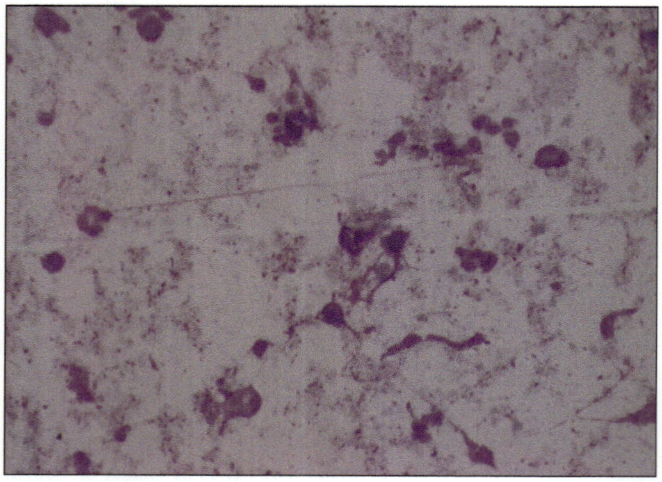

Figure 13.71 Necrosis. A sample taken from the necrotic center of a lung lesion can appear as amorphous, bluish-gray to pink material that may be scattered throughout the smear or concentrated in certain dense aggregates (Diff-Quik: 500× magnification).

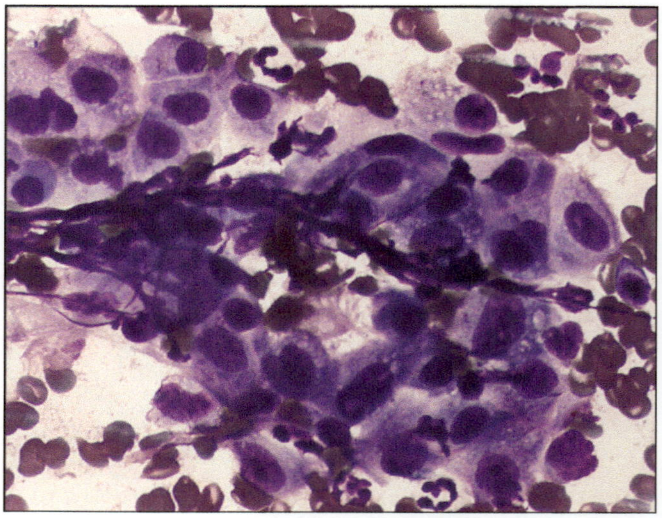

Figure 13.72 Alveolar macrophages. An increased number of alveolar macrophages may be seen with both acute and chronic inflammatory disorders. Similar to macrophages seen in bronchoalveolar washes, they have abundant blue–gray cytoplasm and an eccentrically positioned, round to bean-shaped nucleus (Diff-Quik, 500× magnification).

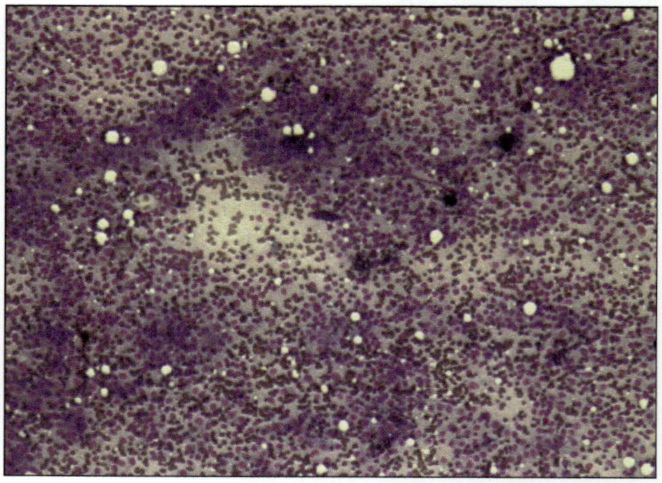

Figure 13.73 Neoplasia. The most common primary tumors of the lung in dogs and cats are epithelial tumors, such as adenocarcinoma, showing typical cell-to-cell adhesion (Diff-Quik, 100× magnification).

Hypersensitivity

A hypersensitivity response or eosinophilic inflammation is present when eosinophils are >10% of the nucleated cell count, especially in the absence of a peripheral eosinophilia. Variable numbers of other leukocytes such as macrophages, neutrophils, and mast cells may also be seen. Causes include allergic or hypersensitivity disorders, eosinophilic bronchopneumopathy, parasite infestation, and some fungal, bacterial, and neoplastic diseases (Clercx *et al.*, 2000; Clercx & Peeters, 2007a; Grimes *et al.*, 2014).

Neoplasia

One of the more important reasons for performing a lung FNA biopsy is to diagnose primary and metastatic pulmonary neoplasia, since neoplastic cells are rarely seen in samples from TTW/BAL unless the tumor has eroded through the bronchial tree. Ultrasound-guided FNA biopsy of focal parenchymal lesions of the lung has been shown to be a very effective tool, with a sensitivity of up to 88% and minimal false-positive diagnoses of neoplasia (McMillan *et al.*, 1988; Wood *et al.*, 1998b). The most common primary tumors of the lung in dogs and cats are epithelial tumors (Ogilvie *et al.*, 1989). Adenocarcinomas of bronchogenic or bronchiolar–alveolar origin are the most common neoplasms of the lung; however, cytologic differentiation is usually not possible (Figures 13.73, 13.74). In addition, differentiating a primary from a metastatic epithelial tumor in the lung is also difficult. Common tumors to metastasize to the lungs include oral and nail bed melanoma, thyroid

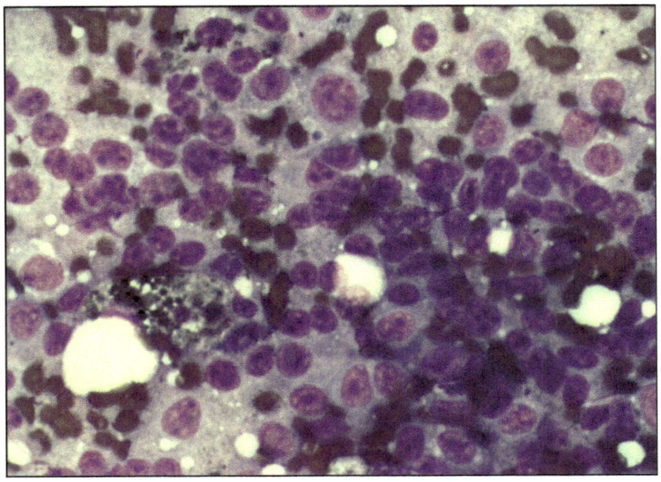

Figure 13.74 Neoplasia. The most common primary tumors of the lung in dogs and cats are epithelial tumors, such as adenocarcinoma, showing typical cell-to-cell adhesion (Diff-Quik, 500× magnification).

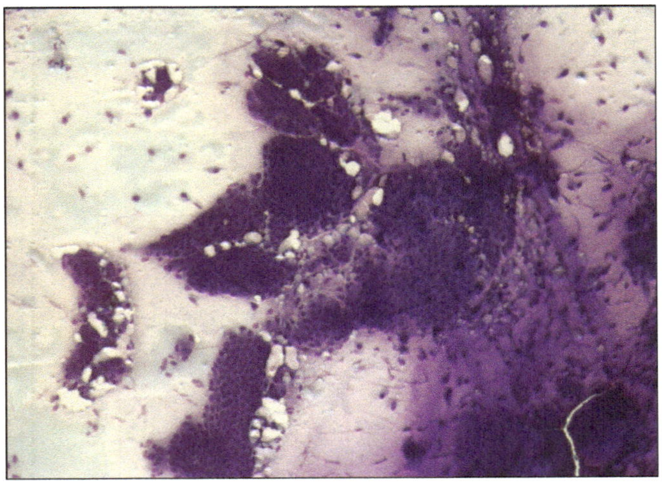

Figure 13.75 Neoplasia. Aspirates of lung carcinomas typically yield highly cellular smears that consist of epithelial cells arranged as cohesive clusters (Diff-Quik, 100× magnification) or three-dimensional balls, with lesser numbers of individualized cells.

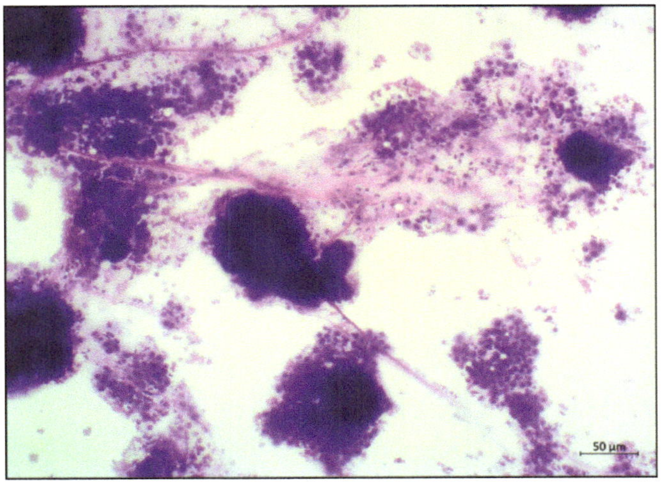

Figure 13.76 Neoplasia. Aspirates of lung carcinomas typically yield highly cellular smears that consist of epithelial cells arranged as cohesive clusters (Wright–Giemsa, 100× magnification) or three-dimensional balls, with lesser numbers of individualized cells.

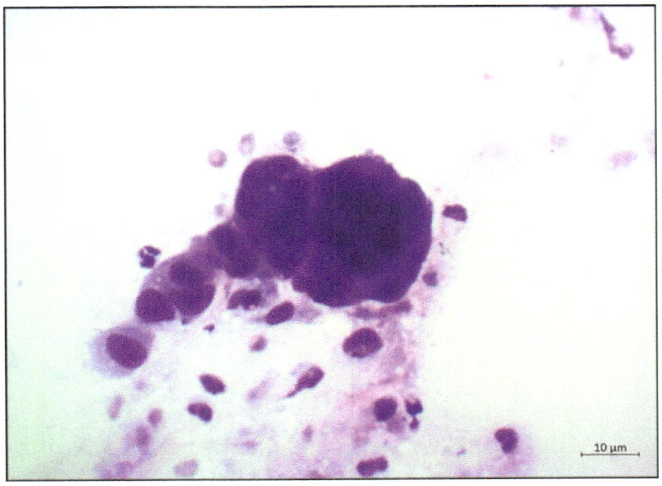

Figure 13.77 Neoplasia. Aspirates of lung carcinomas typically yield highly cellular smears that consist of epithelial cells arranged as cohesive clusters or three-dimensional balls (Wright–Giemsa, 500× magnification), with lesser numbers of individualized cells.

carcinoma, osteosarcoma, mammary carcinoma, and high-grade soft tissue sarcoma (Ogilvie *et al.*, 1989). Aspirates of lung carcinomas typically yield highly cellular smears that consist of epithelial cells arranged as cohesive clusters (Figure 13.75, 13.76) or 3-dimensional balls (Figures 13.77, 13.78), with lesser numbers of individualized cells. Care should be taken not to confuse these individualized cells with discrete cell tumors. Acinar formation indicates glandular origin, suggesting an adenocarcinoma (Figure 13.79). Moderate to marked pleomorphism between cells within the same cluster (Figures 13.80, 13.81), as well as between clumps of cells, is common in pulmonary carcinoma. The neoplastic epithelial cells appear as round to polygonal, basophilic cells displaying various cellular criteria of malignancy including eccentrically placed nuclei with coarsely clumped chromatin and prominent, single to multiple nucleoli; anisokaryosis; and deeply basophilic cytoplasm (Figures 13.82–13.84). Cytoplasmic vacuolation, particularly around the perinuclear region, is frequently prominent (Figure 13.85). Other criteria of malignancy may be seen and include nuclear molding, signet ring cell formation (Figures 13.86, 13.87), nuclear gigantism, and bi- or multinucleated cells (Figure 13.88, 13.89). Necrotic material, with or without inflammation, is also commonly associated with neoplasia. Dysplastic or metaplastic changes to the pulmonary epithelial cells secondary to inflammation can complicate the diagnosis, and histopathologic examination is required to differentiate. Hemolymphatic neoplasia, such as lymphoma and malignant histiocytosis, has been reported to disseminate throughout the lung parenchyma, resulting in diffuse infiltrative disease (Geyer *et al.*, 2010). Canine histiocytic malignancies are aggressive tumors that

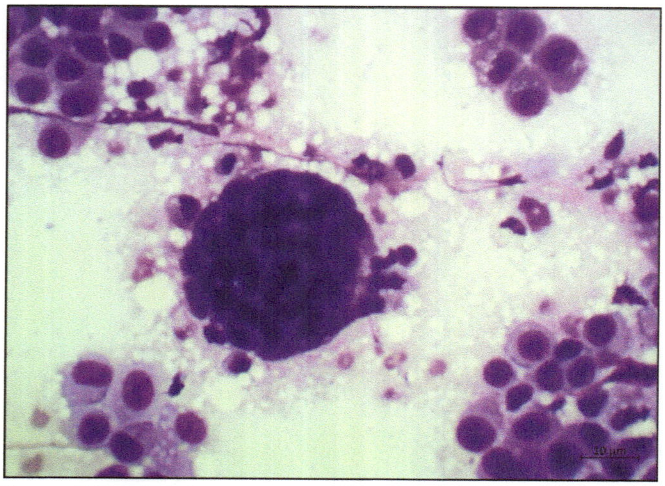

Figure 13.78 Neoplasia. Aspirates of lung carcinomas typically yield highly cellular smears that consist of epithelial cells arranged as cohesive clusters or three-dimensional balls (Wright–Giemsa, 500× magnification), with lesser numbers of individualized cells.

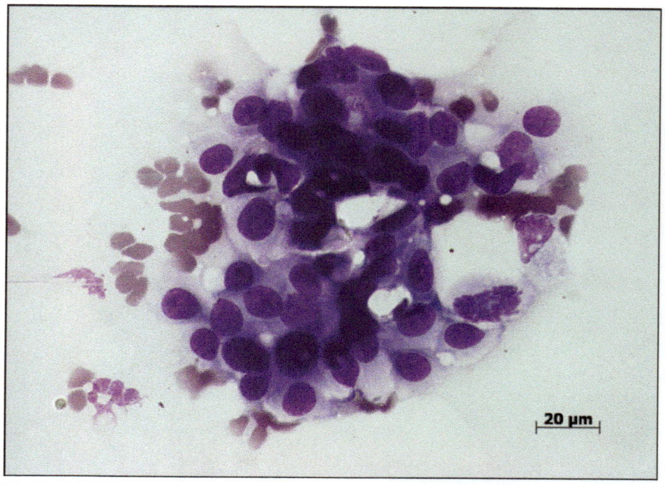

Figure 13.80 Neoplasia. Moderate to marked pleomorphism between cells can be seen within the same cluster of neoplastic epithelial cells sampled from a nodule in the lung (Diff-Quik, 500× magnification for both).

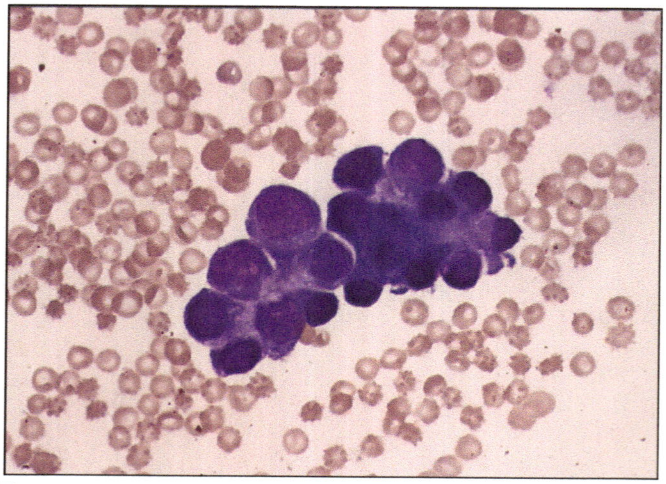

Figure 13.79 Neoplasia. Acinar formation, a cluster of cells that resembles a many-lobed berry, is an indication that the tumor is of glandular origin, suggesting an adenocarcinoma (Diff-Quik, 500× magnification).

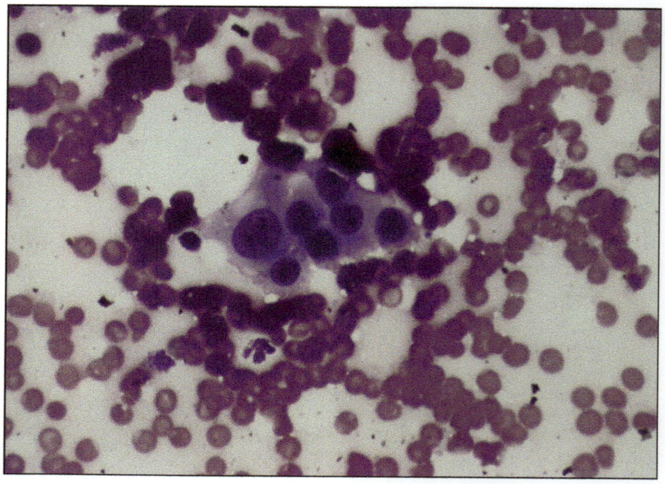

Figure 13.81 Neoplasia. Moderate to marked pleomorphism between cells can be seen within the same cluster of neoplastic epithelial cells sampled from a nodule in the lung (Diff-Quik, 500× magnification for both).

occur with high frequency in Bernese Mountain dogs and flat-coated Retrievers and have been described in the lung parenchyma. Cytologic findings included numerous pleomorphic, large, discrete mononuclear cells with abundant, lightly basophilic, vacuolated, cytoplasm. Nuclei are round to oval to reniform with marked anisokaryosis, and nucleoli are prominent. Multinucleated giant cells are frequently observed (Figures 13.90–13.92) (Brown *et al.*, 1994). A diagnosis of presumptive primary pulmonary mast cell tumor has been described in two dogs, neither of which had a previous history of cutaneous mast cell tumor. Both dogs were presented with a massive solitary pulmonary mast cell tumor (Campbell *et al.*, 2017).

During fluid accumulation in the pleural cavity, the pleural mesothelial cells undergo hypertrophy and hyperplasia, and individual cells exfoliate into the fluid. Cytologic differentiation between these reactive or dysplastic mesothelial cells and carcinoma cells can therefore be difficult. Reactive mesothelial cells can have morphologic features resembling malignancy, especially when they are arranged in large clusters. If present, acinar formation may support a diagnosis of carcinoma or malignant mesothelioma (Hirschberger *et al.*, 1999).

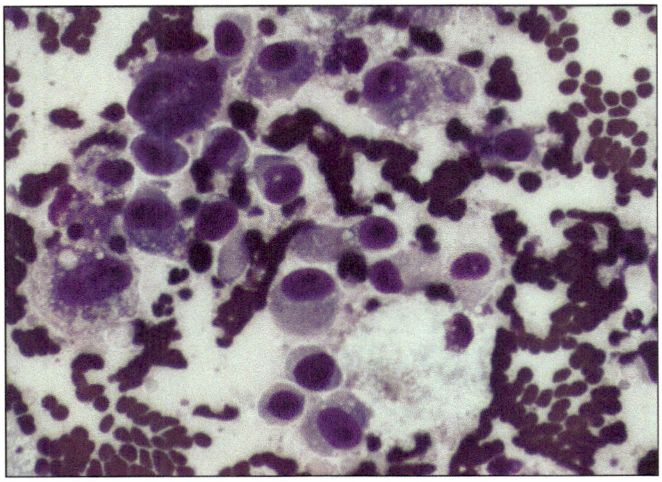

Figure 13.82 Neoplasia. Neoplastic pulmonary epithelial cells appear as round, basophilic cells displaying various malignant criteria such as eccentrically placed nuclei with coarsely clumped chromatin and prominent, single to multiple nucleoli, some with angular shapes; anisokaryosis; multinucleation, some with odd numbers of nuclei per cell, and deeply basophilic cytoplasm (Diff-Quik, 500× magnification).

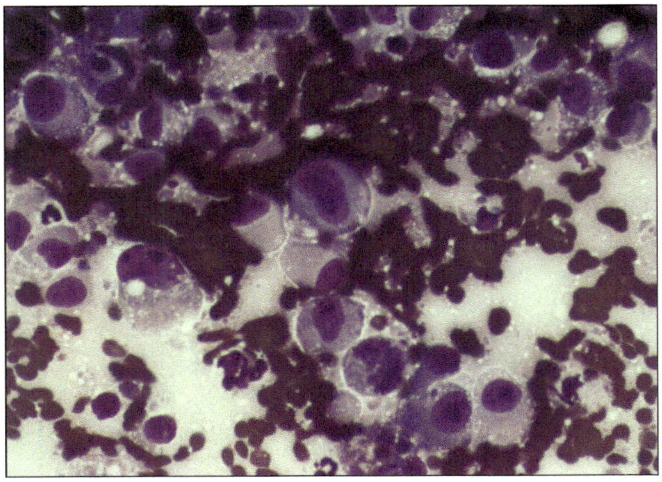

Figure 13.83 Neoplasia. Neoplastic pulmonary epithelial cells appear as round, basophilic cells displaying various malignant criteria such as eccentrically placed nuclei with coarsely clumped chromatin and prominent, single to multiple nucleoli, some with angular shapes; anisokaryosis; multinucleation, some with odd numbers of nuclei per cell, and deeply basophilic cytoplasm (Diff-Quik, 500× magnification).

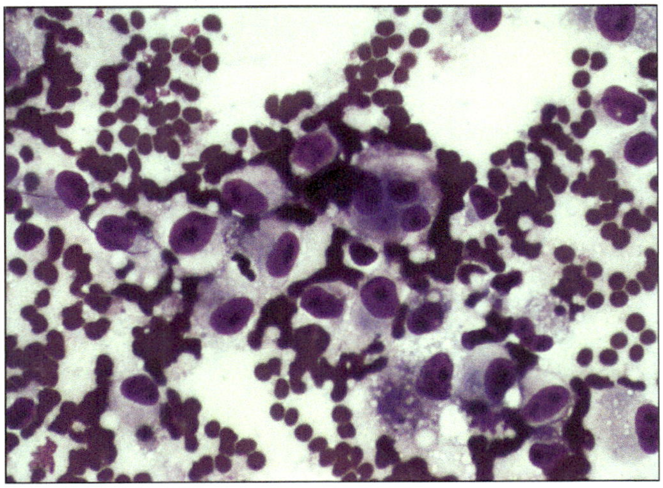

Figure 13.84 Neoplasia. Neoplastic pulmonary epithelial cells appear as round, basophilic cells displaying various malignant criteria such as eccentrically placed nuclei with coarsely clumped chromatin and prominent, single to multiple nucleoli, some with angular shapes; anisokaryosis; multinucleation, some with odd numbers of nuclei per cell, and deeply basophilic cytoplasm (Diff-Quik, 500× magnification).

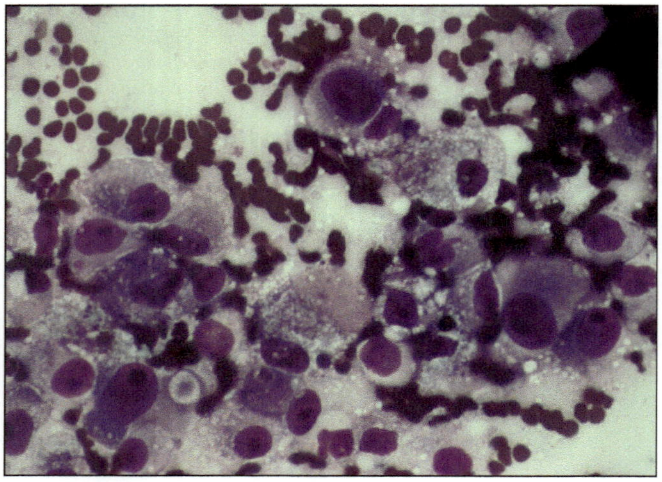

Figure 13.85 Neoplasia. Epithelial cells with cytoplasmic vacuolation, particularly around the perinuclear region, are frequently prominent in pulmonary neoplasia (Diff-Quik, 500× magnification).

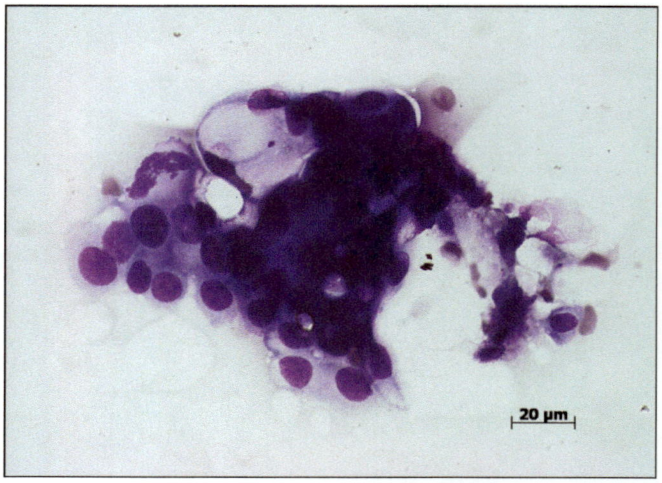

Figure 13.87 Neoplasia. Neoplastic pulmonary epithelial cells displaying malignant criteria such as nuclear molding, signet ring cell formation, nuclear gigantism, and multinucleation (Diff-Quik, 500× magnification).

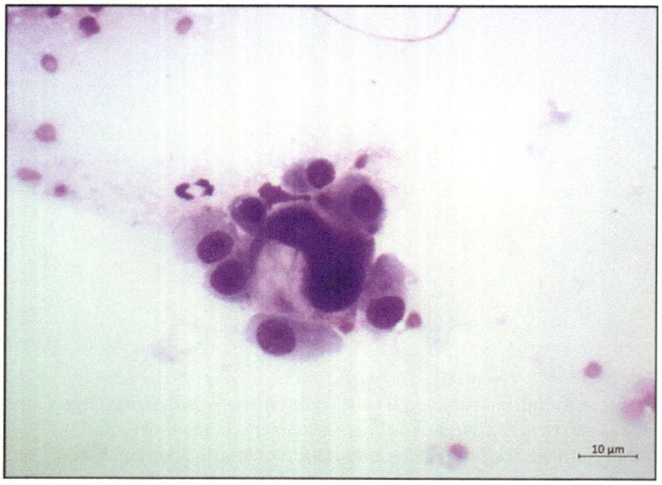

Figure 13.86 Neoplasia. Neoplastic pulmonary epithelial cells displaying malignant criteria such as nuclear molding, signet ring cell formation, nuclear gigantism, and multinucleation (Wright–Giemsa, 500× magnification).

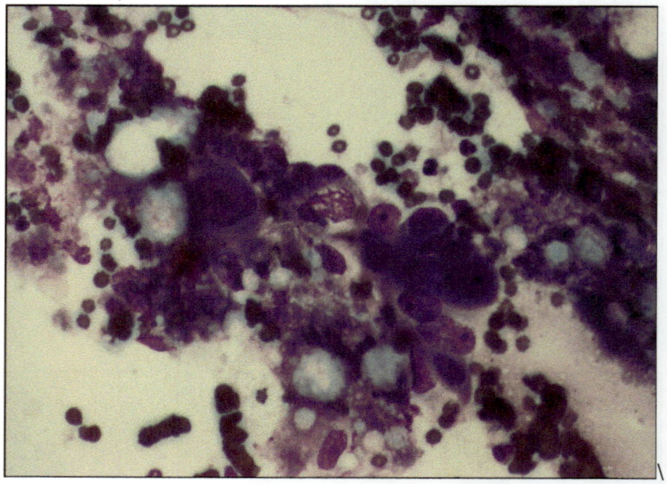

Figure 13.88 Neoplasia. Neoplastic pulmonary epithelial cells displaying malignant criteria such as nuclear molding, signet ring cell formation, nuclear gigantism, and multinucleation (Diff-Quik, 500× magnification).

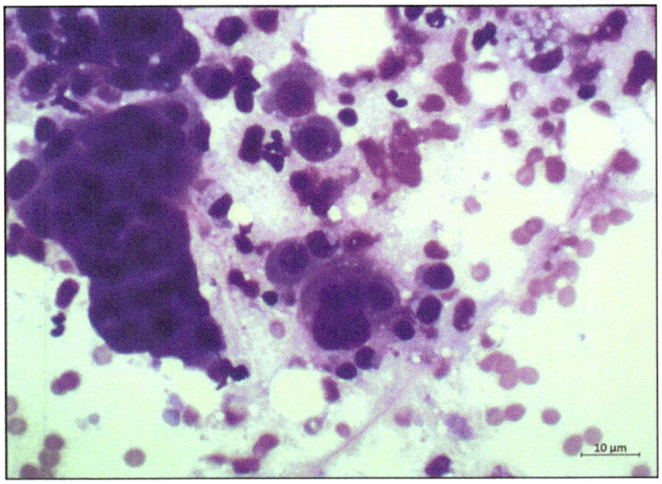

Figure 13.89 Neoplasia. Neoplastic pulmonary epithelial cells displaying malignant criteria such as nuclear molding, signet ring cell formation, nuclear gigantism, and multinucleation (Wright–Giemsa, 500× magnification).

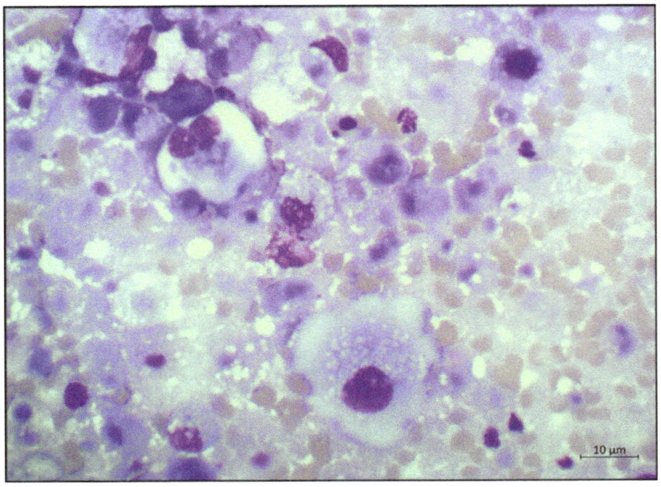

Figure 13.90 Neoplasia. Malignant histiocytic cells displaying marked pleomorphism, with abundant, lightly basophilic, vacuolated, cytoplasm. Nuclei are round to oval to reniform with marked anisokaryosis, and nucleoli are prominent. Multinucleated giant cells are frequently observed (Wright–Giemsa, 500× magnification).

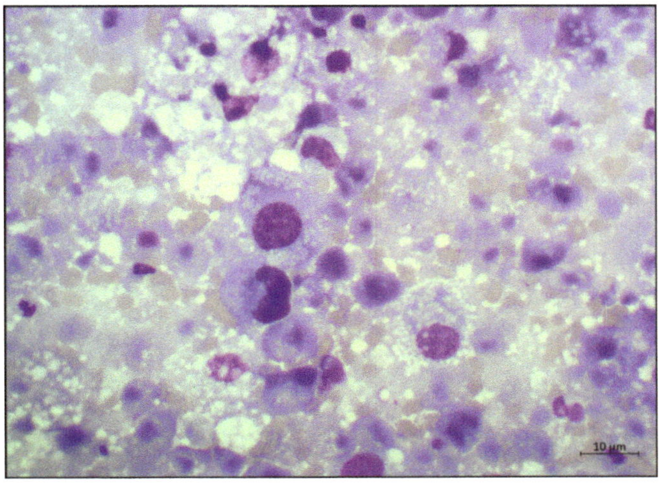

Figure 13.91 Neoplasia. Malignant histiocytic cells displaying marked pleomorphism, with abundant, lightly basophilic, vacuolated, cytoplasm. Nuclei are round to oval to reniform with marked anisokaryosis, and nucleoli are prominent. Multinucleated giant cells are frequently observed (Wright–Giemsa, 500× magnification).

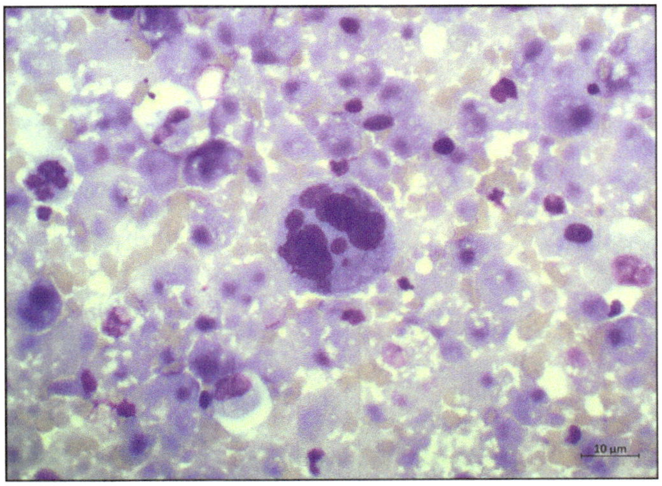

Figure 13.92 Neoplasia. Malignant histiocytic cells displaying marked pleomorphism, with abundant, lightly basophilic, vacuolated, cytoplasm. Nuclei are round to oval to reniform with marked anisokaryosis, and nucleoli are prominent. Multinucleated giant cells are frequently observed (Wright–Giemsa, 500× magnification).

CASES

CASE 1

Signalment/history

A 4-year-old, tortoiseshell domestic shorthair cat. Fully vaccinated; chronic sinusitis unresponsive to antimicrobial therapy; decreased appetite.

Physical examination

Swollen left maxillary sinus; unilateral, mucohemorrhagic discharge from the left nasal passage; inspiratory stridor; FeLV/FIV negative; urinalysis showed concentrated urine.

Computed tomography with contrast of the nasal passages

A CT scan showed a 24 × 22 mm heterogeneously contrast enhancing mass, extending from the left nares caudally to the cribriform plate, eroding the ipsilateral orbital lamina, and invading the orbit ventrally and axially. There was diffuse homogeneous soft tissue opacification of the ipsilateral frontal and sphenoid sinuses as well as the entire nasopharynx (Figure 13.93). The opacification seen within the sinuses did not appear to be a direct extension from the mass itself.

Interpretation: suspected nasal adenocarcinoma with secondary obstructive sinusitis.

Cytology of the nasal mass

A sample of the nasal mass was obtained under general anesthesia through FNA biopsy. The smears were of good diagnostic quality with a high cellularity. There was a moderate blood admixture and many areas with a blue stippled background, consistent with necrosis. High numbers of epithelial cells arranged in papillary or occasionally acinar formations were seen. These cells had a medium to dark blue cytoplasm, often with poorly defined borders (Figure 13.94). Nuclei were round to oval to slightly angular, with a coarse to clumped chromatin pattern and one to multiple prominent and often angular and giant nucleoli. A pronounced anisocytosis, variation in the N:C ratio, anisokaryosis, macronucleosis, nuclear molding, and occasional binucleation were present (Figure 13.95). Very high numbers of degenerate neutrophils and lesser numbers of activated macrophages, small and medium-sized lymphocytes, eosinophils, and plasma cells were seen. High numbers of bacteria were present in the background and phagocytized in the neutrophils.

Interpretation: adenocarcinoma with secondary septic neutrophilic inflammation.

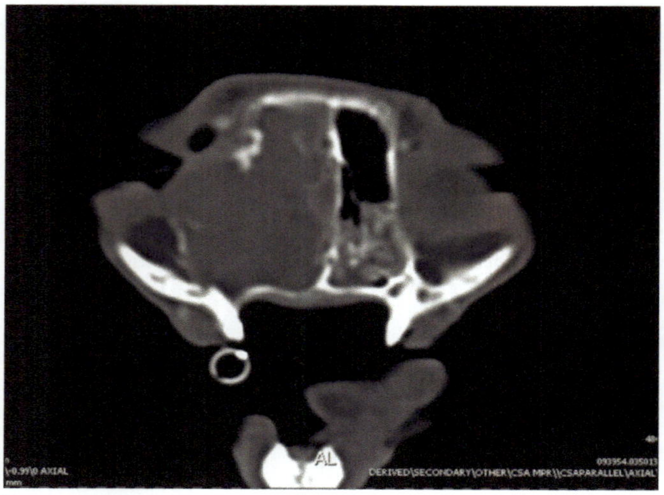

Figure 13.93 Nasal tumor. CT scan showing a mass in the left caudal nasal cavity, eroding the ipsilateral orbital lamina, and invading the orbit ventrally and axially. There was diffuse homogeneous soft tissue opacification of the entire nasopharynx.

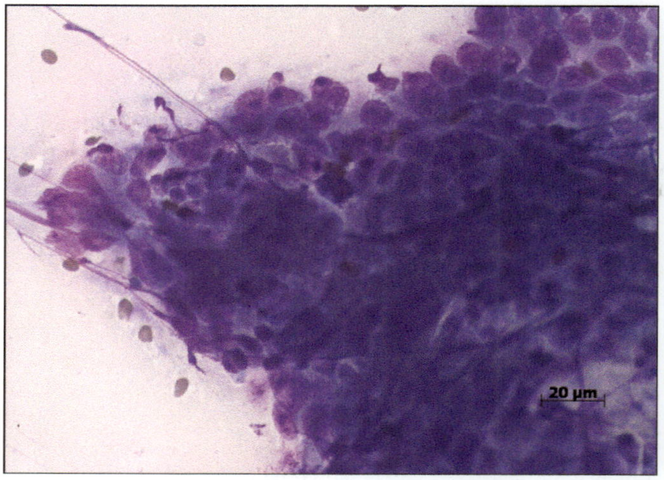

Figure 13.94 Nasal tumor. High numbers of epithelial cells arranged in sheets were seen. The cells had a medium to dark blue cytoplasm, often with poorly defined borders (Diff-Quik, 500× magnification).

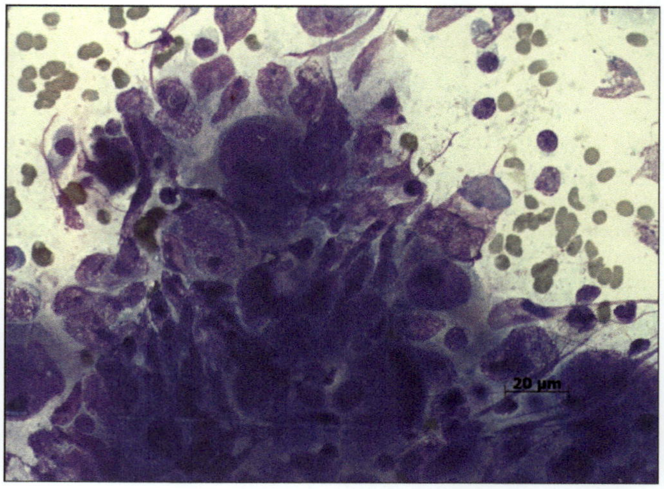

Figure 13.95 Nasal tumor. The nuclei of the neoplastic epithelial cells were round to oval to slightly angular, with a coarse to clumped chromatin pattern and one to multiple prominent and often angular and giant nucleoli. Marked anisocytosis, anisokaryosis, macronucleosis, nuclear molding, and occasional binucleation were present (Diff-Quik, 500× magnification).

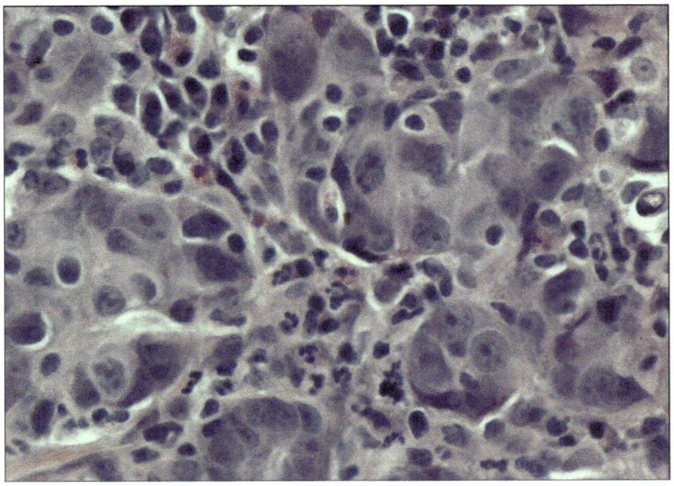
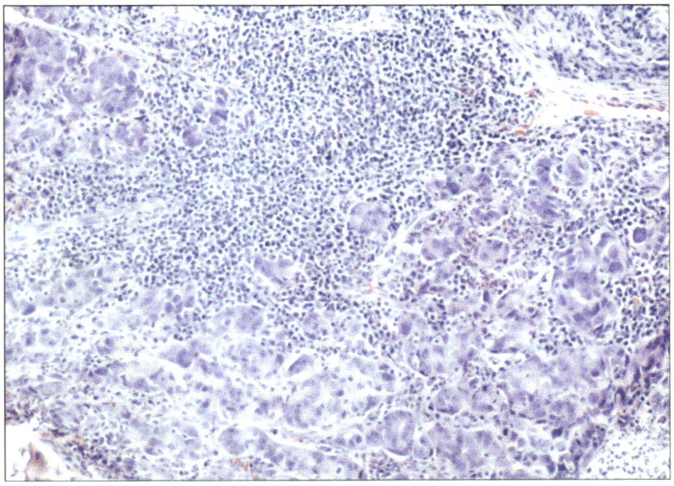

Figures 13.96, 13.97 Nasal tumor. Histopathology of the mass revealed an intact nasal mucosal epithelium. The lamina propria contained extensive areas of tubule-like structures consisting of neoplastic epithelial cells. The cytoplasmic margins of the neoplastic cells were difficult to distinguish, and the cells had a small to moderate amount of homogeneous, eosinophilic cytoplasm. The polygonal, pleomorphic neoplastic cells typically had round to oval nuclei, with prominent and multiple nucleoli, a few of which were macronucleoli and irregularly shaped. The areas surrounding the neoplastic cells consisted of many lymphocytes and plasma cells with fewer macrophages, eosinophils, and neutrophils, with multifocal areas of hemorrhage and necrosis (H&E: 13.81, 500× magnification; 13.82, 50× magnification).

Histopathology of the nasal mass

The sections examined revealed an intact nasal mucosal epithelium. The lamina propria contained extensive areas of tubule-like structures consisting of neoplastic epithelial cells. The neoplastic cells displayed inconspicuous cytoplasmic margins with a small to moderate amount of homogeneous, eosinophilic cytoplasm. The polygonal, pleomorphic neoplastic cells typically had round to oval nuclei, but there were occasional multinucleated, syncytial-like neoplastic cells. Nucleoli were frequently prominent and multiple, a few of which were macronucleoli and irregularly shaped (Figure 13.96). The surrounding areas consisted of many lymphocytes and plasma cells with fewer macrophages, eosinophils, and neutrophils, with multifocal areas of hemorrhage and necrosis (Figure 13.97). The mitotic rate averaged 2–3 mitotic figures per high-power field. Interpretation: high-grade adenocarcinoma.

Follow up/outcome

The owners opted to perform radiation therapy; however, the patient developed severe complications due to the radiation therapy, and a decision was made to euthanize the cat.

Disease pathogenesis

Nasal adenocarcinoma is a malignant neoplasia of glandular cells of the nasal epithelium of dogs and cats. Adenocarcinomas are locally invasive neoplasms and rarely metastasize; occasionally, pulmonary metastasis can be found. Treatment of cats with adenocarcinoma consists of radiation therapy, which provides the most effective treatment at this time. Radiation therapy of the nasal structures can be complicated by cataracts of the eyes forming, blindness due to the radiation, and local skin reactions of the face, which include ulceration and inflammation.

CASE 2

Signalment/history

A 2-year-old, spayed female Dachshund. Chronic intermittent moist cough; referred for suspected cardiac disease.

Physical examination

No abnormalities detected. A mild sinus arrhythmia was present. No abnormal lung sounds were auscultated.

Thoracic radiographs

A standard right lateral thoracic view showed a mild diffuse broncho-interstitial pattern (Figure 13.98).

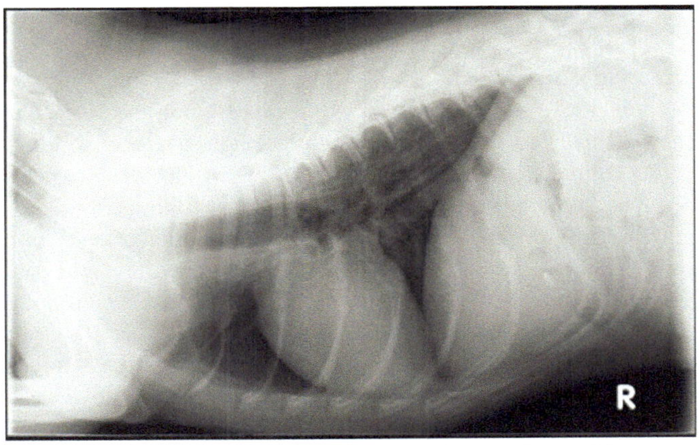

Figure 13.98 Eosinophilic inflammation. Right lateral view of the thoracic cavity showing a mild diffuse bronchointerstitial pattern.

Bronchoalveolar lavage cytology

The smears were of good diagnostic quality and high cellularity with good cell preservation. There was a moderate amount of blue, stringy mucus in the background. The majority of cells present were inflammatory cells, with the population consisting of 59% eosinophils; 27% neutrophils, nondegenerate; 8% small lymphocytes; 6% macrophages, occasionally reactive with cytoplasmic vacuolization (Figure 13.99). Ciliated epithelial cells were present in moderate numbers and squamous epithelial cells were very occasionally seen.

Interpretation: eosinophilic inflammation. Differential diagnoses: eosinophilic bronchopneumopathy secondary to a hypersensitivity reaction or parasites.

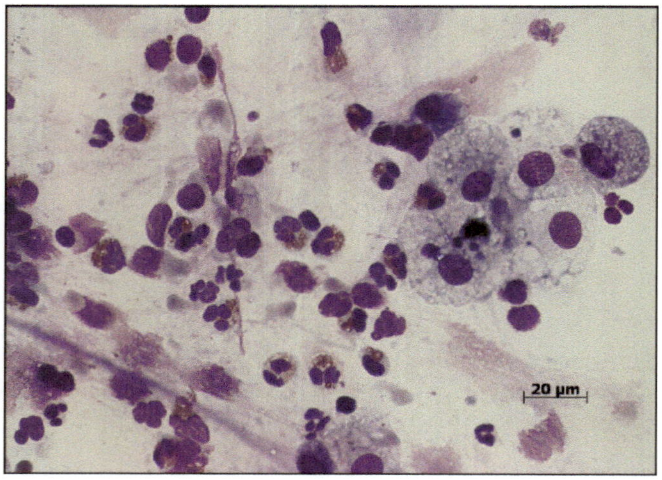

Figure 13.99 **Eosinophilic inflammation. Smears from the bronchoalveolar lavage with high cellularity and a moderate amount of blue, stringy mucus in the background. The majority of nucleated cells present were inflammatory cells, predominated by eosinophils with fewer neutrophils and vacuolated macrophages (Diff-Quik, 500× magnification).**

Follow up

The patient was started on an immunosuppressive dose of corticosteroids, tapered over several weeks. The coughing stopped soon after treatment was initiated.

Disease pathogenesis

Eosinophilic bronchopneumopathy (previously known as pulmonary infiltrates with eosinophils) is a condition that most commonly affects young adult dogs. Females are more frequently affected than males. The most common clinical sign is a harsh cough followed by gagging and retching. The cause of this condition is infiltration of eosinophils into the lungs. Causes of this infiltration of eosinophils can be parasites in the lungs or a hypersensitivity to inhaled allergens. Although peripheral eosinophilia is identified in 50–60% of cases, absence of eosinophilia (as was seen in this case) does not rule the condition out (Clercx *et al.*, 2000; Clercx & Peeters, 2007a). The prognosis is good, and an excellent response is usually seen with corticosteroid treatment. Corticosteroid treatment can often be stopped completely without recurrence of coughing, but it is important to note that a relapse might occur, which will require another course of treatment. In some patients, chronic use of very low dose corticosteroid (e.g. every other day) might be needed.

CASE 3

Signalment/history

A 10-year-old, spayed female Bernese Mountain dog. Anorexia, depression, lethargy.

Physical examination

Mild pyrexia; muffled heart sounds; mild hypoglycemia.

Thoracic radiography

Standard right and left lateral, as well as dorsoventral radiographs were taken. Two well-marginated, round homogeneous soft tissue nodules were noted. The stomach was moderately distended with gas, with lobulated soft tissue opacities noted along the lesser curvature of the stomach (Figures 13.100, 13.101).

Interpretation: suspected primary (with metastatic) or metastatic lung disease. Neoplasia should also be considered for the gastric lesion.

Abdominal ultrasonography

The gastric fundus wall was focally markedly thickened by up to 2 cm with a diffuse hypoechoic appearance devoid of wall layering.

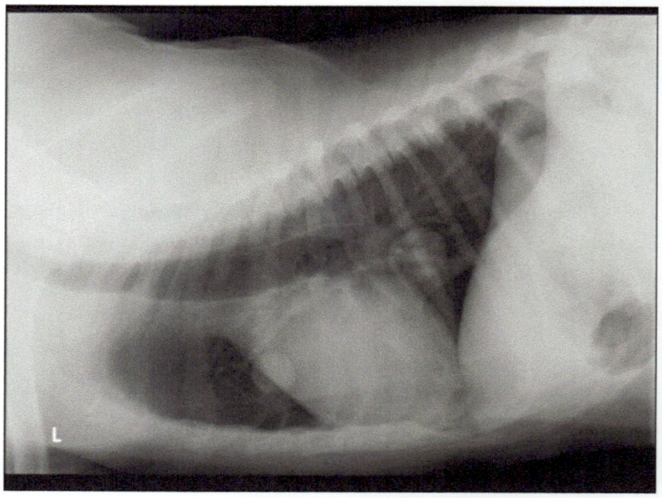

Figure 13.100 **Metastatic lung tumor. Left lateral and dorsoventral radiographs of the thoracic cavity showing two well-marginated, round homogeneous soft tissue nodules. The stomach was moderately distended with gas with lobulated soft tissue opacities noted along the lesser curvature.**

The liver appeared to be normal size but was mild-to-moderately diffusely hypoechoic. The spleen was generous and mildly diffusely hyperechoic. All of the abdominal lymph nodes appeared to be mildly enlarged. There was also a small amount of anechoic free peritoneal fluid noted in the recesses.

Interpretation: suspected gastric adenocarcinoma.

Cytologic examination

Abdominal fluid

The smears were of moderate cellularity and cell preservation was good. There was a moderate blood admixture; moderate numbers of neutrophils and lesser numbers of macrophages and lymphocytes as well as occasional reactive mesothelial cells were present. Moderate numbers of medium to large cells with a medium blue cytoplasm, often with small clear vacuoles, were seen. These cells were present either singly or in small clusters or balls. Nuclei were round to oval with a coarse chromatin pattern and one to multiple small nucleoli. The cell population displayed an anisocytosis, anisokaryosis, increase in N:C variation, multinucleation, nuclear molding, and very occasional irregular mitoses (Figure 13.102).

Interpretation: neoplastic effusion.

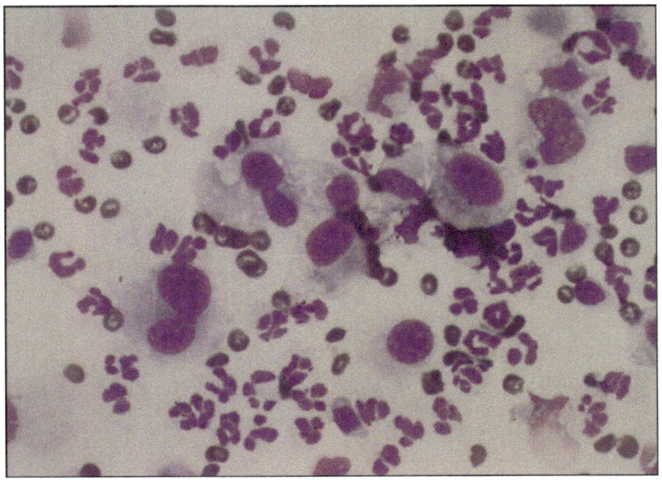

Figure 13.102 Metastatic lung tumor. Abdominal fluid containing moderate numbers of medium to large cells with a medium blue cytoplasm, often with small clear vacuoles. The cells were present either singly or in small clusters. This cell population displayed an anisocytosis, anisokaryosis, increase in nuclear:cytoplasm variation, multinucleation, nuclear molding, very occasional irregular mitoses, round to oval nuclei with a coarse chromatin pattern, and one to multiple small nucleoli (Diff-Quik, 500× magnification).

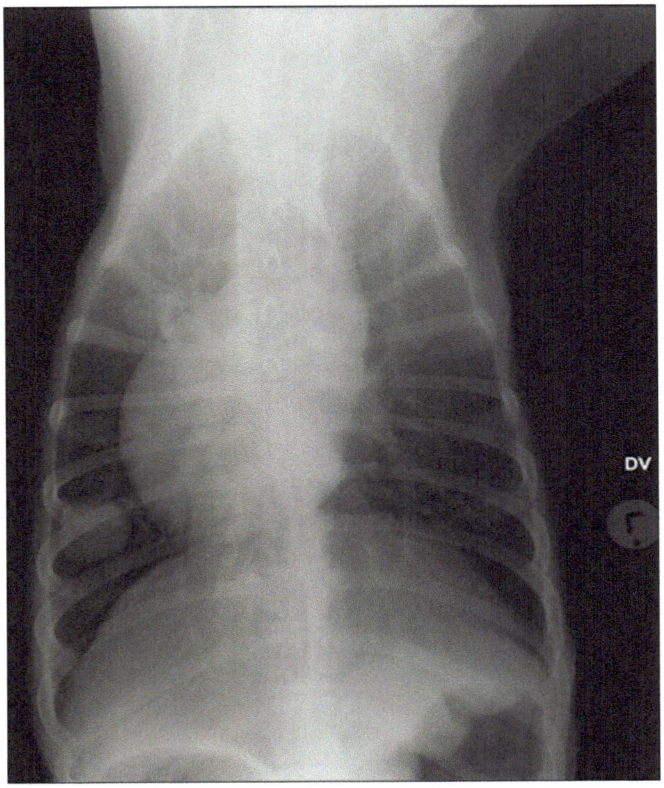

Figure 13.101 Metastatic lung tumor. Left lateral and dorsoventral radiographs of the thoracic cavity showing two well-marginated, round homogeneous soft tissue nodules. The stomach was moderately distended with gas with lobulated soft tissue opacities noted along the lesser curvature.

Gastric wall

One smear of low cellularity with poor cell preservation was examined. There was a marked blood admixture and many platelet clumps containing low numbers of neutrophils were present. Very low numbers of neutrophils and small lymphocytes were present in the bloody background. Very low numbers of discrete cells with a light blue, sometimes finely vacuolated cytoplasm and round to angular nucleus with a coarse chromatin pattern were seen (Figure 13.103). One cell with a small satellite nucleus was noted.

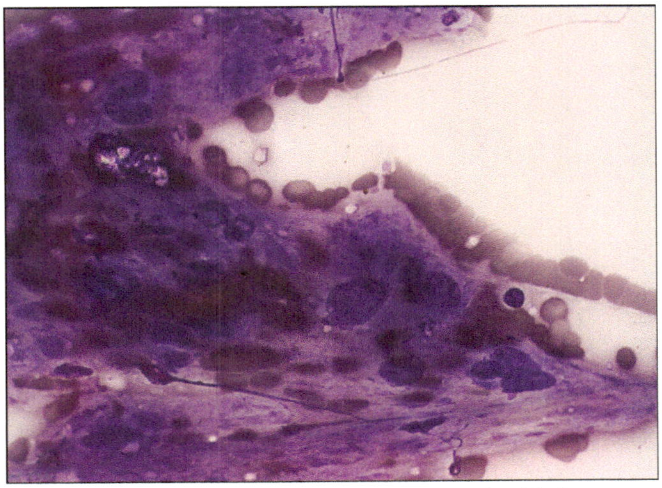

Figure 13.103 Metastatic lung tumor. The FNA sample of the lesion in the gastric mucosa had a marked blood admixture with low cellularity. Very low numbers of neutrophils and small lymphocytes were present in the bloody background, as well as low numbers of discrete cells with a light blue, sometimes finely vacuolated cytoplasm and round to angular nucleus with a coarse chromatin pattern (Diff-Quik, 500× magnification).

Interpretation: peripheral blood and low numbers of atypical cells. Further interpretation was limited due to the low cellularity and poor cell preservation. No normal gastric epithelial cells were seen.

Liver

The smears were of very low cellularity with a severe blood admixture. Occasional hepatocytes in small clusters with a stippled cytoplasm were seen. A few discrete cells with abundant basophilic, sometimes finely vacuolated cytoplasm and round to angular nucleus with a coarse chromatin pattern were seen (Figure 13.104). Low numbers of neutrophils, macrophages, and lymphocytes were also present, especially along the edges of the smears.

Interpretation: peripheral blood with very low numbers of hepatocytes and neoplastic metastasis.

Lung

The smears were of good diagnostic quality and high cellularity with good cell preservation. There was a moderate blood admixture. There were high numbers of epithelial cells arranged in acinar formations (Figure 13.105). These cells were oval to columnar to spindle-shaped with a medium blue cytoplasm, often with numerous small clear vacuoles (Figure 13.106). Nuclei were round to oval with a coarse chromatin pattern and one to two, small, occasionally angular nucleoli. A light pink material was often seen between the cells. Anisocytosis, anisokaryosis, multinucleation, and nuclear molding were present (Figure 13.107). Low numbers of neutrophils and macrophages were also seen.

Interpretation: metastatic adenocarcinoma.

Follow up/outcome

Due to the poor prognosis of the condition, the owners opted for euthanasia.

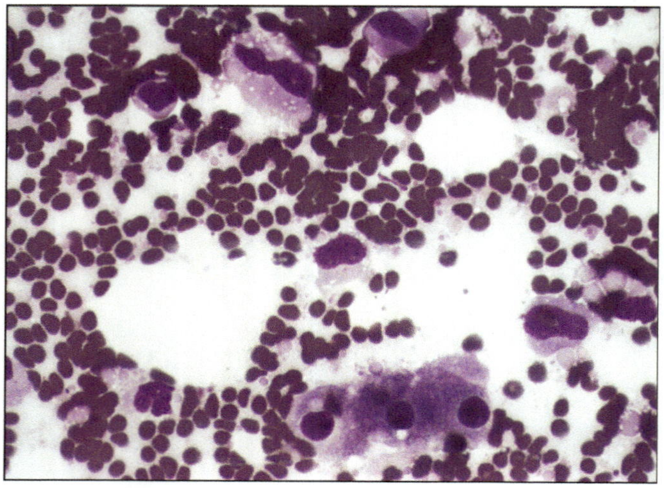

Figure 13.104 Metastatic lung tumor. The smears from the liver were of very low cellularity with a marked blood admixture. Hepatocytes were seen in small clusters. Few discrete cells with abundant basophilic, sometimes finely vacuolated cytoplasm and round to angular nucleus with a coarse chromatin pattern were seen (Diff-Quik, 500× magnification).

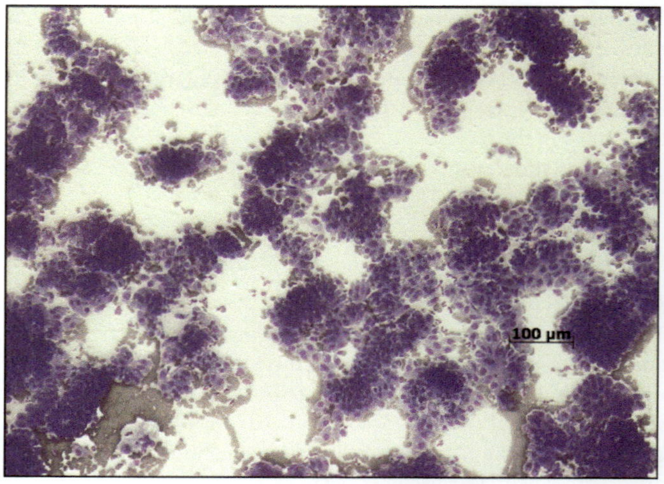

Figure 13.105 Metastatic lung tumor. The aspiration samples of the lung masses showed a moderate blood admixture with high numbers of epithelial cells arranged in acinar formations (Diff-Quik, 100× magnification).

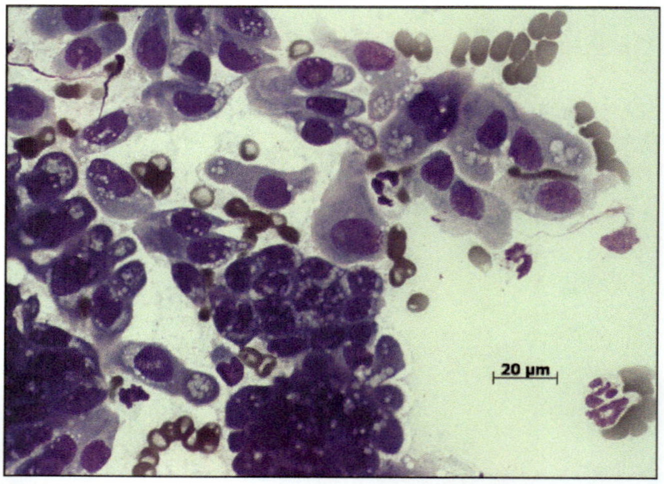

Figure 13.106 Metastatic lung tumor. The epithelial cells from the lung masses were oval to columnar to spindle-shaped with a medium blue cytoplasm, often with numerous small clear vacuoles (Diff-Quik, 500× magnification).

Disease pathogenesis

The pulmonary vascular bed receives a lot of blood coming from the right heart with each cardiac cycle. The lung serves as an ideal location for metastatic disease due to the numerous, well-oxygenated capillary beds through which the blood passes. Cancer cells detach from the primary tumor, enter the blood or lymphatics to be carried to distant sites, migrate from the vessel into the tissue, adhere, and then grow in the new site. Almost all neoplasms can metastasize to the lung but some are more likely to do so, such as oral and nail bed melanoma, thyroid carcinoma, osteosarcoma, and mammary carcinoma.

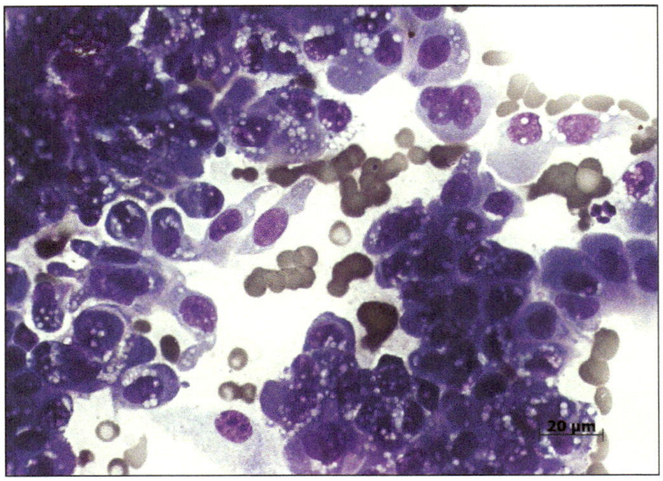

Figure 13.107 Metastatic lung tumor. The neoplastic epithelial cells from the lung mass had round to oval nuclei with a coarse chromatin pattern and one to two, small, occasionally angular nucleoli. Anisocytosis, anisokaryosis, multinucleation, and nuclear molding were present (Diff-Quik, 500× magnification).

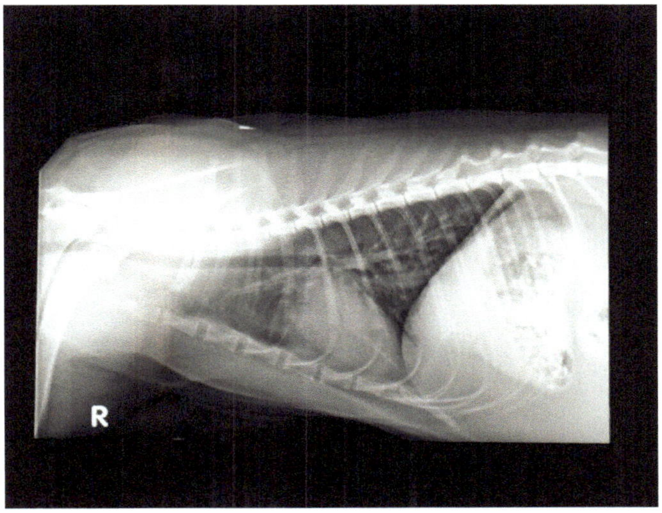

Figure 13.108 Feline asthma. Right lateral and dorsoventral radiographic views of the thoracic cavity showing a diffuse bronchointerstitial lung pattern.

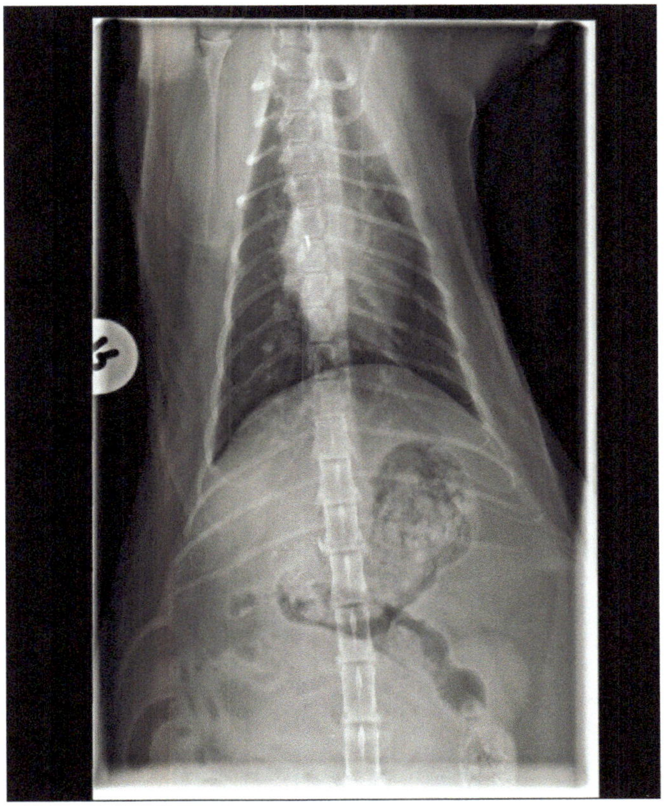

Figure 13.109 Feline asthma. Right lateral and dorsoventral radiographic views of the thoracic cavity showing a diffuse bronchointerstitial lung pattern.

CASE 4

Signalment/history

A 1.5-year-old, sterilized female, Norwegian Forest cat. Fully vaccinated and presented with a history of chronic coughing and wheezing of two months' duration.

Physical examination and minimum database

Bright and alert and normal temperature, heart rate, and respiratory rate. No abnormalities on thoracic auscultation. Mild stress leukogram noted on hematology, mild pre-renal azotemia, and mild hyperalbuminemia due to dehydration.

Thoracic radiography

Standard right and left lateral, as well as dorsoventral radiographs were taken. A broncho-interstitial lung pattern was evident (Figures 13.108, 13.109).

Cytology of the BAL fluid

A large amount of mucoid material was noted on bronchoscopy and submitted for cytologic evailation. The material was very cellular (many clusters of cells, 40–50 cells/50× HPF). There was a mild blood admixture, and the background was highly mucinous (pink granular to fibrillar material with some light blue amorphous material) with some necrosis (degenerate unidentifiable cells). Leukocytes were seen in moderate to high numbers and included 13.5% neutrophils (mostly degenerate), 9% small mononuclear cells (mostly lymphocytes), 16.5% large mononuclear cells (mostly activated macrophages), and 61% eosinophils (Figure 13.110). High numbers of ciliated columnar epithelia cells were present and had medium blue cytoplasm that was sometimes vacuolated, basal oval nuclei with coarse chromatin, and multiple prominent nuclei (Figure 13.111). They showed mild to moderate anisokaryosis and binucleation. No microorganisms were seen.

Interpretation: eosinophilic inflammation with moderate respiratory epithelial hyperplasia and mild necrosis. The epithelial hyperplasia and necrosis were likely due to chronic respiratory inflammation. The presence of copious numbers of respiratory epithelial cells indicates that the sample comes, at least in part, from the upper airways.

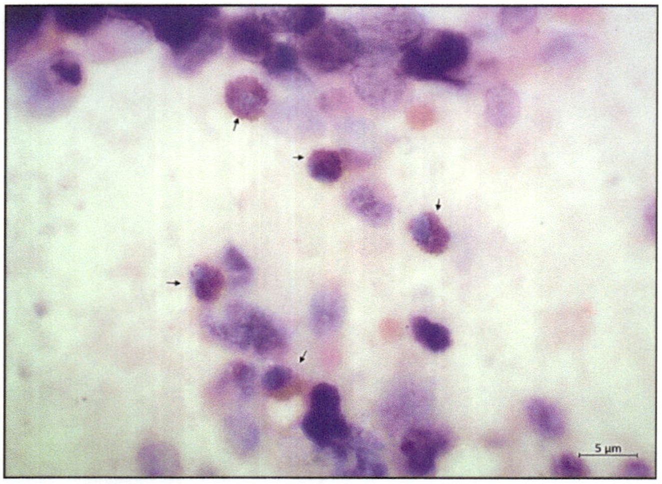

Figure 13.110 **Feline asthma. Bronchoalveolar lavage smear. An increased proportion of eosinophils (arrows) were noted in a moderately mucinous background with a low proportion of ruptured and/or degenerate appearing respiratory epithelial cells (Wright–Giemsa, 1,000× magnification).**

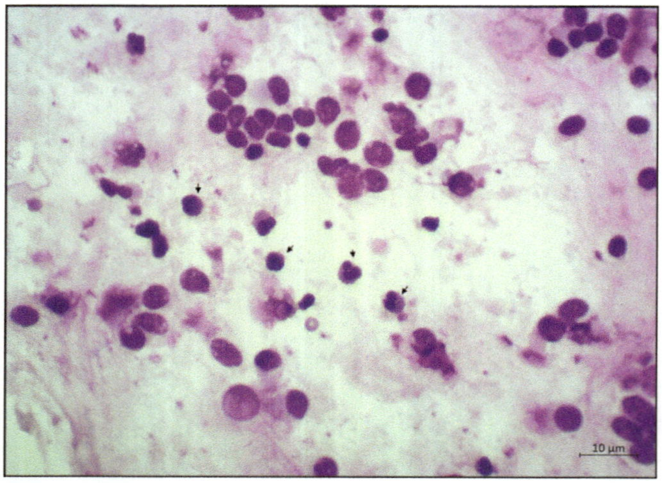

Figure 13.111 **Feline asthma. Bronchoalveolar lavage smear. An increased proportion of eosinophils (arrows) were noted in a moderately mucinous background with a low proportion of ruptured and/or degenerate appearing respiratory epithelial cells (Wright–Giemsa, 500× magnification).**

Eosinophilic inflammation was most likely due to allergic bronchitis/feline asthma, especially given the age of the patient; however, eosinophilic granuloma and parasitic or bacterial infection couldn't be ruled out on cytology.

For the aerobic culture and antimicrobial susceptibility testing of the bronchoalveolar lavage fluid, no growth was noted after 72 hours of incubation.

Follow up/outcome

The patient was diagnosed with feline allergic asthma. The treatment plan included a tapering dosage of oral glucocorticoids and concurrent, chronic inhalant glucocorticoid therapy. A bronchodilator inhaler, deworming, topical parasiticides, and a hypoallergenic diet were also included. The patient responded very well to medication, with no clinical symptoms noted by owners during subsequent follow-up visits.

Disease pathogenesis

Feline asthma is a common lower-airway inflammatory disease in cats affecting approximately 1–5% of the feline population and is thought to be allergic in origin. Generally, clinicopathologic abnormalities of cats with asthma are nonspecific. Common radiographic findings in asthmatic cats include a bronchial or bronchointerstitial lung pattern. Bronchoalveolar lavage fluid sample for cytologic examination can be collected using either bronchoscopy or a blind technique. Eosinophilic inflammation is noted on BAL fluid cytology of asthmatic cats. Adjunctive testing includes culture of the BAL fluid, allergy testing, pulmonary function testing, and biomarkers, for example endothelion-1. The condition is mostly treated with glucocorticoids and bronchodilators. These are effective treatments in many cats; however, some are unresponsive or minimally responsive. Therapies that might help reverse the underlying immunopathology of asthma or could be used as adjuncts in refractory asthma are being investigated in experimental feline asthma models and include allergy-specific immunotherapy, omega-3 fatty acids/nutraceuticals, inhaled lidocaine, tyrosine kinase inhibitors, and stem cells (Trzil, 2020).

CASE 5

Signalment/history

A 3-year-old, intact female, bull terrier. Progressive lethargy, weakness, anorexia, and weight loss were noted in the few weeks prior to presentation. Owners also noted difficulty in breathing, intermittent foaming at the mouth, and a dry cough.

Physical examination and minimum database

The patient was collapsed on presentation, with a poor body condition, and she displayed dyspnea and tachypnea that was characterized by abdominal breathing and abducted elbows. Referred and increased breath sounds were auscultated in all the lung quadrants with increased intensity in the right thoracic area. Hematology revealed a mild stress leukogram and pseudothrombocytopenia due to platelet aggregation and mild hypernatremia on serum biochemistry.

Thoracic radiography

Standard right and left lateral, as well as dorsoventral radiographs were taken. A severe, diffuse broncho-interstitial lung pattern involving all the lung lobes was evident (Figures 13.112–13.114).

Cytology of the BAL

The material was turbid and flocculent and the automated total nucleated cell count was 2,260 cells/µl. The material was moderate cellularity (2 cells/50× HPF). Moderate amounts of mucus were noted in

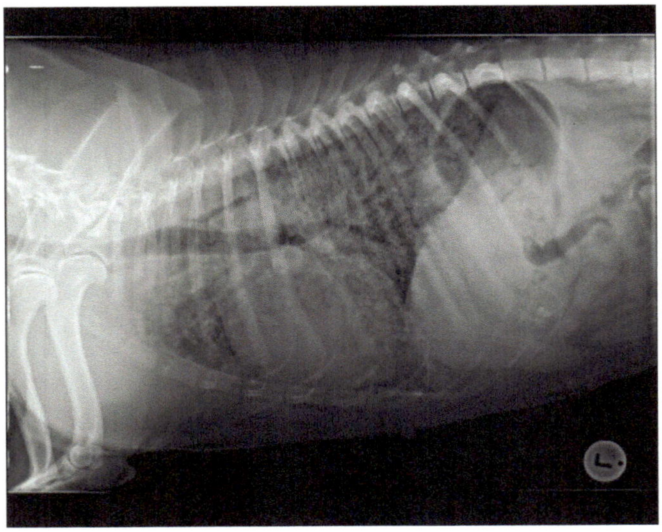

Figure 13.112 Pulmonary neoplasia (carcinoma). Right and left lateral and dorsoventral radiographic views of the thoracic cavity showing a diffuse bronchointerstitial lung pattern.

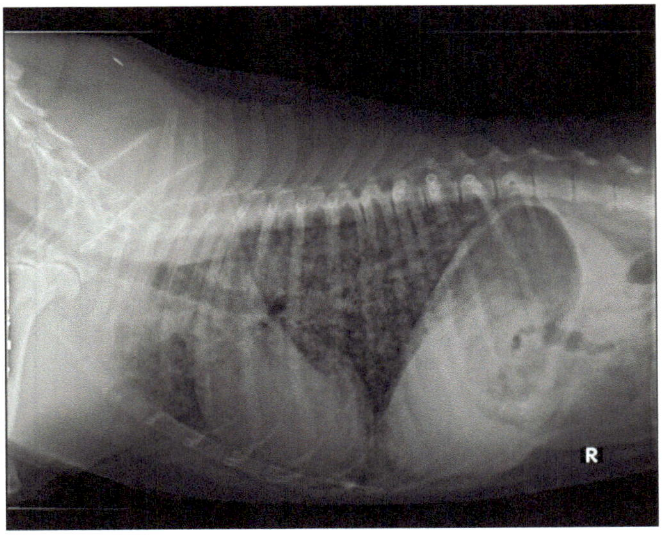

Figure 13.113 Pulmonary neoplasia (carcinoma). Right and left lateral and dorsoventral radiographic views of the thoracic cavity showing a diffuse bronchointerstitial lung pattern.

the background. The nucleated cell count consisted of 83% degenerate neutrophils, 5% lymphoid cells, and 12% macrophages. The macrophages were activated, with vacuolated cytoplasm. In addition, moderate numbers of epithelial cells arranged in tightly cohesive clusters were present (Figure 13.115). These cells were medium sized, round, and had round to oval centrally placed nuclei. The cells displayed intense cytoplasmic basophilia, high N:C ratio, moderate anisocytosis/anisokaryosis, and prominent nucleoli. Occasional multinucleation, with nuclear molding, was also seen (Figure 13.116).

Interpretation: highly suggestive of a carcinoma, with secondary neutrophilic inflammation, and peripheral blood admixture. Histopathology was advised for definitive diagnosis.

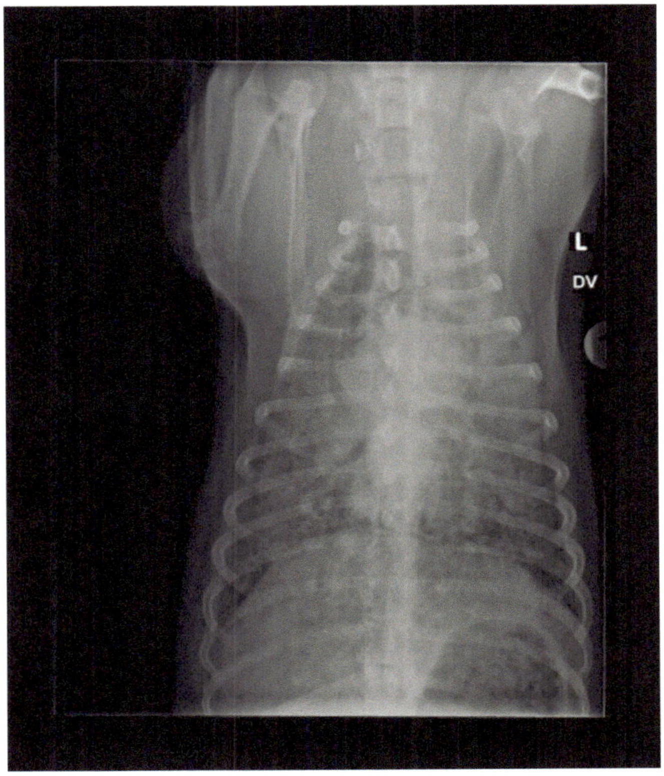

Figure 13.114 Pulmonary neoplasia (carcinoma). Right and left lateral and dorsoventral radiographic views of the thoracic cavity showing a diffuse bronchointerstitial lung pattern.

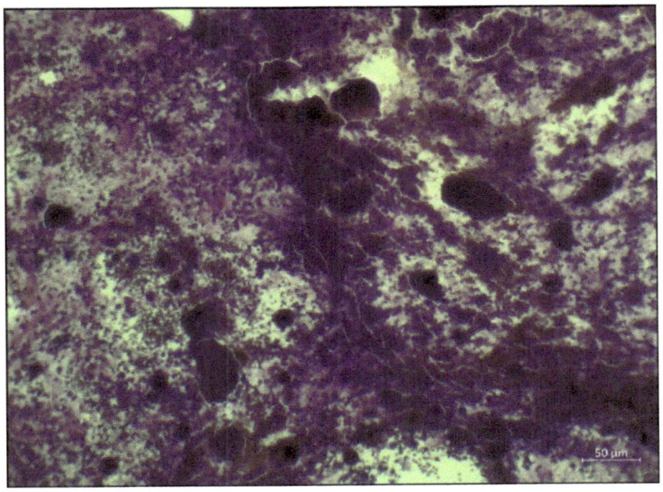

Figure 13.115 Bronchoalveolar lavage smear. Cellular and thick sample with a mild blood admixture and high numbers of tightly cohesive variably sized clusters of epithelial cells and moderate numbers of leukocytes in the background (Wright–Giemsa, 100× magnification).

Outcome

Due to the poor prognosis the owners opted for humane euthanasia. A diagnosis of severe, diffuse primary pulmonary bronchial carcinoma with metastasis to the regional lymph nodes was made on postmortem examination.

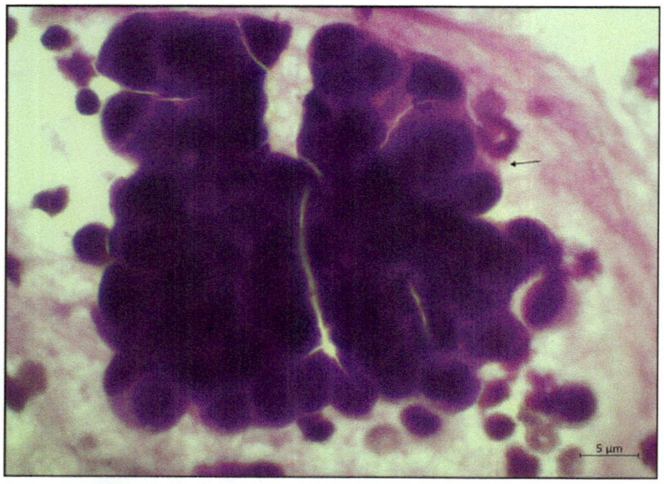

Figure 13.116 Bronchoalveolar lavage smear. A cluster of epithelial cells displaying increased cytoplasmic basophilia, moderate anisocytosis, anisokaryosis, coarse chromatin, multiple nucleoli, bi- and multinucleation with nuclear molding (arrow) (Wright–Giemsa, 1,000× magnification).

Disease pathogenesis

Carcinomas comprise 80% or more of all primary lung tumors in dogs and cats (Hahn *et al.*, 1996; Moulton *et al.*, 1981). Pulmonary epithelial tumors are less common in dogs than in cats, affecting the cranial and caudal lung lobes more equally and often presenting as a single mass. These are often histologic classified as bronchioalveolar, adenocarcinoma, or anaplastic carcinoma; however cytologic differentiation isn't possible (Barrett *et al.*, 2014; Marolf *et al.*, 2011; Burgess & Kerr, 2009). Furthermore, the cytologic preparations from primary and metastatic carcinomas are similar, and the two cannot be definitively differentiated by cytologic evaluation alone. Metastasis of pulmonary carcinomas is less common in dogs compared to cats and a better prognosis is associated with evidence of cell differentiation and the absence of clinical signs (McNiel *et al.*, 1997).

REFERENCES

Alice Defarges Bichot A.D.B. (2021) Lower respiratory tract of the dog and cat. In: *Veterinary Cytology*, First edn. (eds. L.C. Sharkey, M.J. Radin, D. Seelig). Wiley-Blackwell, Hoboken, NJ.

Allerton F.J., Leemans J., Tual C., Bernaerts F., Kirschvink N., Clercx C. (2013) Correlation of bronchoalveolar eosinophilic percentage with airway responsiveness in cats with chronic bronchial disease. *J Small Anim Pract 54*:258–264.

Andreasen C.B. (2003) Bronchoalveolar lavage. *Vet Clin North Am Small Anim Pract 33*:69–88.

Arndt T. (2014) Nasal exudates and masses. In: *Cowell and Tyler's Diagnostic Cytology and Hematology of the Dog and Cat*, 4th edn. (eds. A. Valenciano, R. Cowell) Elsevier Mosby, St. Louis.

Ashbaugh E.A., Mckiernan B.C., Miller C.J., Powers B. (2011) Nasal hydropulsion: A novel tumor biopsy technique. *Journal of the American Animal Hospital Association 47*:312–316.

Baldwin F., Becker A.B. (1993) Bronchoalveolar eosinophilic cells in a canine model of asthma: Two distinctive populations. *Vet Pathol 30*:97–103.

Barachetti L., Mortellaro C.M., Di Giancamillo M., Giudice C., Martino P., Travetti O., Miller P.E. (2009) Bilateral orbital and nasal aspergillosis in a cat. *Veterinary Ophthalmology 12*:176–182.

Barçante J.M., Barçante T.A., Ribeiro V.M., Oliveira-Junior S.D., Dias S.R., Negrão-Corrêa D., Lima W.S. (2008) Cytological and parasitological analysis of bronchoalveolar lavage fluid for the diagnosis of Angiostrongylus vasorum infection in dogs. *Vet Parasitol 158*:93–102.

Barrett L.E., Pollard R.E., Zwingenberger A., Zierenberg-Ripoll A., Skorupski K.A. (2014) Radiographic characterization of primary lung tumors in 74 dogs. *Vet Radiol Ultrasound 55*:480–7.

Barrs V.R., Talbot J.J. (2020) Fungal rhinosinusitis and disseminated invasive aspergillosis in cats. *Veterinary Clinics: Small Animal Practice 50*:331–357.

Benson C.J., Edlund M.B., Gray S., Powell L., Paulin-Curlee G., Armien A., Overmann J.A. (2013) The presence of diatom algae in a tracheal wash from a German Wirehaired Pointer with aspiration pneumonia. *Vet Clin Pathol 42*:221–226.

Black L.J., Hechler A.C., Duffy M.E., Beatty S.S.K. (2017) Presumed lupus erythematosus cells identified in bronchoalveolar lavage fluid from a Mexican Hairless dog. *Vet Clin Pathol 46*:354–359.

Bonfanti U., Bussadori C., Zatelli A., De Lorenzi D., Masserdotti C., Bertazzolo W., Faverzani S., Ghisleni G., Capobianco R., Caniatti M. (2004) Percutaneous fine-needle biopsy of deep thoracic and abdominal masses in dogs and cats. *Journal of Small Animal Practice 45*:191–198.

Brown D.E., Thrall M.A., Getzy D.M., Weiser M.G., Ogilvie G.K. (1994) Cytology of canine malignant histiocytosis. *Vet Clin Pathol 23*:118–123.

Burgess H.J., Kerr M.E. (2009) Cytokeratin and vimentin co-expression in 21 canine primary pulmonary epithelial neoplasms. *J Vet Diagn Invest 21*:815–820.

Burkhard M.J., Millward L. (2010) Respiratory tract. In: *Canine and Feline Cytology. A Color Atlas and Interpretation Guide*, 2nd edn. (eds. R.E. Raskin, D.J. Meyer) Saunders Elsevier, St. Louis.

Campbell O., De Lorimier L.-P., Beauregard G., Overvelde S., Johnson S. (2017) Presumptive primary pulmonary mast cell tumor in 2 dogs. *The Canadian Veterinary Journal 58*:591.

Caniatti M., Cunha N.P.D., Avallone G., Romussi S., Mortellaro C.M., Tranquillo V., Ghisleni G. (2012) Diagnostic accuracy of brush cytology in canine chronic intranasal disease. *Veterinary Clinical Pathology 41*:133–140.

Canonne A.M., Billen F., Tual C., Ramery E., Roels E., Peters I., Clercx C. (2016) Quantitative PCR and cytology of bronchoalveolar lavage fluid in dogs with Bordetella bronchiseptica infection. *J Vet Intern Med 30*:1204–1209.

Clercx C., Peeters D. (2007a) Canine eosinophilic bronchopneumopathy. *Veterinary Clinics of North America: Small Animal Practice 37*:917–935.

Clercx C., Peeters D. (2007b) Canine eosinophilic bronchopneumopathy. *Vet Clin North Am Small Anim Pract 37*:917–35, vi.

Clercx C., Peeters D., Snaps F., Hansen P., Mcentee K., Detilleux J., Henroteaux M., Day M.J. (2000) Eosinophilic bronchopneumopathy in dogs. *Journal of Veterinary Internal Medicine 14*:282–291.

Clercx C., Wallon J., Gilbert S., Snapst F., Coignoul F. (1996) Imprint and brush cytology in the diagnosis of canine intranasal tumours. *Journal of Small Animal Practice 37*:423–427.

Cohn L.A. (2020) Canine nasal disease: An update. *Veterinary Clinics: Small Animal Practice 50*:359–374.

Creevy K.E. (2009) Airway evaluation and flexible endoscopic procedures in dogs and cats: Laryngoscopy, transtracheal wash, tracheobronchoscopy, and bronchoalveolar lavage. *Vet Clin North Am Small Anim Pract 39*:869–880.

Creighton S., Wilkins W.R. (1974) Transtracheal aspiration biopsy: Technique and cytologic evaluation. *J Am Anim Hosp Assoc 10*:219–226.

Damiano V.V., Cohen A., Tsang A.L., Batra G., Petersen R. (1980) A morphologic study of the influx of neutrophils into dog lung alveoli after lavage with sterile saline. *Am J Pathol 100*:349–364.

Day M. (2011) Aspergillosis and penicillosis. In: *Infectious Diseases of the Dog and Cat* 2nd edn (ed. C. Greene) Saunders, St. Louis.

De Lorenzi D., Masserdotti C., Bertoncello D., Tranquillo V. (2009) Differential cell counts in canine cytocentrifuged bronchoalveolar lavage fluid: A study on reliable enumeration of each cell type. *Vet Clin Pathol 38*:532–536.

Deberry J.D., Norris C.R., Sami V.F., Griffrey S.M., Almy F.S. (2002a) Correlation between fine-needle aspiration cytopathology and histopathology of the lung in dogs and cats. *Journal of the American Animal Hospital Association 38*:327.

Deberry J.D., Norris C.R., Samii V.F., Griffey S.M., Almy F.S. (2002b) Correlation between fine-needle aspiration cytopathology and histopathology of the lung in dogs and cats. *J Am Anim Hosp Assoc 38*:327–336.

Defarges Bichot A., Bienzle D. (2021) Lower respiratory tract of the dog and cat. In: *Veterinary Cytology*. (eds. L.C. Sharkey, M.J.Radin, D. Seelig) Wiley, Hoboken, NJ.

Dehard S., Bernaerts F., Peeters D., Detilleux J., Mcentee K., Day M.J., Clercx C. (2008) Comparison of bronchoalveolar lavage cytospins and smears in dogs and cats. *J Am Anim Hosp Assoc 44*:285–294.

Deheer H.L., Mcmanus P. (2005) Frequency and severity of tracheal wash hemosiderosis and association with underlying disease in 96 cats: 2002–2003. *Vet Clin Pathol 34*:17–22.

Duncan C., Stephen C., Lester S., Bartlett K. (2005) Sub-clinical infection and asymptomatic carriage of Cryptococcus gattii in dogs and cats during an outbreak of cryptococcosis. *Medical Mycology 43*:511–516.

Dye J.A., Mckiernan B.C., Rozanski E.A., Hoffmann W.E., Losonsky J.M., Homco L.D., Weisiger R.M., Kakoma I. (1996) Bronchopulmonary disease in the cat: Historical, physical, radiographic, clinicopathologic, and pulmonary functional evaluation of 24 affected and 15 healthy cats. *J Vet Intern Med 10*:385–400.

Elie M., Sabo M. (2006) Basics in canine and feline rhinoscopy. *Clinical Techniques in Small Animal Practice 21*:60–63.

English K. (2014) Transtracheal and bronchoalveolar washes. In: *Cowell and Tyler's Diagnostic Cytology and Hematology of the Dog and Cat* 4th edn. (eds. A.C. Valenciano, R.L Cowell) Elsevier Mosby, St. Louis.

Finke M.D. (2013) Transtracheal wash and bronchoalveolar lavage. *Topics in Companion Animal Medicine 28*:97–102.

French T. (1987) The use of cytology in the diagnosis of chronic nasal disorders. In *The Compendium on Continuing Education for the Practicing Veterinarian (USA)*.

Geyer N.E., Reichle J.K., Valdés-Martínez A., Williams J., Goggin J.M., Leach L., Hanson J., Hill S., Axam T. (2010) Radiographic appearance of confirmed pulmonary lymphoma in cats and dogs. *Veterinary Radiology & Ultrasound 51*:386–390.

Grimes C., Fry M., Leblanc C., Hecht S. (2014) The lung and intrathoracic structures. In: *Cowell and Tyler's Diagnostic Cytology and Hematology of the Dog and Cat*, 4th edn. (eds. A. Valenciano, R. Cowell), Elsevier Mosby, St. Louis.

Hahn F.F., Muggenburg B.A., Griffith W.C. (1996) Primary lung neoplasia in a beagle colony. *Vet Pathol 33*:633–638.

Hawkins E.C., Denicola D.B. (1989) Collection of bronchoalveolar lavage fluid in cats, using an endotracheal tube. *Am J Vet Res 50*:855–859.

Hawkins E.C., Denicola D.B., Kuehn N.F. (1990) Bronchoalveolar lavage in the evaluation of pulmonary disease in the dog and cat. State of the art. *J Vet Intern Med 4*:267–274.

Hawkins E.C., Denicola D.B., Plier M.L. (1995) Cytological analysis of bronchoalveolar lavage fluid in the diagnosis of spontaneous respiratory tract disease in dogs: A retrospective study. *J Vet Intern Med 9*:386–392.

Hawkins E.C., Kennedy-Stoskopf S., Levy J., Meuten D.J., Cullins L., Denicola D., Tompkins W.A., Tompkins M.B. (1994) Cytologic characterization of bronchoalveolar lavage fluid collected through an endotracheal tube in cats. *Am J Vet Res 55*:795–802.

Hawkins E.C., Morrison W.B., Denicola D.B., Blevins W.E. (1993) Cytologic analysis of bronchoalveolar lavage fluid from 47 dogs with multicentric malignant lymphoma. *J Am Vet Med Assoc 203*:1418–1425.

Hawkins E.C., Rogala A.R., Large E.E., Bradley J.M., Grindem C.B. (2006) Cellular composition of bronchial brushings obtained from healthy dogs and dogs with chronic cough and cytologic composition of bronchoalveolar lavage fluid obtained from dogs with chronic cough. *American Journal of Veterinary Research 67*:160–167.

Henderson S., Bradley K., Day M., Tasker S., Caney S., Moore A.H., Gruffydd-Jones T. (2004) Investigation of nasal disease in the cat—A retrospective study of 77 cases. *Journal of Feline Medicine and Surgery 6*:245–257.

Hirschberger J., Denicola D.B., Hermanns W., Kraft W. (1999) Sensitivity and specificity of cytologic evaluation in the diagnosis of neoplasia in body fluids from dogs and cats. *Veterinary Clinical Pathology 28*:142–146.

Hirshman C.A., Austin D.R., Klein W., Hanifin J.M., Hulbert W. (1986) Increased metachromatic cells and lymphocytes in bronchoalveolar lavage fluid of dogs with airway hyperreactivity. *Am Rev Respir Dis 133*:482–487.

Hooi K.S., Defarges A.M., Jelovcic S.V., Bienzle D. (2019) Bronchoalveolar lavage hemosiderosis in dogs and cats with respiratory disease. *Vet Clin Pathol 48*:42–49.

Johnson L.R., Drazenovich T.L. (2007) Flexible bronchoscopy and bronchoalveolar lavage in 68 cats (2001–2006). *J Vet Intern Med 21*:219–225.

Johnson L.R., Queen E.V., Vernau W., Sykes J.E., Byrne B.A. (2013) Microbiologic and cytologic assessment of bronchoalveolar lavage fluid from dogs with lower respiratory tract infection: 105 cases (2001–2011). *J Vet Intern Med 27*:259–267.

Johnson L.R., Vernau W. (2011) Bronchoscopic findings in 48 cats with spontaneous lower respiratory tract disease (2002–2009). *J Vet Intern Med 25*:236–243.

Johnston W.W. (1986) Cytologic diagnosis of lung cancer. Principles and problems. *Pathol Res Pract 181*:1–36.

Kaneko T., Massion P.R., Hara M., Nadel J.A. (1996) Ragweed antigen causes interleukin-8 production in sensitized dog trachea. *Am J Respir Crit Care Med 153*:136–140.

Khoo A., Lane A., Wyatt K. (2017) Intranasal mast cell tumor in the dog: A case series. *The Canadian Veterinary Journal 58*:851.

Kirschvink N., Kersnak E., Leemans J., Delvaux F., Clercx C., Snaps F., Gustin P. (2007) Effects of age and allergen-induced airway inflammation in cats: Radiographic and cytologic correlation. *Vet J 174*:644–651.

Kuehn N.F. (2006) Chronic rhinitis in cats. *Clinical Techniques in Small Animal Practice 21*:69–75.

Lécuyer M., Dubé P.G., Difruscia R., Desnoyers M., Lagacé A. (1995) Bronchoalveolar lavage in normal cats. *Can Vet J 36*:771–773.

Legendre A. (1983) Canine nasal and paranasal sinus tumors. *J. Am. Anim. Hosp. Assoc 19*:115–123.

Lester S.J., Malik R., Bartlett K.H., Duncan C.G. (2011) Cryptococcosis: Update and emergence of Cryptococcus gattii. *Veterinary Clinical Pathology 40*:4–17.

Lobetti R. (2009) A retrospective study of chronic nasal disease in 75 dogs. *Journal of the South African Veterinary Association 80*:224–228.

Marolf A.J., Gibbons D.S., Podell B.K., Park R.D. (2011) Computed tomographic appearance of primary lung tumors in dogs. *Vet Radiol Ultrasound 52*:168–172.

Mccullough S., Brinson J. (1999a) Collection and interpretation of respiratory cytology. *Clinical Techniques in Small Animal Practice 14*:220–226.

Mccullough S., Brinson J. (1999b) Collection and interpretation of respiratory cytology. *Clin Tech Small Anim Pract 14*:220–226.

Mcmillan M.C., Kleine L.J., Carpenter J.L. (1988) Fluoroscopically guided percutaneous fine-needle aspiration biopsy of thoracic lesions in dogs and cats. *Veterinary Radiology 29*:194–197.

Mcniel E.A., Ogilvie G.K., Powers B.E., Hutchison J.M., Salman M.D., Withrow S.J. (1997) Evaluation of prognostic factors for dogs with primary lung tumors: 67 cases (1985–1992). *J Am Vet Med Assoc 211*:1422–1427.

Meler E., Dunn M., Lecuyer M. (2008) A retrospective study of canine persistent nasal disease: 80 cases (1998–2003). *The Canadian Veterinary Journal 49*:71.

Michiels L., Day M., Snaps F., Hansen P., Clercx C. (2003) A retrospective study of non-specific rhinitis in 22 cats and the value of nasal cytology and histopathology. *Journal of Feline Medicine and Surgery 5*:279–285.

Miller C.J. (2007) Approach to the respiratory patient. *Veterinary Clinics of North America: Small Animal Practice 37*:861–878.

Moulton J.E., Von Tscharner C., Schneider R. (1981) Classification of lung carcinomas in the dog and cat. *Vet Pathol 18*:513–528.

Norris A. (1979) Intranasal neoplasms in the dog. *Journal of the American Animal Hospital Association 15*:231–236.

Norris C.R., Decile K.C., Berghaus L.J., Berghaus R.D., Walby W.F., Schelegle E.S., Hyde D.M., Gershwin L.J. (2003) Concentrations of cysteinyl leukotrienes in urine and bronchoalveolar lavage fluid of cats with experimentally induced asthma. *Am J Vet Res 64*:1449–1453.

Nyby M.D., Gregory D.A., Kuhn D.A., Pangborn J. (1977a) Incidence of Simonsiella in the oral cavity of dogs. *Journal of Clinical Microbiology 6*:87–88.

Nyby M.D., Gregory D.A., Kuhn D.A., Pangborn J. (1977b) Incidence of Simonsiella in the oral cavity of dogs. *J Clin Microbiol 6*:87–88.

Ogilvie G., Haschek W., Withrow S., Richardson R., Harvey H., Henderson R., Fowler J., Norris A., Tomlinson J., Mccaw D. (1989) Classification of primary lung tumors in dogs: 210 cases (1975–1985). *Journal of the American Veterinary Medical Association 195*:106–108.

Padrid P.A., Feldman B.F., Funk K., Samitz E.M., Reil D., Cross C.E. (1991) Cytologic, microbiologic, and biochemical analysis of bronchoalveolar lavage fluid obtained from 24 healthy cats. *Am J Vet Res 52*:1300–1307.

Peeters D., Clercx C. (2007) Update on canine sinonasal aspergillosis. *Veterinary Clinics of North America: Small Animal Practice 37*:901–916.

Peeters D.E., Mckiernan B.C., Weisiger R.M., Schaeffer D.J., Clercx C. (2000) Quantitative bacterial cultures and cytological examination of bronchoalveolar lavage specimens in dogs. *J Vet Intern Med 14*:534–541.

Pérez-Arellano J.L., Losa García J.E., García Macías M.C., Gómez Gómez F., Jiménez López A., De Castro S. (1992) Hemosiderin-laden macrophages in bronchoalveolar lavage fluid. *Acta Cytol 36*:26–30.

Rajamäki M.M., Järvinen A.K., Saari S.A., Maisi P.S. (2001a) Effect of repetitive bronchoalveolar lavage on cytologic findings in healthy dogs. *Am J Vet Res 62*:13–16.

Rajamäki M.M., Järvinen A.K., Saari S.A., Maisi P.S. (2001b) Effect of repetitive bronchoalveolar lavage on cytologic findings in healthy dogs. *Am J Vet Res 62*:13–16.

Rakich P.M., Latimer K.S. (1989a) Cytology of the respiratory tract. *Vet Clin North Am Small Anim Pract 19*:823–850.

Rakich P.M., Latimer K.S. (1989b) Cytology of the respiratory tract. *Vet Clin North Am Small Anim Pract 19*:823–850.

Rebar A.H., Denicola D.B., Muggenburg B.A. (1980) Bronchopulmonary lavage cytology in the dog: Normal findings. *Vet Pathol 17*:294–304.

Richard E.A., Depecker M., Defontis M., Leleu C., Fortier G., Pitel P.H., Courouсé-Malblanc A. (2014) Cytokine concentrations in bronchoalveolar lavage fluid from horses with neutrophilic inflammatory airway disease. *J Vet Intern Med 28*:1838–1844.

Roza M.R., Viegas C.A. (2007) The dog as a passive smoker: Effects of exposure to environmental cigarette smoke on domestic dogs. *Nicotine Tob Res 9*:1171–1176.

Spoor M.S., Royal A.B., Berent L.M. (2011) The elusive globule leukocyte. *Vet Clin Pathol 40*:136.

Sykes J.E., Malik R. (2012) Cryptococcosis. In: *Infectious Diseases of the Dog and Cat* 2nd edn. (ed. C. Greene) Saunders, St. Louis.

Tasker S., Knottenbelt C., Munro E., Stonehewer J., Simpson J., Mackin A. (1999) Aetiology and diagnosis of persistent nasal disease in the dog: A retrospective study of 42 cases. *Journal of Small Animal Practice 40*:473–478.

Teske E., Stokhof A., Ingh T.V.D., Wolvekamp W.T.C., Slappendel R., De Vries H. (1991) Transthoracic needle aspiration biopsy of the lung in dogs with pulmonic diseases. *The Journal of the American Animal Hospital Association (USA)*.27. pp. 289–294.

Trzil J.E. (2020) Feline asthma: Diagnostic and treatment update. *Veterinary Clinics of North America: Small Animal Practice 50*:375–391.

Vail D.M., Mahler P.A., Soergel S.A. (1995) Differential cell analysis and phenotypic subtyping of lymphocytes in bronchoalveolar lavage fluid from clinically normal dogs. *Am J Vet Res 56*:282–285.

Warren-Smith C., Roe K., De La Puerta B., Smith K., Lamb C. (2011) Pulmonary adenocarcinoma seeding along a fine needle aspiration tract in a dog. *The Veterinary Record 169*:181.

Windsor R.C., Johnson L.R. (2006) Canine chronic inflammatory rhinitis. *Clinical Techniques in Small Animal Practice 21*:76–81.

Windsor R.C., Johnson L.R., Sykes J.E., Drazenovich T.L., Leutenegger C.M., De Cock H.E. (2006) Molecular detection of microbes in nasal tissue of dogs with idiopathic lymphoplasmacytic rhinitis. *Journal of Veterinary Internal Medicine 20*:250–256.

Withrow S., Susaneck S., Macy D., Sheetz J. (1985) Aspiration and punch biopsy techniques for nasal tumors. *The Journal of the American Animal Hospital Association (USA)*.21: 551–554.

Wood E.F., O'brien R.T., Young K.M. (1998a) Ultrasound-guided fine-needle aspiration of focal parenchymal lesions of the lung in dogs and cats. *J Vet Intern Med 12*:338–342.

Wood E.F., O'brien R.T., Young K.M. (1998b) Ultrasound-guided fine-needle aspiration of focal parenchymal lesions of the lung in dogs and cats. *J Vet Intern Med 12*:338–342.

Woods K.S., Defarges A.M., Abrams-Ogg A.C., Dobson H., Viel L., Brisson B.A., Bienzle D. (2013) Comparison between manual aspiration via polyethylene tubing and aspiration via a suction pump with a suction trap connection for performing bronchoalveolar lavage in healthy dogs. *Am J Vet Res 74*:523–529.

Woods K.S., Defarges A.M., Abrams-Ogg A.C., Dobson H., Brisson B.A., Viel L., Bienzle D. (2014a) Comparison of bronchoalveolar lavage fluid obtained by manual aspiration with a handheld syringe with that obtained by automated suction pump aspiration from healthy dogs. *Am J Vet Res 75*:85–90.

Woods K.S., Defarges A.M., Abrams-Ogg A.C., Viel L., Brisson B.A., Bienzle D. (2014b) Comparison of manual and suction pump aspiration techniques for performing bronchoalveolar lavage in 18 dogs with respiratory tract disease. *J Vet Intern Med 28*:1398–1404.

Ybarra W.L., Johnson L.R., Drazenovich T.L., Johnson E.G., Vernau W. (2012) Interpretation of multisegment bronchoalveolar lavage in cats (1/2001-1/2011). *J Vet Intern Med 26*:1281–1287.

Zhu B.Y., Johnson L.R., Vernau W. (2015) Tracheobronchial brush cytology and bronchoalveolar lavage in dogs and cats with chronic cough: 45 cases (2012–2014). *J Vet Intern Med 29*:526–532.

CHAPTER 14

CENTRAL NERVOUS SYSTEM CYTOLOGY

Chandler C. Carter and Michael F. Rosser

Acknowledgment: this chapter is an updated revision of Central Nervous System Cytology written by A Russell Moore and Anne M. Barger for the 1st edition of *Small Animal Cytologic Diagnosis* (2016).

INTRODUCTION

The central nervous system (CNS) is a complex of different cell types that acts as the conductor of many autonomic functions and allows for higher mentation. Antemortem evaluation of CNS cellularity and structure has historically been hampered by the difficulty of accessing or visualizing the critical structures and the drastic effect of loss of those structures on the individual. Although cerebrospinal fluid (CSF) analysis has become routine, other antemortem modalities, such as CNS cytology, magnetic resonance imaging (MRI), and computed tomography, have only begun to be developed in veterinary species. These modalities used in conjunction have improved the diagnosis and treatment of CNS diseases. This chapter describes CSF analysis and CNS cytology and then provides an overview of how these diagnostic techniques can be used in some of the more commonly encountered diseases.

CEREBROSPINAL FLUID ANALYSIS

CSF was first used as a diagnostic medium more than 100 years ago (Garma-Aviña, 2004). As one of the few readily available means of testing the CNS in a minimally invasive manner, CSF analysis is still commonly employed to better understand the pathology associated with neurologic disorders.

Production and circulation

The role of CSF is to cushion the nervous tissue and provide nutritional support (Elias & Brown, 2008). CSF is an ultrafiltrate of plasma produced by choroid plexus and ependymal cells in the ventricular system of the brain and subarachnoid space (Di Terlizzi & Platt, 2006). Fluid production is dependent on an active transport system and is therefore fairly constant. The pia mater, the layer that forms the CSF–brain interface, is highly permeable and allows easy equilibrium of constituents in the CSF with the interstitial fluid of the nervous system and vice-versa (Bagley, 1996). This allows the CSF to stand as a representative of the CNS parenchyma in some conditions.

Cells lining the arachnoid villus function like valves and allow drainage of CSF into the venous sinuses using transcellular mechanisms (Di Terlizzi & Platt, 2006). Fluid, protein, and even particles as large as red blood cells (RBCs) can be removed from the CSF using this mechanism (Rosenberg *et al.*, 1980). The overall direction of CSF flow in the healthy state is from cranial to caudal (Rosenberg *et al.*, 1980; Elias & Brown, 2008). This has led to the recommendation to collect fluid caudal to the primary lesion (Thomson *et al.*, 1990; Lampe *et al.*, 2020b). Although this is likely a wise choice, diagnostically useful samples can also be obtained cranial to the lesion location.

Indications and contraindications

Indications for collection and evaluation of CSF include clinical suspicion of neoplasia, inflammation, trauma or other causes of hemorrhage, degenerative disorders, or infection within the brain or spinal cord (Elias & Brown, 2008; Di Terlizzi & Platt, 2009).

In one large study, an etiologic diagnosis was provided by CSF analysis in only 2% of 256 canine cases; however, 75% of cases with diseases typically producing CSF abnormalities provided evidence to support the final diagnosis or pathologic process (Bohn *et al.*, 2006). Based on this evidence, CSF analysis should be viewed primarily as a means of furthering understanding of the pathology occurring, with determination of a definitive diagnosis seen as an added bonus. For example, CSF analysis can often be helpful in distinguishing an inflammatory process from a neoplastic one, but only rarely will the cause of the inflammation be evident by CSF analysis alone (Bohn *et al.*, 2006).

With increasing access to advanced diagnostic imaging, MRI techniques are commonly used prior to, or in tandem with, CSF analysis. This combination allows evaluation of the structure (MRI) and biochemical/cellular components (CSF) of the nervous system. Normal imaging findings should not be used as a reason to omit CSF analysis from the diagnostic work up. Abnormal CSF findings can be encountered in cases with normal MRI evaluation. CSF abnormalities are more common than MRI changes in cases of inflammation, degenerative myelopathies, and idiopathic epilepsy/vestibular disease (Bohn *et al.*, 2006; Hugo *et al.*, 2014). Predominant cell types on CSF cytology have been associated with MRI changes, with large mononuclear pleocytosis being almost 23 times more likely to have MRI changes

DOI: 10.1201/9781003258551-14

compared to lymphocytic/small mononuclear or neutrophilic pleocytosis (Hugo *et al.*, 2014). Additionally, CSF analysis may not contribute to a diagnosis when MRI findings provide obvious evidence of intervertebral disk disease (IVDD) or vertebral malformation/instability. However, CSF analysis can aid in the determination of severity and prognosis in these settings (Bohn *et al.*, 2006; Chamisha *et al.*, 2015). CSF analysis has also been recommended prior to contrast studies when meningitis is suspected. Radiopaque contrast medium can exacerbate meningitis-associated clinical signs; a finding supportive of an inflammatory process by CSF could be a contraindication for contrast studies (Wamsley, 2013).

Appropriate timing of sample collection can improve the diagnostic utility of CSF analysis. For example, in dogs with idiopathic epilepsy, both CSF and MRI findings should be normal except, perhaps, following a seizure event (Mellema *et al.*, 1999; Hasegawa *et al.*, 2004; Bohn *et al.*, 2006; Creevy *et al.*, 2013). Therefore, it might be less diagnostically useful to evaluate CSF in a post-ictal patient and pursuing CSF analysis after a seizure-free interval is recommended. As previously mentioned, radiologic contrast dyes will cause an inflammatory response, so sampling after contrast administration would be less diagnostically useful than sampling before contrast administration.

CSF collection in small animals requires general anesthesia. The diagnostic benefits of analysis must be weighed against the anesthetic risk of collection when making diagnostic plans, especially in severely debilitated or compromised patients. Alternative anesthetic protocols, especially ones that do not increase CSF pressure, may be appropriate.

The most common complication associated with CSF collection is hemorrhage. This may be a small amount of hemorrhage associated with transit through a dural or extradural blood vessel, or significant disruption of one of the ramifications of the vertebral plexi. Incidental transit through a dural blood vessel is seen as a flash of blood present at the beginning of sample collection, which clears as CSF is allowed to flow during collection. This amount of hemorrhage is typically not clinically meaningful but can pose a diagnostic challenge in some cases.

Puncture and trauma to the brainstem or spinal cord has been reported, but only rarely (Platt *et al.*, 2005; Luján-Feliu-Pascual *et al.*, 2008). Patients suspected of atlantoaxial subluxation, Chiari-like malformation, or cervical trauma may be at higher risk of trauma due to CSF collection; care should be taken with these cases (Di Terlizzi & Platt, 2009). Additionally, strict compliance to aseptic technique is critical to avoid introduction of infectious agents into the CNS. Bacterial and fungal infections secondary to CSF collection have occurred. As would be expected, CNS complications in these cases can be terminal, although many reported patients have shown gradual recovery.

Respiratory distress due to kinking of endotracheal tubes during positioning for collection is possible. This is essentially only seen with cerebellomedullary collections where the neck must be flexed. Kinking of the tube can be avoided by using a guarded or reinforced tube. Likewise, careful attention to endotracheal cuff pressure during flexion of the neck is recommended to prevent trauma to the trachea.

Increased intracranial pressure (ICP) is often listed as a specific contraindication for CSF collection. ICP can be increased due to intracranial space-occupying lesions (most commonly neoplasia), trauma, hydrocephalus, or inflammatory lesions (Tipold, 2003). Elevation of the head can cause decreased ICP at the cerebellomedullary cistern and increased ICP on lumbar puncture (Carlson *et al.*, 2003). It is believed that the sudden focal release of pressure on puncture of the subarachnoid space for CSF collection can cause herniation and subsequent trauma (Rand *et al.*, 1994b). The true magnitude of this risk has been questioned.

Collection technique

In dogs and cats, CSF can be collected from the cerebellomedullary cistern and the lumbar space. The lumbar space is more likely to have blood contamination. Choice of cerebellomedullary or lumbar puncture should be based on the location of the suspected lesion, an assessment of potential complications, and the comfort of the clinician. Collection as close to and distal to the lesion is recommended (Lampe *et al.*, 2020b). A quick synopsis of CSF collection techniques is provided in Table 14.1.

Table 14.1 **Basic overview of CSF collection techniques**

	Cerebellomedullary cistern	Lumbar space
Patient positioning	Lateral recumbency Spine at edge of table Head flexed at 90° angle Median plane of nose parallel to table	Lateral recumbency Spine at edge of table Pelvis flexed
Puncture location	Atlanto-occipital space	L6–L7 intervertebral space in cats L5–L6 intervertebral space L4–L5 intervertebral space in large dogs
Landmarks (intersection of lines drawn between)	Wings of axis Occipital crest and dorsal arch of axis	Ilial crests Lumbar spinous processes (L6–L7 interspinous space)
Needle position	Perpendicular to spinal cord Bevel facing cranium	45° angle (hub closer to tail) Bevel facing cranium
Collection site	Cerebellomedullary cistern (dorsal to spinal cord)	Ventral subarachnoid space (needle passes through cauda equina)

For collection from both sites, a wide area is clipped and surgically scrubbed. A 22- to 25-gauge 40–90 mm spinal needle can generally be used (Elias & Brown, 2008; Di Terlizzi & Platt, 2009). The stylet included with spinal needles will prevent sampling of tissue during insertion of the needle, but will also block the initial flash of CSF seen on penetration of the dura. This initial flash can be used as a cue that the correct location has been accessed. If a stylet is present, it can be removed after advancing the needle close to the appropriate depth. This will help detect penetration to the correct location and aid the inexperienced collector (Di Terlizzi & Platt, 2009).

Approximately 1–2 ml of CSF should be collected if possible, and is usually sufficient for most diagnostic purposes. As much as 1 ml of CSF for every 5 kg of body weight can be safely collected (Elias & Brown, 2008). CSF should be collected into plain, noncoated, plastic collection tubes. Glass tubes should be avoided as cells tend to adhere to glass. EDTA containing tubes can be used but are typically not needed for anticoagulant purposes; CSF does not routinely clot. Furthermore, EDTA has a bacteriostatic effect that will interfere when culturing the sample and EDTA itself may alter results of other diagnostic testing.

Collection of CSF might not always be achieved on the first try. If bone is encountered, the needle can be pulled back and redirected along a new trajectory until the appropriate space is located. If blood is present in the needle prior to puncture of the cistern, or if frank hemorrhage is encountered, a new needle should be used. If blood is noted after puncture of the cistern, it will often clear if CSF is allowed to flow through the needle. The initial blood-contaminated sample can be collected into an EDTA containing tube to prevent clotting. When blood contamination has visually cleared, a fresh anticoagulant free tube should be used.

Cerebellomedullary cistern

With the patient in lateral recumbency, the area is clipped and scrubbed and the patient positioned with the spine at the edge of the table. This allows sufficient room for CSF to drop out of the needle hub and into the collection tube. Right-handed individuals will typically find it easiest to position the patient with the head to the right. The neck should be flexed until the head is at an approximate right angle to the spine. This will open up the atlanto-occipital space. Padding to keep the median plane of the nose parallel to the table will help prevent axial rotation of the spinal column and ensure proper alignment of nervous tissue structures surrounding the cistern.

The insertion point for the needle is along the midline at the level of a line drawn between the wings of the axis. The midline can be located by palpation of the occipital crest and the dorsal arch of the axis (Figures 14.1a, b). A skin incision with a hypodermic needle or scalpel blade may help in thick skinned animals. The needle is advanced along the median plane with the bevel of the needle facing cranially. In medium to large breed dogs, resistance will be felt during penetration of the dura. After passing through the dura, slight advancement through the meninges will position the needle in the cistern. In smaller animals, resistance at the ligament may not be felt; removal of the stylet from the needle will allow visualization of CSF in the hub on entering the cistern. CSF should begin to flow freely, although sometimes slowly, from the hub and can be caught in a plain,

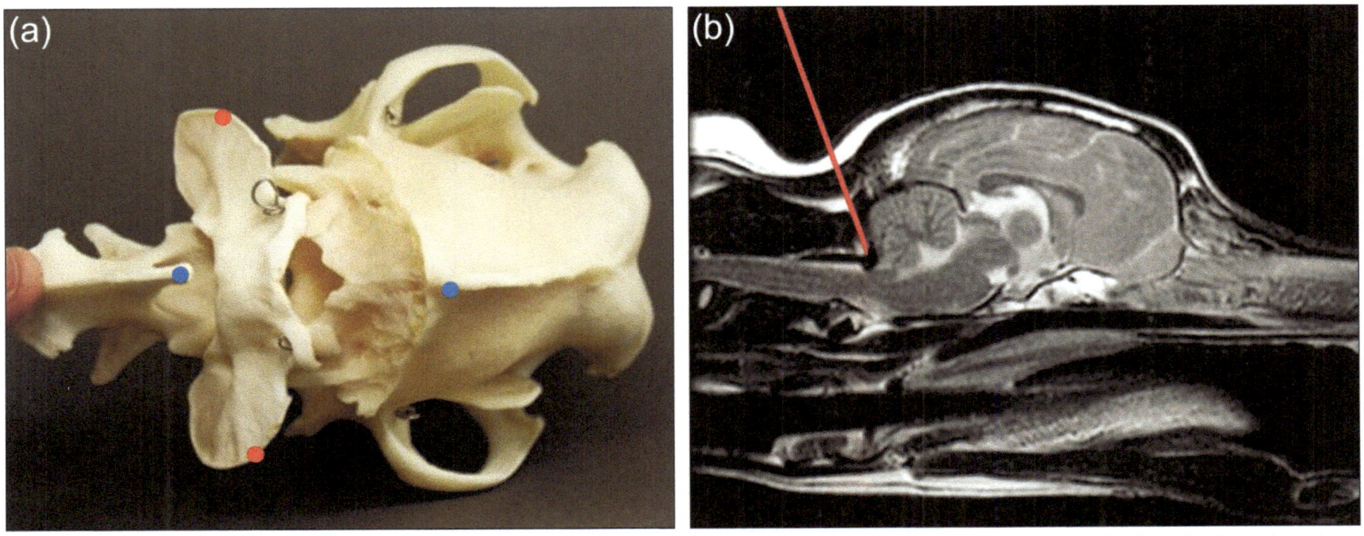

Figures 14.1a, b **Needle placement for a cerebellomedullary cisternal tap. (a) A dorsal view of the caudal aspect of the skull (right), atlas (center), and axis (left) is presented. The neck is in proper flexion for a CSF tap; this opens up the foramen magnum and allows access to the cistern. Red dots indicate the wings of the axis. Blue dots indicate the occipital crest (right) and the spinous process of the axis (left). Needle insertion is approximately at the location where a line connecting the red dots and a line connecting the blue dots would intersect. (Courtesy Neurology Department, College of Veterinary Medicine and Biomedical Sciences, Colorado State University.) (b) T2-weighted mid-sagittal MR image of the head and neck of a dog (rostral is to the right). The red line represents a needle accessing the cerebellomedullary cistern. Note that the bevel is facing cranially. The patient's neck was not maximally flexed when positioning for this image. (MR image obtained and reviewed by a Diplomate of the American College of Veterinary Radiologists at Colorado State University, Fort Collins, Co.)**

additive-free tube. Suction is generally not recommended or needed. If the needle is passed through the cerebellomedullary cistern, it will penetrate the spinal cord and may cause damage.

Lumbar cistern

The clipped and scrubbed patient is placed in lateral recumbency with the spine along the edge of the table. This allows sufficient room for CSF to drop out of the needle hub and into the collection tube. Right-handed individuals will usually find it easiest to position the patient with the head to the right. The pelvis is flexed to help open up the intervertebral spaces.

The insertion point is along the midline at the level of the L6–L7 interspinous space in most patients (Figures 14.2a, b). In larger dogs, the L5–L6 interspinous space may be used. A line drawn between the iliac crests will fall at the level of the L6–L7 interspinous space and can be used as a landmark to help find where to palpate. A skin incision with a hypodermic needle or scalpel blade can be used in thick skinned animals. The needle is advanced along the median plane at a 45° angle to the spine, with the hub of the needle closer to the tail. With skin penetration at the level of the L6–L7 interspinous space and this angle of approach, the needle actually passes through the L5–L6 intervertebral space. Similarly, the L5–L6 interspinous space will allow access to the L5–L4 intervertebral space. The bevel of the needle faces cranially. Because there is less risk of trauma at the lumbar site, the stylet can be left in place until after penetration of the dura. After passing through the dura, the needle typically continues through the cauda equina; this may cause a tail or leg twitch. Although slightly unsettling if it is not expected, this should not lead to significant damage. With a lumbar puncture, CSF is typically collected from the ventral vertebral sinus; if fluid can be obtained from the dorsal space there is less chance of causing trauma. However, sampling from the dorsal space is typically not feasible.

Cerebrospinal fluid handling

Immediately after collection, any tubes containing CSF should be labeled with a minimum of patient ID, sample material (CSF), and volume and type of additive, if used.

CSF is a highly labile material; delays in sample handling can drastically alter test results and should be avoided (Bienzle *et al.*, 2000; Fry *et al.*, 2006). Immediate refrigeration and some form of processing or stabilization of the cellular component of the sample should be instituted within 1 hour of collection (Cook & DeNicola, 1988).

Stabilization of the cellular component of CSF is most important in samples with a protein concentration <50 mg/dl. Cellularity in samples with a protein concentration >50 mg/dl was shown to be fairly stable with just refrigeration for up to 12 hours, while samples with lower protein levels demonstrated an increase in unrecognizable cells and alterations in cell percentages during that same time period and conditions (Fry *et al.*, 2006). Of more concern is the

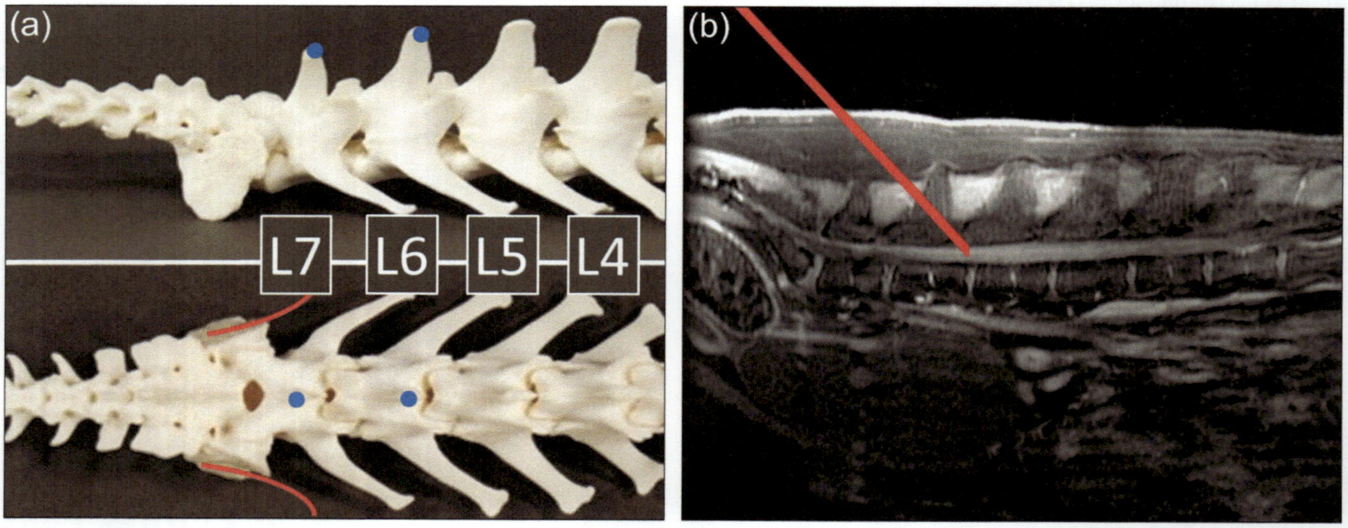

Figures 14.2a, b **Needle placement for a lumbar tap.** (a) Lateral (top) and dorsal (bottom) views of the caudal spine are presented (cranial is to the right). The pelvis has been removed for ease of visualization. The approximate locations of the crests of the ilium are marked with red lines. Blue dots indicate the spinous processes of L6 and L7. Needle insertion is at the L6–L7 interspinous process, approximately at the location where a line connecting the ilial crests and a line connecting the blue dots would intersect. (Courtesy Neurology Department, College of Veterinary Medicine and Biomedical Sciences, Colorado State University.) (b) T2-weighted mid-sagittal MR image of the lumbosacral spinal of a dog (cranial is to the right). The red line represents a needle accessing the vertebral sinus with skin puncture at the level of the L6–L7 interspinous space. The needle travels along a 45° angle with the bevel facing cranially to enter at the L5–L6 intervertebral space. When positioning for a CSF tap, flexing the pelvis will help to open up the intervertebral space. (MR image obtained and reviewed by a Diplomate of the American College of Veterinary Radiologists at Colorado State University, Fort Collins, Co.)

finding that not all cell populations are affected equally by delayed sample handling. Large mononuclear cell percentages decrease and unrecognizable cell percentages increase as early as 2 hours after collection when no preservation other than refrigeration is used (Fry *et al.*, 2006). Small mononuclear cells demonstrate a slower but significant degeneration with prolonged refrigeration. Neutrophils seem least affected by delayed processing. The amount and type of cellular degeneration observed with delayed sample handling will adversely affect the accuracy of the cytologic interpretation. If a sample cannot be analyzed within 24 hours, addition of a preservative is recommended.

Oncotic agents have been recommended as preservatives of the cellular components of CSF samples. Addition of 20% (v/v) fetal calf serum (~3.5 g/dl [35 g/l] protein), a 1:1 volume of hydroxyethyl starch, or three drops of autologous serum for every 0.25 ml of CSF can be recommended (Bienzle *et al.*, 2000; Fry *et al.*, 2006). Serum appears to preserve small and large mononuclear cells better than neutrophils. Hydroxyethyl starch appears to stabilize neutrophils and small mononuclear cells better than large mononuclear cells. CSF samples collected in EDTA tubes have not been shown to influence nucleated cell count or cell preservation (Koch *et al.*, 2019). Addition of 11% autologous serum has shown significant positive results in improving and maintaining cell morphology up to 48–72 hours. Higher concentrations (29%) may create a protein precipitate artifact that could interfere with cytologic evaluation in samples with elevated protein levels. Noted findings include condensation of large mononuclear cells and confusion with small mononuclear cells/lymphocytes, which could affect nucleated cell counts. However, addition of higher concentrations may be helpful for preservation of samples with low protein levels (Bienzle *et al.*, 2000). A recent equine study also confirmed the reliability of autologous serum as a promising preservative up to 96 hours (Quattrini *et al.*, 2023). Studies with larger sample sizes, especially with feline patients, are needed.

Previously, 10% neutral buffered formalin, 50% alcohol, or 90% alcohol have been recommended as preservatives. These agents alter cellular morphology and make cytologic evaluation more challenging. Their use is no longer recommended. A recent study has also revealed the commonly used colloid Vetstarch to be an unreliable stabilizing agent for CSF (Peterson *et al.*, 2020).

Addition of a preservative will have a dilutional effect on the sample. The additive should be reported to the laboratory performing cell counts or other analysis so that proper adjustment for the dilution can be made. As expected, autologous or calf serum will also alter the protein content. A preservative-free aliquot should be submitted concurrently to be used for non-cell related analysis. If an additive is needed, great care should be used to ensure sterility. Considerable bacterial growth can occur during sample transit; such growth will cause alteration in sample cellularity and interpretation (Figure 14.3).

CSF should not be frozen until after evaluation of cellularity has been performed. Freezing will destroy the cells. Freezing can be used as long-term storage for further biochemical testing; however, this is typically only needed in research settings. Unaltered CSF shows no significant change in total protein (TP) when refrigerated at 4°C for up to 48 hours (Fry *et al.*, 2006).

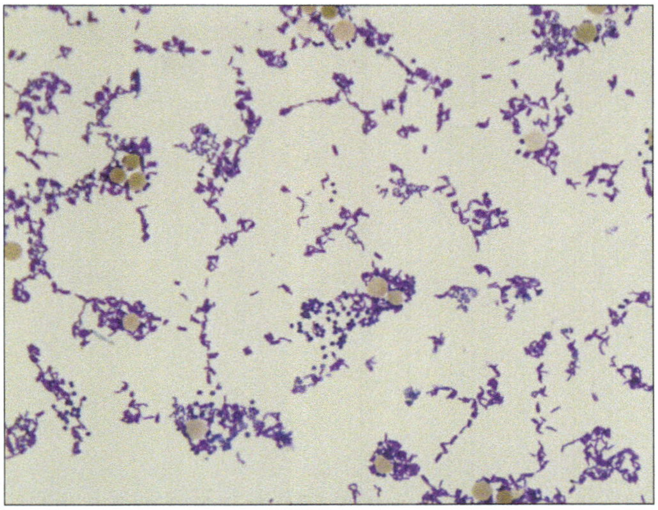

Figure 14.3 **CSF from a 10-year-old Golden Retriever. TNCC = 1 cell/µl, CSF TP = 72 mg/dl. Sample was in transit 3 days before analysis. Note the large number of mixed bacteria present and the lack of an inflammatory population. This is suggestive of bacterial overgrowth; alternatively, it is possible that the inflammatory cells degenerated during shipping (Wright–Giemsa, 1,000× magnification).**

Laboratory analysis

Multiple laboratory tests can be performed on CSF. As reference laboratories become more readily accessible, processing of CSF samples in a clinical setting is becoming a less common event. Often, more advanced analytical techniques can be used in a reference laboratory. Such laboratories also tend to employ more thorough quality control protocols than are practical for in-clinic laboratories. Basic analytical procedures are outlined here to help the reader understand the analytical principles involved and their inherent variability. Some of these techniques can be used in-clinic if needed.

Macroscopic evaluation

Typically, CSF is grossly very bland. Color and turbidity are usually assessed as the first step of analysis. CSF should be clear and colorless.

Turbidity

CSF turbidity is normally graded as clear, turbid, or cloudy (Figure 14.4). Clear CSF means that it is very easy to read newsprint through the sample. Turbid or cloudy CSF can be due to several causes, although it is almost always associated with increased cellularity. Estimates indicate that turbidity is visible when cell counts are >500 cells/µl (0.5×10^9/l) (Di Terlizzi & Platt, 2009).

Color

Visual detection of changes in CSF color is limited. Holding the sample up against a white background can help highlight subtle color deviations in the CSF. Pink to red discoloration may be seen with hemorrhage. Yellow discoloration of CSF is termed xanthochromia

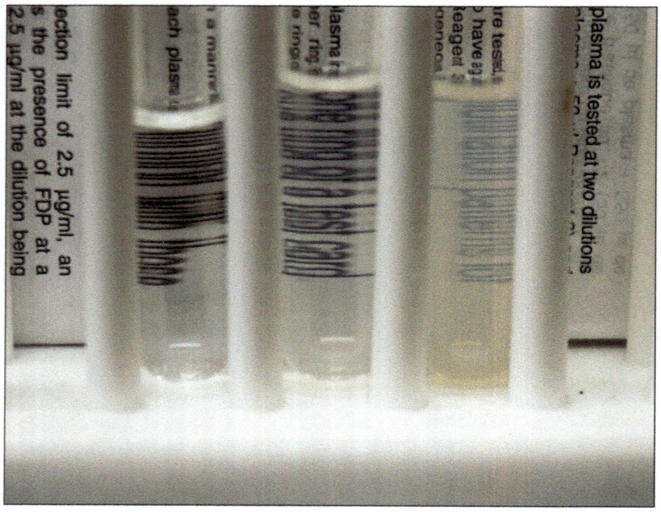

Figure 14.4 The tube to the far left is clear – print can easily be read through the sample. The tube in the middle is turbid – print is readable but hazy. The tube to the far right is cloudy – print is visible through the fluid but not readable.

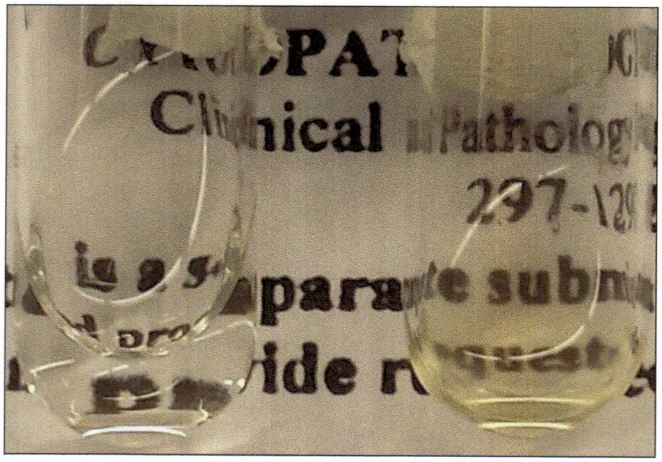

Figure 14.5 The tube on the left contains CSF with normal gross findings: clear and colorless. The tube on the right is both xanthochromic and turbid. Note how the printing on the paper behind the normal sample is crisp, while the printing behind the turbid sample is hazy.

and is typically associated with chronic *in-vivo* hemorrhage (Figure 14.5). As hemoglobin breaks down it first forms oxyhemoglobin and then progresses to bilirubin (Shah & Edlow, 2002). The conversion to oxyhemoglobin can occur both inside and outside the body. The conversion from oxyhemoglobin to bilirubin only occurs *in vivo*. Bilirubin imparts a yellow color to the fluid. Therefore, only pathology that causes red cells to enter the CSF *in vivo* is expected to lead to xanthochromia. Measurement of CSF bilirubin, oxyhemoglobin, and total protein (CSF TP) is used as a more sensitive test for *in-vivo* hemorrhage than visual detection of xanthochromia in human medicine (Falconer *et al.*, 2015).

Serum bilirubin is typically prevented from entering the CNS (Ostrow *et al.*, 2004). However, in extreme hyperbilirubinemia, unconjugated bilirubin can accumulate in nervous tissue. This condition is called kernicterus and causes both bilirubin-associated CNS toxicity and xanthochromia (Belz *et al.*, 2013).

Cell counting

Due to the low cell concentration in most CSF samples, the gold standard for cell counting remains the hemocytometer. This is true in spite of the potentially high variability in repeated measurements of the same sample. One study measuring total nucleated cell count (TNCC) over time with various preservation techniques found a majority of samples had at least one TNCC that was higher 2–48 hours after collection than when the same sample was counted immediately on collection (Fry *et al.*, 2006).

Automated counting techniques have been investigated for CSF (Andrews *et al.*, 2005; Becker *et al.*, 2008; Ruotsalo *et al.*, 2008; Romero-Fernandez *et al.*, 2020; Ortiz-Nisa *et al.*, 2021). These methods have several advantages for highly cellular CSF but have historically had poor performance in samples with low cellularity, which make up the majority of samples. Recent studies on newer generation automated hematology analyzers have shown promising data supporting high sensitivity and specificity in quantification of low cellularity CSF samples in dogs, though they still recommend manual cytologic evaluation to perform differential cell counts (Romero-Fernandez *et al.*, 2020; Ortiz-Nisa *et al.*, 2021). Even studies that advocate counting by automated means provide recommendations for when a hemocytometer count is necessary.

Hemocytometer count

The first step in performing a hemocytometer count is to ensure that the hemocytometer and weighted coverslip are lint free. This is done by rinsing the components with alcohol and allowing the alcohol to evaporate. A humidity chamber is also needed to prevent the sample from drying during preparation. This can be made with a Petri dish lined with a damp sponge or piece of filter paper. A pair of wooden tongue depressors or wooden cotton-tipped swab handles laid over the damp material will elevate the hemocytometer and make sample handing easier (Figure 14.6).

The CSF is gently mixed by inverting the sample tube 15–20 times. Ten µl of CSF is loaded under the coverslip into each side of the hemocytometer. Except in cases of extremely high cell counts, CSF does not need dilution prior to loading in a hemocytometer. After loading, the hemocytometer is allowed to rest in the humidity chamber for 5 minutes so that the cells will settle to the bottom of the counting platform before placing the hemocytometer under a microscope for counting. Turning down the illumination and dropping the condenser will allow easier distinction of the cells and facilitate counting. Nucleated cells and erythrocytes in all nine large squares are counted on both sides of the hemocytometer (Figures 14.7a, b, 14.8a). The mean count of the two sides multiplied by 1.1 will provide the TNCC/µl and RBC/µl of the sample, respectively.

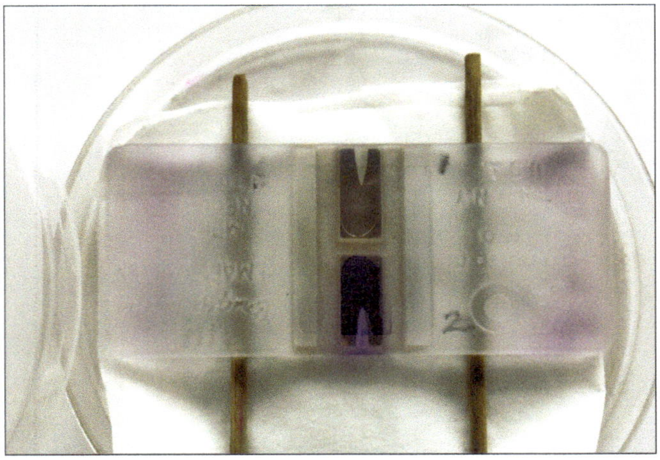

Figure 14.6 A simple humidity chamber for a hemocytometer can be constructed with a Petri dish, absorbent material, and wooden cotton-tipped swab handles. The upper chamber (labeled 1) is loaded with unstained CSF. The lower chamber (labeled 2) is loaded with new methylene blue-stained CSF. Typically, only stained or unstained sample will be used, not both.

A new methylene blue staining technique has been described and can aid in identification of cells during counting (Figure 14.8b; Fry *et al.*, 2006). With this technique, new methylene blue stain is drawn into a microhematocrit tube until one-third of the tube is filled. The stain is then drained out of the tube by blotting on a gauze sponge, essentially removing the major volume of stain and any dilutional effects. The opposite end of the tube is used to draw up CSF until the tube is half filled. The microhematocrit tube is carefully rocked several times to mix the residual stain into the CSF. After 1–5 minutes of incubation, the tube is rocked again to ensure complete mixing of the sample and the hemocytometer can be loaded as usual. With this staining technique, nucleated cells should be easier to distinguish from RBCs; most, but not all, RBCs will not stain while the nucleated cells should stain blue (Becker *et al.*, 2008).

Protein quantification

CSF contains very low amounts of protein. CSF TP is typically measured as mg/dl while serum protein is measured as g/dl. Neither protein determination by refractometer nor the chemical technique used to measure protein in serum is sensitive enough for CSF protein evaluation. For this reason, alternative methods must be used to accurately measure the protein content of CSF. Several dye binding microprotein analytical techniques have been developed but are not usually available outside the reference laboratory. These techniques produce slightly different results from each other and require their own reference intervals for accurate interpretation (Riond *et al.*, 2013). Most, but not all, of these techniques are equally sensitive to both albumin and globulins. This is an advantage. Normal CSF protein is predominantly albumin. Globulin concentrations can increase dramatically secondary to pathology. Differentiation of albumin and globulin has not proven any more sensitive than an accurate TP analysis; therefore, a method that detects both protein groups is recommended (Behr *et al.*, 2006).

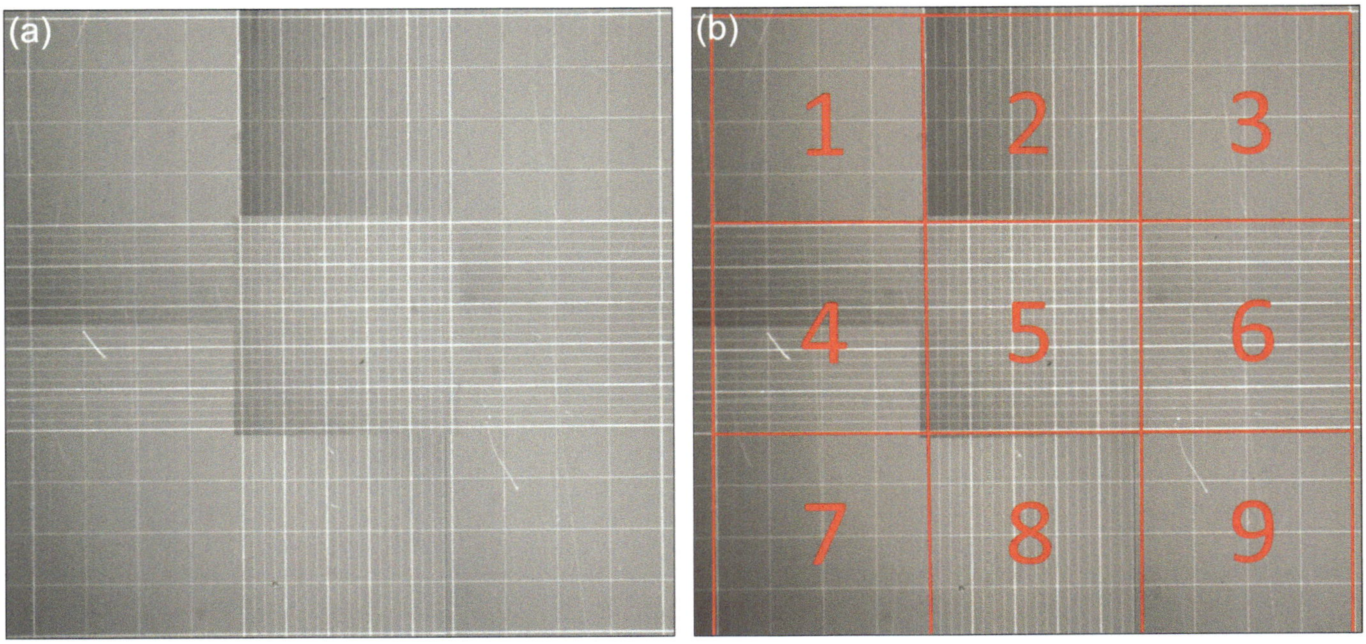

Figures 14.7a, b (a) A hemocytometer grid contains precisely measured lines which, with use of the appropriate weighted coverslip, define the volume of fluid within each square. (b) Each of the outlined and numbered squares contains 0.1 µl of fluid. For CSF cell counting, the number of cells in all nine of the numbered squares is counted and multiplied by 1.1 to adjust to the desired units of cells/µl (1 µl/0.9 µl = 1.1).

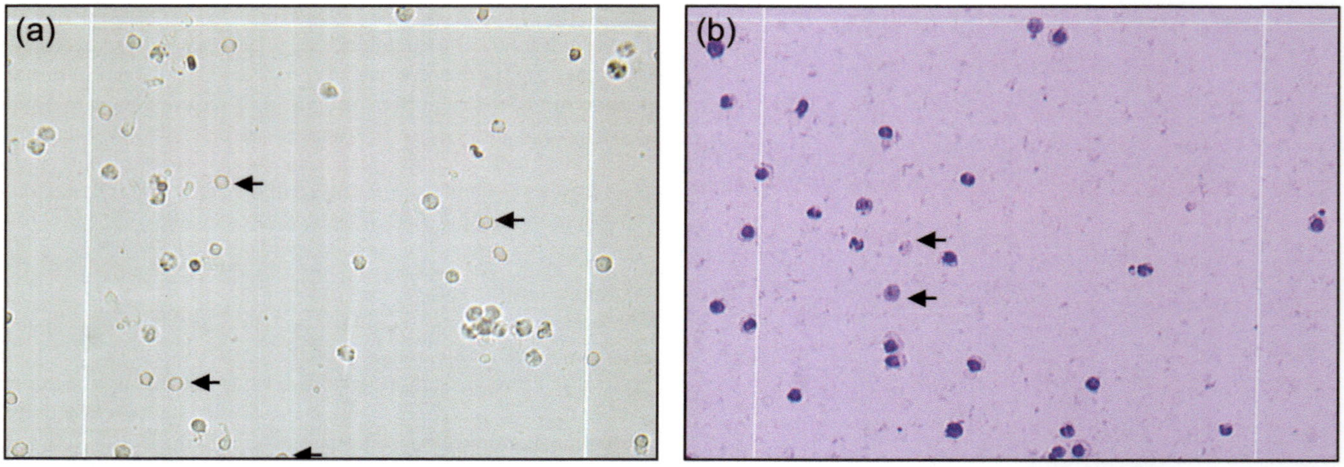

Figures 14.8a, b (a) 200× view of a hemocytometer loaded with unstained CSF. Red blood cells are smaller, round, slightly red, and lack internal structures. Three red blood cells in the image are denoted by arrows; several other red blood cells are present in the field. Nucleated cells are larger and contain an internal structure. (b) 200× view of a hemocytometer loaded with new methylene blue-stained CSF. Two red blood cells are denoted by arrows. They are round, pale blue, and lack nuclear structures. Nuclei stain a deep blue. Although the cell types cannot be differentiated with this technique, distinguishing between red cells and nucleated cells is easier.

A semiquantitative measurement of CSF TP can be made using the protein pad of a urine dipstick (Behr *et al.*, 2003). Most urine dipstick manufactures provide a conversion of the Trace to ++++ scale to a semiquantitative protein value. This method was fairly well correlated with dye binding techniques (Jacobsen *et al.*, 2012). However, urine test strips have their limitations. One study found that test strips were unable to detect globulins when present at 1 g/l, a concentration much greater than would be expected in most abnormal CSF samples (Behr *et al.*, 2003). Ultimately, dipstick measurement is semiquantitative at best and cannot be recommended, except as a screening tool or in an emergency situation.

Historically, qualitative tests such as the Pandy test and the Nonne-Apelt test have been used as more sensitive tests for globulins. Currently, these tests are not routinely used in reference laboratories because of their subjectivity and have largely been replaced by quantitative tests.

Protein electrophoresis

Further classification of CSF protein into albumin and alpha-, beta-, and gammaglobulin fractions can be made using electrophoretic techniques. Both high-resolution electrophoretic techniques and electrophoresis after concentration have been evaluated (Behr *et al.*, 2006; Gama *et al.*, 2007). In a study of 100 high-resolution electrophoretic profiles of canine CSF, electrophoretic evaluation for calculation of albumin quota was highly correlated with TP determination. Significantly, the protein pattern was not associated with any specific pathologic process and albumin quota was no more sensitive for blood–brain barrier dysfunction than CSF TP alone (Behr *et al.*, 2006). These findings suggest that electrophoresis may not be a valuable ancillary diagnostic tool in canine neurologic diseases.

Miscellaneous testing

Many ancillary tests have been proposed for use on CSF. Some of these tests have a clear utility in specific diagnostic settings, while the clinical worth of others is still under investigation. Some of these tests, their potential use, and a limited reference list can be found in Table 14.2.

Cytologic sample preparation and evaluation

Cytologic evaluation of CSF is recommended and may prove useful any time CSF is collected, even when the TNCC is within normal limits (Di Terlizzi & Platt, 2006). Due to the extremely low cellularity of CSF, cell concentration is required. In the reference laboratory setting, this is typically done with a specialized cytocentrifuge and funnels, which remove excess fluid and concentrate the cells into a small area of the slide (Figure 14.9). Unless a clinic performs a large number of fluid analyses, purchasing a specialized cytocentrifuge is not likely to be a wise business decision. Handmade sedimentation chambers can be attempted, but they have shown poor correlation between cellular percentages and may cause decreased cell counts compared to appropriately cytocentrifuged samples (Wamsley, 2013). Utilizing the remaining CSF in the needle shaft and hub to make a direct line smear has shown strong correlation with samples evaluated in a commercial pathology lab and can help provide rapid, clinically meaningful information prior to evaluation by a clinical pathologist (Newton *et al.*, 2017).

Romanowsky-type stains, such as Wright–Giemsa or quick-type Romanowsky stains, have been used for routine cytologic evaluation of CSF. Cells are typically designated as small mononuclear cells, large mononuclear cells, surface epithelial cells, neutrophils, eosinophils, plasma cells, or mast cells.

Table 14.2 **Commonly used or proposed ancillary tests performed with CSF. Diagnostic utility of some of these tests is still under investigation**

Test	Description	Reported utility	References
Albumin quotient	Ratio of CSF albumin to serum albumin: Alb_{CSF}/Alb_{serum}	Detects blood–brain barrier disruption	Sorjonen, 1987; Behr *et al.*, 2006; Pancotto *et al.*, 2010
Neurofilament light chain (NfL)	Neuron-specific cytoskeletal proteins released with axonal damage associated with MUE	Potential biomarker for MUE and evaluating response to therapy	Yun *et al.*, 2021
IgG index	Ratio of the CSF IgG: serum IgG ratio to albumin quotient: eq001	Detects intrathecal production of immunoglobulin; may support encephalic inflammation	Mejias *et al.*, 2008; Tipold & Stein, 2010
IgA	Quantification of IgA in CSF by various methods	High levels are correlated with steroid-responsive meningitis–arteritis	Tipold & Stein, 2010
Autoantibody testing	Detection of various autoantibodies	Can be elevated in GME, NME, and other diseases	Matsuki *et al.*, 2004; Shibuya *et al.*, 2007
Glucose	Direct concentration of CSF glucose or ratio	Decrease may indicate sepsis, neoplasia,	Di Terlizzi & Platt, 2006; Witsberger *et al.*, 2012;
CSF glucose/serum ratio	With serum glucose: $glucose_{CSF}/glucose_{serum}$	or post-ictal states. Increase may indicate disruption of blood–brain barrier or nutraceutical administration	Galan *et al.*, 2013; Tumani *et al.*, 2015
Serology and molecular	Detection of infectious agents (antigen,	Various infectious agents including:	Nghiem & Schatzberg, 2010; Pérez *et al.*, 2011
testing	antibody, or DNA/RNA based tests)	*Toxoplasma*, *Neospora*, *Ehrlichia*, *Anaplasma*, *Rickettsia*, *Coccidiodes*, *Cryptococcus*, *Bartonella*	
Culture	Bacterial and fungal culture	Various agents	Nghiem & Schatzberg, 2010
Flow cytometry	Cytometric evaluation of cells in fluid	Differentiation of the mononuclear cell population. Used for B-cell/T-cell differentiation and characterization in human lymphoma. Questionable use in veterinary medicine	Duque *et al.*, 2012; Pittman *et al.*, 2013; Liu *et al.*, 2015
Matrix metalloproteinase	MMP-9, MMP-2	Concentrations may alter with intracranial	Mariani *et al.*, 2013
		neoplasia	
Neurotransmitters	GABA or glutamate	May be associated with seizure activity	Hasegawa *et al.*, 2004; Creevy *et al.*, 2013; Platt *et al.*, 2013
Fibrinolytic activity	D-dimers	Increased with inflammation. May be marker for steroid-responsive meningitis–arteritis	De la Fuente *et al.*, 2012
Metabolites	Lactate, pyruvate	May be markers for senile dementia or altered metabolism, possibly associated with infectious agents	Pugliese *et al.*, 2005; Joffe, 2007; Galan *et al.*, 2013
Lysosomal storage	Various storage materials	Detect GM-1 gangliosidosis, GM-2	Johnsrude *et al.*, 1996;
disease testing		gangliosidosis, possibly others	Satoh *et al.*, 2011
Enzyme activity	Lactate dehydrogenase, aspartate transferase, various proposed uses		Rand *et al.*, 1994a;
	Creatine kinase		Rand *et al.*, 1994b; Ferreira, 2016; Mariani *et al.*, 2020; Lampe *et al.*, 2020a; Brune *et al.*, 2022
Clusterin	Western blot analysis for clusterin	Chronic spinal cord damage: degenerative myelopathy and chronic IVDD	Shafie *et al.*, 2014

Small mononuclear cells have a scant amount of deeply basophilic cytoplasm and round condensed nucleus; in the normal patient they are small lymphocytes (Figure 14.10). Interestingly, during flow cytometric analysis of normal CSF in the dog, only 60% of the small mononuclear cells that are classified as lymphocytes by cell size and cytoplasm characteristics can be labeled with lymphoid markers (Duque *et al.*, 2012). This may simply reflect a deficiency in our ability to label all canine lymphocytes. Additional immunophenotyping studies with larger sample sizes are needed to further examine the breakdown of normal CSF mononuclear populations.

Large mononuclear cells are morphologically consistent with monocytes from the peripheral blood (Figure 14.11). They have more abundant lightly basophilic cytoplasm, which is often vacuolated, and a round to indented to ameboid nucleus.

'Surface epithelial cells' is a general descriptor for a group of choroid plexus epithelial cells, ependymal cells, endothelial cells, and meningeal cells of mesenchymal origin that look cytologically similar (Figure 14.12; Wessmann *et al* , 2010). They are small uniform cuboidal to columnar cells with moderate to abundant amounts of lightly basophilic finely granular cytoplasm and an eccentrically located small round nucleus with granular to coarse chromatin. Rarely, they are slightly spindloid or are cytologically similar to bland mesothelial cells.

The remaining inflammatory cells look similar in CSF and peripheral tissues (Figures 14.13–14.15). If a cytocentrifuge is used for

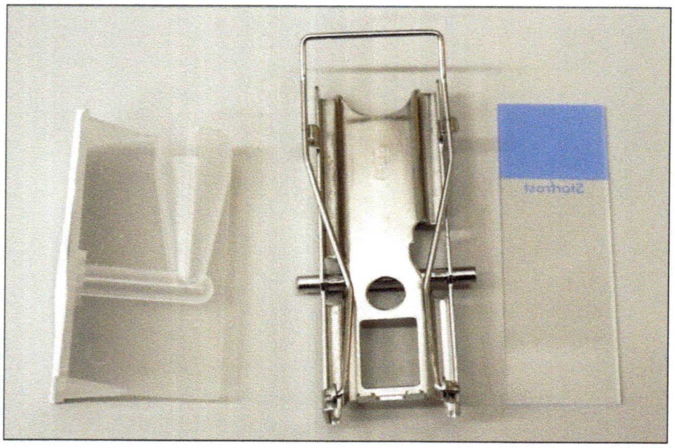

Figure 14.9 The funnel (left) and slide (right) are held together by the clamp (middle). Fluid is loaded into the funnel and then a special centrifuge is used to spin the fluid into a small area on the slide. In the process, excess fluid is absorbed by the pad on the face of the funnel. The end result is considerable concentration of the cellularity into a small area of the slide for cytologic evaluation.

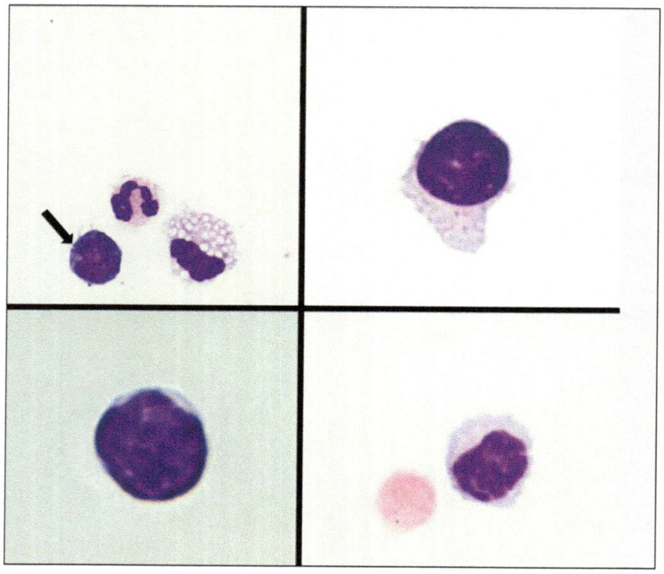

Figure 14.10 Cells counted as small mononuclear cells/lymphocytes have a minimal amount of basophilic cytoplasm, a round nucleus with condensed to clumped chromatin, and lack a visible nucleolus. Nuclei are approximately the size of a red blood cell, as seen in the bottom right image. These cells may also display an increased rim of cytoplasm and contain few punctate, magenta cytoplasmic granules as shown in the top right image. The bottom left image is from a cat, remaining images are from a dog [Wright–Giemsa, 500× magnification (top left image), 1,000× magnification (remaining images)].

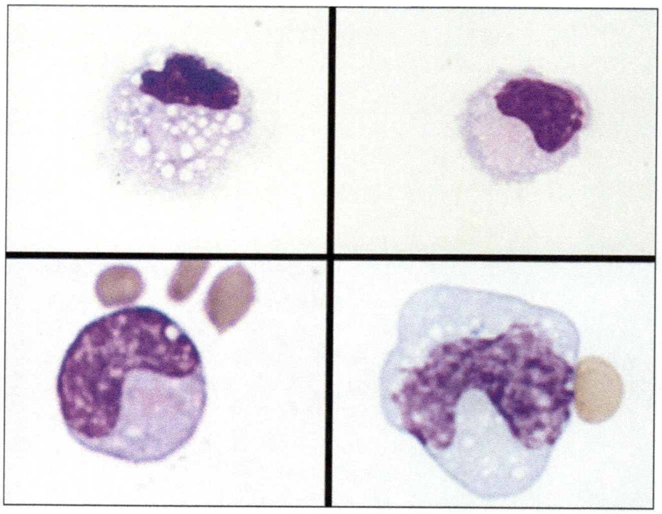

Figure 14.11 Cells counted as large mononuclear cells have an abundant amount of basophilic cytoplasm, an indented to banded to ameboid nucleus, and often contain cytoplasmic vacuoles or a frilled cytoplasmic margin. Cells on the top row from a dog. Cells on the bottom are from a cat (Wright–Giemsa, 1,000× magnification).

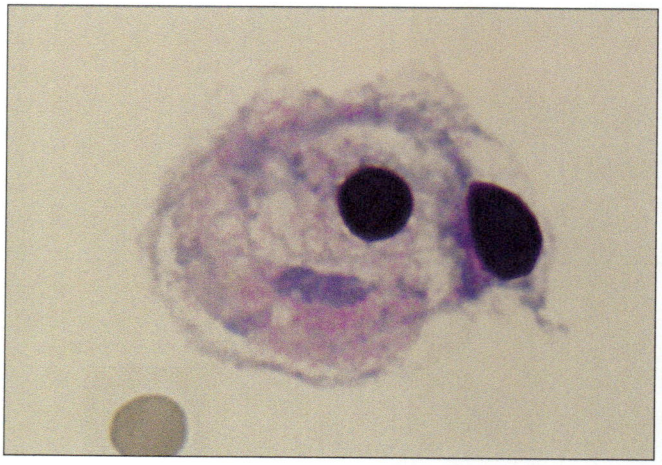

Figure 14.12 Two surface epithelial cells are presented. These cells have basophilic to pink granular cytoplasm and a condensed eccentrically placed nucleus. Surface epithelial cells describe a group of cells that look morphologically similar and typically have no diagnostic significance when found in low numbers (Wright–Giemsa, 1,000× magnification).

preparation, there will be some attenuation, or splattering, of the cells, which may accentuate a dispersed, hypersegmented, or botryoid appearance (Figure 14.16). Similar effects occur with any sample subjected to cytocentrifugation; experienced cytopathologists learn to read through this artifact.

It is best to perform a 100-cell differential count on every case; however, even a concentrated preparation of a very low cellularity fluid may not contain 100 cells for counting. In such situations, counting all of the cells present on the slide and consideration of the limitations associated with counting very few cells in the differential are recommended.

Additional stains can be used in special cases. These include Gram stain for bacteria, new methylene blue for many organisms, and Luxol fast blue for myelin. Prussian blue staining can help to confirm the presence of iron. Rarely, immunocytochemical staining for specific

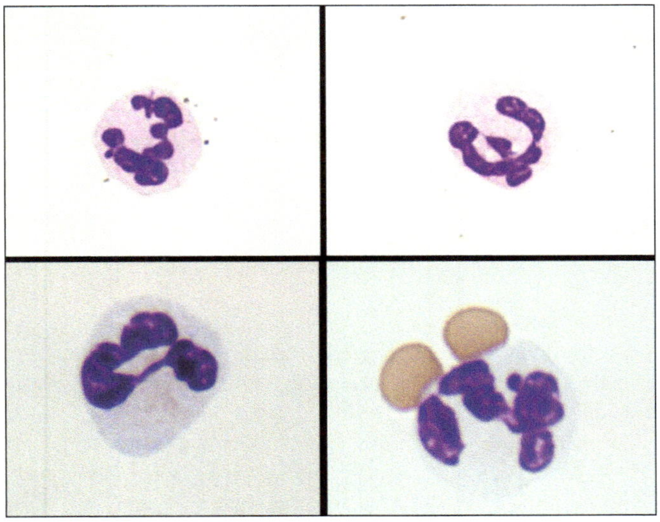

Figure 14.13 Neutrophils in CSF look similar in shape and size to neutrophils found elsewhere in the body. They have a segmented nucleus, moderate amount of pale basophilic cytoplasm, and few fine pink cytoplasmic granules. Cells on the top row are from a dog. Cells on the bottom are from a cat (Wright–Giemsa, 1,000× magnification).

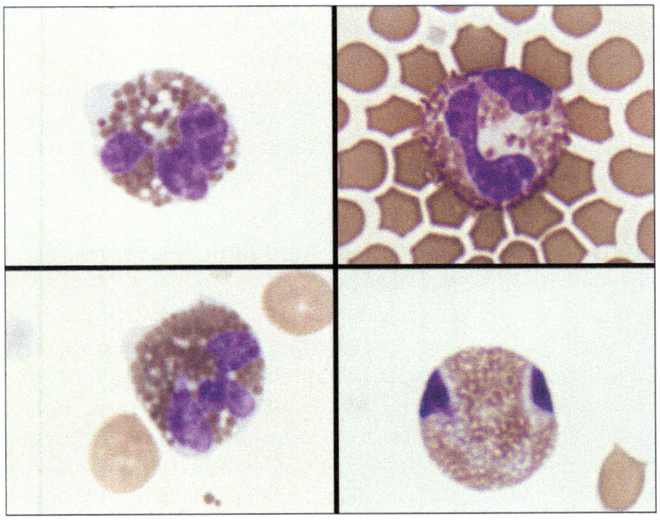

Figure 14.14 Eosinophils are only rarely found in CSF. When present, they have abundant amounts of eosinophilic granules within clear to lightly basophilic cytoplasm, and a lobulated nucleus. Cells on the left are from a dog. Cells on the right are from a cat. Note the distinct variation in granulation between the canine and feline eosinophils (Wright–Giemsa, 1,000× magnification).

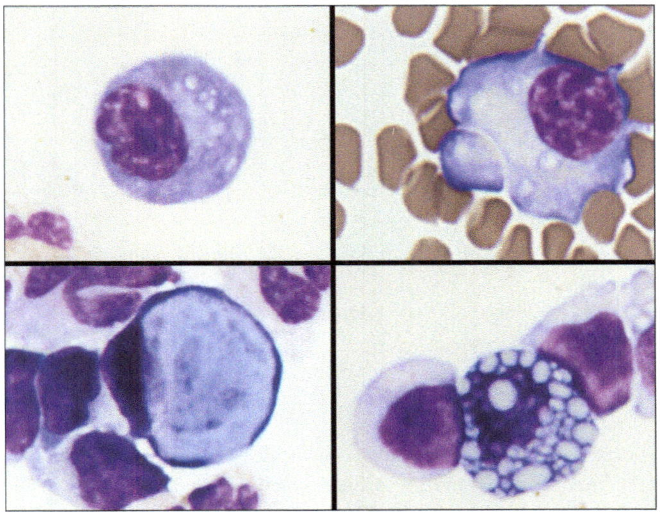

Figure 14.15 Plasma cells can be present when a pathologic process induces intrathecal immunoglobulin production. Two plasma cells are present in the top row of the image; they have small eccentrically placed nuclei with clumped chromatin, basophilic cytoplasm, and a paranuclear clear zone. Two Mott cells with distinct Russell bodies are present in the bottom row. The bottom left Mott cell contains a single large powder blue Russell body, while the bottom right Mott cell displays a more common morphology of multiple smaller Russell bodies. The cell in the upper right corner is from a cat. All other images are from dogs (Wright–Giemsa, 1,000× magnification).

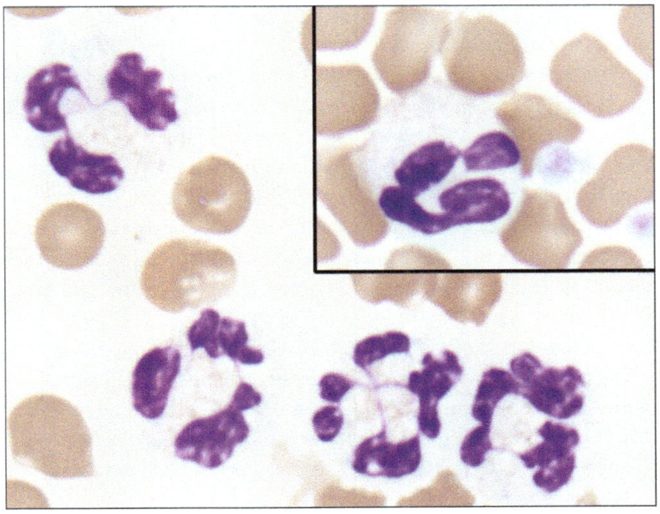

Figure 14.16 Cytocentrifugation concentration techniques often cause mild cell distortion. In this image a peripheral blood neutrophil (upper right) is compared with neutrophils in a cytocentrifuged CSF sample. The attenuated cytoplasm and botryoid nuclear morphology (multiple segments connected by central thin strands of nuclear material) is not uncommon in these types of preparations and should be interpreted carefully. Similar, but less dramatic, distortion can be seen in all cells subjected to cytocentrifugation (Wright–Giemsa, 1,000× magnification).

agents (e.g. feline coronavirus antigen) has been applied to help further identify specific structures or cells in conjunction with other tests (Gruendl *et al.*, 2019).

Normal findings

Due to the slight variations in analytical method, local population, and environment, reference intervals should be established by the

Table 14.3 **Commonly reported normal findings for canine and feline CSF. Reference intervals provided by the laboratory performing the testing are preferred**

Color	Colorless
Clarity	Clear
CSF TP	Cerebellomedullary cistern: <30 mg/dl
	Lumbar space: <45 mg/dl
TNCC	<5 cells/μl
Cellularity	Predominantly small mononuclear cells/lymphocytes and large mononuclear cells; <10% nondegenerate neutrophils, <1% eosinophils.
	Rare surface epithelial cells
RBCs	0

laboratory in which the testing is performed for all clinical pathology tests, including CSF analysis. General recommendations are provided in Table 14.3. These are based on published literature and are likely inferior to laboratory-derived intervals (Chrisman, 1992; Di Terlizzi & Platt, 2009).

Normal CSF is clear, colorless, nonviscous, and does not clot. TP values <30 mg/dl from the cerebellomedullary cistern and <45 mg/dl from a lumbar puncture have been reported as normal (Rand *et al.*, 1990a, b; Chrisman, 1992; Di Terlizzi & Platt, 2009).

RBCs are not expected in CSF *in vivo*. However, the collection process almost always induces at least a few, and sometimes many, RBCs in the final CSF sample. Clinical judgment of the importance of RBC numbers based on how the collection progressed is probably more meaningful than a statistically determined reference interval. Distinguishing blood contamination from true hemorrhage is discussed later in this chapter ('Hemorrhage').

Normal TNCC for both the cerebellomedullary cistern and lumbar punctures are generally cited as <5 cells/μl in both the dog and cat (Cook & DeNicola, 1988; Rand *et al.*, 1990a, b; Chrisman, 1992). On differential count, these are predominantly mononuclear cells comprised of small mononuclear cells consistent with small lymphocytes and large mononuclear cells consistent with monocytoid cells. There have been conflicting reports regarding whether small mononuclear cells or large mononuclear cells predominate in canine and feline CSF (Rand *et al.*, 1990a, b; Chrisman, 1992; Di Terlizzi & Platt, 2009; Duque *et al.*, 2012; Wamsley, 2013). It is generally accepted that up to 8–10% of the cell count can be nondegenerate neutrophils in normal canine and feline samples with minimal blood contamination (Rand *et al.*, 1990a, b; Chrisman, 1992; Rand *et al.*, 1994a). Similarly, eosinophil counts can be as high as 1% in normal CSF samples. Very rare mitotic figures may be seen.

Surface epithelial cells are the most common CNS cells found in CSF cytology samples which may be present in variable numbers depending on the collection technique and other factors (Wessmann *et al.*, 2010). In one retrospective study, the presence of surface epithelial cells was not associated with a specific disease process, TNCC, CSF TP, or inflammatory cell population on cytologic investigation. The suggestion was that these cells are most commonly an incidental finding acquired during needle puncture of the leptomeninges (Wessmann *et al.*, 2010). Surface epithelial cells are usually rare enough that they do not affect the TNCC.

Rarely, myelin, neuropil, or neurons have been observed following puncture at either the cerebellomedullary or lumbar location in patients without degenerative diseases (Fallin *et al.*, 1996; Luján-Feliu-Pascual *et al.*, 2008). A small amount of this material is most suggestive of incidental puncture of the spinal cord and, although not ideal, may not be a pathologic finding.

Contaminants

Post-collection contaminants are often encountered, including desquamated keratin flakes, cytocentrifuge filter fibers, glove powder, dust, and debris (Figures 14.17a, b).

Low numbers of squamous epithelial cells, muscle, or fat are most likely to be contaminants included during collection or sample handling (Figure 14.17c). Large aggregates of anucleate squamous epithelial cells could also suggest an epidermoid cyst (Figure 14.17d).

Aspiration of hematopoietic tissue suggestive of bone marrow has been reported following lumbar puncture in the dog (Christopher, 1992). This could be seen following penetration of the hematopoietic cavity within the vertebral bodies during needle placement. Alternatively, the telencephalon is a site of hematopoiesis during embryogenesis. The choroid plexus is derived from these telencephalic tissues and can host hematopoietic tissues well into adulthood, if the need arises (Bienzle *et al.*, 1995). Collection of myeloid tissue is very rarely seen and inclusion of pieces of vertebral bone or cartilage in the sample is rare.

Categories of cerebrospinal fluid abnormal findings

Elevated cerebrospinal fluid protein

Elevated CSF protein is typically caused by disruption or increased permeability of the blood–brain barrier, including physical damage to the barrier itself, extradural compressive lesions (e.g. IVDD, stenosis), necrosis, exudative processes, or intrathecal production of immunoglobulins (Riond *et al.*, 2013). Protein elevations are suggestive of pathology but not highly sensitive at distinguishing a specific etiology. Dogs with neoplasia, degenerative myelopathy, IVDD, neurovascular disorders, and inflammatory disease have been shown to have higher protein than dogs with idiopathic diseases (Bohn *et al.*, 2006). One study in the cat found that CSF TP 200 mg/dl was highly suggestive for feline infectious peritonitis (FIP) while CSF TP 100 mg/dl was seen with neoplasia, viral disease other than FIP, degenerative disease, and ischemic encephalopathy (Rand *et al.*, 1994a). Iatrogenic hemorrhage during sample collection may also increase CSF protein; this will be discussed later in this chapter (see 'Hemorrhage' section).

Historically, elevated CSF protein without a concurrent increase in cellularity has been termed 'albuminocytologic dissociation'. This term is somewhat misleading in that protein and cells enter the CSF through differing, though often concurrent, mechanisms. Increased

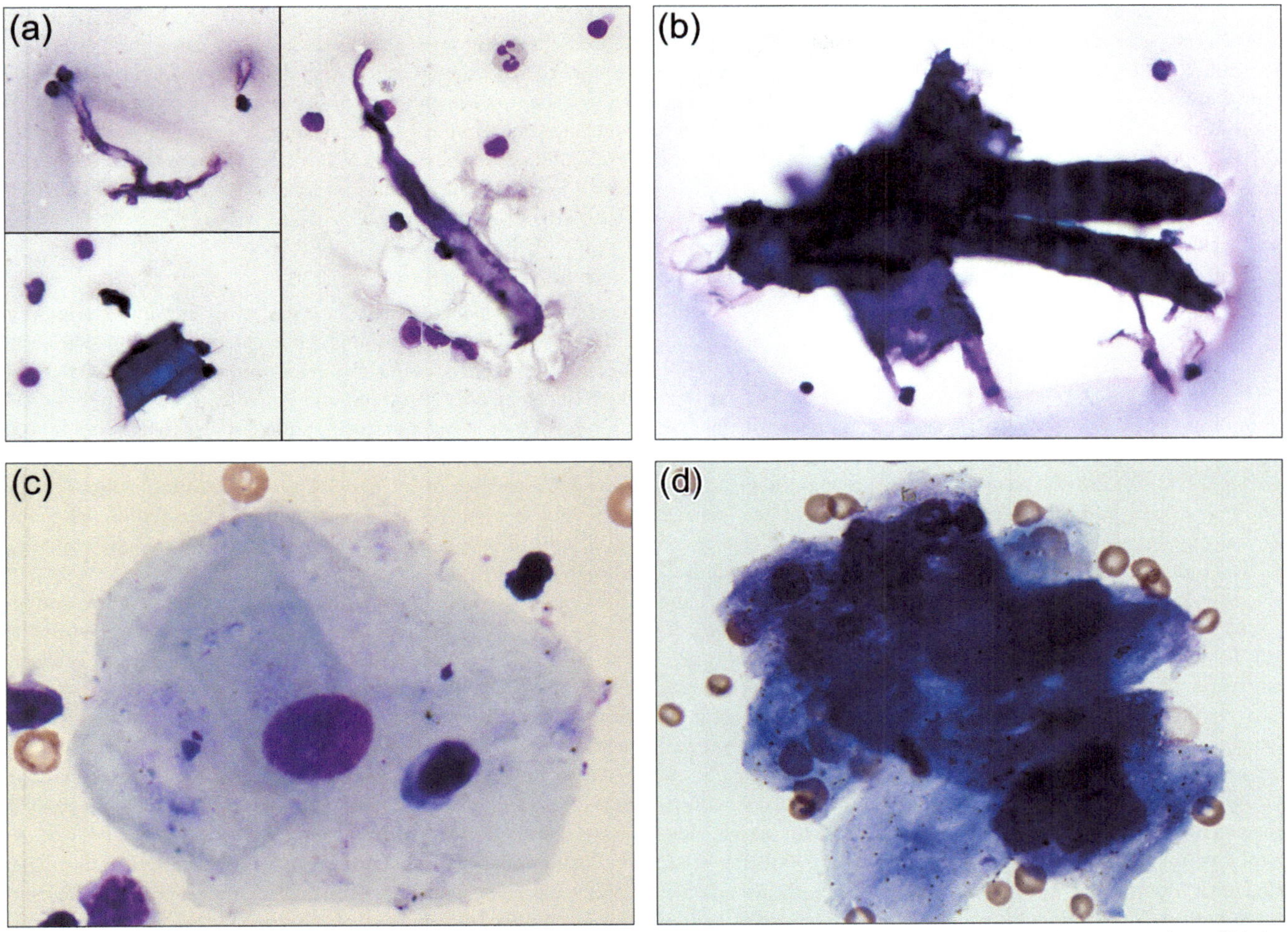

Figures 14.17a–d **Commonly encountered contaminants in CSF preparations. (a, b) Noncellular debris is commonly found in CSF samples and likely originates from lint and particulate matter that fall into the sample or filter fibers that are shed from the sedimentation apparatus. These are post-collection artifacts and can be ignored (Wright–Giemsa, 500× magnification). (c) Cellular components, such as this nucleated keratinocyte, can be included in a CSF sample during either collection or sample processing. Inclusion of this type of material is not completely avoidable, but care should be taken to minimize contamination from any causes (Wright–Giemsa, 500× magnification). (d) A large aggregate of mature keratin debris is present in a patient that does not have evidence of a cystic lesion on imaging. This is most suggestive of surface epithelial cell contamination (Wright–Giemsa, 1,000× magnification).**

CSF protein without increased cellularity would suggest that (1) the insult is not drastic enough to induce diapedesis of cells, (2) disruption of the blood–brain barrier is deep enough in the parenchyma that cells crossing the barrier cannot reach the CSF, or (3) pathologic cells originating within the blood–brain barrier are not superficial enough to slough into the CSF. This is evident in several cases where CSF analysis only found elevated TP and histologic evaluation found CNS disease deep in the nervous tissue (Snyder *et al.*, 2006; Lane, 2012b). If a sophisticated single word term for increased CSF protein is desired, the term proteinorrhacia could be accurately used. A recent retrospective study of 497 dogs found 16.5% of dogs met criteria for albuminocytological dissociation or proteinorrhacia, which were most commonly associated with cranial nerve neuropathies, underlying brain neoplasms, brain vascular events, and idiopathic vestibular disease. (Suñol *et al.*, 2021).

Altered cell percentages

Occasionally, the TNCC will be within normal limits but the percentages of cell types will be outside the expected ratio. If a sufficient number of cells are available to provide an accurate differential and there are no concerns over sample handling or peripheral blood contamination, the increased percentage of a specific cell type may be suggestive of a similar pathology, such as a true pleocytosis of that cell type. It should be remembered, however, that a delay in sample processing will cause changes in cell percentages, even when preservative agents are used.

Pleocytosis

The Greek-derived term 'pleocytosis' is used to describe an increased cell count in the CSF; it means an increase in cells. Pleocytosis is typically categorized based on the major cell type, or combination of cell types, causing the increase. This type of categorization helps to narrow down the pathologic process in play but is rarely definitive for a specific etiology. For example, a neutrophilic pleocytosis is the most common finding with IVDD. However, large mononuclear, eosinophilic, or even lymphocytic pleocytosis can be found in some patients with IVDD. Additionally, a neutrophilic pleocytosis is commonly found in neoplastic and infectious diseases.

A typical progression of the predominant inflammatory cell population occurs in the CSF as elsewhere in the body. A more acute or ongoing inflammatory process is likely to contain neutrophils. With chronicity, there is a shift to large mononuclear cells and small mononuclear cells/lymphocytes.

Neutrophilic pleocytosis

Neutrophilic pleocytosis, or an increased number of neutrophils in the CSF, is seen in cases with an acute inflammatory process (Figure 14.18). Possible causes include nervous tissue trauma (including IVDD and fibrocartilaginous embolus), hemorrhage, infectious agents, neoplasia, steroid-responsive meningitis–arteritis (SRMA), and necrotizing vasculitis. Infectious agents include bacterial (*Pseudomonas* spp., *Streptococcus* spp., *Mycobacteria* spp., and *Bartonella henselae* and related species), rickettsial (*Rickettsia rickettsii, Ehrlichia canis, E. ewingii*), fungal (*Aspergillus* spp., *Cryptococcus neoformans, Blastomyces dermatitidis, Fusarium solani*, and causes of phaeohyphomycosis), parasitic (*Cuterebra* spp.), and viral (canine distemper virus and FIP) causes among others. Although protozoal infections are typically expected to produce an eosinophilic pleocytosis, *Neospora caninum* in dogs and feline protozoal diseases (such as sarcocystosis and toxoplasmosis) have presented with marked neutrophilic or mixed pleocytosis (Lavely & Lipsitz, 2005; Bisby *et al.*, 2010; Gunn-Moore Reed, 2011). Additionally, a suppurative reaction to myelography dyes commonly occurs 24 hours after administration (Widmer *et al.*, 1992).

As would be expected, a neutrophilic pleocytosis was observed in a study of seven dogs with spinal epidural empyema (Lavely *et al.*, 2006). All CSF samples collected in this study had evidence of disease, independent of which location the sample was collected from. This indicates that sampling CSF cranial to a lesion can be diagnostically useful. However, the mean TNCC of cerebellomedullary samples was much lower than that found on lumbar punctures (15.3 cells/μl and 212.5 cells/μl, respectively).

Eosinophilic pleocytosis

Eosinophilic pleocytosis has been described in both veterinary and human medicine when eosinophil percentages are >10%, irrespective of what cell type makes up the predominant cell population (Figure 14.19; Levine *et al.*, 2014). In human medicine, >10 eosinophils/μl is seen as an indication of an eosinophilic process (Hughes *et al.*, 2003). This is not to imply that all cases with an eosinophilic pleocytosis will have a low number of eosinophils. Eosinophil percentages as high as 95% with mean TNCC of 84 cells/μl and a maximum cell count of 4,740 cells/μl have been reported in dogs with eosinophilic meningoencephalitis (Windsor *et al.*, 2009).

Because low numbers of eosinophils are seen as more significant than low numbers of other cells, care should be taken to ensure that the eosinophils present in a CSF sample are not simply a reflection of peripheral blood contamination. In one study of neurologically healthy cats, eosinophil numbers in CSF were associated with CSF RBC numbers and likely only represented peripheral blood contamination (Chrisman, 1992). In the dog, an association between peripheral eosinophilia and CSF eosinophilia was not found, but likely still exists (Smith-Maxie *et al.*, 1989).

Eosinophilic pleocytosis has been identified with infectious agents, IVDD, paraneoplastic processes, and idiopathic eosinophilic meningoencephalitis. Infectious agents reported in the dog include bacteria,

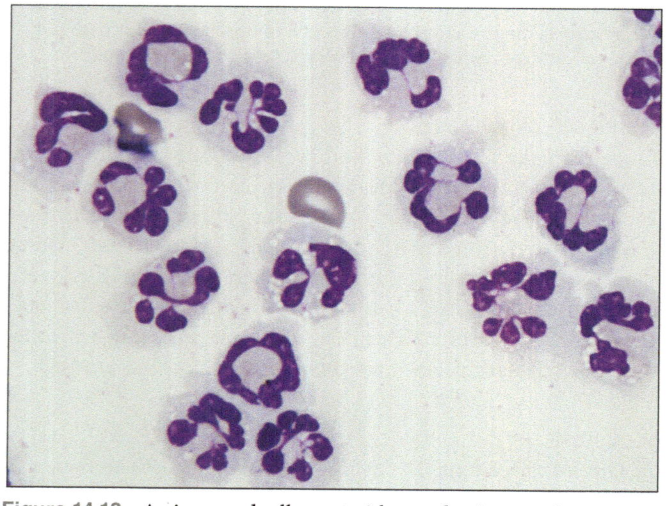

Figure 14.18 An increased cell count with a predominance of neutrophils is termed a neutrophilic pleocytosis (Wright–Giemsa, 1,000× magnification).

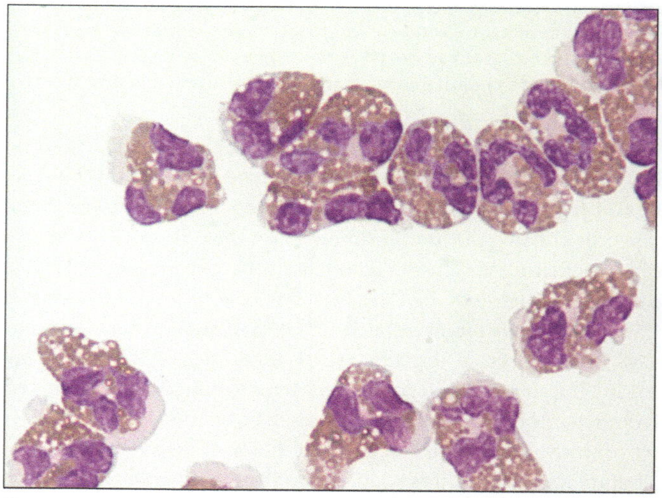

Figure 14.19 Increased number or percentage of eosinophils, which cannot be explained by peripheral blood contamination, is a significant finding, even if the eosinophil population is not the predominant cell type, as in this image (Wright–Giemsa, 1,000× magnification).

Cryptococcus neoformans, *Neospora caninum*, *Balisascaris procyonis*, *Spirocerca lupi*, *Toxoplasma gondii*, *Angiostrongylus cantonensis*, *Prototheca zopfii*, canine distemper virus, and rabies virus (Windsor *et al.*, 2009; Galgut *et al.*, 2010; Lane *et al.*, 2012a; Lunn *et al.*, 2012; Miglio *et al.*, 2013; Chai *et al.*, 2018). Steroid-responsive meningoencephalomyelitis with a predominance of eosinophils has been described in both the dog and the cat (Chrisman, 1992). Eosinophilic meningoencephalitis has been reported in the cat (Rand *et al.*, 1994a). Eosinophil activity has been implicated in autoimmune-mediated neurologic processes and may be the underlying cause of idiopathic eosinophilic meningoencephalitis (Correale Fiol, 2004; Windsor *et al.*, 2009). One case of persistent eosinophilic pleocytosis in a dog with primary intracranial histiocytic sarcoma has been described (Corsini *et al.*, 2022). Lymphoma/leukemia, carcinoma, and several drug reactions have been reported to cause eosinophilic pleocytosis in human medicine (Hughes *et al.*, 2003).

Large mononuclear pleocytosis

Cells counted in the large mononuclear category are largely members of the monocyte/macrophage lineage (Figure 14.20). A large mononuclear pleocytosis therefore is typically seen in cases with a chronic disease process. Bacterial meningitis usually presents initially with a neutrophilic pleocytosis, which may progress to a large mononuclear pleocytosis as antibiotic therapy is instituted and healing begins. It should also be noted that several primary CNS tumors, such as astrocytomas, liberate cells that are cytologically very similar to macrophages and can be misclassified as large mononuclear cells.

Potential causes of a large mononuclear pleocytosis include chronic trauma (including IVDD), infectious agents, inflammatory processes (granulomatous meningoencephalitis [GME], necrotizing meningoencephalitis [NME], and necrotizing leukoencephalitis [NLE]), and neoplasia. Infectious etiologies reported to produce a large mononuclear pleocytosis include chronic/healing bacterial meningitis and fungal (*Histoplasma capsulatum* and *Blastomyces dermatitidis*) agents (Bromel *et al.*, 2005; Lavely & Lipsitz, 2005).

Small mononuclear/lymphocytic pleocytosis

Cells classified as small mononuclear cells visually resemble small lymphocytes (Figure 14.21). Indeed, most are lymphoid in origin. Very rarely, normal CNS cells and neoplastic cells will have a 'lymphoid' appearance in CSF (Spriggs, 1954). For most cases, classifying an increase in small mononuclear cells as a lymphocytic pleocytosis is appropriate, although the rare exception should be remembered.

A lymphocytic/small mononuclear pleocytosis can be seen with traumatic (including IVDD), infectious, or inflammatory (GME, NME, and NLE) processes. Infectious causes include viral (canine distemper virus, rabies virus, Borna disease, feline leukemia virus, and others), bacterial (after institution of antibiotics), rickettsial (*Ehrlichia* spp.), fungal (*Coccidiodes immitis*), and protozoal (*Trypanosoma evansi* and possibly *Hepatozoon canis*) agents (Chrisman, 1992; Lavely & Lipsitz, 2005; Marchetti *et al.*, 2009; Gunn-Moore Reed, 2011; Defontis *et al.*, 2012).

Mixed cell pleocytosis

A mixed cell pleocytosis by definition does not have a specific cell type that is most predominant. It is typically a mixture of neutrophils, large mononuclear cells, and small mononuclear cells, and possibly includes plasma cells or eosinophils (Figure 14.22). This mixture of cells usually denotes either a transition from an acute to chronic inflammatory process or a process that has been present for an extended period of time but which is still active.

Common causes of a mixed pleocytosis include trauma (IVDD and other spinal cord insults), infectious agents, neoplasia, vascular diseases/infarction, hemorrhagic myelomalacia, and inflammation

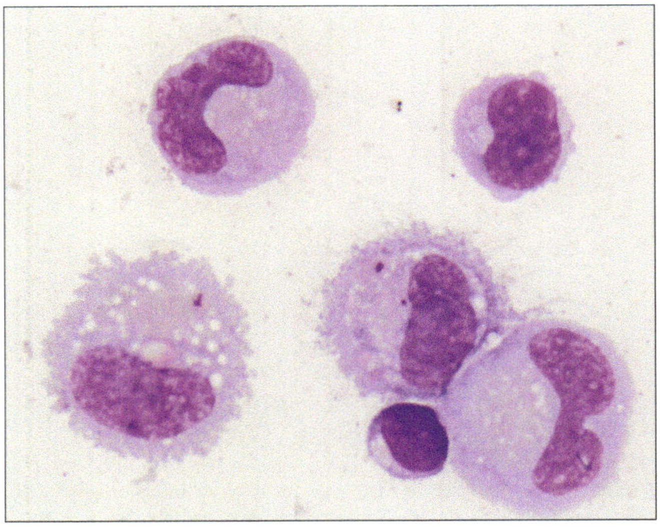

Figure 14.20 A large mononuclear pleocytosis is diagnosed when the predominant cell type is large mononuclear cells (Wright–Giemsa, 1,000× magnification).

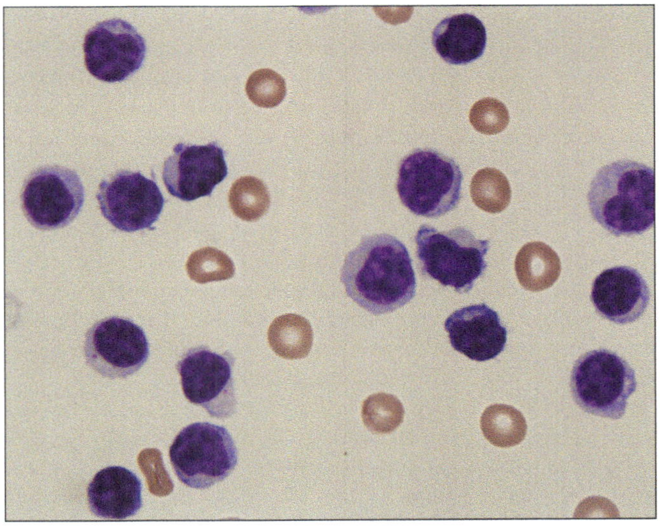

Figure 14.21 When small mononuclear cells consistent with lymphocytes are the most common cell seen, a lymphocytic pleocytosis should be diagnosed (Wright–Giemsa, 1,000× magnification).

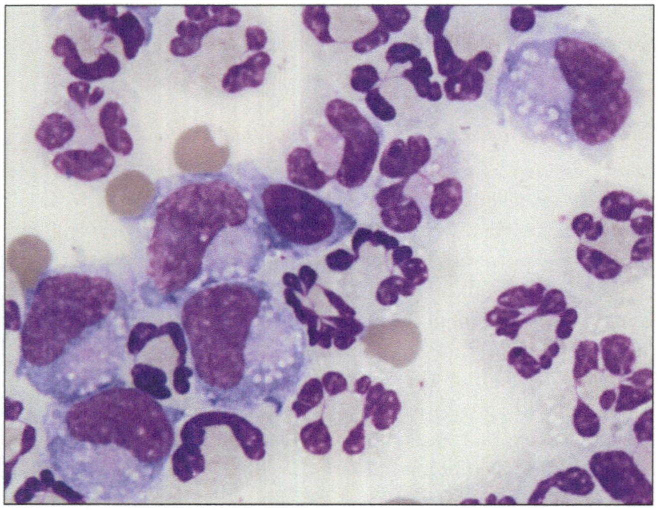

Figure 14.22 **A mixed pleocytosis is defined by an increased cell count that lacks a single predominant cell type. In this image, neutrophils, small mononuclear, and large mononuclear cells are present. Plasma cells and eosinophils, among others, can also be found in a mixed pleocytosis (Wright–Giemsa, 1,000× magnification).**

(GME and steroid-responsive meningoencephalomyelitis). Infectious agents include fungal (*Cryptococcus neoformans*, *Coccidiodes immitis*, *Blastomyces dermatitidis*, and *Aspergillus* spp.), protozoal (*Toxoplasma gondii*, *Neospora caninum*, *Babesia* spp., and *Leishmania* spp.) and viral (canine distemper virus and FIP virus) etiologies (Chrisman, 1992; Lavely & Lipsitz, 2005; Lester *et al.*, 2011; Márquez *et al.*, 2013). Bacterial meningitis can rarely display a mixed pleocytosis if the patient is sampled during the transition from a neutrophilic to large mononuclear phase. One such case involving *Mycobacterium haemophilum* has recently been described in a dog (De New *et al.*, 2023).

Nervous tissue

Sampling of the solid components of the CNS and its supporting structures during CSF collection is very rare but can occur, either as an incidental, pathologic, or iatrogenic event. As stated previously, surface epithelial cells are the most common CNS cells found and are usually not indicative of pathology.

Myelin-like material has been reported in 20% of canine CSF cases (Figures 14.23a, b; Luján-Feliu-Pascual *et al.*, 2008; Zabolotzky *et al.*, 2010). After Romanowsky-type staining, this material is a pink to purple extracellular foamy to frothy material. It can contain internal circular structures or long ribbon-like filaments that may represent damaged cytoplasmic membranes (Figure 14.23c). Myelin should stain positive with Luxol fast blue stains.

The significance of myelin on a cytologic preparation is somewhat ambiguous. Intracellular and extracellular myelin has been reported in a few cases with histologically confirmed degenerative myelopathy, myelomalacia, and IVDD (Fallin *et al.*, 1996; Mesher *et al.*, 1996; Bauer *et al.*, 2006). A much larger retrospective study of 98 dogs found no correlation with any specific disease (Zabolotzky *et al.*, 2010). Instead, extracellular myelin was more commonly found

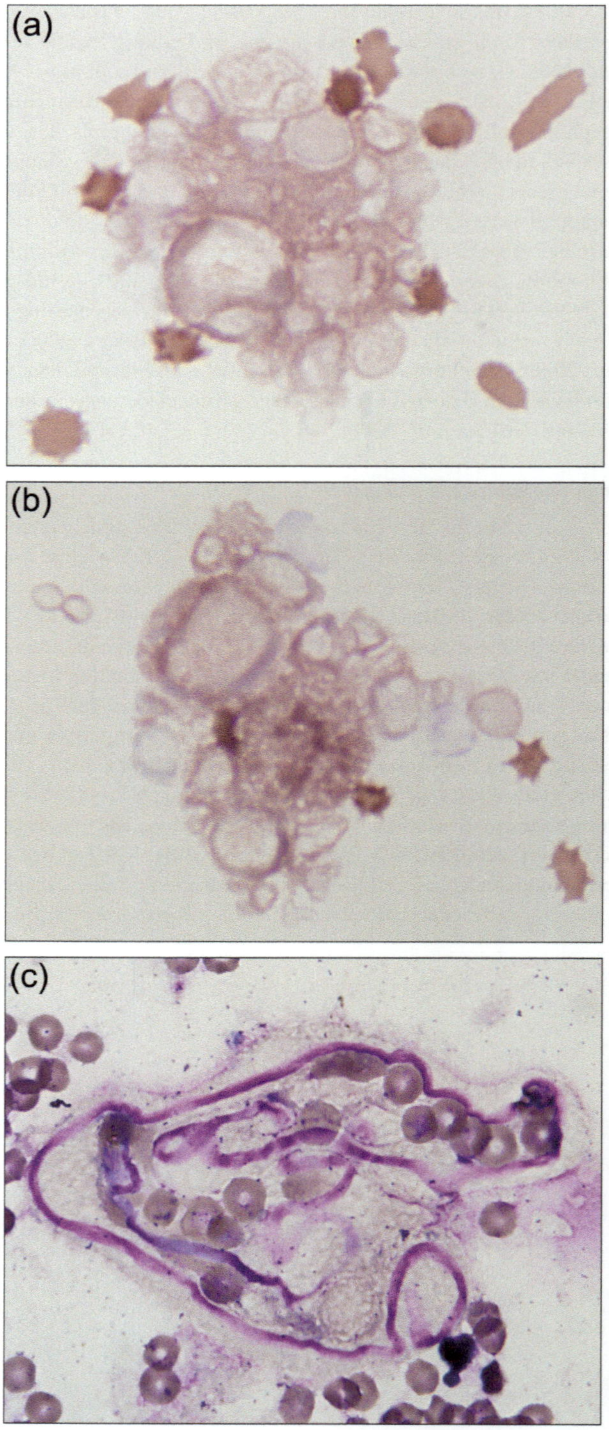

Figures 14.23a–c **(a, b) The large aggregate of pink to purple extracellular material is myelin. Note the many round inclusions and lack of overt cellular structure. Crenated red blood cells are also present in the images. (c) Pink to purple ribbon-like material and lighter pink foamy material supportive of myelin are present entrapping red blood cells (Wright–Giemsa, 1,000× magnification).**

in lumbar punctures and from smaller dogs that showed clinical recovery atypical of myelomalacia. This could suggest that most often extracellular myelin is an artifact. A larger group of dogs with imaging, with or without histologic confirmation of myelomalacia, did not describe myelin specifically, but did indicate that most cases had xanthochromia (Okada *et al.*, 2010). Myelomalacia caused by fibrocartilaginous embolism in five cats failed to show myelin figures; instead a neutrophilic pleocytosis was present in some of the cases (Mikszewski *et al.*, 2006).

Neurons and neuropil can occasionally be present in CSF samples (Fallin *et al.*, 1996). These look similar in CSF cytology to their appearance on cytologic smears of brain tissue (see 'Central Nervous System Cytology' for a detailed description of these structures). Inclusion of neuropil in the CSF sample is most often an iatrogenic event; however, degenerative and traumatic causes could also be considered. Although significant complications have been observed in some patients when nervous tissue is present in CSF, the presence of these structures should not be equated with 'pithing' the patient, as many cases never develop clinical changes following collection (Luján-Feliu-Pascual *et al.*, 2008).

Hemorrhage

Increased RBC numbers or RBC breakdown products in a CSF sample can be caused by iatrogenic/collection-associated hemorrhage, trauma, cerebrovascular accidents, or other pathologic processes that cause extravasation of erythrocytes such as neoplasia, vasculitis, and infectious diseases such as leptospirosis, toxoplasmosis, and cryptococcosis. By far the most common cause is contamination during collection. Several clues can help distinguish the presence of RBCs due to peripheral blood contamination from true hemorrhage.

A traumatic CSF tap can cause the CSF to appear visually discolored in the needle hub. Often this small amount of hemorrhage will resolve if CSF is allowed to continue to flow out of the needle. If the initial fluid obtained after puncture is red or discolored, collection into at least two tubes is recommended. CSF analysis should be performed on the final tube collected.

As mentioned previously, xanthochromia is predominantly caused by *in-vivo* hemorrhage and should not occur outside the body; a xanthochromic sample can support a diagnosis of hemorrhage in a patient that does not have peripheral hyperbilirubinemia (see Figure 14.5).

The presence of erythrophagocytosis, hemosiderin, or hematoidin has been suggested as confirmation of *in-vivo* hemorrhage (Figures 14.24a, b). Sample handling and time between collection and slide preparation should be considered when using these clues. Erythrophagia, hemosiderin, and hematoidin formation can occur in a very short period of time. Prussian blue staining can be used to confirm the presence of iron and hemosiderin. Interestingly, neither evidence of erythrophagocytosis nor xanthochromia was noted in cats with known, or suspected, CNS trauma (Rand *et al.*, 1994b). Instead, increased numbers of erythrocytes and a mild neutrophilic pleocytosis were noted. A recent case report noted significant evidence of hematoidin and hemorrhage associated with cerebral vascular hamartoma in a 9-week-old Irish Setter puppy (Williams *et al.*, 2023).

Attempts to quantify the effects of hemorrhage on other components of the CSF analysis have been contradictory. One retrospective study did not find a correlation between the number of RBCs and TNCC or TP in samples with iatrogenic blood presence in neurologically normal dogs (Hurtt & Smith, 1997). A more recent study in dogs found that serial dilutions with whole blood up to 8,500 RBC/μL did not cause any significant changes in TNCC or protein concentration,

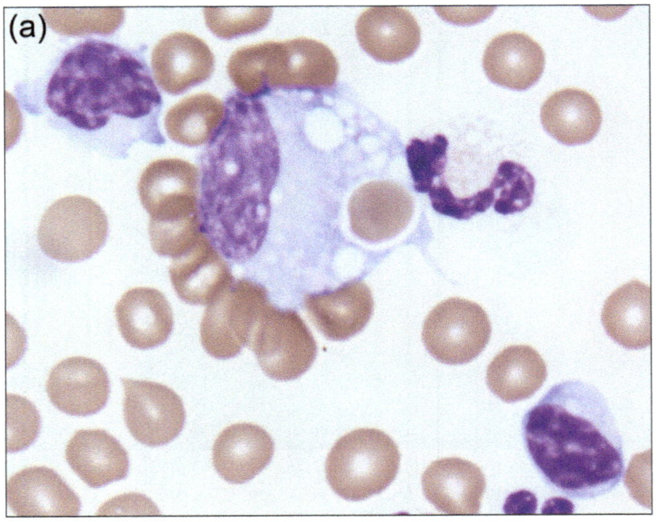

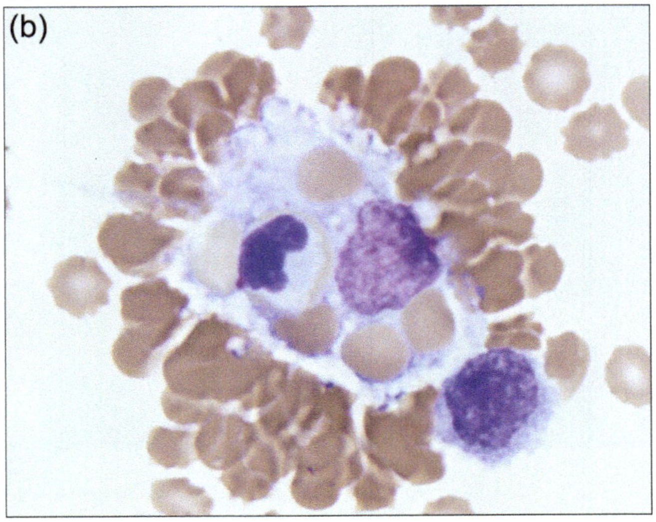

Figures 14.24a, b (a) The central large mononuclear cell is erythrophagocytic. Note how the red cell is within a distinct vacuole. (b) This large mononuclear cell displayed erythrophagia and leukophagia (Wright–Giemsa, 1,000× magnification). (Note: erythrophagocytosis can be used to support a diagnosis of *in-vivo* hemorrhage. However, if a delay in sample handling occurs, erythrophagocytosis by itself could be caused by collection-associated blood contamination and *ex-vivo* phagocytosis.)

and no correlations were appreciated retrospectively in blood contaminated samples up to 210,000 RBC/μL (MacNeill *et al.*, 2018). Other studies support alterations in TNCC or the cellular differential count with much lower degrees of blood contamination (Becker *et al.*, 2008; Doyle & Solano-Gallego, 2009). Several formulae to predict the effect of RBC contamination on cellularity and CSF TP have been suggested (Rand *et al.*, 1994a). Given the apparently poor correlation between RBC counts in blood-contaminated CSF samples, TNCC, and TP across studies, use of correction formulas is not currently recommended (MacNeill *et al.*, 2018). Iatrogenic blood contamination may also affect CSF enzyme concentrations (e.g. LDH, CK) (Brune *et al.*, 2023).

Infectious agents

Direct observation of infectious agents on cytologic samples is both very exciting (for the microscopist) and imminently useful (for the clinician). Bacteria (*Streptococcus* spp., *Staphylococcus* spp., *Mycobacterium* spp.), fungi (*Blastomyces dermatitidis*, *Histoplasma capsulatum*, *Cryptococcus neoformans*, and *Aspergillus* spp.), protozoa (*Toxoplasma gondii*, *Sarcocystis neurona*, and *Neospora caninum*), and parasites (*Angiostrongylus cantonensis*, *Dirofilaria immitis*, *Balisascaris procyonis*, *Taenia* spp., *Spirocerca lupi*, and *Cuterebra* spp.) have been found on cytologic preparations of CSF (Figures 14.25a–d). These structures look cytologically similar independent of where they are found in the body. As with much of cytology, failing to

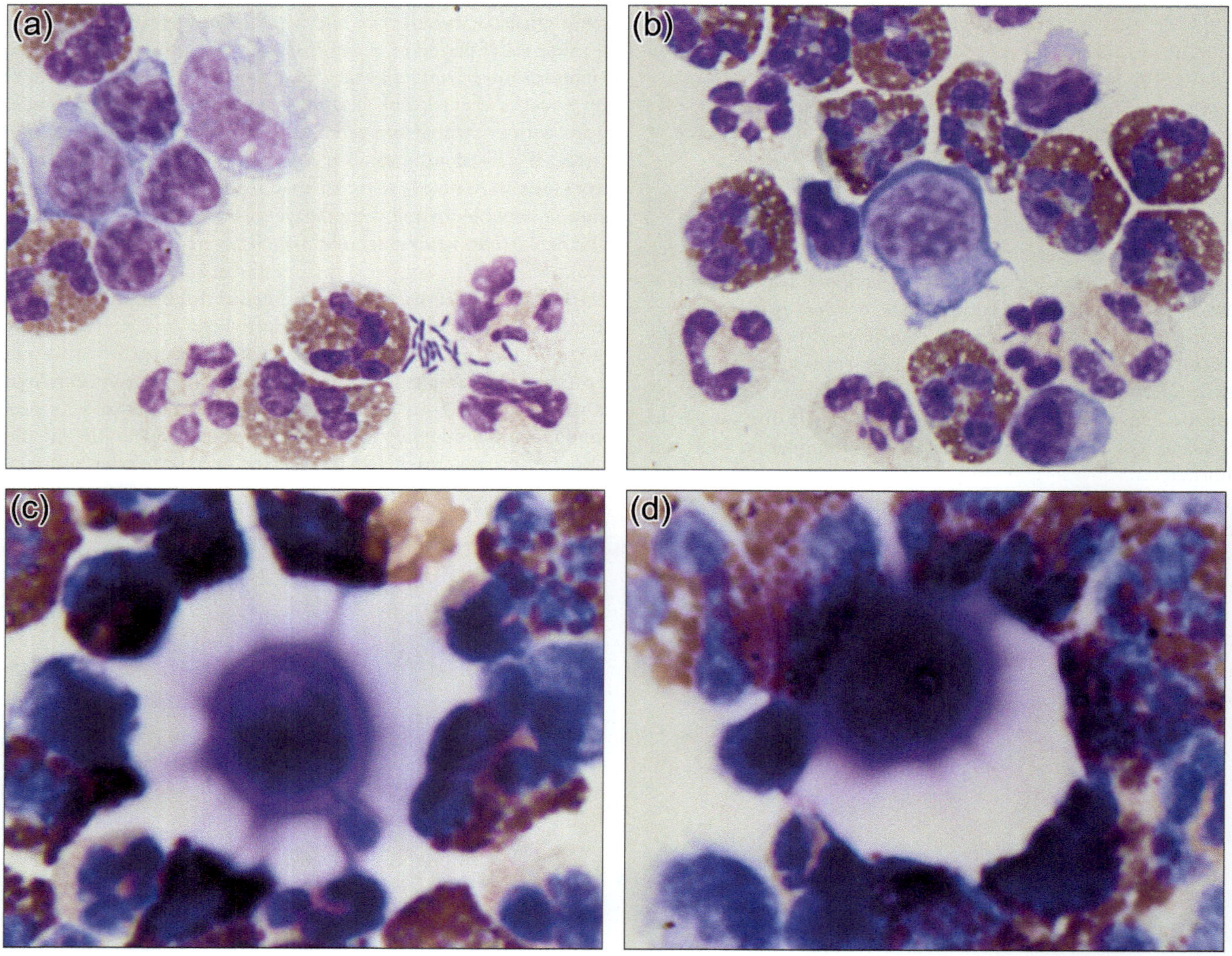

Figures 14.25a–d CSF from a 3-year-old, spayed female yellow Labrador Retriever. TNCC = 4,100 cells/μl, CSF TP = 147 mg/dl. (a, b) A mixed pleocytosis consisting of neutrophils, eosinophils, large mononuclear, and small mononuclear cells was found on CSF evaluation. Intracellular and extracellular rod-shaped bacteria are present in the lower right corner of both of these images. The eosinophil population is not commonly encountered in a sample with only bacteria present (Wright–Giemsa, 1,000× magnification). (c, d) A thorough evaluation of the preparation found the cause of the eosinophilia. Large yeasts with narrow based budding and thick mucoid capsule, consistent with *Cryptococcus neoformans*, were present (Wright–Giemsa, 1,000× magnification; additional digital enlargement used to help display cytologic features of the yeast).

visualize the organism does not rule out the diagnosis. If post-collection contamination can be ruled out, observation of organisms can be diagnostically useful.

Neoplastic cells in cerebrospinal fluid/neoplastic pleocytosis

CSF abnormalities are seen in approximately 90% of cases with intracranial tumors (Platt *et al.*, 2002). A neoplastic population, or suspected neoplastic population, is occasionally found on CSF cytology evaluation. More commonly, an increased CSF TP, inflammatory pleocytosis, and a conspicuous lack of a neoplastic cell population are found in cases with proven CNS neoplasia. Care should be taken not to confuse normal surface epithelium present in low numbers with a neoplastic cell population.

Neoplastic cells in fluid can look like they do in their primary site. For example, large cohesive clusters containing up to 200 cells have been observed in CSF with choroid plexus carcinoma (Pastorello *et al.*, 2010). Also, psammoma bodies are found in CSF of some cases with meningioma (Wessmann *et al.*, 2010). Lymphoma in CSF looks similar to lymphoma diagnosed elsewhere in the body although it may not exfoliate as well into CSF, with a recent study revealing that only few CSF samples confirm CNS lymphoma (Durand *et al.*, 2022).

However, neoplastic cells in fluid will often take on an altered appearance. Some of the cellular signaling pathways that lead to cytoplasmic differentiation are dependent on interaction with extracellular structures such as basement membranes, stroma, or surrounding cells. Cells deprived of these location-based signals often lose some of their cytoplasmic differentiation. Cytologically, this means that neoplastic cells in fluid are often rounded and occasionally can only accurately be described as discrete cells of unknown origin (Behling-Kelly *et al.*, 2010). A definitive diagnosis of the tissue of origin or possible cell lineage can sometimes be very challenging without immunocytochemical staining for specific cell structures and receptors (Stowe *et al.*, 2012; Cian *et al.*, 2013). Even in cases where many cells are rounded and fairly nondescript, very occasional cell–cell junctions or other cytologic clues can be found that hint at a possible histogenesis. It is wise to carefully evaluate a suspect population.

Neoplastic pleocytosis from meningioma, choroid plexus carcinoma, histiocytic sarcoma, lymphoma, and ependymoma have been reported in dogs and cats, among others (Rand *et al.*, 1994b; Dickinson *et al.*, 2006; Harms *et al.*, 2009; Pastorello *et al.*, 2010; Toyoda *et al.*, 2020; Durand *et al.*, 2022). Meningioma is the most prevalent primary intracranial tumor and appears to be the most common cause of a neoplastic pleocytosis. This may not reflect how readily the cells shed into the CSF; in humans, gliomas, including anaplastic astrocytoma and glioblastoma multiforme, are more likely to exfoliate than meningiomas (Chhieng *et al.*, 2002). Additionally, metastatic cancers can be found on CSF evaluation. Further examples of specific CNS neoplasms will be discussed in detail later in this chapter.

CENTRAL NERVOUS SYSTEM CYTOLOGY

Cytology of CNS parenchyma is becoming increasingly utilized in veterinary medicine, as it can be used to good effect in conjunction with imaging to diagnose and plan treatment in patients with CNS lesions (Powell, 2005). Fine needle aspiration (FNA) is an excellent modality for deep-seated tumors where direct visual access would require disruption of a large amount of normal nervous tissue. Although the acquisition of samples and the practice of CNS cytology are highly specialized, a basic overview is included to help guide diagnostic procedures and patient care.

Sampling

CNS biopsy can be obtained through less invasive ultrasound or CT-guided (either free-hand or stereotactic) FNAs or by more invasive open craniotomy accessed FNA or incisional biopsy techniques (Platt *et al.*, 2002). The exact procedure for acquiring these samples is complex, necessitates specialized imaging and equipment, and is outside the scope of this text. Consultation with a neurologist or surgeon with experience in CNS cytologic collection is recommended.

The basic principles that need to be observed include preparation of a fresh sample that is thin enough for cytologic evaluation.

CNS cells deteriorate quite rapidly, causing a loss of cellular structure and differential staining. Sample processing is often expedited for intraoperative samples by including the cytologist in scheduling the surgery and staining samples quickly. Samples collected postmortem need special care. Although a delay of hours is acceptable for histologic evaluation, it will likely significantly affect cytologic evaluation and should be avoided.

Sample thickness is another concern. Much of the CNS lacks significant fibrous connective tissue in health. This makes it very soft and makes a squash type preparation of material collected by FNA, at surgery, or at gross necropsy very easy. One exception to this rule is a sample with large numbers of glial cells; these can be more challenging to spread and produce an even distribution of cells (Lee & Tihan, 2015). Less than a cubic millimeter of tissue is needed for a high-quality squash preparation. Multiple thin smears are preferred to a single dense sample. Touch imprints of samples collected for histopathology can be used to produce an interpretation (Powell, 2005).

Several staining techniques can be used for CNS cytology. Alcohol fixed wet slides can be stained with hematoxylin and eosin (Iqbal *et al.*, 2006). Although this is not a commonly used cytologic stain, it has the main advantage of being quick. The sample is alcohol fixed when still wet and immediately stained; this allows a diagnosis within 10 minutes of sample collection in some cases. Romanowsky-type stains can be used on dried slides and are more commonly utilized.

Indications and contraindications

The same basic principles outlined for CSF collection hold true for indications and contraindications of CNS cytology. One obvious caveat is that the lesions must be physically within the reach of the cytology needle or the surgeon's scalpel. Additionally, important, uninvolved structures cannot lie along the path of needle insertion or significant complications can arise. Tumor seeding along the sampling tract has been reported in human medicine; the occurrence of iatrogenic tumor spread in veterinary medicine is unknown (Patrick *et al.*, 2006).

One common use for intraoperative cytologic evaluation of CNS samples is to determine the diagnostic adequacy of a sample collected for histologic evaluation. In human medicine it has been noted that only one-third of the first samples collected by stereotactic techniques are diagnostic. A quick review of a smear can indicate that more samples are needed to reach a diagnosis before the patient leaves the operating room (Lee & Tihan, 2015).

Cytologic evaluation of a series of ten canine brain tumors with concurrent histologic evaluation found that the two modalities shared only 50% agreement for a specific diagnosis, although all FNA samples were confirmatory for neoplasia (Platt *et al.*, 2002). In human medicine, where the technique is used much more frequently, a lack of agreement is only found in 3% of cases (Lee & Tihan, 2015). Given the diagnostic benefits, the economic cost, and the minimally invasive nature of CNS FNA cytology, even the authors that found a poor agreement between cytology and histopathology still advocate FNA of intracranial lesions. Additionally, cytologic evaluation of samples obtained at necropsy can be a quick and inexpensive way to identify underlying pathology. A better description of the pathologic process that led to the demise of a beloved pet can sometimes help in the acceptance of pet loss.

Normal cytologic findings

The CNS is composed of a multitude of cells, each with their own specialized function and form. Within the category of neuroepithelial cells are neurons and glial cells. The glia can be further stratified into astrocytes, oligodendrocytes, Schwann cells, ependymal cells, and choroid plexus cells. Neuroepithelial cells derive from the neuroectoderm. CNS cells derived from the mesenchyme include meningeal cells and microglia.

Neuropil

Neuropil is a meshwork of axons, dendrites, synaptic junctions, and glial fibrillary processes. As such, it is made of parts of neurons, astrocytes, oligodendrocytes, microglial cell membranes, and extracellular matrix (Miller & Zachary, 2017). Cytologically, neuropil appears as a fine eosinophilic felt-like meshwork interwoven with nuclei from neurons and glial cells (Figures 14.26a–d).

Neurons

Larger neurons will often have a triangular shape, ample amounts of basophilic, somewhat granular cytoplasm, a large nucleus, and a large prominent nucleolus (Figures 14.26a–d, 14.27; Lee & Tihan, 2015). The long cytoplasmic processes of the neuron will often produce a pink, amorphous to faintly fibrillar appearance surrounding the neuron. This fibrillary material can also be seen arrayed around glial cells as part of their glial fibrillary processes. The inner granular layer of the cerebellum is composed of much smaller neurons, which produce a population of small round basophilic cells. These cells can be mistaken for glial cells if the location of the sample site is not known or if the significance of interspersed large neurons, such as Purkinje cells, is overlooked (Lee & Tihan, 2015).

Astrocytes

Astrocytes are glial cells that form the blood–brain barrier and participate in repair and support of the CNS (Figures 14.26a–d). To do this they maintain foot processes along the blood vessel and surrounding axon. Astrocytes make up the predominant cell type in the CNS (Miller & Zachary, 2017).

They are basophilic cells smaller than large neurons and have open chromatin on cytology; their finer processes are not commonly appreciated. Histologically, they are divided into protoplasmic astrocytes which have short cellular processes and fibrous astrocytes which have long branching processes. The protoplasmic astrocytes are found within the gray matter while fibrous astrocytes are found within the white matter.

Oligodendrocytes

Oligodendrocytes play a role in myelination of axons (Figures 14.26a–d). To do this they have a large amount of cytoplasm, which extends out in thin processes and wraps around nearby neurons. A single oligodendrocyte can interact with up to 50 neurons. However, most of this cytoplasm is not directly around the nucleus, leading to frequent confusion of oligodendrocyte nuclei and lymphocytes.

Microglia

Microglia are thought to be the CNS resident component of the monocyte–macrophage system. Their primary role is the removal of cellular debris and fluid via phagocytosis and pinocytosis. Interestingly, although microglia are the resident monocyte–macrophage population, up to 70% of the macrophages in an inflammatory or degenerative response within the CNS are derived from blood monocytes. Although several histologic forms occur, including amoeboid and ramified microglia, on cytologic evaluation they are typically smaller cells with round to rod-shaped nuclei and scant cytoplasm. Microglial cells appear similar to macrophages located elsewhere, with foamy, lipid filled cytoplasm (Figure 14.28).

Meningeal cells

There are three layers in the meninges: the dura mater, arachnoid membrane, and pia mater (Miller & Zachary, 2017). The pia mater is closely adhered to the brain and spinal cord. It is a layer of fibroblasts that can be as thin as a single cell layer. The pia mater forms fibrous connections with the arachnoid membrane. The arachnoid membrane is a multilayered mesenchymal tissue. Nerve bundles and blood vessels are found in the space between the arachnoid membrane and the pia mater. This subarachnoid space is also the location most commonly accessed for collection of CSF. Together the arachnoid and pia mater are referred to as the leptomeninges. Lining the outer surface of the arachnoid membrane and inner surface of the dura mater is a single layer of mesothelial-like cells whose function is similar to mesothelium in the abdomen and thorax; it allows frictionless movement of the brain and spinal cord within the bony vault of the calvarium and spinal canal. The dura mater is a dense collagenous membrane. It is bilayered and acts as the inner periosteal layer of the calvarium

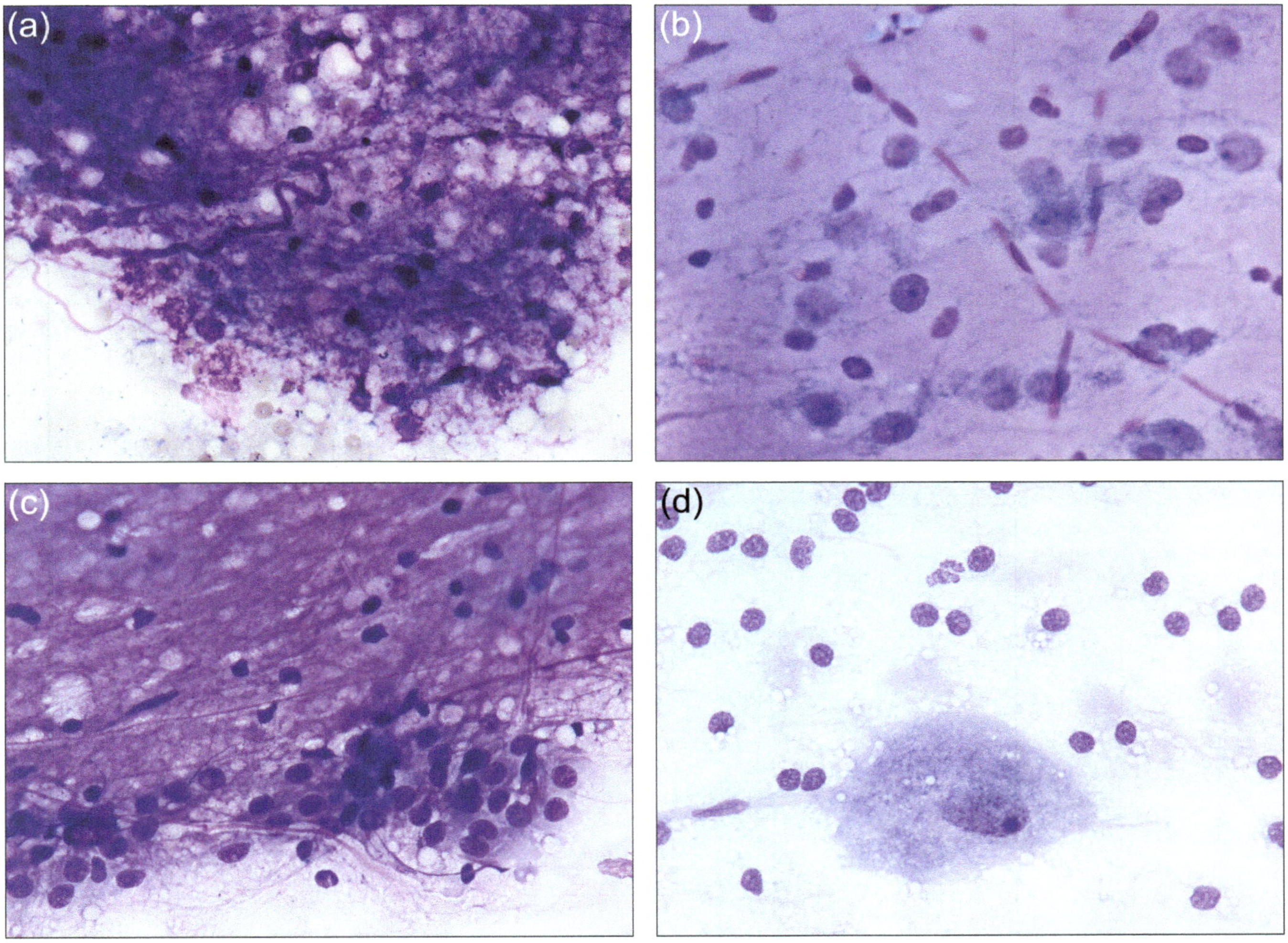

Figures 14.26a–d Squash preparations of normal CNS tissue in dogs. (a) A frothy pink to purple extracellular material with interspersed small, condensed nuclei on CSF analysis is consistent with neuropil. Note how both diffuse material and long ribbon-like structures are present (Wright–Giemsa, 500× magnification). (b) A preparation of gray matter from the cerebral cortex shows many fine capillaries filled with red blood cells. The smallest, condensed nuclei are most consistent with oligodendrocytes. These cells have a large amount of cytoplasm; however, it is found distant to the nuclei, wrapped around neuronal processes. The nuclei located next to the vasculature, with open chromatin and moderate poorly discernible basophilic cytoplasm, are most consistent with astrocytes. The larger nuclei with a distinct nucleolus and more abundant cytoplasm belong to neurons (Wright–Giemsa, 1,000× magnification). (c) A preparation of white matter from the cerebral cortex has more prominent felt-like neuropil. The more condensed round nuclei causing nonstaining defects in the neuropil are most consistent with oligodendrocytes. In this location astrocytes are classified as fibrous astrocytes; they have smaller nuclei and sparsely branched processes. Significant numbers of neuron cell bodies are not expected in the white matter; however, neuronal dendrites and axons contribute to the felt-like network in the neuropil. The cuboidal to columnar cells along the bottom of the image are cytologically consistent with ependymal or choroid plexus cells; in this location they are expected to be ependymal in origin (Wright–Giemsa, 1,000× magnification). (d) An imprint from canine cerebellum. The single large neuron in the lower half of the image has abundant amounts of granular basophilic cytoplasm, few clear cytoplasmic vacuoles, and a large ovoid nucleus with stippled chromatin and single large nucleolus. Given the location, this large neuron is a Purkinje cell and the smaller round cells in the image are likely a combination of glial cells and neurons from the inner granular layer. The background consists of wispy fibrillar cell processes from neurons and glial cells (Wright–Giemsa, 1,000× magnification).

and spinal canal. The bilayer splits in the spinal canal and creates the extradural space.

Cytologically, meningeal cells can be found in sheets or individually; they have moderate amounts of faintly eosinophilic cytoplasm and nuclei that are variably round to ovoid to elongate (Figures 14.29a, b). The cytoplasmic borders are often ill defined; however, storiform or pseudoacinar arrangements can be seen.

Ependymal cells

Ependymal cells are cuboidal to columnar epithelial cells that have basally located nuclei and apical cilia (Miller & Zachary, 2017). Their primary function is the movement of CSF through the ventricular system. Ependymal cells are joined by gap junctions. This allows transfer of proteins and fluid from the CSF, around the ependymal cells and into the extracellular spaces of the brain. Ependymal

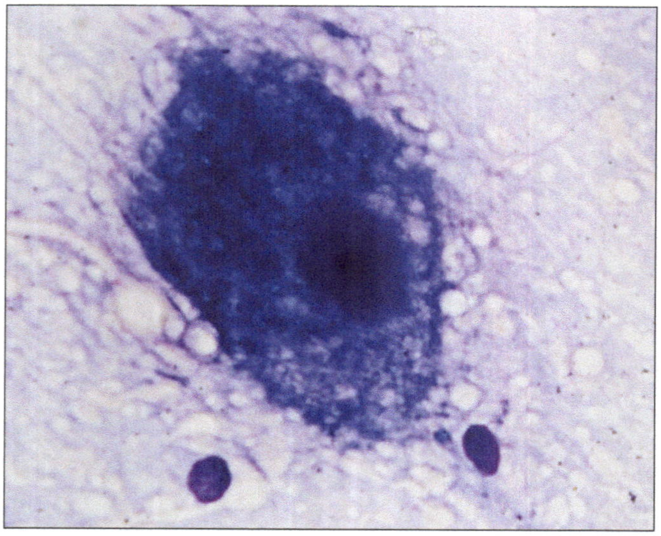

Figure 14.27 A large neuron with abundant granular basophilic cytoplasm, large nucleus, and prominent nucleolus is present in an imprint of gray matter from the cerebral cortex (Wright–Giemsa, 1,000× magnification).

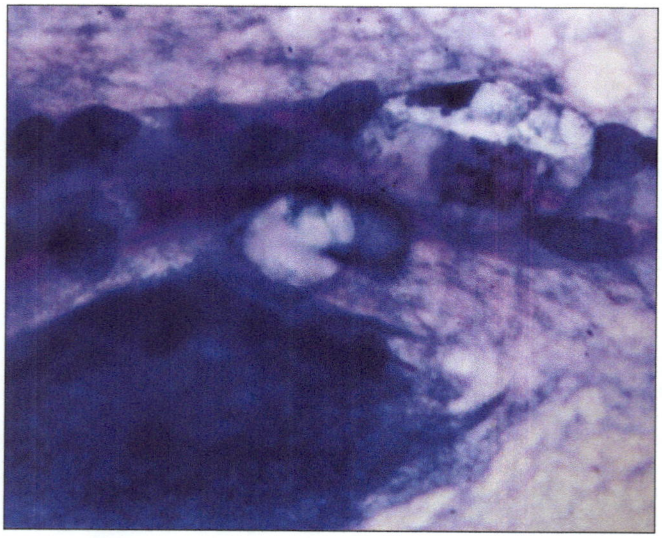

Figure 14.28 A red blood cell filled vessel runs horizontally through the image. Two microglial cells are associated with the vessel. They have foamy clear cytoplasm and rod-like nuclei. A neuron cell body is present in the lower left of the image (Wright–Giemsa, 1,000× magnification).

cells are found in the ventricles, the mesencephalic aqueduct, and the central canal of the spinal cord. Cytologically, it is challenging to distinguish ependymal cells from choroid plexus cells (Figure 14.26c).

Choroid plexus cells

In situ, choroid plexus cells are specialized ependymal cells arranged in fronds. They produce approximately 90% of the CSF volume. Choroid plexus cells are cuboidal epithelial cells that are distinct from other ependymal cells. Among other features, choroid plexus cells have apical microvilli while ependymal cells are ciliated.

An excellent review of choroid plexus cells in multiple species has been published (Garma-Aviña, 2004). This study found four subtypes of choroid plexus cells. In the dog, most (~75%) choroid plexus cells are large polygonal cells measuring 15–20 µm. These cells are termed alpha cells and are characterized by countless basophilic granules and small, round highly regular nuclei lacking obvious nucleoli (Figure 14.30a). Approximately 25% of the cells are similarly sized to alpha cells but have gray to faintly acidophilic granules and are called beta cells (Figures 14.30b, c). Sometimes, a few tiny round clear vacuoles can be noted in beta cells. Their nuclei are slightly larger and paler with finer chromatin than alpha cells. Both alpha and beta cells are positive for pancytokeratin. A third type of cell, the gamma cell, is characterized by the presence of large membrane bound cytoplasmic vesicles that measure between 3 and 30 µm (Figure 14.30d). Pancytokeratin can stain fine linear structures within these vesicles; however, the majority of the cell is pancytokeratin negative. This cell type makes up about 1–3% of cells in the dog. Less than 1% of cells in normal canine choroid plexus are epiplexus macrophages, also called Kolmer cells. These large cells are interposed between the other cell types and have copious pale cytoplasm. Nuclei can be round, oval, or bi-lobed and the cytoplasm often contains fine clear vacuoles.

PATHOLOGY OF THE CENTRAL NERVOUS SYSTEM

Infectious lesions

Bacterial meningitis

Bacterial meningitis typically presents in a patient who is reluctant to move and extremely painful but otherwise does not show specific, focal neurologic lesions (Table 14.4). Bacteria may access the CNS by direct implantation (trauma, CSF tap), local spread (diskospondylitis), or hematogenous spread from bacteremia. Common bacterial causes include *Staphylococcus* spp., *Escherichia coli*, *Pasteurella multocida*, *Actinomyces* spp., *Nocardia* spp., *Streptococcus* spp., and, rarely, some anaerobic entities (Tipold & Stein, 2010).

CSF analysis most commonly reveals a neutrophilic pleocytosis with increased CSF TP (Figures 14.31a–d, 14.32). With chronicity or antibiotic therapy, a mixed or mononuclear pleocytosis may occur. Direct observation of bacteria in the cytologic preparation is rare but can occur (Radaelli & Platt, 2002). In cases with a high index of suspicion, collection in a non-EDTA containing tube for bacterial culture or polymerase chain reaction (PCR) is appropriate, independent of what is found on cytologic evaluation of the sample. One report of necropsy confirmed bacterial meningitis in the dog found that only one in eight CSF samples grew bacteria on routine cultures (Radaelli & Platt, 2002).

Prognosis with bacterial meningitis is variable, depending on the exact etiology, underlying patient factors, and the clinician's ability to institute appropriate early antimicrobial therapy (Muñana, 1996).

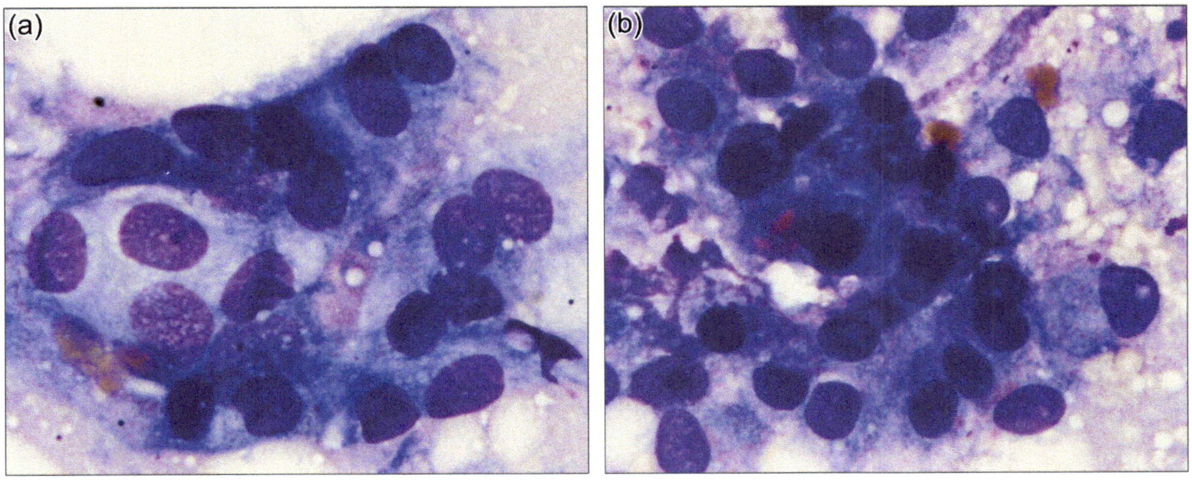

Figures 14.29a, b Imprint of the dura. (a) Meningeal cells are present in a sheet of polygonal to spindloid cells with poorly distinct cell borders and round to oval nuclei. (b) A pseudoacinar arrangement is present in the center bottom of the field (Wright–Giemsa, 1,000× magnification).

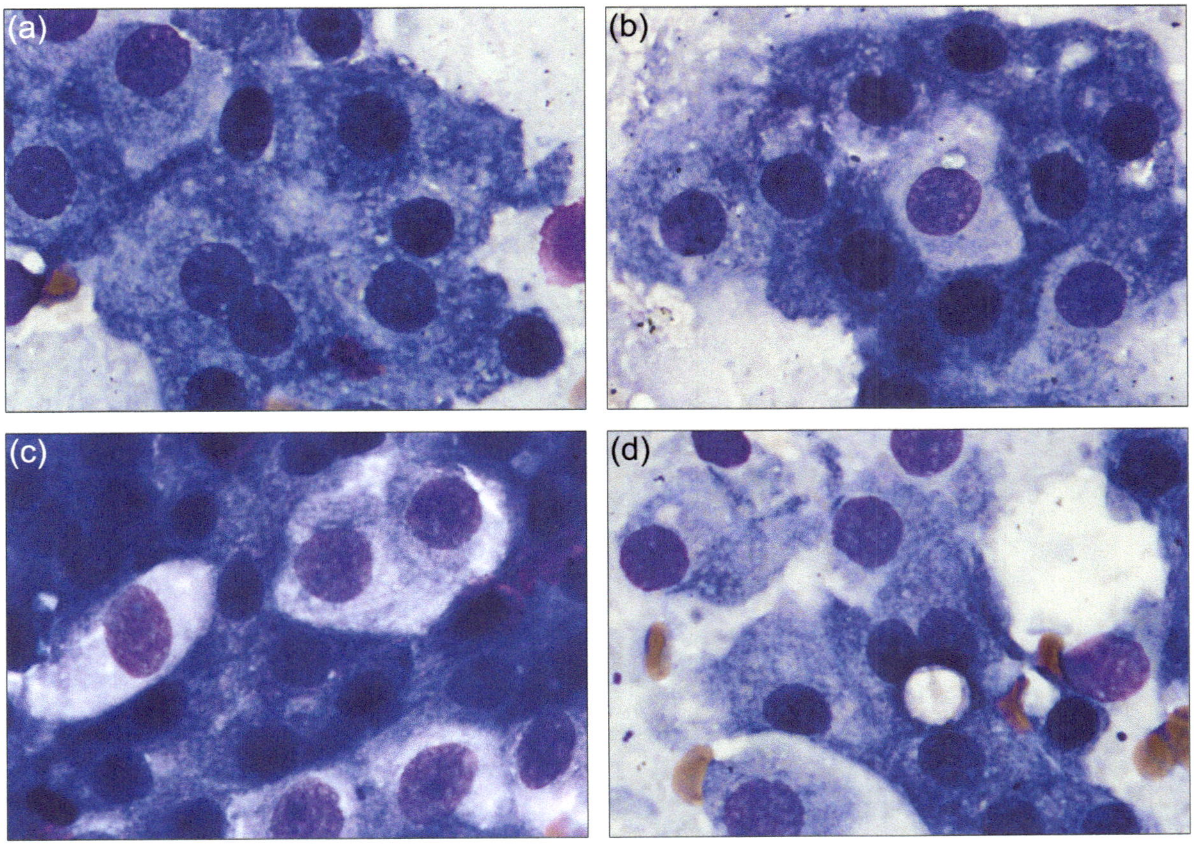

Figures 14.30a–d Cytologic imprints of the choroid plexus. (a) Seventy-five percent of the cells are polygonal cells with basophilic granules and small round nuclei. These have been called alpha cells. (b) A beta cell is seen in the center of the image; it is roughly the same size as the surrounding alpha cells and has a slightly larger, more open nucleus and eosinophilic to gray cytoplasmic granules. (c) Four beta cells are present in a dense cluster of alpha cells. (d) Very rarely, cells with a large membrane bound vesicle can be found in the choroid plexus. These are called gamma cells. Gamma cell vesicles were found extracellularly in the preparation (not shown) (Wright–Giemsa, 1,000× magnification).

Table 14.4 **A summary of the significant diagnostic findings with bacterial meningitis**

Signalment	Any
Clarity	Clear to turbid
Color	Possible red/xanthochromia
CSF TP	Mild to marked increase
CSF cellularity	Acute: mild to marked neutrophilic pleocytosis
	Chronic: mixed or mononuclear pleocytosis
CNS cytology	Not commonly performed
Ancillary testing	Culture, PCR
Notes	Bacteria are not commonly observed on CSF even when culture positive

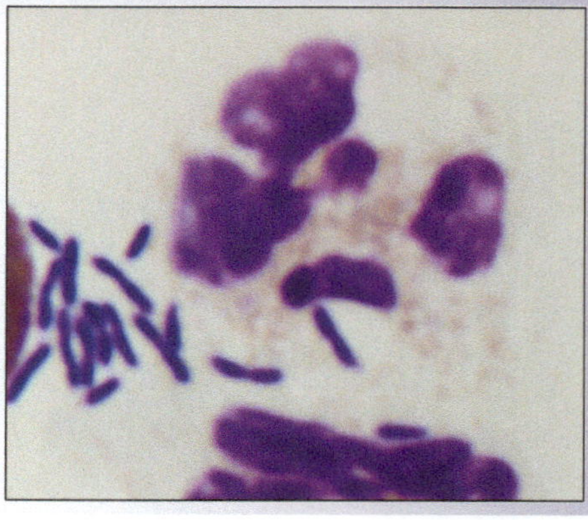

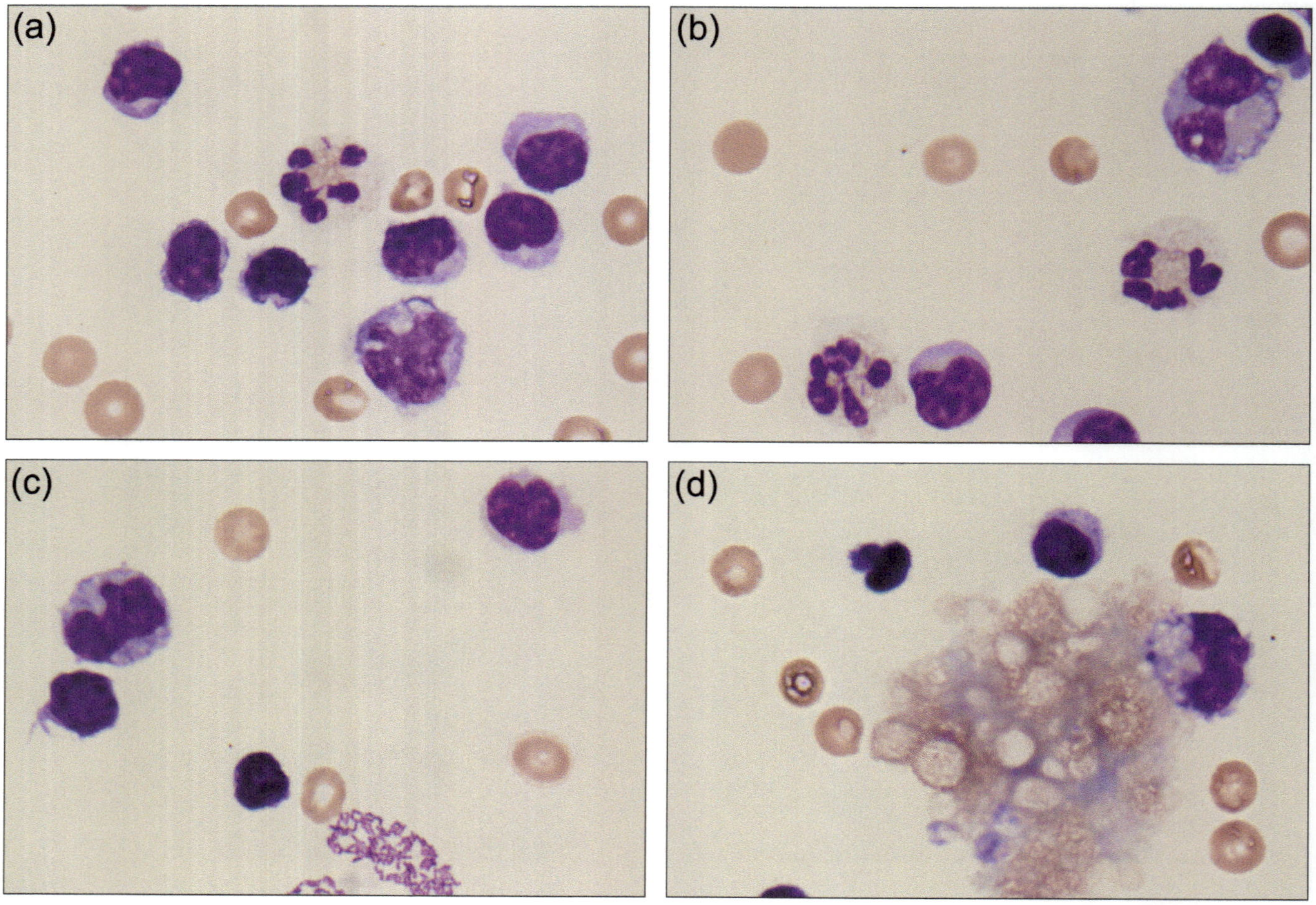

Figure 14.31a–d CSF from an 8-year-old Jack Russell Terrier. TNCC = 286 cells/µl, CSF TP = 472 mg/dl. (a, b) A mixed pleocytosis with small mononuclear cells, large mononuclear cells, and neutrophils is present. Note the small rod-shaped bacteria within the neutrophils. (c) Large mats of rod-shaped bacteria are also present extracellularly. (d) An aggregate of myelin with small round structures inside foamy eosinophilic to basophilic material is present. Although this can be an incidental finding, given the history and cytologic findings, myelomalacia is a more likely cause (Wright–Giemsa, 1,000× magnification). The patient was diagnosed with bacterial meningitis. She responded well to medical management.

Canine distemper virus encephalitis

With adequate vaccination, canine distemper virus (CDV) encephalitis is less common than in years past and vaccine-associated cases are rarely seen (Table 14.5). Classic clinical signs of CDV encephalitis include chewing gum seizures, myoclonus (rhythmic muscle jerking), vestibular signs, and circling or dementia, depending on the immunocompetence and age at onset of signs (Thomas, 1998).

CSF findings with CDV encephalitis are dependent on age (Thomas, 1998). Younger dogs typically have a mild neutrophilic pleocytosis with mildly increased CSF TP. Mature dogs have a moderate mononuclear pleocytosis with moderate elevations of CSF TP. Increased CSF TP without concurrent elevations in TNCC are seen (Koutinas *et al.*, 2002). CSF antibody titers IgG index, and RT-PCR have been used to help support a CDV encephalitis diagnosis.

Feline infectious peritonitis meningoencephalitis/meningomyelitis

CNS involvement of the coronavirus infection FIP is typically seen in cats <4 years old (Table 14.6; Rand *et al.*, 1994a). It presents with neurologic signs suggesting multifocal lesions referable to the cerebellum, brainstem, thalamocortex, or spinal cord.

On CSF analysis there is a markedly increased CSF TP. Rand *et al.* (1994a) found that cats with CNS involvement of FIP had a mean CSF TP of 368 mg/dl and none of the cats had a CSF TP 200 mg/dl. All cases with other causes of inflammatory disease had CSF TP 200 mg/dl. Hence it has been suggested that a CSF TP 200 mg/dl may be an appropriate indicator of FIP. In these same cats, the mean TNCC was 510 cells/μl characterized as a neutrophilic pleocytosis with neutrophil percentages over 80%. A more recent study, however, reported that only 25% of cats with CNS FIP had an increased CSF TP and 67% had a pleocytosis (Steinberg *et al.*, 2008). Testing of the CSF for anti-corona antibodies or direct detection of coronavirus has been utilized (Boettcher *et al.*, 2007). RT-PCR of CSF has excellent specificity and positive predictive value for the detection of FCoV RNA, although sensitivity in cats without clinical signs of neurologic disease is limited (Doenges *et al.*, 2016).

In contrast, non-FIP viral disease in the cat typically presents with a less impressive pleocytosis. Six of nine cats in one study had a normal TNCC; the remaining three had a TNCC just over the reference interval (Rand *et al.*, 1994a). Nucleated cellularity was most

Table 14.5 A summary of the significant diagnostic findings with canine distemper virus encephalitis

Signalment	Dogs; all ages
Clarity	Clear
Color	Colorless
CSF TP	Mild to marked increase
CSF cellularity	Young dogs: mild neutrophilic pleocytosis Older dogs: moderate mononuclear pleocytosis
CNS cytology	Not commonly performed
Ancillary testing	CSF antibody titer, IgG index, RT-PCR
Notes	Younger dogs: chewing gum seizures, vestibular dysfunction, myoclonus Older dogs: encephalitis

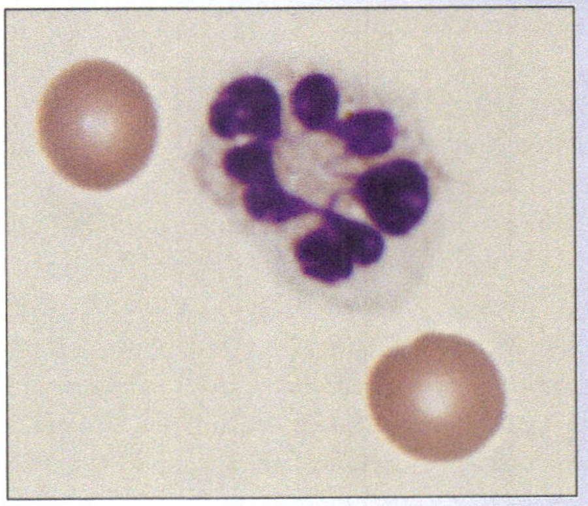

Table 14.6 A summary of the significant diagnostic findings with feline infectious peritonitis meningoencephalitis/meningomyelitis

Signalment	Cats; <4 years old
Clarity	Clear to turbid
Color	Colorless
CSF TP	Marked increase (>200 mg/dl)
CSF cellularity	Marked neutrophilic pleocytosis
CNS cytology	Not commonly performed
Ancillary testing	Anti-corona antibodies, detection of corona virus, RT-PCR
Notes	May present without pleocytosis or increased CSF TP

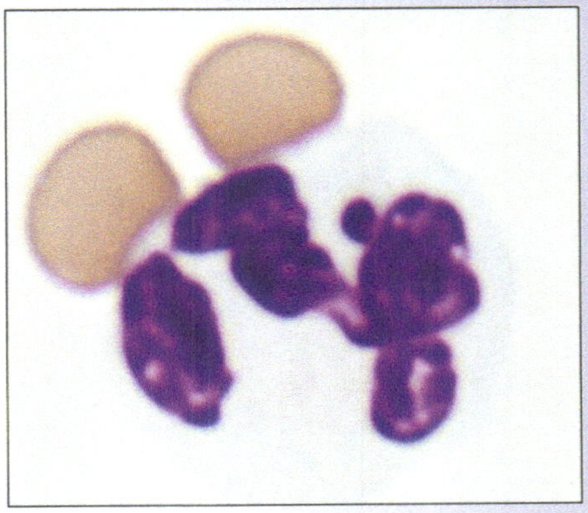

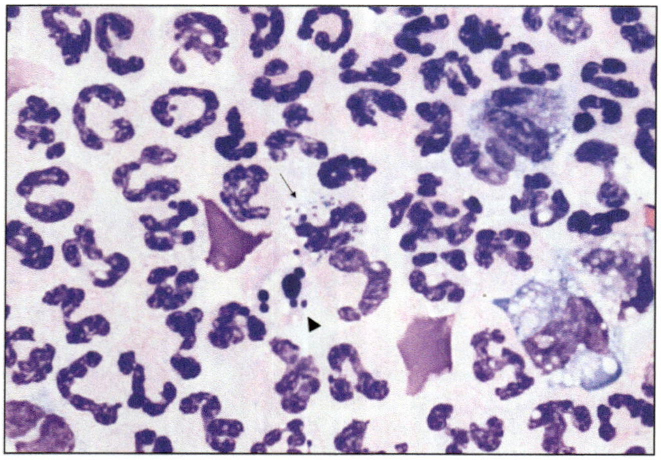

Figure 14.32 CSF from a 12-year-old mixed breed dog. TNCC = 157,830 cells/μl, CSF TP = 4,158 mg/dl. A marked neutrophilic pleocytosis is present with many neutrophils appearing degenerate. Rare neutrophils contain intracellular cocci bacteria arranged in pairs (thin arrow). A leukocyte undergoing karyorrhexis is also shown (arrowhead), which should not be mistaken for intracellular bacteria or fungal yeast (Wright–Giemsa, 1,000× magnification). The patient had concurrent septic peritonitis, a hepatic abscess, and suspected bacteremia.

commonly small mononuclear cells and CSF TP was normal to mildly increased with a mean of 28 mg/dl.

Inflammatory lesions

Steroid-responsive meningitis–arteritis

Steroid-responsive meningitis-arteritis (SRMA) is a systemic autoimmune disorder with primary inflammatory lesions in the leptomeninges and vasculature (hence meningitis–arteritis) of young-adult dogs (Table 14.7; Tipold & Stein, 2010). It is suspected to have an infectious origin. Widespread T-cell activation is noted and suggests a superantigen (Tipold & Stein, 2010). A genetic component is also suspected as Bernese Mountain Dogs, Boxers, Beagles, and Nova Scotia Duck Tolling Retrievers appear to have a breed or familial predisposition. Other medium to large breed dogs have been diagnosed with SRMA.

CSF examination typically reveals a turbid sample with a marked neutrophilic pleocytosis, occasionally >1,000 cells/μl. Evidence of hemorrhage, including xanthochromia and erythrophagocytosis, is common (Figures 14.33a–d). Elevated immunoglobulin levels, typically IgA, are reported prominent findings. Elevated CSF IL-8, matrix metalloproteinases, and CD11a have been noted in the CSF and could be the cause of the marked pleocytosis. An altered B-cell/T-cell ratio in the blood and CSF, leading to a Th2 response and autoantibody production, can be seen as well. A concurrent peripheral leukocytosis is common (Tipold & Stein, 2010).

As the name implies, the disease commonly requires immunosuppressive doses of glucocorticoids or other immunosuppressive drugs to attain remission. Because the clinical pathology findings with the disease are not highly specific for SRMA, exclusion of other causes of a marked neutrophilic pleocytosis is warranted. Of special note is that many SRMA cases look similar to bacterial meningitis on CSF analysis. Since cytologic detection of bacteria in CSF is not 100% sensitive, culture or other appropriate infectious disease testing before starting immunosuppressive therapy may be warranted in case of suspected SRMA.

Meningoencephalitis of unknown etiology

As definitive diagnosis of immune-mediated inflammatory disease of the CSF requires histopathologic diagnosis, patients with compatible clinical signs, CSF, and imaging findings are often placed under the umbrella diagnosis of meningoencephalitis of unknown etiology (MUE). Histopathologic subtypes of MUE include granulomatous meningoencephalomyelitis (GME), necrotizing leukoencephalitis (NLE), and necrotizing meningoencephalitis (NME). A T-cell mediated immune-mediated pathogenesis has been proposed for these conditions, although the trigger of this response has not yet been determined (Vitale & Foss, 2019).

Granulomatous meningoencephalomyelitis

Granulomatous meningoencephalomyelitis (GME) is an autoimmune inflammatory disease of the canine CNS that accounts for 5–25% of CNS disorders in the dog (Table 14.8; Suzuki *et al.*, 2003; Adamo *et*

Table 14.7 **A summary of the significant diagnostic findings with steroid-responsive meningitis–arteritis**

Signalment	Bernese Mountain Dog, Boxer, Beagle, Nova Scotia Duck Tolling Retriever. Young adults
Clarity	Clear to turbid
Color	Possible red/xanthochromia
CSF TP	Mild to marked increase
CSF cellularity	Marked neutrophilic pleocytosis
CNS cytology	Not commonly performed
Ancillary testing	Elevated immunoglobulin. Concurrent peripheral lymphocytosis
Notes	Consider ruling out infectious agents before treatment

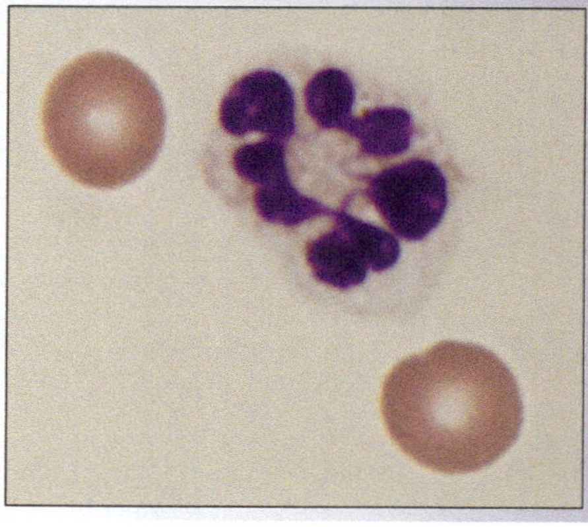

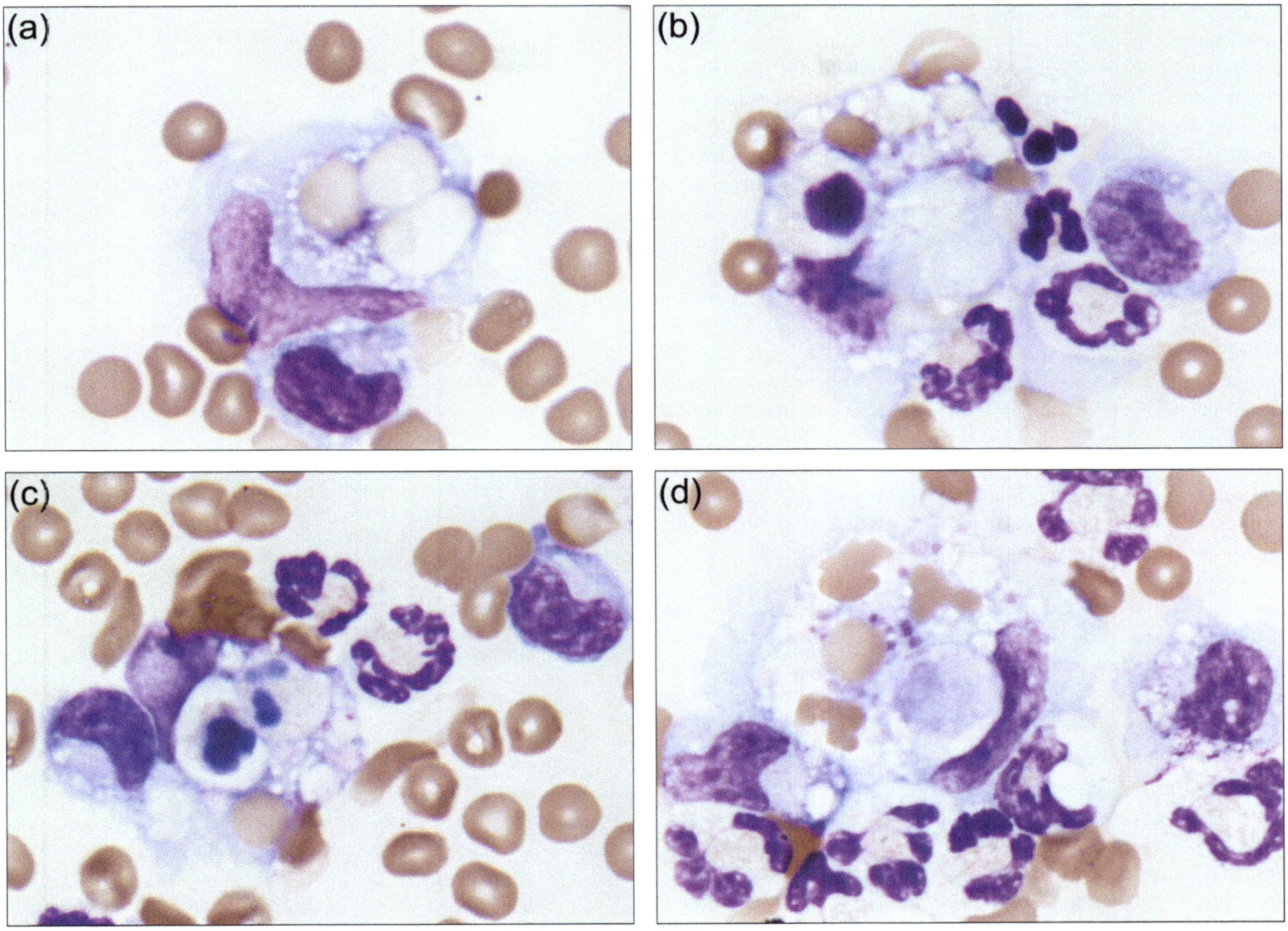

Figures 14.33a–d CSF from a 1-year-old, spayed female German Shorthaired Pointer. TNCC = 4,060 cells/µl, CSF TP = 320 mg/dl. (a) Large mononuclear cells in the sample display pronounced erythrophagocytosis. (b–d) Many large mononuclear cells have phagocytized cellular debris (Wright–Giemsa, 1,000× magnification). Evaluation of synovial fluid from the right carpus and both stifle joints suggested a concurrent immune-mediated polyarthritis; the inflammatory lesions in the CSF are interpreted as part of a systemic autoimmune disease. The infectious agent profile was negative; the patient responded well to prolonged immunosuppression.

Table 14.8 A summary of the significant diagnostic findings with granulomatous meningoencephalomyelitis

Signalment	Small breed dogs, especially toy breeds and terriers. Possible female bias
Clarity	Clear to turbid
Color	Possible red/xanthochromia
CSF TP	Moderate to marked increase
CSF cellularity	Moderate to marked mononuclear pleocytosis Rarely, neutrophilic pleocytosis
CNS cytology	Mononuclear inflammation
Ancillary testing	CSF-based autoantibody testing is possible
Notes	Necrosis is present but most often not seen

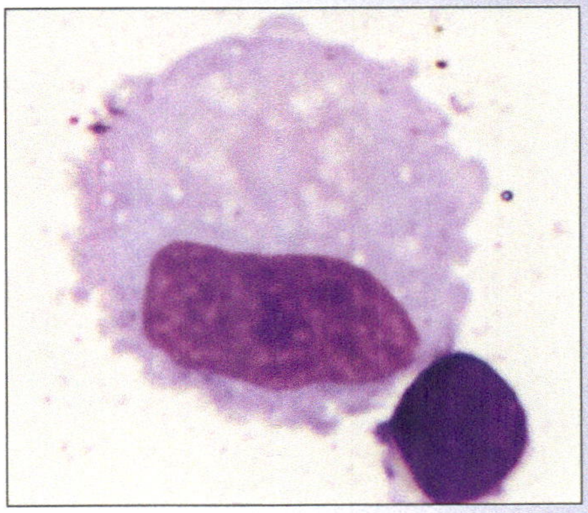

al., 2007; Talarico & Schatzberg, 2010). The exact instigator of the autoimmune response is unknown. It presents as large accumulations of mononuclear cells cuffing small blood vessels in the parenchyma and meninges of the cerebrum, brainstem, spinal cord, or rarely cerebellum (Higginbotham *et al.*, 2007). Ocular, focal, or disseminated forms of GME occur; rarely, the focal lesions can appear mass-like on imaging and can be found in the cerebrum with smaller disseminated lesions (Thomas, 1999). GME is typically seen in small breed dogs, especially toy breed and terriers. Females may be overrepresented (Higginbotham *et al.*, 2007).

CSF findings typically include a lymphocytic/small mononuclear pleocytosis (TNCC = 50–900 cells/μl) and increased protein (CSF TP = 40–400 mg/dl) (Figure 14.34; Adamo *et al.*, 2007). A neutrophilic or large mononuclear pleocytosis may also occur; one study found that 17% of GME patients had a neutrophilic pleocytosis. Confirmed cases of GME have even been found to have normal CSF (Bailey & Higgins, 1986). FNA might be utilized in cases with a focal/mass-type lesion. An inflammatory population would be expected on CNS cytology based on histologic biopsies of GME; however, this has not been reported in the literature.

As with SRMA, immunosuppression is a mainstay of GME treatment. CSF analysis and fine needle cytology are not sensitive enough for detection of infectious agents; culture or other diagnostic techniques should be used prior to immunosuppression.

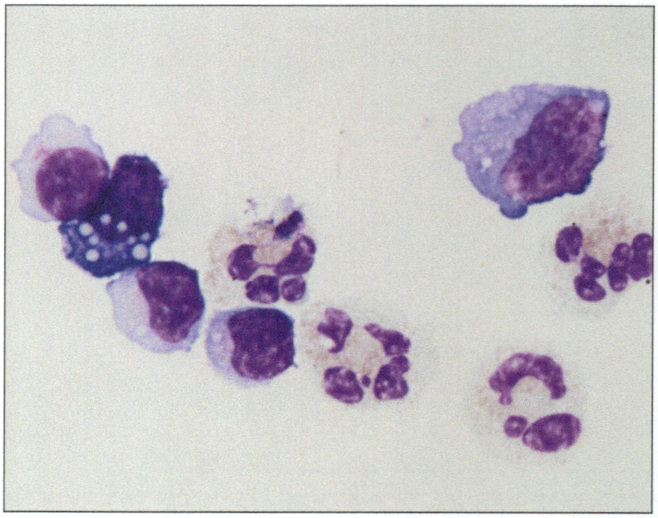

Figure 14.34 CSF from a 12-year-old mixed breed dog. TNCC = 426 cells/μl, CSF TP = 136 mg/dl. There is a mixed pleocytosis with small and large mononuclear cells most predominant and lower numbers of neutrophils. Plasma cells, including Mott cells, are also present in the sample and suggest intrathecal immunoglobulin production (Wright–Giemsa, 1,000× magnification). Infectious disease testing was negative. The clinical diagnosis was granulomatous meningoencephalomyelitis. Neurologic signs responded well to immune suppression.

Necrotizing leukoencephalitis

Originally named necrotizing encephalitis and described in the Yorkshire Terrier, necrotizing leukoencephalitis (NLE) has been reported in young (average 4.5 years old) dogs of other breeds as well (Table 14.9; Higginbotham *et al.*, 2007). It can be found in the cerebrum and brainstem with clinical signs associated with the location of the lesion. The inciting cause is unknown.

Histologically, NLE presents as a focal area of necrosis in the white matter of the cerebrum and thalamus. This necrosis is often not observed in CSF analysis; instead there is a mild, typically mixed pleocytosis and mild to moderate CSF TP elevations.

Necrotizing meningoencephalitis

Necrotizing meningoencephalitis (NME) has historically been called pug-dog encephalitis. Similar findings have been reported in non-pug dogs; most are juvenile to young adults (Table 14.10; Higginbotham *et al.*, 2007). An autoimmune process is suspected (Suzuki *et al.*, 2003; Talarico & Schatzberg, 2010). Like NLE, NME consists of focal lesions with a necrotic center. In NME the lesion is typically restricted to the cerebrum.

Another distinction between NME and NLE is the decidedly lymphocytic/small mononuclear pleocytosis found in most cases of NME (Higginbotham *et al.*, 2007). Sixteen of 17 cases with histologic

Table 14.9 A summary of the significant diagnostic findings with necrotizing leukoencephalitis

Signalment	Yorkshire Terriers, other dogs. Young adults
Clarity	Clear
Color	Colorless
CSF TP	Mild to moderate increase
CSF cellularity	Mild mixed pleocytosis
CNS cytology	Not commonly performed
Ancillary testing	CSF-based autoantibody testing is possible
Notes	Necrosis is not commonly apparent on CSF

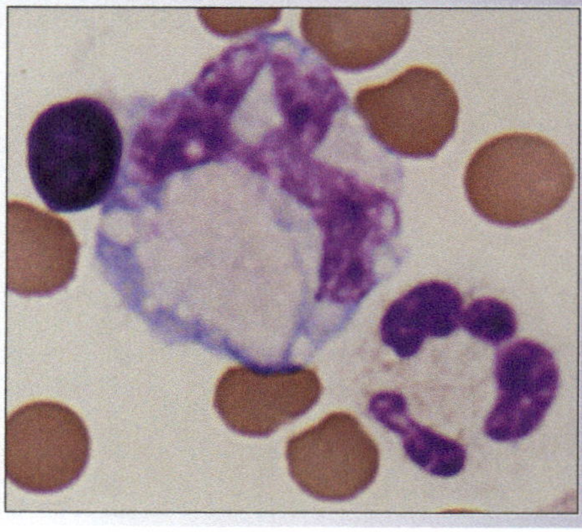

Table 14.10 A summary of the significant diagnostic findings with necrotizing meningoencephalitis

Signalment	Pugs and other dog breeds. Juvenile to young adults
Clarity	Clear
Color	Colorless
CSF TP	Mild to moderate elevations
CSF cellularity	Moderate small mononuclear pleocytosis
CNS cytology	Not commonly performed
Ancillary testing	CSF-based autoantibody testing is possible
Notes	Previously called pug-dog encephalitis

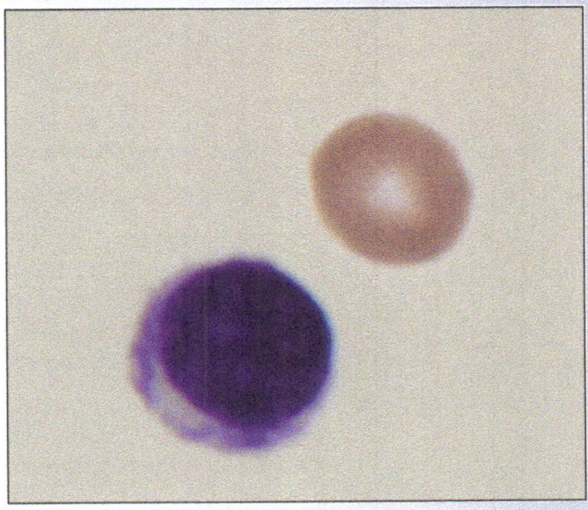

Table 14.11 A summary of significant diagnostic findings with cerebrovascular accidents (strokes)

Signalment	Dogs and cats. Cavalier King Charles Spaniel, Greyhounds may be predisposed
Clarity	Clear to turbid
Color	Possible red/xanthochromia
CSF TP	Mild to moderate increase
CSF cellularity	Normal to marked neutrophilic or large mononuclear pleocytosis
CNS cytology	Not commonly performed
Ancillary testing	Diagnosis by imaging. Glutamate quantification may be helpful
Notes	Ischemic and hemorrhagic forms exist

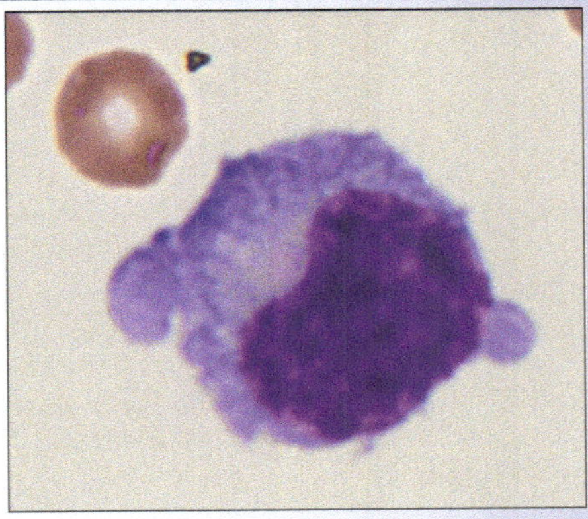

confirmation of NME had a small mononuclear predominance with a mean percentage of 90% small mononuclear cells. Neutrophilic, large mononuclear, or mixed pleocytosis, or even normal CSF cell counts can be observed. Otherwise presentation is similar to NLE.

Cerebrovascular accidents/stroke

Previously, it was believed that cerebrovascular accidents (CVAs) did not routinely occur in dogs and cats. However, they are increasingly being recognized in veterinary medicine (Table 14.11; Garosi *et al.*, 2006). Mean age for dogs with a CVA is 8 years, although patients as young as 18 months have been reported. One study found eight of 40 (20%) dogs were Cavalier King Charles Spaniels and another 12% were Greyhounds, which probably is an overrepresentation of these breeds, although a breakdown of the common breeds at the reporting institution was not included to help support or refute this assumption (Garosi *et al.*, 2006). Underlying causes of CVAs in veterinary medicine have not been well documented. Lesions can be located in the telencephalon, thalamus/midbrain, cerebellum, and multifocally. CVAs can be further classified as either ischemic (infarction due to obstruction) or hemorrhagic (due to rupturing of vasculature) events.

CVAs show signs of hemorrhage on CSF, including increased CSF protein, mild neutrophilic or mononuclear pleocytosis (TNCC <30 cells/μl), xanthochromia, and hemosiderosis (Garosi *et al.*, 2006). Some work has suggested that CSF glutamate concentrations may be a marker for CVAs, although sensitivity and specificity have not yet been evaluated (Platt *et al.*, 2013). Commonly, patients with CVAs have normal CSF and must be diagnosed by clinical signs and advanced imaging (Gonçalves *et al.*, 2011).

Central nervous system trauma

External trauma as a primary cause of CNS disease is typically apparent based on physical and neurologic examinations (Table 14.12). CSF evaluation is often not needed but may reveal considerable amounts

Table 14.12 A summary of the significant diagnostic findings with CNS trauma

Signalment	Any
Clarity	Clear to turbid
Color	Possible red/xanthochromia
CSF TP	Possible increase (commensurate with hemorrhage)
CSF cellularity	Leukocytes consistent with blood contamination Possible myelin or neuropil
CNS cytology	Not commonly performed
Ancillary testing	In acute phase, changes can be ascribed to hemorrhage
Notes	CSF analysis typically not needed

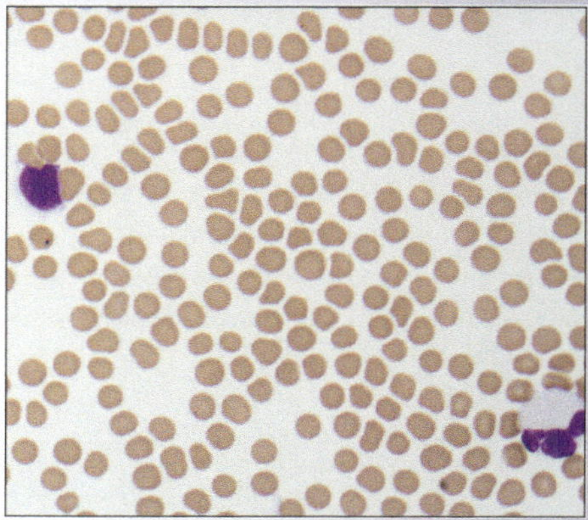

Table 14.13 A summary of the significant diagnostic findings with intervertebral disk disease

Signalment	Dachshunds, chondrodystrophic dogs. Rarely occurs in cats
Clarity	Clear
Color	Colorless
CSF TP	Approximately one-half have mild increase
CSF cellularity	Acute cases: mild to moderate neutrophilic pleocytosis Chronic cases: mild to moderate mononuclear pleocytosis
CNS cytology	Not commonly performed
Ancillary testing	Diagnosis made by imaging Myelin basic protein and creatinine kinase may predict return to function
Notes	Macrophage:monocyte ratio >0.7 and deep pain negative may be highly sensitive indicator of a negative outcome

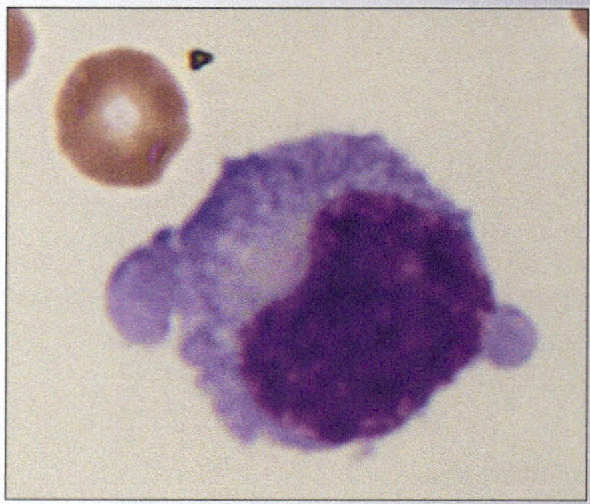

of hemorrhage and possibly myelin, neuropil, or other nervous tissue. Because of the mixing of peripheral blood into the CSF, TNCC and CSF TP are typically elevated, especially in the initial phases of trauma.

Technically, trauma is the direct pathologic mechanism causing neurologic signs in IVDD and other degenerative diseases. The underlying cause may be a degenerative weakness of the disks in IVDD; however, it is the explosion of disk material impacting the spinal cord that determines the severity and extent of the neurologic deficits.

Congenital or degenerative lesions

Intervertebral disk disease

Intervertebral disk disease (IVDD) is a degenerative process caused by a combination of factors, including age, genetic, and environmental components, that lead to a degeneration and herniation of disk material into the spinal canal (Table 14.13). Common locations for disk herniation are within the cervical region and near the thoracolumbar junction. Herniation can occur as a sudden event or as a slower, less traumatic process. IVDD is uncommon in cats; reported incidence is 0.02–0.12% in the cat, compared with 2% in dogs (Marioni-Henry, 2010). Dachshunds are at significantly higher risk than other dog breeds. Other chondrodystrophic breeds are also at a higher risk.

Because of the variable pathology associated with IVDD, CSF findings can be variable. In a series of 30 dogs with IVDD, a median CSF TP of 24.1 mg/dl was reported and 43% had a mild increase in CSF TP (Chamisha *et al.*, 2015). Mild to moderate pleocytosis was seen in 51% of dogs. The incidence of pleocytosis could be further broken down into 23% of cervical cases and 61% of thoracolumbar cases showing pleocytosis (Brisson, 2010). Median TNCC was 52 cells/µl, with various forms of pleocytosis noted (Chamisha *et al.*, 2015). Erythrophagia was noted in only 19% of cases. In other reports, myelin figures have been seen in the CSF of patients with IVDD (Fallin *et al.*, 1996).

Most commonly, CSF analysis does not significantly add to the diagnosis of IVDD; radiographic techniques are sufficiently informative to allow a diagnosis. However, once the diagnosis of IVDD has been made, evaluation of the CSF can be prognostic. A neutrophilic pleocytosis typically is found in acute cases of IVDD. Cases with fewer neutrophils, more large mononuclear cells, lower TP, and lower RBC counts likely have had sufficient time to progress from an acute inflammatory response to a more chronic state and therefore are more likely to have a worse outcome (Srugo *et al.*, 2011; Levine *et al.*, 2014). Recent studies have evaluated several biomarkers and visually determined macrophage:monocyte ratios in CSF as potential prognostic markers in IVDD (Bittermann *et al.*, 2019; Chamisha *et al.*, 2015; Levine *et al.*, 2010). Although results from these studies are somewhat conflicting, myelin basic protein and creatine kinase concentrations have been shown to be highly predictive of return to ambulatory function. (Olby *et al.*, 2020). Further evaluation of the clinical utility of these biomarkers is needed.

Fibrocartilaginous embolus

Fibrocartilaginous emboli (FCE) most commonly, but not exclusively, occur in large and giant breed dogs and domestic shorthair cats (Table 14.14; De Risio & Platt, 2010). Median age in the dog is 5–6 years. The history usually includes a peracute nonprogressive myelopathy that is not painful after the first 24 hours. The lesion is an embolism in the intra-parenchymal spinal cord arteries of material chemically and histologically similar to the nucleus pulposus of intervertebral disks. Several theories have been proposed to explain how this happens. MRI is the preferred diagnostic tool and will demonstrate a focal spinal cord swelling.

CSF analysis usually is employed to exclude other causes. CSF abnormalities are found in 45–75% of cases with FCE and include mildly elevated CSF TP, mild to moderate pleocytosis (TNCC = 7–84 cells/μl), and xanthochromia (De Risio & Platt, 2010).

Cystic lesions/hydrocephalus

Cystic structures are occasionally observed during imaging techniques of the neurologic patient (Table 14.15). Subarachnoid cysts are commonly seen in the dorsal subarachnoid space at the first or third cervical vertebrae of younger large breed dogs or caudal thoracic vertebrae of older small breed dogs (Skeen *et al.*, 2003). These structures are typically an intradural outpouching of arachnoid membranes. They may communicate with the CSF (Gnirs *et al.*, 2002).

Hydrocephalus can be caused by obstruction of CSF flow, and can be classified as either internal (within the ventricular system) or external (within the subarachnoid space). The end result of both types of obstruction is the retention of CSF. CSF overproduction is very rarely a cause of hydrocephalus.

Neither of these lesions are truly cysts, in that they are not epithelial lined structures. Aspiration of the fluid areas in cases of subarachnoid cysts or hydrocephalus will produce material similar to normal CSF (Thomas, 1999; Gnirs *et al.*, 2002).

Epidermoid cysts are typically seen in the fourth ventricle in the dog. They are true cysts, being lined by stratified squamous epithelium, and are filled with desquamated cells (Spoor *et al.*, 2013). On cytology, epidermoid cysts have large aggregates of anucleate squamous epithelial cells, which could be mistaken for post-collection artifact of surface epidermal keratin. Epidermoid cysts are congenital lesions representing aberrant location of ectoderm in the neural tube. These structures may develop in the spinal cord and have been reported following spinal trauma or repeated CSF collection. If cysts also contain adnexal differentiation, they are termed dermoid cysts.

Rarely, meningeal carcinomatosis will produce cystic structures (Mateo *et al.*, 2010). Samples from these tumors could contain neoplastic cells on cytologic evaluation of the CSF. Finally, the choroid plexus can form cysts that are either symptomatic or asymptomatic (Galano *et al.*, 2002).

Lysosomal storage diseases

Lysosomal storage diseases are a group of congenital diseases caused by a metabolic deficiency in a catabolic pathway (Table 14.16; Miller & Zachary, 2017). Usually they are the result of a single gene deficiency. On a cellular basis this leads to an inability to break down a specific metabolite, which then builds up in the lysosomes. Typically,

Table 14.14 **A summary of the significant diagnostic findings with fibrocartilaginous embolism**

Signalment	Large and giant breed dogs, 5–6 years old. Domestic shorthair cats
Clarity	Clear
Color	Possible xanthochromia
CSF TP	Mild increase
CSF cellularity	Mild to moderate neutrophilic pleocytosis
CNS cytology	Not commonly performed
Ancillary testing	Diagnosis made by imaging
Notes	Peracute history of severe pain/neurologic deficits that becomes pain free after 24 hours

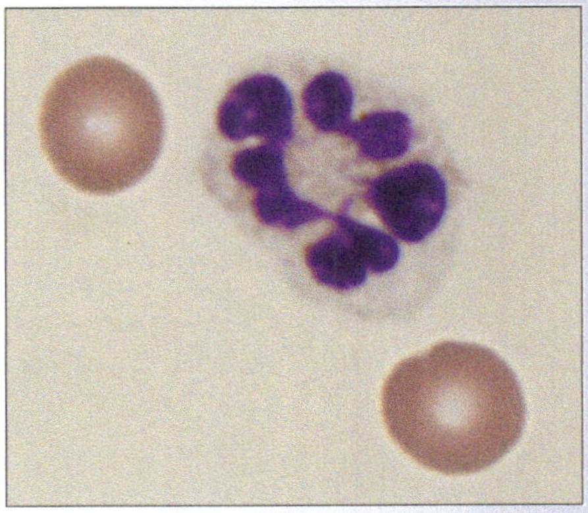

the patient presents early in life with a multitude of defects, both within and outside the CNS, depending on the type of lysosomal storage disease. Multiple types of storage disease occur, not all of which are expected to display neurologic effects. GM-1 and GM-2 gangliosidosis, ceroid lipofuscinosis, globoid cell leukodystrophy (Krabbe's-like disease), mucopolysaccharidosis, and Neimann–Pick type C have been reported to involve the CNS of dogs and cats. Alpha mannosidosis is seen in the cat but has not yet been reported in the dog.

One of the defining cytologic findings of lysosomal storage diseases is an abundance of blue, metachromatic, or pink cytoplasmic material (Figures 14.35a, b, 14.36). This is found within the nervous tissue itself but can also be seen in the large mononuclear population in the CSF and peripheral blood. Special staining of the cells, including periodic acid–Schiff, T-blue, and Luxol fast blue, can be used. Urine oligosaccharide profiles can be used as a screening test. CSF and peripheral blood testing for the retained metabolite or genetic testing for the specific gene defect are commonly used to provide an antemortem diagnosis. Electron microscopy and special staining can be used on histologic samples.

Neoplasia

Intracranial neoplasia has been reported in up to 3% of canine cases. In one series of 173 canine primary brain tumors, tumor types with the highest incidence included meningioma (45% of cases), astrocytoma (17%), oligodendroglioma (14%), choroid plexus tumors (7%), and primary CNS lymphoma (4%) (Snyder *et al*., 2006). Meningioma is the most common intracranial tumor reported in the cat. It accounted for 58.1% of feline primary intracranial tumors; lymphoma (14.4%), pituitary tumors (8.8%), astrocytoma (2.8%), and oligodendroglioma (2.4%) made up the other more populated categories in a series of 160 cats (Troxel *et al*., 2003). Metastasis and direct extension of extracranial neoplasms occurred in only 5% and 4% of feline intracranial neoplasm cases, respectively. Meningioma is the most common primary spinal cord lesion in the dog (José-López *et al*., 2013). Other primary tumor types rarely found in the CNS of the dog and cat include primitive neuroectodermal tumors, glioblastomas, olfactory neuroblastomas, histiocytic sarcomas, and vascular tumors (Figures 14.37a, b).

Neoplasia is commonly associated with a neutrophilic pleocytosis or increased neutrophil percentage. However, a neutrophilic

Table 14.15 **A summary of the significant diagnostic findings with cystic lesions and hydrocephalus**

Signalment	Various
Clarity	Clear
Color	Colorless
CSF TP	Within reference limits
CSF cellularity	Within reference limits
CNS cytology	Not commonly performed
Ancillary testing	Diagnosis made by imaging
Notes	Rarely, congenital malformations or neoplasms can produce cysts

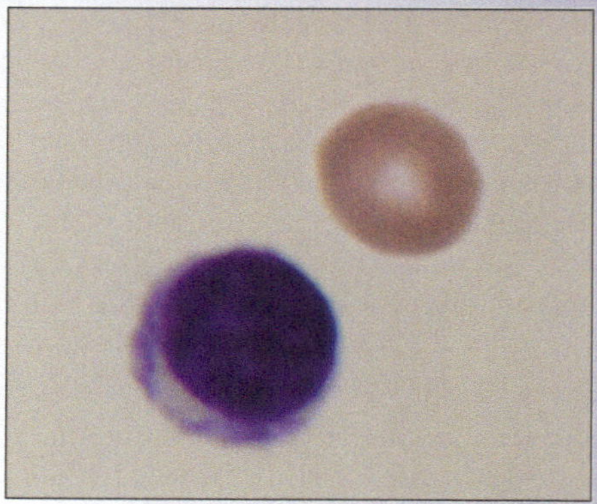

Table 14.16 **A summary of the significant diagnostic findings with lysosomal storage diseases**

Signalment	Various breeds of dogs and cats. Typically younger
Clarity	Clear
Color	Colorless
CSF TP	Normal to mild increase
CSF cellularity	Purple to pink granules noted within cells
CNS cytology	Not commonly performed
Ancillary testing	Storage material observed in peripheral blood cells. Urine mucopolysaccharidosis screen. Testing for specific metabolite or genetic defect
Notes	Multiple forms, most with concurrent congenital malformations

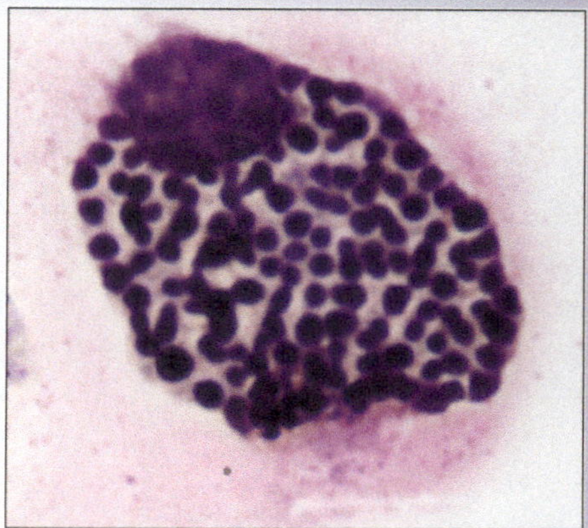

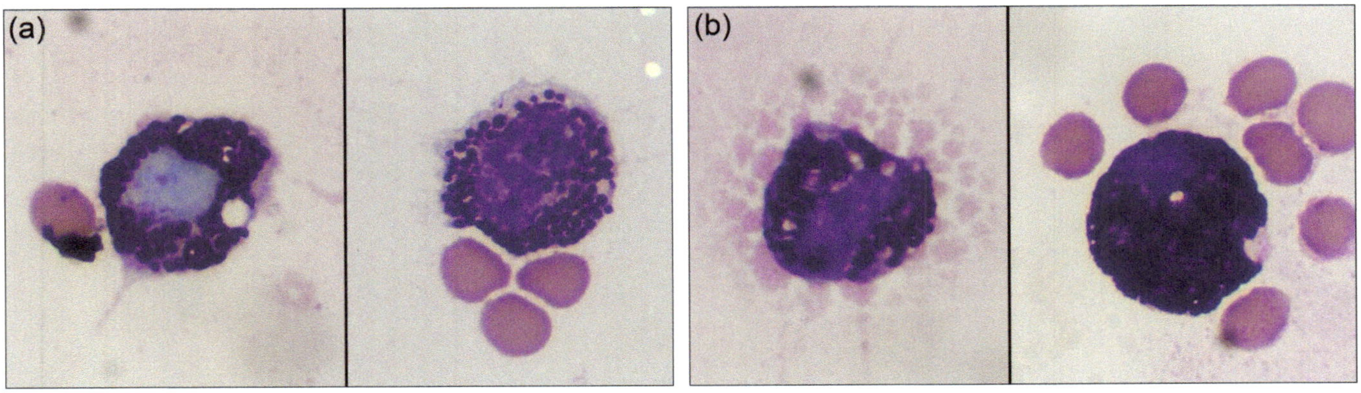

Figures 14.35a, b CSF from an 8-month-old, spayed female Boston Terrier presenting for pain when jumping and not being active as a puppy. TNCC = 1 cell/μl, RBC = 300 cells/μl, CSF TP = 49.5 mg/dl. Most of the mononuclear cells had variably sized magenta granules, which often distended the nucleus (Wright–Giemsa, 1,000× magnification). A urine screening was positive for mucopolysaccharidosis. Further characterization of the genetic disorder was not attempted. (Courtesy Dr. Seung Yoo.)

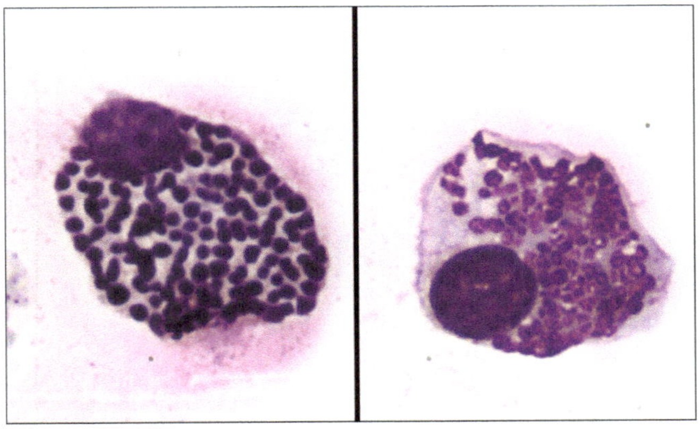

Figure 14.36 CSF from a 1-year-old, intact male Staffordshire Terrier with presenting complaints of ataxia, tetraparesis, and intermittent mental dullness. MRI changes were consistent with C2-C3 disk protrusion secondary to trauma or traumatic exacerbation of a congenital malformation. TNCC = 2 cells/μl, CSF TP = 64 mg/dl. Low numbers of large mononuclear cells (probably macrophages) are present. They have a small eccentrically placed round nucleus and abundant magenta cytoplasmic globular inclusions (Wright–Giemsa, 1,000× magnification). Further investigation showed strong positive mucopolysaccharidosis in urine and an underlying lysosomal storage disease was suspected. (Courtesy Dr. Laura Brandt.)

pleocytosis should not always be expected. One theory to explain the lack of pleocytosis states that some tumor locations are distant enough from the site of sampling or deep enough to prevent significant cellular shedding into the collected CSF. In a series of meningiomas, tumors in the caudal portion of the cranial fossa had higher cell counts, while those in more rostral locations commonly had lower counts (Dickinson *et al.*, 2006). Necrosis inducing inflammation has been used to explain neutrophilic pleocytosis associated with neoplasia; it could also be posited that less necrotic lesions would result in fewer neutrophils being present.

Patients with intracranial tumors are commonly presented when the owner notices a neurologic defect. Often the neurologic defects are the result of the space-occupying effects of the mass on surrounding tissue and not a primary effect of the tumor. A thorough neurologic examination is recommended to localize the lesion. In human medicine, lesion localization is commonly used to narrow down the differential list prior to cytologic evaluation (Powell, 2005). Similarly, lesion location and other magnetic resonance imaging features in dogs may help to prioritize likely differentials for intracranial tumors (Miller *et al.*, 2019b).

Meningiomas account for 45% and 85% of primary intracranial tumors and 22.3% and 59% of all intracranial tumors in dogs and cats, respectively (Table 14.17; Motta *et al.*, 2012). There is a breed predilection in Boxers and dolichocephalic breeds, including German Shepherd Dogs, Golden Retrievers, and Labrador Retrievers. Meningiomas seem more common in domestic shorthair cats. Most canine cases are over 7 years old at diagnosis and most cats are over 9 years old.

Meningioma

Meningiomas are intradural and extramedullary lesions. In the dog they are commonly diagnosed in the olfactory/frontal region, optic chiasm, suprasellar and parasellar regions, or cervical spinal cord. In the cat, the most common locations include the tela choroidea of the third ventricle, the supratentorial meninges, and the cerebellar meninges. Concurrent meningioma and another intracranial neoplasm were found in 13.9% of feline and 19% of canine meningioma patients (Motta *et al.*, 2012).

The most recent veterinary classification system of meningiomas describes nine variants (Koestner *et al.*, 1999). These include benign, slow growing tumors (including meningothelial, fibroblastic, transitional, psammomatous, angiomatous, papillary, granular, and myxoid subtypes) and more aggressive anaplastic tumors. However, multiple case reports and veterinary texts describe histologic subtypes not included in this classification. Tumor grading following the more recent WHO classification for central nervous system tumors has also been proposed (Belluco *et al.*, 2022). In both the human and veterinary classification systems, meningiomas are graded into three histologic

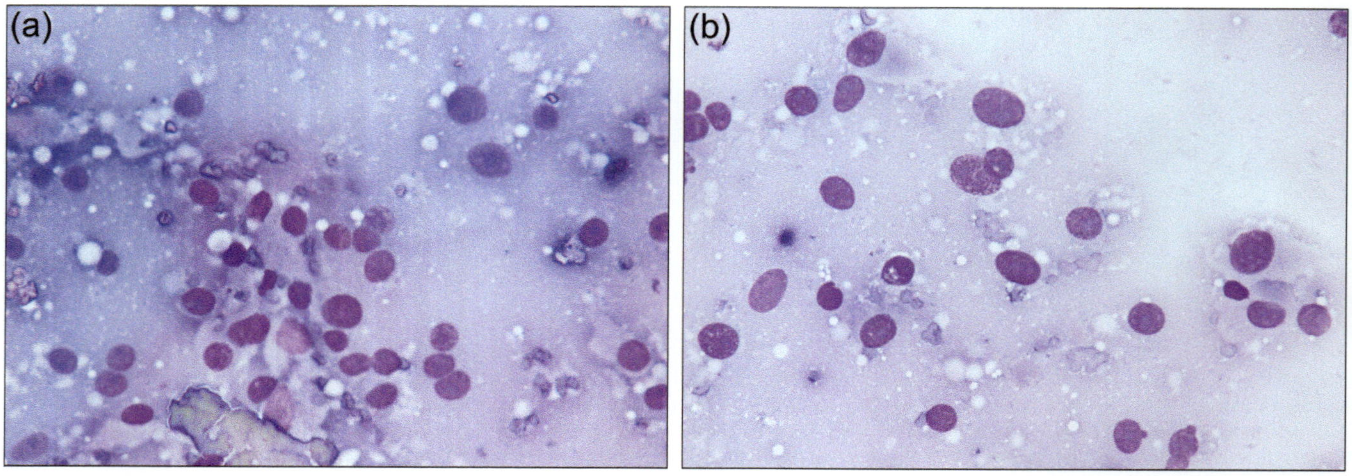

Figures 14.37a,b CNS cytology from a dog. (a) A neoplastic population of neurons. The cells resemble large pyramidal cells found in the cerebellum with many ruptured cells present (Wright–Giemsa, 500× magnification). (b) Where the cells are well intact, they are roughly triangular with basophilic faintly granular cytoplasm, a large eccentrically located ovoid nucleus with stippled chromatin and single large distinct nucleolus. This morphology is suggestive of a ganglioneuroma (Wright–Giemsa, 1,000× magnification). The cytologic diagnosis was confirmed by histopathology.

Table 14.17 A summary of the significant diagnostic findings with meningioma

Signalment	Boxers, German Shepherd Dogs, Golden Retrievers, Labrador Retrievers. Domestic shorthair cats
Clarity	Clear
Color	Colorless
CSF TP	Possible increase
CSF cellularity	Normal to moderate neutrophilic pleocytosis. Rarely, neoplastic cells seen
Lesion location	Intradural, extramedullary. Dog: olfactory, frontal, suprasellar, parasellar region, optic chiasm, cervical spinal cord. Cat: 3rd ventricle, supratentorial and cerebellar meninges
CNS cytology	Moderately-sized cohesive cells, intranuclear cytoplasmic inclusions, folded nuclei
Ancillary testing	Positive: CD-18, actin. Negative: S-100, CD3, CD79a, PAX5, cytokeratin, GFAP
Notes	Multiple histologic types described

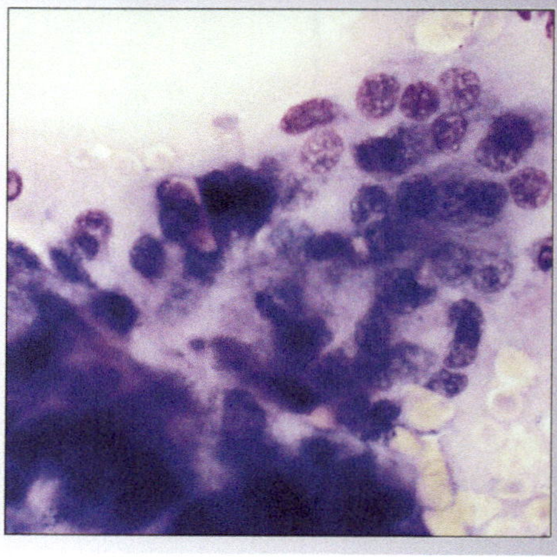

grades (I–III; or benign, atypical, and anaplastic). Classification and grading of meningiomas has prognostic value in human medicine, although the prognostic significance of grade or subtype of meningiomas in veterinary medicine is still uncertain (José-López *et al.*, 2013). Recommendations for standardization of canine meningioma grading have recently been proposed to improve intra-observer agreement (Belluco *et al.*, 2022). Metastasis has been reported in the dog and cat but does not appear common.

Although it has been reported that meningiomas often have a neutrophilic pleocytosis, multiple retrospective studies report that the majority of cases had a TNCC <5 cells/μl (Dickinson *et al.*, 2006; Toyoda *et al.*, 2020). CSF TP increases were found in most meningioma cases; all cases with a pleocytosis and 61% of canine meningioma cases lacking pleocytosis had elevated protein.

FNA or intraoperative biopsy smears often contain clusters and cohesive groups of cells that lack prominent vasculature (Figures 14.38–14.40). The neoplastic cells appear closely adherent to vascular walls. The cells have variable amounts of spindloid to wispy cytoplasm, a round to elongate nucleus, punctate chromatin, and a small prominent nucleolus. Intranuclear cytoplasmic pseudoinclusions and nuclear folding have been described in meningiomas in both the dog and cat (Harms *et al.*, 2009). Intranuclear cytoplasmic pseudoinclusions are round basophilic vacuolated intranuclear structures, which appear to be a bleb of cytoplasm within the nucleus. They have been found in normal hepatocytes, meningiomas, Leydig cell tumors, melanomas, and papillary thyroid carcinomas, among others. Papanicolaou staining may help highlight these inclusions, but they have been reported with Wright–Giemsa staining alone.

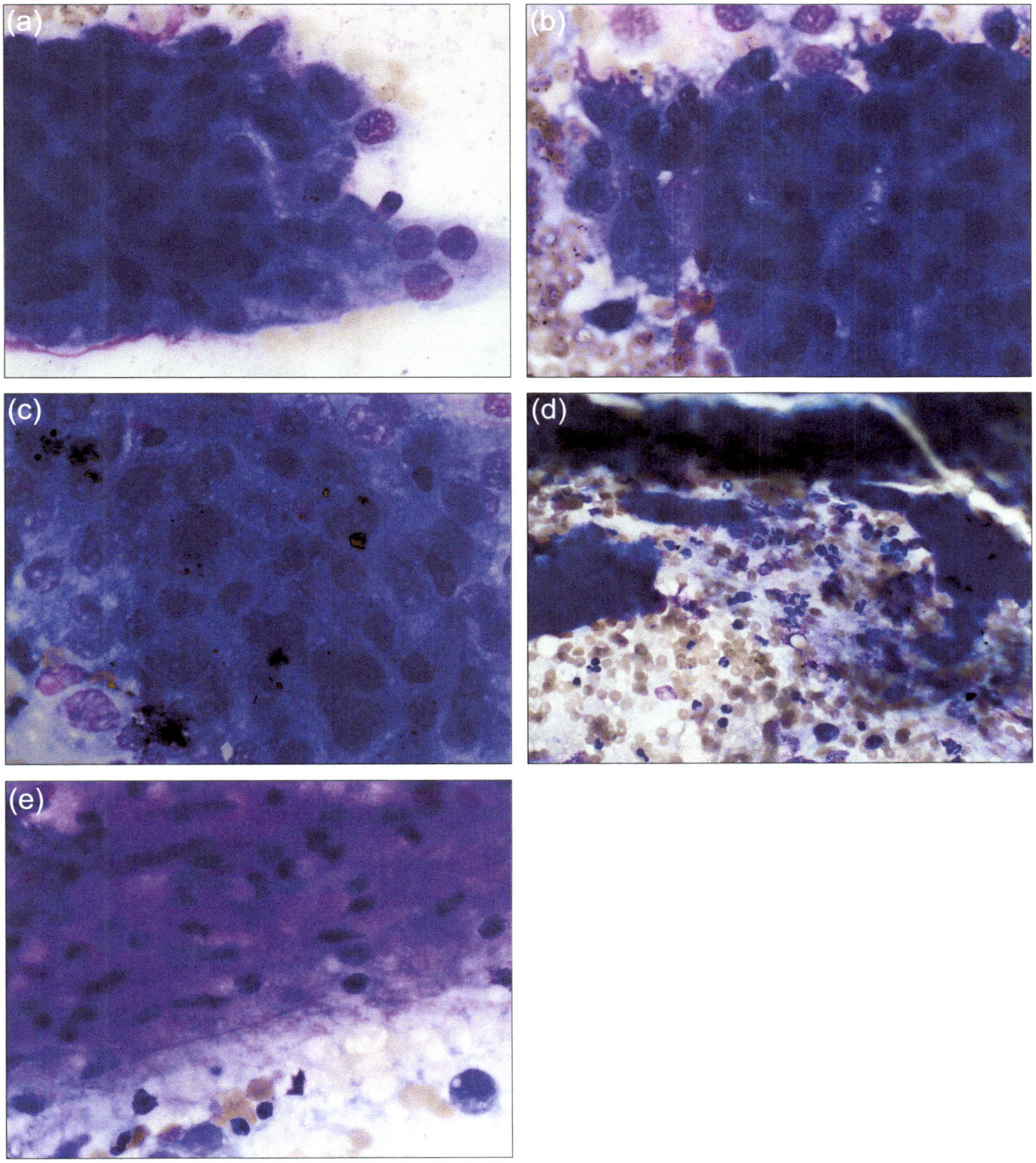

Figures 14.38a–e Aspirate of a mass in the forebrain of a dog. (a) Sheets of cohesively clustered polygonal cells with moderate amounts of basophilic cytoplasm and round to ovoid nuclei are present (Wright–Giemsa, 1,000× magnification). (b) Note the minimal to moderate anisocytosis and anisokaryosis in the cell population (Wright–Giemsa, 1,000× magnification). (c) Hematoidin crystals and aggregates of blue–black granular material (likely hemosiderin) are present and suggest chronic hemorrhage (Wright–Giemsa, 500× magnification). (d) Several areas of the slide had increased numbers of nondegenerate neutrophils and cellular debris (Wright–Giemsa, 500× magnification). (e) The pink extracellular felt-like material is a dense aggregate of neuropil. Nuclei of glial cells are present within the neuropil (Wright–Giemsa, 1,000× magnification).

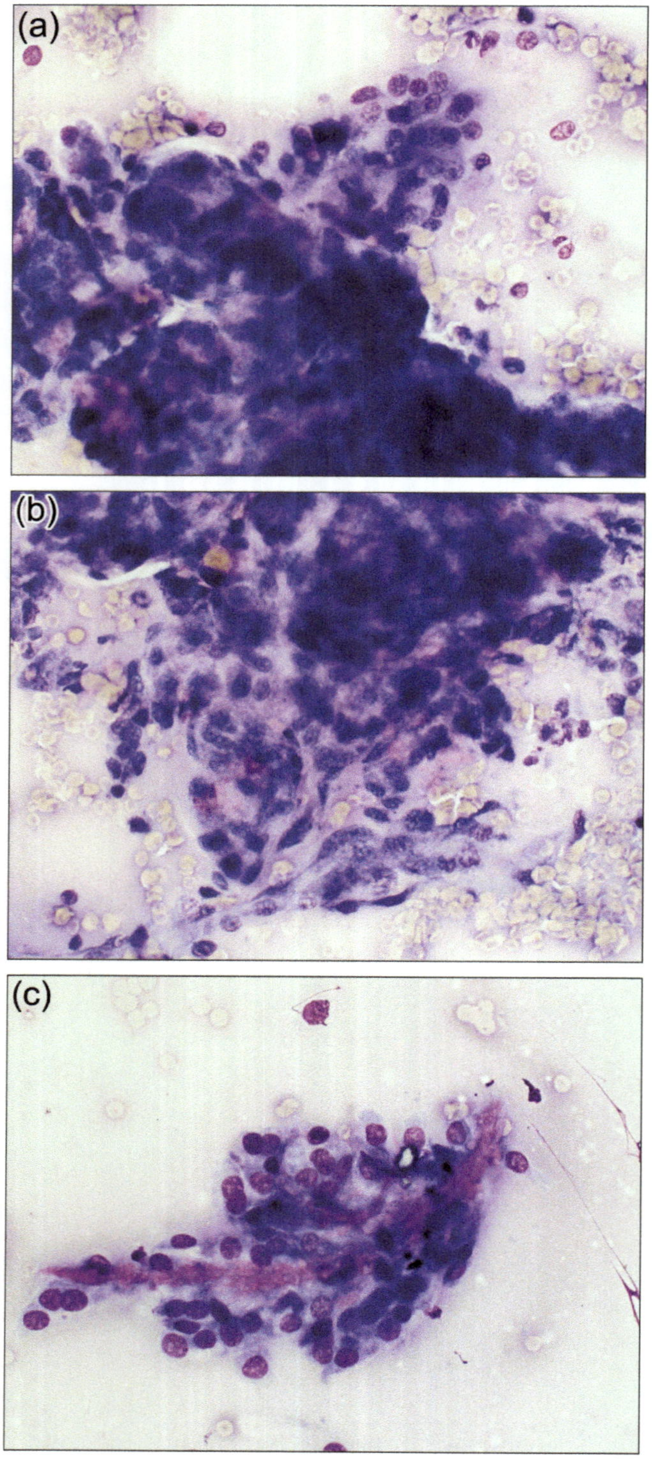

Figures 14.39a–c CNS cytology from a dog. (a) Large aggregates of spindloid cells are present. (b) Nucleoli are round with granular chromatin and poorly distinct nucleoli. (c) There is a lack of vasculature; however, minimal pink fibrillar extracellular material is present (Wright–Giemsa, 500× magnification).

Neoplastic cells do not appear to be a common finding in CSF samples but have been reported; the presence of neoplastic cells may be related to the location of the primary lesion (Harms *et al.*, 2009). When present, meningiomas appear as aggregated and individualized cells with moderate amounts of basophilic, finely granulated cytoplasm, a paranuclear clear zone, round to oval nuclei, finely stippled chromatin, indistinct nucleoli, and rare erythrophagocytosis. Most cells are polygonal, although rare spindloid cells can be present.

Cytologically, distinction of the subtypes of meningioma is often not possible. However, occasional whorling arrangements of epithelial-like cells around a central hyalinized necrotic mineral core (psammoma body) suggest a psammomatous meningioma, and spindle cells in a storiform pattern can suggest a fibroblastic meningioma (Motta *et al.*, 2012). The presence of magenta cytoplasmic granules within neoplastic meningeal cells may support a granular-type meningioma (Figure 14.41).

There is a reported overlap of morphologies between meningiomas and astrocytomas; both can appear as spindloid cells and they have been grouped in some studies (Platt *et al.*, 2002). Meningiomas should stain positive with patchy areas for CD-18 and actin. They should also be negative for S-100, lymphoid markers, cytokeratin, and glial fibrillary acidic protein (GFAP).

Astrocytoma

In the dog, Boxers and Boston Terriers are more likely to have astrocytomas (Table 14.18; Figures 14.42a, b; Snyder *et al.*, 2006). Astrocytomas make up about 17% of intracranial tumors in the dog and 2.8% of intracranial tumors in the cat. They are commonly found in the telencephalon, diencephalon, and cerebellum and are intra-axial lesions (Lee & Tihan, 2015).

Smears of astrocytomas are slightly more cellular than normal brain. In keeping with the astrocyte's role of providing nutritional support to neurons and forming part of the blood–brain barrier, astrocytomas typically have thin-walled, demarcated, and branching blood vessels with streams of elongate tumor cells radiating from the vessel margins and possessing long, thin cytoplasmic processes (Vernau *et al.*, 2001). Their cytoplasm is faintly eosinophilic with an extensive network of randomly criss-crossing eosinophilic fibrillary cytoplasmic processes. Cytologically, low-grade astrocytomas on CSF have been described as appearing similar to histiocytes, monocytes, or foamy macrophages. Astrocytomas are vimentin, S-100, and GFAP positive (Cantile & Youssef, 2015).

Oligodendroglioma

Oligodendrogliomas have been reported in older domestic shorthair and Maine Coon cats, with a mean age of 9 years (Table 14.19; Troxel *et al.*, 2003). In dogs, Boxers and Boston Terriers are more likely to have oligodendrogliomas (Snyder *et al.*, 2006). They make up approximately 2.4% of intracranial tumors in the cat and 14% of intra-cranial tumors in the dog. These tumors are often located in the temporal lobe or prosencephalon as intra-axial lesions.

Oligodendrocytes are glial cells responsible for myelination of neurons. As such, they have a soft, gelatinous to mucoid texture

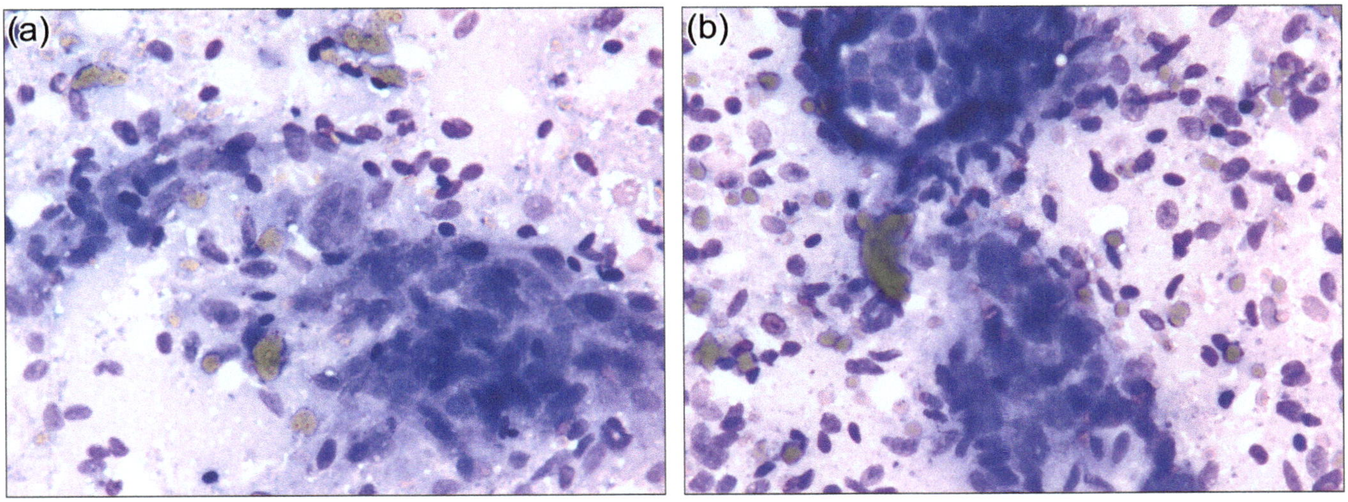

Figures 14.40a, b Imprint of a mass from a mixed breed dog. Dense aggregates of pleomorphic meningeal cells are present, which have poorly distinct cell borders that give the impression of a spindloid cell, ovoid nucleoli, and, where visible, a poorly distinct single nucleolus (Wright–Giemsa, 500× magnification).

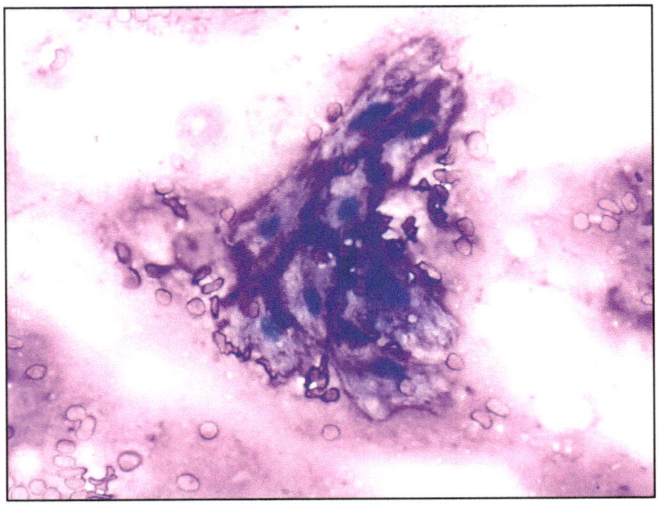

Figure 14.41 Imprint of an intradural extramedullary mass extending from L4 to the caudal aspect of L5 in an 8-year-old spayed female domestic shorthair cat. Dense aggregates of meningeal cells are present which are polygonal to spindloid in shape with uniform round to oval nuclei and moderate amounts of pale basophilic cytoplasm containing bright magenta granulation. Aggregates of cells are closely associated with copious amounts of bright pink extracellular matrix material. Histopathologic evaluation confirmed a granular-type meningioma with coexpression of cytokeratin and vimentin (Wright–Giemsa, 500× magnification).

that can be appreciated during smear preparation and have a honeycombed appearance on histopathology (Figures 14.43a–d; Vernau *et al.*, 2001). Many vascular structures with glomeruloid capillary tufts are observed in these tumors. Cytology smears are often highly cellular, with many closely packed cells that have a round nucleus and fine, granular chromatin. When present, nucleoli are small and single. This morphology does not appear to be retained in fluid preparations. When they are visible on cytologic preparations of CSF, oligodendrogliomas have been described as large cells with a round nucleus and abundant deeply basophilic cytoplasm, which often have globular projections (Dickinson *et al.*, 2000). Rare neoplastic cells in pairs or aggregates and occasional mitotic figures have been noted. Oligodendrogliomas are GFAP negative (Cantile & Youssef, 2015).

Ependymoma

Ependymoma is rarely seen. Several cases have been well described (Rand *et al.*, 1994b; Vernau *et al.*, 2001; Vural *et al.*, 2006; Traslavina *et al.*, 2013; Woolford *et al.*, 2013; Gibson *et al.*, 2021). The mean age in a group of 18 cats with ependymoma was 9 years; a clear breed predisposition was not evident (Table 14.20). Ependymomas in dogs have a less predictable age distribution and may affect young to middle-aged dogs. These tumors tend to arise in the lateral, third, or fourth ventricle and form an intraventricular mass when intracranial but may also originate from the spinal cord (Pancotto *et al.*, 2013; Miller *et al.*, 2019a; Gibson *et al.*, 2021). They are typically well-demarcated lesions.

Ependymomas have been reported to smear easily on cytologic preparation (Vernau *et al.*, 2001). One case affecting the spinal cord of a dog exfoliated for fine needle aspiration (Gibson *et al.*, 2021). Consistent, but not pathognomonic, histologic and cytologic features of ependymomas are branching papillary structures, pseudorosettes, and true rosette formations (Figures 14.44a, b; Woolford *et al.*, 2013). Pseudorosettes are palisading layers of ependymal cells with their ependymal processes facing inward around a blood vessel. A true rosette is a tubular formation of ependymal cells around an empty cavity. Nuclei are eccentrically placed, round to ovoid, and have a cribriform chromatin pattern. The cytoplasm is eosinophilic with distinct borders. Necrotic cells seem to be a common feature. Ultrastructural demonstration of cilia can help confirm a diagnosis of ependymoma (Cheville, 2009). These tumors should stain positive for GFAP in the cat. GFAP staining appears inconsistent in the dog;

Table 14.18 **A summary of the significant diagnostic findings with astrocytoma**

Signalment	Boxers, Boston Terriers
Clarity	Clear
Color	Colorless
CSF TP	Possible increase
CSF cellularity	Normal to moderate neutrophilic pleocytosis. Rarely, can find neoplastic cells which look similar to monocytes
Lesion location	Intra-axial. Telencephalon, diencephalon, cerebellum
CNS cytology	Elongate tumor cells arranged around thin-walled vessels
Ancillary testing	Positive: vimentin, S-100, GFAP
Notes	Can look like monocyte/macrophage or meningioma on cytology

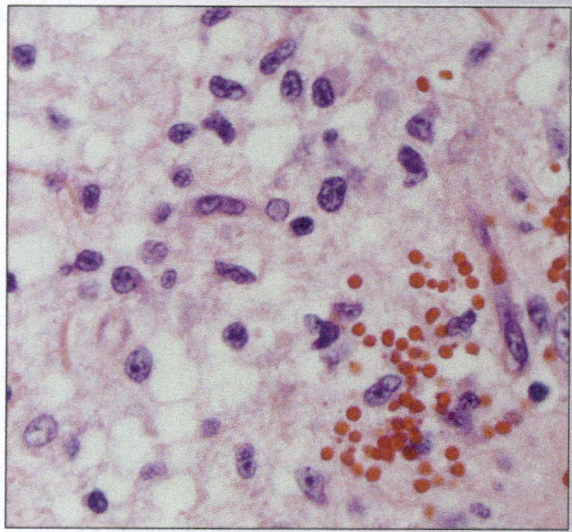

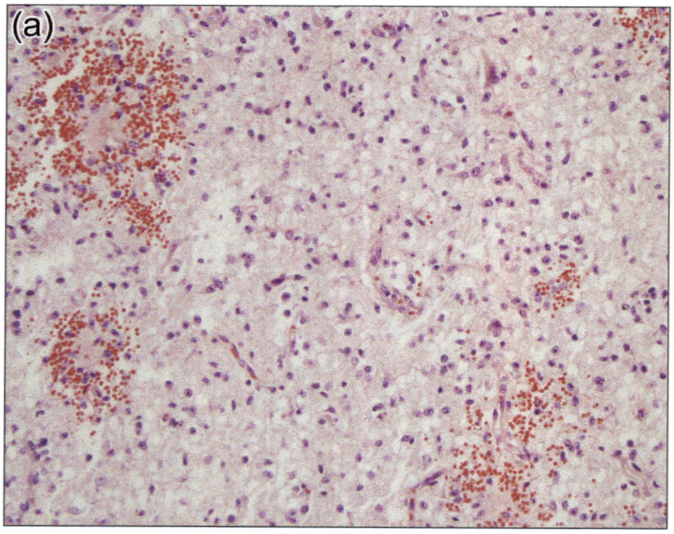

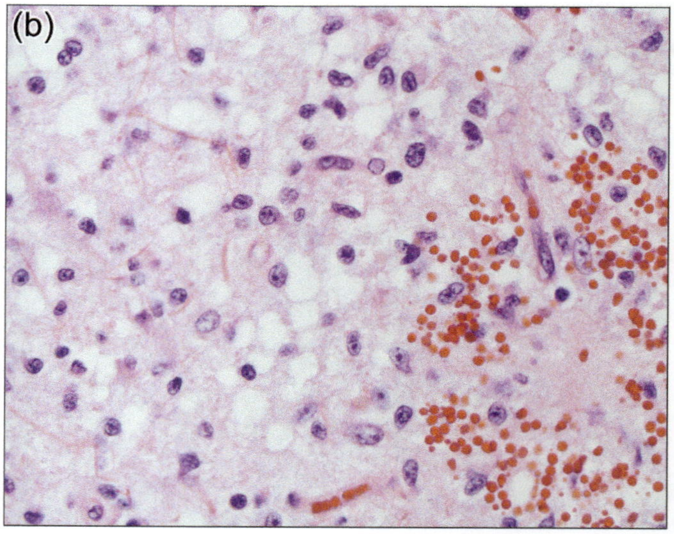

Figures 14.42a, b **Tissue from a 10-year-old, neutered male Boxer with a 1-day history of seizures. On necropsy a red mass was present in the base of the left piriform lobe. (a) The neoplastic cells have scant cytoplasm and abundant fibrillary processes. Several areas of hemorrhage and pseudopalisading around necrotic areas are present along the left side of the image (H&E, 200× magnification). (b) A closer image (500× magnificaion) helps to demonstrate the fibrillary processes (upper left) and an area of hemorrhage (lower right). The amount of hemorrhage is not uncommon; it imparted a red color to the lesion grossly. Diagnosis of this mass was a fibrous astrocytoma. (Case courtesy Dr. Greta Krafsur.)**

most documented cases are GFAP negative, although GFAP staining within pseudorosettes and/or rosettes has been reported in canine ependymomas (Cantile & Youssef, 2015; Miller *et al.*, 2019a).

Choroid plexus tumors

Choroid plexus tumors in the dog make up approximately 7–10% of all primary intracranial CNS tumors, but they are only rarely found in the cat (Table 14.21). The masses arise from choroid plexus epithelium found in the lateral, third, and fourth ventricles or the lateral apertures and are the most common tumors found in an intraventricular location (Westworth *et al.*, 2008; Miller *et al.*, 2019b). Both choroid plexus papillomas and choroid plexus carcinomas have been described, with more cases being carcinomas than papillomas (64% and 36%, respectively). Choroid plexus tumors commonly occur in middle-aged dogs, with a mean age of 6 years. Golden Retrievers may be overrepresented.

On intraoperative cytology, choroid plexus tumors are grossly soft and friable and spread easily into smears (Figures 14.45a, b; Vernau *et al.*, 2001). They have abundant blood vessels, which often branch into papillary and medusoid-shaped fronds. There are large numbers of cells in sheets and clusters. Occasionally, cells are individualized. When in sheets and clusters, the epithelial cells

Table 14.19 A summary of the significant diagnostic findings with oligodendroglioma

Signalment	Boxers, Boston Terriers. Domestic shorthair and Maine Coon cats
Clarity	Clear
Color	Colorless
CSF TP	Possible increase
CSF cellularity	Normal to moderate neutrophilic pleocytosis. Rarely, can find neoplastic cells, which are large round cells with abundant cytoplasm and globular projections
Lesion location	Intra-axial. Temporal lobe, prosencephalon
CNS cytology	Honeycombed, glomerular tufts of capillaries, tightly packed cells with fine granular chromatin. Mucoid material common
Ancillary testing	Negative: cytokeratin, GFAP
Notes	Mass is grossly gelatinous/mucoid

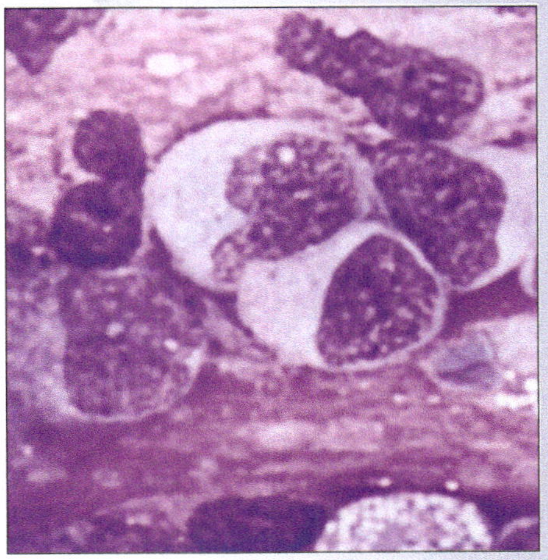

Table 14.20 A summary of the significant diagnostic findings with ependymoma

Signalment	Dog and cat
Clarity	Clear
Color	Colorless
CSF TP	Possible increase
CSF cellularity	Normal to moderate neutrophilic pleocytosis. Rarely, neoplastic cells seen
Lesion location	Intraventricular or spinal cord
CNS cytology	Ciliated columnar cells with pseudorosette and true rosette formation
Ancillary testing	Cat: positive GFAP. Dog: equivocal GFAP
Notes	Confirm cilia on electron microscopy if needed

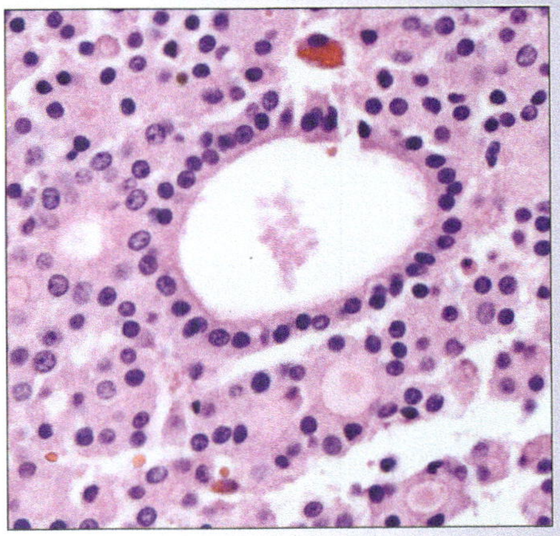

are columnar with a basally located nucleus. The individualized cells are small with plentiful eosinophilic cytoplasm that does not form extended processes. Nuclei are round to ovoid with finely granular chromatin, a dark-staining nuclear border, and one or more prominent nucleoli. Carcinomas have been reported to display more prominent anisokaryosis, but were otherwise similar to papillomas.

Reports in the veterinary literature suggest that choroid plexus cells should be cytokeratin positive and GFAP negative (Cantile & Youssef, 2015). Interestingly, human choroid plexus cells are positive for vimentin as well as cytokeratin and are GFAP negative (Sarnat, 1998).

There is the suggestion that the CSF TP content is higher in choroid carcinomas than papillomas: median 108 mg/dl compared with 34 mg/dl, respectively (Westworth *et al.*, 2008). Neoplastic cells are found in the CSF of approximately half of the cases. Choroid plexus carcinomas have been described as moderately sized cells, with abundant slightly granular, vacuolated, and basophilic cytoplasm and round to oval nuclei with coarse chromatin and irregular nucleoli (Pastorello *et al.*, 2010). Occasional mitotic figures are also seen. Intraventricular or subarachnoid metastasis has been noted on MRI and can help to support the malignant nature of choroid plexus tumors (Westworth *et al.*, 2008). A case of a choroid plexus papilloma and concurrent meningioma has been reported in a 7-year-old female English Cocker Spaniel (Espino *et al.*, 2009).

Primary CNS lymphoma has been described in both dogs and cats (Table 14.22). Retrospective studies suggest that it is more common in the cat than the dog, although both are at a low incidence rate (Troxel

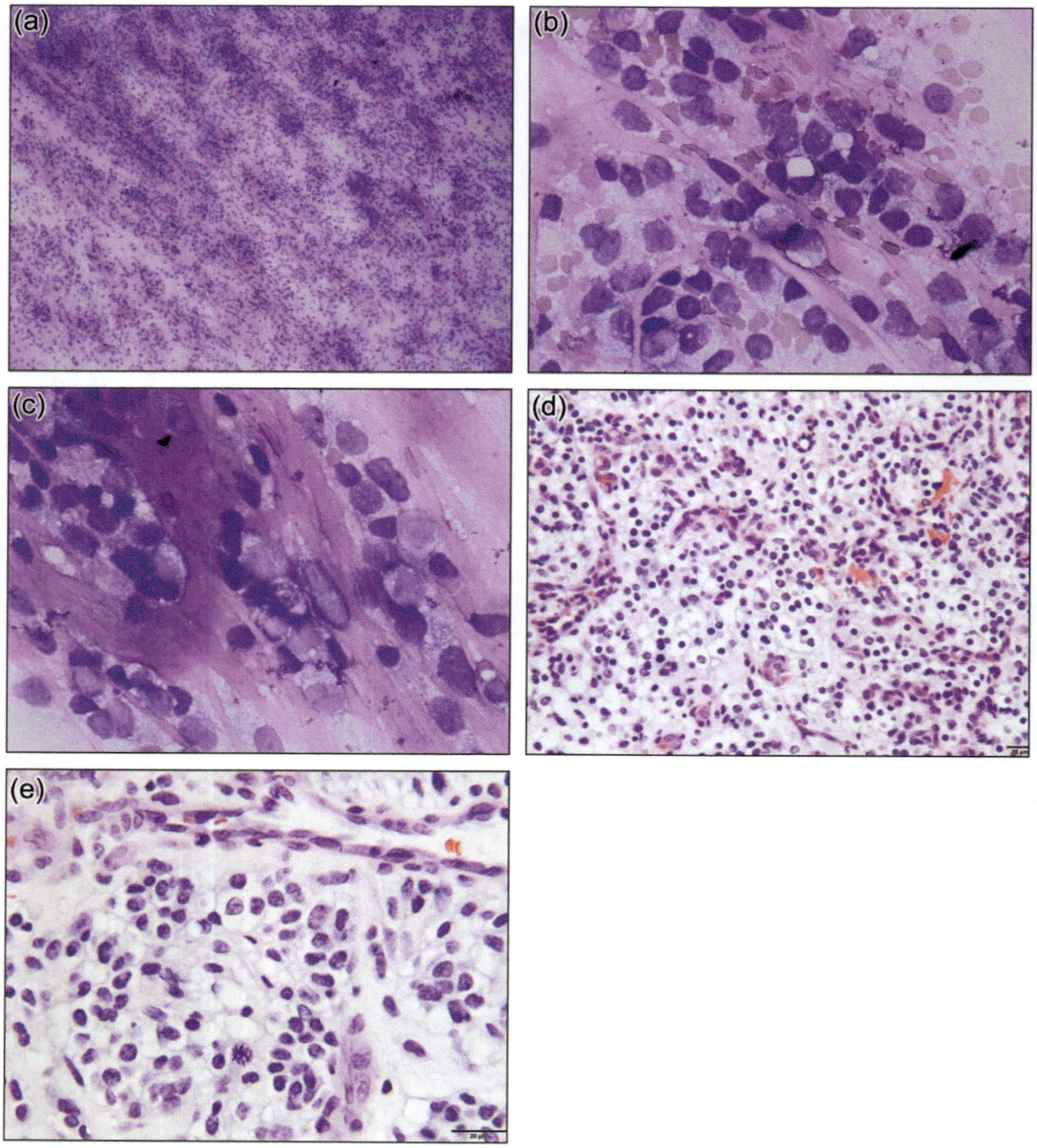

Figures 14.43a–e Canine oligodendroglioma. (a) The specimen is highly cellular and has many branching capillaries and abundant pink extracellular material. Cells are sometimes arranged in linear arrays separated by strands of extracellular material (Wright–Giemsa, 100× magnification). (b) Nucleated cells are predominantly round cells that have large, variably shaped nuclei and a moderate amount of pale gray–blue cytoplasm. Anisocytosis and anisokaryosis are mild. The nuclei have stippled chromatin and usually lack appreciable nucleoli. The cytoplasm often has low to moderate numbers of small clear vacuoles and/or a small amount of very fine pink granular material. Thin strands of pink extracellular matrix material separate neoplastic cells. (c) Extracellular matrix material may also more abundant, forming thick branching structures (Wright–Giemsa, 500× magnification). (a–c courtesy Dr. Sara Connolly.) (d) Neoplastic cells have hyperchromatic round nuclei with moderate atypia, rare mitoses, pale eosinophilic to vacuolated cytoplasm, and distinct cellular borders. There is pronounced microvascular proliferation (H&E, 200× magnification). (e) Higher magnification of the neoplastic population illustrating mitotic figures and microvascular proliferation (H&E, 400× magnification). (c, d courtesy Dr. J. M. Jankovsky.)

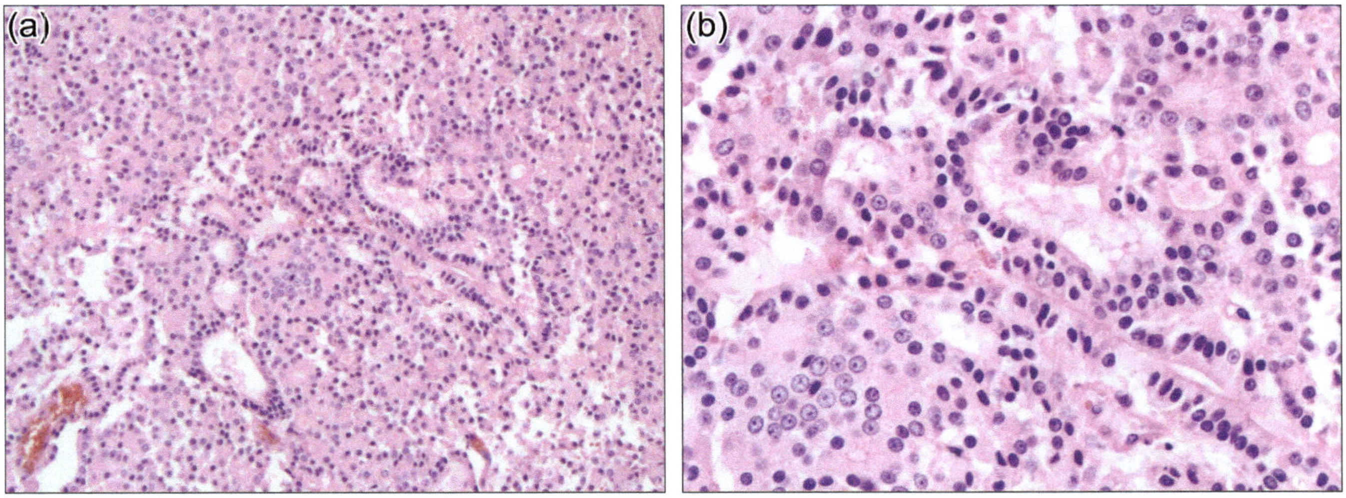

Figures 14.44a, b Feline ependymoma. (a) Histologically, there is a population of large cuboidal to columnar cells. Several true rosettes (cells arranged around an open space) and pseudorosettes (cells arranged around a blood vessel) are present (H&E, 200× magnification). (b) A close-up image of branching tubular structures. Note the barely discernible ciliated apical surface of the columnar cells lining the tubules (H&E, 500× magnification). (Case courtesy Dr. Sushan Han.)

Table 14.21 **A summary of the significant diagnostic findings with choroid plexus tumors**

Signalment	Golden Retrievers, 6 years old. Rare in cats
Clarity	Clear
Color	Colorless
CSF TP	Possible increase
CSF cellularity	Normal to moderate neutrophilic pleocytosis One-half of cases have neoplastic cells: moderately-sized cells, abundant granular cytoplasm, oval nuclei, and irregular nucleoli
Lesion location	Intraventricular. Lateral, 3rd, 4th ventricle
CNS cytology	Papillary and medusoid-shaped fronds, sheets and clusters of columnar cells with basal nuclei
Ancillary testing	Positive: cytokeratin and GFAP
Notes	Carcinomas may have more anisokaryosis

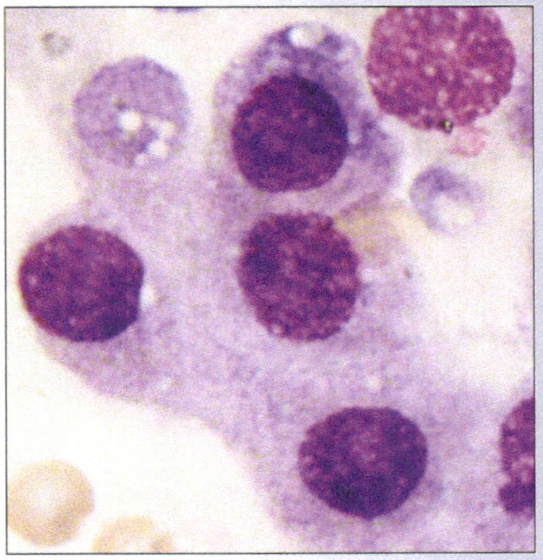

et al., 2003; Snyder *et al.*, 2006). CNS lymphoma is more likely to be a component of multicentric lymphoma than a primary disease; only eight of 23 (34.8%) cats with intracranial lymphoma had primary CNS lymphoma. In cats, diffuse cerebral or brainstem involvement on MRI was predictive of lymphoma (Troxel *et al.*, 2003). Both T- and B-cell primary CNS lymphomas have been described in the dog and cat; most cases tend to be T-cell in origin (Koestner *et al.*, 1999), although a retrospective study involving mostly FeLV+ cats showed a B-cell predominance (Mello *et al.*, 2019). In humans, a quarter of human immunodeficiency virus-positive patients with neurologic signs have primary CNS lymphoma. A specific association between feline immunodeficiency virus and primary CNS lymphoma has not been found.

Primary central nervous system lymphoma

On intraoperative smear preparations there are few prominent and branched vessels, with many individualized round cells morphologically similar to lymphomatous cells noted elsewhere in the body (Vernau *et al.*, 2001; Lee & Tihan, 2015). Primary CNS lymphoma can produce cytologic smears that are highly cellular with an angiocentric arrangement. The smears can often be devoid of intermingled brain tissue.

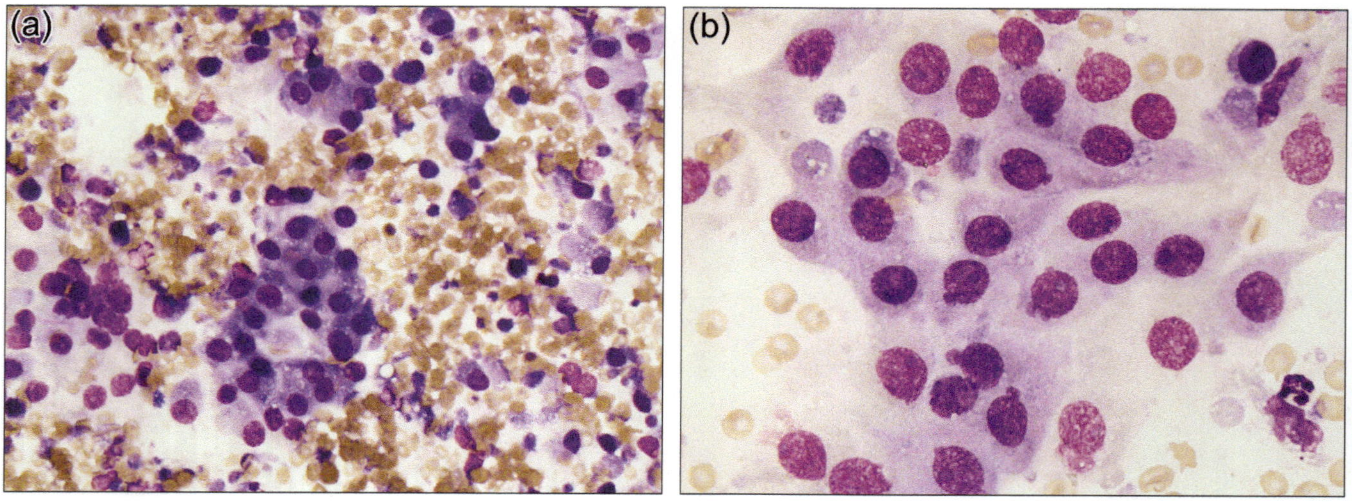

Figures 14.45a, b Cytology from an extra-axial mass in the area of the 4th ventricle with involvement of the vermis, brainstem, and pons of an 8-year-old English Bulldog. (a) Large cohesive clusters of cells are present and are associated with abundant red blood cells (Wright–Giemsa, 500× magnification). (b) Polygonal to elongate cells with lightly basophilic cytoplasm and a round nucleus are present. There is minimal anisocytosis and anisokaryosis (Wright–Giemsa, 1,000× magnification). Histologic evaluation confirmed the tissue was from the choroid plexus and suggested it was a papilloma.

Table 14.22 **A summary of the significant diagnostic findings with primary CNS lymphoma**

Signalment	Dog and cat
Clarity	Clear
Color	Colorless
CSF TP	Moderate increase
CSF cellularity	Mild pleocytosis, most commonly mononuclear or mixed. Possible neoplastic lymphocytes
Lesion location	Diffuse or mass lesion. Diffuse cerebral or brainstem involvement on MRI is predictive
CNS cytology	Discrete cells with minimal cytoplasm and high N:C ratio
Ancillary testing	Immunocytochemistry or immunohistochemistry. PARR, or flow cytometry may be a low yield test
Notes	More commonly is component of multicentric lymphoma

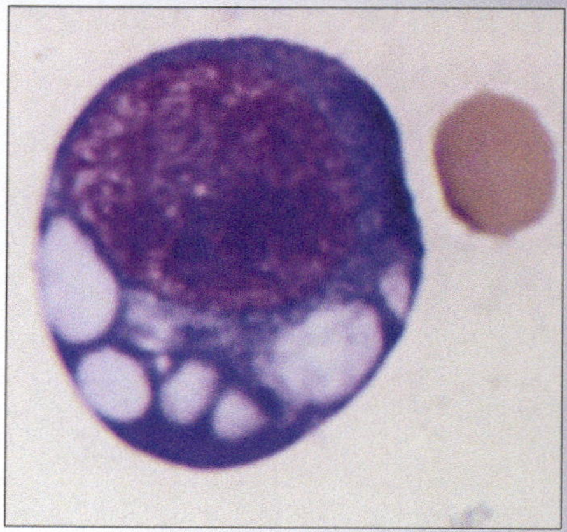

Given how highly exfoliative lymphoma is elsewhere in the body, it would be expected that lymphoma would be easily detected on CSF cytology. However, lymphoma was diagnosed on CSF cytology in only 20% of cats with confirmed intracranial or spinal lymphoma in a recent study (Durand *et al.*, 2022). This is consistent with previous studies that showed CS Flymphoma to be poorly exfoliative in the CSF for both cats and dogs (Troxel *et al.*, 2003; LaRue *et al.*, 2018). 65% of cats in the Durand study had a mild pleocytosis without overtly neoplastic cells (median TNCC = 16.5 cells/ µl) with mononuclear or mixed pleocytosis being most common. A concurrent increase in total protein is another commonly reported finding, with mean values ranging from 54.5 to 93 mg/dL across retrospective studies (Troxel *et al.*, 2003; Durand *et al.*, 2022).

As with lymphoma elsewhere in the body, neoplastic lymphocytes are easiest to detect cytologically when they present with typical lymphoid nuclear to cytoplasmic ratio, deeply basophilic cytoplasm, and large round nuclei with nucleoli (Figures 14.46a, b). They can also present as less pleomorphic small cells, granular lymphocytes, or highly pleomorphic cells that do not resemble lymphocytes at all (Figures 14.47a–d; Fernandez *et al.*, 2013).

Flow cytometry and PCR for antigen receptor rearrangements (PARR) in lymphocytes to support a diagnosis of lymphoma can be used on dog and cat CSF samples. Based on anecdotal experiences and well-established facts from analysis outside the CNS, several limitations to the technique should be recognized. Flow cytometry studies require a fairly large number of viable cells for evaluation. One human study

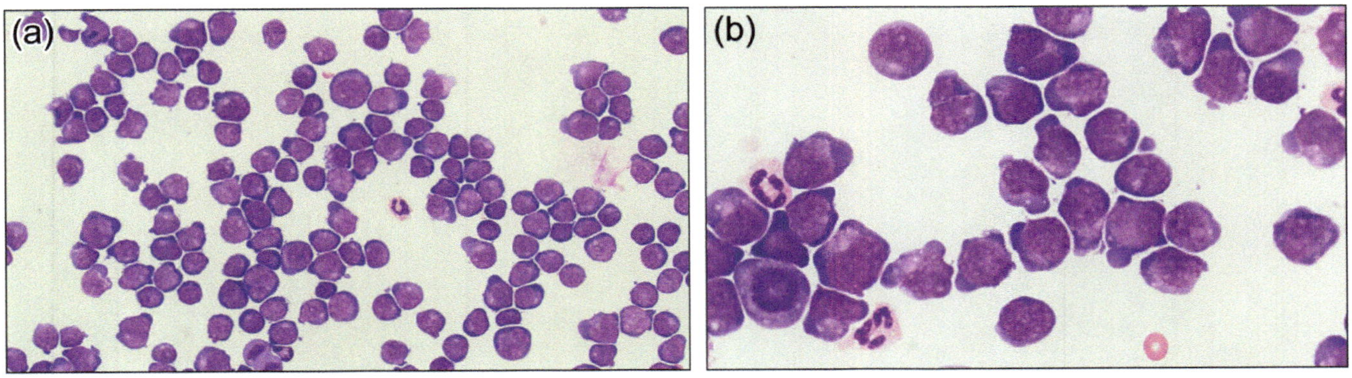

Figures 14.46a, b **CSF from a dog, TNCC and TP unavailable. (a) There is a population of individualized round cells with a high nuclear to cytoplasmic ratio. Nuclei appear round to slightly indented with finely stippled chromatin. Cytoplasm is deeply basophilic and often contains a zone of perinuclear cytoplasmic clearing. These cells measure 1.5–2× the diameter of a neutrophil, consistent with a large-cell lymphoma. The cells were CD3+ and CD79a- on immunocytochemistry, which confirmed the diagnosis of T-cell lymphoma (Wright–Giemsa, 500× magnification). (b) Closer evaluation reveals one to multiple prominent nucleoli per nucleus. Rare cells contain cleaved nuclei. Note the mitotic figure at the bottom right of the image (Wright–Giemsa, 1,000× magnification).**

found that a full flow cytometry evaluation had higher likelihood of being inconclusive when CSF cellularity was <100,000 cells/µl (Pittman *et al.*, 2013). Similarly, PARR performed on a sample with a pleocytosis seems reasonable when cells present on the sample have a suspicious morphology. However, the practical limitations on the amount of recovered DNA from a sample with a cell count of 50 cells/µl is self-evident. Flow cytometry and PCR techniques are commonly used in human medicine to diagnose and further identify lymphoma, with a large number of inconclusive cases (Pittman *et al.*, 2013; Liu *et al.*, 2015). A thorough study of the utility of CSF PARR or flow cytometric analysis has not been conducted in veterinary medicine, although confirmatory diagnoses using both methods have been reported (LaRue *et al.*, 2018). Until such studies are performed in veterinary medicine, use of PARR or flow cytometry on CSF samples may be attempted as long as the high rate of inconclusive findings is acceptable.

Histiocytic sarcoma

Histiocytic sarcoma may occur as a primary intracranial or spinal neoplasm, or may metastasize to the central nervous system in cases of disseminated disease (Table 14.23). Disease distribution within the CNS may vary, although the majority of tumors have a rostrotentorial component (Toyoda *et al.*, 2020). Breed predispositions include Bernese Mountain dogs, Golden Retrievers, Shetland sheepdogs, Rottweilers, and Corgis. Interestingly, Rottweilers had exclusively disseminated disease in a recent retrospective study, whereas Corgis and Shetland sheepdogs typically had primary CNS tumors (Toyoda *et al.*, 2020). Overall, intracranial histiocytic sarcoma is relatively rare, comprising approximately 2–3% of primary intracranial tumors in dogs (Snyder *et al.*, 2006). Intracranial histiocytic sarcoma has been described in cats but appears rare (Riker *et al.*, 2023; Monteiro *et al.*, 2021).

MRI features of histiocytic sarcomas and meningiomas may be similar, with both tumor types appearing as extra-axial masses with uniform contrast enhancement (Ishikawa *et al.*, 2016). A recent retrospective study compared CSF findings in dogs with confirmed meningiomas and intracranial histiocytic sarcomas (Toyoda *et al.*, 2020; Table 14.23). In this study, median CSF TNCC was significantly higher in dogs with primary intracranial histiocytic sarcoma (170 cells/µL) compared to dogs with disseminated histiocytic sarcoma affecting the CNS or meningioma, which both had median TNCC within the normal range. Neoplastic cells were identified in 52% of CSF samples from dogs with either primary or disseminated CNS histiocytic sarcoma.

Cytologically, histiocytic sarcoma in the CNS appears similarly to other sites, comprised of individualized to aggregated, rounded to stellate cells with a histiocytic morphology. Significant cellular pleomorphism is expected in these cells, including frequent mitotic activity, anisokaryosis, and prominent or bizarrely shaped nucleoli. Positive immunocytochemical staining for CD1 and CD11c may serve as confirmation in suspect cases (Cluzel *et al.*, 2016).

Pituitary tumors

Pituitary tumors are reported as the third most common primary intracranial tumor in the cat, with an incidence of approximately 9% (Troxel *et al.*, 2003). They have been reported in domestic shorthair and domestic longhair cats. They commonly cause endocrine abnormalities, including acromegaly, poorly regulated diabetes mellitus, pituitary dependent hyperadrenocorticism, hypoadrenocorticism, and hyperthyroidism (Troxel *et al.*, 2003).

Descriptions of pituitary tumors by cytology or CSF analysis are very limited in veterinary literature. This is probably due to the deep location of the pituitary gland, the small tumor size (median 1.3 cm^2), and the diagnostic utility of clinical signs associated with endocrine dysfunction. In human literature, pituitary tumors are described with a classic neuroendocrine appearance: intact nuclei within a pool of cytoplasm that lacks distinct cellular borders (Powell, 2005).

Granular cell tumors

Granular cell tumors are rare neoplasms in dogs and cats with a controversial histogenesis. These tumors most commonly arise within

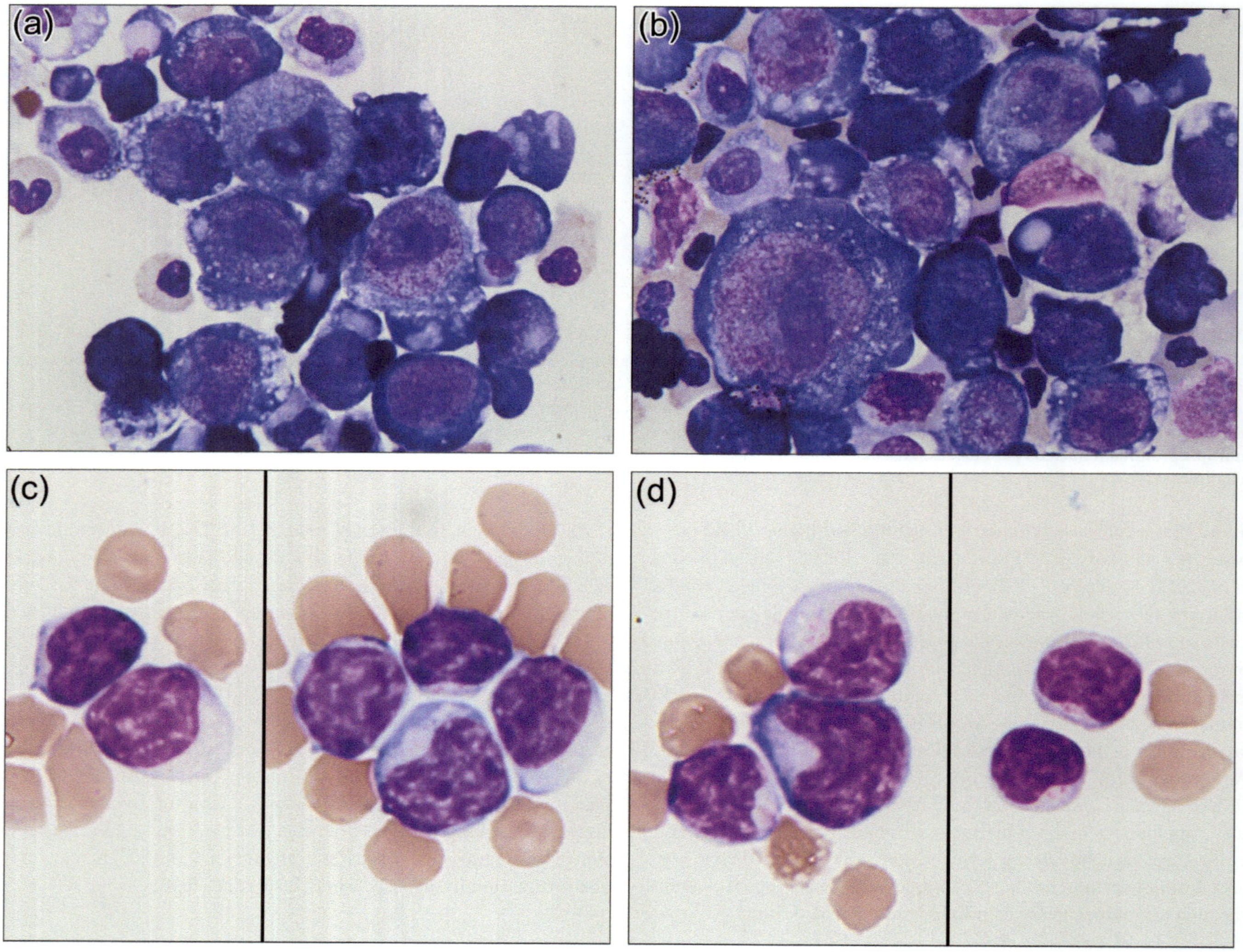

Figures 14.47a–d Cytomorphology in CNS lymphoma can also be variable. CSF from a 9-year-old Boxer. TNCC = 4,200 cells/µl, CSF TP = 330 mg/dl (a, b); CSF from a 10-year-old mixed breed dog with diffuse lesions in the CNS on MRI. TNCC = 13 cells/µl, CSF TP = 149 mg/dl (c, d). (a) There is a pleomorphic population of large mononuclear cells that have minimal amounts of deeply basophilic cytoplasm, round nucleus, stippled chromatin, and one to several prominent nucleoli. Note the mitotic figure in the upper center of the image. (b) The neoplastic cells occasionally have clear cytoplasmic vacuoles (right side of image). The cytomegalic cell in the lower left corner has an oblong nucleolus, which is larger than the adjacent small mononuclear cell (Wright–Giemsa, 1,000× magnification). Flow cytometry was requested but could not be performed. PCR for lymphoma found a clonal rearrangement of the T-cell receptor, supporting a diagnosis of T-cell lymphoma. (c) The predominant cell type is small mononuclear cells, which have minimal amounts of basophilic cytoplasm and a round to indented nucleus with clumped chromatin. Nuclei measure approximately 1.5 times the size of a red blood cell. The morphology is most suggestive of a small to intermediate-sized lymphocyte. (d) Most of these cells had few small pink cytoplasmic granules located beside the nucleus. The large number of granulated lymphocytes was interpreted as evidence of lymphoma (Wright–Giemsa, 1,000× magnification).

the oral cavity, although laryngeal, periocular, visceral, and rarely intracranial granular cell tumors have been reported (Patnaik, 1993; Levitin *et al.*, 2019). A recent case series highlighted the utility of intraoperative impression smear cytology of these lesions (Levitin *et al.*, 2019). Cytologic preparations are typically highly cellular and consist of individualized, round to polygonal to rarely spindloid cells with eosinophilic cytoplasmic granules on Wright–Giemsa stain (Figure 14.48a, b). PAS-positivity to the cytoplasmic granules and cytoplasmic S-100 immunoreactivity are expected findings on histopathology of these tumors.

Metastatic and invasive neoplasia

Metastatic neoplasia to the CNS is fairly common, occurring in up to 8.8% of extra-neural malignant neoplasms in one study (Heck *et al.*, 2018). Most often these tumors look cytologically similar to their appearance outside the nervous system.

Carcinomas of mammary, intestinal, urothelial, prostatic, and cutaneous squamous cell origin have produced meningeal carcinomatosis in dogs (Figures 14.49a, b; Mateo *et al.*, 2010; Pancotto et al., 2013). Metastatic hemangiosarcoma, lymphoma, melanoma, and less commonly osteosarcoma or histiocytic sarcoma have also been described in dogs (Heck *et al.*, 2018).

Lymphoma and osteosarcoma are the most common forms of metastatic spinal neoplasia in the cat (Marioni-Henry, 2010). These are also relatively common differentials for feline intracranial metastatic tumors; others include pulmonary adenocarcinoma, squamous cell carcinoma, fibrosarcoma, hemangiosarcoma, myxosarcoma, pleomorphic or unclassified sarcoma, and unclassified carcinoma (Troxel *et al.*, 2003).

Table 14.23 **A summary of the significant diagnostic findings with CNS histiocytic sarcoma**

Signalment	Bernese Mountain dogs overrepresented. Primary in Shetland sheepdogs and Corgis, Disseminated in Rottweilers. Rare in cats.
CSF TP	Moderate to marked increase
CSF cellularity	Moderate to marked pleocytosis in primary cases, may be normal in disseminated cases. Neoplastic cells present in 52% of cases
Lesion location	May vary but often rostrotentorial. Extra-axial and uniformly contrast enhancing on MRI.
CNS cytology	Discrete cells with marked atypia and frequent mitoses
Ancillary testing	CD1 and CD11c immunocytochemistry

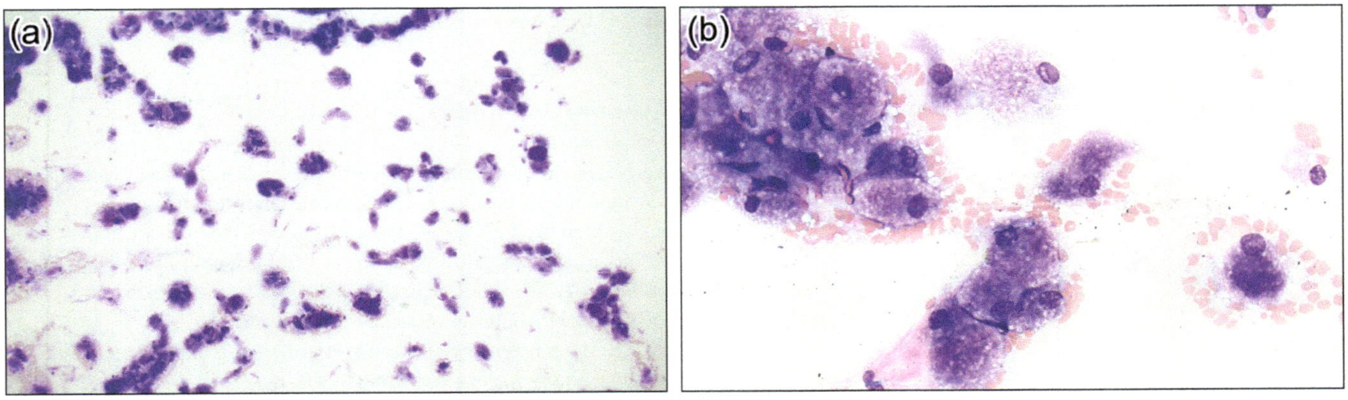

Figures 14.48a, b Impression smear of an extensive intracranial mass with extra- and intra-axial components in a 7-year-old castrated male Chihuahua. Cytologic and histopathologic findings were consistent with a meningeal granular cell tumor. (a) A population of rounded to polygonal to rarely spindloid cells are arranged both individually and in clusters (Wright–Giemsa, 100× magnification). (b) The neoplastic cells have round to ovoid nuclei which are often eccentrically located. Bright pink cytoplasmic granules are prominent, along with variably distinct cytoplasmic vacuolation. Significant anisocytosis and mild to moderate anisokaryosis are present (Wright–Giemsa, 500× magnification).

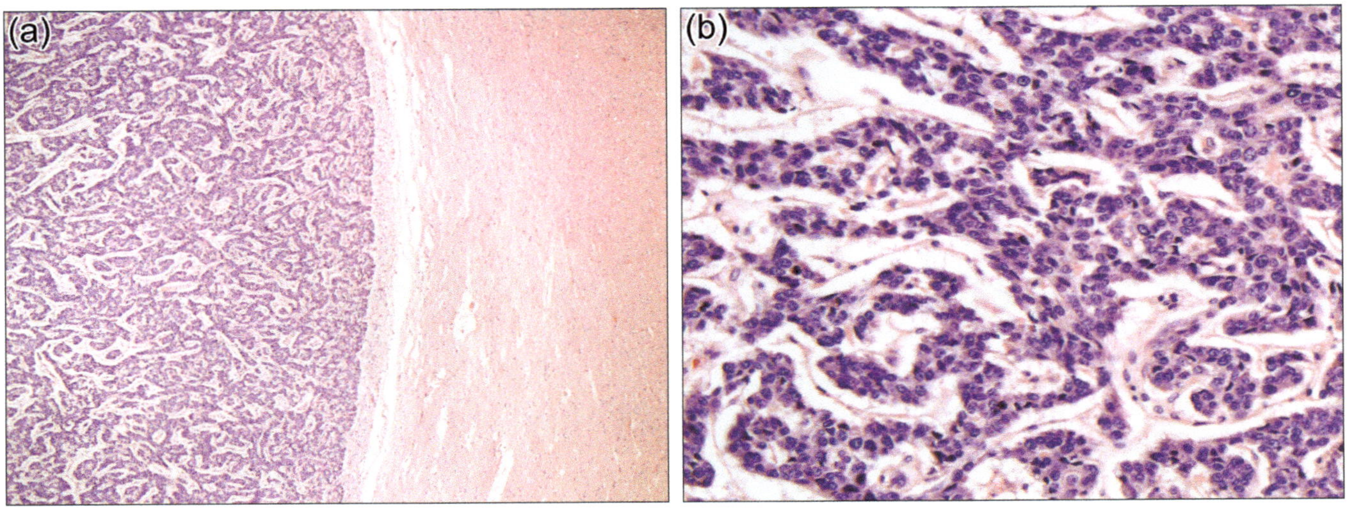

Figures 14.49a, b Cortex, metastatic mammary tumor. (a) The neoplastic tissue (left) compresses the adjacent nervous tissue (right). This mass-effect on normal tissue is the most common cause of clinical signs (H&E, 50× magnification). (b) At higher power, neoplastic epithelial cells form ribbons and indistinct tubular structures reminiscent of normal mammary gland (H&E, 200× magnification). (Case courtesy Dr. Paula Schaffer.)

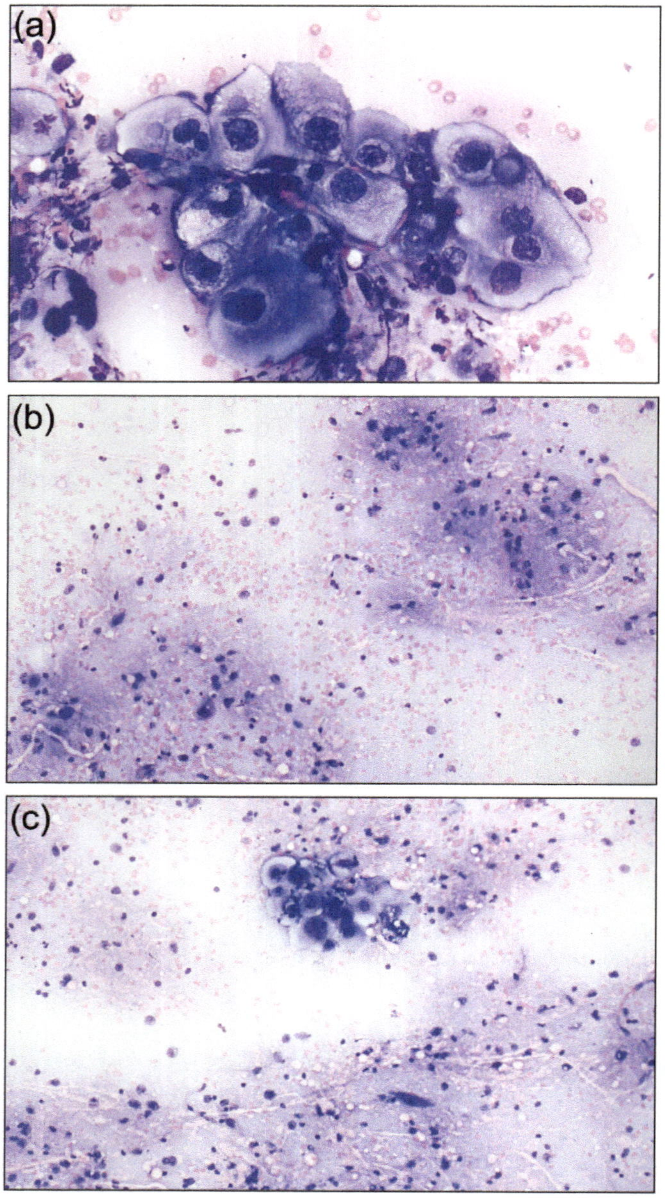

Figures 14.50a–c Post-mortem FNA of a right mandibular mass in a 14-year-old spayed female Bichon Frise with a history of oral squamous cell carcinoma. MRI revealed lysis of the right mandible and calvarium with extension of the mass into the cerebral cortex. (a) Cohesive clusters of rounded to polygonal squamous epithelial cells are present, which often contain many punctate, perinuclear cytoplasmic vacuoles. Moderate to marked anisocytosis and anisokaryosis, dyskeratosis, prominent and variably sized nucleoli, and occasional binucleation or multinucleation support a squamous cell carcinoma (Wright–Giemsa, 500× magnification). (b) Areas of the same slide contain frothy, pink to purple extracellular material with embedded nuclei and pale-pink ribbon-like structures, compatible with neuropil (Wright–Giemsa, 200× magnification). (c) Individualized and clustered malignant squamous epithelial cells are closely associated with aggregates of neuropil. The cytologic features supported the MRI findings of tumor extension into the cerebrum (Wright–Giemsa, 200× magnification).

Several tumors arising from locations outside the CNS may impinge on or invade neural tissue, including vertebral osteosarcomas or nasal tumors (Cantile & Youssef, 2015). Cytologic evaluation of these lesions should not involve intentional sampling of the CNS, although evidence of neural tissue may rarely be identified incidentally or during post-mortem examination (Figure 14.50a–c).

CASES

CASE 1

Signalment/history

Nine-year-old, intact male Dandie Dinmont Terrier. The patient presented with a several-month history of listlessness, which progressed to depression and inability to rise. CBC, biochemical panel, and urinalysis were unremarkable.

Examination findings

On physical examination there was marked muscle atrophy of the left and right supraspinatus and left biceps muscles. There was moderate bilateral hindlimb ataxia and moderate left forelimb lameness. A mild right-sided head tilt was also noted. On neurologic examination, conscious proprioception was decreased in all four limbs but was more pronounced on the hindlimbs. There was moderate decreased panniculus at L3 and mild rotational nystagmus.

An MR study showed a contrast enhancing heterogeneous region in the axilla. Adjacent to the fourth ventricle in the vermis was an area of contrast enhancement (Figure 14.51).

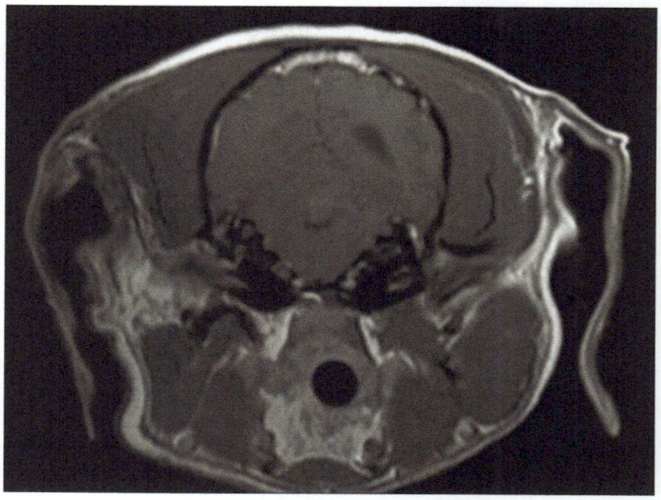

Figure 14.51 A T1-weighted post-contrast MR image from a 9-year-old Dandie Dinmont Terrier. An area of mild hyperintensity is present in the vermis adjacent to the fourth ventricle. (Image obtained and reviewed by a Diplomate of the American College of Veterinary Radiologists at Colorado State University, Fort Collins, Co.)

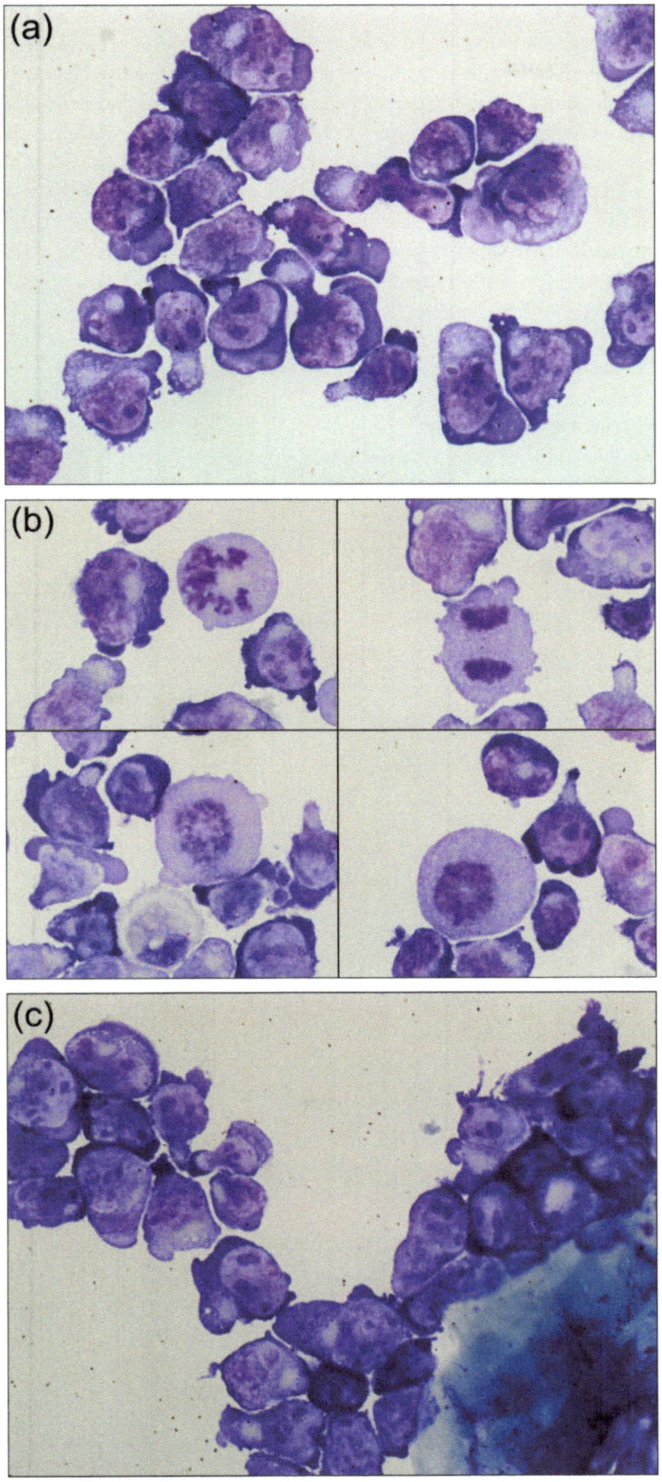

Figures 14.52a–c Cytocentrifuged preparations of CSF from a 9-year-old Dandie Dinmont Terrier (Wright–Giemsa: b, 200× magnification; a and c, 1,000× magnification).

CSF analysis

A CSF sample was collected from the cerebellomedullary cistern and submitted for evaluation. The sample was clear and cloudy. It had a CSF TP = 46 mg/dl (normal <30 mg/dl), TNCC = 806 cells/µl (normal <5 cells/µl), RBCs = 0/µl. Images from the cytocentrifuged preparation of the CSF are shown (Figures 14.52a–c).

CSF cytology description

A highly cellular cytocentrifuged sample is examined. The cells are almost entirely highly pleomorphic large mononuclear cells, most consistent with large lymphocytes (Figure 14.52a). The cells have moderate amounts of basophilic cytoplasm with lobulated edges and a distinct paranuclear clear zone. Nuclei are round to lobular to cerebriform, with stippled chromatin and 1–5 distinct nucleoli. Many mitotic figures are present including atypical mitotic figures (Figure 14.52b). Occasional keratin flakes are noted (Figure 14.52c).

Interpretation: neoplastic pleocytosis, consistent with lymphoma; increased CSF protein.

Outcome

PCR for lymphoma was performed and revealed a monoclonal T-cell population. This confirms the diagnosis of lymphoma. The patient was discharged to his owners pending a decision regarding treatment and was subsequently lost to follow-up.

CASE 2

Signalment/history

Eight-year-old, neutered male Labrador Retriever. The patient had a 3-month history of pacing and walking in circles to the right. Three weeks prior to presentation, he had a seizure. An MRI evaluation was performed at that time and found a right cerebral mass. The dog was started on a course of prednisolone. He presented for further evaluation of the mass and discussion of treatment options.

Examination findings

On neurologic examination the patient had proprioceptive ataxia; conscious proprioception was decreased in the left fore- and hindlimbs. CBC found a mild neutrophilia (12.4×10^3/µl [RI 2.6–11]) and lymphopenia (0.4×10^3/µl [RI 1–4.8]). MRI revealed an extra-axial mass with a cystic center present cranial to the cerebellum (Figure 14.53). A biopsy was performed (Figures 14.54a–d).

Cytology description

Much of the sample is very dense, preventing complete evaluation of the cytologic features (Figure 14.54a). There are cohesively clustered polygonal cells with basophilic slightly granular cytoplasm, an eccentrically located ovoid to round nucleus with stippled chromatin, and rarely a poorly distinct nucleolus (Figures 14.54b, c). There is minimal anisocytosis present. Aggregates of myelin are present (Figure 14.54d).

Interpretation: neoplasia; suspect choroid plexus tumor or meningioma.

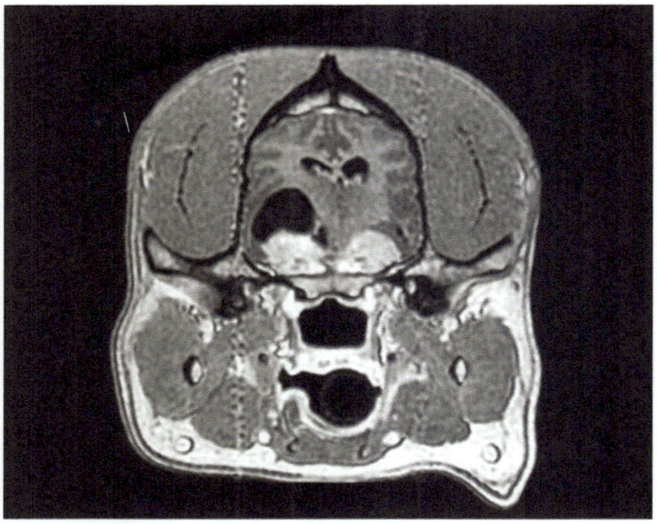

Figure 14.53 A T1-weighted MR image from an 8-year-old Labrador Retriever. A large cystic mass is present just cranial to the cerebellum, which causes compression of the right temporal lobe. (Image obtained and reviewed by a Diplomate of the American College of Veterinary Radiologists at Colorado State University, Fort Collins, Co.)

Outcome

On histopathology, there was a solid, multilobular neoplasm of polygonal cells and minimal stroma (Figures 14.55a–d). The cells had eosinophilic cytoplasm, indistinct cell borders, round nuclei with smudged chromatin and 1–2 prominent nucleoli. Rarely, cells had intranuclear cytoplasmic pseudoinclusions; folded nuclei were found (Figure 14.55d). There was mild anisocytosis and anisokaryosis and a low mitotic index. The histologic diagnosis was meningothelial meningioma. The patient was started on a course of stereotactic radiation therapy and is progressing appropriately at the time of writing.

CASE 3

Signalment/history

Two-year-old, spayed female German Shepherd. The patient had a 1-week history of inability to stand, acute blindness, and collapse episodes.

Examination findings

On neurological examination, the patient had a dull mentation with non-ambulatory tetraparesis and ventroflexion of the head and neck. Pupillary light response was absent on the left and decreased on the

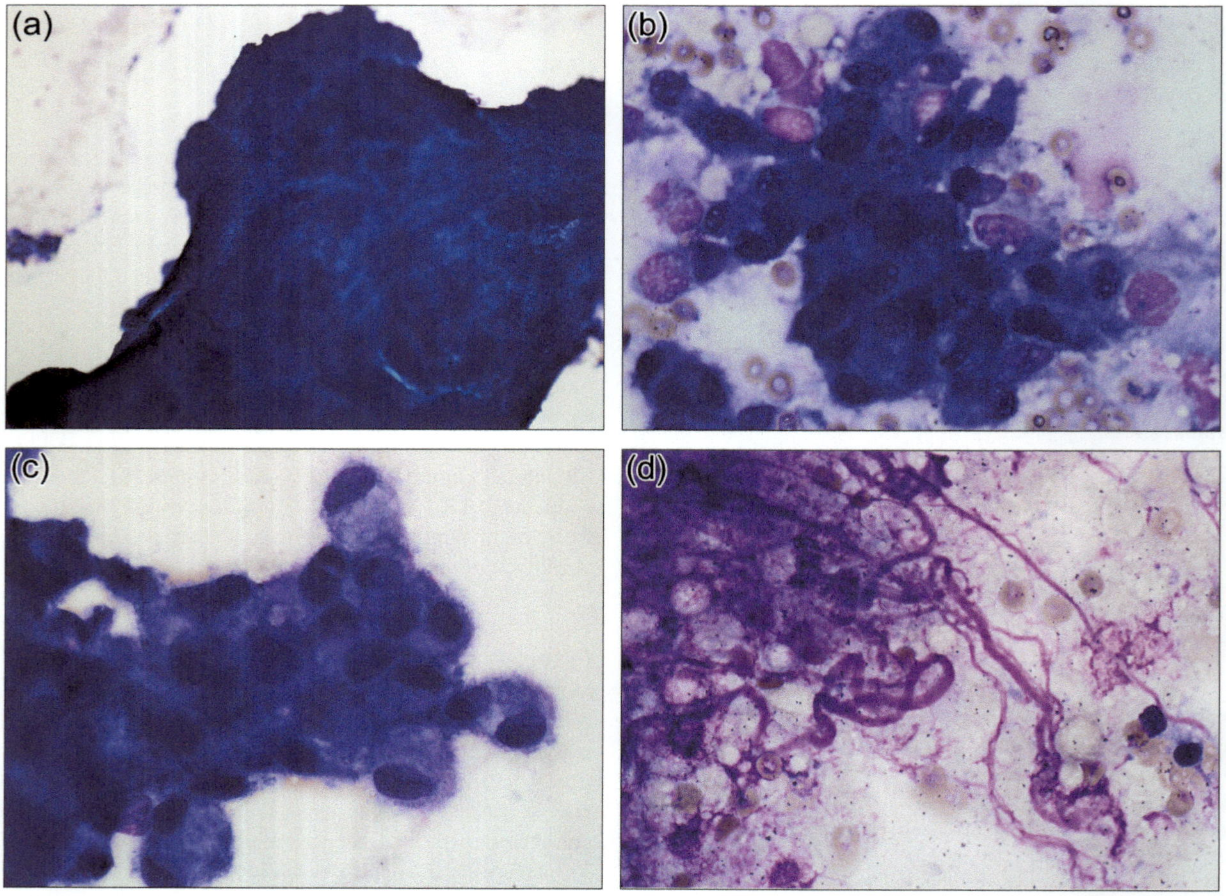

Figures 14.54a–d CNS biopsy of a cystic extra-axial mass near the cerebellum (Wright–Giemsa: a, 500× magnification; b–d, 1,000× magnification).

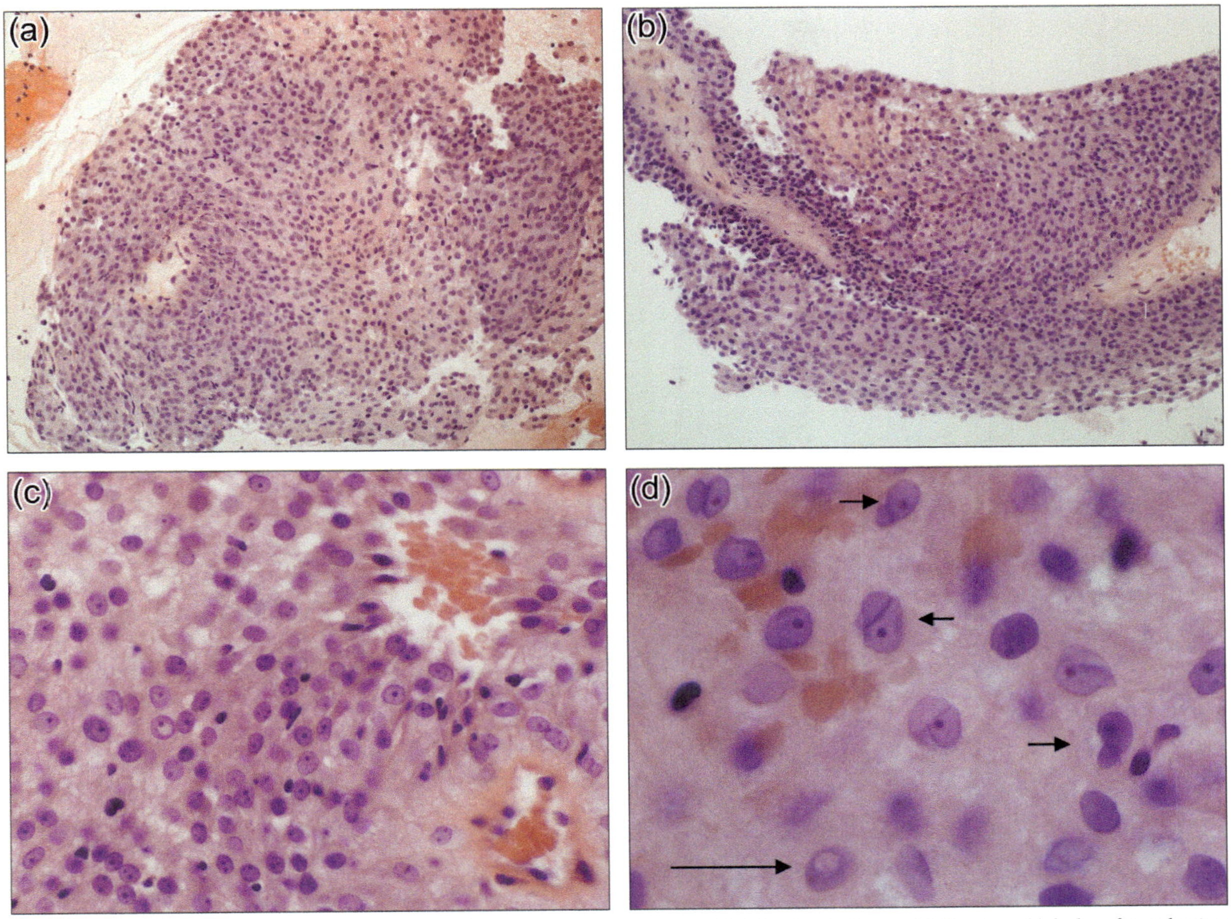

Figures 14.55a–d Histologic sections of a meningothelial meningioma in an 8-year-old Labrador Retriever. (a) Sheets and lobules of neoplastic cells are present; fibrin and red blood cell clumps are seen along the edge of the image. (b) Note how the neoplastic cells are arranged around the blood vessel. (c) The neoplastic cells are polygonal with poorly distinct cell margins, eosinophilic cytoplasm, round nuclei, peripheralized chromatin, and one to several nucleoli. (d) Two of the characteristic findings in this tumor type are displayed: intranuclear cytoplasmic pseudoinclusions (long arrow) and folded nuclei (short arrows) (H&E: (a) and (b), 200× magnification; c, 500× magnification; d, 1,000× magnification).

right with possible swelling of the left optic nerve on fundic examination. Postural reflexes were abnormal with mildly delayed placing in the forelimbs and absent placing in the pelvic limbs. Decreases in withdrawal reflexes in all limbs, perineal reflex, and patellar reflexes were noted. These findings indicated multifocal disease involving the brainstem, cerebellum, and peripheral nervous system (nerve, muscle, and/or neuromuscular junction). MRI revealed right oliquus capitis caudalis and lateral pterygoid muscle changes consistent with polymyositis, mild lateral ventricular asymmetry, and mild medial retropharyngeal lymphadenopathy.

CSF analysis

A CSF sample was collected from the cerebellomedullary cistern and submitted for evaluation. The sample was clear and colorless. It had a CSF TP = 46.7 mg/dl (normal <30 mg/dl), TNCC = 128 cells/mm^3 (normal <5 cells/mm^3), RBCs = 67/μl. During hemocytometry, numerous round structures with a smooth contour and an apparent 'halo' or pericellular clearing were identified, which ranged from 1 to 2× the diameter of an erythrocyte (Figure 14.56). Images from the cytocentrifuged preparation of the CSF are shown (Figures 14.57a–c).

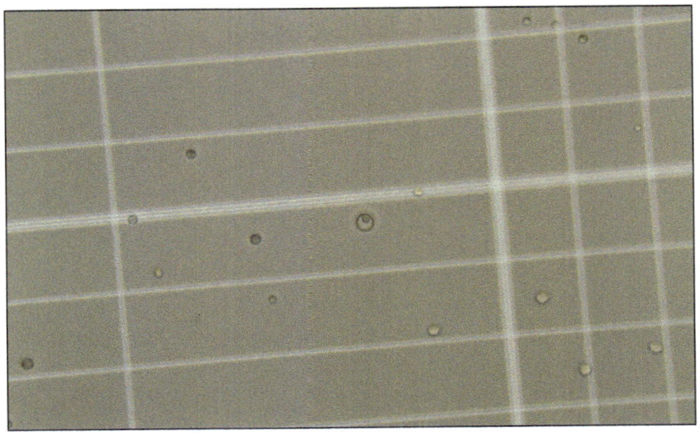

Figure 14.56 200× view of a hemocytometer loaded with unstained CSF.

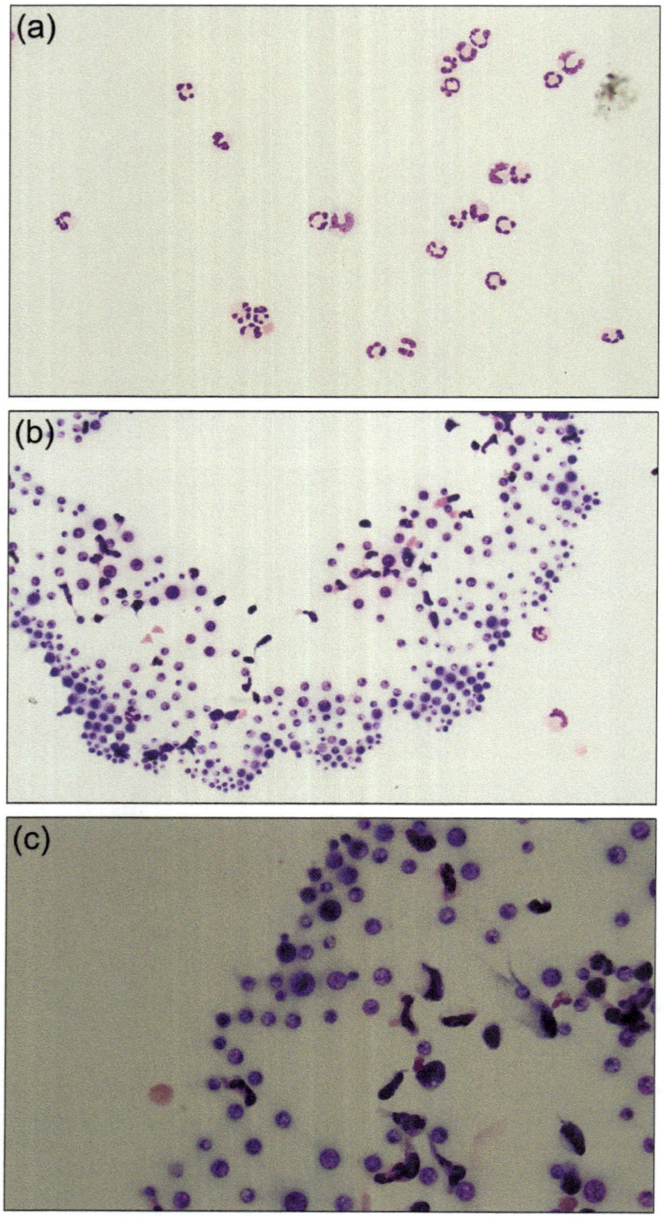

Figures 14.57a–c Cytocentrifuged preparations of CSF from a 2-year-old German shepherd (Wright–Giemsa: a and b, 500× magnification, c 1,000× magnification).

CSF cytology description

A highly cellular cytocentrifuged sample is examined. A 100-cell differential count yielded 74% moderately degenerate neutrophils, 24% large mononuclear cells, and 2% small mononuclear cells/lymphocytes (Figure 14.57a). Many fungal yeast organisms were identified, which had a round, pink to purple granular contour and a nonstaining capsule of variable thickness, consistent with *Cryptococcus* spp. (Figure 14.57b). These organisms were variable in size and seldom displayed narrow-based budding (Figure 14.57c). Low numbers of erythrocytes and bare nuclei were noted in the background. Given these findings, the unknown structures seen on hemocytometry were also interpreted as *Cryptococcus* spp. yeast.

Interpretation: neutrophilic pleocytosis with *Cryptococcus* spp. yeast; increased CSF protein.

Outcome

Unfortunately, the patient's status declined during recovery from anesthesia; she did not regain consciousness and lost the ability to breathe spontaneously. Humane euthanasia was elected, and a necropsy was not performed.

REFERENCES

Adamo P.F., Adams W.M., Steinberg H. (2007) Granulomatous meningoencephalomyelitis in dogs. *Comp Contin Educ Pract Vet 29(11)*:678–690.

Andrews J., Setran E., McDonnel L. et al. (2005) An evaluation of the Cell-Dyn 3200 for counting cells in cerebrospinal and other body fluids. *Lab Hematol 11(2)*:98–106.

Bagley R.S. (1996) Pathophysiologic sequelae of intracranial disease. *Vet Clin North Am Small Anim Pract 26(4)*:711–733.

Bailey C.S., Higgins R.J. (1986) Characteristics of cerebrospinal fluid associated with canine granulomatous meningoencephalomyelitis: A retrospective study. *J Am Vet Med Assoc 188(4)*:418–421.

Bauer N.B., Bassett H., O'Neill E.J. et al. (2006) Cerebrospinal fluid from a 6-year-old dog with severe neck pain. *Vet Clin Pathol 35(1)*:123–125.

Becker M., Bauer N., Moritz A. (2008) Automated flow cytometric cell count and differentiation of canine cerebrospinal fluid cells using the ADVIA 2120. *Vet Clin Pathol 37(3)*:344–352.

Behling-Kelly E., Petersen S., Muthuswamy A. et al. (2010) Neoplastic pleocytosis in a dog with metastatic mammary carcinoma and meningeal carcinomatosis. *Vet Clin Pathol 39(2)*:247–252.

Behr S., Trumel C., Palanché F. et al. (2003) Assessment of a Pyrogallol Red technique for total protein measurement in the cerebrospinal fluid of dogs. *J Small Anim Pract 44(12)*:530–533.

Behr S., Trumel C., Cauzinille L. et al. (2006) High resolution protein electrophoresis of 100 paired canine cerebrospinal fluid and serum. *J Vet Intern Med 20(3)*:657–662.

Belz K.M., Specht A.J., Johnson V.S. et al. (2013) MRI findings in a dog with kernicterus. *J Am Anim Hosp Assoc 49(4)*:286–292.

Belluco S., Marano G., Baiker K. et al. (2022) Standardisation of canine meningioma grading: Inter-observer agreement and recommendations for reproducible histopathologic criteria. *Vet Comp Oncol 20(2)*:509–520.

Bienzle D., Kwiecien J.M., Parent J.M. (1995) Extramedullary hematopoiesis in the choroid plexus of five dogs. *Vet Pathol 32(4)*:437–440.

Bienzle D., McDonnell J.J., Stanton J.B. (2000) Analysis of cerebrospinal fluid from dogs and cats after 24 and 48 hours of storage. *J Am Vet Med Assoc 216(11)*:1761–1764.

Bisby T.M., Holman P.J., Pitoc G.A. et al. (2010) *Sarcocystis* sp. encephalomyelitis in a cat. *Vet Clin Pathol 39(1)*:105–112.

Bittermann S., Schild C., Marti E. et al. (2019) Analysis of blood degradation products and ferritin in the cerebrospinal fluid of dogs with acute thoracolumbar disk extrusion, a prospective pilot study. *BMC Vet Res 15*:148.

Boettcher I.C., Steinberg T., Matiasek K. et al. (2007) Use of anti-coronavirus antibody testing of cerebrospinal fluid for diagnosis of feline infectious peritonitis involving the central nervous system in cats. *J Am Vet Med Assoc 230(2)*:199–205.

Bohn A.A., Wills T.B., West C.L. et al. (2006) Cerebrospinal fluid analysis and magnetic resonance imaging in the diagnosis of neurologic disease in dogs: A retrospective study. *Vet Clin Pathol 35(3)*:315–320.

Brisson B.A. (2010) Intervertebral disc disease in dogs. *Vet Clin North Am Small Anim Pract 40(5)*:829–858.

Bromel C., Sykes J.E., Brömel C. (2005) Epidemiology, diagnosis, and treatment of blastomycosis in dogs and cats. *Clin Tech Small Anim Pract 20(4)*:233–239.

Brune J.E., Chen A.V., Coffey T. (2023) Determination of the effect of iatrogenic blood contamination on lactate dehydrogenase and creatine kinase activity in canine cerebrospinal fluid. *Vet Clin Pathol 52(1)*:64–70.

Cantile C., Youssef S. (2015) Neoplastic diseases of the nervous system. In: *Jubb, Kennedy & Palmer's Pathology of Domestic Animals*, 6th edn. (ed. M.G. Maxie) Saunders Elsevier, St. Louis, pp. 396–406.

Carlson G.D., Oliff H.S., Gorden C. et al. (2003) Cerebral spinal fluid pressure: Effects of body position and lumbar subarachnoid drainage in a canine model. *Spine 28(2)*:119–122.

Chai O., Yas E., Brenner O., Rojas A. et al. (2018) Clinical characteristics of Spirocerca lupi migration in the spinal cord. *Vet Parasitol* 253:16–21.

Chamisha Y., Aroch I., Kuzi S. et al. (2015) The prognostic value of cerebrospinal fluid characteristics in dogs without deep pain perception due to thoracolumbar disc herniation. *Res Vet Sci 100*:189–196.

Cheville N.F. (2009) The neoplastic cell. In: *Ultrastructural Pathology: The Comparative Cellular Basis of Disease*, 2nd edn. (ed. N. Cheville) Wiley-Blackwell, Ames, pp. 756–793.

Chhieng D.C., Elgert P., Cohen J.-M. et al. (2002) Cytology of primary central nervous system neoplasms in cerebrospinal fluid specimens. *Diagn Cytopathol 26(4)*:209–212.

Chrisman C.L. (1992) Cerebrospinal fluid analysis. *Vet Clin North Am Small Anim Pract 22(4)*:781–810.

Christopher M.M. (1992) Bone marrow contamination of canine cerebrospinal fluid. *Vet Clin Pathol 21(3)*:95–98.

Cian F., Palus V., Cherubini G.B. et al. (2013) What is your diagnosis? Cerebrospinal fluid from a dog. *Vet Clin Pathol 43(1)*:115–116.

Cluzel C., Aboulmali A.A., Dugas S. et al. (2016) Diffuse leptomeningeal histiocytic sarcoma in the cerebrospinal fluid of 2 dogs. *Vet Clin Pathol 45(1)*:184–190.

Cook J.R., DeNicola D.B. (1988) Cerebrospinal fluid. *Vet Clin North Am Small Anim Pract 18(3)*:475–499.

Correale J., Fiol M. (2004) Activation of humoral immunity and eosinophils in neuromyelitis optica. *Neurology 63(12)*:2363–2370.

Corsini G., Sanchez-Masian D., Verin R. et al. (2022) Persistent marked cerebrospinal fluid eosinophilia in a dog with primary central nervous system histiocytic sarcoma. *Vet Clin Pathol.* doi: 10.1111/vcp.13183

Creevy K.E., Gagnepain J.F., Platt S.R. et al. (2013) Comparison of concentrations of γ-aminobutyric acid and glutamate in cerebrospinal fluid of dogs with idiopathic epilepsy with and without seizure-related magnetic resonance imaging hyperintense areas in the limbic system. *Am J Vet Res 74(8)*:1118–1125.

De la Fuente C., Monreal L., Cerón J.J. et al. (2012) Fibrinolytic activity in cerebrospinal fluid of dogs with different neurological disorders. *J Vet Intern Med 26(6)*:1365–1373.

De New K.M., Coates J.R., Wellehan J. et al. (2023) Mycobacterium haemophilum infection in canine cerebrospinal fluid. *Vet Clin Pathol.* doi: 10.1111/vcp.13206

De Risio L., Platt S.R. (2010) Fibrocartilaginous embolic myelopathy in small animals. *Vet Clin North Am Small Anim Pract 40(5)*:859–869.

Defontis M., Richartz J., Engelmann N. et al. (2012) Canine *Trypanosoma evansi* infection introduced into Germany. *Vet Clin Pathol 41(3)*:369–374.

Di Terlizzi R., Platt S. (2006) The function, composition and analysis of cerebrospinal fluid in companion animals: Part I – function and composition. *Vet J 172(3)*:422–431.

Di Terlizzi R., Platt S.R. (2009) The function, composition and analysis of cerebrospinal fluid in companion animals: part II - analysis. *Vet J 180(1)*:15–32.

Dickinson P.J., Keel M.K., Higgins R.F. et al. (2000) Clinical and pathologic features of oligodendrogliomas in two cats. *Vet Pathol 37(2)*:160–167.

Dickinson P.J., Sturges B.K., Kass P.H. et al. (2006) Characteristics of cisternal cerebrospinal fluid associated with intracranial meningiomas in dogs: 56 cases (1985–2004). *J Am Vet Med Assoc 228(4)*:564–567.

Doenges S.J., Weber K., Dorsch R. et al. (2016) Detection of feline coronavirus in cerebrospinal fluid for diagnosis of feline infectious peritonitis in cats with and without neurological signs. *J Feline Med Surg 18(2)*:104–109.

Doyle C., Solano-Gallego L. (2009) Cytologic interpretation of canine cerebrospinal fluid samples with low total nucleated cell concentration, with and without blood contamination. *Vet Clin Pathol 38(3)*:392–396.

Duque C., Parent J., Bienzle D. (2012) The immunophenotype of blood and cerebrospinal fluid mononuclear cells in dogs. *J Vet Intern Med 16(6)*:714–719.

Durand A., Keenihan E., Schweizer D. et al. (2022) Clinical and magnetic resonance imaging features of lymphoma involving the nervous system in cats. *J Vet Intern Med 36(2)*:679–693.

Elias A., Brown C. (2008) Cerebellomedullary cerebrospinal fluid collection in the dog. *Lab Anim 37(10)*:457–458.

Espino L., Suarez M., Santamarina G. et al. (2009) First report of the simultaneous occurrence of choroid plexus papilloma and meningioma in a dog. *Acta Vet Hung 57(3)*:389–397.

Falconer H.L., Walker S.A., Ashby J.P. (2015) Specificity of elevated cerebrospinal fluid bilirubin in the investigation of subarachnoid haemorrhage. *Ann Clin Biochem 54*:404–406.

Fallin C.W., Raskin R.E., Harvey J.W. (1996) Cytologic identification of neural tissue in the cerebrospinal fluid of two dogs. *Vet Clin Pathol 25(4)*:127–129.

Ferreira A. (2016) Diagnostic value of creatine kinase activity in canine cerebrospinal fluid. *Can Vet J 57(10)*:1081–1086.

Fernandez N.J., Davies J.L., Diaz J. et al. (2013) What is your diagnosis? Cerebrospinal fluid from a dog. *Vet Clin Pathol 42(2)*:244–245.

Fry M.M., Vernau W., Kass P.H. et al. (2006) Effects of time, initial composition, and stabilizing agents on the results of canine cerebrospinal fluid analysis. *Vet Clin Pathol 35(1)*:72–77.

Galan A., Carletti B.E., Morgaz J. et al. (2013) Comparative study of select biochemical markers in cerebrospinal fluid of healthy dogs before and after treatment with nutraceuticals. *Vet Clin Pathol 43(1)*:72–77.

Galano H.R., Platt S.R., Neuwirth L. et al. (2002) Choroid plexus cyst in a dog. *Vet Rad Ultrasound 43(4)*:349–352.

Galgut B.I., Janardhan K.S., Grondin T.M. et al. (2010) Detection of *Neospora caninum* tachyzoites in cerebrospinal fluid of a dog following prednisone and cyclosporine therapy. *Vet Clin Pathol 39*(*3*):386–390.

Gama F.G., Santana A.E., Filho E.C. et al. (2007) Agarose gel electrophoresis of cerebrospinal fluid proteins of dogs after sample concentration using a membrane microconcentrator technique. *Vet Clin Pathol 36*(*1*):85–88.

Garma-Aviña A. (2004) Cytology of the normal and abnormal choroid plexi in selected domestic mammals, wildlife species, and man. *J Vet Diag Invest 16*(*4*):283–292.

Garosi L., McConnell J.F., Platt S.R. et al. (2006) Clinical and topographic magnetic resonance characteristics of suspected brain infarction in 40 dogs. *J Vet Intern Med 20*(*2*):311–321.

Gibson A.M., Rosser M.F., de Oliveira C.R. et al. (2021) Magnetic resonance imaging findings and antemortem cytologic diagnosis of intramedullary spinal cord ependymoma in a dog. *J Am Vet Med Assoc 259*(*12*):1446–1451.

Gnirs K., Ruel Y., Blot S. et al. (2002) Spinal subarachnoid cysts in 13 dogs. *Vet Rad Ultrasound 44*(*4*):402–408.

Gonçalves R., Carrera I., Garosi L. et al. (2011) Clinical and topographic magnetic resonance imaging characteristics of suspected thalamic infarcts in 16 dogs. *Vet J 188*(*1*):39–43.

Gruendl S., Matiasek K., Matiasek L. et al. (2017) Diagnostic utility of cerebrospinal fluid immunocytochemistry for diagnosis of feline infectious peritonitis manifesting in the central nervous system. *J Feline Med Surg 19*(*6*):576–585.

Gunn-Moore D.A., Reed N. (2011) CNS disease in the cat: Current knowledge of infectious causes. *J Feline Med Surg 13*(*11*):824–836.

Harms N.J., Dickinson R.M., Nibblett B.M.D. et al. (2009) What is your diagnosis? Intracranial mass in a dog. *Vet Clin Pathol 38*(*4*):537–540.

Hasegawa D., Matsuki N., Fujita M. et al. (2004) Kinetics of glutamate and gamma-aminobutyric acid in cerebrospinal fluid in a canine model of complex partial status epilepticus induced by kainic acid. *J Vet Med Sci 66*(*12*):1555–1559.

Heck L.C., Cony F.G., Bianchi M.V. et al. (2018) Pathological features of 78 metastatic or multicentric neoplasms involving the central nervous system in dogs. *Pesqui Vet Bras 38*(*10*):1989–1998.

Higginbotham M.J., Kent M., Glass E.N. (2007) Noninfectious inflammatory central nervous system diseases in dogs. *Comp Contin Educ Vet 29*(*8*):488–497; quiz 497, 501.

Hughes P.A., Magnet A.D., Fishbain J.T. (2003) Eosinophilic meningitis: a case series report and review of the literature. *Mil Med 168*(*10*):817–821.

Hugo T.B., Heading K.L., Labuc R.H. (2014) Canine cerebrospinal fluid total nucleated cell counts and cytology associations with the prevalence of magnetic resonance imaging abnormalities. *Vet Med (Auckl) 18*(*5*):75–84.

Hurtt A.E., Smith M.O. (1997) Effects of iatrogenic blood contamination on results of cerebrospinal fluid analysis in clinically normal dogs and dogs with neurologic disease. *J Am Vet Med Assoc 211*(*7*):866–867.

Iqbal M., Shah A., Wani M.A. et al. (2006) Cytopathology of the central nervous system. Part I. Utility of crush smear cytology in intraoperative diagnosis of central nervous system lesions. *Acta Cytol 50*(*6*):608–616.

Ishikawa C., Ito D., Kitagawa M. et al. (2016) Comparison of conventional magnetic resonance imaging and nonenhanced three dimensional time-of-flight magnetic resonance angiography findings between dogs with meningioma and dogs with intracranial histiocytic sarcoma: 19 cases (2010–2014). *J Am Vet Med Assoc 248*(*10*):1139–1148.

Jacobsen E.A., Helmers R.A., Lee J.J. et al. (2012) The expanding role(s) of eosinophils in health and disease. *Blood 120*(*19*):3882–3890.

Joffe A.R. (2007) Lumbar puncture and brain herniation in acute bacterial meningitis: A review. *J Intensive Care Med 22*(*4*):194–207.

Johnsrude J.D., Alleman A.R., Schumacher J. et al. (1996) Cytologic findings in cerebrospinal fluid from two animals with GM2-gangliosidosis. *Vet Clin Pathol 25*(*3*):80–83.

José-López R., de la Fuente C., Pumarola M. et al. (2013) Spinal meningiomas in dogs: Description of 8 cases including a novel radiological and histopathological presentation. *Can Vet J 54*(*10*):948–954.

Koch B.C., Daniels L.O., Thomsen L.T. et al. (2019) Collection of cerebrospinal fluid into EDTA versus plain tubes does not affect the standard analysis in dogs. *Acta Vet Scand 61*(*1*):23. doi: 10.1186/s13028-019-0457-1

Koestner A., Bilzer T., Fatzer R. et al. (1999) Lymphomas and hematopoietic tumors. In: *Histologic Classification of Tumors of the Nervous System of Domestic Animals*. Armed Forces Institute of Pathology, Washington DC, pp. 30–32.

Koutinas A.F., Polizopoulou Z.S., Baumgaertner W. et al. (2002) Relation of clinical signs to pathological changes in 19 cases of canine distemper encephalomyelitis. *J Comp Pathol 126*(*1*):47–56.

Lampe R., Foss K.D., Hague D.W. et al. (2020a) Comparison of creatine kinase in cerebrospinal fluid collected from the cerebellomedullary and lumbar cisterna in 10 dogs with neurologic disease. *Vet Clin Pathol 49*(*3*):436–439.

Lampe R., Foss K.D., Vitale S. et al. (2020b) Comparison of cerebellomedullary and lumbar cerebrospinal fluid analysis in dogs with neurological disease. *J Vet Intern Med 34*(*2*):838–843.

Lane L.V., Meinkoth J.H., Brunker J.D. et al. (2012a) Disseminated protothecosis diagnosed by evaluation of CSF in a dog. *Vet Clin Pathol 41*(*1*):147–152.

Lane L.V., Meinkoth J.H., Stern A.W. et al. (2012b) Pathology in practice. Nonepitheliotropic B-cell lymphoma of the nasal cavity with associated suppurative rhinitis and epidermal ulceration and lymphoma of the right kidney. *J Am Vet Med Assoc 240*(*6*):677–679.

LaRue M.K., Taylor A.R., Back A.R. et al. (2018) Central nervous system lymphoma in 18 dogs (2001 to 2015). *J Small Anim Pract 59*(*9*):547–552.

Lavely J.A., Lipsitz D. (2005) Fungal infections of the central nervous system in the dog and cat. *Clin Tech Small Anim Pract 20*(*4*):212–219.

Lavely J.A., Vernau K.M., Vernau W. et al. (2006) Spinal epidural empyema in seven dogs. *Vet Surg 35*(*2*):176–185.

Lee H.S., Tihan T. (2015) The basics of intraoperative diagnosis in neuropathology. *Surg Pathol Clin 8*(*1*):27–47.

Lester S.J., Malik R., Bartlett K.H. et al. (2011) Cryptococcosis: Update and emergence of *Cryptococcus gattii*. *Vet Clin Pathol 40*(*1*):4–17.

Levine G.J., Cook J.R., Kerwin S.C. et al. (2014) Relationships between cerebrospinal fluid characteristics, injury severity, and functional outcome in dogs with and without intervertebral disk herniation. *Vet Clin Pathol 43*(*3*):437–446.

Levine G.J., Levine J.M., Witsberger S.C. et al. (2010) Cerebrospinal fluid myelin basic protein as a prognostic biomarker in dogs with thoracolumbar intervertebral disk herniation. *J Vet Intern Med 24*(*4*):890–896.

Levitin H.A., Foss K.D., Hague D.W. et al. (2019) The utility of intraoperative impression smear cytology of intracranial granular cell tumors: Three cases. *Vet Clin Pathol 48*(*2*):282–286.

Liu L., Cao F., Wang S. et al. (2015) Detection of malignant B lymphocytes by PCR clonality assay using direct lysis of cerebrospinal fluid and low volume specimens. *Int J Lab Hematol 37*(*2*):165–173.

Luján-Feliu-Pascual A., Garosi L., Dennis R. et al. (2008) Iatrogenic brainstem injury during cerebellomedullary cistern puncture. *Vet Rad Ultrasound 49*(*5*):467–471.

Lunn J.A., Lee R., Smaller J. et al. (2012) Twenty two cases of canine neural angiostronglyosis in eastern Australia (2002–2005) and a review of the literature. *Parasit Vectors* 5:70.

MacNeill A.L., Andre B.G., Zingale Y. et al. (2018) The effects of iatrogenic blood contamination on total nucleated cell counts and protein concentrations in canine cerebrospinal fluid. *Vet Clin Pathol 47*(*3*):464–470.

Marchetti V., Lubas G., Baneth G. et al. (2009) Hepatozoonosis in a dog with skeletal involvement and meningoencephalomyelitis. *Vet Clin Pathol 38(1)*:121–125.

Mariani C.L., Boozer L.B., Braxton A.M. et al. (2013) Evaluation of matrix metalloproteinase-2 and –9 in the cerebrospinal fluid of dogs with intracranial tumors. *Am J Vet Res 74(1)*:122–129.

Mariani C.L., Nye C.J., Ruterbories L. et al. (2020) Cerebrospinal fluid lactate concentrations in dogs with seizure disorders. *J Vet Intern Med 34(6)*:2562–2570.

Marioni-Henry K. (2010) Feline spinal cord diseases. *Vet Clin North Am Small Anim Pract 40(5)*:1011–1028.

Márquez M., Pedregosa J.R., López J. et al. (2013) *Leishmania* amastigotes in the central nervous system of a naturally infected dog. *J Vet Diag Invest 25(1)*:142–146.

Mateo I., Lorenzo V., Muñoz A. et al. (2010) Meningeal carcinomatosis in a dog: Magnetic resonance imaging features and pathological correlation. *J Small Anim Pract 51(1)*:43–48.

Matsuki N., Fujiwara K., Tamahara S. et al. (2004) Prevalence of autoantibody in cerebrospinal fluids from dogs with various CNS diseases. *J Vet Med Sci 66(3)*:295–297.

Mejías M., Molina M.C., Ferreira A. (2008) Assessment of the IgG index in dogs by indirect immunoenzimatic assays as diagnostic tool for inflammatory diseases of central nervous system. *Res Vet Sci 84(3)*:335–340.

Mellema L.M., Koblik P.D., Kortz G.D. et al. (1999) Reversible magnetic resonance imaging abnormalities in dogs following seizures. *Vet Rad Ultrasound 40(6)*:588–595.

Mello L.S., Leite-Filho R.V., Panziera W. et al. (2019) Feline lymphoma in the nervous system: Pathological, immunohistochemical, and etiological aspects in 16 cats. *Pesq Vet Bras 39(6)*:393–401.

Mesher C.I., Blue J.T., Guffroy M.R.G. et al. (1996) Intracellular myelin in cerebrospinal fluid from a dog with myelomalacia. *Vet Clin Pathol 25(4)*:124–126.

Miglio A., Antognoni M.T., Mangili V. (2013) What is your diagnosis? Bronchoalveolar lavage and cerebrospinal fluid from a dog in Italy. *Vet Clin Pathol 42(1)*:109–110.

Mikszewski J.S., Van Winkle T.J., Troxel M.T. (2006) Fibrocartilaginous embolic myelopathy in five cats. *J Am Anim Hosp Assoc 42(3)*:226–233.

Miller A.D, Koehler J.W., Donovan T.A. et al. (2019a) Canine ependymoma: Diagnostic criteria and common pitfalls. *Vet Path 56(6)*:860–867.

Miller A.D., Miller C.R., Rossmeisl J.H. (2019b) Canine primary intracranial cancer: A clinicopathologic and comparative review of glioma, meningioma, and choroid plexus tumors. *Front Oncol 9*:1151.

Miller A.D., Zachary J.F. (2017) Nervous system. In: *Pathologic Basis of Veterinary Disease* (ed. J.F. Zachary) Elsevier, St. Louis, pp. 805–907.

Monteiro S., Hughes K., Genain M.A. et al. (2021) Primary histiocytic sarcoma in the brain with renal metastasis causing internal ophthalmoparesis and external ophthalmoplegia in a Maine Coon cat. *JFMS Open Rep 25(7)*. doi: 10.1177/20551169211038515.

Motta L., Mandara M.T., Skerritt G.C. (2012) Canine and feline intracranial meningiomas: An updated review. *Vet J 192(2)*:153–165.

Muñana K.R. (1996) Encephalitis and meningitis. *Vet Clin N Am 26(4)*:857–874.

Newton P.L., Fry D.R., Best M.P. (2017) Comparison of direct in-house cerebrospinal fluid cytology with commercial pathology results in dogs. *J Small Anim Pract 58(12)*:694–702.

Nghiem P.P., Schatzberg S.J. (2010) Conventional and molecular diagnostic testing for the acute neurologic patient. *J Vet Emerg Crit Care 20(1)*:46–61.

Okada M., Kitagawa M., Ito D. et al. (2010) Magnetic resonance imaging features and clinical signs associated with presumptive and confirmed progressive myelomalacia in dogs: 12 cases (1997–2008). *J Am Vet Med Assoc 237(10)*:1160–1165.

Olby N.J., da Costa R.C., Levine J.M. et al. (2020) Prognostic factors in canine acute intervertebral disc disease. *Front Vet Sci 7*:590569.

Ortiz-Nisa S., Sanz A., Pastor J. et al. (2021) Performance of the Sysmex XN-V body fluid module for canine cerebrospinal fluid cell count. *Vet Clin Pathol 50(3)*:359–368.

Ostrow J.D., Pascolo L., Brites D. et al. (2004) Molecular basis of bilirubin-induced neurotoxicity. *Trends Mol Med 10(2)*:65–70.

Pancotto T., Rossmeisl J.H., Panciera D.L. et al. (2010) Blood-brain-barrier disruption in chronic canine hypothyroidism. *Vet Clin Pathol 39(4)*:485–493.

Pancotto T., Rossmeisl J.H., Zimmerman K. et al. (2013) Intramedullary spinal cord neoplasia in 53 dogs (1990–2010): Distribution, clinicopathologic characteristics, and clinical behavior. *J Vet Intern Med 27(6)*:1500–1508.

Pastorello A., Constantino-Casas F., Archer J. (2010) Choroid plexus carcinoma cells in the cerebrospinal fluid of a Staffordshire Bull Terrier. *Vet Clin Pathol 39(4)*:505–510.

Patnaik A.K. (1993) Histologic and immunohistochemical studies of granular cell tumors in seven dogs, three cats, one horse, and one bird. *Vet Pathol 30(2)*:176–185.

Patrick T., Giannini C., Ebersold M.J. et al. (2006) Iatrogenic cerebellar implantation of a vestibular schwannoma. Case report. *J Neurosurg 104(3)*:452–456.

Pérez C., Maggi R.G., Diniz P.P. et al. (2011) Molecular and serological diagnosis of *Bartonella* infection in 61 dogs from the United States. *J Vet Intern Med 25(4)*:805–810.

Peterson L.N., Christian J.A., Bentley R.T. et al. (2020) Evaluation of the hydroxyethyl starch stabilizing agent, Vetstarch, in the preservation of canine cerebrospinal fluid samples. *Vet Clin Pathol. 49(1)*:95–99.

Pittman M., Treese S., Chen L. et al. (2013) Utility of flow cytometry of cerebrospinal fluid as a screening tool in the diagnosis of central nervous system lymphoma. *Arch Pathol Lab Med 137(11)*:1610–1618.

Platt S.R., Alleman A.R., Lanz O.I. et al. (2002) Comparison of fine-needle aspiration and surgical-tissue biopsy in the diagnosis of canine brain tumors. *Vet Surg 31(1)*:65–69.

Platt S.R., Coates J.R., Eifler D.M. et al. (2013) Effect of treatment with simvastatin and cyclosporine on neurotransmitter concentrations in cerebrospinal fluid after subarachnoid hemorrhage in dogs. *Am J Vet Res 74(8)*:1111–1117.

Platt S.R., Dennis R., Murphy K. et al. (2005) Hematomyelia secondary to lumbar cerebrospinal fluid acquisition in a dog. *Vet Rad Ultrasound 46(6)*:467–471.

Powell S.Z. (2005) Intraoperative consultation, cytologic preparations, and frozen section in the central nervous system. *Arch Pathol Lab Med 129(12)*:1635–1652.

Pugliese M., Carrasco J.L., Andrade C. et al. (2005) Severe cognitive impairment correlates with higher cerebrospinal fluid levels of lactate and pyruvate in a canine model of senile dementia. *Prog Neuropsychopharmacol Biol Psychiatry 29(4)*:603–610.

Quattrini C., Scalco R., Vernau W. et al. (2023) Effect of time and autologous serum addition on the analysis of cerebrospinal fluid in horses. *J Vet Intern Med 37(2)*:713–717.

Radaelli S.T., Platt S.R. (2002) Bacterial meningoencephalomyelitis in dogs: A retrospective study of 23 cases (1990–1999). *J Vet Intern Med 16(2)*:159–163.

Rand J.S., Parent J., Jacobs R. (1990a) Reference intervals for feline cerebrospinal fluid: Biochemical and serologic variables, IgG concentration, and electrophoretic fractionation. *Am J Vet Res 51(7)*:1049–1054.

Rand J.S., Parent J., Jacobs R. et al. (1990b) Reference intervals for feline cerebrospinal fluid: Cell counts and cytologic features. *Am J Vet Res 51(7)*:1044–1048.

Rand J.S., Parent J., Percy D. et al. (1994a) Clinical, cerebrospinal fluid, and histological data from twenty-seven cats with primary inflammatory disease of the central nervous system. *Can Vet J 35(2)*:103–110.

Rand J.S., Parent J., Percy D. et al. (1994b) Clinical, cerebrospinal fluid, and histological data from thirty-four cats with primary noninflammatory disease of the central nervous system. *Can Vet J 35(3)*:174–181.

Riker J., Clarke L.L., Demeter E.A. et al. (2023) Histiocytic sarcoma with central nervous system involvement in 6 cats. *J Vet Diagn Investig 35(1)*:87–91.

Riond B., Steffen F., Schmied O. et al. (2013) Total protein measurement in canine cerebrospinal fluid: Agreement between a turbidimetric assay and 2 dye-binding methods and determination of reference intervals using an indirect a posteriori method. *Vet Clin Pathol 43(1)*:78–88.

Romero-Fernandez N., Ives E.J., Fraser A.R. et al. (2020) Evaluation of the Idexx ProCyte Dx® for analysis of canine cerebrospinal fluid. *J Small Anim Pract. 61(2)*:110–115.

Rosenberg G.A., Kyner W.T., Estrada E. (1980) Bulk flow of brain interstitial fluid under normal and hyperosmolar conditions. *Am J Physiol 238(1)*:F42–49.

Ruotsalo K., Poma R., da Costa R.C. et al. (2008) Evaluation of the ADVIA 120 for analysis of canine cerebrospinal fluid. *Vet Clin Pathol 37(2)*:242–248.

Sarnat H.B. (1998) Histochemistry and immunocytochemistry of the developing ependyma and choroid plexus. *Microsc Res Tech 41(1)*:14–28.

Satoh H., Yamauchi T., Yamasaki M. et al. (2011) Rapid detection of GM1 ganglioside in cerebrospinal fluid in dogs with GM1 gangliosidosis using matrix-assisted laser desorption ionization time-of-flight mass spectrometry. *J Vet Diag Invest 23(6)*:1202–1207.

Shafie I.N., McLaughlin M., Burchmore R. et al. (2014) The chaperone protein clusterin may serve as a cerebrospinal fluid biomarker for chronic spinal cord disorders in the dog. *Cell Stress Chaperones 19(3)*:311–320.

Shah K.H., Edlow J.A. (2002) Distinguishing traumatic lumbar puncture from true subarachnoid hemorrhage. *J Emerg Med 23(1)*:67–74.

Shibuya M., Matsuki N., Fujiwara K. et al. (2007) Autoantibodies against glial fibrillary acidic protein (GFAP) in cerebrospinal fluids from pug dogs with necrotizing meningoencephalitis. *J Vet Med Sci 69(3)*:241–245.

Skeen T.M., Olby N.J., Muñana K.R. et al. (2003) Spinal arachnoid cysts in 17 dogs. *J Am Anim Hosp Assoc 39(3)*:271–282.

Smith-Maxie L.L., Parent J.P., Rand J. et al. (1989) Cerebrospinal fluid analysis and clinical outcome of eight dogs with eosinophilic meningoencephalomyelitis. *J Vet Intern Med 3(3)*:167–174.

Snyder J.M., Shofer F.S., Van Winkle T.J. et al. (2006) Canine intracranial primary neoplasia: 173 cases (1986–2003). *J Vet Intern Med 20(3)*:669–675.

Sorjonen D.C. (1987) Total protein, albumin quota, and electrophoretic patterns in cerebrospinal fluid of dogs with central nervous system disorders. *Am J Vet Res 48(2)*:301–305.

Spoor M.S., Spagnoli S.T., Burton E.N. et al. (2013) What is your diagnosis? Cystic mass in the fourth ventricle of the brain of a dog. *Vet Clin Pathol 42(3)*:387–388.

Spriggs A.I. (1954) Malignant cells in cerebrospinal fluid. *J Clin Pathol 7(2)*:122–130.

Srugo I., Aroch I., Christopher M.M. et al. (2011) Association of cerebrospinal fluid analysis findings with clinical signs and outcome in acute nonambulatory thoracolumbar disc disease in dogs. *J Vet Intern Med 25(4)*:846–855.

Steinberg T.A., Boettcher I.C., Matiasek K. et al. (2008) Use of albumin quotient and IgG index to differentiate blood- vs brain-derived proteins in the cerebrospinal fluid of cats with feline infectious peritonitis. *Vet Clin Pathol 37(2)*:207–216.

Stowe D.M., Escobar C., Neel J.A. (2012) What is your diagnosis? Cerebrospinal fluid from a dog. *Vet Clin Pathol 41(3)*:429–430.

Suñol A., Garcia-Pertierra S., Faller K.M.E. (2021) Cerebrospinal fluid analysis in dogs: Main patterns and prevalence of albuminocytological dissociation. *Vet Rec 188(5)*:e27. doi: 10.1002/vetr.272021.

Suzuki M., Uchida K., Morozumi M. et al. (2003) A comparative pathological study on canine necrotizing meningoencephalitis and granulomatous meningoencephalomyelitis. *J Vet Med Sci 65(11)*:1233–1239.

Talarico L.R., Schatzberg S.J. (2010) Idiopathic granulomatous and necrotising inflammatory disorders of the canine central nervous system: A review and future perspectives. *J Small Anim Pract 51(3)*:138–149.

Thomas W.B. (1998) Inflammatory diseases of the central nervous system in dogs. *Clin Tech Small Anim Pract 13(3)*:167–178.

Thomas W.B. (1999) Nonneoplastic disorders of the brain. *Clin Tech Small Anim Pract 14(3)*:125–147.

Thomson C.E., Kornegay J.N., Stevens J.B. (1990) Analysis of cerebrospinal fluid from the cerebellomedullary and lumbar cisterns of dogs with focal neurologic disease: 145 cases (1985–1987). *J Am Vet Med Assoc 196(11)*:1841–1844.

Tipold A. (2003) Cerebrospinal fluid. In: *Braund's Clinical Neurology in Small Animals: Localization, Diagnosis and Treatment* (ed. C.H. Vite) International Veterinary Information Service, Ithaca. www.ivis.org. Accessed 4/8/2023.

Tipold A., Stein V.M. (2010) Inflammatory diseases of the spine in small animals. *Vet Clin North Am Small Anim Pract 40(5)*:871–879.

Toyoda I., Vernau W., Sturges B.K. et al. (2020) Clinicopathological characteristics of histiocytic sarcoma affecting the central nervous system in dogs. *J Vet Intern Med 34(2)*:828–837.

Traslavina R.P., Kent M.S., Mohr F.C. et al. (2013) Clear cell ependymoma in a dog. *J Comp Pathol 149(1)*:53–56.

Troxel M.T., Vite C.H., Van Winkle T.J. et al. (2003) Feline intracranial neoplasia: Retrospective review of 160 cases (1985–2001). *J Vet Intern Med 17(6)*:850–859.

Tumani H., Jobs C., Brettschneider J. et al. (2015) Effect of epileptic seizures on the cerebrospinal fluid – A systematic retrospective analysis. *Epilepsy Res 11*:423–431.

Vernau K.M., Higgins R.J., Bollen A.W. et al. (2001) Primary canine and feline nervous system tumors: Intraoperative diagnosis using the smear technique. *Vet Pathol 38(1)*:47–57.

Vitale S., Foss K. (2019) Immune-mediated central nervous system disease – Current knowledge and recommendations. *Top Companion Anim Med 34*:22–29.

Vural S.A., Besalti O., Ilhan F. et al. (2006) Ventricular ependymoma in a German shepherd dog. *Vet J 172(1)*:185–187.

Wamsley H.L. (2013) Clinical pathology. In: *BSAVA Manual of Canine and Feline Neurology* (eds. S.R. Platt, N.J. Olby) British Small Animal Veterinary Association, Gloucester, pp. 36–58.

Wessmann A., Volk H.A., Chandler K. et al. (2010) Significance of surface epithelial cells in canine cerebrospinal fluid and relationship to central nervous system disease. *Vet Clin Pathol 39(3)*:358–364.

Westworth D.R., Dickinson P.J., Vernau W. et al. (2008) Choroid plexus tumors in 56 dogs (1985–2007). *J Vet Intern Med 22(5)*:1157–1165.

Widmer W.R., DeNicola D.B., Blevins W.E. et al. (1992) Cerebrospinal fluid changes after iopamidol and metrizamide myelography in clinically normal dogs. *Am J Vet Res 53(3)*:396–401.

Williams M.J., Baughman B.S., Shores A. et al. (2023) CSF from a puppy with a cerebral vascular hamartoma. *Vet Clin Pathol 52(1)*:97–101.

Windsor R.C., Sturges B.K., Vernau K.M. et al. (2009) Cerebrospinal fluid eosinophilia in dogs. *J Vet Intern Med 23*(*2*):275–281.

Witsberger T.H., Levine J.M., Fosgate G.T. et al. (2012) Associations between cerebrospinal fluid biomarkers and long-term neurologic outcome in dogs with acute intervertebral disk herniation. *J Am Vet Med Assoc 240*(*5*):555–562.

Woolford L., de Lahunta A., Baiker K. et al. (2013) Ventricular and extraventricular ependymal tumors in 18 cats. *Vet Pathol 50*(*2*):243–251.

Yun T., Koo Y., Chae Y. et al. (2021) Neurofilament light chain as a biomarker of meningoencephalitis of unknown etiology in dogs. *J Vet Intern Med 35*(*4*):1865–1872.

Zabolotzky S.M., Vernau K.M., Kass P.H. et al. (2010) Prevalence and significance of extracellular myelin-like material in canine cerebrospinal fluid. *Vet Clin Pathol 39*(*1*):90–95.

CHAPTER 15

BODY CAVITY EFFUSIONS

Ilse Schwendenwein

INTRODUCTION

An effusion is an abnormal accumulation of fluid within a body cavity (Beatty & Barrs, 2010; Dempsey & Ewing, 2011; Gavazza *et al.*, 2013; Valenciano *et al.*, 2013) (Table 15.1). In health, a small amount of fluid between the parietal and visceral surfaces of body cavities acts as a lubricant to facilitate the motion of internal organs against each other and the body cavity walls (Dempsey Ewing, 2011). Within the pleural space, fluid-mediated adhesion of lungs to the chest wall allows mechanical coupling for a direct transmission of forces for normal respiration (Dempsey Ewing, 2011). Visceral and parietal surfaces are lined with mesothelial cells. Mesothelial cells are arranged in a pavement-like monolayer on a basal membrane. They play a pivotal role in fluid and cell transport across the serosal cavities, antigen presentation, inflammation, tissue repair, coagulation and fibrinolysis, and tumor cell adhesion. Mesothelial cells are derived from the mesoderm but exhibit mesenchymal and epithelial characteristics by expressing desmin, cytokeratin, and vimentin intermediate filaments (Mutsaers, 2004; Reggeti et al., 2005). They typically develop epithelial or fibroblast morphology and phagocytic activity with specific inflammatory stimulation (Reggeti *et al.*, 2005). In health only 0.16–0.5% of cells undergo mitosis at any one time, but in cases of injury, the mitotic rate increases dramatically by up to 30–80% on the wound edge. Mesothelial healing is different from other true epithelial surfaces as it occurs diffusely across the wound and not continually from the wound margins toward the center (Mutsaers, 2004). The mesothelium provides a protective barrier against physical damage and invading organisms. Mesothelial cells are connected by tight junctions and secrete glycosaminoglycans, predominantly hyaluronan, which forms a protective coat against microorganisms and tumor cells (Mutsaers, 2004; Dempsey & Ewing, 2011). They also have fibrinolytic activities to prevent the formation of fibrous adhesions (Mutsaers, 2004; Dempsey & Ewing, 2011).

Normal body cavity fluid is a clear, colorless to yellowish, low protein plasma dialysate with a low cellularity. Its formation is regulated by a delicate balance between hydrostatic and oncotic forces within the capillary bed, interstitial fluid, mesothelial and endothelial permeability, and integrity of lymphatic drainage. The lymphatic vessels communicate directly with body cavities through openings, called stomata (mouths), which are the only openings wide enough to allow cells and larger molecules to exit the vessels.

The chemical composition of body cavity fluids is determined by the permeability of capillary walls, which can be passed by nonprotein solutes such as glucose, urea, creatinine, electrolytes, bicarbonate, calcium, and phosphate. The small amount of protein in normal body fluids is derived from interstitial fluid. Protein concentration in interstitial fluid varies between tissues. It is lowest in skeletal muscle (1.5 g/dl [15 g/l]) and highest within the liver (6 g/dl [60 g/l]). Normal body cavity fluid has a protein concentration <2.5 g/dl (25 g/l). The concentration of cells is low ($<1.5 \times 10^3/\mu l$) in dogs and cats and they consist of mesothelial cells, small lymphocytes, macrophages, and a few nondegenerate neutrophils. As it is difficult to collect enough pleural or peritoneal fluid from healthy dogs and cats, reference intervals for physiologic pleural and abdominal fluid in these species are scarce and vary widely.

PATHOPHYSIOLOGY OF EFFUSIONS

Mechanisms involved in the build-up of effusions are transudative, exudative, blocked lymphatic drainage, hemorrhage, lymphorrhage, ruptured viscera or torsion of organs, and/or neoplasia. In many cases a combination of these mechanisms is present at the time of diagnosis. Body cavity effusions can also be symptoms of anaphylaxis (Summers *et al.*, 2021) or chronic infectious disease such as Leishmaniasis (Sebastián-Marcos *et al.*, 2019) or systemic inflammatory disease (Covey & Connolly, 2018). Removal and diagnostic evaluation of body cavity fluids is not only useful in establishing a diagnosis but also a therapeutic measure. The availability of ultrasound diagnostics allows the early detection of small fluid accumulations, which can be safely sampled under visual control for diagnostic purposes even if therapeutic removal is not warranted.

Transudation is the passage of fluid due to hydrostatic or oncotic forces, whereas exudation means fluid accumulation due to a change in vascular permeability owing to inflammation. This allows for increased protein concentration in exudates. For practical reasons the term modified transudate has been introduced, which describes a transudate with increased protein concentration. Some authors discourage the use of this term and suggest its replacement by 'protein-rich transudate', which describes the pathophysiologic mechanisms more appropriately (Stockham & Scott, 2013). Differentiation between transudative and exudative effusions is highly relevant because exudates are commonly produced by local inflammatory processes within the respective body cavity, whereas transudation is commonly elicited by systemic disease or mechanical obstruction.

DOI: 10.1201/9781003258551-15

Table 15.1 **Classification of effusions**

Effusion	Appearance	TP	TNCC	Cytology	Other tests
Normal fluid	Light yellow, clear	<2.5 g/dl	<5 × 10³/μl		
Transudate	Light yellow, clear	<2.5 g/dl	<5 × 10³/μl		
Protein-rich transudate	Yellow, clear	2.6–3.5 g/dl	<5 × 10³/μl		
(Modified transudate)	Yellow, clear	>3.5 g/dl	>5 × 10³/μl		
Exudate	Yellow, turbid	>3.5 g/dl	>5 × 10³/μl		
Nonseptic exudate	Yellow, high viscosity, turbid	>3.5 g/dl	>5 × 10³/μl		Low glucose concentration
Septic exudate	Beige, brown to green, flocculent, smelly	>3.5 g/dl	>5 × 10³/μl	Degenerate neutrophils; infectious agents visible	Low glucose concentration
FIP-associated exudate	Yellow, clear, high viscosity, tends to clot	>3.5 g/dl, usually much higher	Low	Protein precipitates with cracked glass-like appearance; cells do not spread so identification is difficult	High globulin concentration; low albumin:globulin ratio
Hemorrhage (acute)	Shades of red	Usually >3.5 g/dl	Comparable to peripheral blood	Platelets absent	
Hemorrhage (chronic)	Shades of red	Variable, depending on dilution	Variable	Platelets absent	
Chylous (early)	Milky, white opaque	>3.5 g/dl	>5 × 10³/μl	Small well-differentiated lymphocytes; cytoplasmic lipid vacuoles in all types of cells but predominantly in macrophages presence of chylomicrons	Triglyceride concentration > 100 mg/dl
Chylous (late)	Milky, white opaque	>3.5 g/dl	>5 × 10³/μl	Increasing number of neutrophils and macrophages exceeding the small well-differentiated lymphocytes; cytoplasmic lipid vacuoles in all types of cells but predominantly in macrophages Presence of chylomicrons	Triglyceride concentration > 100 mg/dl
Lymph	Clear slightly turbid	Variable higher than transudate	Variable but increased	Predominantly small lymphocytes	Absence of chylomicrons
Pseudochylous	Stable turbidity, slightly yellow	Variable but higher than transudates	Variable but mostly increased	Pyknotic cells	Cholesterol concentration > plasma cholesterol
Bilious effusion	Green to yellow orange, mucinous strands	Variable but higher than transudates	Variable but mostly increased	Bilious mucus and biliary pigment; variable inflammatory cells	Bilirubin concentration > plasma bilirubin
Uroperitoneum (early)	Yellow, clear	Low	Low		
Uroperitoneum (late)	Yellow, clear	Low	Low	Unremarkable	Creatinine >> plasma creatinine
Viscous rupture	Turbid, flocculent, odorous			Mixed bacterial population may be present; feed material may be detected	
Neoplastic	Variable	Variable	Variable	Tumor cells present	None

TP, total protein; TNCC, total nucleated cell count.

The dichotomous differentiation into exudates and transudates is intended to give guidelines for further diagnostic measures. Other types of effusion, such as bilious, hemorrhagic, chylous, organ torsion, viscous or urinary bladder rupture, and neoplastic, are varieties and/or combinations of transudative and exudative processes and should be addressed as such when identified. These terms are self-explaining with respect to etiology; their classification as transudates or exudates adds diagnostic value only indirectly by indicating the duration in some cases. Effusions such as long-standing low protein (pure) transudates, long-standing modified transudates, chylic or bilious effusions and ascites caused by urinary bladder rupture elicit local inflammatory reactions so that transudates mature into exudates (Thompson & Rebar, 2016).

The conventional approach to differentiate transudates from exudates by fluid total protein concentration and nucleated cell count and/or neutrophil concentration (percentage) has been challenged by recent research because evidence-based data for the conventional approach are lacking (Zoia, Petini *et al.*, 2020). The respective cut-offs for TP and TNCC differ markedly among references and contradictory results such as a high TNCC combined with a low protein concentration are common. Particles such as cell aggregates or coagulated material either present within the effusion or forming when diluted with hematology analyzer reagents might interfere with automated cell counts. (Giordano *et al.*, 2015) Therefore some authors consider chemical assays to be more sensitive in identifying exudates, but as such less specific, than conventional classification schemes. 'Light's criteria', a dichotomous classification system based solely on biochemical tests, has been adopted from human medicine and applied to canine and feline pleural effusions (Zoia & Drigo, 2016; Zoia, Petini *et al.*, 2020). In human medicine Light's criteria are used to differentiate between transudative or exudative pleural fluid which is of imminent importance in detecting tuberculosis-associated pleural effusions. Light's criteria combine measurements of lactate dehydrogenase activity (LDH) and total protein (TP) concentration in simultaneously collected samples of the effusion and patient's serum/plasma. A ratio (LDHr) is calculated by dividing $LDH_{effusion}$ by the LDH activity of serum. An LDHr > 0.6 indicates an exudative effusion. The rationale behind LDH activity measurement is the ubiquitous activity of LDH within all cells; it is as such a surrogate marker for cellularity. Serum should be preferred because high LDH activity within platelets might falsely increase LDH activity in plasma samples. Other preanalytical conditions such as even minor blood contamination of body cavity fluid by sampling or micro- (invisible) hemolysis of serum samples might yield erroneous results in LDH measurements. A TPr (TP concentration of the effusion divided by serum protein concentration) is calculated accordingly to differentiate a protein-rich transudate caused by increased hydrostatic pressure from a pure transudate caused by decreased oncotic pressure. In protein-rich transudates the TPr exceeds 0.5. Light's criteria have been applied in their original as well as modified versions or combined with other tests. Acquisition of simultaneous serum samples might restrict their clinical usefulness. Performance of single or combined biochemical measurands such as lactate dehydrogenase activity (LDH) (Smuts *et al.*, 2016), cholesterol and albumin concentrations (Alonso, Mattoso *et al.*, 2021), or lipoprotein profiles (Alonso, Behling-Kelly *et al.*, 2022) have also been investigated to aid differentiation between exudates, pure transudates, and protein-rich transudates. However, lipoprotein profiles did not add much value to the total protein measurement (Alonso, Behling-Kelly *et al.*, 2022). A correct diagnosis can only be established when clinical data, patient history/medication, and laboratory test results are reasonably combined and should not be based solely on isolated laboratory test results. A case-oriented holistic approach where all these previously mentioned factors are considered will yield more accurate results than strictly following the conventional classification scheme of transudates, protein-rich transudates, and exudates (Athanasiou, 2019).

Transudates

Transudates form because of an increased hydrostatic pressure with or without a decreased oncotic pressure (hypoproteinemia/hypalbuminemia) and/or blocked lymphatic drainage (Stockham & Scott, 2013). Increased hydrostatic pressure can occur because of congestive and, especially, right-sided heart failure or mechanical obstruction of the venous outflow. The amount of protein spilling into the body cavity depends on the protein content of the interstitial fluid of the organ, which is mainly affected by the increase of hydrostatic pressure (see above). An increase in post-sinusoidal hydrostatic pressure leads to the formation of a protein-rich transudate, because the protein concentration in hepatic interstitial fluid almost meets serum plasma protein concentration. Protein-rich transudates are most commonly caused by congestive heart failure (mostly right-sided heart failure in dogs). In cases of severe hypoproteinemia (e.g. hepatic fibrosis or protein-losing pathologies), even a post-sinusoidal transudate will have a low protein concentration, which complicates its identification as such (Stockham & Scott, 2013).

Disorders resulting in portal hypertension represent another mechanism for transudate formation. These diseases can be classified by overlapping systems. The vascular system identifies the lesions as pre-sinusoidal, sinusoidal, and post-sinusoidal, and the anatomic system classifies them as luminal (e.g. thrombosis) or extraluminal (Stockham & Scott, 2013). In dogs, the most common causes for the formation of protein-poor transudates are hepatic fibrosis and protein-losing diseases (more commonly nephropathies than enteropathies). Another mechanism for transudate formation is a decrease or cessation of lymphatic drainage. This might occur with protein-losing enteropathies or diseases of internal lymph nodes.

The body cavity fluid from healthy animals is a clear, light yellow, low protein plasma dialysate, which contains only a few nucleated cells consisting of mononuclear cells such as macrophages, small lymphocytes, and mesothelial cells, and a few nondegenerate neutrophils. Transudates are of similar composition, but cellularity is probably at least in the beginning lower due to dilution. When serum protein concentration is within the reference interval for the species, the increase of hydrostatic pressure will incite transudation, whereas the protein content of the transudate will be influenced by the protein concentration of the interstitial fluid of the organ in which the hydrostatic pressure is increased (see above).

Exudates

Exudates form as a sequela of increased vascular and mesothelial permeability caused by inflammation. This type of effusion is rich in proteins and cells, predominantly neutrophils, which permeate the capillary walls and invade the respective body cavity.

Septic exudates

Septic exudates are caused by bacterial, viral, fungal, or protozoal infections. The detection of infectious agents by microscopic evaluation can be difficult; therefore cytologic features such as the presence of degenerate neutrophils should be complemented by bacterial culture. Depending on the type of bacteria involved and their toxin production, degenerate neutrophils will occur (Figures 15.1–15.5). Some bacteria species such as *Nocardia* or *Actinomyces* cause only mild degeneration of neutrophils in close proximity (Thompson & Rebar, 2016). Phagocytized bacteria will be most readily detected in the marginal areas of a cytospin preparation or feathered edge of a smear. In septic effusions the background might change from clear to smudged,

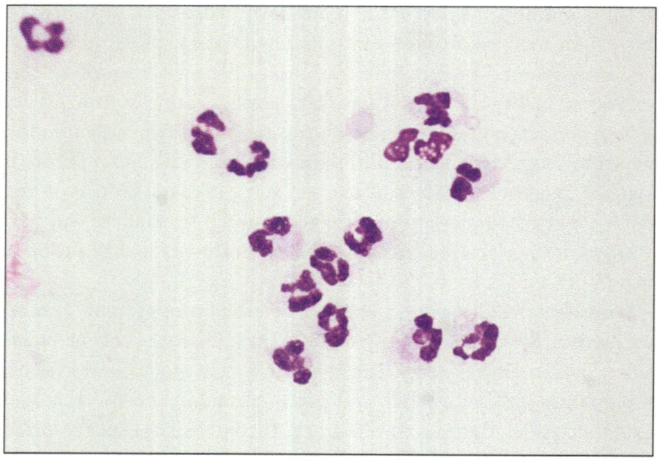

Figure 15.1 Septic exudate from a dog, containing high numbers of degenerate neutrophils. The chromatin is smudged with nuclear swelling with cytoplasmic vacuolization (Hemafix™, 1,000× magnification).

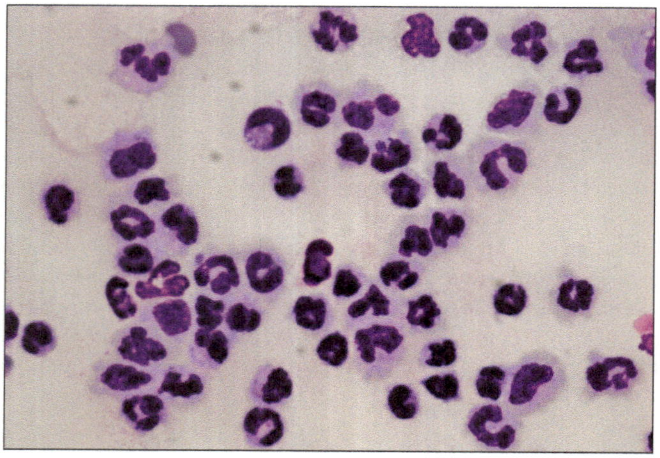

Figure 15.2 Septic exudate from a dog. Degenerate neutrophils and many intra- and extracellular rod-shaped bacteria are observed (Hemafix™, 1,000× magnification).

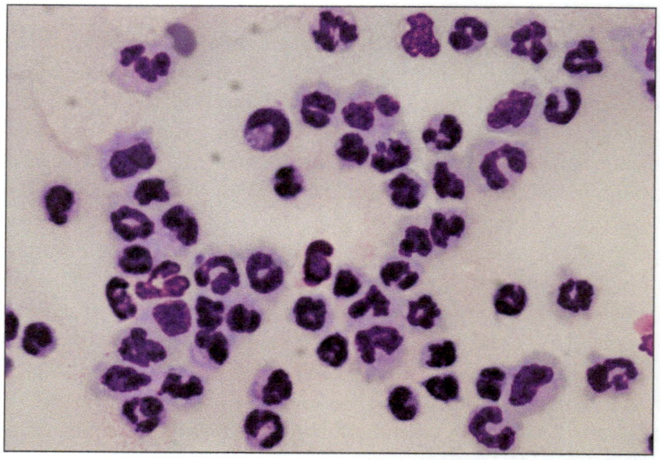

Figure 15.3 Septic exudate from a dog. Rare intracellular rod-shaped bacteria are present (center, top, right) (Hemafix™, 1,000× magnification).

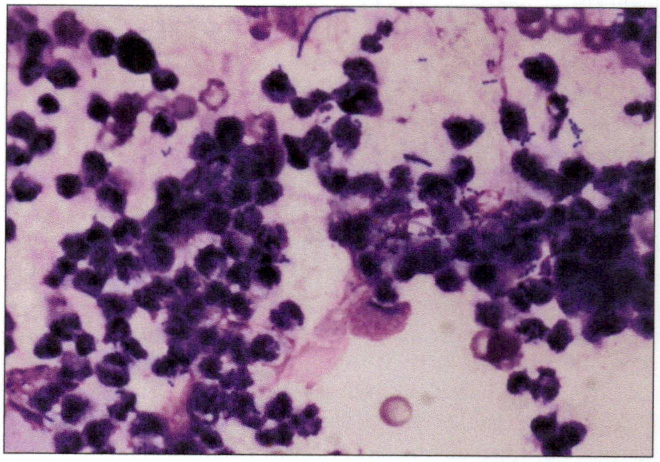

Figure 15.4 Abdominal effusion from a dog. Many degenerate neutrophils are observed with a mixed population of rod and cocci bacteria. Because of the mixed population of bacteria, there is concern for gastrointestinal perforation or leakage (Hemafix™, 1,000× magnification).

with an increase of precipitates and cellular debris. Bacterial peritonitis can be categorized into primary and secondary forms (Culp *et al.*, 2009). Primary bacterial peritonitis is defined by infection of the peritoneal cavity without an identifiable intraperitoneal source of infection, whereas in secondary bacterial peritonitis a penetrating injury can be confirmed (Culp *et al.*, 2009). Bacterial translocation penetrating a functionally defective intestinal wall is theorized as an inciting mechanism for primary septic peritonitis. In dogs and cats with primary bacterial peritonitis, mostly Gram-positive bacteria and often only a single species were cultured in the majority of cases, whereas Gram-negative and multi-species culture predominated in secondary bacterial peritonitis (Culp *et al.*, 2009). *Bartonella* spp. are bacteria that do not conform to the paradigm of septic exudates, as they produce protein-rich transudates by damaging endothelial cells and thus increasing capillary permeability (Cherry et al., 2009). These organisms require advanced culture technique or molecular methods for detection and should be considered as a differential, when no other cause for an effusion can be identified.

Nonseptic exudates

Nonseptic exudates can form because of necrosis due to ischemia, anatomic dislocations, irritating sterile body fluids due to rupture of viscera (bile, urine), sterile foreign bodies (surgical sponges), or neoplasia.

Feline infectious peritonitis

Feline infectious peritonitis (FIP)-associated effusions are high-protein exudates with low cellularity (Figures 15.6, 15.7). They are caused by a viral-induced vasculitis, which allows large proteins to enter the

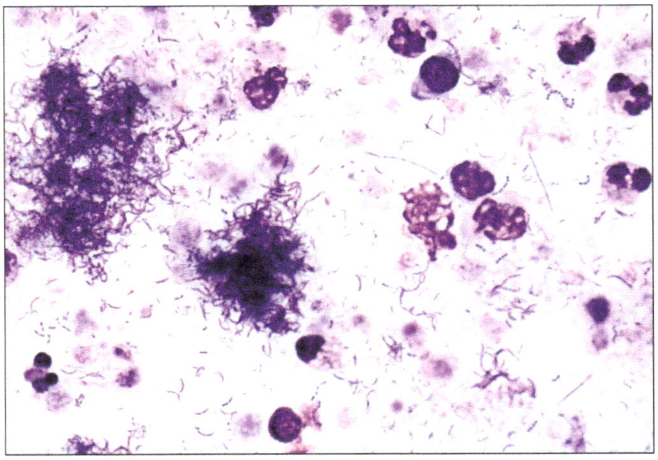

Figure 15.5 Direct smear from an abdominal effusion from a dog. Note the mixed bacterial population within the background. Rods, cocci, and filamentous rods are observed (Hemafix™, 1,000× magnification).

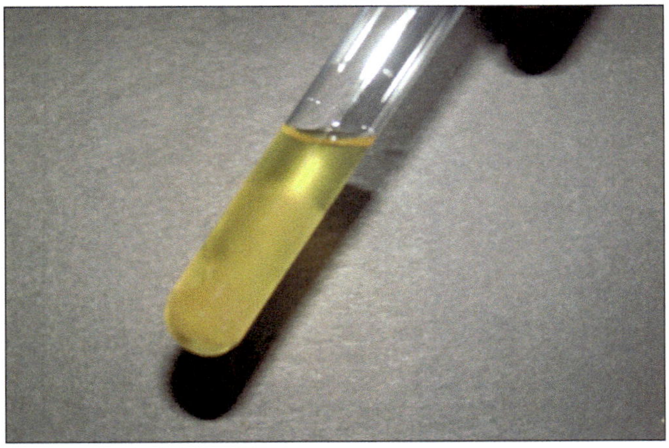

Figure 15.6 Abdominal effusion from a cat infected with FIP virus. Note the large fibrin clot in the sample.

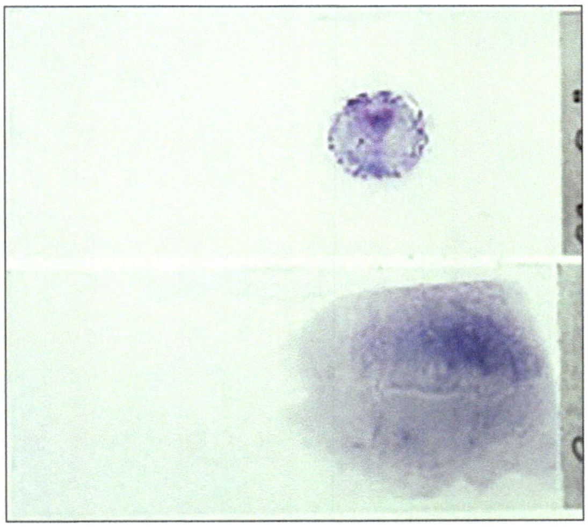

Figure 15.7 Direct smear and cytospin preparation from an effusion from a cat with FIP. The high protein concentration of the effusion results in the gelatinous appearance of the sample.

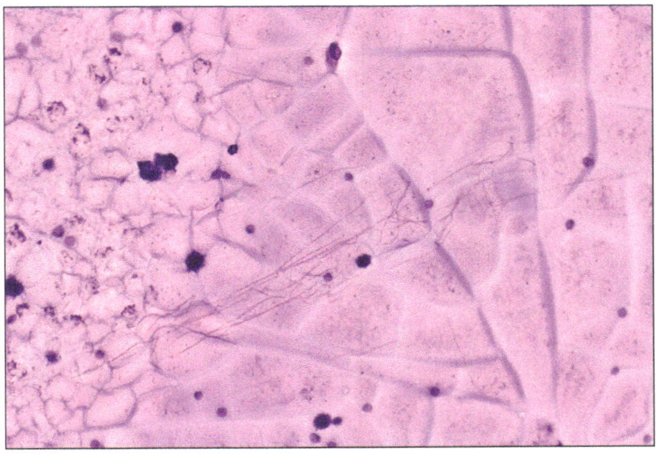

Figure 15.8 FIP virus-associated effusion from a cat. The background is filled with stippled eosinophilic proteinaceous material, so thick that it often appears to have glass-like 'cracks' (Hemafix™, 500× magnification).

body cavity fluid, whereas the cells remain within the tissue forming the characteristic perivascular granulomas. Vascular endothelial growth factor produced by FIP virus-infected macrophages/monocytes increases vascular permeability and correlates with the amount of fluid produced in the course of the disease (Takano *et al.*, 2011). A pinkish background with cracks resembling broken glass and cells that are not spread out well, so that it is difficult to recognize the segmented nuclei of neutrophils, is a typical finding in FIP-associated effusions (Figures 15.8, 15.9). The Rivalta test, a simple protein precipitation test, has been proven useful in indicating suspect FIP in effusions (Fischer, Sauter-Louis *et al.*, 2012; Fischer, Weber *et al.*, 2013; Barker & Tasker, 2020). In a large study of 851 feline patients from which 782 had conclusive test results, a diagnostic sensitivity of 0.91 and a specificity of 0.66 were reported (Fischer, Sauter-Louis *et al.*, 2012). Briefly 20 µL of 100% acetic acid are added to 7 mL of distilled water and thoroughly mixed. 20 µL of the effusion collected into EDTA tubes are layered on the surface of this solution. A positive test result is issued when the drop of the effusion stays on the surface, or forms a tailed sinking drop or forms an inverted jelly fish drifting down to the bottom of the test tube (Fischer, Weber *et al.*, 2013). The test result is negative when the drop resolves or the precipitate disappears and the mixture stays clear (Fischer, Weber *et al.*, 2013). Determination of the effusion's LDH/TNCC ratio might be another feasible tool to decide whether the effusion is FIP associated or not. LDH activity in FIP-associated effusions is usually high despite a low TNCC thus yielding a high fluid LDH/TNCC ratio. In a study including 648 animals, LDH/TNCC ratios > 7.54 increased the probability of an effusion being FIP associated by about 6.59 times (Romanelli *et al.*, 2022). Measuring α1-acid-glycoprotein in feline effusions is also helpful in classifying them as FIP associated; a concentration of >1550 µg/mL yielded a sensitivity and specificity of 93% each (Hazuchova *et al.*, 2017). Otherwise, viral-induced effusions are rare.

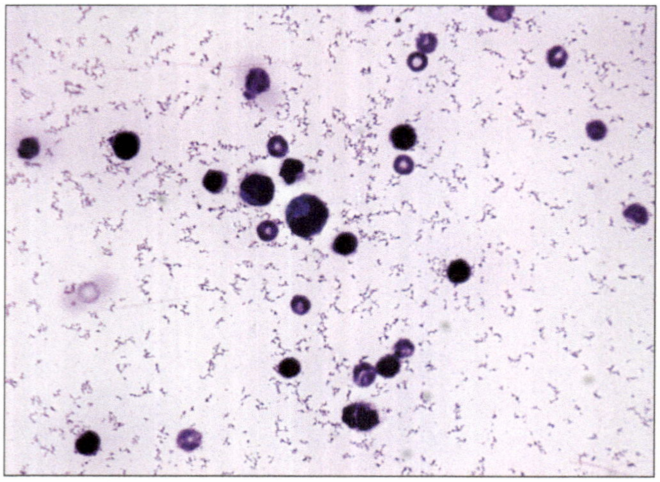

Figure 15.9 FIP virus-associated effusion from a cat. The sample is of low cellularity with few nucleated cells and erythrocytes. The nucleated cells are difficult to evaluate due to the thick proteinaceous background material (Hemafix™, 1,000× magnification).

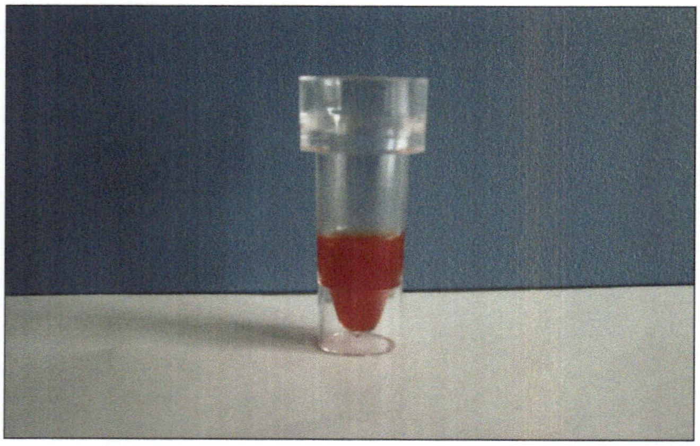

Figure 15.10 Effusion from a dog. (15.11) The fluid is red and was cytologically consistent with a hemorrhagic effusion. (15.11) Post-centrifugation. Note the red cell pellet and clearing of the supernatant.

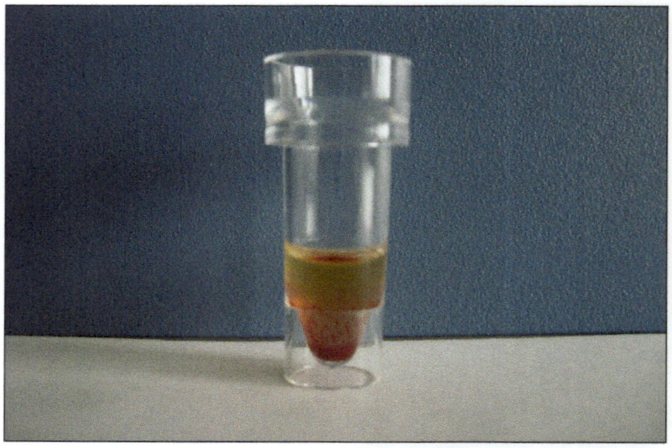

Figure 15.11 Effusion from a dog. The fluid is red and was cytologically consistent with a hemorrhagic effusion. Post-centrifugation. Note the red cell pellet and clearing of the supernatant.

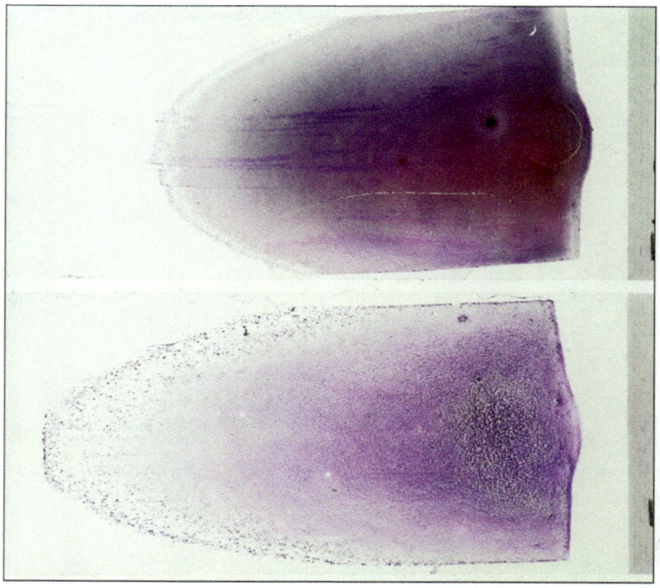

Figure 15.12 Direct smears from two separate effusions. The slide on the top represents a hemorrhagic effusion, the slide below a neoplastic effusion with hemorrhage. The basophilic speckles at the feathered edge likely represent neoplastic clusters of cells.

Hemorrhagic effusions

An effusion is called hemorrhagic when the effusion is mainly composed of blood (Figures 15.10–15.12). In severe hemorrhage, the composition of the effusion will initially be similar to the animal's peripheral blood, but will change rapidly due to the reabsorption of fluids, solutes, and cells. Platelets disintegrate and disappear quickly, and fluid will be reabsorbed. Due to fibrinolytic activity of mesothelial cells, a hemorrhagic effusion will not clot when transferred into a native test tube. Reabsorption of fluids occurs more rapidly than absorption of cells, so that the hematocrit of the effusions will soon exceed the hematocrit of peripheral blood. There is no evidence-based fixed threshold for when to address an effusion as hemorrhagic; some authors suggest hemorrhage when the hematocrit of the effusion is more than 25–50% of the hematocrit in peripheral blood (Dempsey & Ewing, 2011; Stockham & Scott, 2013; Epstein & Balsa, 2020); others suggest an RBC concentration above $500 \times 10^3/\mu L$ (Bohn, 2017) or a PCV above 10% (Athanasiou, 2019).

Minor hemorrhage usually accompanies effusions caused by inflammation when vascular permeability is increased. Sampling can cause iatrogenic hemorrhage into a body cavity effusion. Differentiation between iatrogenic and pathologic hemorrhage is important and can be attempted by evaluating the following indicators:

- The clinician taking the sample should be observant if only the first portion of the tap shows bloody discoloration. If so, fractionated sampling should be carried out, where another test tube is

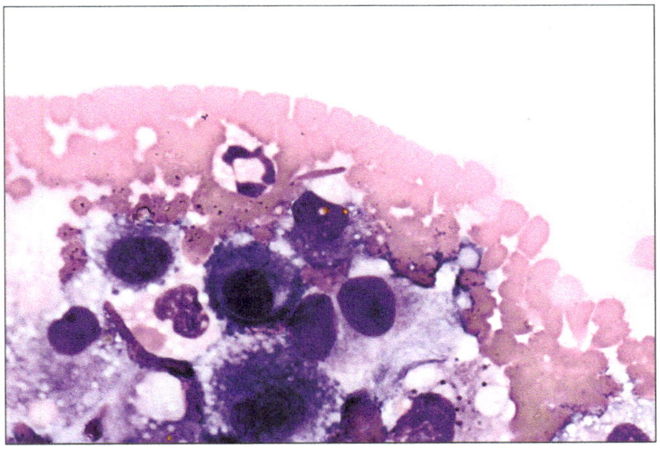

Figure 15.13 **Pericardial effusion from a dog. Pictured are macrophages and reactive mesothelial cells and few orange hematoidin crystals (Hemafix™, 1,000× magnification).**

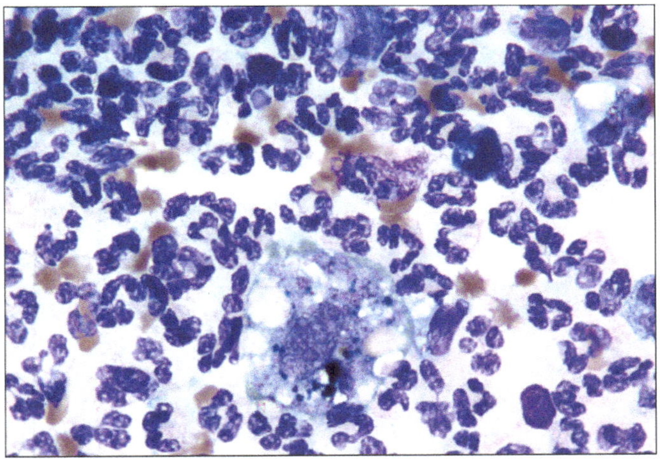

Figure 15.14 **Abdominal fluid from a dog. This sample is cellular and consists of neutrophils with a few macrophages. The macrophage pictured contains bluish-green to black pigment consistent with hemosiderin (Hemafix™, 1,000× magnification).**

filled with the non-bloody fraction of the tap. The non-contaminated fluid is diagnostically more relevant than the first portion.
- Iatrogenic hemorrhagic effusions clot when transferred into a test tube without an anticoagulant. Microscopic evaluation will reveal platelets in traumatic taps, whereas erythrophagocytosis and crystals such as hematoidin (Figure 15.13) and hemosiderin (Figure 15.14), which indicate hemoglobin degradation, are missing. Platelets and platelet clumps usually accumulate in the feathered edge of the smear. As mentioned above, true hemorrhagic effusions do not clot, platelets are usually not visible, and erythrophagocytosis and hemoglobin degradation products can be detected.
- The composition of hemorrhagic effusions changes depending on the cause, amount, frequency, and time course of vascular injury. When frequent minor hemorrhages occur, the oncotic pressure gradient is disrupted with the result that water will spill into the

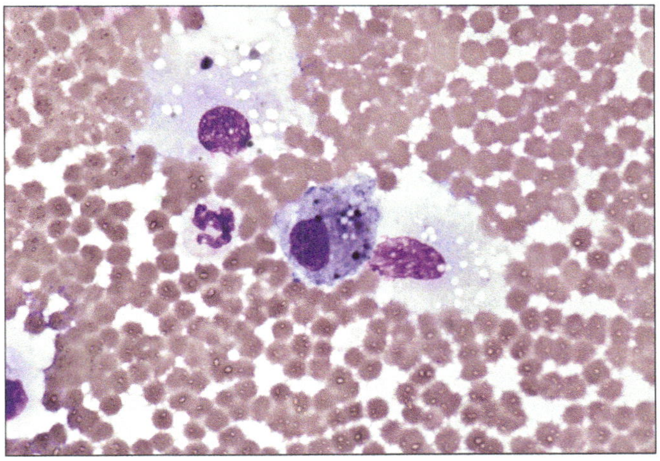

Figure 15.15 **Pericardial fluid from a dog. Pictured is a macrophage containing bluish-black pigment consistent with hemosiderin (Hemafix™, 1,000× magnification).**

effusion and dilute its content. Hemoglobin will be degraded and form hematoidin or hemosiderin, and macrophages will engulf erythrocytes and/or pigment. Hematoidin crystals (Figure 15.13) are brightly orange rhomboids; hemosiderin appears as blue–green to brown pigment (Figures 15.14, 15.15). Also, when hematopoietic cells are detected in a hemorrhagic abdominal effusion, accidental sampling of the spleen or splenic rupture should be considered.

Hemorrhagic effusions can be caused by a variety of events including trauma, coagulation disorders, inflammation, or neoplasia. Packed cell volume and protein content are highly variable depending on the amount and time course of the hemorrhagic event. Acute high volume hemorrhage might result in an effusion in which the hematocrit will be higher than in peripheral blood and will have a high protein concentration. Chronic intermittent bleeding will cause a variable packed cell volume and protein concentration depending on the reabsorption of cells and fluid.

Pericardial effusions are almost always hemorrhagic. Indeed, cytologic evaluation of hemorrhagic pericardial effusion is of limited diagnostic value because it is nondiagnostic in the majority of cases (Cagle *et al.*, 2014). The diagnostic utility was considerably higher when the hematocrit of the fluid was <10% (0.1 l/l) (Cagle *et al.*, 2014). However, in the author's opinion, a cytologic examination should never be omitted, because a positive finding will substantially support diagnosis. Screening for tumor cells in severely hemorrhagic effusions is cumbersome, as they might be overlooked when only a few are present. This happens with tumors that do not exfoliate readily (e.g. hemangiosarcoma). Preparation of native smears with a feathered edge, and thorough evaluation of this area, are recommended as tumor cells often accumulate in this area.

Lymphorrhagic effusion

Lymphorrhage describes the leakage of lymphatic fluids into a body cavity (Gavazza *et al.*, 2013; Stockham Scott, 2013). This can be caused

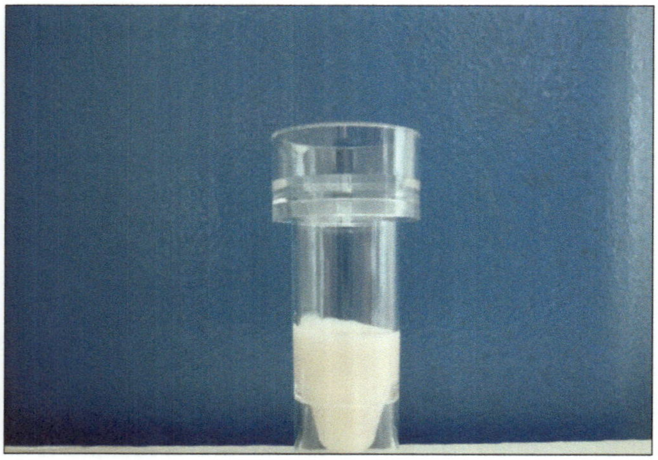

Figure 15.16 Chylous effusion from a cat. The fluid is white and turbid.

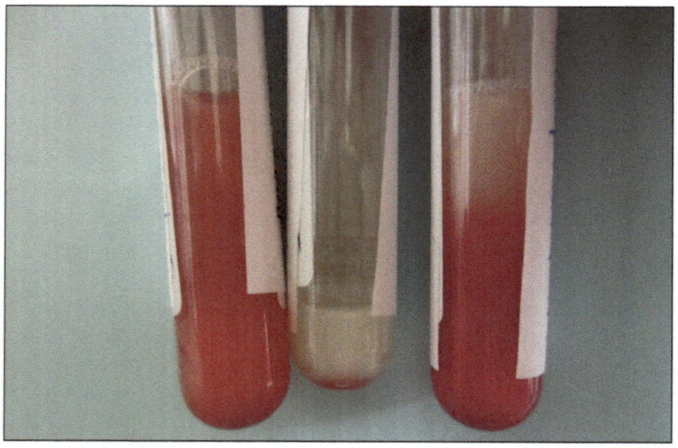

Figure 15.17 Chylous effusion from a cat. This fluid has blood contamination, giving it a 'strawberry milkshake' appearance.

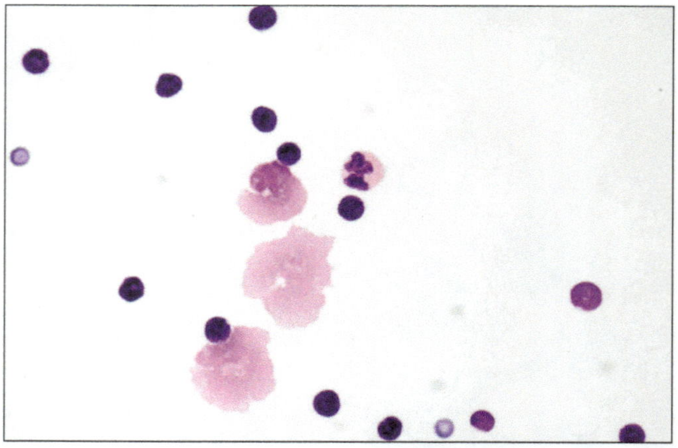

Figure 15.18 Acute chylothorax in a cat. Small lymphocytes predominate. The triglyceride concentration of the fluid was 1,350 mg/dl (15.2 mmol/l) and the cholesterol was 120 mg/dl (1.36 mmol/l) (Hemafix™, 1,000× magnification).

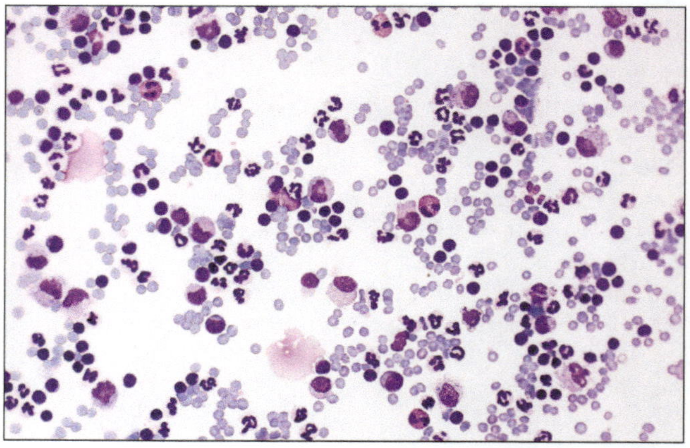

Figure 15.19 Chronic chylothorax in a cat. Small lymphocytes are prominent but a much higher number of neutrophils are present. Vacuolated macrophages are also observed. The triglyceride concentration of the fluid was 1,932 mg/dl (21.8 mmol/l) and the cholesterol 158 mg/dl (1.8 mmol/l) (Hemafix™, 400× magnification).

by traumatic or nontraumatic events such as stasis of lymph, lymphatic hypertension, compromised lymphatic valve function (due to dilatation of lymphatic vessels and increased permeability), or neoplastic occlusion. The presence of chylomicrons defines a lymphorrhagic effusion as chylous.

Chylomicrons are formed in the intestinal mucosa cells and transported via lymphatic vessels and the thoracic duct to the blood stream. Chylous pleural or abdominal effusions indicate a rupture of lymphatic vessels on the way from the intestines to the thoracic duct and cranial vena cava. Chylomicrons might be absent when food intake has ceased or a low-fat diet was consumed. Chylothorax is relatively common in cats but rare in dogs. Chylous effusions can occur in all body cavities but they usually affect the thoracic cavity. The causes of chylous effusions include trauma, idiopathic, or cardiac or tumor associated. The effusion is creamy white (Figures 15.16, 15.17) and chylomicrons form a lipid layer on top of the fluid when allowed to stand at 4°C. The concentration of triglycerides in the effusion usually exceeds the serum triglyceride concentration. Effusions with a triglyceride concentration >100 mg/dl (1.13 mmol/l) are defined as chylous (Birchard *et al.*, 1995; Dempsey Ewing, 2011; Valenciano et al., 2013). In recently formed chylous effusions, small lymphocytes are the predominant cell type (Figure 15.18). In chronic cases, neutrophils and macrophages migrate into the effusion and a mixed inflammatory cell population is present (Figure 15.19). Pink, homogeneous, round precipitates of chylomicrons and lipid-filled cytoplasmic vacuoles in macrophages, neutrophils, and lymphocytes are other diagnostic features. Chylomicrons can be stained with Sudan red (Figure 15.20). Chyloabdomen is a rare finding in dogs and cats, but might occur as a symptom of lymphangiectasia in protein-losing enteropathies in dogs. In cats neoplasia was identified as the most common cause for chyloabdomen in a recent study(Hatch, Jandrey *et al.*, 2018). Nonchylous lymphorrhagic effusions occur when nonintestinal lymphatic vessels are affected by hypertension, rupture, or inflammation, food intake has ceased, and/or chylomicrons have been destroyed. The predominant

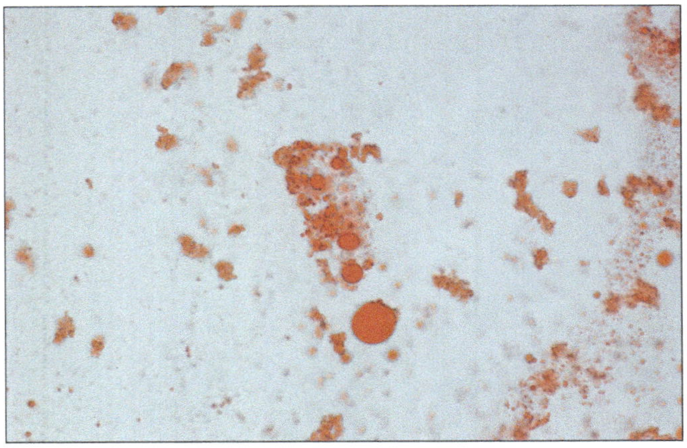

Figure 15.20 **Sudan red staining of a chylous effusion can be performed to identify the chylomicrons (Hemafix™, 400× magnification).**

cell type is also the small lymphocyte. Protein concentration in chylous and lymphorrhagic effusion is usually > 2.5 g/dl (25 g/l).

Pseudochylous

Pseudochylous effusions are yellowish to creamy turbid fluids, and no lipid layer forms when the effusion is left standing (Figures 15.21, 15.22). Turbidity is caused by low-density cholesterol-rich lipoproteins. The cholesterol concentration of the fluid exceeds plasma cholesterol concentration, whereas the triglyceride concentration is low. The high cholesterol concentration is caused by disintegrating cell walls being trapped in the body cavity. Cholesterol concentration is much higher in pseudochylous effusions than in plasma. Cellular composition is variable depending on the cause. This type of effusion is not very common in veterinary medicine.

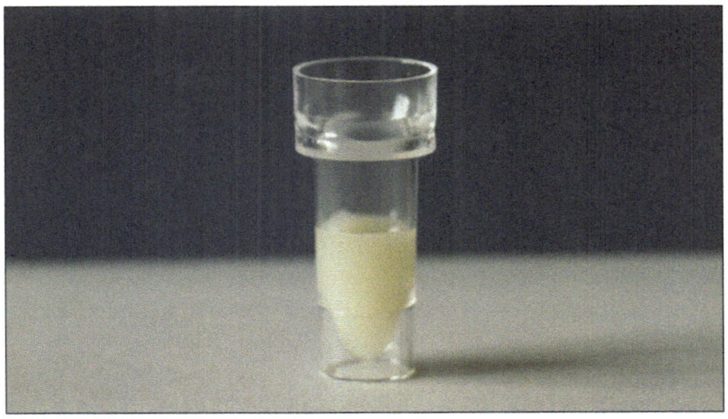

Figure 15.21 **Pleural fluid from a pseudochylous effusion. The fluid is white and turbid, similar to a true chylous effusion.**

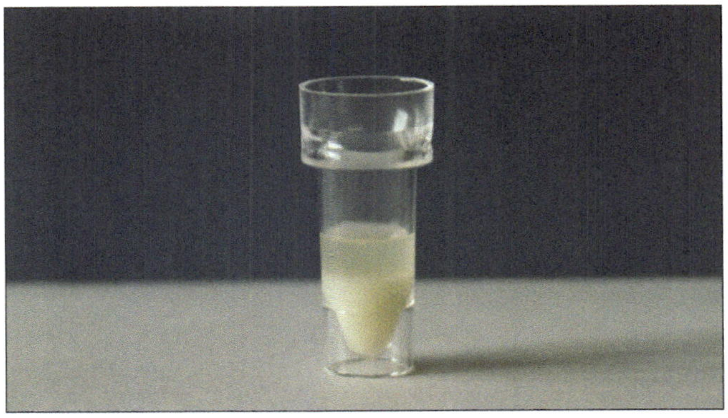

Figure 15.22 **Pleural fluid from a pseudochylous effusion. Post-centrifugation. Note the presence of a whitish sediment after centrifugation.**

Effusions caused by rupture of a hollow organ or tissue

Uroabdomen

Uroabdomen occurs when urine spills into the abdominal cavity subsequent to trauma, urolithiasis, or neoplasia (Stockham & Scott, 2013). Early uroperitoneum will resemble a transudate unless trauma has caused hemorrhage. Total nucleated cell count and protein concentration are low. Differential cell count will be unaltered in early lesions unless they are caused by neoplasia. Fluid creatinine concentration at least double the plasma creatinine concentration has been applied as a rule of thumb to define uroperitoneum. A recent study suggests a body cavity fluid creatinine concentration ≥2.1 mg/dL (88.42 μmol/L) and a $creatinine_{fluid}$ to $creatinine_{serum}$ ratio ≥1.25 as diagnostic cut-offs yielding a diagnostic accuracy of 99% for uroabdomen in dogs (Paes *et al.*, 2022). Eventually, even sterile urine elicits an inflammatory response within the abdominal cavity, so that the protein and cell concentrations may change to an exudate. In suspect cases, comparison between plasma creatinine and fluid creatinine concentration is useful. Determination of urea concentration is less useful, because urea is a small molecule that can diffuse freely, so that it equilibrates much more readily with plasma urea than creatinine. In cases of long-standing uroperitoneum, when the patient is unable to excrete urine, the difference between fluid creatinine concentration and plasma creatinine decreases. If renal function is undisturbed and at least some urine can be voided, the difference remains detectable. Bacteria might be present, if the patient has a concurrent urinary tract infection.

Bile peritonitis

Bile peritonitis occurs when bilious fluid leaks into the abdominal cavity; it can be induced by trauma, inflammation, obstruction, or neoplasia. In rare cases, bile can also leak into the thoracic cavity, for example caused by a fistulous tract from the diaphragmatic surface of the gallbladder (Wustefeld-Janssens *et al.*, 2011). In dogs, the most common cause is a gallbladder rupture due to an undetected and untreated gallbladder mucocele, which is an accumulation of mucus within the gallbladder leading to gallbladder distention and eventual rupture (Thompson & Sherman, 2021). The formation of a mucocele is not completely understood but hypersecretion of mucus from the gallbladder lining epithelium is one of the main mechanisms. The amount of bile lost into the abdominal cavity will not cause a clinically detectable effusion, but due to its irritant properties, bile elicits an inflammatory response. A greenish to brownish, sometimes orange, discoloration of the fluid might give a first hint, followed by microscopic detection of bilirubin crystals or bilious mucus. The diagnosis can be confirmed by comparing fluid and plasma bilirubin concentrations, with fluid bilirubin concentration exceeding plasma concentration. Blood supply for the gallbladder and common bile duct depends on a single artery branching from the proper hepatic artery, making it extremely susceptible to necrosis after trauma (Center, 2009). In cytologic preparations, bilirubin crystals and amorphous blue bilious mucus can be seen (Figures 15.23, 15.24). White bile (representing only mucus secreted by the gallbladder; Figure 15.25) is encountered when bile pigment is trapped within liver parenchyma during cholestatic disease and gallbladder content oozes into the abdominal cavity.

Leakage of gastric or intestinal contents

Leakage of gastric or intestinal contents might be caused by foreign bodies, ischemia, severe gastrointestinal inflammatory disease, or neoplasia. Again, the amount of material leaking into the body cavity might be negligible, but it will induce a severe inflammatory response and cause a septic exudate. Leakage of chyme influences the gross appearance of the fluid, causing changes in color, odor, and viscosity. Food particles might be detected by gross examination but also by microscopy (Figure 15.26). A mixed bacterial population is typical for secondary septic peritonitis.

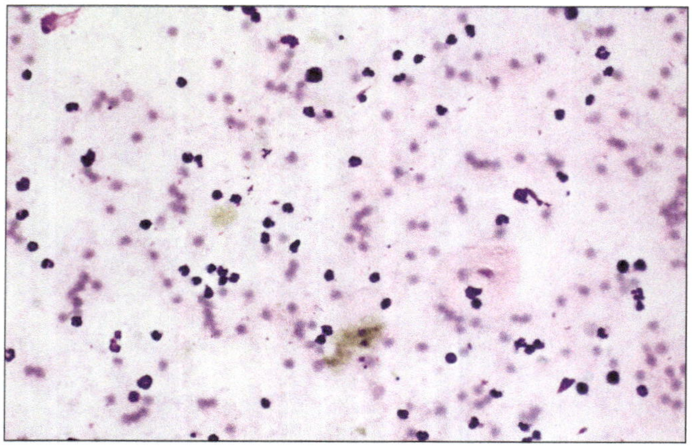

Figure 15.23 Abdominal fluid from a dog. The sample is cellular. Direct smears reveal a smudged background consisting of red blood cells, pyknotic cells, neutrophils, and pigmented precipitate (Hemafix™, 400× magnification).

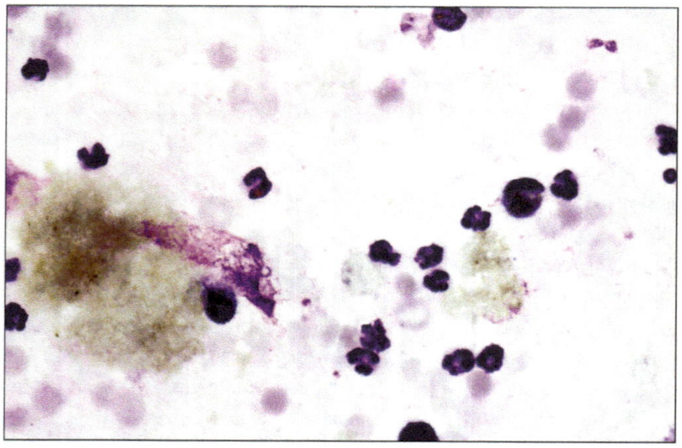

Figure 15.24 Abdominal fluid from a dog. Aggregates of greenish-gold pigmented material consistent with bile (Hemafix™, 1,000× magnification).

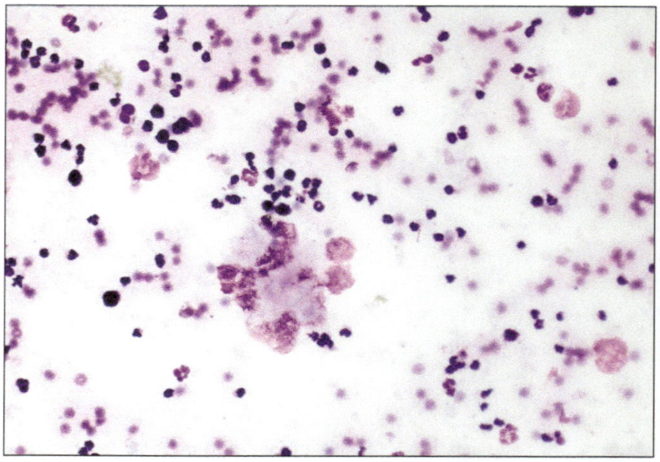

Figure 15.25 Direct smear from bile peritonitis from a dog. The sample is cellular and consists of neutrophils with a smudged background, pink mucinous material, or 'white bile' (Hemafix™, 400× magnification).

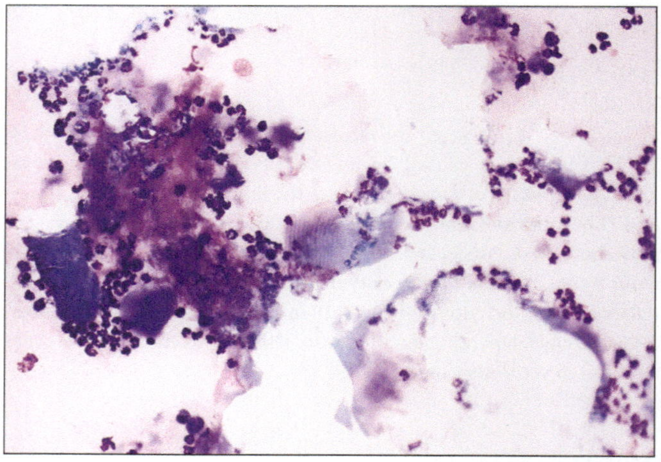

Figure 15.26 Abdominal fluid from a dog with a penetrating foreign body. Striated skeletal muscle is observed (Hemafix™, 400× magnification).

Neoplastic effusions

Tumor-associated effusions

Tumor-associated effusions show a high variability in their composition. An effusion is classified as tumor associated when tumor cells can be identified during microscopic examination. However, not all tumor-associated effusions yield a sufficient number of tumor cells; therefore complementary diagnostic imaging is needed to establish a diagnosis. Tumors might cause transudation by obstructing venous or lymphatic drainage; they can elicit exudation by inciting an inflammatory reaction or rupture of an internal organ or cause hemorrhage, or a combination of those mechanisms. Cytology is an excellent but not overall sensitive tool to identify tumor-associated effusions. Sensitivity and specificity of cytology were 65% and 99%, respectively, for dogs and 61% and 100% for cats (Hirschberger *et al.*, 1999). In severely hemorrhagic effusion the diagnostic sensitivity for detecting neoplastic cells is considered low (Cagle *et al.*, 2014). Diagnosis is facilitated when tumor cells exfoliate into the effusion and can be differentiated from reactive mesothelial cells, but absence of tumor cells does not rule out neoplasia. Detection of a mass by diagnostic imaging and directly obtaining a sample from the lesion might be a more efficient approach. Determination of the origin of neoplastic cells with Romanowsky-type stains is often difficult and has to be complemented by special stains. Reactive mesothelial cells are especially difficult to differentiate from epithelial neoplasia, as they also show criteria of malignancy as indicators of proliferative activity in terms of healing or inflammatory stimulation. As always, severe inflammation is a complicating factor in the interpretation of cytopathologic criteria of malignancy. However, cytology is still an excellent tool in identifying neoplastic effusions (Hirschberger *et al.*, 1999). Special cytochemical stains for identifying tissue-specific intermediate filaments, such as cytokeratin, vimentin, and desmin, are useful for establishing a definitive diagnosis. Cytologic preparations are stable at room temperature for at least 24 hours prior to staining (Przeździecki & Sapierzyński, 2013). Preparation of cell blocks from effusions is a feasible alternative to preserve effusion-derived cells for additional cytochemical staining, thus aiding the identification of cells (Melega *et al.*, 2020).

Lymphoma-associated effusions

Lymphoma-associated effusions are relatively common when internal lymph nodes or organs are affected. Microscopic evaluation reveals a variable number of immature lymphoid round cells. Small-cell lymphoma might be difficult to diagnose by cytology alone, so complementary diagnostic testing, such as clonality testing by polymerase chain reaction, is warranted. When cell concentrations are determined by advanced laser-based flow cytometry, characteristic cytograms are generated, which have to be confirmed by microscopic evaluation (Figures 15.27–15.30) (Bauer & Moritz, 2005).

Mast cell tumor

Mast cell-associated effusions are more common in cats than in dogs because in this species internal organs are more often affected by mast cell tumors (Valenciano *et al.*, 2013). Mast cells exfoliate readily into the effusion and can be identified by their variable content of magenta to purple colored granules (Figures 15.31–15.35). As in other lesions, mast cells in effusions can be accompanied by eosinophilia.

Other round cell tumors

Other round cell tumors, such as multiple myeloma (Figures 15.36, 15.37) or malignant histiocytosis (Figures 15.38, 15.39), might also exfoliate into body cavity effusions, thus indicating the etiology.

Sarcomas

Sarcomas such as hemangiosarcoma are not easily detected by cytologic evaluation of body cavity effusions as they do not exfoliate well.

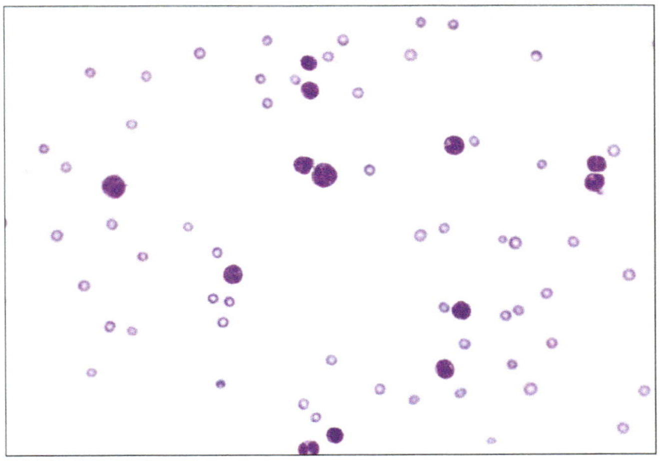

Figure 15.27 Pleural fluid from a dog with a mediastinal mass. Large round cells are observed with round to occasionally lobulated nuclei and smooth chromatin. The mass is a lymphoma (Hemafix™, 400× magnification).

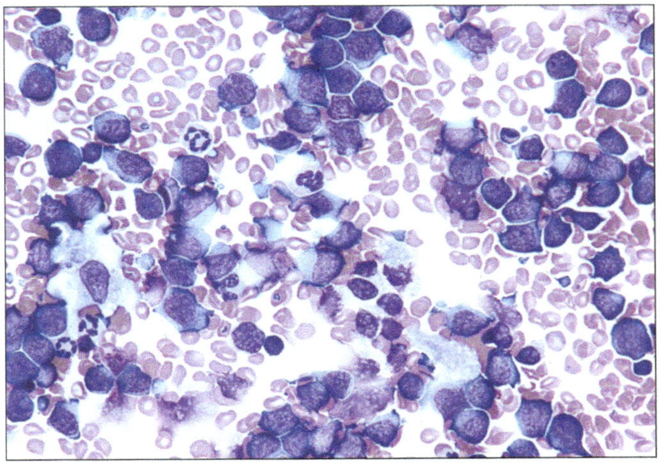

Figure 15.28 Pleural fluid from a dog with lymphoma: cytospin preparation. The sample consists of a population of large lymphocytes. These cells are round with a scant rim of basophilic cytoplasm and large prominent nucleoli (Hemafix™, 1,000× magnification).

Rupture of the tumor and formation of a hemorrhagic effusion raise suspicion; however, even tumor rupture does not yield a high number of tumor cells in the effusion. Inspection of the feathered edge or buffy coat preparations increases the sensitivity for detection of mesenchymal tumor cells (Figures 15.40, 15.41) (Valenciano *et al.*, 2013). Detection of canine prostate specific membrane antigen (cPMSA), which is expressed by endothelial cells in canine hemangiosarcomas, in hemorrhagic effusions might help to establish a final diagnosis of this tumor type (Dowling *et al.*, 2019).

Mesotheliomas

Mesotheliomas (Figures 15.42–15.44) are uncommon tumors in small animals and, as mentioned above, difficult to differentiate from

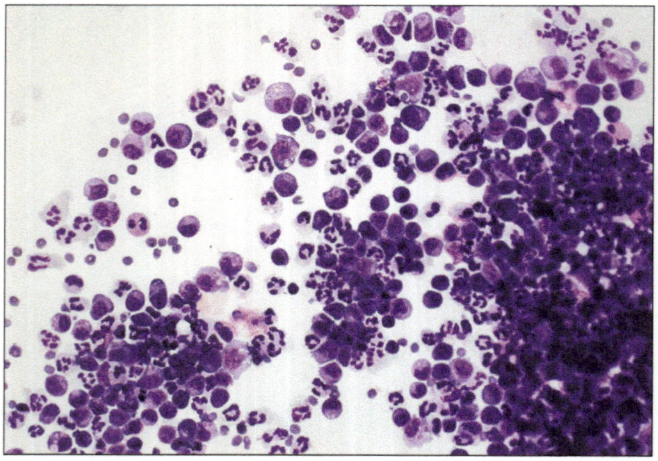

Figure 15.29 Abdominal fluid from a cat with large granular cell lymphoma. The there is a population of large round cells containing variable numbers of pink cytoplasmic granules. The nuclei are round with prominent nucleoli (Hemafix™, 400× magnification).

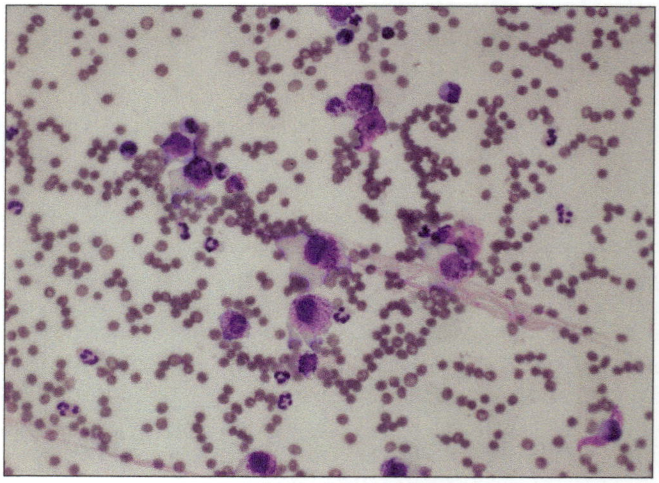

Figure 15.31 Abdominal fluid from a dog with mast cell neoplasia. Variably sized mast cells are observed (Hemafix™, 400× magnification).

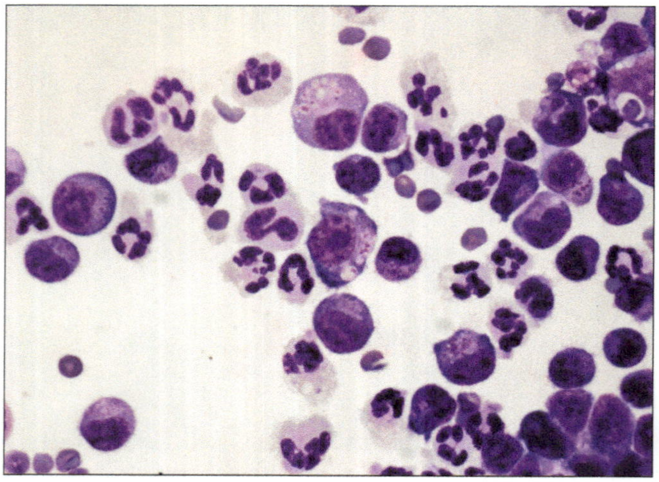

Figure 15.30 Abdominal fluid from a cat with large granular cell lymphoma. The granulation is quite prominent in some cells and the granules are variably sized (Hemafix™, 1,000× magnification).

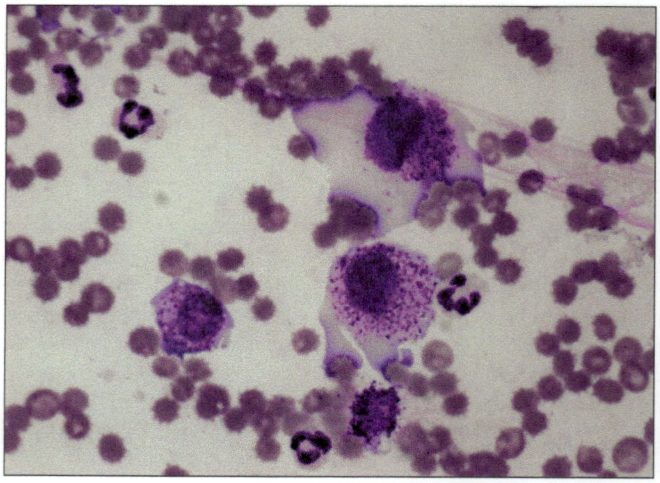

Figure 15.32 Abdominal fluid from a dog with mast cell neoplasia. Because of the intermediate amount of granulation, nuclear features can be easily evaluated and include anisokaryosis and prominent, irregular nucleoli (Hemafix™, 1,000× magnification).

carcinoma or adenocarcinoma (Valenciano *et al.*, 2013). Development of these tumors has been associated with exposure to asbestos, aluminum oxide, or simian virus 40, and in young animals, where congenital forms seem to exist (Martins *et al.*, 2011). The identification of a primary tumor by diagnostic imaging might suggest carcinoma or adenocarcinoma. Otherwise, immunohistochemistry is useful to distinguish between carcinomas/adenocarcinomas and mesothelioma (Reggeti *et al.*, 2005; Bacci *et al.*, 2006; Al-Dissi & Philibert, 2011). Mesothelial cells stain positive for cytokeratin, vimentin, and desmin, defining a characteristic pattern for cells of mesothelial origin (Przeździecki & Sapierzyński, 2013). Double staining protocols for Romanowsky stained slides with Wilms-tumor antigen (WT-1) and cytokeratin to identify reactive mesothelial cells are useful in differentiating them from carcinoma cells (Marrinhas *et al.*, 2022). By histopathology, the differentiation of epithelioid from mesenchymal types of mesothelioma and mixed types can be achieved (Valenciano et al., 2013). Electron microscopy might be another useful tool in establishing a diagnosis of mesothelioma. Mesothelial cells have unique long, often branching, microvilli, a continuous basement membrane, and prominent desmosomes that can be visualized by that technique (Bacci et al., 2006; Al-Dissi & Philibert, 2011). Diagnosis of mesothelioma by cytology alone is discussed controversially yielding a highly variable sensitivity from 4 to 77% (Milne *et al.*, 2021). Immunohistochemistry on cell block preparations is useful in differentiating mesothelial

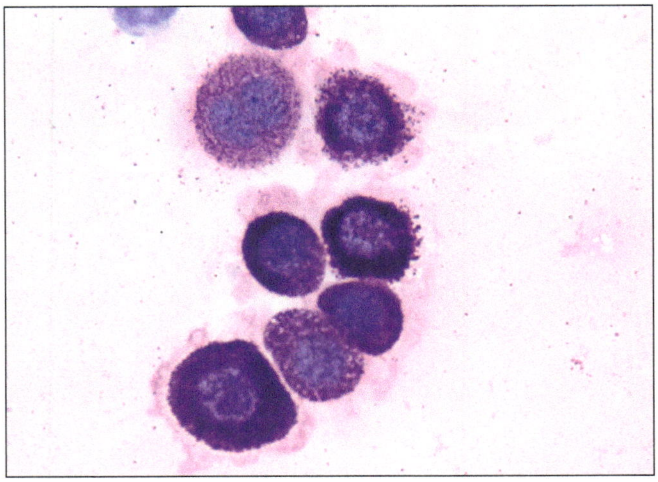

Figure 15.33 Cytospin preparation from abdominal fluid from a dog with visceral mast cell neoplasia (Hemafix™, 1,000× magnification).

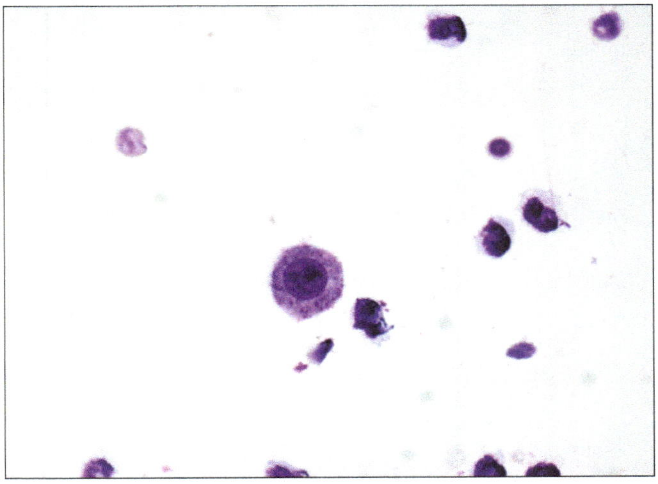

Figure 15.34 Abdominal fluid from a dog with splenic masses. The fluid is of low cellularity. Poorly differentiated mast cells with minimal granulation can be difficult to identify (Hemafix™, 1,000× magnification).

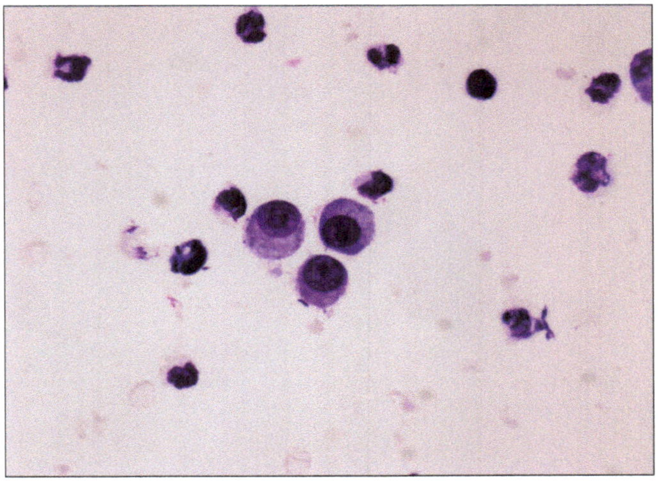

Figure 15.35 Abdominal fluid from a dog with splenic masses. Round cells are observed; only the cell on the left has a few tiny metachromatic granules (Hemafix™, 1,000× magnification).

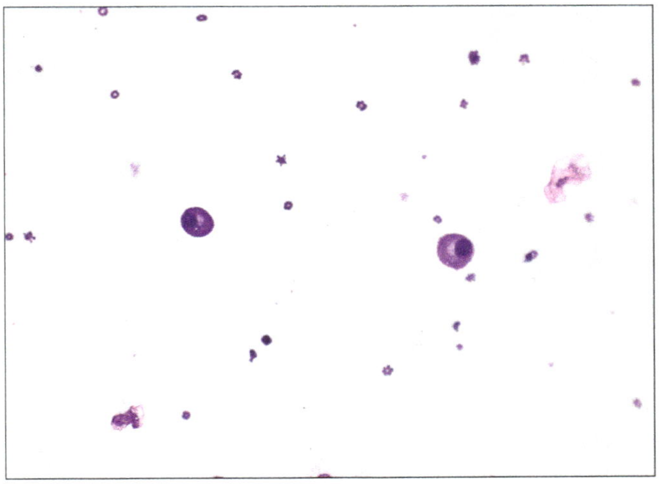

Figure 15.36 Pleural fluid from a cat with multiple myeloma. Well-differentiated plasma cells are identified with eccentrically located nuclei and perinuclear clear areas. The total protein in the effusion was 7.5 g/dl (75 g/l) (Hemafix™, 400× magnification).

hyperplasia, mesothelioma, and carcinoma in dogs when compared with biopsy results (Milne *et al.*, 2021). A panel of cytokeratin, WT-1, desmin, and m-RNA binding protein 3 (IMP3) appeared to be most useful in distinguishing reactive mesothelial cells, mesothelioma, and carcinoma (Milne *et al.*, 2021).

Carcinomas and adenocarcinomas

Carcinomas and adenocarcinomas exfoliate in clusters (Figures 15.45–15.51). Demonstration of strong nuclear criteria of malignancy should elicit diagnostic imaging to identify an eventual primary tumor, which can be accessed for fine needle aspiration (Valenciano *et al.*, 2013). Cytologic evaluation of the effusion alone cannot reliably identify the tissue of origin. Thus, immunocytochemistry is useful to classify the cells as epithelial by a positive staining for cytokeratin.

SAMPLING TECHNIQUES

The collection of body cavity effusions for fluid evaluation is not only a diagnostic but also a therapeutic measure. When available, ultrasound-guided aspiration is recommended but not strictly required. Light sedation and/or local anesthesia are recommended for thoraco- and pericardiocentesis in noncooperative patients. Sedation is usually preferred as the application of local anesthetic is sometimes more irritating than the sampling procedure. The hair at the puncture site is clipped and the skin surgically scrubbed. Sterile conditions should be pursued to prevent contamination of the body cavity. Eighteen- to 20-gauge hypodermic needles or butterfly cannulas (preferred) are

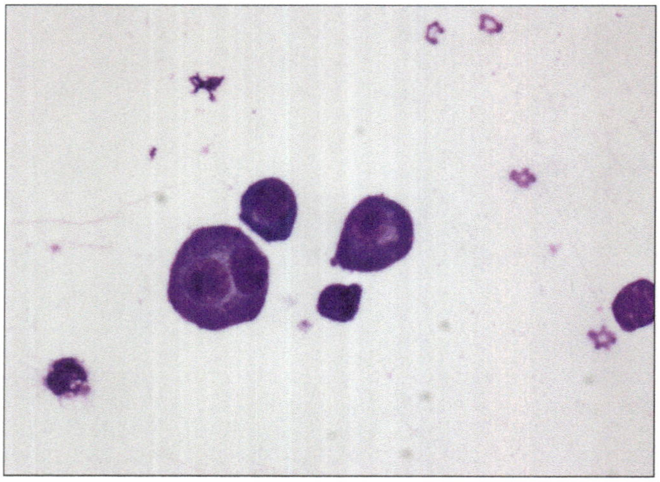

Figure 15.37 Pleural fluid from a cat with multiple myeloma. Atypical plasma cells are also noted, with binucleation and prominent, irregular nucleoli (Hemafix™, 1,000× magnification).

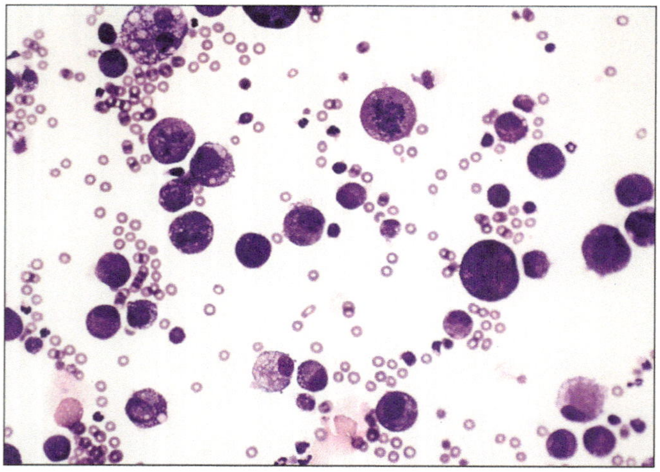

Figure 15.38 Abdominal fluid from a Bernese Mountain Dog with histiocytic neoplasia. The sample is cellular and consists of a population of large neoplastic round cells. Anisocytosis, anisokaryosis, and atypical mitotic figures are observed (Hemafix™, 400× magnification).

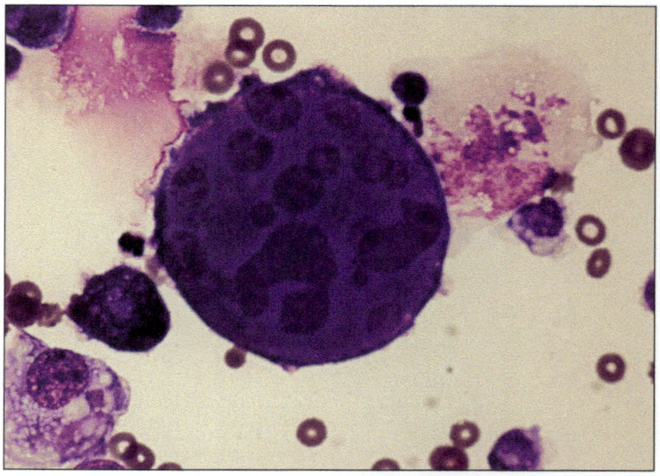

Figure 15.39 Abdominal fluid from a Bernese Mountain Dog with histiocytic neoplasia. Marked atypia is observed in this sample, with bizarre ballooning giant cells, anisokaryosis, and irregular nucleoli (Hemafix™, 1,000× magnification).

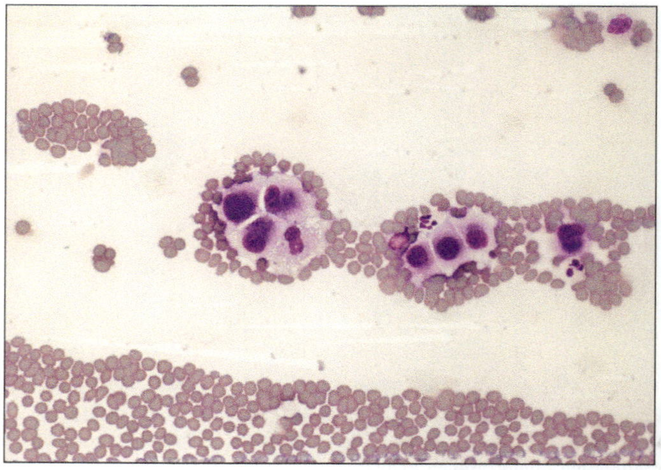

Figure 15.40 Pericardial effusion from a dog with hemangiosarcoma. Low numbers of pleomorphic plump mesenchymal cells are noted (Hemafix™, 400× magnification).

most useful (Alleman, 2003). For the removal of larger amounts of fluid from the pleural or pericardial space, over-the-needle catheters have also been recommended. When a needle is used, the bevel of the needle should always face the parietal side of the body cavity to prevent irritation of internal organs by suctioning them into the needle lumen. A minimum of at least two EDTA-containing test tubes, a sterile plain tube, and a heparin-coated tube should be ready at hand before the sampling procedure is started. It is important to have more than one tube ready to allow fractionated sampling in cases of traumatic puncture.

Thoracocentesis

Thoracocentesis requires special equipment such as tubing and a three-way stopcock to allow the removal of large amounts of fluid and prevent the formation of pneumothorax. The animal is held either standing or in sternal recumbency. Lateral recumbency should be avoided because it can aggravate respiratory distress. As the mediastinum is fenestrated in most dogs and cats, pleural effusions are usually present on both sides unless fibrotic pouches were formed. Therefore, diagnostic imaging prior to or during sampling is useful to assess the amount and localization of the fluid accumulation. The skin over the puncture site should be gently drawn forward before inserting the needle so that intact skin will seal the puncture site when the needle is removed. Usually the 7th or 8th intercostal space at the costochondral junction is punctured. Make sure to enter the pleural cavity always on the cranial aspect of the rib to avoid injuries to intercostal blood vessels and nerves, which are located caudally.

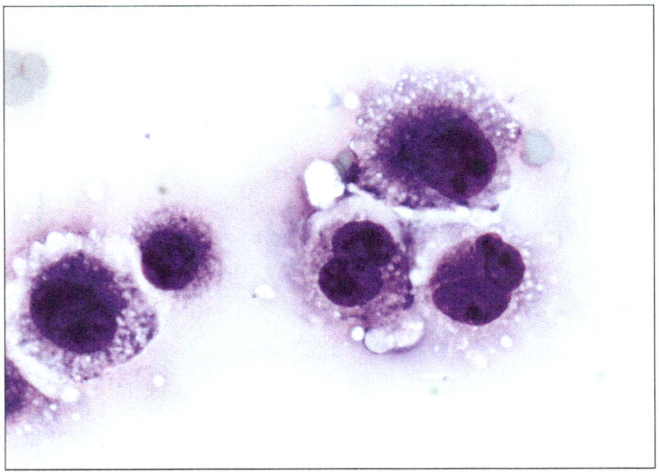

Figure 15.41 Pericardial effusion from a dog with hemangiosarcoma. The nuclei contain prominent irregular nucleoli. Variation in the nucleoli is observed (Hemafix™, 1,000× magnification).

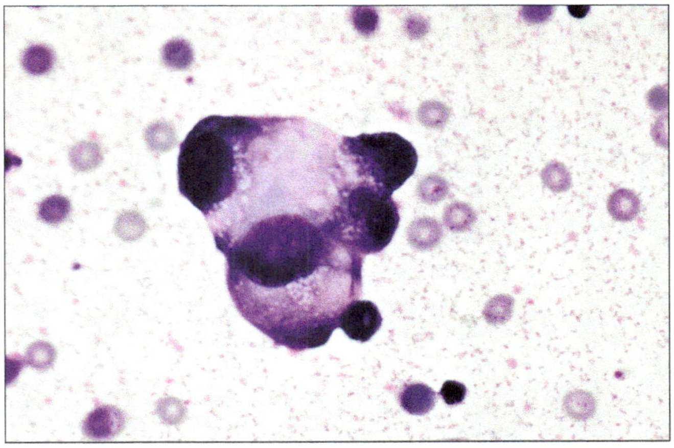

Figure 15.43 Pleural fluid from a Bernese Mountain Dog with malignant mesothelioma. Bizarre ballooning cells, marked anisocytosis and anisokaryosis, and macronuclei with inconspicuous nuclei (Hemafix™, 1,000× magnification).

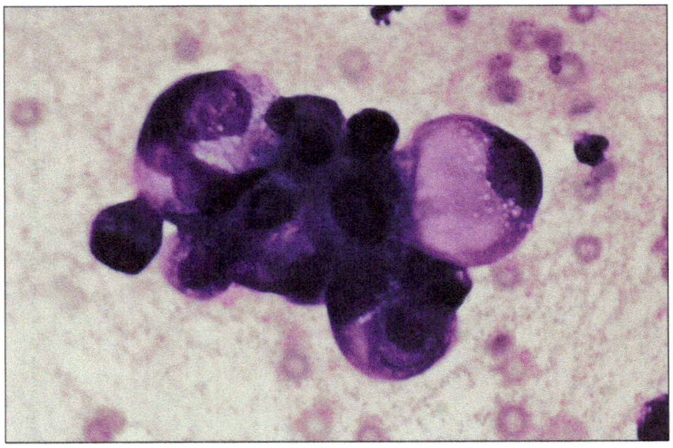

Figures 15.42 Pleural fluid from a Bernese Mountain Dog with malignant mesothelioma. A cluster of neoplastic cells exhibiting basophilic cytoplasm and in other cells ballooning pink cytoplasm, large nuclei with coarse chromatin. Mesothelioma was confirmed at necropsy (Hemafix™, 1,000× magnification).

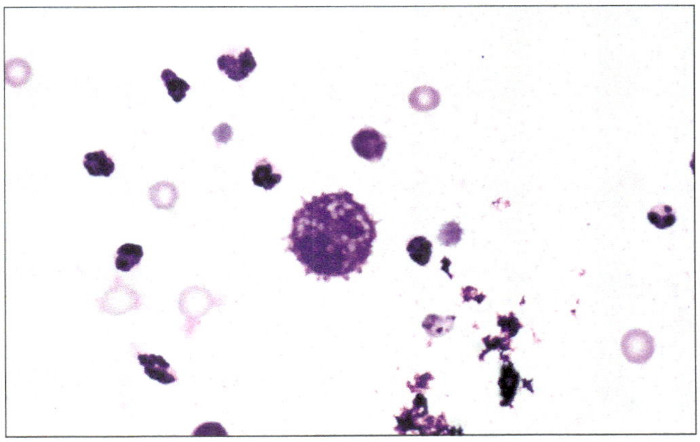

Figure 15.44 Pleural fluid from a Bernese Mountain Dog with malignant mesothelioma. Note the single mesothelial cell arranged in a background of thick stippled proteinaceous material (Hemafix™, 1,000× magnification).

Pericardiocentesis

Pericardiocentesis also requires special equipment to allow the removal of large amounts of fluid and prevent the formation of pneumothorax. The procedure is usually performed from the right side in the 4th to 5th intercostal space where cardiac palpitations can be felt through the chest wall. Electrocardiographic monitoring and/or ultrasound guidance is recommended during pericardiocentesis, as premature ventricular contractions might occur. Also, the pericardium has to be punctured by a closed system to avoid the formation of pneumothorax.

Abdominocentesis

Abdominocentesis can be performed with a needle alone; the fluid is allowed to drain spontaneously. The urinary bladder should be emptied before the procedure. The patient should be in a standing position or fixed in lateral recumbency. The puncture site is either at the point of maximal dependency or 2–3 cm caudal to the umbilicus just beside the midline. Penetration of the abdominal wall through the musculature is enough to seal the puncture site.

Diagnostic peritoneal lavage is sometimes recommended for the detection of peritonitis, but it is strictly contraindicated in suspected neoplasia. A fenestrated large bore (10–14 G) over-the-needle catheter is inserted and fixed to the abdominal wall. Next, 20 ml/kg body weight of prewarmed buffered saline or Ringer's solution is instilled. The animal is then rolled from side to side and the fluid removed for evaluation. Usually, only a small amount of fluid can be drained.

HANDLING OF SAMPLES

For determination of cell concentration (cell counts) and cytologic evaluation, fluid should be collected into EDTA tubes (lavender

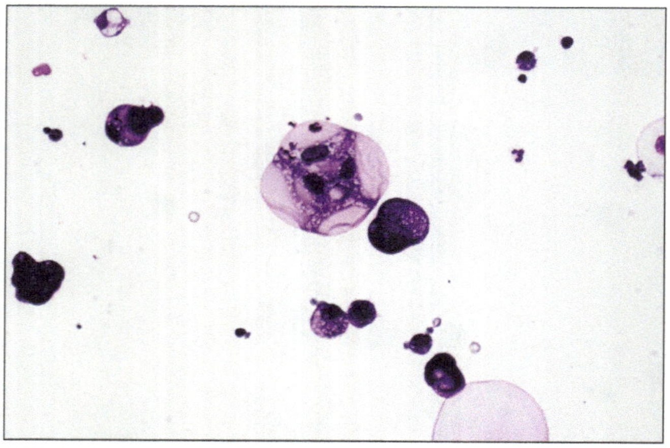

Figures 15.45 **Pleural fluid from a dog with a history of a primary lung carcinoma. Clusters and individualized epithelial cells are observed. The individualized cells have ballooning cytoplasm and one cell has a signet ring appearance (Hemafix™, 400× magnification).**

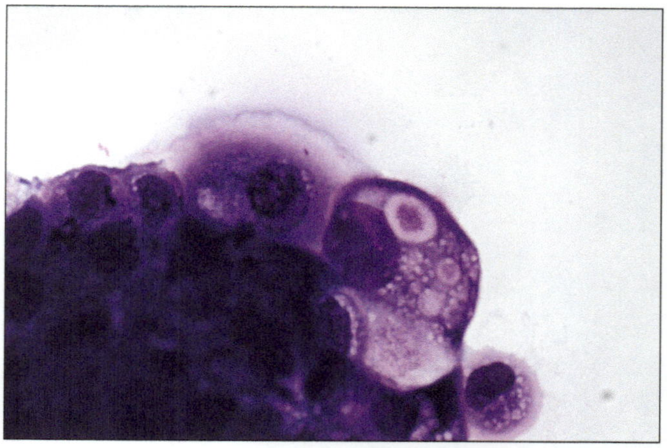

Figure 15.47 **Pleural fluid from a dog with a history of a primary lung carcinoma. Higher magnification. The cytoplasm contains eosinophilic granular to globular material. Prominent nucleoli are visualized (Hemafix™, 1,000× magnification).**

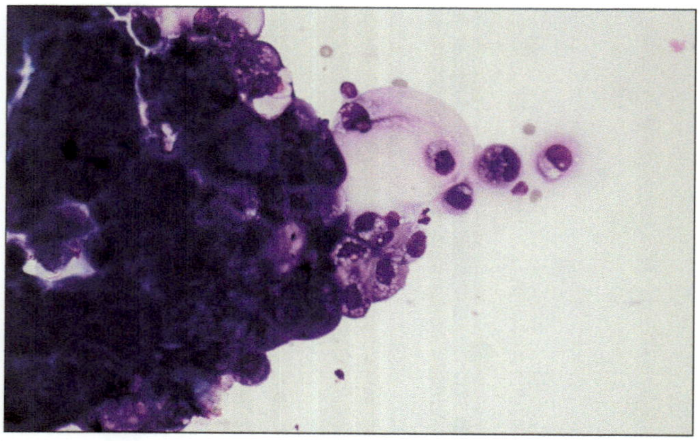

Figure 15.46 **Pleural fluid from a dog with a history of a primary lung carcinoma. A large cluster of irregular epithelial cells exhibiting marked anisocytosis, anisokaryosis, perinuclear vacuolization, and occasionally ballooning cytoplasm are pictured (Hemafix™, 400× magnification).**

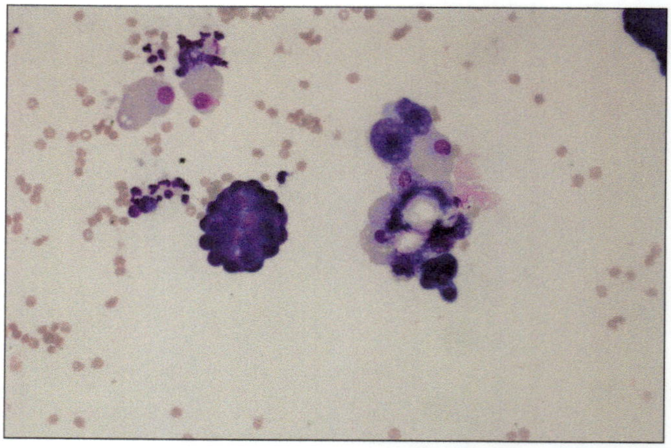

Figure 15.48 **Abdominal fluid from a Yorkshire Terrier with a history of ovarian carcinoma. Dense clusters of neoplastic epithelial cells are observed, occasionally exhibiting a papillary cluster (Hemafix™, 200× magnification).**

stopper). This prevents clot formation so that accurate cell counts and adequate slides for microscopic evaluation can be prepared. Total protein, creatinine, bilirubin, triglycerides, and cholesterol can be measured in EDTA-plasma by most assays; only measurement of lipase and lactate dehydrogenase activity is confounded by EDTA, therefore heparinized or native fluid is required. A sterile plain tube should be available when bacterial culture is necessary.

Evaluation of the sample should be performed as soon as possible. If samples are submitted to a referral laboratory, native smears and smears of a sediment preparation should be prepared to provide adequate sample quality for cytologic evaluation. If a smear was prepared from a concentrated fluid and submitted, it should be labeled as such. If collection was not sterile, *in-vitro* growth of bacteria can lead to erroneous results. The samples should be stored at 4°C until evaluation.

LABORATORY EVALUATION

The clinician should measure and report the amount of fluid removed from the body cavity and comment on possible iatrogenic hemorrhage. Gross examination evaluates color, turbidity, odor, and viscosity. This should be done by the clinician when the sample is submitted, because color might change during storage and transport. Gross examination must not be neglected as it often yields valuable information regarding the underlying disease (Figures 15.6, 15.10, 15.11, 15.16, 15.17, 15.21, 15.22, 15.52–15.57).

Physiologic fluids and/or transudates are usually clear, colorless to slightly yellowish fluids with a low viscosity and without a discerning odor (Figure 15.52). Blood (Figures 15.10, 15.11), chylous lymph (Figure 15.16), bile, urine, and septic and nonseptic inflammation can

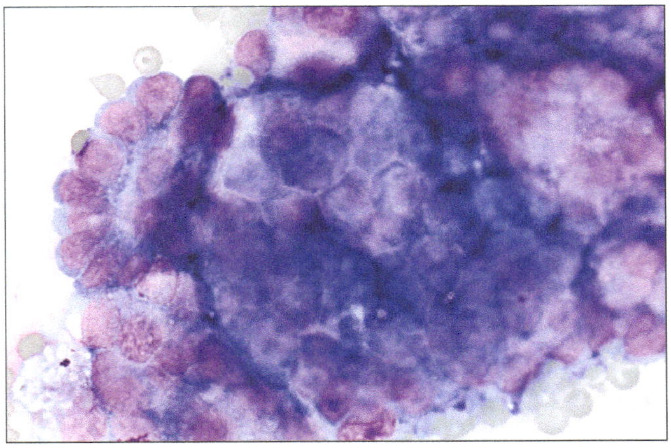

Figure 15.49 Abdominal fluid from a Yorkshire Terrier with a history of ovarian carcinoma. Higher magnification revealing a globoid cohesive epithelial cluster exhibiting anisocytosis and anisokaryosis (Hemafix™, 1,000× magnification).

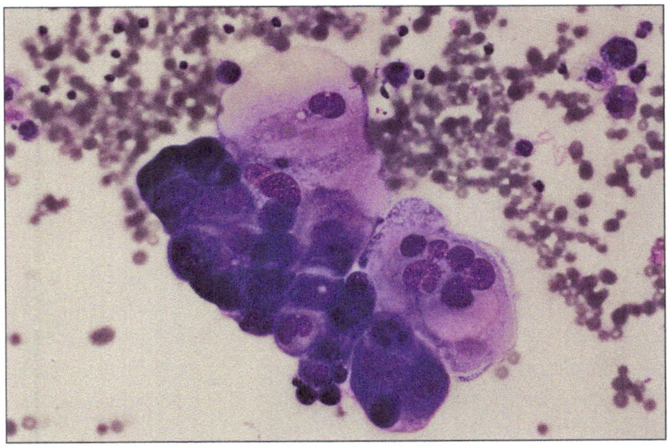

Figure 15.50 Abdominal fluid from a dog with prostatic carcinoma. A cluster of cells with multinucleation and marked anisocytosis and anisokaryosis are observed (Hemafix™, 400× magnification).

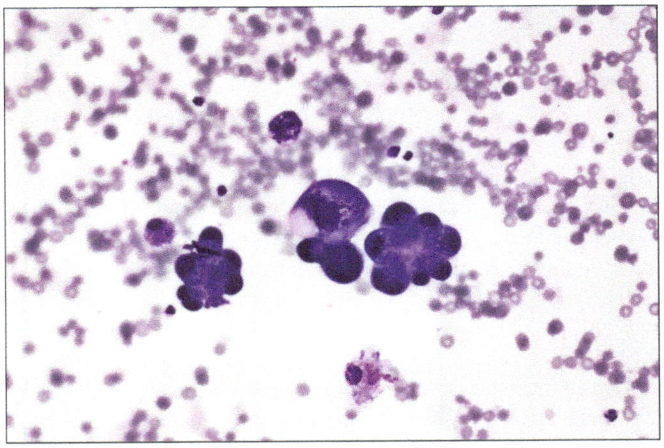

Figure 15.51 Abdominal fluid from a dog with prostatic carcinoma. Acinar structures are observed with a multinucleated cell (Hemafix™, 400× magnification).

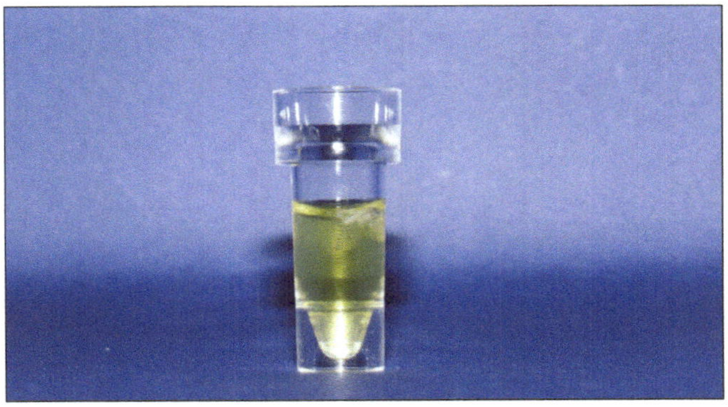

Figure 15.52 Transudate from a dog. The fluid is pale yellow and clear.

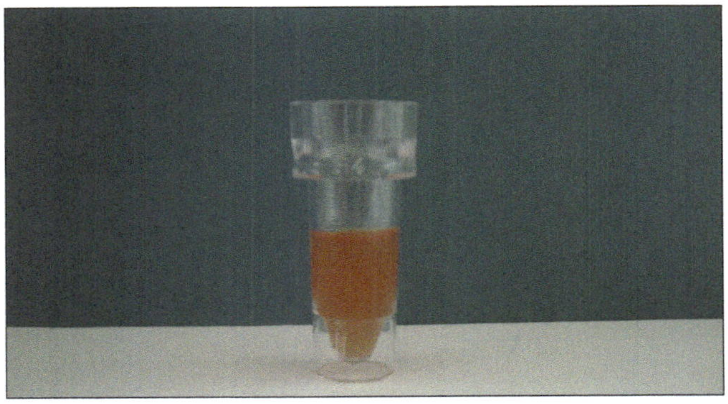

Figure 15.53 Effusion from a dog. This fluid is an exudate. Exudates have a high cell count and protein concentration and are therefore often turbid.

cause a multitude of color changes. All shades of red to pink signal hemorrhage. As long as the red blood cells (RBCs) remain intact, the supernatant is clear; in cases of hemolysis the supernatant will be reddish. Beige to creamy or reddish-brown coloration is often seen in septic exudates (Figures 15.53–15.55).

Turbidity is caused by light diffraction, which can be elicited by particles, such as cells (Figures 15.53, 15.54), or cholesterol-containing lipids or chylous fluid. The presence of chylomicrons causes a milky white opaque appearance (Figures 15.16, 15.17). When chylous fluid is allowed to stand, a creamy layer is formed on top (Figure 15.17). Turbid samples with high cellularity clear when cells follow gravity and sink or are spun down by centrifugation. Turbidity caused by cholesterol-rich lipids does not clear when allowed to stand or centrifuged.

Viscosity is due to the friction between neighboring particles in a fluid, which are moving at different velocities. Viscosity in effusions can change due to an increase in inflammatory proteins or increased cellularity. FIP-associated exudates are typical examples (Figure 15.6). Coagulated material might cause a flocculent appearance. 'Sulfur granules' (yellow grains in reddish brown turbid exudates) are a typical finding in septic exudates caused by *Nocardia* or *Actinomyces* spp. (Figures 15.56, 15.57). A foul odor can also occur with septic inflammation.

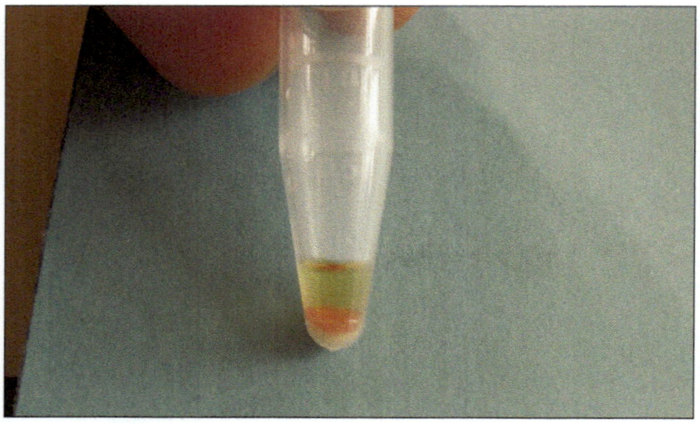

Figure 15.54 **Effusion from a dog. The sample was centrifuged. Note the thick cell pellet post-centrifugation.**

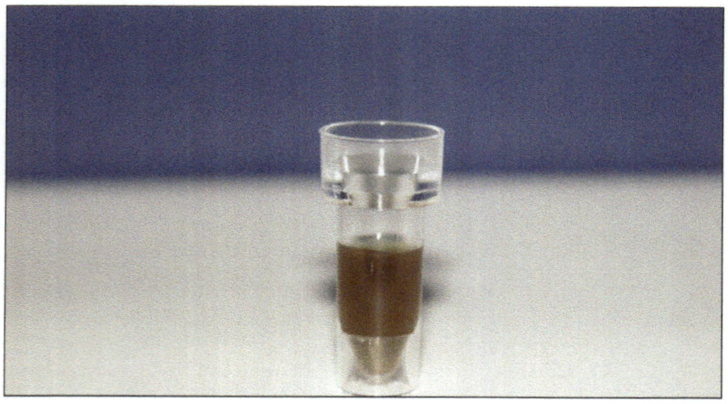

Figure 15.55 **Effusion from a dog. This patient had a penetrating foreign body. The sample is markedly turbid and brown.**

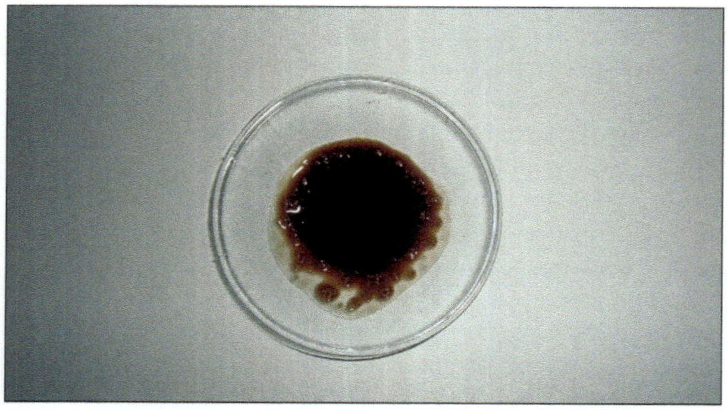

Figure 15.56 **Pleural effusion from a cat. This patient had a septic pleuritis with *Nocardia* spp. Note the sulfur granules.**

Microbiologic cultures

Fluid samples collected into sterile tubes without anticoagulant (EDTA can be bacteriostatic) may be submitted for bacterial and fungal cultures. The reference laboratory should be contacted for special culture conditions when indicated. Fluids should be cultured for both anaerobic and aerobic bacteria.

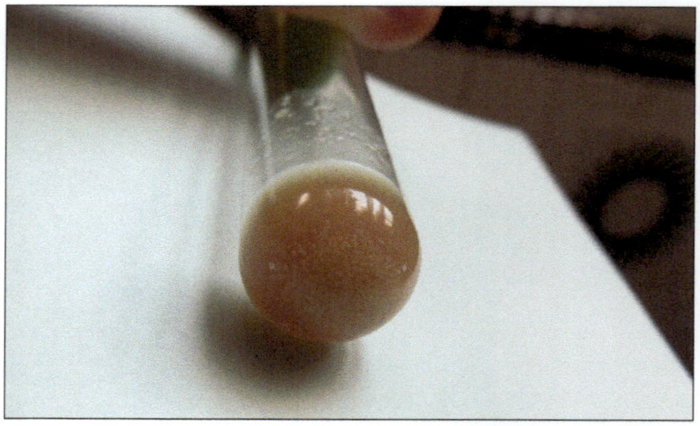

Figure 15.57 **Pleural effusion from a cat. This patient had septic pleuritis with *Actinomyces* spp. Again, note the sulfur granules.**

Biochemistry analytes

A variety of clinical chemistry analytes are helpful in determining the nature of an effusion. Measurement of total protein concentration is always performed to differentiate between transudates and other types of effusion. The other biochemistry tests are only required in specific clinical situations. Different brands of benchtop analyzers might vary considerably in their analytical performance when used for the analysis of body cavity effusions (Hetzel *et al.*, 2012). This is not surprising because the expected concentrations of some analytes in body cavity effusions are beyond or close to the analytical range of various assay systems. Therefore, very often numerical results cannot be obtained.

Total protein concentration can reliably be determined by refractometry, the biuret method, and urine test strips (Braun *et al.*, 2001; Papasouliotis *et al.*, 2002). The measurement should be made from the supernatant of a centrifuged sample to avoid measurement errors. However, it has to be kept in mind that refractometry measurements for concentrations of 2.5 g/dl (25 g/l) are less accurate than photometric testing by the biuret method. The protein test pad on commercial urine test strips can also be used for a semiquantitative protein assessment (Braun et al., 2001). Effusions with a protein concentration of 2.5 g/dl (25 g/l) are categorized as transudates; when the protein concentration lies between 2.5 and 3.5 g/dl (25 and 35 g/l) and cellularity is low, the effusion is categorized as a protein-rich transudate (previously described as modified transudate), whereas effusions with high cellularity and protein concentration are exudates.

Triglyceride concentration is measured to confirm the nature of a chylous effusion. A concentration of >100 mg/dl (11.3 mmol/l) is considered diagnostic. However, in anorectic animals, the concentration might be lower. In those cases, comparison with blood triglyceride concentration might be helpful (Dempsey & Ewing, 2011; Valenciano *et al.*, 2013).

Cholesterol concentration in effusions exceeding plasma cholesterol concentration aids the identification of pseudochylous effusions.

Glucose concentration determination and calculating the difference between blood glucose concentration and glucose concentration in the body cavity fluid have been considered helpful in differentiating septic from nonseptic effusions (Bonczynski *et al.*, 2003). A difference in glucose concentration between blood and effusion above 20 mg/dL has been suggested as highly suspect for a septic process (Dempsey & Ewing, 2011). Accordingly, the concentration of fluid lactate and the difference from blood lactate have been used for the same purpose. These data were based on a low case number, and a later study demonstrated them to be unreliable (Szabo et al., 2011). This is not surprising as all cells consume glucose, so highly cellular effusions will always have a decreased glucose concentration. However, glucose/lactate measurements give just a quick orientation and cannot replace cytologic evaluation and culture testing to confirm a septic process.

Creatinine concentrations at least double the plasma creatinine concentration are expected in cases of uroperitoneum. Sample dilution for creatinine measurement might be warranted to obtain a numerical result. More recently a fluid-creatinine to serum-creatinine ratio of ≥1.25 has been suggested to confirm uroabdomen in dogs (Paes *et al.*, 2022).

Bilirubin concentration is measured in effusions to confirm leakage of bile into an effusion; the bilirubin concentration of the fluid in the effusion exceeds the plasma concentration.

Measurement of bile acid concentration in abdominal effusions is useful to diagnose anicteric gall-bladder rupture, when bilirubin concentrations are inconclusive (Pascual *et al.*, 2022).

Lipase activity measurement can be helpful in establishing a diagnosis of pancreatitis-associated effusion; the enzyme activities in the effusion are higher than in plasma (de Arespacochaga *et al.*, 2006).

Lactate dehydrogenase (LDH) activity measurement has been used in humans to differentiate between benign and malignant ascites caused by ovarian tumors and to differentiate between benign and malignant pleural effusions (Halperin *et al.*, 1998; Bielsa *et al.*, 2008). However, LDH is an enzyme present in most cells, so its activity is correlated with cellularity. LDH measurement is also a component of Light's criteria, a classifications system established in human medicine to differentiate between exudates and transudates which has been evaluated for veterinary patients (Zoia, Slater *et al.*, 2009; Zoia, Petini *et al.*, 2020; Alonso, Mattoso *et al.*, 2021).

Plasma cardiac troponin I was found to be helpful in differentiating dogs with cardiac hemangiosarcoma from dogs with hemangiosarcoma of other sites or other tumors, and dogs with pericardial effusions of other than neoplastic origin (Chun *et al.*, 2010). However, there was an overlap of values between the groups, so this test might be of limited value in the assessment of a single patient, without specific findings of a cardiac mass in diagnostic imaging.

Plasma or effusion fluid N-terminal pro brain natriuretic peptide (NT-proBNP) is useful in identifying congestive processes which contribute to the formation of effusions, especially in cats (Humm *et al.*, 2013; Wurtinger *et al.*, 2017; O'Shaughnessy *et al.*, 2022). In dogs with cardiac tamponade, an increase of NT-proBNP has been observed after removal of the pericardial fluid, probably due to improved ventricular filling pressure (Baumwart *et al.*, 2017).

Acid–base status, electrolytes, glucose, and lactate concentration in blood and pericardial effusion were considered diagnostic in differentiating dogs with neoplastic from those with nonneoplastic pericardial effusions. The overlap between the two groups is wide, so diagnostic use of these tests for categorizing a single patient is fairly limited (de Laforcade *et al.*, 2005).

Under field conditions, measurement of leukocyte esterase in peritoneal fluid of dogs might be useful to rule out bacterial peritonitis, because a negative test result has a high specificity (Thomovsky *et al.*, 2014).

Coagulation testing in peripheral blood is routinely performed to investigate the cause of hemorrhagic effusions. Measurements of fibrinogen degradation products (FDPs), D-dimer, fibrinogen concentration in effusions and peripheral blood, and viscoelastic measurements in dogs with all types of cavitary effusion indicate enhanced fibrinolytic activity. (Zoia, Drigo *et al.*, 2022). This is caused by proteins involved in hemostasis that spill into cavitary effusions regardless of their mechanism of formation into a milieu in which the actions of these proteins are not well regulated, owing to the lack of other constituents of the hemostatic system such as platelets or vascular endothelium. (Zoia, Drigo *et al.*, 2022).

Cell concentrations are usually determined by electronic cell counters or a hemocytometer (Bauer & Moritz, 2005; Pinto da Cunha *et al.*, 2009; Stockham Scott, 2013). Cell clumping, cell fragmentation, and noncellular debris can cause erroneous cell counts (Cowell et al., 1987; Pinto da Cunha *et al.*, 2009). Advanced hematology analyzers might provide additional information regarding the cellular composition, such as indicating tumor cells (Bauer & Moritz, 2005); however, microscopic slide evaluation must not be omitted. Malodorous, flocculent effusions (Figures 15.55–15.57) should not be introduced into an electronic counter, because they might block and contaminate tubing. In these cases, estimation of cellularity by evaluation of an appropriately prepared direct smear suffices.

SLIDES FOR CYTOLOGIC EVALUATION

Preparation

A direct smear from a well-mixed sample should always be prepared and evaluated to verify the electronic cell count. Effusions with low cellularity ($<5 \times 10^3/\mu l$) require concentration techniques for assessment of their cellular composition. A standardized volume of fluid (e.g. 1 ml) should be centrifuged in a tipped test tube at 150–350 g (this is 1,500 rpm when the radius is 15 cm) for 5 minutes. The supernatant is decanted into another tube for chemical analyses and the cell pellet is gently mixed with the fluid that has remained within the tip of the tube due to capillary forces. A drop of this cell suspension is used for the smear preparation.

The preparation of a concentration line (Figures 15.58, 15.59) by a special smear technique is another way to increase cellularity for evaluation purposes. A drop of well-mixed effusion is planted on a dust-free clean slide (the carrier slide) and a spreading slide is then put in front of the drop at an angle of 55°. The liquid is allowed to spread along the edge of the spreading slide and the spreading slide is dragged along two-thirds of the carrier slide. The spreading slide is then lifted abruptly, creating a concentration line.

Cytospin preparations use a cytocentrifuge to deposit cells directly onto a glass slide to yield high-quality preparations (Figures 15.60–15.62). A glass slide is covered by filter paper, which has a central hole in the diameter of the sedimentation chamber's opening that is lined by a sealing rubber ring. The sedimentation chamber is fixed onto the filter paper-covered slide by a clamp. The filter paper is intended to absorb the fluid. Then the sedimentation chamber is loaded with a standardized amount of well-mixed fluid (100 µl) and introduced into the centrifuge with special swinging buckets and spun at 150–350 g. After that, the clamp, sedimentation chamber, and filter paper are removed. The slide is then dried and can be stained (Figure 15.59).

Cell block preparations

Cell block preparations of cytologic fluid specimens are a useful complementary tool, when additional tests such as immuno- or histochemical stains, in-situ hybridization tests, cytogenetics, or polymerase chain reaction tests are required or the cells have to be preserved for further investigations (Marcos *et al.*, 2017, Melega *et al.*, 2020; Shidham, 2021, Walsh & Patel, 2020; Milne *et al.*, 2021). Another major advantage of cell block preparations is the preservation of

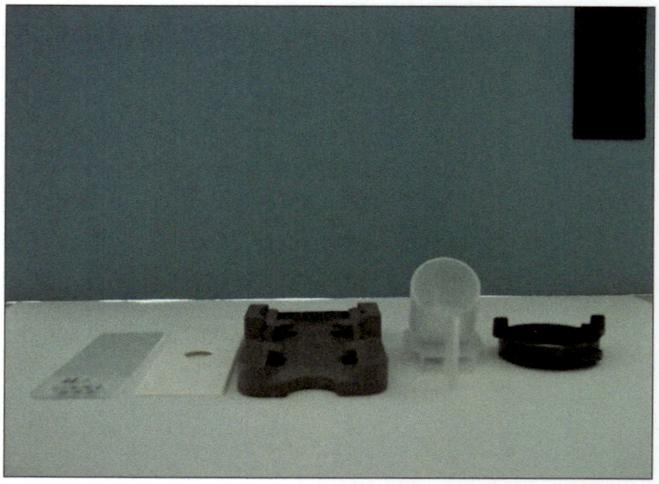

Figure 15.60 Cytospin preparation. From left to right: glass slide, filter card with central hole, slide carrier, angular sedimentation chamber, and fixation clamp.

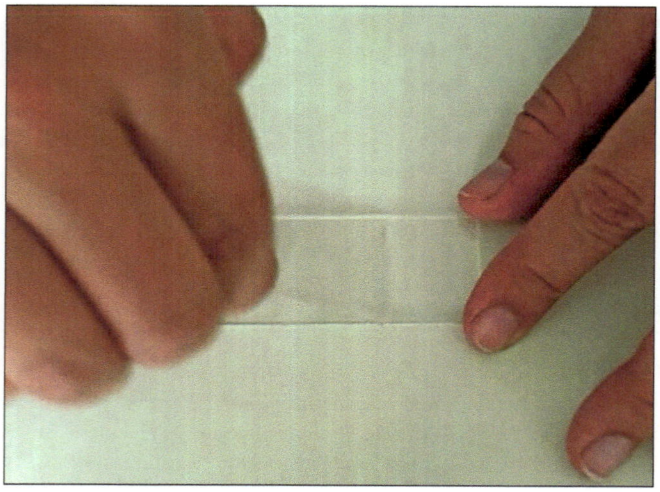

Figure 15.58 Preparation of a concentration line. A spreader slide is positioned at a 55° angle, drawn quickly along two-thirds of the slide, and abruptly lifted.

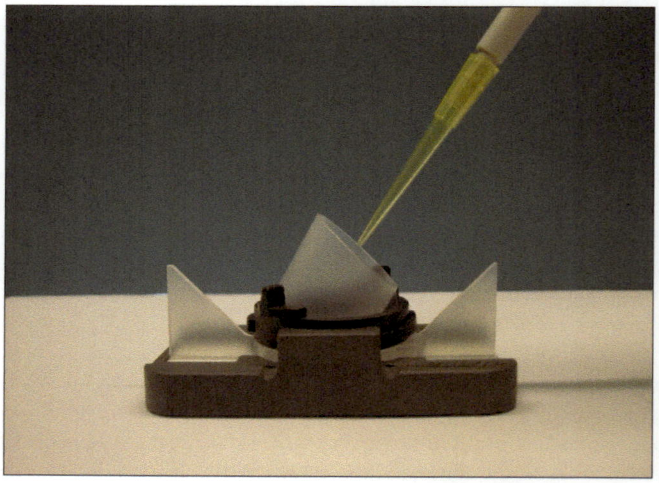

Figure 15.61 Cytospin preparation. Adjusted sedimentation chamber being filled with the fluid specimen.

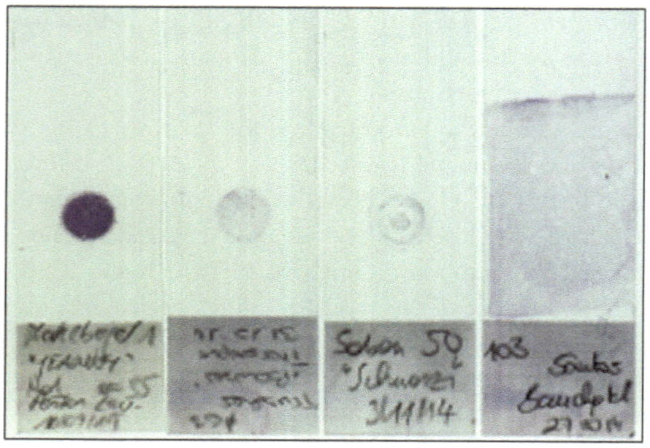

Figure 15.59 Cytospin preparations of different concentrations and a concentration line smear. (Courtesy Dr. M. Bernkopf.)

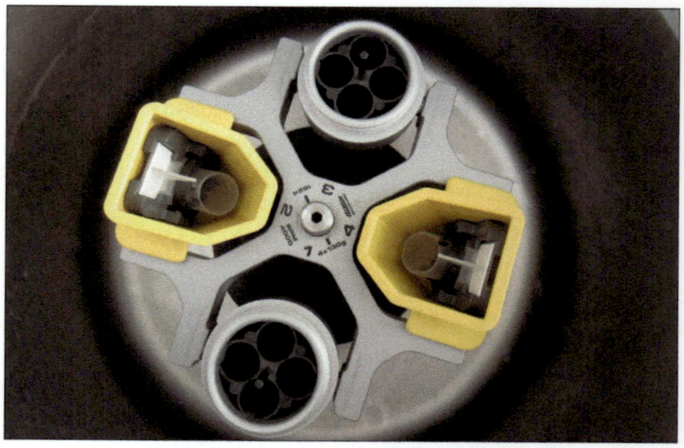

Figure 15.62 Cytospin preparation. The centrifuge rotor is loaded with the cytospin elements.

residual tissue architecture from minimally invasively sampled specimens (Walsh & Patel, 2020). The concentration of infectious agents and as such increasing sensitivity is another useful aspect (Walsh & Patel, 2020). Cell blocks can be prepared in clinic laboratories without special appliances. Embedding, cutting, and staining for slide preparation require histology equipment. Cell tube preparation and agar-based cell blocks have been evaluated yielding comparable results. Cell tube preparation allowed a better separation from red blood cells, was easier to standardize, and cellularity was higher than in agar-based cell blocks, but laboratory processing was slightly more demanding (Melega *et al.*, 2020). Evaluation of cell block preparations needs expertise merging cytology and histopathology.

Staining

Slides are stained with Romanowsky-type stains for first assessment (Figure 15.59). When required, other stains such as Gram stain, Sudan red (Figure 15.20), or toluidine blue stains (Figure 15.63) can be useful. When indicated, the staining times should be adapted to low protein concentrations (decreased) to avoid overstaining of the cells.

Macroscopic evaluation

The cellularity of the slides can be crudely estimated by macroscopic evaluation (Figures 15.7, 15.12, 15.64, 15.65). Highly cellular fluids yield dense smears, whereas fluids of low cellularity appear more translucent. FIP-associated effusions are of gelatin-like appearance (Figure 15.7). Septic exudates can produce flocculent smears (Figure 15.64). Hemorrhagic fluids produce smears resembling blood smears (Figure 15.12). Small clumps in the feathered edge of native smears can indicate tumor cell clusters (Figure 15.65) (Gupta *et al.*, 2011).

Microscopic evaluation

A variety of cells can be detected in body cavity fluids. Mesothelial cells from the visceral and parietal linings exfoliate in health together with a low number of macrophages, small lymphocytes, and neutrophilic granulocytes. The appearance of tumor cells depends on the exfoliative properties of the tumor in question.

Mesothelial cells (Figures 15.66–15.78), which cover the visceral and parietal sides of the mesothelium, appear in small numbers in normal body cavity fluids. They exfoliate either in clusters or as single round cells. Mesothelial cells are typically large (2–3 RBCs in diameter). They contain one or two centrally positioned round to slightly oval nuclei. The nuclear chromatin has a fine reticular structure and one or two round nucleoli of similar size can be visible. The cytoplasm is basophilic. Sometimes mesothelial cells have a pink 'flaming' ring with small cilia-like projections (Figures 15.67, 15.75). This is the glycocalyx halo of recently exfoliated mesothelial cells (Villiers Blackwood, 2005). The nature of mesothelial cells in terms of malignancy can be difficult to assess, as these cells exhibit prominent signs of malignancy when stimulated by fluid accumulation or inflammatory processes.

Low numbers of neutrophils are present in almost all effusions, and the number of neutrophils increases with inflammation. Neutrophils can be differentiated into nondegenerate and degenerate forms:

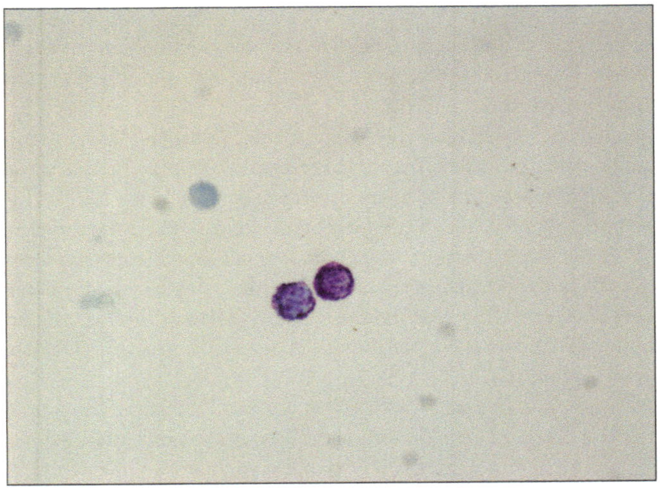

Figure 15.63 Mast cells stained with toluidine blue stain (Hemafix™, 600× magnification).

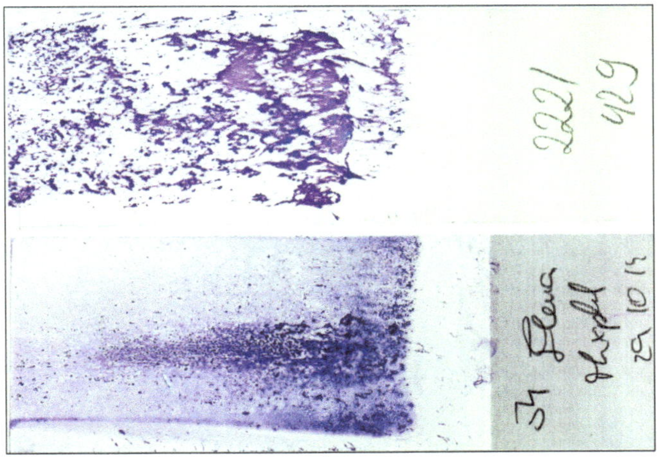

Figure 15.64 Slide preparations from septic exudates. The slide on top is a mixed bacterial infection. The bottom slide is from a sample with *Actinomyces* spp. It is a squash preparation of a sulfur granule.

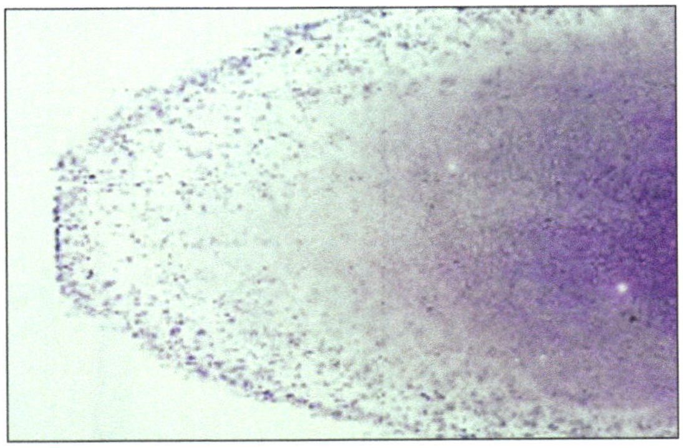

Figure 15.65 Direct smear of a neoplastic effusion. The tiny speckles at the feathered edge represent tumor cell clusters.

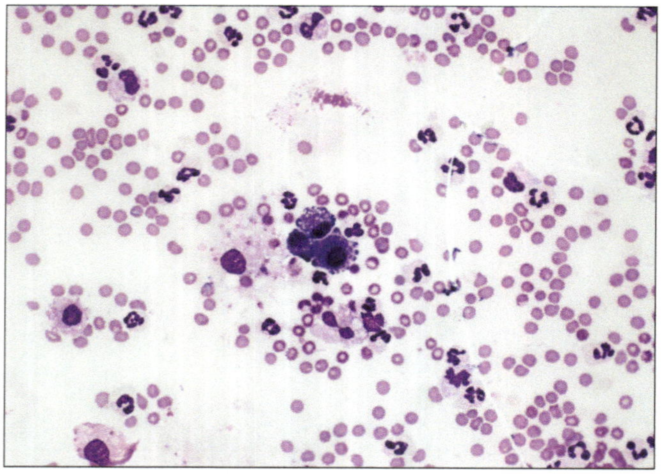

Figure 15.66 The center of the slide shows a cluster of mesothelial cells. The 'ear-like' protrusions are a drying artifact. Note the different positions of the nucleus, which is round to oval with a smooth chromatin pattern (Hemafix™, 400× magnification).

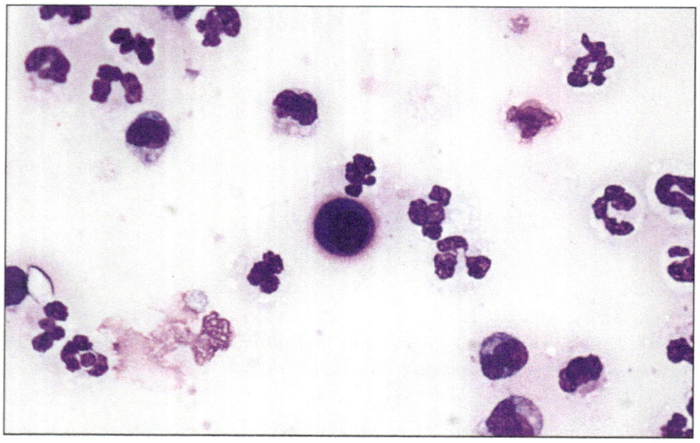

Figure 15.67 This mesothelial cell has a cytoplasmic fringe (glycocalyx), coarse nuclear chromatin, and discrete nucleoli (Hemafix™, 1,000× magnification).

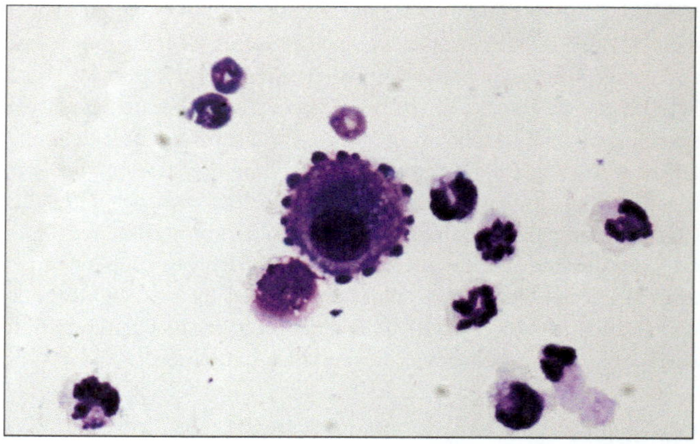

Figure 15.68 This mesothelial cell has a round nucleus with smooth chromatin and abundant cytoplasm with ear-like protrusions (Hemafix™, 1,000× magnification).

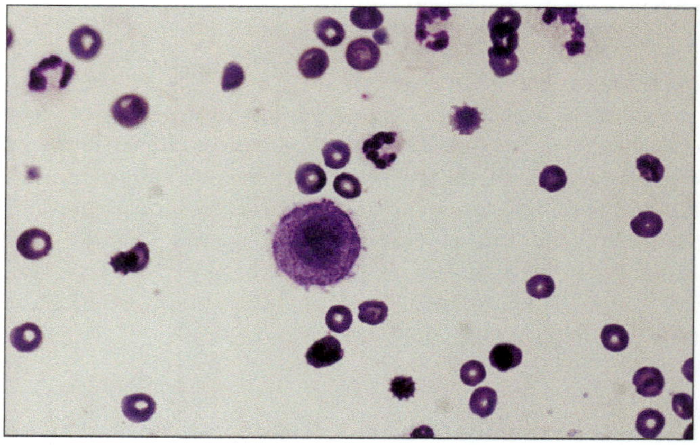

Figure 15.69 The nuclei of mesothelial cells can vary in shape and occasionally will be cleaved or bean-shaped (Hemafix™, 1,000× magnification).

- Nondegenerate neutrophils (Figures 15.79–15.81) resemble those seen in peripheral blood, with basophilic clumped chromatin and segmented nuclei. They are suggestive of nonseptic inflammation. Hypersegmentation and pyknosis of the nucleus is a common finding in aging neutrophils (Figures 15.82, 15.83). Aging neutrophils and nuclear remnants are often phagocytized by macrophages.
- Degenerate neutrophils (Figures 15.1–15.4) have undergone hydropic degeneration induced by bacterial toxins, which alter membrane permeability. Water diffuses into the cells and nuclei and causes swelling of the nucleus, which fills more cytoplasm. Nuclear chromatin becomes homogeneous and stains pink.

Macrophages (Figures 15.84–15.86) are also present in effusions and resemble tissue macrophages. They are large round cells with a bean-shaped amoeboid nucleus with a condensed reticular chromatin pattern. Cytoplasm is pale gray, often vacuolated, and might contain phagocytized material.

Small well-differentiated lymphocytes are commonly seen in small numbers in all effusions, except in lymphatic/chylous effusions where they are often the predominant cell type (Figures 15.10, 15.18). They are similar to lymphocytes in peripheral blood, with a round nucleus with a dense chromatin pattern and a small blue cytoplasmic rim. Reactive lymphocytes are slightly larger; the cytoplasm is deep blue, more abundant, and can show ear-like projections. These cells are common in inflammatory effusions. Occasionally, plasma cells can be found (Figure 15.87).

Eosinophils (Figures 15.88, 15.89) are readily recognized as they resemble those in peripheral blood. They can be increased in neoplastic disease (mast cell tumors, lymphoma), parasite infestation, or allergic reactions. Repeated removal of fluid from body cavities might also cause an influx of eosinophils.

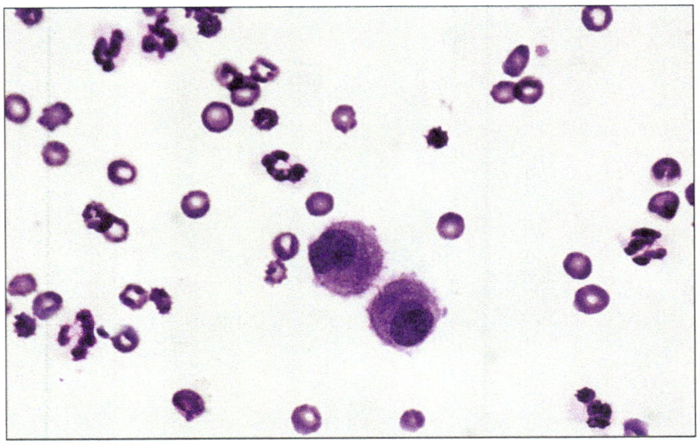

Figure 15.70 These mesothelial cells exhibit dense chromatin and prominent nucleoli (Hemafix™, 1,000× magnification).

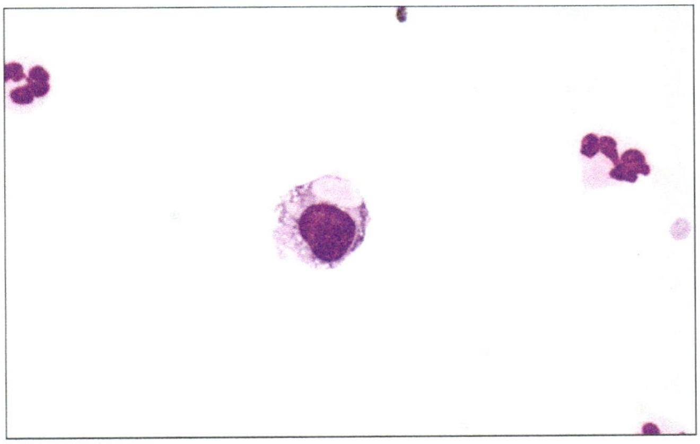

Figure 15.71 Mesothelial cells can occasionally have discrete cytoplasmic vacuoles (Hemafix™, 1,000× magnification).

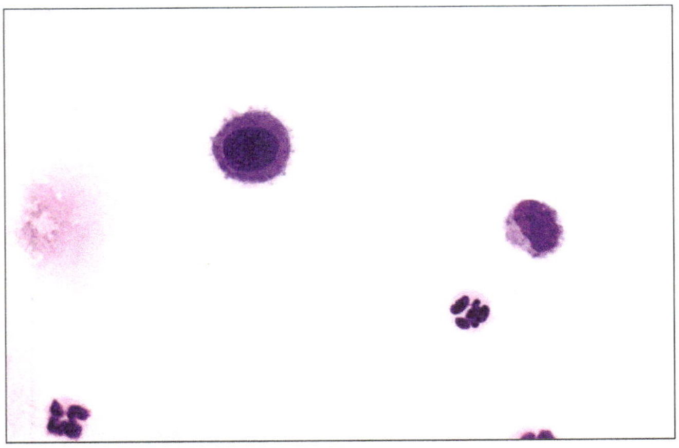

Figure 15.72 These mesothelial cells have discrete oval nuclei (Hemafix™, 1,000× magnification).

Mast cells are inflammatory cells and can be found in low numbers in body cavity effusions. They are round cells with a round centrally positioned nucleus, which is often obscured by magenta to purple colored granules. In mast cell tumor-associated effusions, they occur in

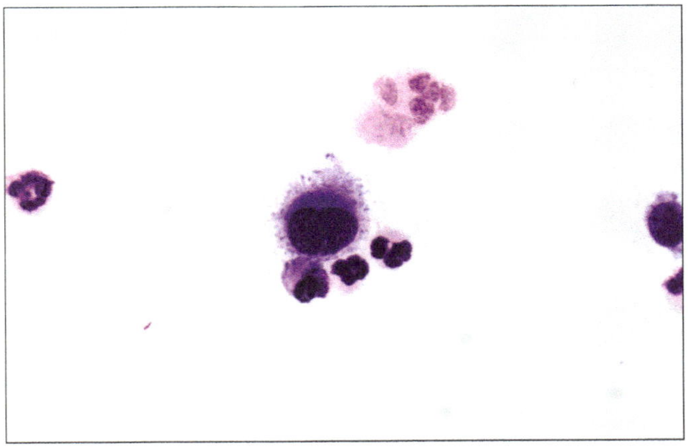

Figure 15.73 Mesothelial cells are commonly binucleate (Hemafix™, 1,000× magnification).

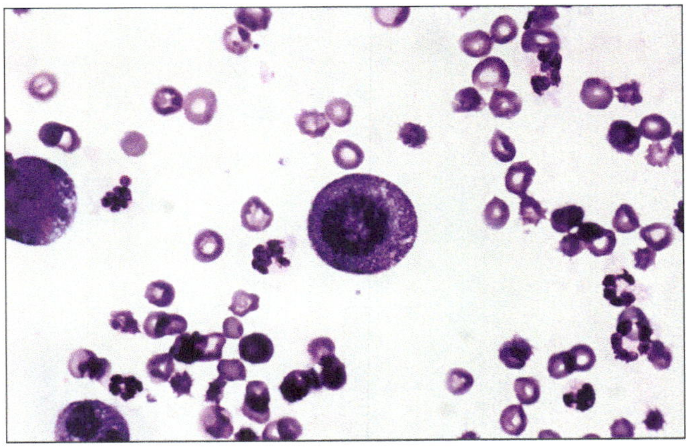

Figure 15.74 Mitotic figures are occasionally observed in the mesothelial population (Hemafix™, 1,000× magnification).

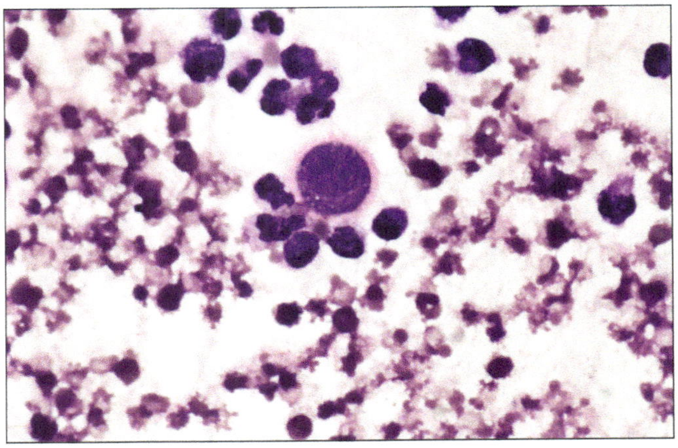

Figure 15.75 A mesothelial cell surrounded by degenerate neutrophils, with a round nucleus and cytoplasmic fringe (Hemafix™, 1,000× magnification).

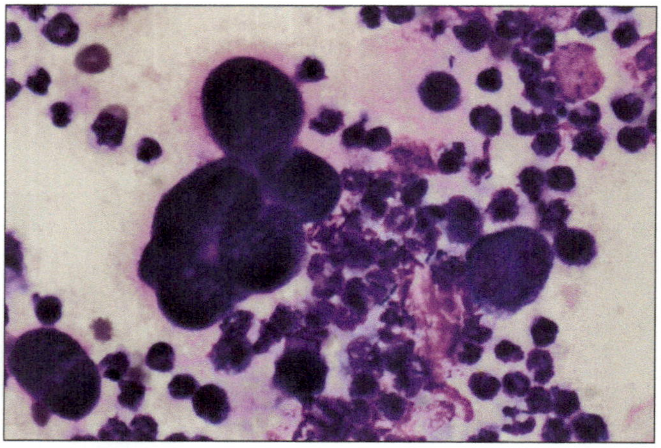

Figure 15.76 Reactive mesothelial cells from a septic exudate. The mesothelial cells have variability in the nuclear to cytoplasmic ratio, vacuolated cytoplasm, and anisocytosis (Hemafix™, 1,000× magnification).

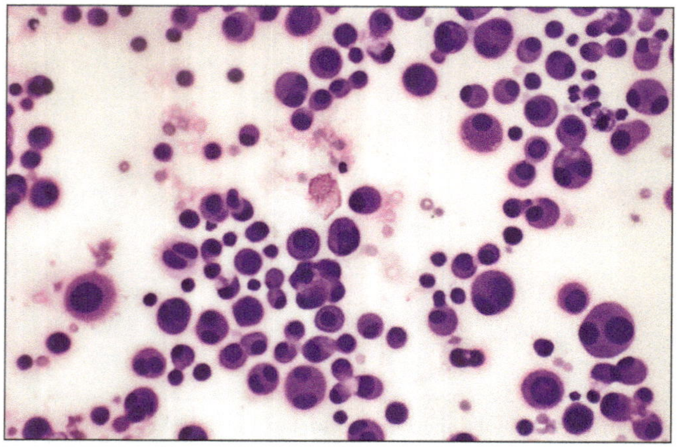

Figures 15.77 Recurrent pericardial effusion from a Wire-haired Pointer. The mesothelial cells are reactive and pleomorphic with marked anisocytosis and anisokaryosis (Hemafix™, 400× magnification).

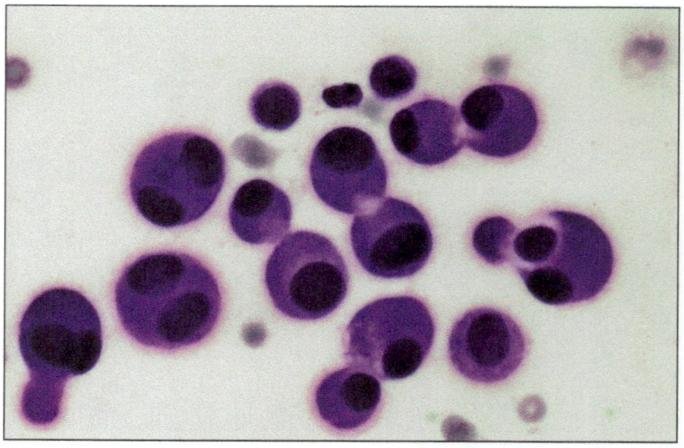

Figure 15.78 Recurrent pericardial effusion from a Wire-haired Pointer. Clusters of hyperplastic mesothelial cells exhibit anisocytosis and anisokaryosis but have a smooth chromatin pattern (Hemafix™, 1,000× magnification).

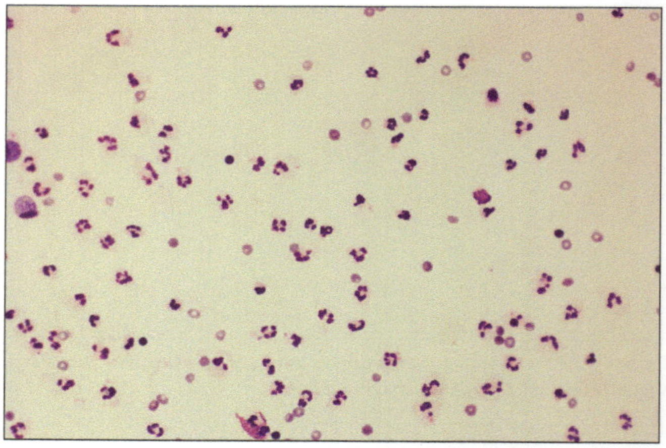

Figure 15.79 Cytospin preparation of a transudate. Nondegenerate neutrophils are occasionally hypersegmented (Hemafix™, 400× magnification).

high concentration and can also exhibit high variability in size and granularity (Figures 15.31, 15.32, 15.34, 15.35, 15.63).

Erythrocytes are also present in effusions due either to hemorrhage or contamination. They deteriorate and hemoglobin degradation products such as hematoidin (orange rhomboid crystals; Figure 15.13) or hemosiderin (blue to greenish pigment; Figure 15.15) are formed and can be detected within macrophages. Bacteria (Figures 15.5, 5.90, 15.91) and parasites (Figure 15.92) can also be detected by microscopic examination. Phagocytized bacteria are more readily detected in the feathered edge or margins. Their staining properties in Romanowsky stains vary from blue to pinkish and do not reflect their Gram staining properties.

Neoplastic cells of all types can be observed in effusions. Carcinoma and adenocarcinoma of various origins (Figures 15.45–15.51), mesothelioma (Figures 15.42–15.44), and round cell tumors such as lymphoma (Figures 15.27–15.30), mastocytoma (Figures 15.31, 15.32, 15.34, 15.35, 15.63), multiple myeloma (Figures 15.36, 15.37), and malignant histiocytosis (Figures 15.38, 15.39) or ectopic thyroid carcinomas (Figures 15.93, 15.94) readily exfoliate into body cavity effusions. Mesenchymal tumors such as hemangiosarcomas (Figures 15.40, 15.41) may shed only a few cells and the associated effusions are usually hemorrhagic; thus tumor cells can be easily overlooked. Malignant melanoma can also metastasize and form a tumor-associated effusion (Figures 15.95, 15.96). As mentioned above, differentiation between different types of carcinomas and mesothelioma is often impossible unless a primary tumor is identified or special stains are performed. Considering the high variability in the morphology of reactive mesothelial cells, at least four to five cytomorphologic criteria of malignancy as well as adequate cellularity should be present in a suspect cell population before an effusion is considered to be neoplastic. A few criteria of malignancy in a low number of cells, especially in combination with an inflammatory reaction, must not be overinterpreted. Absence of tumor cells in an

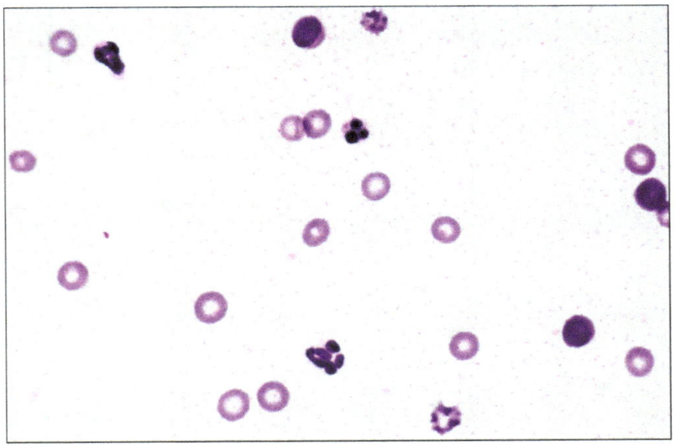

Figure 15.80 A pyknotic cell is pictured in the top center (Hemafix™, 1,000× magnification).

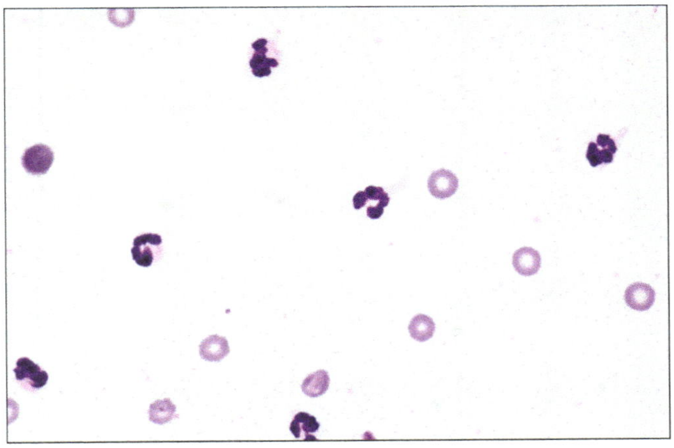

Figure 15.81 Cytospin preparation consisting of nondegenerate neutrophils (Hemafix™, 1,000× magnification).

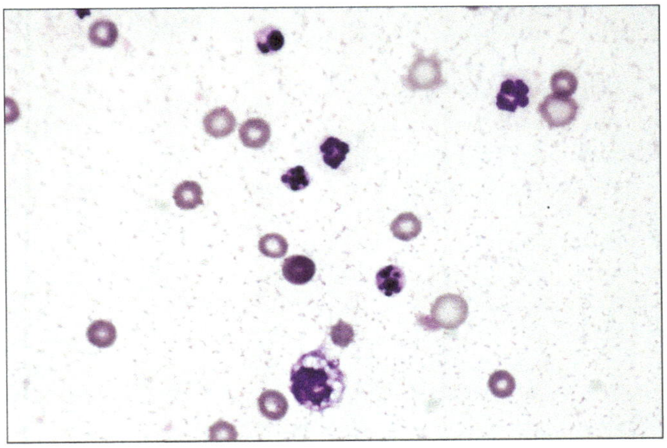

Figure 15.82 Aging neutrophils can appear as pyknotic and/or karyorrhectic cells (Hemafix™, 1,000× magnification).

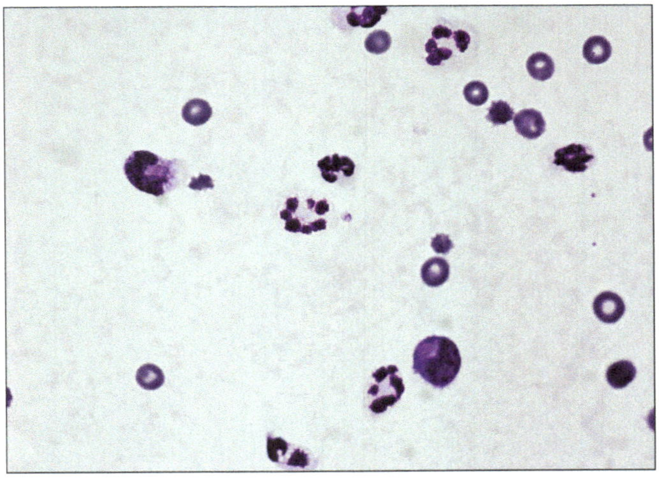

Figure 15.83 Hypersegmented neutrophils are arranged in a background of proteinaceous material and few red blood cells (Hemafix™, 1,000× magnification).

effusion, as in any cytologic preparation, never rules out neoplasia. However, cytologic evaluation should never be omitted as a positive result provides a quick result and makes a substantial contribution to diagnosis.

CASES

CASE 1

Signalment/history

A 4-year-old, neutered male Labrador Retriever was hit by a car 3 days previously and presented for abdominal pain and lethargy.

Physical examination

On physical examination, the patient was febrile and tachycardic with severe abdominal pain. Abdominal radiographs revealed abundant amounts of peritoneal fluid.

Diagnostic tests

A sample was taken and protein and cell concentrations were determined: protein, 3.8 g/dl (38 g/l); nucleated cell count, 6.5×10^3 cells/µl; red blood cell count, 45×10^3 cells/µl.

The fluid was characterized as an exudate. Cytologically, a mixed inflammatory population was observed, predominated by neutrophils with lesser numbers of vacuolated macrophages containing a greenish-black pigment suggestive of bile (Figures 15.97, 15.98). The total bilirubin was measured in the effusion and compared with serum: serum total bilirubin, 1.5 mg/dl (25.7 µmol/l); fluid total bilirubin, 6.5 mg/dl (111.2 µmol /l).

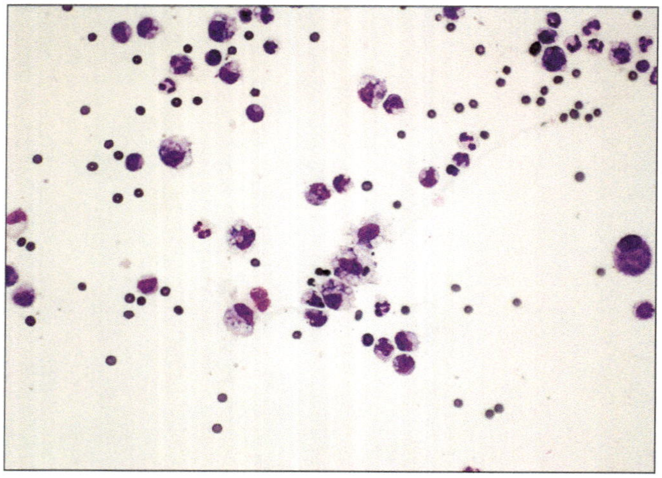
Figure 15.84 Activated macrophages have vacuolated cytoplasm (Hemafix™, 400× magnification).

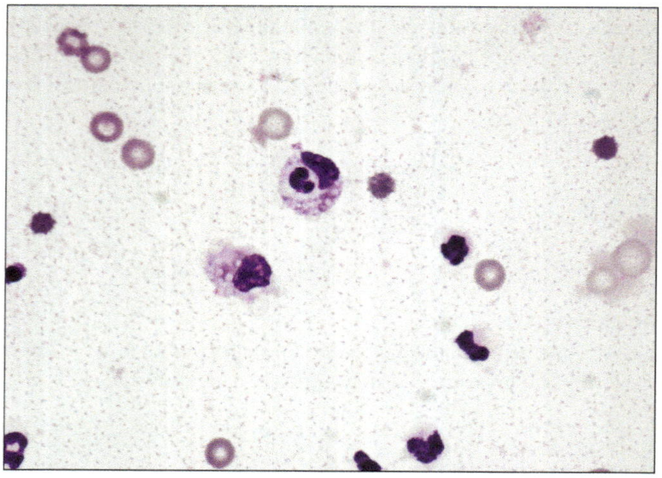
Figure 15.85 Activated macrophage that has phagocytized a neutrophil (leukophagia) (Hemafix™, 1,000× magnification).

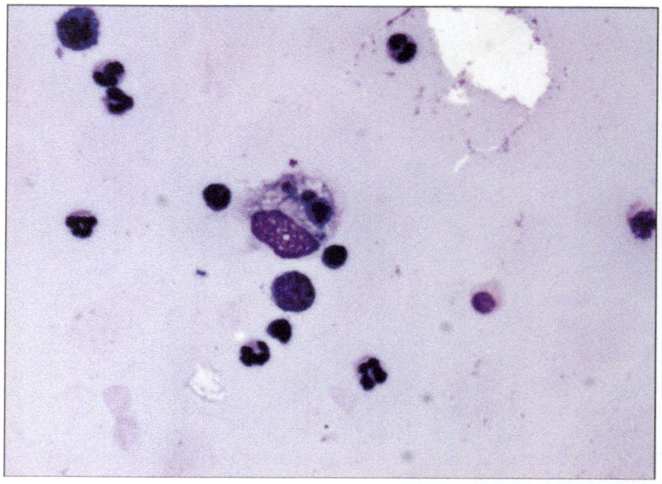
Figure 15.86 Macrophage phagocytizing pyknotic cells (Hemafix™, 1,000× magnification).

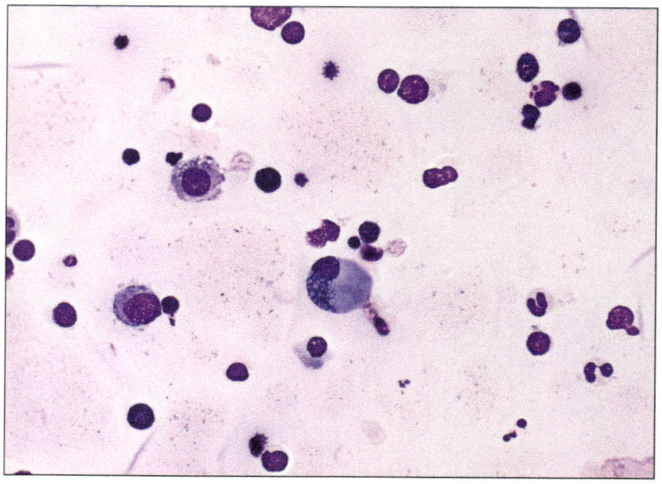
Figure 15.87 Pleural fluid from a cat. In the center is a Mott cell (Hemafix™, 1,000× magnification).

Diagnosis

Bile peritonitis.

Management

An emergency exploratory laparotomy was performed, and a ruptured gallbladder was identified and removed.

CASE 2

Signalment/history

A female spayed Bichon Frisè, 11 years old, was on a hypoallergenic diet because of chronic diarrhea varying in severity suspected of inflammatory bowel disease. She was referred because of labored breathing for 2 days and coughing. The dog has been eating well most of the time; now she has no appetite.

Physical examination

On physical exam, body condition score 2/5; muffled heard sounds, abdominal distention with undulation. Diagnostic imaging: liquidothorax and mild ascites. Gastric and intestinal biopsies were taken by endoscopy.

Diagnostic tests

Bloodwork revealed mild thrombocytosis, neutrophilia, increased C-reactive protein (102 mg/L; RI: <5mg/L), increased DGGR-Lipase activity 1,525 U/L (RI: <125 U/L). severe hypoproteinemia (TP 3.06g/dL; RI: 6.0–7.5 g/dL), hypalbuminemia (0.85 g/dL; RI: 2.58–4.73 g/dL), and hypocholesterolemia (84 mg/dL; RI 125–250 mg/dL). Urine was unremarkable and negative for proteinuria (urine protein/creatinine ratio: <0.5).

Thoracic fluid: colorless, clear, NCC 290/μL; total protein concentration: 0.1g/dL; cytology (Figures 15.99, 15.100, 15.101): clear

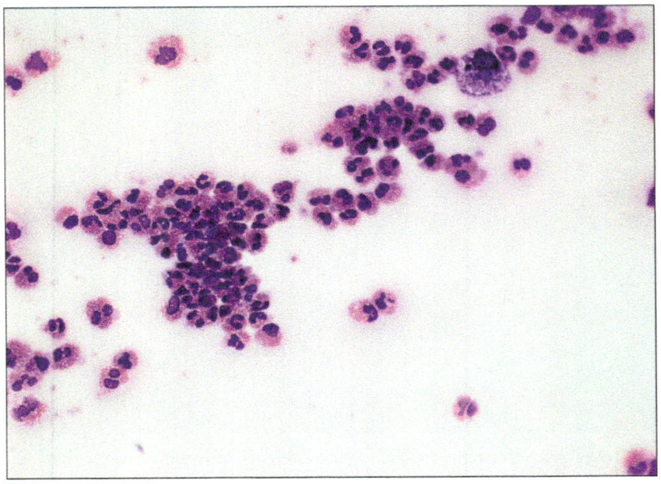

Figure 15.88 Abdominal fluid from a domestic shorthair cat. Activated macrophages and many eosinophils are observed (Hemafix™, 400× magnification).

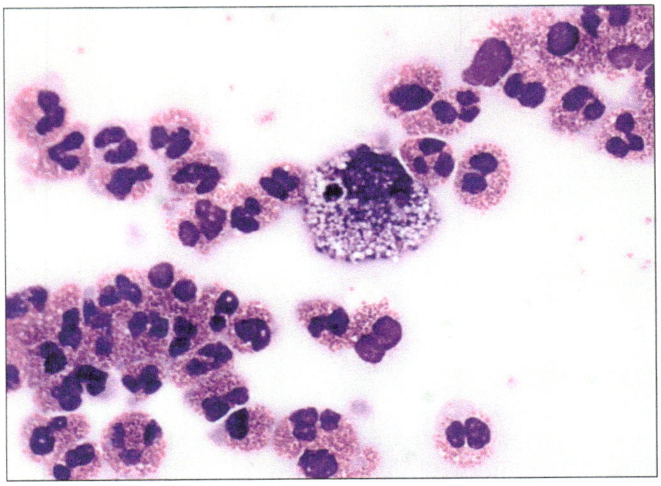

Figure 15.89 Abdominal fluid from a domestic shorthair cat. Many eosinophils and a vacuolated macrophage are pictured. The cat was diagnosed with intestinal eosinophilic granulomatosis (Hemafix™, 1,000× magnification).

background, predominance of reactive mesothelial cells accompanied by few non-degenerate neutrophils. Pure transudate.

Diagnosis

Thoracic and abdominal transudation due to protein-losing enteropathy confirmed by severe hypoproteinemia and hypocholesterolemia. Biopsies revealed blocked lymphatic vessels within the mucosa accompanied by a lymphoplasmacytic inflammation.

CASE 3

Signalment/history

A domestic shorthair cat, spayed female, 9 years old, was presented because of worsening dyspnea and loss of appetite over the last 4 days.

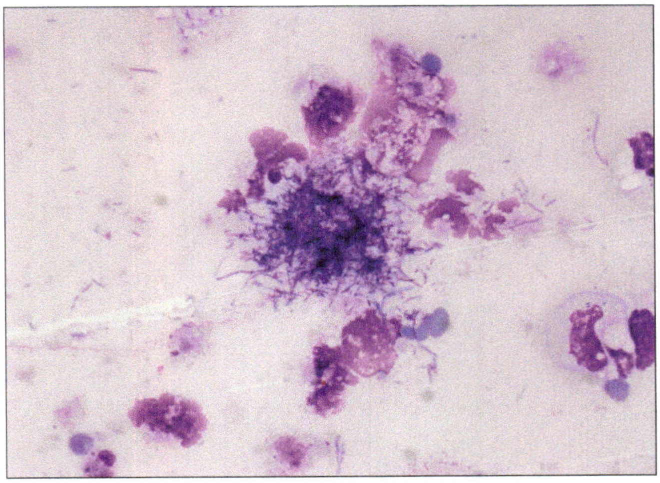

Figure 15.90 Sulfur granule from a patient infected with *Nocardia* spp. or *Actinomyces* spp. (Hemafix™, 1,000× magnification).

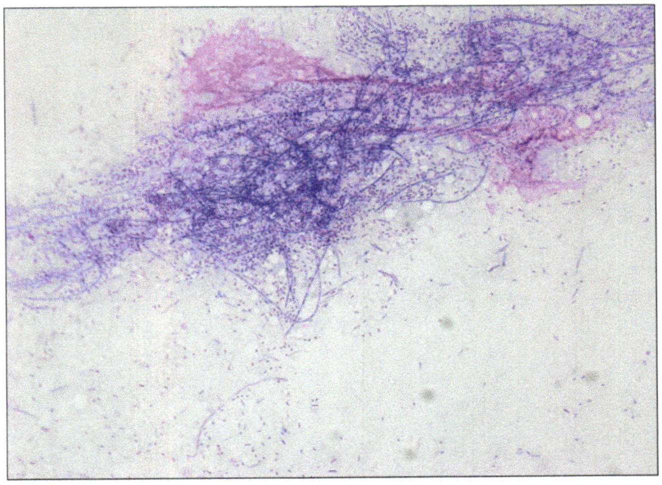

Figure 15.91 A squash preparation of pleural fluid reveals a mold of filamentous septated bacteria. Culture revealed *Actinomyces* spp. (Hemafix™, 1,000× magnification).

The cat has been treated with antibiotics due to suspect pneumonia without improvement of the cat's condition.

Physical examination

Physical exam revealed an enucleated left eye, tachypnoea, and tachycardia with muffled heart sounds.

Diagnostic tests

Thoracic radiographs showed an effusion, which was sampled for diagnostic and therapeutic reasons.

The thoracic fluid was red and turbid with a few clots. The NCC was $4.7 \times 10^3/\mu L$; however, due to clots, this number may be unreliable. The total protein was 4.7 g/dl. Cytologic evaluation revealed many round cells with black fine granules consistent with melanin. Criteria

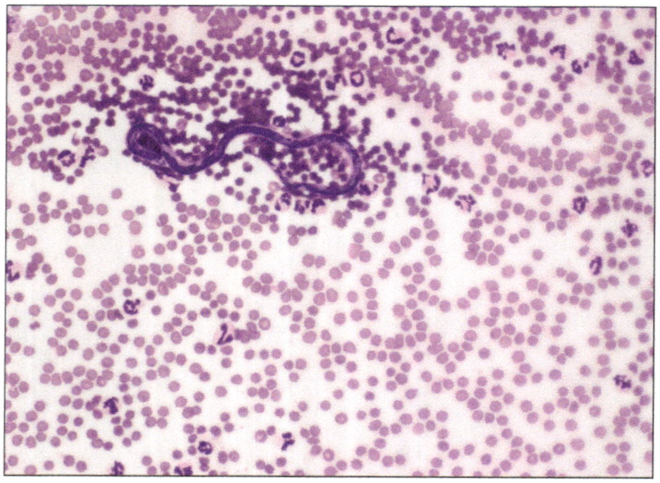

Figure 15.92 Hemorrhagic abdominal fluid from a dog. Rarely, parasites may be observed in samples containing blood. A microfilarial parasite (*Dirofilaria repens*) is shown in this image. This patient had a history of blunt abdominal trauma, which caused the hemorrhagic effusion. The organism was an incidental finding in this case (Hemafix™, 400× magnification).

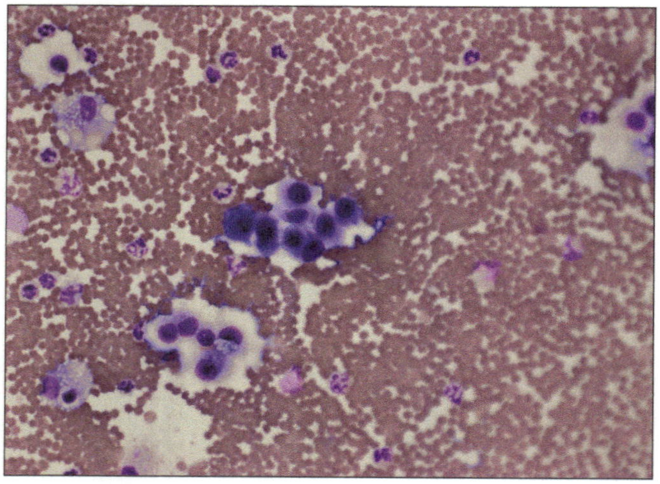

Figure 15.93 Pericardial fluid from a Border Collie with ectopic thyroid carcinoma. Clusters of round, slightly polygonal cells with faint tight junctions, coarse chromatin, and irregular nucleoli (Hemafix™, 400× magnification).

of malignancy were noted and included anisocytosis, anisokaryosis (occasionally noted in multinucleated cells), and atypical mitotic figures. Occasional inflammatory cells were also noted. (Figures: 15.102, 15.103, 15.104, 15.105, 15.106, 15.107, 15.108.)

Diagnosis

The interpretation of the fluid was malignant melanoma. When the owner was informed about the result, he reported that the left eye had been enucleated two years ago because of an iris melanoma. At the time of surgery no metastatic disease was detected.

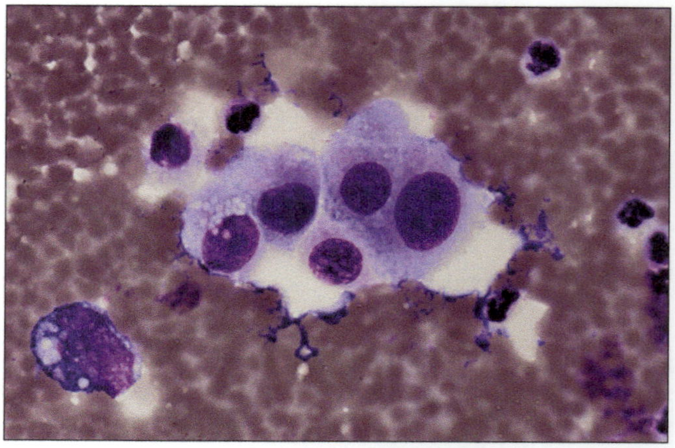

Figure 15.94 Pericardial fluid from a Border Collie with ectopic thyroid carcinoma. The neoplastic cells are large with large prominent nucleoli (Hemafix™, 1,000× magnification).

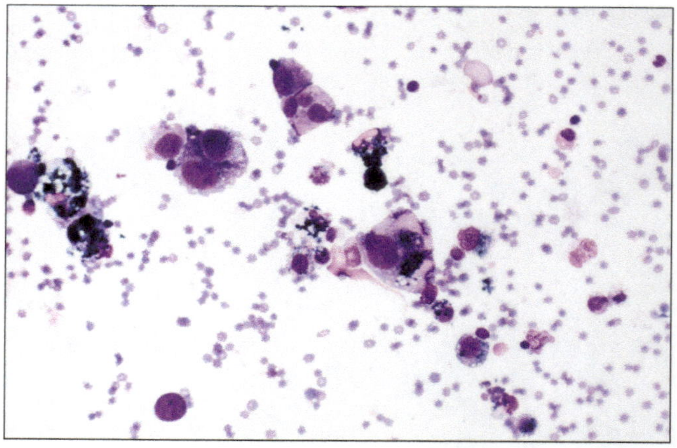

Figure 15.95 Pleural fluid from a cat with a history of uveal malignant melanoma. Pleomorphic mesenchymal cells exhibiting multiple criteria of malignancy and fine black pigment granules (Hemafix™, 400× magnification).

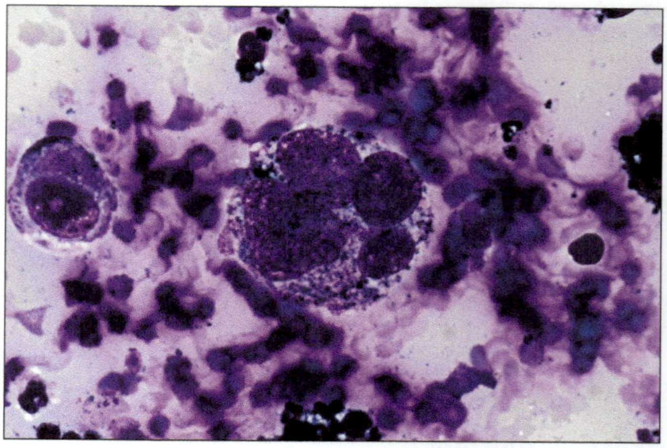

Figure 15.96 Pleural fluid from a cat with a history of uveal malignant melanoma. Multinucleated giant cell containing blue–black melanin granules (Hemafix™, 1,000× magnification).

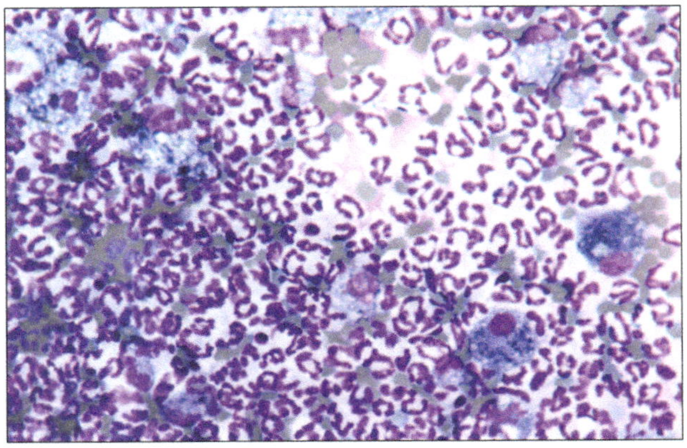

Figure 15.97 Abdominal fluid from the patient presented in case 1. The sample is cellular and consists of neutrophils with fewer macrophages containing pigmented material within the cytoplasm (Hemafix™, 400× magnification).

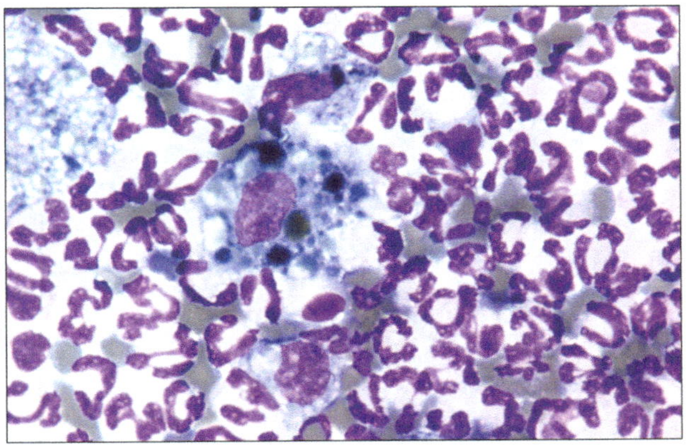

Figure 15.98 Within the cytoplasm of the macrophage, pigmented material consistent with bile is visualized (Hemafix™, 1,000× magnification).

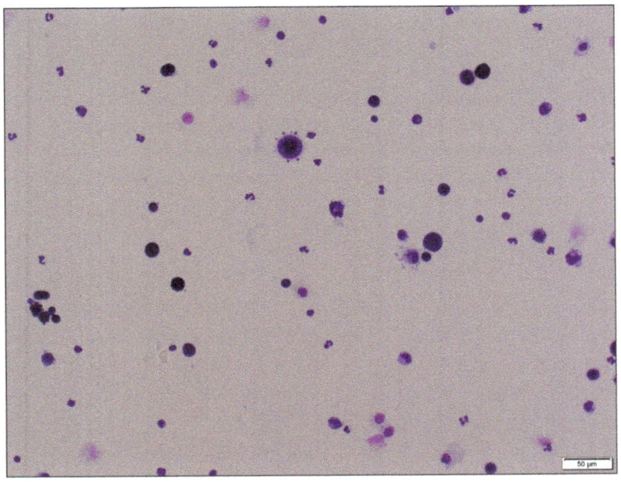

Figure 15.99 Clear background, predominantly mesothelial cells and a few non-degenerate neutrophils. Note the blue overstaining because of the low protein concentration (cytospin preparation, Hemafix™, 200× magnification).

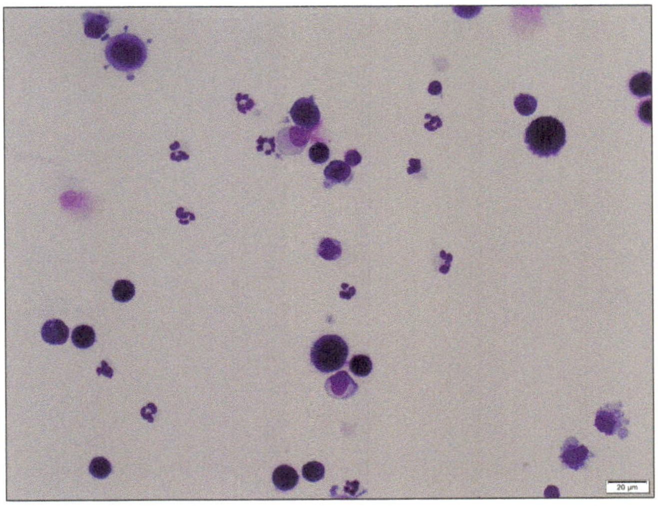

Figure 15.100 Clear background, non-degenerate neutrophils and mesothelial cells (cytospin preparation, Hemafix™, 400× magnification).

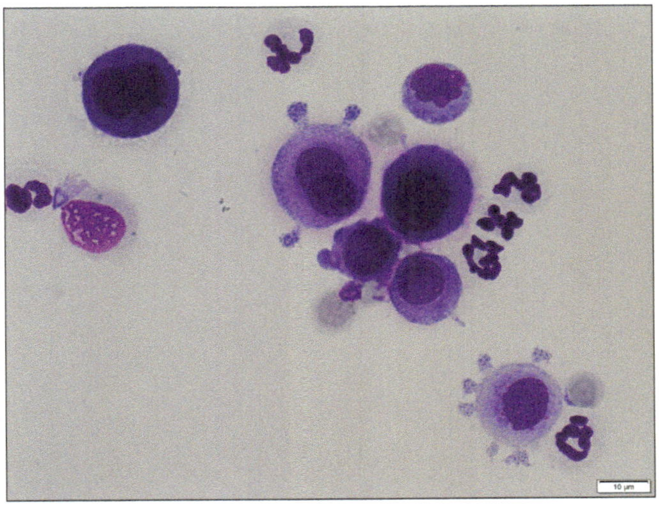

Figure 15.101 Mesothelial cells of varying size and staining intensity and non-degenerate neutrophils (cytospin preparation, Hemafix™, 1,000× magnification).

CASE 4

Signalment/history

A Norwegian Forest cat, castrated male, 4 years old, an indoor cat living in an apartment with a balcony, was presented because of lethargy, decreased appetite, and worsening dyspnea over the last 3 days.

Physical examination

Physical examination revealed an accelerated pulse and respiratory rate with muffled heart and lung sounds with occasional wet rales.

Figure 15.102 Corpus of a smear with a concentration line – note the clear background with erythrocytes – no tumor cells are visible in this area (Hemafix™, 100× magnification).

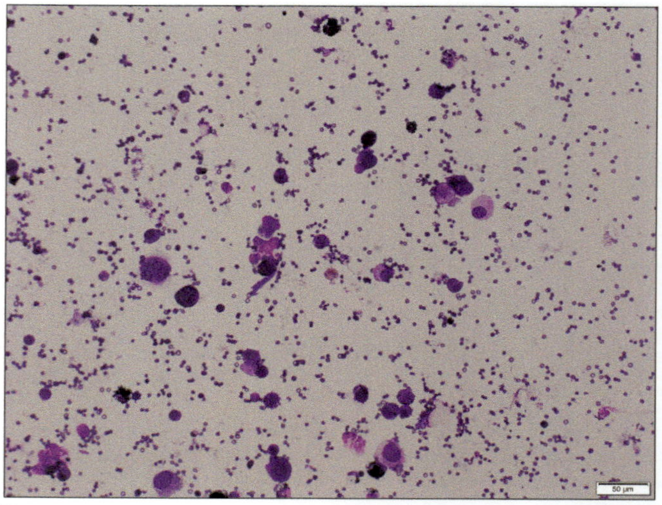

Figure 15.104 Clear background, erythrocytes, lytic cells and round cells of variable size, black pigment (Hemafix™, 200× magnification).

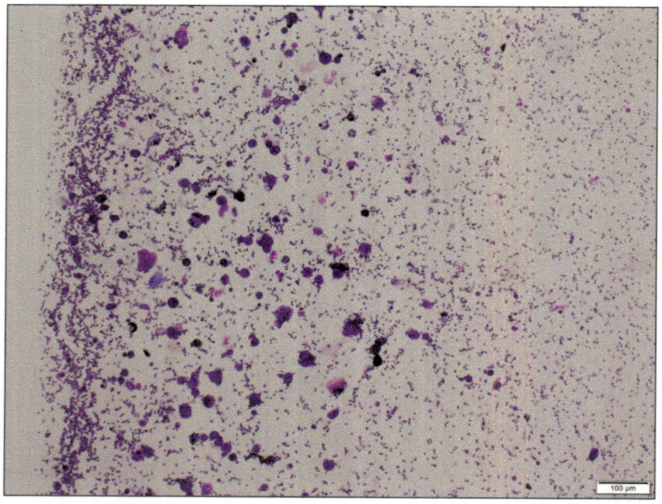

Figure 15.103 Concentration line – note pleiomorphic round cells and chunks of black pigment (Hemafix™; 100× magnification).

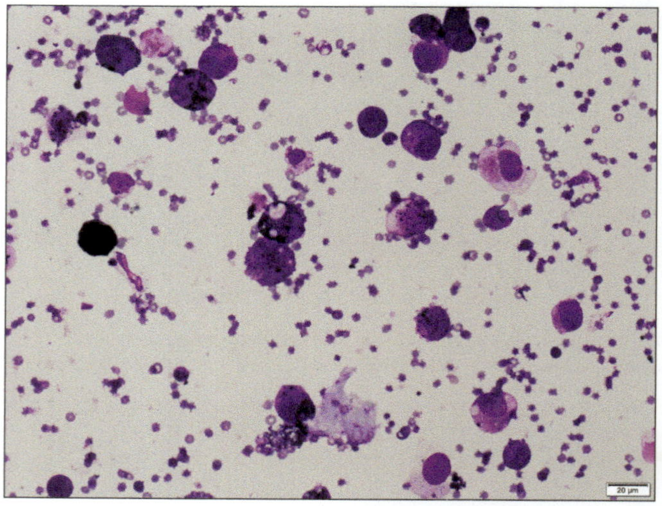

Figure 15.105 Clear background, erythrocytes and round cells exhibiting anisocytosis, anisokaryosis, and different amounts of black pigment, sometimes dust-like and sometimes chunky (Hemafix™, 400× magnification).

Diagnostic tests

The first thoracic ultrasound examination revealed a pleural effusion and echogenic nodular infiltrates in the heart base and right ventricular wall. NT-pro-BNP and troponin I showed abnormal concentrations in peripheral blood. The pleural effusion was light yellow and clear and categorized as protein-rich transudate (TP: 3.4 g/dL; 34g/L), with a nucleated cell count of $0.83 \times 10^3/\mu L$ consisting mainly of macrophages (70%), small lymphocytes (10%), non-degenerate neutrophils (10%), and 10% of atypical large immature lymphocytes with hand mirror-like protrusions of the basophilic cytoplasm. The concentration of these cells was considered too low for successful clonality testing. After 3 days of conservative therapy with furosemide and therapeutic removal of pleural fluid, a pericardial effusion developed and was sampled.

Pericardial fluid

Color: light red

Turbidity +++

Total protein concentration: 3.8 g/dL (38 g/L)

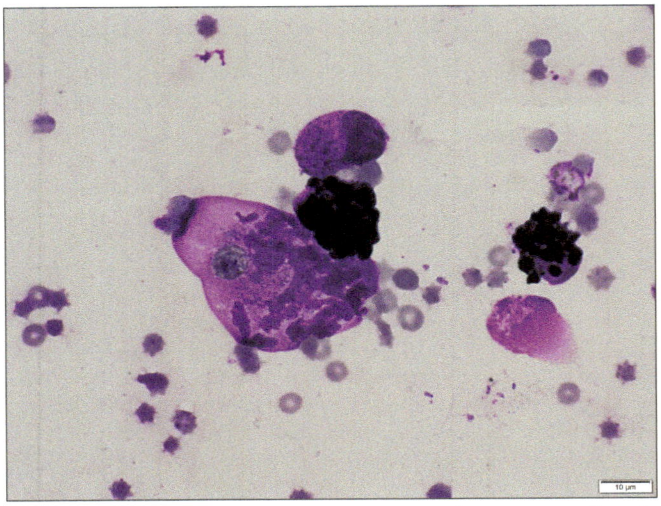

Figure 15.106 Irregular mitosis within a giant cell, two tumor cells with dense melanin aggregates, and on top a tumor cell with dust-like granules (Hemafix™, 1,000× magnification).

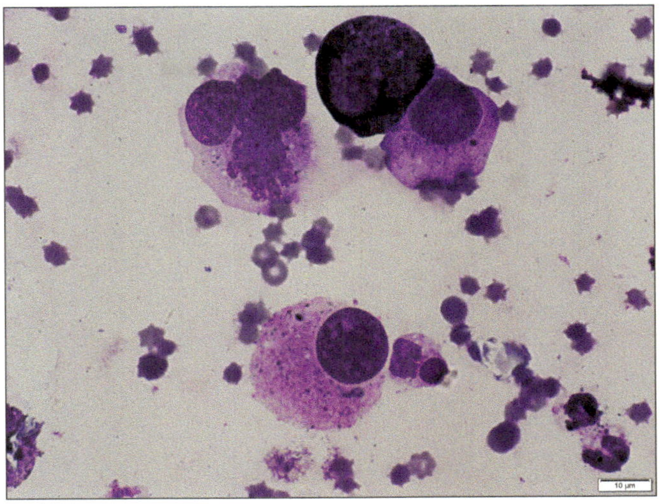

Figure 15.107 Large melanoma cells with variable amounts of granules (Hemafix™, 1,000× magnification).

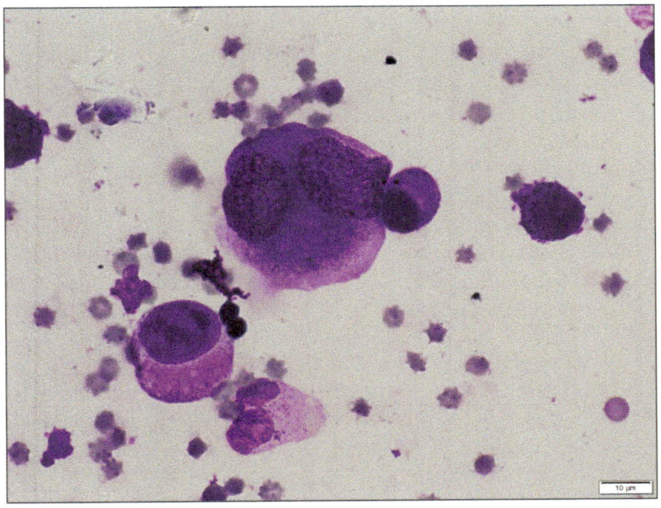

Figure 15.108 Binucleated giant melanoma cell with faint shadows of melanin (Hemafix™, 1,000× magnification).

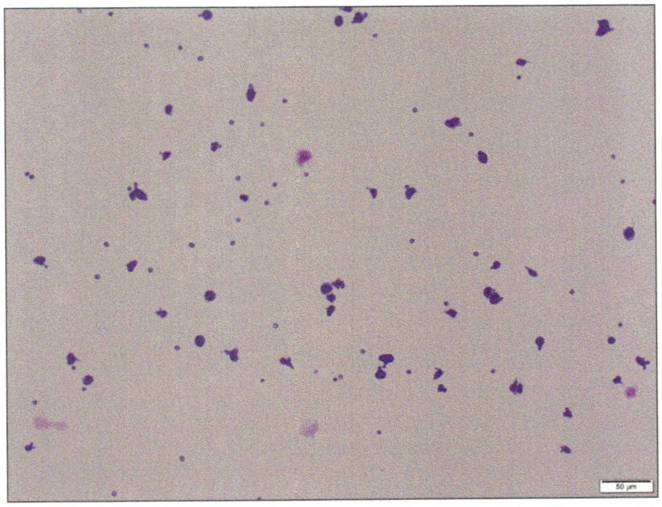

Figure 15.109 Clear background, some erythrocytes, and a pleiomorphic population of lymphoid cells exhibiting mirror-like cytoplasmic protrusions. Monolayer of native smear (Hemafix™, 200× magnification).

Total nucleated cell concentration: $38 \times 10^3/\mu L$

Cytology: Clear background, pleiomorphic population of immature lymphoid cells of variable size, immature nuclear chromatin, sometimes cleaved nuclei, and sometime faint nucleoli. High mitotic rate. The amount of dark blue cytoplasm is highly variable and hand-mirror-like protrusions are common. (Figures 15.109, 15.110, 15.111, 15.112.)

Diagnosis

Highly suspect for lymphoma-associated effusion – the high mitotic rate indicates high-grade disease.

Due to the deteriorating condition and the poor prognosis, the patient was humanely euthanized. Necropsy confirmed malignant lymphoma with positive immunostaining for CD 20, indicating a B-cell lymphoma. Involved were heart, lung, and mediastinal lymph nodes. The tumor spread was localized within the thoracic cavity.

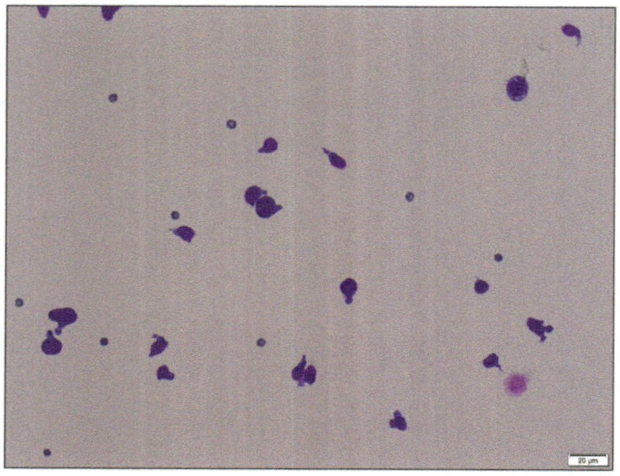

Figure 15.110 Pleiomorphic lymphoid round cells of variable size and hand mirror-like cytoplasmic protrusions. Note the mitosis top right (Hemafix™, 400× magnification).

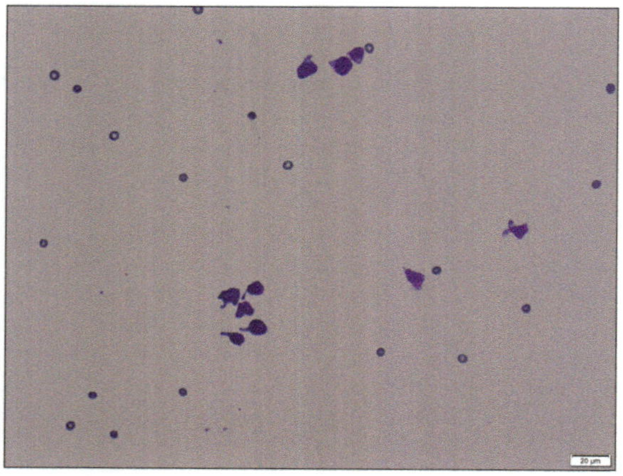

Figure 15.111 Pleiomorphic lymphoid round cells and cytoplasmic protrusions (Hemafix™, 400× magnification).

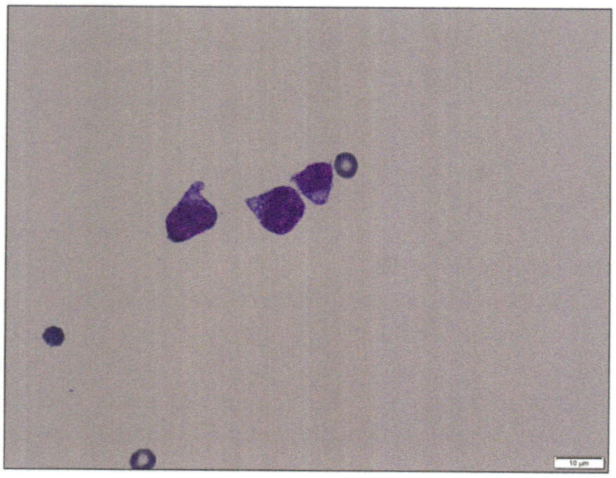

Figure 15.112 Pleiomorphic lymphoid round cells and cytoplasmic protrusions and clod-like nuclear chromatin (Hemafix™, 1,000× magnification).

REFERENCES

Al-Dissi A.N., Philibert H. (2011) A case of biphasic mesothelioma with osseous and chondromatous differentiation in a cat. *Can Vet J 52*:534.

Alleman A.R. (2003) Abdominal, thoracic, and pericardial effusions. *Vet Clin North Am Small Anim Pract 33*(*1*):89–118.

Alonso F.H., Behling-Kelly E., Borjesson D.L. (2022) Lipoprotein profile of pleural and peritoneal transudates in dogs and cats. *Journal of Veterinary Internal Medicine 36*(2):464–472.

Alonso F.H., Mattoso C.R., Leme F.O. et al. (2021) Evaluation of a new multiple regression model based on biochemical parameters for the distinction of canine exudates and transudates. *Veterinary Clinical Pathology 50*(3):394–403.

Athanasiou L.V., Spyropoulou M., Meichner K. (2019) The laboratory diagnostic approach to thoracic and abdominal effusions in the dog, cat, and horse. *Journal of the Hellenic Veterinary Medical Society 70*(3):1589–1602.

Bacci B., Morandi F., De Meo M. et al. (2006) Ten cases of feline mesothelioma: An immunohistochemical and ultrastructural study. *J Comp Pathol 134*:347–354.

Barker E. and S. Tasker (2020) Update on feline infectious peritonitis. *In Practice 42*(7):372–383.

Bauer N., Moritz A. (2005) Flow cytometric analysis of effusions in dogs and cats with the automated haematology analyser ADVIA 120. *Vet Rec 156*:674–678.

Baumwart R.D., Hanzlicek A.S., Lyon S.D. et al. (2017) Plasma N-terminal pro-brain natriuretic peptide concentrations before and after pericardiocentesis in dogs with cardiac tamponade secondary to spontaneous pericardial effusion. *Journal of Veterinary Cardiology 19*(5):416–420.

Beatty J., Barrs V. (2010) Pleural effusion in the cat: A practical approach to determining aetiology. *J Feline Med Surg 12*:693–707.

Bielsa S., Salud A., Martínez M. et al. (2008) Prognostic significance of pleural fluid data in patients with malignant effusion. *Eur J Intern Med 19*:334–339.

Birchard S., McLoughlin M., Smeak D. (1995) Chylothorax in the dog and cat: A review. *Lymphology 28*:64–72.

Bohn A.A. (2017) Analysis of canine peritoneal fluid analysis. *Veterinary Clinics: Small Animal Practice 47*(1):123–133.

Bonczynski J.J., Ludwig L.L., Barton L.J. et al. (2003) Comparison of peritoneal fluid and peripheral blood pH, bicarbonate, glucose, and lactate concentration as a diagnostic tool for septic peritonitis in dogs and cats. *Vet Surg 32*:161–166.

Braun J.P., Guelfi J.F., Pagès J.P. (2001) Comparison of four methods for determination of total protein concentrations in pleural and peritoneal fluid from dogs. *Am J Vet Res 62*:294–296.

Cagle L.A., Epstein S.E., Owens S.D. et al. (2014) Diagnostic yield of cytologic analysis of pericardial effusion in dogs. *J Vet Intern Med 28*:66–71.

Center S.A. (2009) Diseases of the gallbladder and biliary tree. *Vet Clin North Am Small Anim Pract 39*:543–598.

Cherry N.A., Diniz P.P.V.P., Maggi R.G. et al. (2009) Isolation or molecular detection of *Bartonella henselae* and *Bartonella vinsonii* subsp. *berkhoffii* from dogs with idiopathic cavitary effusions. *J Vet Intern Med 23*:186–189.

Chun R., Kellihan H.B., Henik R.A. et al. (2010) Comparison of plasma cardiac tro-ponin I concentrations among dogs with cardiac hemangiosarcoma, noncardiac hemangiosarcoma, other neoplasms, and pericardial effusion of nonhemangiosarcoma origin. *J Am Vet Med Assoc 237*:806–811.

Covey H.L., Connolly D.J. (2018) Pericardial effusion associated with systemic inflammatory disease in seven dogs (January 2006–January 2012). *Journal of Veterinary Cardiology 20*(2):123–128.

Cowell R., Tyler R., Clinkenbeard K. et al. (1987) Collection and evaluation of equine peritoneal and pleural effusions. *Vet Clin North Am Equine Pract* 3:543–561.

Culp W.T.N., Zeldis T.E., Reese M.S. et al. (2009) Primary bacterial peritonitis in dogs and cats: 24 cases (1990–2006). *J Am Vet Med Assoc* *234*:906–913.

de Arespacochaga A.G., Hittmair K.M., Schwendenwein I. (2006) Comparison of lipase activity in peritoneal fluid of dogs with different pathologies: A complementary diagnostic tool in acute pancreatitis? *J Vet Med Series A 53*:119–122.

de Laforcade A.M., Freeman L.M., Rozanski E.A. et al. (2005) Biochemical analysis of pericardial fluid and whole blood in dogs with pericardial effusion. *J Vet Intern Med 19*:833–836.

Dempsey S.M., Ewing P.J. (2011) A review of the pathophysiology, classification, and analysis of canine and feline cavitary effusions. *J Am Anim Hosp Assoc 47*:1–11.

Dowling M., Samuelson J., Fadl-Alla B. et al. (2019) Overexpression of prostate specific membrane antigen by canine hemangiosarcoma cells provides opportunity for the molecular detection of disease burdens within hemorrhagic body cavity effusions. *Plos one 14*(1): e0210297.

Epstein S.E., Balsa I.M. (2020) Canine and feline exudative pleural diseases. *Veterinary Clinics: Small Animal Practice 50*(2):467–487.

Fischer Y., Sauter-Louis C., Hartmann K. (2012) Diagnostic accuracy of the Rivalta test for feline infectious peritonitis. *Veterinary Clinical Pathology 41*(4):558–567.

Fischer Y., Weber K., Sauter-Louis C., Hartmann K. (2013) The Rivalta's test as a diagnostic variable in feline effusions–evaluation of optimum reaction and storage conditions. *Tierärztliche Praxis Ausgabe K: Kleintiere/ Heimtiere 41*(05):297–303.

Gavazza A., Turinelli V., Lubas G. (2013) Effusion in the cat: Classification of 396 fluids according to a problem-oriented scheme. *Comp Clin Pathol 22*:517–521.

Giordano A., Stranieri A., Rossi G. et al. (2015) High diagnostic accuracy of the Sysmex XT-2000iV delta total nucleated cells on effusions for feline infectious peritonitis. *Veterinary Clinical Pathology 44*(2):295–302.

Gupta A., Banajee K., Gaunt S. et al. (2011) Guessing game: 1× cytologic 'diagnoses'. *Vet Clin Pathol 40*:1.

Halperin R., Hadas E., Bukovsky I. et al. (1998) Peritoneal fluid analysis in the differentiation of ovarian cancer and benign ovarian tumor. *Eur J Gynaecol Oncol 20*:40–44.

Hatch A., Jandrey K.E., Tenwolde M.C., Kent M.S. (2018) Incidence of chyloabdomen diagnosis in dogs and cats and corresponding clinical signs, clinicopathologic test results, and outcomes: 53 cases (1984–2014). *Journal of the American Veterinary Medical Association 253*(7):886–892.

Hazuchova K., Held S., Neiger R. (2017) Usefulness of acute phase proteins in differentiating between feline infectious peritonitis and other diseases in cats with body cavity effusions. *Journal of feline medicine and surgery 19*(8):809–816.

Hetzel N., Papasouliotis K., Dodkin S. et al. (2012) Biochemical assessment of canine body cavity effusions using three bench-top analysers. *J Small Anim Pract 53*:459–464.

Hirschberger J., DeNicola D.B., Hermanns W. et al. (1999) Sensitivity and specificity of cytologic evaluation in the diagnosis of neoplasia in body fluids from dogs and cats. *Vet Clin Pathol 28*:142–146.

Humm K., Hezzell M., Sargent J. et al. (2013) Differentiating between feline pleural effusions of cardiac and non-cardiac origin using pleural fluid NT-proBNP concentrations. *J Small Anim Pract 54*:656–661.

Marcos R., Santos M., Marrinhas C. et al. (2017) Cell tube block: A new technique to produce cell blocks from fluid cytology samples. *Veterinary Clinical Pathology 46*(1):195–201.

Marrinhas C., Lopes C., Santos M. et al. (2022) Mesothelial cells: The messed-up cells that make a confusion out of an effusion. *Vet Clin Pathol 51*:194–195.

Martins D., Souza G., Pedrozo J.S.R. et al. (2011) Thoracic and abdominal mesothelioma in a dog: A cytologist's view. *Comp Clin Pathol 20*:289–293.

Melega M., Santos M., Caniatti M. et al. (2020) Cell blocks in veterinary medicine: A comparison of two methods (cell tube and agar) in 52 effusions from dogs and cats. *Veterinary Clinical Pathology 49*(4):632–639.

Milne E.M., Piviani M., Hodgkiss-Geere H.M. et al. (2021) Comparison of effusion cell block and biopsy immunohistochemistry in mesothelial hyperplasia, mesothelioma, and carcinoma in dogs. *Veterinary Clinical Pathology 50*(4):555–567.

Mutsaers S.E. (2004) The mesothelial cell. *Int J Biochem Cell Biol 36*:9–16.

O'Shaughnessy S., Crawford I., Arsevska E. et al. (2022) Clinical findings associated with N-terminal pro-B-type natriuretic peptide measurement in dogs and cats attending first opinion veterinary practices. *Veterinary Record 191*(2): e945

Paes P.R., Alonso F.H., Chaves N.G. et al. (2022) Laboratory diagnosis of canine uroperitoneum based on cellular and biochemical characteristics of serum and abdominal fluid. *Veterinary Clinical Pathology 51*(1):107–111.

Papasouliotis K., Murphy K., Dodkin S. et al. (2002) Use of the Vettest 8008 and refractometry for determination of total protein, albumin, and globulin concentrations in feline effusions. *Vet Clin Pathol 31*:162–166.

Pascual M., Fauchon E., Monti P. et al. (2022) Anicteric Gallbladder Rupture with Elevated Bile Acids in Abdominal Effusion in a Dog with Cholecystitis. *Journal of the American Animal Hospital Association 58*(3):146–151.

Pinto da Cunha N., Giordano A., Caniatti M. et al. (2009) Analytical validation of the Sysmex XT-2000iV for cell counts in canine and feline effusions and concordance with cytologic diagnosis. *Vet Clin Pathol 38*:230–241.

Przeździecki R., Sapierzyński R. (2013) Using of immunocytochemistry in differential diagnosis of neoplasms of serosal cavities in dogs. *Pol J Vet Sci 17*:149–159.

Reggeti F., Brisson B., Ruotsalo K. et al. (2005) Invasive epithelial mesothelioma in a dog. *Vet Pathol Online 42*:77–81.

Romanelli P., Paltrinieri S., Bonfanti U. et al. (2022) Utility of the Ratio between Lactate Dehydrogenase (LDH) Activity and Total Nucleated Cell Counts in Effusions (LDH/TNCC Ratio) for the Diagnosis of Feline Infectious Peritonitis (FIP). *Animals 12*(17):2262.

Sebastián-Marcos P., Santarelli G., Gómez S. et al. (2019) Canine leishmaniasis associated with pericardial effusion in a 4-year-old dog. *Journal of veterinary cardiology 23*:32–37.

Shidham V.B., Layfield L.J. (2021) Cell-blocks and immunohistochemistry. *Cytojournal 18*.

Smuts C.M., Mills J.N., Gaál T. (2016) Transudate or exudate: Can lactate dehydrogenase activity in canine and feline effusions help to differentiate between the 2? *Veterinary Clinical Pathology 45*(4):680–688.

Stockham S.L., Scott M.A. (2013) *Fundamentals of Veterinary Clinical Pathology* 2nd edn. Wiley-Blackwell, Ames.

Summers A.M., Culler C., Cooper E. (2021) Spontaneous abdominal effusion in dogs with presumed anaphylaxis. *Journal of Veterinary Emergency and Critical Care 31*(4):483–489.

Szabo S.D., Jermyn K., Neel J. et al. (2011) Evaluation of postceliotomy peritoneal drain fluid volume, cytology, and blood-to-peritoneal fluid lactate and glucose differences in normal dogs. *Vet Surg 40*:444–449.

Takano T., Ohyama T., Kokumoto A. et al. (2011) Vascular endothelial growth factor (VEGF), produced by feline infectious peritonitis (FIP) virus-infected monocytes and macrophages, induces vascular permeability and effusion in cats with FIP. *Virus Res 158*:161–168.

Thomovsky E.J., Johnson P.A., Moore G.E. (2014) Diagnostic accuracy of a urine reagent strip to identify bacterial peritonitis in dogs with ascites. *Vet J 202*(3):640–642.

Thompson C.A., Rebar A.H. (2016) Body cavity fluids. *Canine and feline cytology* 191.

Thompson B.J., Sherman R.A. (2021) Comprehensive Review of Biliary Peritonitis. *Topics in companion animal medicine 44*:100532.

Valenciano A.C., Arndt T.P., Rizzi T.E. (2013) Effusions: Abdominal, thoracic, and pericardial. In: *Cowell and Tyler's Diagnostic Cytology and Hematology of the Dog and Cat*, 4th edn. (eds. Valenciano A.C., Cowell R.L.) Elsevier Health Sciences, St. Louis, pp. 244–265.

Villiers E., Blackwood L. (2005) *BSAVA Manual of Canine and Feline Clinical Pathology*. British Small Animal Veterinary Association, Gloucester.

Walsh K.A., Patel R.T. (2020) Cell Block Preparation Techniques and Applications in Veterinary Medicine. *Veterinary Cytology*:73–78.

Wurtinger G., Henrich E., Hildebrandt N. et al. (2017) Assessment of a bedside test for N-terminal pro B-type natriuretic peptide (NT-proBNP) to differentiate cardiac from non-cardiac causes of pleural effusion in cats. *BMC veterinary research 13*(1):1–7.

Wustefeld-Janssens B.G., Loureiro J.F., Dukes-McEwan J. et al. (2011) Biliothorax in a Siamese cat. *J Feline Med Surg 13*:984–987.

Zoia A., Slater L.A., Heller J. et al. (2009) A new approach to pleural effusion in cats: Markers for distinguishing transudates from exudates. *Journal of feline medicine and surgery 11*(10):847–855.

Zoia A., Drigo M. (2016) Diagnostic value of Light's criteria and albumin gradient in classifying the pathophysiology of pleural effusion formation in cats. *Journal of feline medicine and surgery 18*(8):666–672.

Zoia A., Petini M., Righetti D. et al. (2020) Discriminating transudates and exudates in dogs with pleural effusion: Diagnostic utility of simplified Light's criteria compared with traditional veterinary classification. *Veterinary Record 187*(1): e5–e5.

Zoia A., Drigo M., Caldin M. et al. (2022) Fibrinolysis in Dogs with Intracavitary Effusion: A Review. *Animals 12*(19):2487.

CHAPTER 16

CYTOLOGY OF ENDOCRINE TISSUES

Sara Connolly

INTRODUCTION

The endocrine system is a group of organs responsible for the production of hormones and proteins that contribute to and control metabolic body functions. Microscopically, these organs are primarily composed of epithelial cells; however, cytology from the endocrine organs is often distinctly different from cytology of other epithelial organs. These organs have been given their own cytologic pattern termed 'neuroendocrine' or 'naked nuclei' because distinct borders between cells are often absent (Figure 16.1). Another common cytologic trait among these organs is that the malignant forms of neoplasia do not often show many criteria of malignancy, which makes a diagnosis of malignant endocrine neoplasia difficult by cytology alone. A diagnosis of carcinoma in these organs often requires histologic evaluation and the documentation of capsular and vascular invasion. Knowledge of common tumor types found within these organs in the dog and cat is helpful when cytologic findings are equivocal. Organs that will be discussed in this chapter include the thyroid gland (follicular and medullary portions), parathyroid gland, endocrine pancreas, adrenal gland (cortex and medulla), chemoreceptor organs, and a special group of endocrine neoplasia found in multiple locations, neuroendocrine carcinoma or carcinoids.

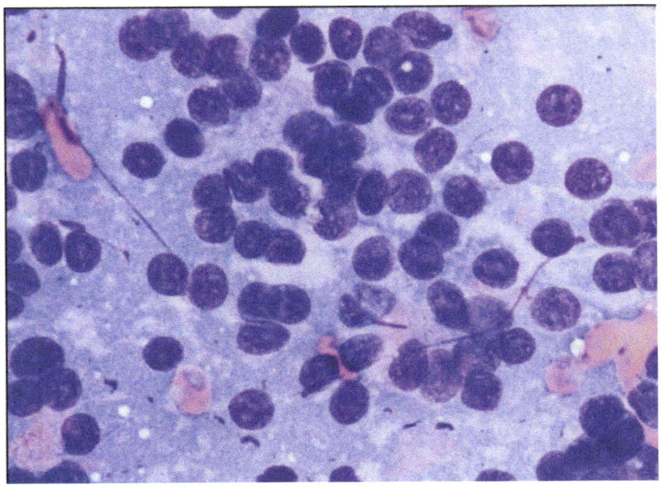

Figure 16.1 Bare nuclei. Dog. This figure shows the classic bare or 'naked' nuclei appearance noted on cytology of many endocrine tissues (Wright–Giemsa, 1,000× magnification).

DOI: 10.1201/9781003258551-16

THYROID GLAND

Normal thyroid gland

The thyroid gland is composed of primarily thyroid follicular cells, which line the thyroid follicles. Cytologically, these cells are seen in sheets that often have poorly distinct cell borders and appear as nuclei on a background of light blue to light purple cytoplasm. If intact cell borders are present, the cells should have a high to rarely moderate nuclear to cytoplasmic (N:C) ratio and a round, central nucleus. The nuclei have finely stippled to reticular chromatin and inconspicuous nucleoli. A variable amount of colloid may be present. Colloid appears as amorphous, eosinophilic, extracellular material on cytology.

Thyroid medullary cells (also called parafollicular cells or C cells) are the second main cellular component of the thyroid gland. A cytologic description of these cells has not been previously documented. These cells may have a similar cytologic appearance to thyroid follicular cells, as the histologic findings in these cell populations are similar and they often require additional special stains for differentiation (Feldman *et al.*, 2005). Thyroid medullary cells make up approximately 9% of the cells within the canine thyroid gland (Sokolowska *et al.*, 2022).

Thyroid gland inflammation

Although inflammation does occur in the thyroid gland and is thought to be one of the main causes of hypothyroidism in dogs, cytologic evidence of inflammation is not common because the inflammation does not often lead to gland enlargement to a significant degree. Inflammation that leads to hypothyroidism is composed of predominantly lymphocytes, with plasma cells and macrophages occasionally noted on histology (Miller, 2017).

Thyroid gland neoplasia

The thyroid gland is often sampled for cytology when a mass is palpated in the ventral neck during a physical examination. The specific causes for neoplastic thyroid lesions in the dog and cat are different, but cytologic findings are often similar. Thyroid adenomatous hyperplasia and thyroid adenomas are much more common in the cat. In two studies, <10% of thyroid tumors in cats were diagnosed as thyroid carcinoma (Leav *et al.*, 1976; Naan et al., 2006). In cats, proliferations of thyroid follicular cells are often functional, which leads to clinical

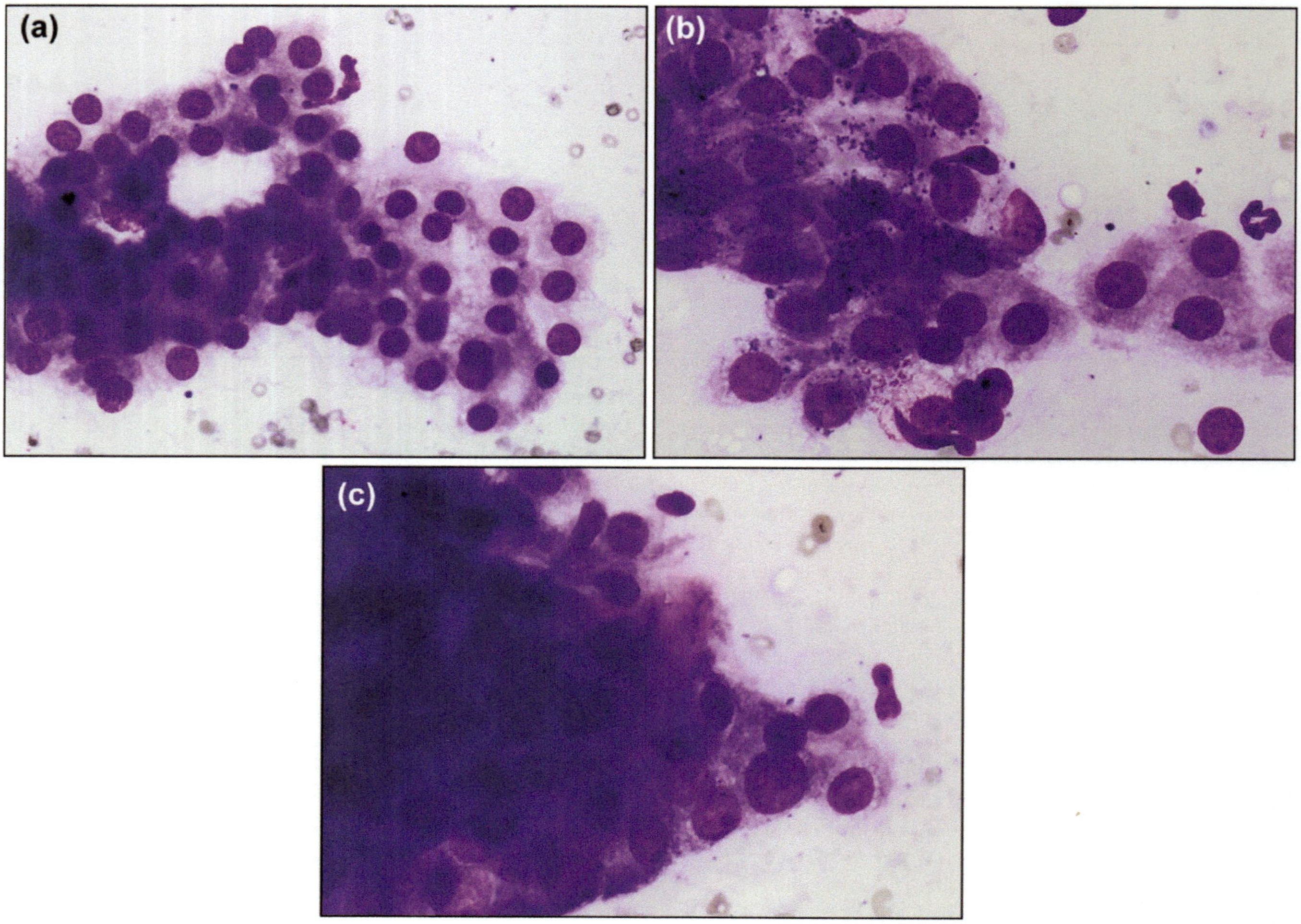

Figures 16.2a–c Thyroid. Cat. Aspirates from a bilateral mass palpated in the area of the thyroid (Wright–Giemsa: a, 1,000× magnification; b, c, 1,500× magnification).

signs of hyperthyroidism including increased appetite, weight loss, ill-thrift, and increased activity/restless behavior. Not all thyroid nodules may be functional when first palpated, but they may later develop into functional lesions (Norsworthy *et al.*, 2002). The average age for feline thyroid adenomas and thyroid carcinomas was found to be 12.4 years and 15.8 years, respectively (Leav *et al.*, 1976). The following should increase suspicion for feline thyroid carcinoma prior to histopathologic examination: recurring hyperthyroidism despite previous radioiodine therapy; multiple palpable cervical nodules; and cervical nodules that are firmly attached to underlying structures (Waters Scott-Moncrieff, 2002). Aspiration of an area of thyroid hyperplasia or a thyroid adenoma will show increased sheets and clusters of epithelial cells with poorly distinct cell borders (Figure 16.2a). Intact cells will have a high N:C ratio and a small amount of lightly basophilic cytoplasm. The cells will have a round, central nucleus with finely stippled to reticular chromatin and often inconspicuous nucleoli. Overall, this population will exhibit minimal anisocytosis and anisokaryosis. Cells may contain fine, blue–black, intracytoplasmic granules, thought to be tyrosine granules (Figures 16.2b, 16.3). Rarely, a small amount of

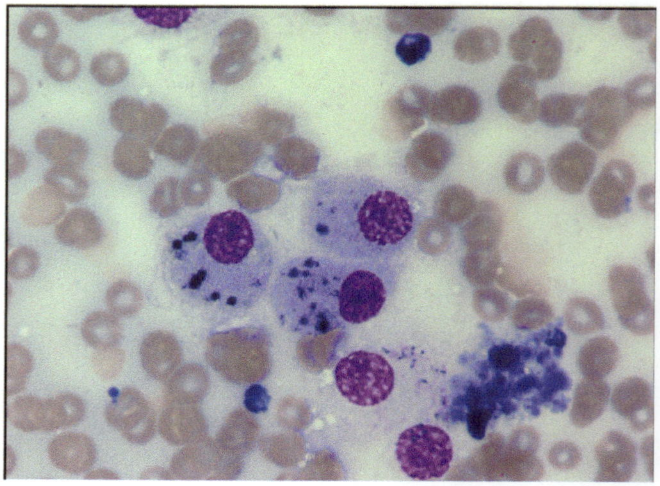

Figure 16.3 Thyroid. Another example of the intracytoplasmic pigment occasionally noted in thyroid cytology (Wright–Giemsa, 1,000× magnification).

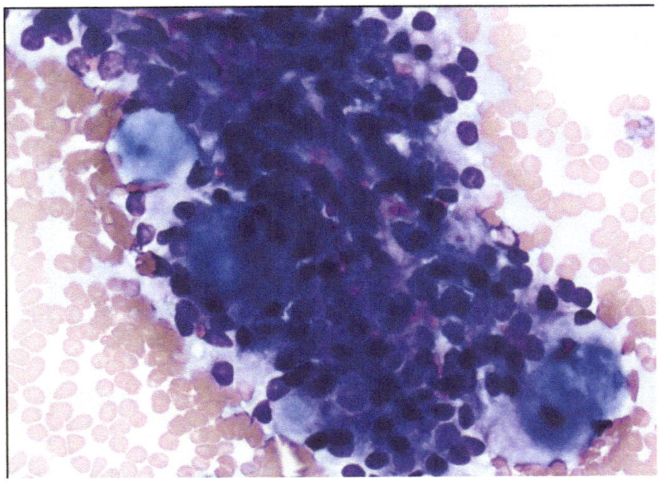

Figure 16.4 **Thyroid. Dog. Another example of extracellular protein material rarely noted in thyroid cytology. The blue staining to the protein is not typical (Wright–Giemsa, 500× magnification).**

extracellular pink (Figure 16.2c) or less commonly blue (Figure 16.4) material is seen that is thought to be thyroglobulin protein. Clinical suspicion for thyroid adenomatous hyperplasia versus thyroid adenoma may be possible depending on the type of lesion palpated. A diffusely enlarged gland would be more consistent with thyroid adenomatous hyperplasia, and a distinct nodule or mass would be more consistent with thyroid adenoma. Histopathology would need to be performed to definitively determine the cause of gland enlargement.

Thyroid neoplasia accounts for approximately 1% of all canine neoplasms and 90–100% are due to thyroid carcinoma (Wucherer & Wilke, 2010; Campos *et al.*, 2014). Thyroid adenomas make up 10–30% of canine thyroid tumors and are often incidental findings discovered at necropsy (Leav *et al.*, 1976; Wucherer Wilke, 2010). Thyroid cystadenomas have also recently been reported in dogs that presented as a ventral cervical mass lesion. Cytologic findings were variable and consisted primarily of proteinaceous fluid and cellular debris with only one case containing cells consistent with thyroid. Measurement of total T4, which was markedly increased, in the aspirated fluid was used to confirm thyroid origin (Maurin *et al.*, 2019). Breeds reported to be overrepresented with thyroid neoplasia include Golden Retrievers, Beagles, Siberian Huskies (Wucherer Wilke, 2010), and Boxers (Leav *et al.*, 1976). A sex predilection is not described and animals older than 10 years of age are at higher risk (Wucherer Wilke, 2010), with the average age for canine thyroid adenomas and carcinomas reported as 10.7 years and 9.0 years, respectively (Leav *et al.*, 1976). Thyroid follicular carcinoma is more common than thyroid medullary carcinoma and accounts for 50–88% of canine thyroid neoplasms (Campos *et al.*, 2014; Soares et al., 2020). Cytologic findings for follicular thyroid tumors are similar to those described above for thyroid adenomatous hyperplasia and thyroid adenoma, with possibly slightly more evidence of anisocytosis and anisokaryosis (Thompson *et al.*, 1980) (Figures 16.5a–c). Thyroid carcinomas are often locally invasive with evidence of metastasis frequently noted at the time dogs are presented for a palpable mass in the cervical region (Leav *et al.*, 1976). The most common sites for metastasis are the lungs and regional lymph nodes (Leav *et al.*, 1976; Giannasi et al., 2021; Skinner et al., 2021). Approximately one-third of thyroid follicular carcinomas in the dog are functional (Campos *et al.*, 2014); therefore signs of hyperthyroidism may be present. Familial forms of thyroid follicular cell carcinoma have been described in the dog and associated with genetic mutations (Yu *et al.*, 2021, 2022). Thyroid carcinosarcoma is an uncommon form of thyroid neoplasia that has previously been described in the dog (Grubor Haynes, 2005; Almes et al., 2008; Cook *et al.*, 2022) and cat (Rich *et al.*, 2019). These neoplasms contain malignant epithelial and mesenchymal cells which may or may not both be noted on cytology (Cook *et al.*, 2022). Histopathology is needed to confirm the diagnosis with immunohistochemistry often being helpful (Grubor Haynes, 2005; Rich *et al.*, 2019; *Cook et al.*, 2022). Thyroid mixed medullary and follicular cell carcinoma has also been described in a dog with cytologic findings consistent with aspiration of the thyroid gland (Newman *et al.*, 2022). Histopathologic evaluation with immunohistochemistry was needed to make a definitive diagnosis (Newman *et al.*, 2022). Sampling of incidental thyroid nodules noted on ultrasound or CT is recommended as occasionally these nodules are noted to be malignant (Pollard *et al.*, 2015; Bertolini *et al.*, 2017).

Thyroid C cells (or thyroid medullary cells) are also found within the thyroid gland and can lead to neoplasia. The incidence of this tumor in dogs has previously been described as low, but thyroid medullary carcinoma was found to represent approximately one-third of canine thyroid neoplasms in a previous study (Campos *et al.*, 2014). Adenomas and carcinomas of thyroid medullary origin can produce amyloid (Patnaik Lieberman, 1991), which would appear cytologically as amorphous, fluffy, dark pink material in close association with the medullary neoplastic cells. The amyloid is thought to be produced locally, unlike with systemic diseases that cause amyloidosis of multiple organs. Confirmation of amyloid can be achieved by staining with Congo red and then using a polarizing filter to detect birefringence. Adenomas may occur as single or multiple lesions (Miller, 2017). Carcinomas are more likely to be multinodular in origin and more likely to lead to irregular enlargement of one or both lobes of the thyroid gland (La Perle, 2011). Carcinomas also have the potential to metastasize, with the most common locations of metastasis being the cranial cervical lymph nodes and the lungs. A unique case of multiple bone metastasis of medullary thyroid carcinoma has been reported in the dog (Renzi *et al.*, 2022) Cytochemical and immunocytochemical stains/labeling antibodies that may be most beneficial for establishing a diagnosis of thyroid medullary carcinoma include Grimelius stain, neuron-specific enolase, synaptophysin, and calcitonin (Patnaik Lieberman, 1991) with cytokeratin-19 and thyroglobulin being beneficial to determine follicular origin (Ciaputa *et al.*, 2014). Special staining may be the only way to distinguish a medullary neoplasm, as microscopic findings are similar to those of follicular neoplasms (Feldman *et al.*, 2005). Prognostic factors have recently been described for thyroid carcinoma of either follicular or medullary origin regarding increased likelihood of local invasiveness (tumor diameter, tumor volume, tumor fixation, ectopic location, follicular cell origin) and presence of distant metastasis (tumor diameter, tumor volume, bilateral location) (Campos *et al.*, 2014).

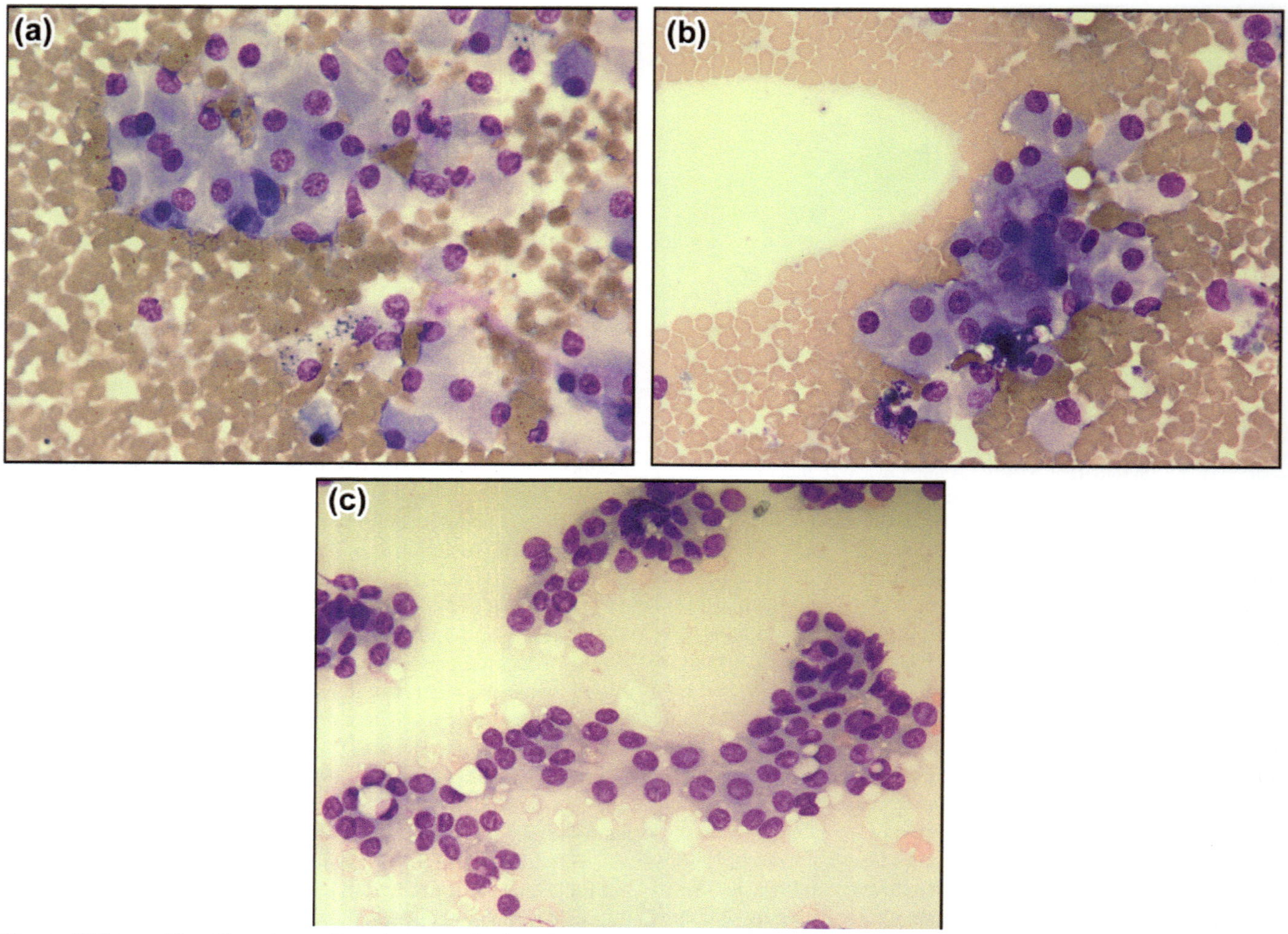

Figures 16.5a–c Thyroid carcinoma. Dog. Aspirates of a thyroid carcinoma confirmed on histopathology. Note that only 16.5c shows evidence of moderate anisokaryosis (Wright–Giemsa, 500× magnification).

Ectopic thyroid tissue is common due to the complex embryogenesis of this organ. This tissue is usually found in the mediastinum but can be found anywhere from the base of the tongue to the diaphragm (Miller, 2017). Thyroid neoplasms due to accessory thyroid tissue have been reported in the dog (Almes *et al.*, 2008; Boes *et al.*, 2009a; Lyssens *et al.*, 2020), but not the cat, and are an important differential to remember for lesions in the thoracic cavity with cytologic findings of endocrine origin. Sublingual ectopic thyroid neoplasia was found to make up 7.5% of thyroid neoplasia in a retrospective canine study (Broome *et al.*, 2014).

Thyroid cysts

Thyroglossal duct cysts, thyroid cystic lesions, and parathyroid cystic lesions are also possible in the area of the thyroid (Swainson *et al.*, 2000; Phillips *et al.*, 2003). Thyroglossal duct cysts occur due to remnants of the thyroglossal duct (Miller, 2017). These types of lesions could lead to palpation and sampling of a mass. Cysts are epithelial-lined structures; however, the epithelial cells rarely exfoliate on cytology. This leads to aspiration of low cellularity fluid as the most common cytologic finding. For cysts/cystic lesions of the thyroid, cytologic findings are consistent with those of a seroma or hematoma including removal of brown to serosanguinous to orange, slightly cloudy fluid with an often low total nucleated cell count, variable but often elevated protein, and a mixed cellular makeup (Figure 16.6; Hofmeister *et al.*, 2001; Phillips *et al.*, 2003; Miller et al., 2017). Measurement of total T4 and parathyroid hormone (PTH) in the cyst fluid may be beneficial to help determine the origin of the lesion (Phillips *et al.*, 2003). Thyroid cystadenomas and cystic carcinomas have been described in the cat; therefore, additional testing may be needed when a cystic lesion is suspected to rule out thyroid neoplasia (Miller *et al.*, 2017).

Thyroid goiters

Goitrous hypothyroidism leading to a palpable ventral cervical mass has been reported in both dogs and cats and can occur secondary to congenital thyroid dyshormonogenesis in young animals (Peterson,

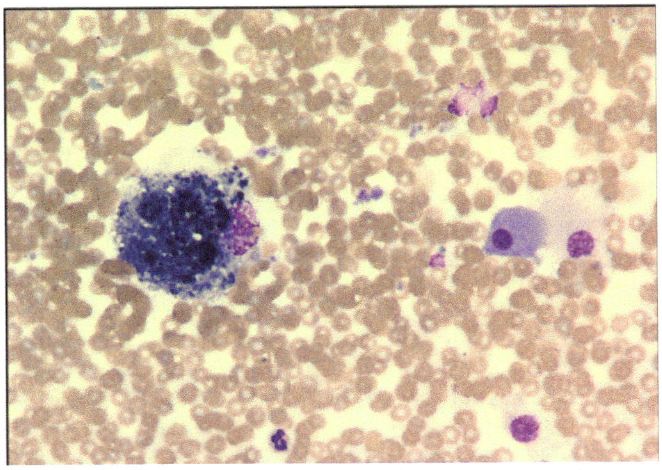

Figure 16.6 Thyroid cyst. Aspirate of fluid from a thyroid cyst showing moderate blood contamination and a macrophage that contains amorphous debris (Wright–Giemsa, 500× magnification).

2015) or as spontaneous cases in adults (Galgano *et al.*, 2014). These cases are often diagnosed by clinical signs (small stature, dull mentation, weakness/inactivity, weight gain, poor hair coat) and evaluation of thyroid hormones (Peterson, 2015; Galgano *et al.*, 2014). Cytology is not often a component of the case workup.

PARATHYROID GLAND

Normal parathyroid gland

The parathyroid gland is composed almost exclusively of chief cells (also called principal cells). These cells are noted in sheets with poorly distinct cell borders and a high N:C ratio. There is a small amount of eosinophilic cytoplasm and a round, central nucleus. Nuclei have reticular to ropey chromatin and low numbers of small nucleoli. The parathyroid gland is a highly vascularized organ, so blood contamination may be frequent.

Parathyroid gland inflammation

Parathyroid gland inflammation has been described histologically but not cytologically. Immune-mediated lymphocytic parathyroiditis leads to diffuse destruction of chief cells and glandular fibrosis. The inflammatory infiltrate is composed of lymphocytes and plasma cells and will eventually lead to hypoparathyroidism (Miller, 2017).

Parathyroid gland neoplasia

Chief cells of the parathyroid gland can form cancerous and hyperplastic lesions, which may lead to a palpable mass in the ventral neck (Kallet *et al.*, 1991) and subsequent aspiration; however, the masses that develop are often too small to be palpated (Feldman *et al.*, 2005; Gear *et al.*, 2005) and are sampled for cytology only after surgical removal. If a cystic lesion is noted within the mass, evaluation of fluid parathyroid hormone levels may be helpful to determine parathyroid origin (Lamoureux *et al.*, 2019; Virtanen *et al.*, 2020). These lesions are often functional, leading to the release of increased amounts of PTH. Common presenting complaints include polyuria and polydipsia, listlessness, muscle weakness, and inappetence (Berger Feldman, 1987). Hypercalcemia (total and ionized) is a common finding with hyperplasia, adenomas, and carcinomas and is often used along with serum phosphorus and measurement of serum PTH to aid in diagnosis (Coady *et al.*, 2019). The median age for diagnosis of primary hyperparathyroidism in the dog is 11.2 years and most dogs diagnosed with hyperparathyroidism are over 8 years of age (Feldman *et al.*, 2005). Keeshonds are overrepresented in case series of canine primary hyperparathyroidism (Berger Feldman, 1987). Middle-aged cats from 8 to 15 years of age are most commonly diagnosed with primary hyperparathyroidism with no breeds reported as overrepresented (Parker *et al.*, 2015).

Adenomas are more common than hyperplasia or carcinomas (Gear *et al.*, 2005; Parker *et al.*, 2015) and often lead to enlargement of a single parathyroid gland; however, bilateral disease has been documented (Kallet *et al.*, 1991). Lesions are often found in the ventral neck within the thyroid gland and are less common in the cranial mediastinum (Feldman *et al.*, 2005). Cytologically, these lesions contain sheets of cells with poorly distinct cell borders and a high N:C ratio. The cells have a small amount of lightly eosinophilic cytoplasm and a round, central nucleus. Small needle-like, eosinophilic, cytoplasmic granules can be seen but with unknown frequency and unknown significance (Soo Choi Arndt, 2016). The nuclei have lacey to ropey chromatin and occasionally up to three small nucleoli. Only mild anisocytosis and anisokaryosis are observed. Increased nuclear pleomorphism is expected in a parathyroid carcinoma, but overall atypia is still mild.

Parathyroid carcinomas are uncommon. In one study done in collaboration between six veterinary universities, only 25 canine cases were identified over a 20-year period for which complete surgical excision was the treatment of choice (Sawyer *et al.*, 2011). In another collaborative, multi-institutional study, 100 cases were identified over a 10-year period (Erickson *et al.*, 2021). Feline cases are documented only as single case reports or in a small case series (Kallet *et al.*, 1991; Phillips *et al.*, 2003; Cavana *et al.*, 2006; Virtanen et al., 2020). Parathyroid carcinomas rarely lead to a palpable lesion and are often diagnosed after investigation of a persistent hypercalcemia or clinical signs associated with hypercalcemia (Sawyer *et al.*, 2011). Lesions are often identified via cervical ultrasound, and a definitive diagnosis is made via histopathology.

ENDOCRINE PANCREAS

Normal endocrine pancreas

Endocrine cells of the pancreas are found in small islets that contain multiple types of cells. The most common cell in these islets is the β cell responsible for the production of insulin. Other cells found in the islets include cells responsible for the production of glucagon, δ cells, which produce somatostatin, and F-cells, which secrete pancreatic polypeptide. Normal endocrine pancreas may be sampled for cytology when collecting fine-needle aspirates or impression smears of the exocrine pancreas. These samples would likely contain low to very low numbers of endocrine pancreatic cells. Endocrine pancreas would be identified as groups of cell-free nuclei on a background of lightly basophilic cytoplasm. The nuclei would be round, exhibit minimal anisocytosis, and have finely stippled chromatin and a single prominent nucleolus. Intact cells should have a high N:C ratio and similar nuclear findings.

Endocrine pancreas inflammation

Cytologic inflammation of the endocrine pancreas has not been described. Histologically, inflammation can be observed in the endocrine pancreas secondary to exocrine pancreatitis or immune-mediated isletitis. Immune-mediated disease would be characterized by an infiltrate of lymphocytes and plasma cells (Miller, 2017). A study characterizing pancreatic islet findings noted lymphocytes more frequently in cats with diabetes mellitus compared to controls (Zi *et al.*, 2016).

Endocrine pancreas neoplasia

Tumors of the endocrine pancreas are most likely to originate from the β islet cells, the most numerous endocrine cells in pancreatic islets (Hawkins *et al.*, 1987), responsible for the production of insulin causing an insulinoma. These lesions are most common in older dogs, average age 9 years. They are found with equal frequency in both limbs of the pancreas and carcinomas are more common than adenomas (Hawkins *et al.*, 1987). Frequency in the cat is extremely rare (Jackson *et al.*, 2009; Gifford *et al.*, 2020). Diagnosis is often made based on clinical signs, serum biochemistry results, and abdominal imaging. Proliferation of the endocrine pancreatic cells often leads to increased insulin production, which causes clinical signs associated with hypoglycemia (weakness/lethargy, generalized muscle twitching, ataxia, mental confusion, seizures). Serum biochemistry results often include hypoglycemia and hyperinsulinemia (Hawkins *et al.*, 1987) and a presumptive diagnosis is made based on the finding of hypoglycemia during observation of clinical signs and resolution with dextrose therapy. Observation of hyperinsulinemia at the same time as hypoglycemia is also used to make a presumptive diagnosis. Abdominal radiography is often unrewarding due to small tumor size. Abdominal ultrasound may be more beneficial but still not very sensitive, with only 36% tumor identification (Robben *et al.*, 2005). The use of contrast enhanced ultrasonography may be helpful to confirm lesions within the pancreas (Cervone *et al.*, 2019; Burti *et al.*, 2022); however, computed tomography with contrast enhancement has the best sensitivity, 71–96%, to detect primary insulinoma lesions (Buishand, 2022). Adenomas are often found as single lesions 3 cm in size, but cases of multiple adenomas have been reported (La Perle, 2011). Carcinomas are often larger than adenomas, may be multilobular in appearance, and invade the surrounding parenchyma (Miller, 2017).

Cytologic findings include a highly cellular sample composed of sheets of nuclei on a lightly basophilic background of cytoplasm and occasional distinct, rounded epithelial cells (Figures 16.7a–c). Intact cells have a moderate N:C ratio, a moderate amount of lightly basophilic cytoplasm with occasional punctate cytoplasmic vacuoles, and a round, often eccentrically placed nucleus. The punctate vacuoles are also noted in the background cytoplasm. The nuclei have finely stippled chromatin and a single, prominent nucleolus. A higher degree of cellular atypia is expected in a β-cell carcinoma as compared with a β-cell adenoma, but the presence of marked atypia and mitotic figures is rare (Miller, 2017).

Common sites for metastasis include the liver and regional lymph nodes (Hawkins *et al.*, 1987) and metastasis can be present in up to 50% of patients at the time of diagnosis (Lurye Behrend, 2001). The presence of metastatic disease makes resolution difficult even though surgical excision of the primary lesion is still recommended. Removal of the primary tumor and debulking of metastatic disease may be enough to cause resolution or lessening of clinical signs (Lurye Behrend, 2001). Prognosis is highly dependent on the presence or absence of metastatic lesions at the time of diagnosis for dogs treated surgically (Lurye Behrend, 2001). Lack of hypoglycemia has been documented in 50% of dogs with no evidence of metastatic disease for up to 14 months after surgery. During the same time frame, lack of clinical signs was documented in 20% of dogs with metastatic disease (Caywood *et al.*, 1988). A median survival of 74 days is reported in dogs undergoing medical management (Tobin *et al.*, 1999).

Immunocytochemical staining with insulin will help to confirm the diagnosis of insulinoma; however, the intensity of staining does not correlate with tumor hormone production, degree of hypoglycemia, or degree of hyperinsulinemia (Hawkins *et al.*, 1987). Endocrine neoplasia of the other pancreatic islet cells has been reported in small animals, but the reports are sparse and cytologic findings are not confirmed.

CHEMORECEPTOR ORGANS

Chemoreceptor tissue is found in multiple locations throughout the body, but tissue in the carotid body and aortic bodies is the most likely to form a mass lesion that may be sampled by cytology. These tissues are responsible for detecting changes in blood carbon dioxide content, pH, and oxygen tension, and changing respiration and blood flow accordingly.

Chemoreceptor organ neoplasia

Canine breeds overrepresented in case series reports for chemoreceptor organ neoplasia include the English Bulldog, Boston Terrier, and Boxer (Hayes & Sass, 1988). Aortic body tumors occur more frequently in dogs, which is in contrast to humans where carotid body tumors are more frequent (Hayes & Sass, 1988; Brown *et al.*, 2003). In a study of 111 cardiac tumors, 31 aortic body tumors (27.9%) were identified (Janus *et al.*, 2016). Aortic body (Buergelt Das, 1968) and carotid body (Yates et al., 1980) tumors have also been described in the cat.

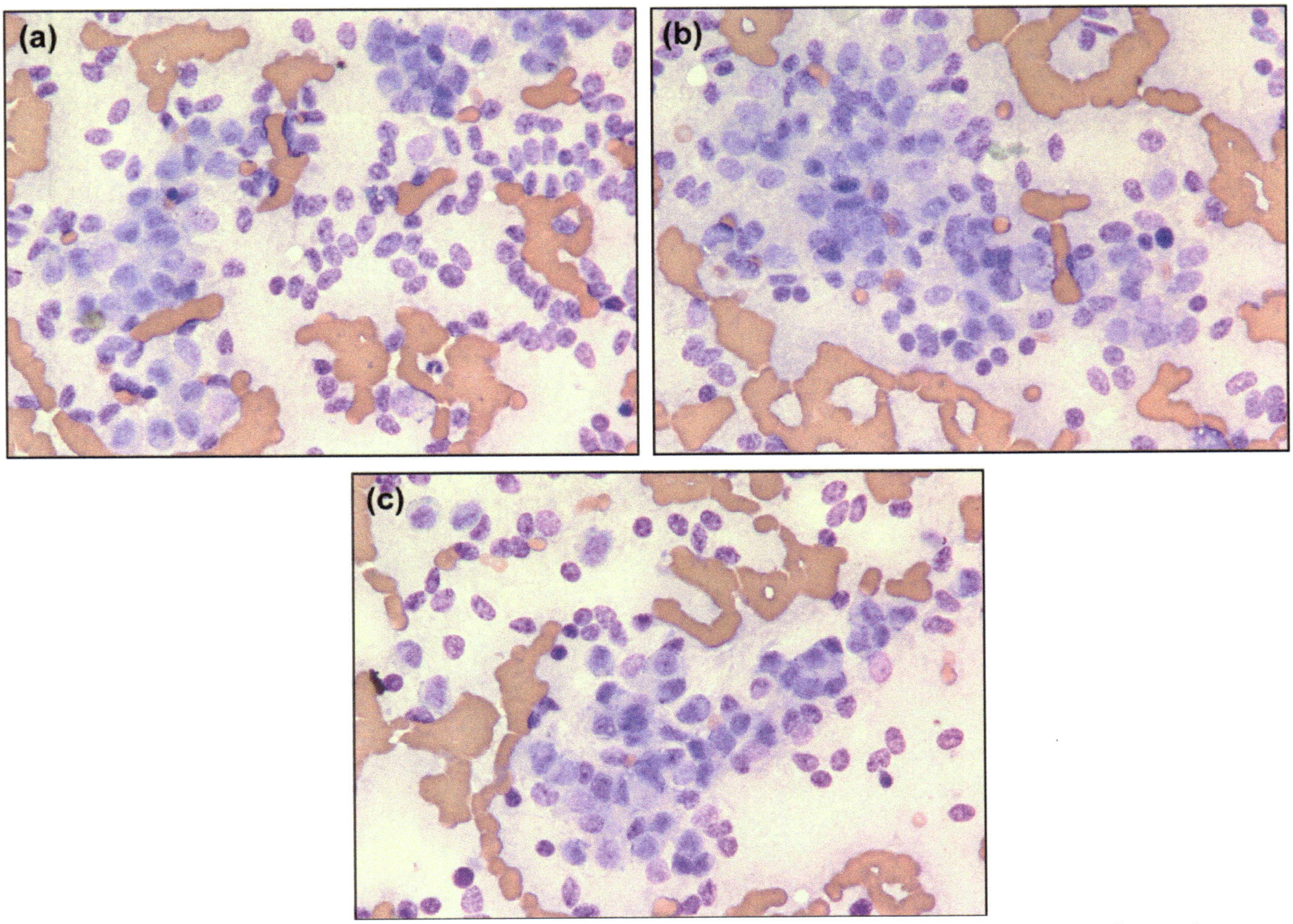

Figures 16.7a–c **Insulinoma. Aspirates of an insulinoma confirmed on histopathology. Note the classic bare nuclei appearance and minimal anisocytosis (Wright–Giemsa, 500× magnification).**

Aortic body tumors appear as a single mass or multilobulated lesion at the base of the heart (~90%) and are less likely to be of mediastinal or sternal/hilar lymph node origin (~10%) (Brown *et al.*, 2003). They may cause clinical signs associated with cardiac compromise and, less likely, respiratory signs associated with deviation/compression of the trachea. In dogs, aortic body adenomas are more common than carcinomas, and criteria for differentiation include tumor size and infiltrative behavior.

Carotid body tumors occur at or near the bifurcation of the common carotid artery, leading to a mass in the cranial cervical or retropharyngeal region. These lesions usually occur in older dogs, with a median age of 10 years (Obradovich *et al.*, 1992). As with aortic body tumors, the distinction between an adenoma and a carcinoma is based on tumor size and local infiltration. Metastasis is common in carotid body carcinomas (up to one-third of cases), and occurs most frequently to the lungs, kidneys, liver, pancreas, and tracheobronchial and mediastinal lymph nodes (La Perle, 2011). A case of metastasis to the submucosal area near the pharynx has also been described in the dog (Hardcastle *et al.*, 2013).

Cytologically, chemodectomas often appear as large numbers of nuclei on a background of basophilic cytoplasm with rare intact cells seen (Figures 16.8a–d). The cells appear to have a small to moderate amount of lightly basophilic cytoplasm with rare punctate cytoplasmic vacuoles and a round, variably placed nucleus. The nuclei have finely stippled to ropey chromatin and one to three small nucleoli. Anisocytosis and anisokaryosis are often mild or, rarely, moderate (Hardcastle *et al.*, 2013). Low numbers of spindle-shaped mesenchymal cells may also be seen. This population exhibits minimal anisocytosis and anisokaryosis. The cells have a small amount of basophilic cytoplasm and an elongate, central nucleus. The nuclei have finely stippled chromatin and inconspicuous nucleoli. Rarely, a small to abundant amount of extracellular, pink, fibrillar matrix may be identified, which may lead to a misdiagnosis of ectopic thyroid tissue or thyroid neoplasia (see Figure 16.5b). Immunochemical stains that may be helpful to confirm the diagnosis of an aortic or carotid body tumor in the dog and cat include neuron-specific enolase, synaptophysin, S-100, and chromogranin A (Brown *et al.*, 2003; Paltrinieri *et al.*, 2004; Aresu *et al.*, 2006). Neuron-specific enolase

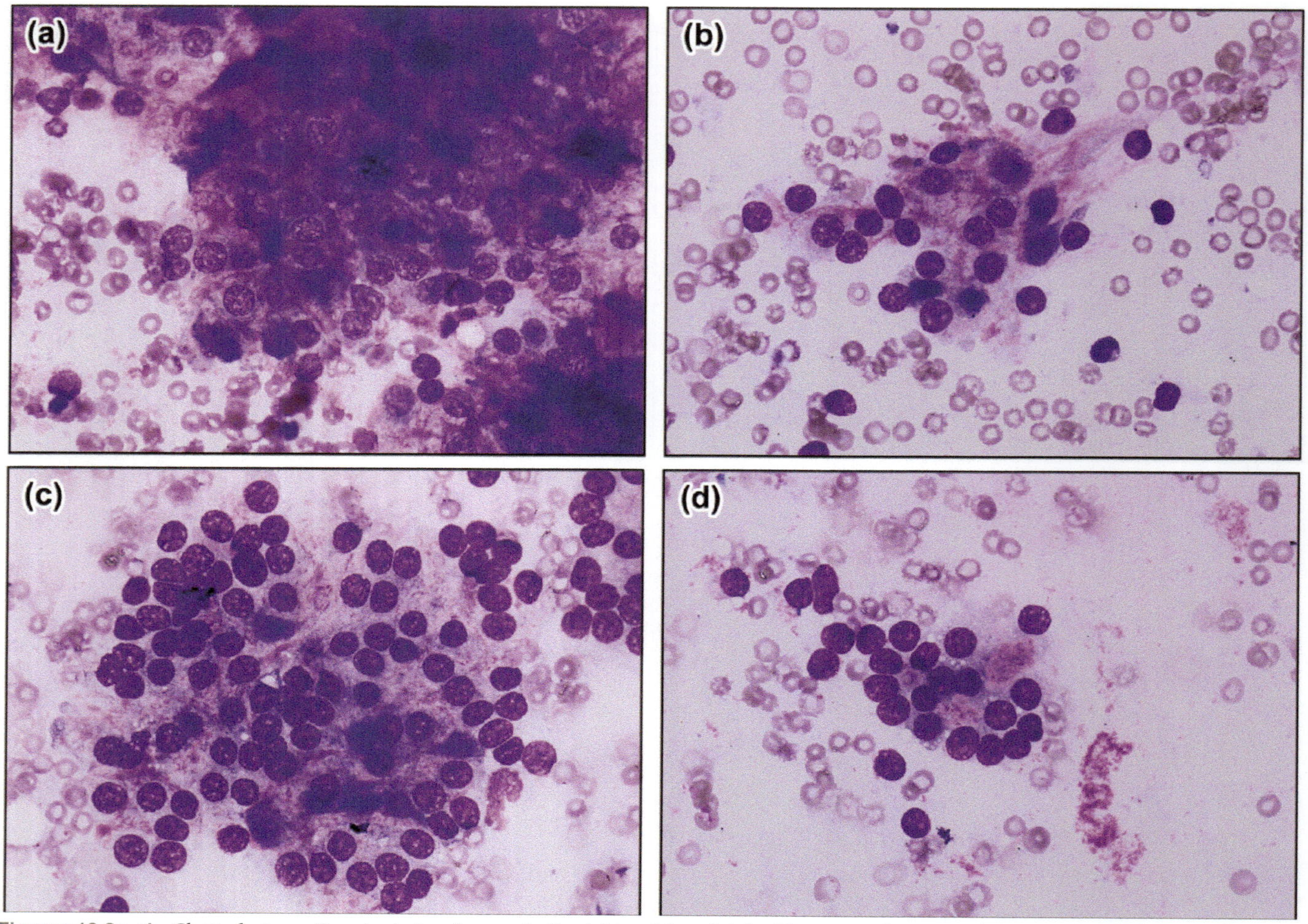

Figures 16.8a–d **Chemodectoma. Dog. Aspirates of a mass in the right auricle and right side aortic arch. Histopathology confirmed chemodectoma (Wright–Giemsa, 1,000× magnification).**

and synaptophysin staining was not found to correlate with histologic grade, but chromogranin A and S-100 staining intensity and density were found to decrease with increasing tumor grade (Brown *et al.*, 2003; Aresu *et al.*, 2006).

ADRENAL GLAND

Normal adrenal gland

The adrenal gland is divided into two distinct regions, which appear cytologically different. The adrenal cortex is comprised of the zona glomerulosa, zona fasciculata, and zona reticularis. Cells of this layer are derived from coelomic epithelium during development, which may be the reason for increased numbers of intact cells on cytology compared with other endocrine organs (La Perle, 2011). Distinction between the layers is not possible on cytology. Normal adrenal cortex cells will appear as large numbers of cell-free nuclei on a background of lightly basophilic cytoplasm with many distinct lipid vacuoles (Figures 16.9a–c). Intact cells have a moderate to low N:C ratio. The nuclei are round, variably placed, and have coarse chromatin and a single, small nucleolus.

Adrenal medullary cells have a classic endocrine appearance as they are derived from ectoderm of the neural crest (La Perle, 2011). Normal adrenal medulla will be highly cellular and contain cell-free nuclei on a background of basophilic cytoplasm. Intact cells have a high to moderate N:C ratio and a round, central nucleus. The nuclei have finely stippled chromatin and inconspicuous nucleoli.

Adrenal gland inflammation

Inflammation within either portion of the adrenal gland has not been previously described cytologically. Pathologically, the adrenal cortex is a common place for inflammation during systemic infections (Miller, 2017). Adrenal gland abscessation has been reported in the dog (Vuong & Aoki, 2021). Lymphoplasmacytic inflammation has been documented in the adrenal glands of dogs and cats with

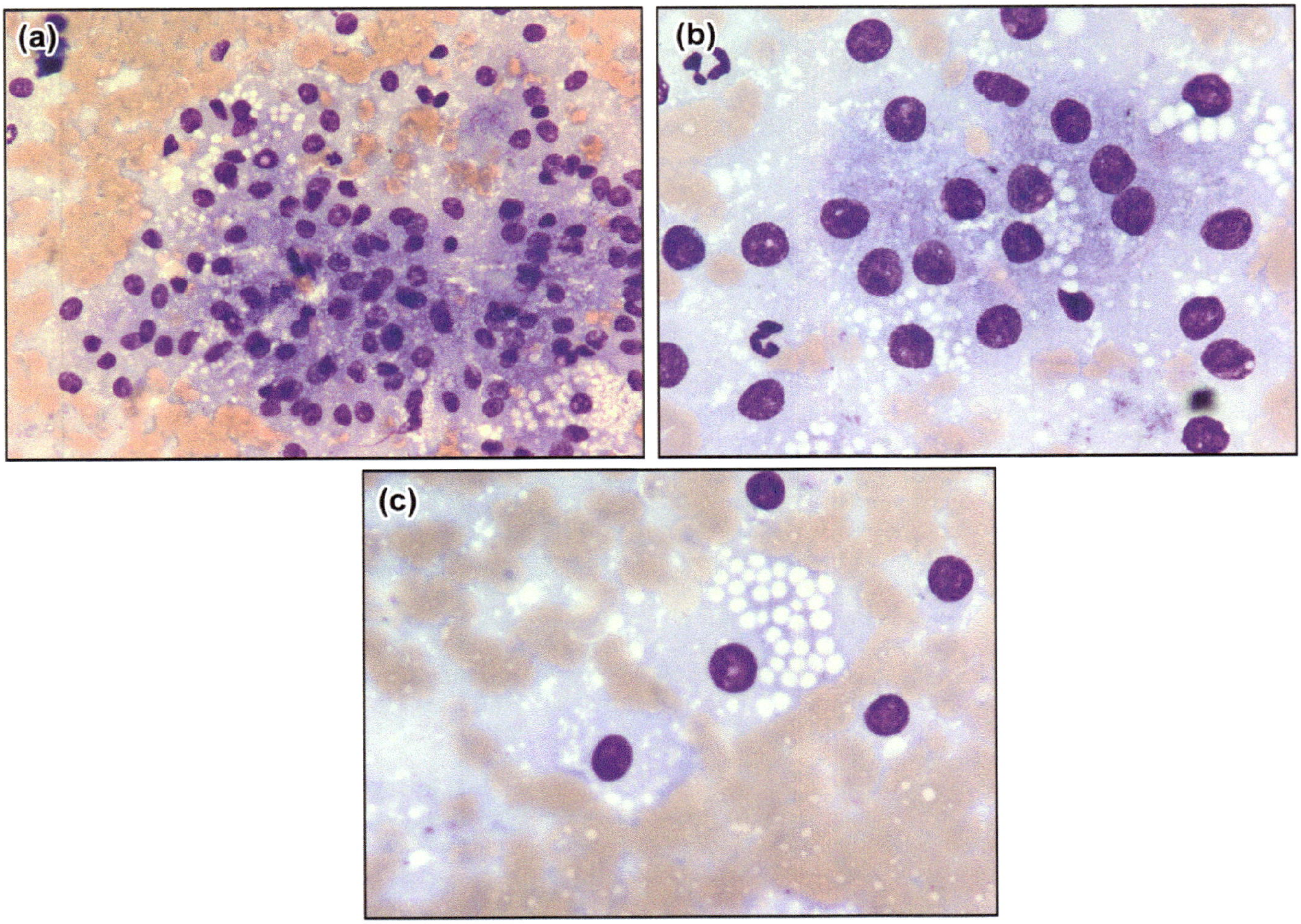

Figures 16.9a–c **Normal adrenal cortex. Impression smears of normal adrenal cortex. Note the distinct cytoplasmic vacuoles in many cells, consistent with lipid (Wright–Giemsa: a, 500× magnification; b and c, 1,000× magnification).**

hypoadrenocorticism, with the inflammatory response thought to represent autoimmune disease (Friedenberg *et al.*, 2018; Roberts & Dobromylskyj, 2022).

ADRENAL GLAND NEOPLASIA

Hyperplastic and neoplastic lesions that may lead to enlargement of the adrenal glands and sampling for cytology may occur in the adrenal cortex or adrenal medulla. These lesions are often not palpated but are discovered during ultrasonography after patients are presented for clinical signs associated with hyperadrenocorticism or, less likely, clinical signs associated with hyperaldosteronism, hyperestrogenemia, or pheochromocytomas. A retrospective study of dogs undergoing abdominal computed tomography showed 9.3% of dogs had incidental adrenal gland masses (Baum *et al.*, 2016). Cytologic ability to differentiate adrenocortical neoplasia and pheochromocytoma has been found to have a high specificity and sensitivity (Bertazzolo *et al.*, 2014), but differentiation between benign and malignant lesions is difficult. Fine-needle aspiration of the adrenal gland is a relatively safe procedure with a rare incidence of complications (Sumner *et al.*, 2018; Pey *et al.*, 2020). Hyperadrenocorticism may be suspected in dogs and cats that present for polyuria/polydipsia, polyphagia, a pot-bellied appearance, and poor hair coat, which are all secondary to increased glucocorticoid production. Clinical laboratory testing often shows no changes on the complete blood count, common serum biochemistry changes (hyperglycemia, increased alkaline phosphatase), and likely decreased urine specific gravity. Approximately 80–100% of cats with hyperadrenocorticism also have diabetes mellitus, which is often the initial diagnosis. Concurrent hyperadrenocorticism should be further investigated in cats for which large doses of insulin do not lead to control of clinical signs of diabetes mellitus (Waters Scott-Moncrieff, 2002). Since adrenal lesions in cats more commonly cause hyperaldosteronism, clinical signs may involve muscle weakness, plantigrade stance, problems jumping, and neck ventroflexion secondary to hypokalemia or signs of hypertension such as blindness due to retinal detachment or intraocular hemorrhage (Kooistra, 2020). At this point, advanced diagnostic testing, including dexamethasone suppression tests, adrenocorticotropic hormone (ACTH) stimulation test, and abdominal ultrasound, may be performed. There are two main causes for hyperadrenocorticism: a functional pituitary adenoma and a functional adrenal gland neoplasm of the adrenal cortex, located primarily in the zona fasciculata. A pituitary adenoma would lead to bilateral enlargement of the adrenal cortices secondary to continuous stimulation by ACTH. These types of lesions are often measured via ultrasonography but not sampled for cytology.

Functional adrenal neoplasia only accounts for a small number of cases of hyperadrenocorticism (10–15%) in the dog (La Perle, 2011), with nonfunctional adrenal tumors and adrenal tumors that produce aldosterone also reported (Renschler & Dean, 2009). Functional adrenal tumors in cats typically produce aldosterone with those that produce cortisol or sex hormones (Guerios *et al.*, 2015; Nadolski *et al.*, 2016; Griffin, 2021) also possible. The median age for diagnosis of adrenal tumors is around 10.5–12 years in the dog (Labelle *et al.*, 2004; Arenas *et al.*, 2013). Adenomas are more frequent than carcinomas in dogs and often occur as single unilateral nodules (Miller, 2017). The literature on whether adenomas or carcinomas are more frequent in cats is conflicting (Daniel *et al.*, 2016; Boland & Barrs, 2017) with adrenal neoplasia being extremely uncommon in cats (Griffin, 2021). Carcinomas are usually larger than adenomas and may be bilateral. The criteria that may be helpful to diagnose an adrenal carcinoma are tumor size >2 cm, increased cellular pleomorphism, hemorrhage, necrosis, capsular invasion, surrounding structure invasion, and vascular invasion (Labelle *et al.*, 2004).

If an adrenal mass is noted, cytologic findings that would indicate adrenal cortical origin include a variable number of cell-free nuclei on a light purple background with a moderate amount of cell-free lipid. Increased numbers of intact cells are noted compared with other endocrine neoplasms. The cells have a low to moderate N:C ratio and exhibit mild to rarely moderate anisocytosis and anisokaryosis. The cells have a moderate to abundant amount of lightly basophilic cytoplasm with variable numbers of punctate cytoplasmic vacuoles and a round, variably placed nucleus. The nuclei have coarse chromatin and a single small nucleolus. Adrenocortical carcinomas may show slightly more atypia, but well-differentiated lesions are also possible. The most common locations for metastasis of adrenocortical carcinoma are the liver and lungs (Labelle *et al.*, 2004).

Adrenal medullary lesions are often due to benign or malignant neoplastic proliferations of chromaffin cells, which are termed pheochromocytomas. Median age for occurrence of these tumors in dogs is 10.5 years, there is no breed or sex predilection, and approximately 50–60% are an incidental finding (Gilson *et al.*, 1994; Barthez *et al.*, 1997). Clinical signs suggestive of a functional pheochromocytoma are related to increased release of catecholamines (norepinephrine, epinephrine), leading to tachycardia, hypertension, and possibly neurologic abnormalities. The most common presenting complaints for dogs with a definitive diagnosis of pheochromocytoma include weakness/lethargy, polyuria/polydipsia, collapse, and vomiting; however, these findings may or may not be directly related to the tumor, as up to 50% of dogs have concurrent neoplasms (Barthez *et al.*, 1997). Pheochromocytomas may also produce clinical signs secondary to a large, space-occupying mass in approximately 10% of cases including ascites, limb edema, abdominal pain, abdominal distension, and a palpable abdominal mass (Barthez *et al.*, 1997). Measurement of plasma-free metanephrines, free metanephrine, and free normetanephrine may be appropriate, noninvasive diagnostic tests to help with the diagnosis of pheochromocytoma as well as the measurement of urine metanephrines (Gostelow *et al.*, 2013; Salesov *et al.*, 2015).

Adrenal medullary lesions are often large (>10 cm) single masses that may compress or completely replace the surrounding adrenal cortex (La Perle, 2011). Rare bilateral lesions are reported (Barthez *et al.*, 1997). Criteria for diagnosis of malignant lesions are the same as those for carcinoma in other endocrine tumors (capsular and vascular invasion). The incidence of locally invasive lesions is reported as 39–50%, and metastasis is reported in 13–28% of cases (Gilson *et al.*, 1994; Barthez *et al.*, 1997). Previously reported metastatic sites in the dog include the liver, lungs, regional and distant lymph nodes, spleen, kidney, prostate, bone, pancreas, peritoneum, spinal canal, brain, caudal vena cava, heart, and jejunum (Gilson *et al.*, 1994; Barthez *et al.*, 1997; Boes *et al.*, 2009b; Machida Machida, 2020; Gregor *et al.*, 2022). Cytologic findings include a highly cellular sample composed of sheets of rounded cells with poorly distinct cell borders and large numbers of cell-free nuclei (Figures 16.10a–d). The cells have a rarely moderate to high N:C ratio and exhibit mild to rarely moderate anisocytosis and anisokaryosis. The cells have a small to rarely moderate amount of lightly basophilic cytoplasm and a round, central nucleus. The nuclei have finely stippled to rarely reticular chromatin and occasionally a single small nucleolus. Immunocytochemical staining that may be beneficial to confirm the chromaffin origin of cells from an adrenal mass include chromogranin A and synaptophysin, although not all tumors may stain with both markers (Barthez *et al.*, 1997).

Other than tumors of the predominant cellular components of the adrenal gland, few reports of other primary lesions and metastatic lesions within the adrenal gland have been published. Additional primary adrenal gland neoplasms that have been previously described include myelolipomas (Tursi *et al.*, 2005), neuroblastomas (Marcotte *et al.*, 2004; Mestrinho et al., 2019), lymphoma (Romine *et al.*, 2016) malignant peripheral nerve sheath tumor (Ichikawa *et al.*, 2018), and ganglioneuromas (Miller, 2017). The rate of metastasis to the adrenal gland in the dog has been documented as 21% and in the cat as 14.8% (Labelle De Cock, 2005). In terms of metastatic lesions accounting for adrenal tumors, they make up 26.7% of adrenal tumors in the dog and 60% in the cat (Labelle De Cock, 2005). The metastatic lesions are bilateral in approximately 50% of cases in dogs and cats (Labelle De Cock, 2005).

CARCINOIDS (NEUROENDOCRINE CARCINOMA)

Carcinoids are tumors of neuroendocrine cell origin that arise in multiple places throughout the body. They arise from enterochromaffin cells, which are present in the gastrointestinal (GI) tract, tracheobronchial tree, pancreatic ducts, biliary tree, and genitourinary tract (Giles *et al.*, 1974). In the GI tract, neuroendocrine cells are scattered throughout the mucosa and are normally responsible for the production of digestive hormones including secretin, somatostatin, and cholecystokinin, or they produce serotonin as part of the amine precursor

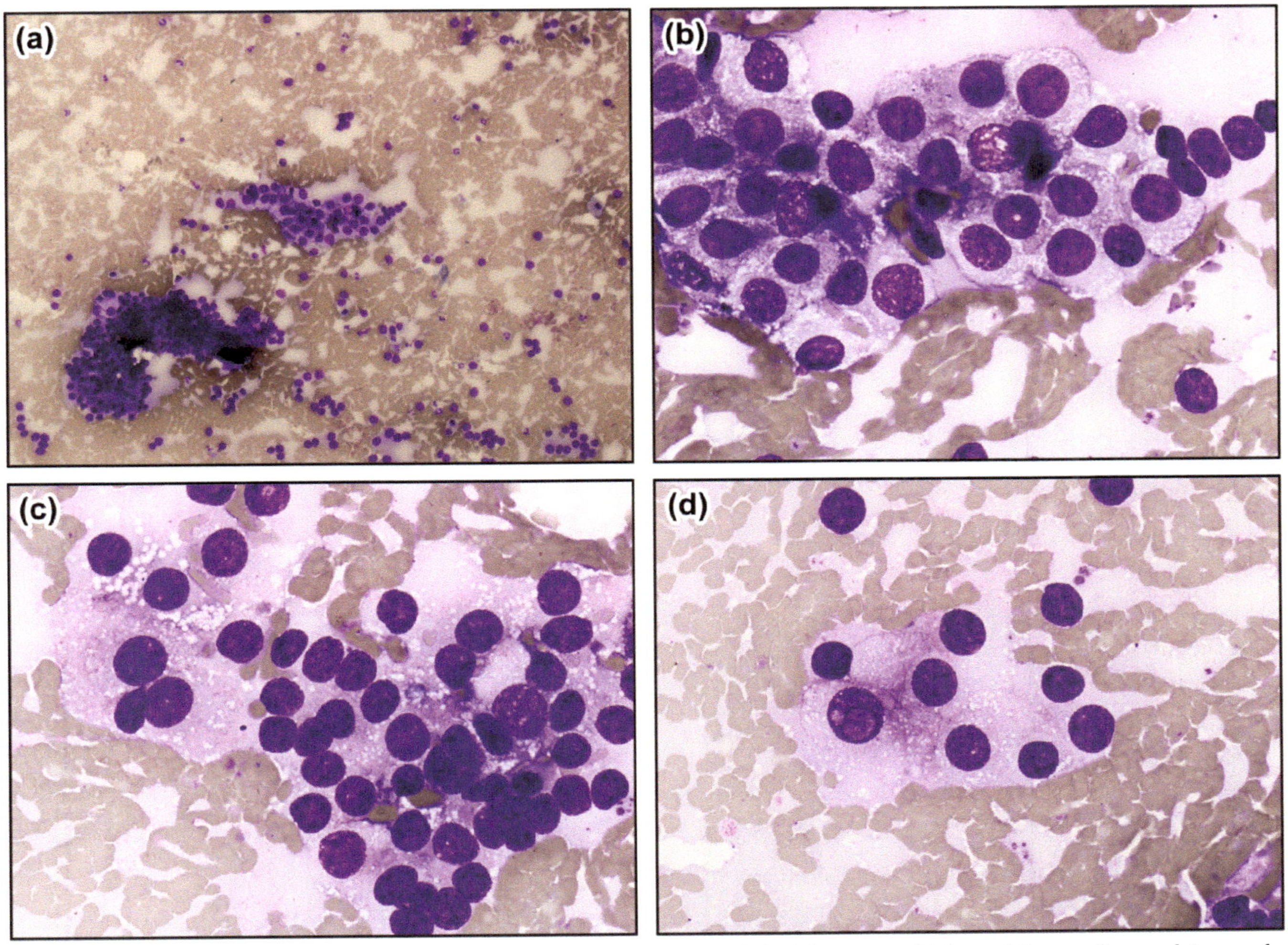

Figures 16.10a–d **Adrenal medullary mass. Cat. Aspirates of a mass in the left adrenal gland that measured 2.6 cm × 2.5 cm on ultrasound. Increased levels of normetanephrine and metanephrine were documented (Wright–Giemsa: a, 100× magnification; b–d, 1,000× magnification).**

uptake decarboxylation (APUD) group (Uzal *et al.*, 2015). Neoplasms due to these cells are seen most commonly in the dog but have also been described in the cat; however, these are uncommon tumors in both species. GI carcinoids in dogs and cats have been described in the stomach, duodenum, jejunum, ileocecal junction, cecocolic junction, colon, and rectum (Giles *et al.*, 1974; Patnaik *et al.*, 1980a; Patnaik Lieberman, 1981; Sykes Cooper, 1982; Rossmeisl et al., 2002; Sako et al., 2003). Rectal carcinoids are occasionally seen as pedunculated lesions protruding from the rectum or anus, so they may be visualized during a physical examination or palpated during a rectal examination (Sykes Cooper, 1982). Metastatic lesions from GI carcinoids have been documented in the liver, lungs, heart, trachea, tonsils, pancreas, and mesenteric lymph nodes (Giles *et al.*, 1974; Patnaik et al., 1980; Sako et al., 2003). Carcinoids in dogs and cats have also been described in the pancreas (Carakostas et al., 1979; Michishita *et al.*, 2017) and in the gallbladder of dogs (O'Brien *et al.*, 2021).

Liver carcinoids make up approximately 13–14% of primary liver neoplasms in the dog. These lesions are often diffuse in dogs and cats, affecting multiple liver lobes, and >70% occur in dogs under 10 years of age (Patnaik *et al.*, 1980; Patnaik, 1992). Metastasis is reported in up to 93% of cases of hepatocellular carcinoid. When these lesions are found to have metastasized, the most common locations are the abdominal lymph nodes and peritoneum (Patnaik *et al.*, 1980). Liver carcinoids have also been described in cats but with very low frequency (Patnaik, 1992; Meachem *et al.*, 2016). Extrahepatic biliary carcinoids have also been described in dogs and cats (Patnaik, 1992; Morrell *et al.*, 2002).

Another location for carcinoid formation is the lungs, with rare canine reports available in the literature (Soo Choi *et al.*, 2008) and a multi-institutional study showing these tumors make up 1.5% of primary lung tumors in dogs (McPhetridge *et al.*, 2022). The most recent of these reports described cytologic findings that included large numbers of cell-free nuclei on a pale, basophilic background with a low number of intact, rounded cells (Figures 16.11a, b). The intact cells exhibit mild to rarely moderate anisocytosis, anisokaryosis, and variability in N:C ratio. The cells have a small to rarely moderate amount of lightly

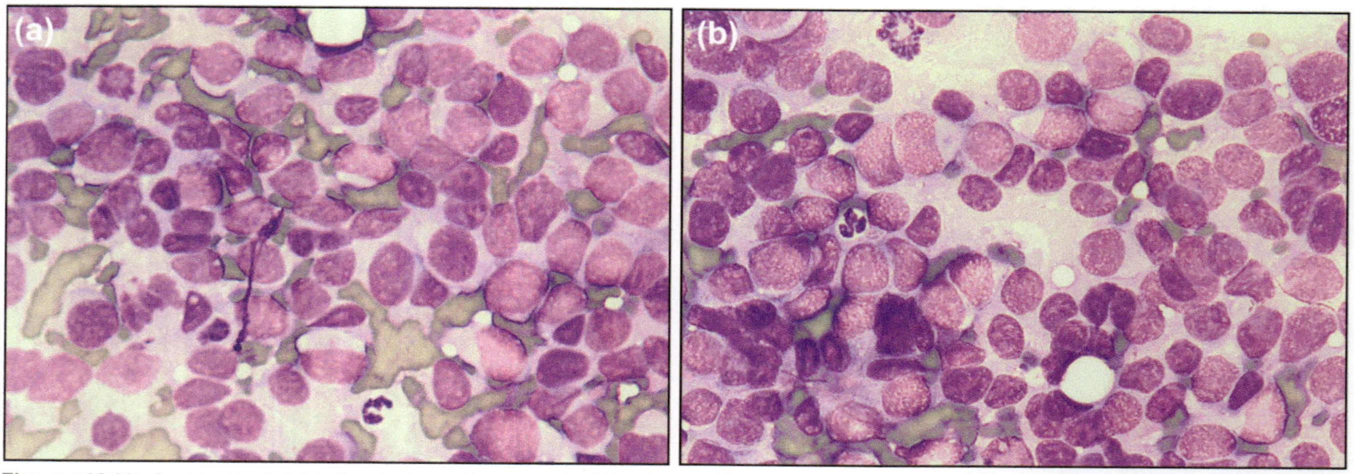

Figures 16.11a, b **Carcinoid. Note the classic poorly preserved cell borders, mild anisocytosis and anisokaryosis, and the high nuclear to cytoplasmic ratio of the cells (Wright–Giemsa, 700× magnification).**

basophilic cytoplasm and a round, variably placed nucleus. The nuclei have finely stippled to reticular chromatin and inconspicuous nucleoli. In this report, the intact cells rarely had low numbers of small, basophilic cytoplasmic granules and a small amount of eosinophilic extracellular and intracellular material was noted (Soo Choi *et al.*, 2008).

Neuroendocrine carcinomas have also been described in the perianal region in a cat (Joudrey *et al.*, 2015), mammary gland of dogs (Nakahira *et al.*, 2015; Nakagaki *et al.*, 2021, 2022), kidney of a dog (Sozmen *et al.*, 2020), and frontal sinus in a dog (Baek *et al.*, 2019). Occasionally, neuroendocrine carcinomas are productive leading to clinical signs consistent with the overproduction of the associated hormone including a gastrinoma in a cat (Lane *et al.*, 2016) and an ACTH producing sinusoidal neuroendocrine tumor in a dog (Baek *et al.*, 2019).

Once histologic sections have been obtained, staining with specific silver stains to confirm the presence of argyrophil granules and/or argentaffin granules may be beneficial to obtain the diagnosis (Giles *et al.*, 1974). Basic neuroendocrine markers, nonspecific enolase, chromogranin A, and synaptophysin may also be helpful (Patnaik, 1992; Sako *et al.*, 2003; Soo Choi *et al.*, 2008).

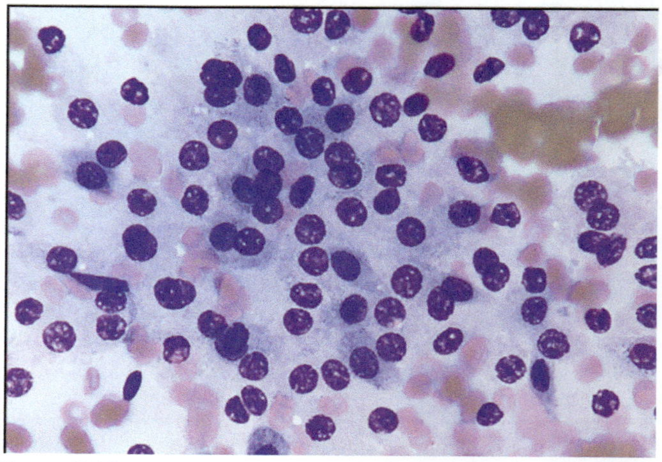

Figure 16.12 **Aspirate from the ventral neck mass. A cluster of neoplastic epithelial cells is present with indistinct cytoplasmic borders. The overall cell population is fairly uniform with only mild anisokaryosis (Wright–Giemsa, 700× magnification).**

CASES

CASE 1

Signalment/history

A 10-year-old, spayed female mixed-breed dog presented with a palpable ventral neck mass.

Cytology

The mass was aspirated. The sample was markedly hemodiluted. Clusters of neoplastic epithelial cells were observed. These cells were round with a moderate amount of basophilic cytoplasm and indistinct cell borders (Figure 16.12). The nuclei were round with coarsely stippled chromatin pattern and small but prominent nucleoli. A few cells contained pigmented granular material within the cytoplasm (Figure 16.13). Cytologically, this sample was consistent with thyroid neoplasia. Although the cells do not exhibit many criteria of malignancy, thyroid carcinoma is likely.

Management

The mass was surgically excised and diagnosed as a thyroid carcinoma.

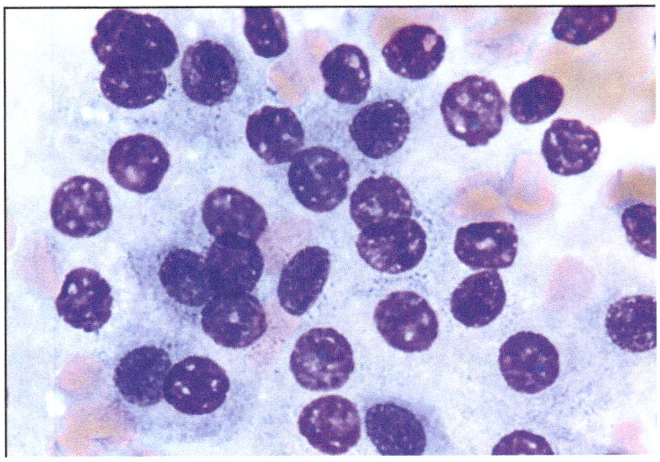

Figure 16.13 Occasionally, cells contained a few basophilic granular structures within the cytoplasm (Wright–Giemsa, 1,500× magnification).

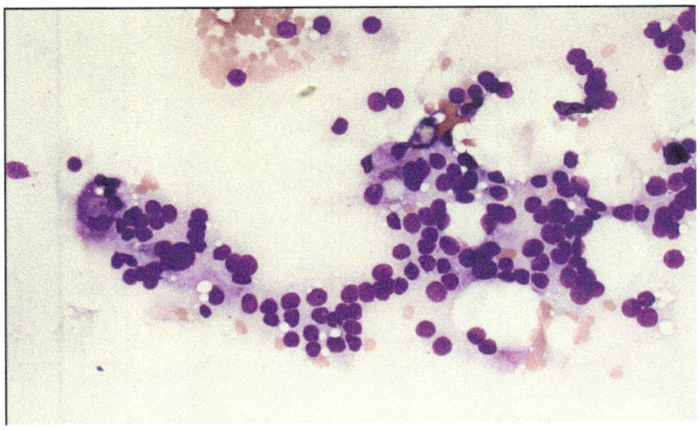

Figure 16.14 Aspirate from an intraluminal gallbladder mass. A loosely cohesive sheet of neoplastic cells is present with indistinct cell borders and mild anisokaryosis (Wright–Giemsa, 500× magnification, courtesy of Dr. Michael Rosser and Dr. Taylor Hanson).

CASE 2

Signalment/history

A 6-year-old, male castrated English Bulldog presented for a suspected gallbladder mucocele. The dog had a three-week history of intermittent anorexia, vomiting, and melena. The referring veterinarian identified a gallbladder mass on abdominal ultrasound.

Cytology

The mass was aspirated. The smears were very low in nucleated cellularity with mild to moderate blood contamination. One smear was moderately cellular and contained several cohesive sheets of cells with poorly distinct cell borders and mild to rarely moderate anisokaryosis. The nuclei were round with lacy chromatin and inconspicuous nucleoli. The cells have a moderate amount of basophilic cytoplasm (Figure 16.14).

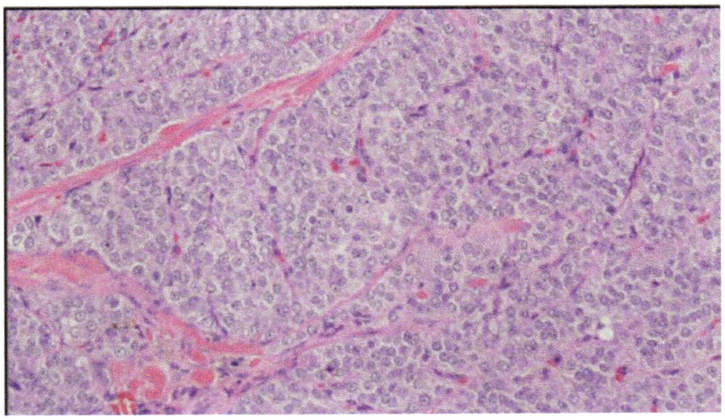

Figure 16.15 Histopathology of a gallbladder mass. The cells are arranged in nests, packets, and sheets and show mild anisocytosis and anisokaryosis (hematoxylin and eosin, 100× magnification, courtesy of Dr. Patrick Roady).

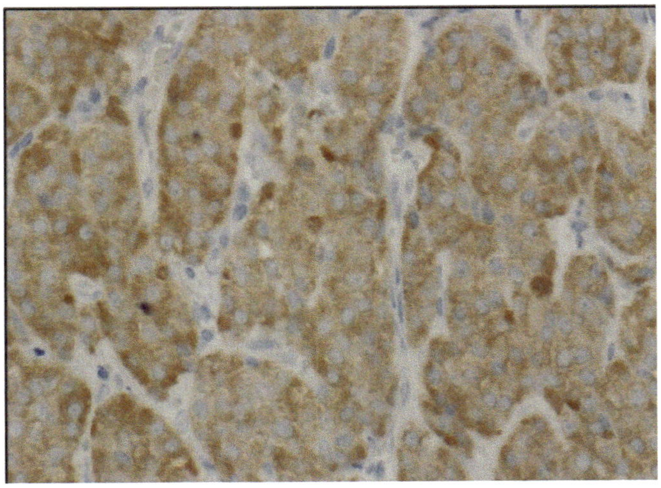

Figure 16.16 Histopathology of a gallbladder mass. The cells label positive for synaptophysin which is indicative of neuroendocrine origin (HRP polymer mouse monoclonal antibody with DAB chromogen and hematoxylin counter stain, 400× magnification, courtesy of Dr. Patrick Roady).

Management

The patient underwent surgery, and the entire gallbladder was removed and submitted for histopathology. Histopathologic evaluation showed an unencapsulated and invasive mass expanding and effacing the gallbladder submucosa. The mass was composed of cells in nests, packets, and sheets suggestive of an epithelial tumor (Figure 16.15). Additional immunostaining was performed with synaptophysin, which was positive (Figure 16.16), and cytokeratin, which was negative. These results indicated a neuroendocrine carcinoma.

REFERENCES

Almes K.M., Heaney A.M., Andrews G.A. (2008) Intracardiac ectopic thyroid carcinosarcoma in a dog. *Vet Pathol* 45:500–504.

Arenas C., Pérez-Alenza D., Melián C. (2013) Clinical features, outcome and prognostic factors in dogs diagnosed with non-cortisol-secreting adrenal tumours without adrenalectomy: 20 cases (1994–2009). *Vet Rec 173*:501.

Aresu L., Tursi M., Iussich S. et al. (2006) Use of S-100 and chromogranin A antibodies as immunohistochemical markers on detection of malignancy in aortic body tumors in dogs. *J Vet Med Sci 68*:1229–1233.

Baek Y., Ang M.J., Park J. et al. (2019) Canine adrenocorticotrophic hormone-producing sinusoidal neuroendocrine tumor associated with Cushing's disease. *J Vet Med Sci 81*:1863–1867.

Barthez P.Y., Marks S.L., Woo J. et al. (1997) Pheochromocytomas in dogs: 61 cases (1984–1995). *J Vet Intern Med 11*:272–278.

Baum J.I., Boston S.E., Case J.B. (2016) Prevalence of adrenal gland masses as incidental findings during abdominal computed tomography in dogs: 270 cases (2013–2014). *J Am Vet Med Assoc 249*:1165–1169.

Berger B., Feldman E.C. (1987) Primary hyperparathyroidism in dogs: 21 cases (1976–1986). *J Am Vet Med Assoc 191*:350–356.

Bertazzolo W., Didier M., Gelain M.E. et al. (2014) Accuracy of cytology in distinguishing adrenocortical tumors from pheochromocytoma in companion animals. *Vet Clin Pathol 43*:453–459.

Bertolini G., Drigo M., Angeloni L. et al. (2017) Incidental and nonincidental canine thyroid tumors assessed by multidetector row computed tomography: A single-centre cross sectional study in 4520 dogs. *Vet Radiol Ultrasoun 58*:304–314.

Boes K., Messick J., Green H. et al. (2009a) What is your diagnosis? Impression smear from an intracardiac mass in a dog. *Vet Clin Pathol 39*:119–120.

Boes K., Zimmerman K., Saunders G. et al. (2009b) What is your diagnosis? Shoulder mass in a dog with lameness. *Vet Clin Pathol 38*:511–515.

Boland L.A., Barrs V.R. (2017) Peculiarities of feline hyperadrenocorticism update on diagnosis and treatment. *J Feline Med Surg 19*:933–947.

Broome M.R., Peterson M.E., Walker J.R. (2014) Clinical features and treatment outcomes of 41 dogs with sublingual ectopic thyroid neoplasia. *J Vet Intern Med 28*:1560–1568.

Brown P.J., Rema A., Gartner F. (2003) Immunohistochemical characteristics of canine aortic and carotid body tumours. *J Am Vet Med Assoc 50*:140–144.

Buergelt C.D., Das K.M. (1968) Aortic body tumor in a cat: A case report. *Vet Pathol 5*:84–90.

Buishand F.O. (2022) Current trends in diagnosis, treatment and prognosis of canine insulinoma. *Vet Sci 9*:540.

Burti S., Zotti A., Rubini G. et al. (2022) Contrast-enhanced ultrasound findings of focal pancreatic lesions in dogs. *Vet Rec 191*:e2080.

Campos M., Ducatelle R., Rutteman et al. (2014) Clinical, pathologic, and immunohistochemical prognostic factors in dogs with thyroid carcinoma. *J Vet Intern Med 28*(6):1805–1813.

Carakostas M.C., Kennedy G.A., Kittleson M.D. et al. (1979) Malignant foregut carcinoid tumor in a domestic cat. *Vet Pathol 16*:607–609.

Cavana P., Vittone V., Capucchio M.T. et al. (2006) Parathyroid adenocarcinoma in a nephropathic Persian cat. *J Feline Med Surg 8*:340–344.

Caywood D.D., Wilson J.W., Hardy R.M. et al. (1988) Pancreatic insulin-secreting neoplasms: Clinical, diagnostic, and prognostic features in 73 dogs. *J Am Anim Hosp Assoc 24*:577–584.

Cervone M., Harel M., Ségard-Weisse E. et al. (2019) Use of contrast-enhanced ultrasonography for the detecting of a feline insulinoma. *J Feline Med Surg Open Rep*:1–7.

Ciaputa R., Nowak M., Kandefer-Gola M. et al. (2014) Morphological and immunohistochemical characteristics of follicular-compact thyroid carcinoma in dog. *Folia Histochem Cyto 52*:157–161.

Coady M., Fletcher D.J., Goggs R. (2019) Severity of ionized hypercalcemia and hypocalcemia is associated with etiology in dogs and cats. *Front Vet Sci 6*:276.

Cook M.R., Gasparini M., Cianciolo R.E. et al. (2022) Clinical outcomes of thyroid tumours with concurrent epithelial and mesenchymal components in 14 dogs (2006–2020). *Vet Med Sci 8*:509–516.

Daniel G., Mahony O.M., Markovich J.E. et al. (2016) Clinical findings, diagnostics and outcome in 33 cats with adrenal neoplasia (2002–2013). *J Feline Med Surg 18*:77–84.

Erickson A.K., Regier P.J., Watt M.M. et al. (2021) Incidence, survival time, and surgical treatment of parathyroid carcinomas in dogs: 100 cases (2010–2019). *J Am Vet Med Assoc 259*:1309–1317.

Feldman E.C., Hoar B., Pollard R. et al. (2005) Pretreatment clinical and laboratory findings in dogs with primary hyperparathyroidism: 210 cases (1987–2004). *J Am Vet Med Assoc 227*:756–761.

Friedenberg S.G., Brown D.L., Meurs K.M. et al. (2018) Lymphocyte subsets in the adrenal glands of dogs with primary hypoadrenocorticism. *Vet Pathol 55*:177–181.

Galgano M., Spalla I., Callegari C. et al. (2014) Primary hypothyroidism and thyroid goiter in an adult cat. *J Vet Intern Med 28*:682–686.

Gear R.N.A., Neiger R., Skelly B.J.S. et al. (2005) Primary hyperparathyroidism in 29 dogs: Diagnosis, treatment, outcome and associated renal failure. *J Small Anim Pract 46*:10–16.

Giannasi C., Rushton S., Rook A. et al. (2021) Canine thyroid carcinoma prognosis following the utilisation of computed tomography assisted staging. *Vet Rec* e55. 189(1): e55.

Gifford C.H., Morris A.P., Kenney K.J. et al. (2020) Diagnosis of insulinoma in a Maine Coon cat. *J Feline Med Surg Open Rep*:1–10.

Giles R.C., Hildebrandt P.K., Montgomery C.A. (1974) Carcinoid tumor in the small intestines of a dog. *Vet Pathol 11*:340–349.

Gilson S.D., Withrow S.J., Wheeler S.L. et al. (1994) Pheochromocytoma in 50 dogs. *J Vet Intern Med 8*:228–232.

Gostelow R., Bridger N., Syme H.M. (2013) Plasma-free metanephrine and free normetanephrine measurement for the diagnosis of pheochromocytoma in dogs. *J Vet Intern Med 27*:83–90.

Gregor K.M., Knebel A., Haverkamp A. et al. (2022) Metastatic canine phaeochromocytoma with unusual manifestation. *J Comp Path 192*:33–40.

Griffin S. (2021) Feline abdominal ultrasonography: What's normal? What's abnormal The adrenal glands. *J Feline Med Surg 23*:33–49.

Grubor B., Haynes J.S. (2005) Thyroid carcinosarcoma in a dog. *Vet Pathol 42*:84–87.

Guerios S.D., de Melo Souza C.H., Bacon N.J. (2015) Adrenocortical tumor in a cat secreting more than one type of corticosteroid. *J Feline Med Surg Open Rep*:1–5.

Hardcastle M.R., Meyer J., McSporran K.D. (2013) Pathology in practice. *J Am Vet Med Assoc 242*:175–177.

Hawkins K.L., Summers B.A., Kuhajda F.P. et al. (1987) Immunocytochemistry of normal pancreatic islets and spontaneous islet cell tumors in dogs. *Vet Pathol 24*:170–179.

Hayes H.M., Sass B. (1988) Chemoreceptor neoplasia: A study of the epidemiological features of 357 canine cases. *J Vet Med Series A 35*:401–408.

Hofmeister E., Kippenes H., Mealey K.L. et al. (2001) Functional cystic thyroid adenoma in a cat. *J Am Vet Med Assoc 219*:190–193.

Ichikawa M., Suzuki S., Tei M. et al. (2018) Malignant peripheral nerve sheath tumor originating from the adrenal gland in a dog. *J Vet Med Sci 80*:1572–1575.

Jackson T.C., Debey B., Lindbloom-Hawley S. et al. (2009) Cellular and molecular characterization of a feline insulinoma. *J Vet Intern Med 23*:383–387.

Janus I., Nowak M., Noszczyk-Nowak A. et al. (2016) Epidemiological and pathological features of primary cardiac tumors in dogs from Poland in 1970–2014. *Acta Vet Hung 64*:90–102.

Joudrey S.D., Robinson D.A., Blair R. et al (2015) Perianal neuroendocrine tumor with suspected lymph node metastasis causing colonic compression and subsequent megacolon. *Can Vet J 56*:240–244.

Kallet A.J., Richter K.P., Feldman E.C. et al. (1991) Primary hyperparathyroidism in cats: Seven cases (1984–1989). *J Am Vet Med Assoc 199*:1767–1771.

Kooistra H.S. (2020) Primary hyperaldosteronism in cats an underdiagnosed disorder. *Vet Clin North Am Small Anim Pract 50*:1053–1063.

La Perle K.M.D. (2011) Endocrine system. In: *Pathologic Basis of Veterinary Disease*, 5th edn. (eds. M.D. McGavin, J.F. Zachary) Mosby Elsevier, St. Louis, pp. 660–697.

Labelle P., De Cock H.E.V. (2005) Metastatic tumors to the adrenal glands in domestic animals. *Vet Pathol 42*:52–58.

Labelle P., Kyles A.E., Farver T.B. et al. (2004) Indicators of malignancy of canine adrenocortical tumors: Histopathology and proliferation index. *Vet Pathol 41*:490–497.

Lamoureux A., Fournet A., Hahn H.M. et al. (2019) Primary hyperparathyroidism due to cystic parathyroid adenoma in a cat. *Open Vet J 9*:109–113.

Lane M., Larson J., Hecht S. et al. (2016) Medical management of gastrinoma in a cat. *J Feline Med Surg Open Rep.* 2(1): 1–7.

Leav I., Schiller A.L., Rijnberk A. et al. (1976) Adenomas and carcinomas of the canine and feline thyroid. *Am J Pathol 83*:61–122.

Lurye J.C., Behrend E.N. (2001) Endocrine tumors. *Vet Clin North Am Small Anim Pract 31*:1083–1110.

Lyssens A., van den Berg M.F., Peremans K. et al. (2020) ^{131}treatment in dogs with hyperthyroidism cause by a non-resectable ectopic thyroid tumour: 5 cases (2008–2019). *J Small Anim Pract 62*:137–144.

Machida T., Machida N. (2020) Invasion of pheochromocytoma from the caudal vena cava to the right ventricular cavity in a dog. *Case Rep Vet Med 2020*:5382687.

Marcotte L., McConkey S.E., Hanna P. et al. (2004) Malignant adrenal neuroblastoma in a young dog. *Can Vet J 45*:773–776.

Maurin M., Davies D., Jahns H. et al. (2019) Non-functional thyroid cystadenoma in three boxer dogs. *BMC Vet Res 15*:228.

McPhetridge J.B., Scharf V.F., Regier P.J. et al. (2022) Distribution of histopathologic types of primary pulmonary neoplasia in dogs and outcome of affected dogs: 340 cases (2010–2019). *J Am Vet Med Assoc 260*:234–243.

Meachem M.D., Wobeser B.K. (2016) What's your diagnosis? Multiple hepatic masses in a cat. *Vet Clin Pathol 45*:509–510.

Mestrinho L.A., Marques M.I., Jesus S. et al. (2019) Surgical excision of an adrenal neuroblastoma in a dog. *Front Vet Sci 6*:161.

Michishita M., Takagi M., Kishimoto T.E. et al. (2017) Pancreatic neuroendocrine carcinoma with exocrine differentiation in a cat. *J Vet Diagn Invest 29*:325–330.

Miller M.A. (2017) Endocrine system. In: *Pathologic Basis of Veterinary Disease*, 6th edn. (ed. J.F. Zachary) Elsevier, St. Louis, pp. 682–723.

Miller M.L., Peterson M.E., Randolph J.F. et al. (2017) Thyroid cysts in cats: A retrospective study of 40 cases. *J Vet Intern Med 31*:723–729.

Morrell C.N., Volk M.V., Mankowski J.L. (2002) A carcinoid tumor in the gallbladder of a dog. *Vet Pathol 39*:756–758.

Naan E.C., Kirpensteijn J., Kooistra H.S. et al. (2006) Results of thyroidectomy in 101 cats with hyperthyroidism. *Vet Surg 35*:287–293.

Nadolski A.C., Markovich J.E., Jennings S.H. et al. (2016) Mammary development, hyperestrogenemia, and hypocortisolemia in a male cat with an adrenal cortical carcinoma. *Can Vet J 57*:1077–1080.

Nakahira R., Michishita M., Yoshimura H. et al. (2015) Neuroendocrine carcinoma of the mammary gland in a dog. *J Comp Pathol 152*:188–191.

Nakagaki K.Y.R., Nunes M.M., Garcia A.P.V. et al. (2021) Neuroendocrine carcinomas of the canine mammary gland: Histopathological and immunohistochemical characteristics. *Front Vet Sci 7*:621714.

Nakagaki K.Y.R., Nunes M.M., Garcia A.P.V. et al. (2022) Solid carcinoma of the canine mammary gland: A histological type or tumor cell arrangement? *J Comp Pathol 190*:1–12.

Newman S.J., Yanez R.A., Kiupel M. (2022) Mixed medullary and follicular cell thyroid carcinoma in a dog. *J Vet Diagn Invest 34*:960–963.

Norsworthy G.D., Adams V.J., McElhaney M.R. et al. (2002) Palpable thyroid and parathyroid nodules in asymptomatic cats. *J Feline Med Surg 4*:145–151.

Obradovich J.E., Withrow S.J., Powers B.E. et al. (1992) Carotid body tumors in the dog: Eleven cases (1978–1988). *J Vet Intern Med 6*:96–101.

O'Brien K.M., Bankoff B.J., Rosenstein P.K. et al. (2021) Clinical, histopathologic and immunohistochemical features of 13 cases of canine gallbladder neuroendocrine carcinoma. *J Vet Diagn Invest 33*:294–299.

Paltrinieri S., Riccaboni P., Rondena M. et al. (2004) Pathologic and immunohistochemical findings in a feline aortic body tumor. *Vet Pathol 41*:195–198.

Parker V.J., Gilor C., Chew D.J. (2015) Feline hyperparathyroidism pathophysiology, diagnosis and treatment of primary and secondary disease. *J Feline Med Surg 17*:427–439.

Patnaik A.K. (1992) A morphologic and immunocytochemical study of hepatic neoplasms in cats. *Vet Pathol 29*:405–415.

Patnaik A.K., Hurvitz A.I., Johnson G.F. (1980a) Canine intestinal adenocarcinoma and carcinoid. *Vet Pathol 17*:149–163.

Patnaik A.K., Hurvitz A.I., Lieberman P.H. (1980b) Canine hepatic neoplasms: A clinicopathologic study. *Vet Pathol 17*:553–564.

Patnaik A.K., Lieberman P.H. (1981) Canine goblet-cell carcinoid. *Vet Pathol 18*:410–413.

Patnaik A.K., Lieberman P.H. (1991) Gross, histologic, cytochemical and immunocytochemical study of medullary thyroid carcinoma in sixteen dogs. *Vet Pathol 28*:223–233.

Peterson M.E. (2015) Primary goitorous hypothyroidism in a young adult domestic longhair cat: Diagnosis and treatment monitoring. *J Feline Med Surg Open Rep.* 1(2) : 1–7.

Pey P., Diana A., Rossi F. et al. (2020) Safety of percutaneous ultrasound-guided fine-needle aspiration of adrenal lesions in dogs: Perception of the procedure by radiologists and presentation of 50 cases. *J Vet Intern Med 34*:626–635.

Phillips D.E., Radlinsky M.G., Fischer J.R. et al. (2003) Cystic thyroid and parathyroid lesions in cats. *J Am Anim Hosp Assoc 39*:349–354.

Pollard R.E., Bohannon L.K., Feldman E.C. (2015) Prevalence of incidental thyroid nodules in ultrasound studies of dogs with hypercalcemia (2008–2013). *Vet Radiol Ultrasoun 56*:63–67.

Renschler J.S., Dean G.A. (2009) What is your diagnosis? Abdominal mass aspirate in a cat with an increased Na:K ratio. *Vet Clin Pathol 38*:69–72.

Renzi A., Sabattini S., D'Annunzio G. et al. (2022) Multiorgan metastases with massive bone involvement of a medullary thyroid carcinoma in a dog. *Vet Clin Pathol*:1–5.

Rich A.F., Piviani M., Swales H. et al. (2019) Bilateral thyroid carcinosarcoma in a cat. *J Comp Pathol 171*:24–29.

Robben J.H., Pollak Y.W., Kirpensteijn J. et al. (2005) Comparison of ultrasonography, computed tomography, and single-photon emission computed tomography for detection and localization of canine insulinoma. *J Vet Intern Med 19*:15–22.

Roberts E., Dobromylskyj M.J. (2022) Histopathological evaluation of the adrenal glands in a cat with primary hypoadrenocorticism and multiple endocrine disease. *J Feline Med Surg Open Rep*:1–5.

Romine J.F., Kozicki A.R., Elie M.S. (2016) Primary adrenal lymphoma causing hypoaldosteronism in a cat. *J Feline Med Surg Open Rep.* 2(2): 1–6.

Rossmeisl J.H., Forrester S.D., Robertson J.L. et al. (2002) Chronic vomiting associated with a gastric carcinoid in a cat. *J Am Anim Hosp Assoc 38*:61–66.

Sako T., Uchida E., Okamoto M. et al. (2003) Immunohistochemical evaluation of a malignant intestinal carcinoid in a dog. *Vet Pathol 40*:212–215.

Salesov E., Boretti F.S., Sieber-Ruckstuhl N.S. et al. (2015) Urinary and plasma catecholamines and metanephrines in dogs with pheochromocytoma, hypercortisolism, nonadrenal disease and in healthy dogs. *J Vet Intern Med 29*:597–602.

Sawyer E.S., Northrup N.C., Schmiedt C.W. et al. (2011) Outcome of 19 dogs with parathyroid carcinoma after surgical excision. *Vet Comp Oncol 10*:57–64.

Skinner O.T., Souza C.H.deM., Kim D.Y. (2021) Metastasis to ipsilateral medial retropharyngeal and deep cervical lymph nodes in 22 dogs with thyroid carcinoma. *Vet Surg 50*:150–157.

Soares L.M.C., Pereira A.H.B., de Campos C.G. et al. (2020) Histopathological and immunohistochemical characteristics of thyroid carcinoma in the dog. *J Comp Pathol 177*:34–41.

Sokolowska J., Cywińska A., Puchalska M. (2022) Comparative histology of C thyrocytes in four domestic animal species: Dog, pig, horse and cattle. *Animals 12*:1324.

Soo Choi U., Alleman A.R., Choi J. et al. (2008) Cytologic and immunohistochemical characterization of a lung carcinoid in a dog. *Vet Clin Pathol 37*:249–252.

Soo Choi U., Arndt T. (2016) Endocrine/Neuroendocrine system. In *Canine and Feline Cytology: A Color Atlas and Interpretation Guide*. 3rd edn. (eds. R.E. Raskin, D.J. Meyer) Elsevier, St. Louis, pp. 430–452.

Sozmen M., Devrim T., Kuruca N. et al. (2020) Primary unilateral small cell neuroendocrine carcinoma of the kidney in a dog. *J Comp Pathol 176*:71–75.

Sumner J.A., Lacorcia L., Rose A.M. et al. (2018) Clinical safety of percutaneous ultrasound-guided fine-needle aspiration of adrenal gland lesions in 19 dogs. *J Small Anim Pract 59*:357–363.

Swainson S.W., Nelson O.L., Niyo Y. et al. (2000) Radiographic diagnosis: Mediastinal parathyroid cyst in a cat. *Vet Radiol Ultrasound 41*:41–43.

Sykes G.P., Cooper B.J. (1982) Canine intestinal carcinoids. *Vet Pathol 19*:120–131.

Thompson E.J., Stirtzinger T., Lumsden J.H. et al. (1980) Fine needle aspiration cytology in the diagnosis of canine thyroid carcinoma. *Can Vet J 21*:186–188.

Tobin R.L., Nelson R.W., Lucroy M.D. et al. (1999) Outcome of surgical versus medical treatment of dogs with beta cell neoplasia: 39 cases (1990–1997). *J Am Vet Med Assoc 215*:226–230.

Tursi M., Iussich S., Prunotto M. et al. (2005) Adrenal myelolipoma in a dog. *Vet Pathol 42*:232–235.

Uzal F.A., Plattner B.L., Hostetter J.M. (2015) Alimentary system. In: *Jubb, Kennedy and Palmer's Pathology of Domestic Animals*, Vol. 2, 6th edn. (ed. M.G. Maxie) Elsecier, St. Louis, pp. 1–257.

Virtanen J.K., Mölsä S.H., Hagner K.A. et al. (2020) Primary hyperparathyroidism caused by bilateral parathyroid cystic carcinoma in a cat. *J Feline Med Surg Open Rep.* 6(2): 1–6.

Vuong K.S., Aoki K. (2021) A multi-organ infection involving a left adrenal gland abscess in a diabetic dog. *Can Vet J 62*:154–159.

Waters C.B., Scott-Moncrieff J.C.R. (2002) Cancer of endocrine organs. In: *Cancer in Dogs and Cats: Medical and Surgical Management*, 2nd edn. (ed. W.B. Morrison) Teton NewMedia, Jackson, pp. 573–609.

Wucherer K.L., Wilke V. (2010) Thyroid cancer in dogs: An update based on 638 cases (1995–2005). *J Am Anim Hosp Assoc 46*:249–254.

Yates W.D.G., Lester S.J., Mills J.H.L. (1980) Chemoreceptor tumors diagnosed at the Western College of Veterinary Medicine 1967–1979. *Can Vet J 21*:124–129.

Yu Y., Bovenhuis H., Wu Z. et al. (2021) Deleterious mutations in the TPO gene associated with familial thyroid follicular cell carcinoma in Dutch German longhaired pointers. *Genes 12*:997.

Yu Y., Krupa A., Keesler R.I. et al. (2022) Familial follicular cell thyroid carcinomas in a large number of Dutch German longhaired pointers. *Vet Comp Oncol 20*:227–234.

Zi E., Lunardi F., Zanetti R. et al. (2016) Endocrine pancreas in cats with diabetes mellitus. *Vet Pathol 53*:136–144.

CHAPTER 17

OCULAR CYTOLOGY

Anne M. Barger and Samantha Lee

INTRODUCTION

Ocular cytology can be very useful to the clinician in establishing a diagnosis, determining if a patient is responding appropriately to therapy, or determining the necessity for additional diagnostic testing. The clinician's familiarity with the appearance of normal tissue and resident cell types is essential for accurate interpretation of a cytologic specimen. Before a pathologic process can be identified, an understanding of what is normal is critical. Each ocular structure has a distinct histology. Normal cytology will be reviewed in each section and followed by cytologic appearance of pathologic processes.

EYELIDS

Comprised of a dorsal and ventral lid connected by medial and lateral canthi, the eyelids serve as an extension of haired skin for protection and lubrication of the cornea. Typical structures identified in the skin elsewhere are also found in the eyelid; however, unique sebaceous glands, the meibomian glands and glands of Zeis, positioned on the inner surface of the eyelid along the palpebral conjunctiva, create an additional site for pathology to occur. Common lesions of cytologic importance in the dog and cat include infectious and noninfectious inflammation, non-neoplastic masses, and neoplasia.

INFLAMMATION

Inflammation of the eyelid, termed blepharitis, may involve one or both eyelids and can present as focal or diffuse lesions. The inflammatory populations that occur in the eyelid parallel those found in the skin of other parts of the body and follow a similar algorithm of differentials. Certain diseases may only involve the eyelids, while others, such as demodectic and sarcoptic mange, include the eyelids in addition to other lesions on the face and body (Aroch *et al.*, 2008). Infectious, immune-mediated, and foreign body reactions should be considered if suppurative inflammation is present. Primary bacterial blepharitis in adult dogs is often caused by *Staphylococcus* spp. and *Streptococcus* spp., and many degenerate neutrophils are typical on cytologic examination (Stiles, 2012). Juvenile cellulitis (also known as puppy pyoderma or puppy strangles), a presumed immune-mediated condition that causes severe sterile abscessation and edema of the muzzle and mandibular lymph nodes in puppies, often involves the eyelids (Bassett *et al.*, 2005). Cytology of pustules reveals aseptic suppurative to pyogranulomatous inflammation.

Eosinophilic inflammation alone or as part of a mixed inflammatory population may result as part of a hypersensitivity response to insect stings or bites. Additionally, immune-mediated eosinophilic plaques may involve the eyelids and reveal marked eosinophilic inflammation with or without lower numbers of other inflammatory cells. Pyogranulomatous inflammation secondary to fungal infections (dermatophytes, *Blastomyces dermatitidis*) and foreign body reactions may also occur (Figure 17.1). Patients infected with *Leishmania infantum* often develop eyelid lesions, which can vary in presentation including dry dermatitis and alopecia, blepheredema, ulcers, and discrete granulomas (Pena *et al.*, 2000). Cytology of granulomas reveals numerous macrophages with or without neutrophils, and in many cases *Leishmania infantum* amastigotes are present (Pena *et al.*, 2000).

Common non-neoplastic masses that occur on the eyelid include the chalazion, hordeolum, and cystic structures. Chalazion is a lipogranuloma of the meibomian gland, and build-up of the secretory product leads to granulomatous inflammation (Figure 17.2; Stades & van der Woerdt, 2013). Many macrophages and lower numbers of multinucleated giant cells and small lymphocytes are most commonly seen on cytology. Hordeolum is focal abscessation of the sebaceous glands of the eyelid, including the meibomian glands and glands of

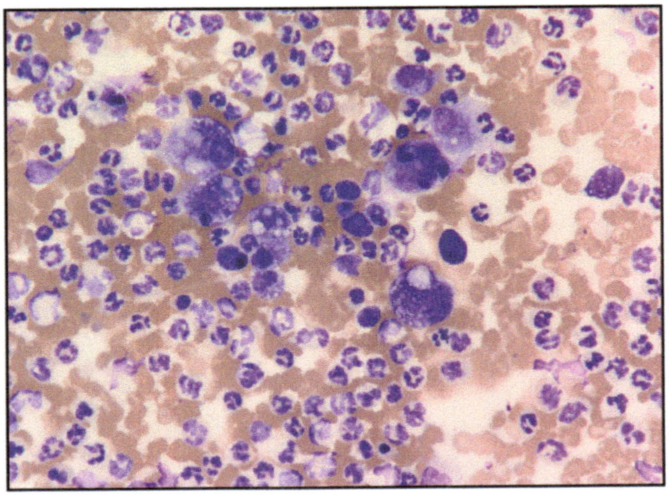

Figure 17.1 FNA of an eyelid mass from a dog. Many vacuolated macrophages and low numbers of multinucleated macrophages are present (Wright–Giemsa, 500× magnification).

DOI: 10 1201/9781003258551-17

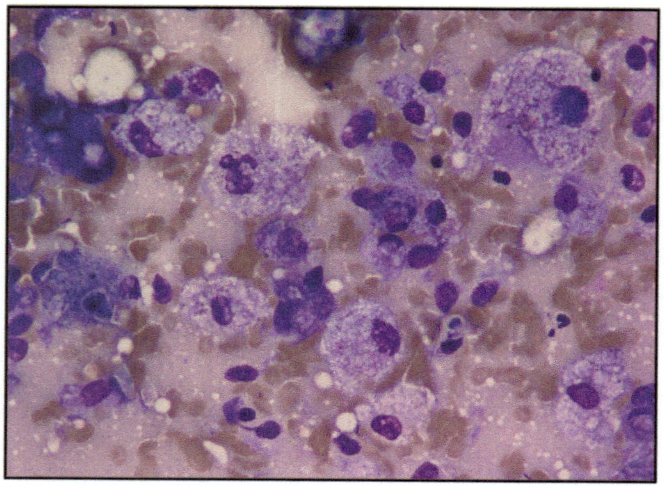

Figure 17.2 FNA of an eyelid mass from a dog. Note the abundance of vacuolated macrophages with low numbers of multinucleated giant cells. No infectious organisms were identified (Wright–Giemsa, 1,000× magnification).

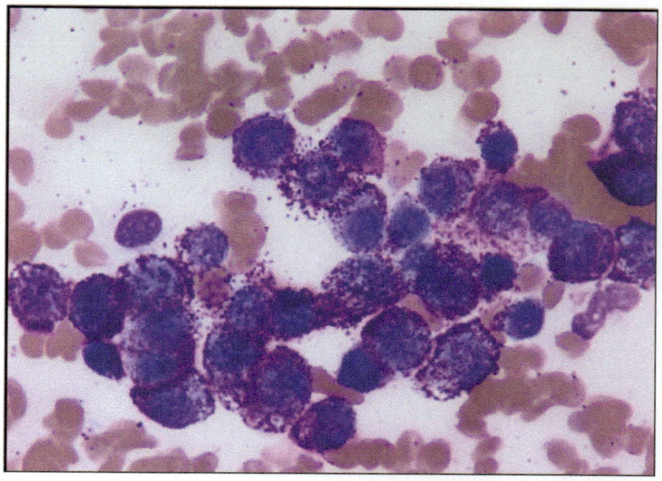

Figure 17.3 FNA of an eyelid mass from a dog. Many mast cells are present, which contain many dark purple cytoplasmic granules (Wright–Giemsa, 1,000× magnification).

Zeis, and aspiration will reveal suppurative inflammation. Lastly, Meibomian cysts can occur and typically consist of foamy macrophages and cholesterol crystals in highly proteinaceous material on cytologic examination.

Neoplasia

Neoplastic masses of the eyelid are most often benign (Krehbiel & Langham, 1975). The most common tumor is the meibomian adenoma, with meibomian adenocarcinoma being far less common (Krehbiel & Langham, 1975). Meibomian adenomas appear cytologically similar to aspiration of any other sebaceous glandular tissue, with many clusters of epithelial cells filled with discrete clear cytoplasmic vacuoles. Melanomas are the second most common tumor of the eyelid and appear cytologically similar to melanomas of other sites but are typically less aggressive. Fibroma, fibrosarcoma, papilloma, squamous cell carcinoma (SCC), mast cell tumor (Figure 17.3), lipoma, granular cell tumor, histiocytoma, and meibomian gland epithelioma (Figures 17.4a, b) are all less common but reported (Krehbiel & Langham, 1975; Lu & Dubielzig, 2012). Histiocytosis of Bernese Mountain Dogs frequently involves the eyelids, and aspiration of the nodules reveals neoplastic histiocytes with marked criteria of malignancy (Moore, 1984).

Conjunctiva

The conjunctiva is a mucous membrane that lines the inner surface of the eyelids and nictitating membrane and then reflects back onto the anterior portion of the globe. The palpebral conjunctiva consists of pseudostratified epithelium with goblet cells and lymphoid follicles. The bulbar conjunctiva consists of nonkeratinized squamous

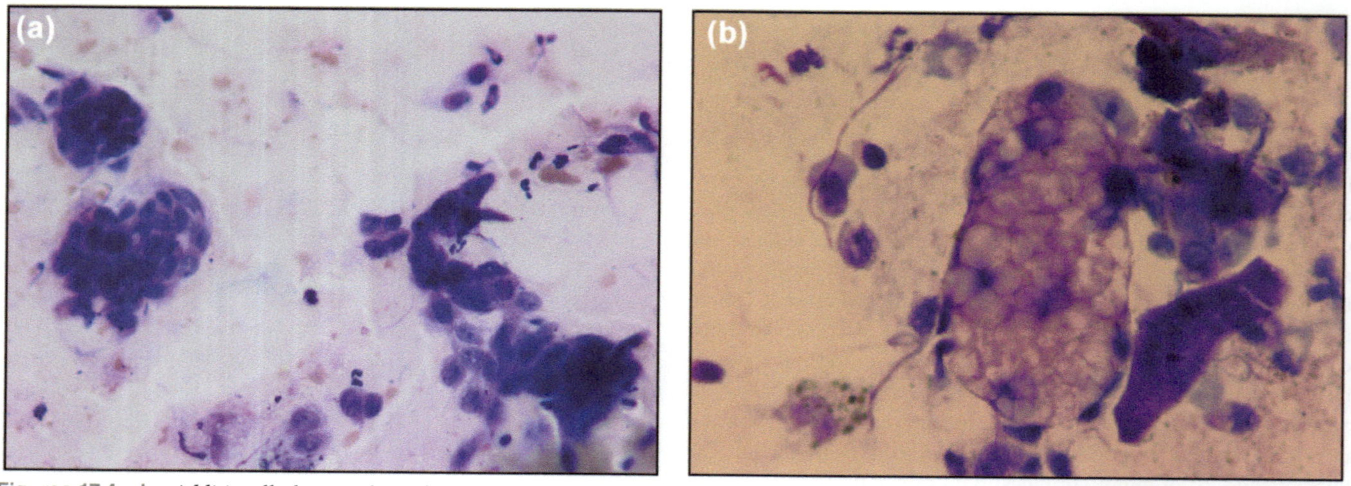

Figures 17.4a, b Additionally, low numbers of epithelial clusters with abundant cytoplasmic clear vacuolation consistent with benign sebaceous epithelial cells are present (Wright–Giemsa: a, 500× magnification; b, 1,000× magnification). Many cohesive clusters of benign epithelial cells with a small amount of basophilic cytoplasm, round nuclei, and indistinct nucleoli are present.

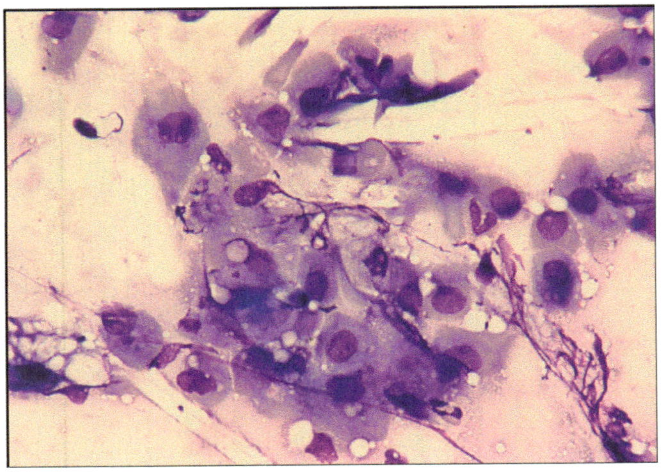

Figure 17.5 **Conjunctival scrape from a dog. One cluster of nonkeratinized squamous epithelial cells is present. The cells have abundant amounts of basophilic cytoplasm and a single round nucleus (Wright–Giemsa, 1,000× magnification).**

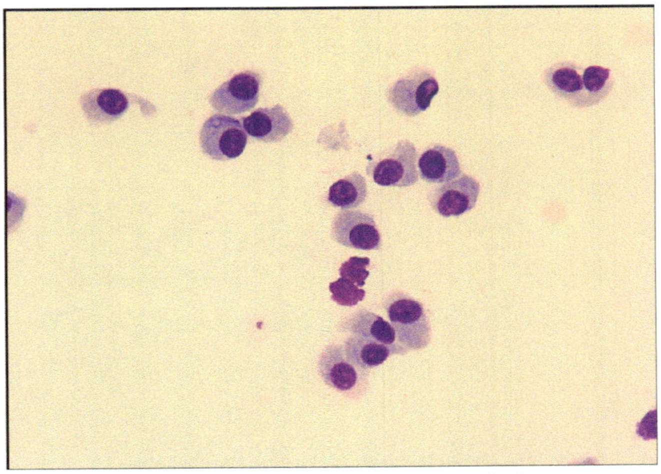

Figure 17.7 **Conjunctival scrape from a dog. Scattered columnar epithelial cells are observed. These cells are rectangular to spindle in shape with single round nuclei (Wright–Giemsa, 1,000× magnification).**

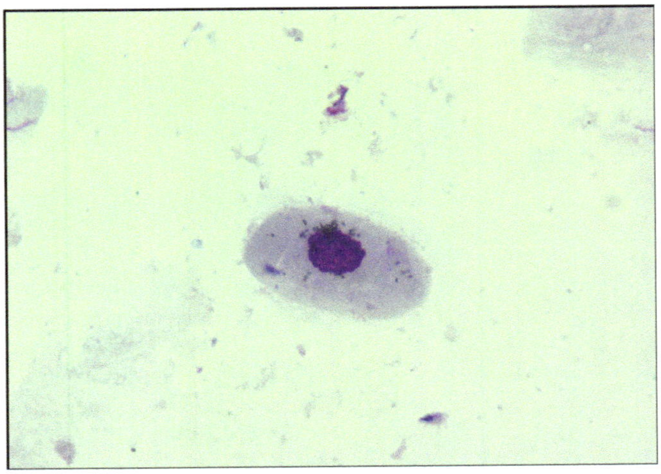

Figure 17.6 **Conjunctival swab from a dog. A single squamous epithelial cell coated in melanin granules is present (Wright–Giemsa, 1,000× magnification).**

epithelium (Figure 17.5; Raskin, 2010). As this tissue approaches the limbus it is common to see melanin granules coating the epithelial cells (Figure 17.6; Young & Prasse, 2007). The melanin granules are easy to confuse with bacteria. Melanin granules have a brownish-gold staining with most Romanowsky stains while bacteria will stain pale to deeply basophilic. Epithelial cells from most tissues are cohesive and can be found in sheets and clusters; however, squamous epithelial cells can be more individualized. Columnar epithelial cells are elongate and on cytology can appear similar to spindle cells. The other types of epithelial cells are more likely to be round with a centrally placed nucleus and variable amounts of cytoplasm depending on the location within the conjunctiva (Figure 17.7). Goblet cells have voluminous amounts of cytoplasm, which is filled with eosinophilic globular material. Cytologically, lymphoid follicles will consist of a mixed lymphoid population, predominated by small lymphocytes with few large lymphocytes and plasma cells.

Cytologic samples of conjunctiva can be obtained by multiple techniques, including swabs, scrapes, and imprints (Bauer and Speiss, 1996). The sampling technique will impact the types of epithelial cells observed. An imprint will likely sample the surface epithelium and result in squamous epithelial cells being the most prominent. A scrape will sample deeper areas of the tissue, so goblet cells and small lymphocytes will also be observed in addition to epithelial cells. The epithelial cells from the deeper layers are more likely to have a centrally placed nucleus and a moderate rim of pale basophilic cytoplasm (Bolzan *et al.*, 2005). Common findings from cytology from healthy conjunctiva include a predominance of epithelial cells with a small amount of mucus and few small lymphocytes (Lavach et al., 1977). Impression cytology, performed by applying a cellulose filter to the superficial layers of epithelial cells, produces cellular samples while also preserving tissue architecture (Perazzi *et al.*, 2017).

Inflammation

Cytologically, inflammation of the conjunctiva is characterized by the type of inflammatory cells seen (e.g. >85% neutrophils is consistent with suppurative inflammation). Nonspecific changes that may accompany inflammation include lymphoid hyperplasia, epithelial hyperplasia, and squamous metaplasia with keratinization of squamous epithelial cells (Wilcock, 2007). Excessive mucus is often produced resulting in thick eosinophilic strands of mucinous material (Figure 17.8). Conjunctivitis can be primary or secondary. Cytologically, unless the causative agent is identified, the underlying cause is often difficult to discern. Neutrophils are commonly associated with bacterial, viral, and fungal infections but can also be seen secondary to keratoconjunctivitis sicca and allergic disease. The condition of the neutrophils should be evaluated. If the neutrophils are undergoing karyolysis or appear degenerate, this can

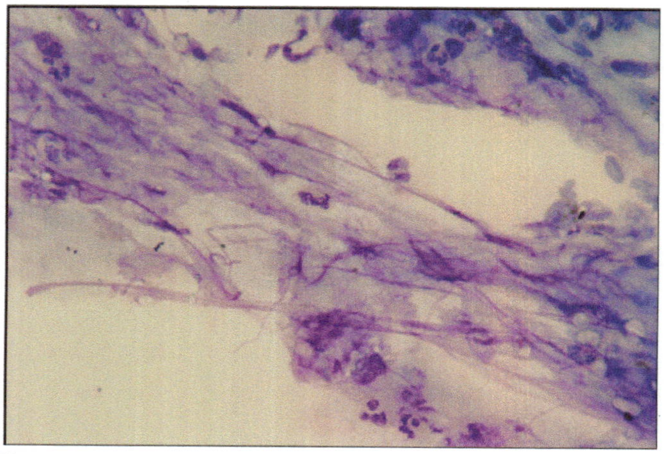

Figure 17.8 Conjunctival swab from a dog. Several thick strands of eosinophilic mucinous material are observed, admixed with scattered neutrophils (Wright–Giemsa, 1,000× magnification).

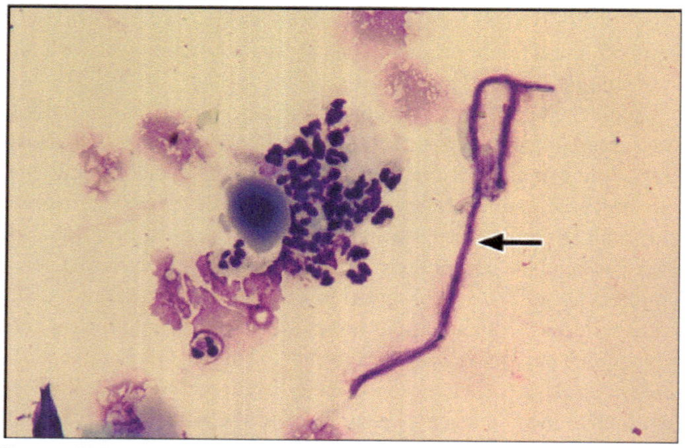

Figure 17.9 Conjunctival scrape from a dog. A group of degenerate neutrophils are surrounding a squamous epithelial cell. The epithelial cell has a 'fried egg' appearance with a centrally placed nucleus and a moderate rim of basophilic cytoplasm. A fungal hyphal structure (indicated by an arrow) is also observed (Wright–Giemsa, 500× magnification).

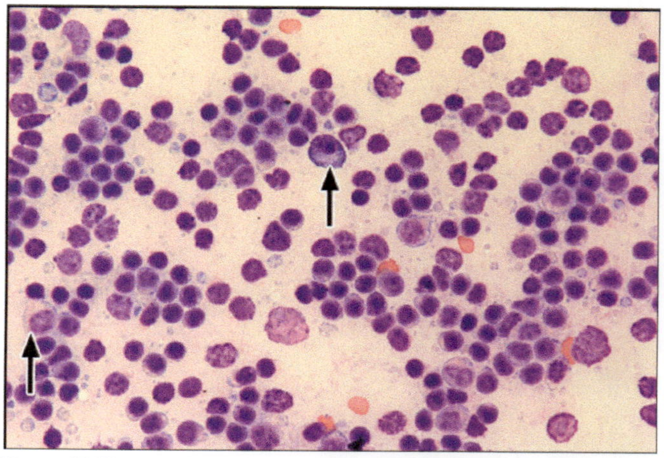

Figure 17.10 Conjunctival scrape from a dog with lymphoplasmacytic conjunctivitis. The sample is cellular, and a mixed lymphoid population predominated by small lymphocytes with few plasma cells (indicated by arrows) is observed. Note the perinuclear clearing or prominent Golgi apparatus in the cytoplasm of the plasma cells (Wright–Giemsa, 500× magnification).

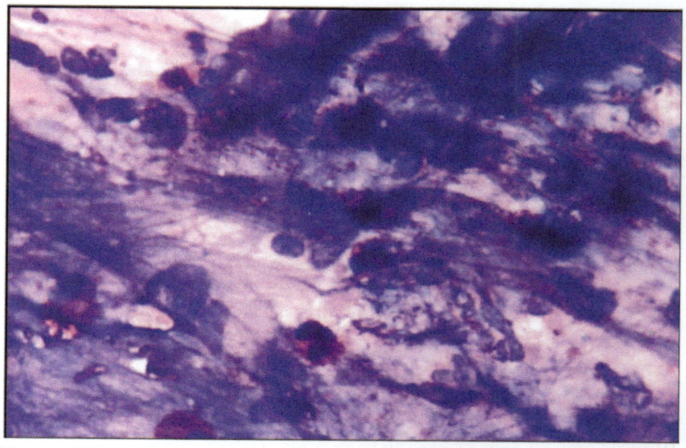

Figure 17.11 Conjunctival swab from a cat with allergic conjunctivitis. The sample is cellular. A mixed inflammatory population, predominantly neutrophils with many eosinophils, is observed embedded in a thick mat of eosinophilic mucinous material (Wright–Giemsa, 1,000× magnification).

be associated with bacterial infection. Degenerate neutrophils have pale swollen nuclei that are starting to lose the filamentous structure connecting the lobules of the nucleus (Figure 17.9). Fungal conjunctivitis has been reported in cats, including primary conjunctival sporotrichosis (Spinelli *et al.*, 2021) and disseminated histoplasmosis with conjunctival and/or nictitating membrane involvement (Ewald *et al.*, 2020). Small numbers of lymphocytes and plasma cells can be observed in normal conjunctiva but also can be associated with inflammation or immune stimulation. In true lymphoplasmacytic inflammation, the lymphoid inflammatory cell population predominates over the epithelial cells. Immune-mediated diseases, such as pannus, medial canthal blepharitis of Long-haired Dachshunds, and follicular conjunctivitis, will have a very cellular infiltrate predominated by small lymphocytes with many plasma cells (Figure 17.10; Raskin, 2010). In other immune-mediated diseases, such as pemphigus, neutrophils and eosinophils are the primary inflammatory cells. Allergic conjunctivitis can result in a mixed cellular infiltrate with a high number of eosinophils and scattered mast cells (Figure 17.11).

Cellular inclusions may be observed in conjunctival specimens. These inclusions can be identified in inflammatory cells and conjunctival epithelial cells and may be intracytoplasmic or intranuclear. Infectious organisms such as *Chlamydia* spp., *Mycoplasma* spp., or distemper virus can be found in the cytoplasm of epithelial cells (Figures 17.12a, b). However, more commonly the cytoplasmic inclusions are benign structures such as melanin granules or ophthalmic ointment (Figure 17.13), which are easy to misinterpret as an infectious etiology (Young & Taylor, 2006). Viral inclusions have been

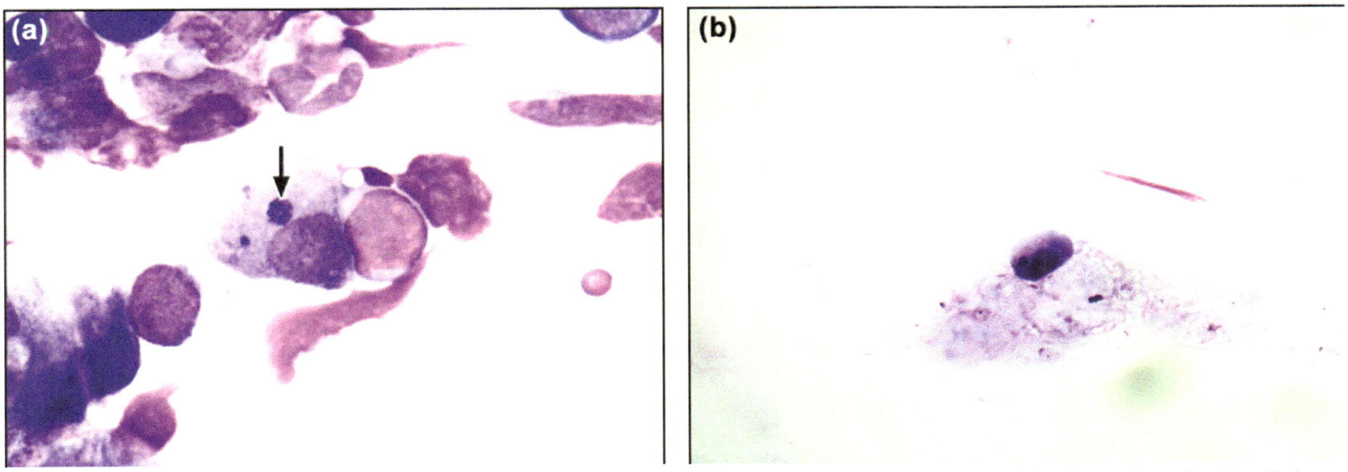

Figures 17.12a, b Conjunctival swab from a cat with an ocular discharge. (a) A large epithelial cell with a chlamydial inclusion (arrow) is identified (Wright–Giemsa, 1,000× magnification). (Courtesy Dr. Richard Meadows.) (b) Conjunctival scrape from a dog with a bilateral ocular discharge, nasal discharge, and a fever. One epithelial cell is observed containing a single basophilic cytoplasmic inclusion consistent with canine distemper virus (Wright–Giemsa, 400× magnification).

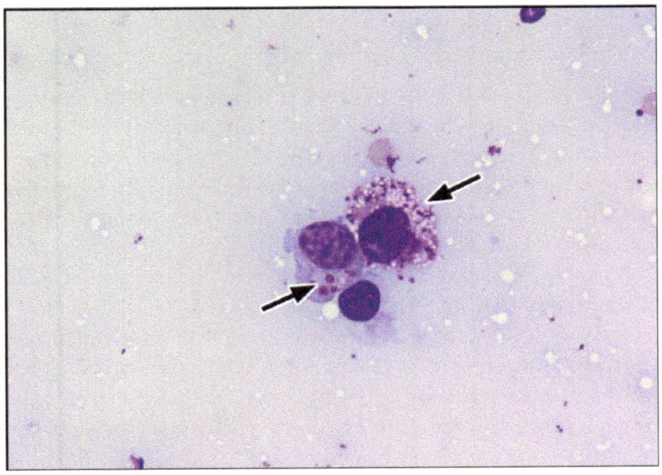

Figure 17.13 Conjunctival swab from a dog. The patient had been receiving ophthalmic ointment in both eyes for 1 week prior to sampling. A single epithelial cell containing several eosinophilic inclusions consistent with ophthalmic ointment is indicated by the arrow on the left. A single mast cell is also present (right arrow) (Wright–Giemsa, 1,000× magnification).

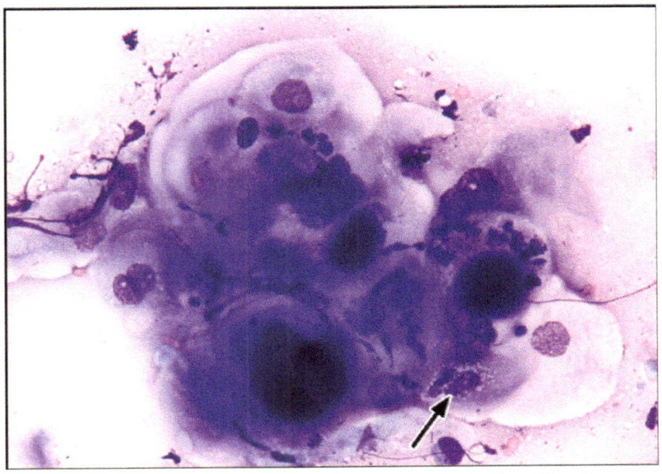

Figure 17.14 Conjunctival aspirate from a conjunctival swelling in a cat with squamous cell carcinoma. A cluster of neoplastic squamous epithelial cells, occasionally coated in neutrophils. The arrow indicates a perinuclear ring of cytoplasmic vacuoles (Wright–Giemsa, 1,000× magnification).

reported to occur (Raskin, 2010) with feline herpesvirus and canine distemper, but are infrequently encountered in cytologic specimens (Hillström *et al.*, 2012).

Neoplasia

Conjunctival neoplasia may appear as a discrete mass or an irregular thickening of the conjunctiva. If a mass is identified, fine needle aspiration (FNA) is the most efficient method to obtain a cytologic sample; however, conjunctival scrapes can also be beneficial. Many tumors have been described and include mast cell tumor, lymphoma, melanoma, hemangioma, hemangiosarcoma, and SCC, with SCC as the most common (Pirie *et al.*, 2006; Maggs, 2008; Schobert *et al.*, 2010; Fife et al., 2011; Olbertz *et al.*, 2012). Cytologically, SCCs appear similar regardless of the location. The cells are round to polygonal with varying amounts of pale basophilic to keratinized cytoplasm. The nuclei vary greatly in size with a coarsely stippled to pyknotic chromatin. A ring of perinuclear vacuoles can be observed (Figure 17.14). Occasionally, neutrophils can be seen coating the cytoplasm. It is not uncommon to have a significant suppurative inflammatory response accompanying the tumor. The presence of inflammation makes SCC difficult to differentiate from squamous dysplasia secondary to inflammation.

Mast cell tumors (MCTs) can be readily diagnosed with cytology via FNA (Fife *et al.*, 2011). MCTs are round cell tumors and the

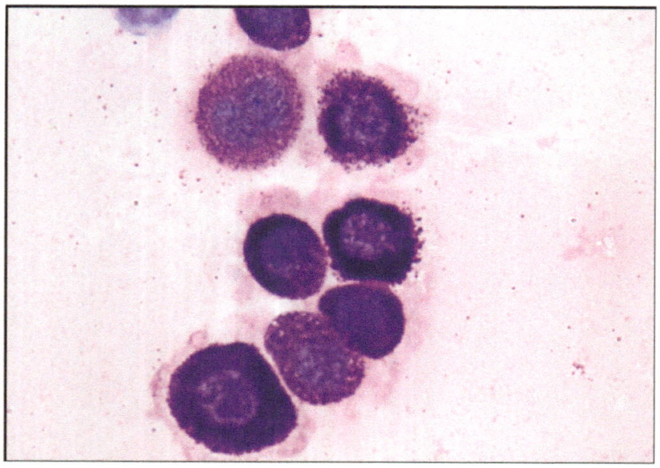

Figure 17.15 Conjunctival scrape from a dog with conjunctival swelling with mast cell neoplasia. Highly granular mast cells are identified (Wright–Giemsa, 1,000× magnification).

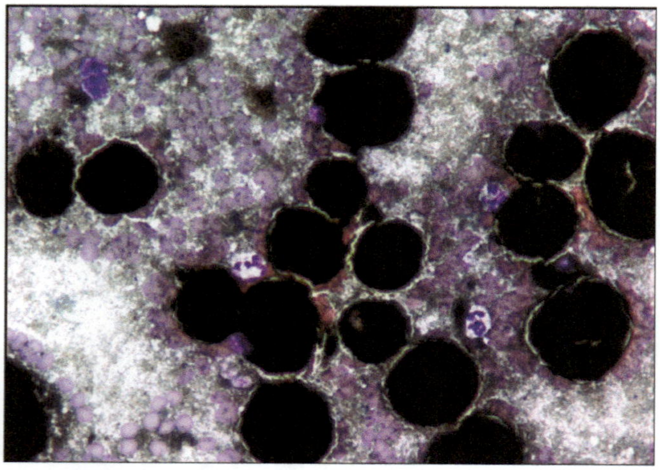

Figure 17.16 Conjunctival aspirate from a mass in a cat with a conjunctival melanoma. The sample is highly cellular with many highly granular neoplastic melanocytes. The cells are so granular, the nuclear detail cannot be visualized. Melanin granules and red blood cells are present in the background (Wright–Giemsa, 1,000× magnification).

neoplastic cells are typically individualized and round. Mast cells have a moderate amount of cytoplasm filled with dark purple granules (Figure 17.15). Stains such as Diff-Quik® do not consistently stain the granules, which may decrease the diagnostic yield of in-house cytology.

Conjunctival melanomas typically consist of very cellular samples often containing high numbers of melanin granules, although amelanotic melanomas have been reported (Schobert *et al.*, 2010). Amelanotic melanoma can be difficult to diagnose cytologically without immunocytochemical or immunohistochemical staining. Melanotic melanomas are relatively easy to diagnose with cytology since the cells are frequently heavily pigmented (Figure 17.16). This abundance of pigment may obscure nuclear detail.

NICTITATING MEMBRANE

The nictitating membrane (third eyelid) has a T-shaped cartilage with a large gland at its base and is covered in nonkeratinized stratified squamous epithelium (Samuelson, 2007; Raskin, 2010). Lymphoid tissue is also present on the bulbar conjunctiva of the third eyelid. The presence of this normal tissue should be considered when diagnosing inflammatory disease within the third eyelid.

Inflammatory disorders of the third eyelid are characterized cytologically by the cells that are identified. These can be an extension of conjunctivitis or follicular hyperplasia accompanying lymphoplasmacytic inflammation.

Neoplasms of the nictitating membrane are similar to those described in the conjunctiva but should also include adenocarcinoma. Adenocarcinoma is one of the most common tumors at this location (Raskin, 2010). These cells will exhibit prominent criteria of malignancy such as anisocytosis and anisokaryosis. The cells are glandular in origin so they will often contain multiple discrete vacuoles within the cytoplasm.

SCLERA

The sclera consists of three layers: the lamina fusca, which communicates with the outer choroid; the sclera proper, which is composed of connective tissue; and the episclera, which consists of loose connective tissue and is highly vascular (Samuelson, 2007). Sampling of normal sclera will be of low cellularity because healthy connective tissue does not exfoliate very well.

Scleral inflammation can be primary or secondary to other ocular inflammatory diseases. Primary canine episcleritis has been characterized immunohistochemically as a mixture of T and B lymphocytes and $CD18^{+}$ histiocytic cells (Breaux *et al.*, 2007). Cytologically, there will be a mixed inflammatory population predominated by small lymphocytes with high numbers of vacuolated macrophages. Low numbers of neutrophils can be observed.

CORNEA

The cornea is the transparent anterior portion of the fibrous ocular tunic. It is composed of multiple layers. The most anterior layer consists of nonkeratinized squamous epithelial cells. The stroma consists of mesenchymal cells, primarily fibrocytes (also called corneal keratocytes) admixed with collagen bundles (Young & Prasse, 2007). The posterior cornea consists of a single-layered corneal endothelium and its basement membrane, Descemet's membrane (Samuelson, 2007). Cytologically, the most anterior surface of the cornea is generally what is sampled, so nonkeratinized squamous epithelial cells are the most frequent cells seen, occasionally admixed with a few spindle-shaped cells. With corneal injury, some general changes that can occur include keratinization of the squamous epithelial cells and the presence of more basal appearing epithelial cells. These cells are smaller with larger nuclei and a scant to moderate rim of basophilic

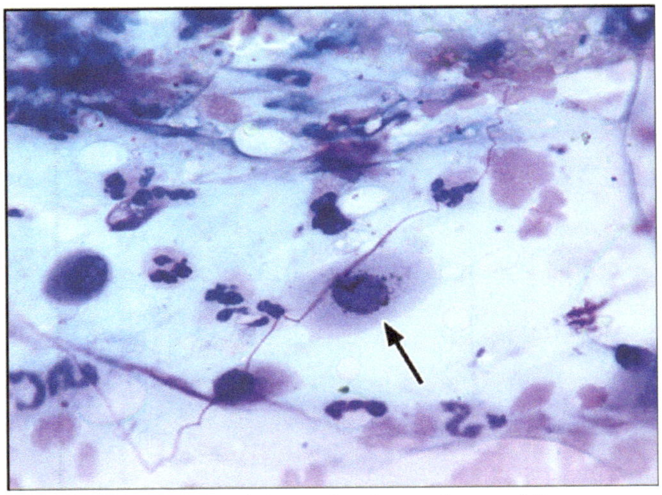

Figure 17.17 **Corneal swab from a dog. Scattered neutrophils are observed in a background of mucus. A nonkeratinized squamous epithelial cell coated in melanin granules is indicated by an arrow (Wright–Giemsa, 1,000× magnification).**

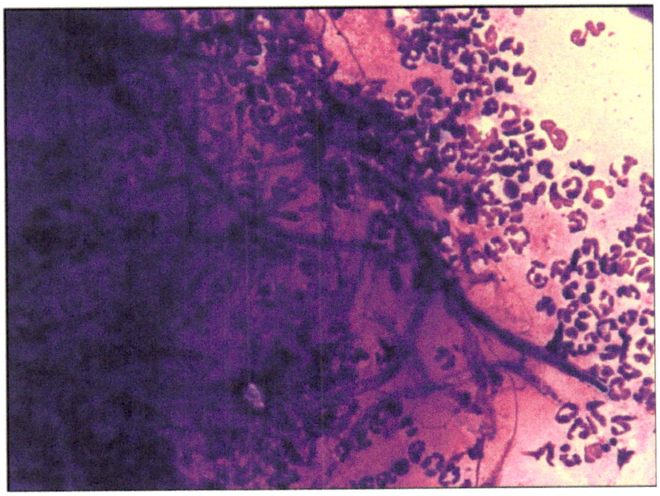

Figure 17.18 **Corneal swab from an ulcerative lesion from a feline cornea with fungal keratitis. Neutrophils are observed surrounding fungal hyphae. Septation and branching are noted. Culture revealed *Aspergillus flavus* (Wright–Giemsa, 1,000× magnification).**

cytoplasm. Additionally, cells from the limbus and conjunctiva can be recruited to the cornea (Wilcock, 2007). These cells are often coated in pigmented granules (Figure 17.17).

Inflammation

Inflammation of the cornea can occur secondary to physical or chemical damage, infectious organisms, immune-mediated corneal disease, uveitis, and elevated ocular pressures (Wilcock, 2007). Bacterial and fungal keratitis often causes a suppurative inflammatory response. Fungal keratitis is commonly seen in horses (Cutler, 2004) but has also been reported in dogs and cats (Labelle *et al.*, 2009; Binder et al., 2011; Pucket et al., 2012; Nevile et al., 2016). Fungal organisms are readily identified in corneal swabs or scrapes. The morphology depends on the type of fungus, but some general features include septation and branching and uniform parallel walls (Figure 17.18). Cytologic specimens from bacterial keratitis are typically highly cellular. Many neutrophils are observed and the neutrophils are often degenerate. Intracytoplasmic bacterial organisms are also seen (Figure 17.19). Recognition of the organisms within the cytoplasm of neutrophils is important to truly recognize them as pathogens rather than contaminants. Within the background are thick strands of mucinous material, which should be differentiated from fungal hyphae. Common bacterial pathogens reported in canine bacterial keratitis include *Streptococcus* and *Pseudomonas* spp. (Hindley *et al.*, 2016). The most frequent bacteria isolated from feline bacterial keratitis include the *Staphylococcus* genus (Golreich *et al.*, 2020).

Eosinophilic keratitis has been reported in cats. Feline herpesvirus-1 has been suggested as but not confirmed as a possible etiology (Naisse *et al.*, 1998). Cytologically, eosinophils are seen in high numbers with a mixture of mature squamous epithelial cells, mucinous material, and low numbers of neutrophils (Figures 17.20a, b). Granules from eosinophils are commonly seen in the background.

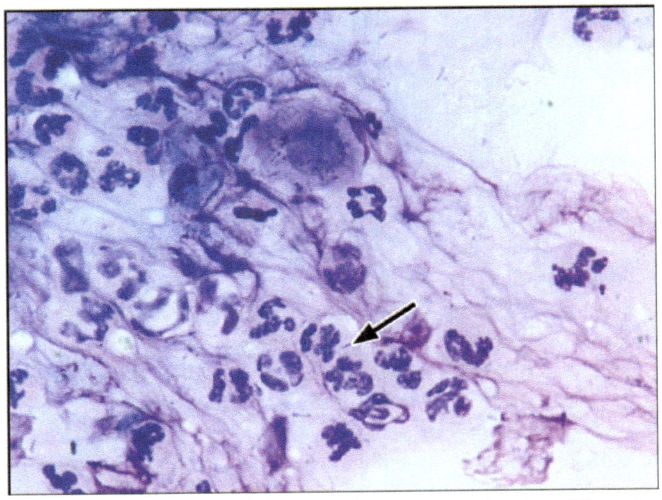

Figure 17.19 **Corneal swab from an ulcerative lesion in a dog with septic suppurative keratitis. The sample is cellular, many neutrophils are observed, rarely containing phagocytized rod-shaped bacteria (arrow). Extracellular bacteria are also observed (Wright–Giemsa, 1,000× magnification).**

Mast cells, small lymphocytes, and plasma cells have also been reported in low numbers (Prasse & Winston, 1996; Lucyshyn *et al.*, 2021).

Pannus (also called chronic superficial keratitis) is an immune-mediated disease diagnosed most commonly in German Shepherd Dogs and sighthounds. The distinctive clinical appearance in affected breeds includes corneal pigmentation, vascularization, and crystalline degeneration. Because the clinical appearance is highly suggestive of a diagnosis of pannus, cytology is rarely performed in these cases. When cytologic specimens are obtained from the affected areas of the cornea, an inflammatory population consisting of lymphocytes, plasma cells, and few macrophages can be observed.

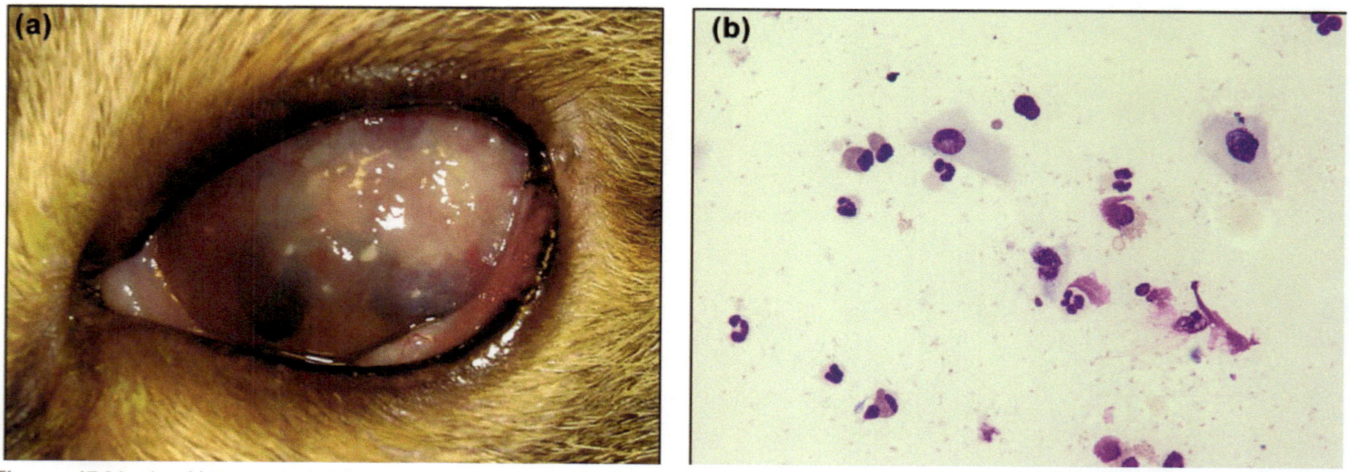

Figures 17.20a, b **(a) Domestic shorthair cat with a severe corneal lesion, left eye. (Courtesy Dr. Amber LaBelle.) (b) Corneal swab from the same cat. Fairly equal numbers of eosinophils and neutrophils are observed. A few eosinophils are ruptured, resulting in free granules in the background (Wright–Giemsa, 1,000× magnification).**

Neoplasia

Primary neoplasia of the cornea is fairly uncommon; however, SCC, hemangiosarcoma, and melanoma have been reported in multiple species (Kaps *et al.*, 2005; Cazalot et al., 2011; Takiyama et al., 2010; Dreyfus et al., 2011). These tumors exfoliate well and consist of clusters of neoplastic epithelial cells, similar to those diagnosed in the conjunctiva (Figure 17.14). Hemangiosarcoma has been rarely reported (Cazalot *et al.*, 2011). Cytologically, these tumors do not exfoliate well from any tissue, including the cornea, making biopsy a more useful diagnostic tool in these cases. Hemangiosarcoma cells are often spindle-shaped with large round to oval nuclei with prominent nucleoli. Epithelioid variants have been reported with cells described as cohesive (Warren Summers, 2007). Additionally, erythrophagia has been described as a cytologic feature of these tumors (Barger *et al.*, 2012).

Epithelial inclusion cysts have been reported and can be congenital or secondary to previous ocular injury (Simonazzi *et al.*, 2009). Clinically, they appear as white to yellow to tan smooth masses on the corneal surface associated with variable corneal vascularization. Aspiration of these structures reveals aggregates of mature keratinized epithelial cells, primarily anucleate with aggregates of keratinaceous debris. Cytologically, these greatly resemble follicular cysts of the dermis (see Chapter 4).

INTRAOCULAR STRUCTURES

Aspiration of intraocular structures may be deliberate or unintentional. Aspirates of aqueous and vitreous humors are useful diagnostic tools.

Aqueous humor

Aqueous humor is a clear and colorless fluid that has been described as acellular and of low protein concentration in multiple species (Hazel *et al.*, 1985). Anterior uveitis results in breakdown of the blood–aqueous barrier and transudation of inflammatory cells into the aqueous humor, increasing the cellularity and protein concentration. The ciliary body and iris contain melanocytes, so during an inflammatory process melanin granules and melanophages may exfoliate into the aqueous humor (Raskin, 2010). Causes of uveitis are numerous, including neoplasia, metabolic derangements (diabetes mellitus, systemic hypertension), immune-mediated, infectious (bacterial, protozoal, fungal, parasitic), viral (canine distemper virus, feline infectious peritonitis), traumatic, and idiopathic. Cytologic evaluation of aqueous fluid can aid in the diagnosis of inflammatory uveitis and lymphoma (Wiggans *et al.*, 2013; Wegg *et al.*, 2020). Additional diagnostic tests, such as immunocytochemical staining for feline coronavirus antigen or PCR testing for viral or infectious disease, can be beneficial in obtaining a definite diagnosis (Felten *et al.*, 2018; Wiggans et al., 2013). Neoplasms of the anterior uvea (iris and ciliary body) can be aspirated; however, this type of diagnostic sampling is infrequently performed. Melanoma is a common anterior uveal tumor (Grahn *et al.*, 2006) and consists of individualized and aggregates of highly pigmented neoplastic melanocytes. Ciliary body tumors are most frequently ciliary body adenoma and adenocarcinoma (Wilcock, 2007). These cells appear distinct from melanoma because they exfoliate in tightly cohesive clusters and are not pigmented. The adenocarcinomas will exhibit obvious cellular criteria of malignancy including large prominent nucleoli (Hendrix Donnell, 2007; Ferreria *et al.*, 2019).

Vitreous humor

Vitreous humor is a gelatinous fluid of low cellularity, which often contains melanin granules. Inflammation can result in a decreased viscosity of the fluid. Posterior uveitis caused by organisms such as *Blastomyces dermatitidis* causes severe inflammation, primarily neutrophilic. The fluid is highly cellular and organisms are readily identified (Figure 17.21a). Protothecosis (Figure 17.21b), histoplasmosis, and cryptococcocus can also result in severe uveitis (Schultze *et al.*, 1998; Wilcock, 2007; Raskin, 2010). When aspirating vitreous, other structures in the globe can be aspirated, especially in patients with intraocular diseases such as uveitis, rupture of the lens capsule, or retinal detachment.

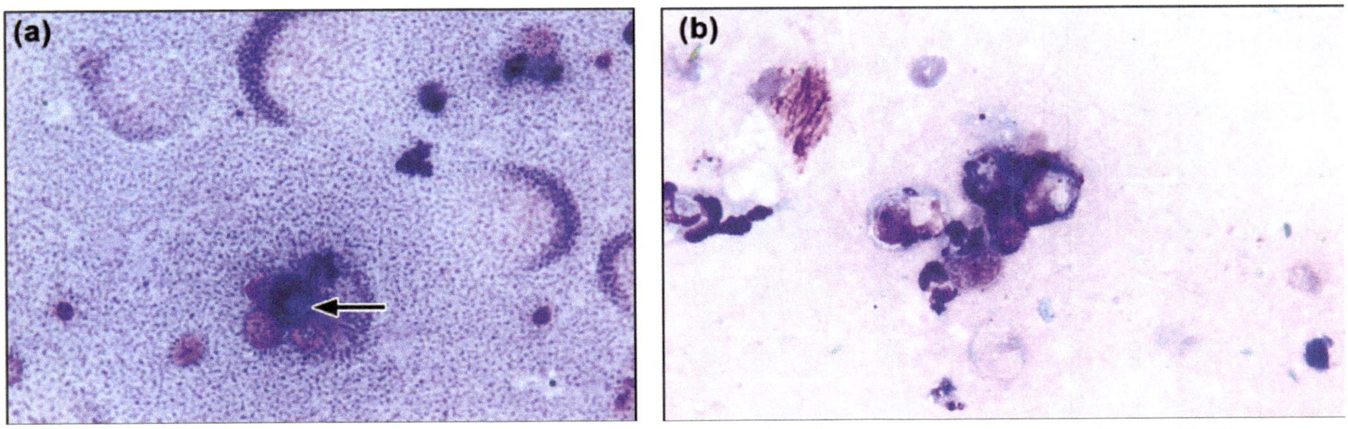

Figures 17.21a, b (a) Vitreous aspirate from a dog with uveitis of both eyes. A fungal yeast organism (arrow) consistent with *Blastomyces dermatitidis* is pictured. The background consists of thick stippled proteinaceous material, consistent with vitreous. (b) Vitreous aspirate from a dog with retinal prothecosis. Organisms are noted with few neutrophils (Wright–Giemsa: both, 1,000× magnification). (Courtesy Dr. Reema Patel.)

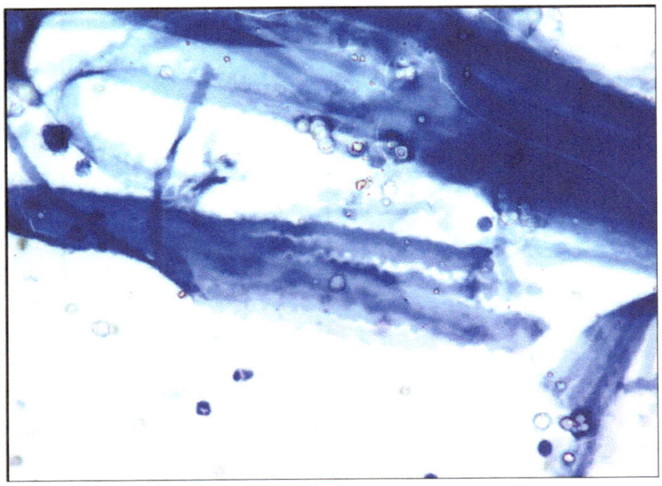

Figure 17.22 Vitreous aspirate from a dog with a luxated lens. Many lens fibers with scalloped edges are present (Wright–Giemsa, 500× magnification).

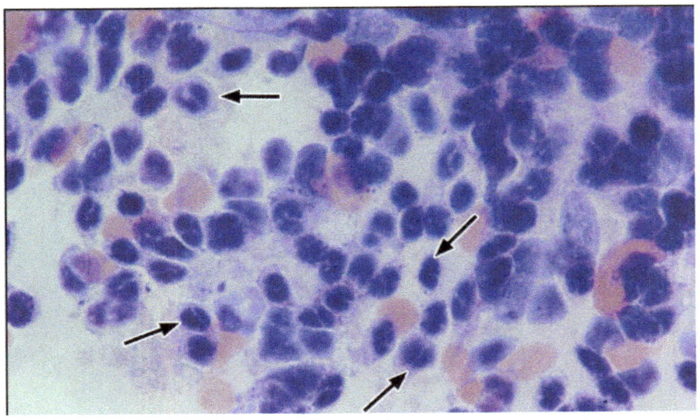

Figure 17.23 Vitreous aspirate from a dog with uveitis caused by *Blastomyces dermatitidis*. The patient had a detached retina of the right eye. Aspiration of the retina was performed and characteristic photoreceptor nuclei are observed (arrows) (Wright–Giemsa, 1,000× magnification).

Lens

The lens consists of an elastic capsule, tightly adherent squamous to cuboidal epithelial cells, and lens fibers (Samuelson, 2007). The lens fibers are elongate structures with scalloped edges that resemble lasagna noodles (Figure 17.22). Aspiration of the lens results in the aspiration of many of these fibers. The retina, especially when detached, can be easily aspirated.

Retina

The retina consists of ten layers: retinal pigmented epithelial layer, photoreceptor layer, external limiting membrane, outer nuclear layer, outer plexiform layer, inner nuclear layer, inner plexiform layer, ganglion cell layer, nerve fiber layer, and internal limiting membrane. Aspiration of the retina often reveals a disorganized arrangement of cells. Distinguishing features of retinal cells include the unique shape of the photoreceptor nuclei (Figure 17.23) and the rod-shaped melanin granules of the retinal pigmented epithelium (Figure 17.24). Occasionally, these granules are phagocytized by macrophages or observed in the background (Figure 17.25). Recognition of these structures is very important so that appropriate interpretation of these findings can be made.

RETROBULBAR SPACE

The retrobulbar space lies caudal to the globe and contains the zygomatic salivary gland, masticatory and extraocular muscles, nerves, blood vessels, and the lacrimal gland (Winer *et al.*, 2018). Due to the close proximity of these structures to the globe, primary retrobulbar pathology commonly causes ocular signs such as exophthalmos.

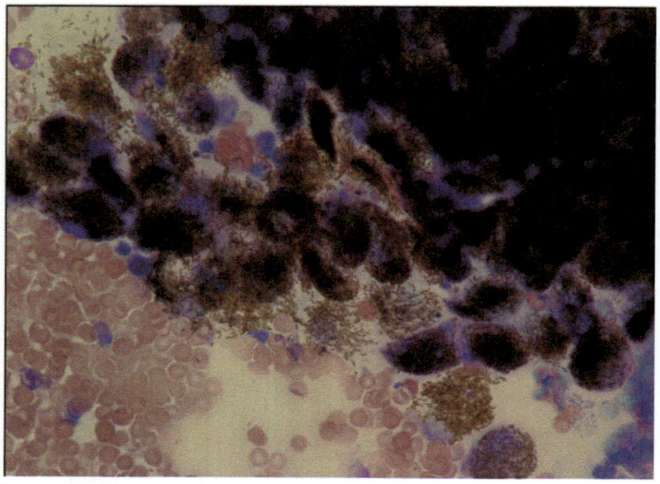

Figure 17.24 Retinal pigmented epithelium from the same sample as in Figure 17.19 (Wright–Giemsa, 500× magnification).

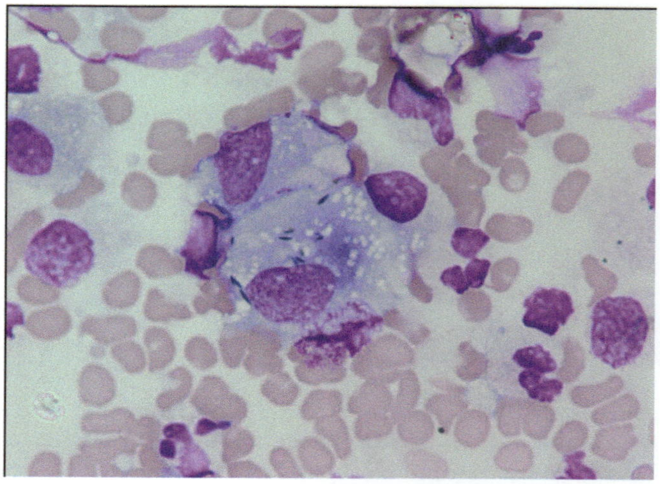

Figure 17.25 Vitreous aspirate from a dog with uveitis. A macrophage, containing many pigment granules likely from the retinal pigmented epithelium, is observed (Wright–Giemsa, 1,000× magnification).

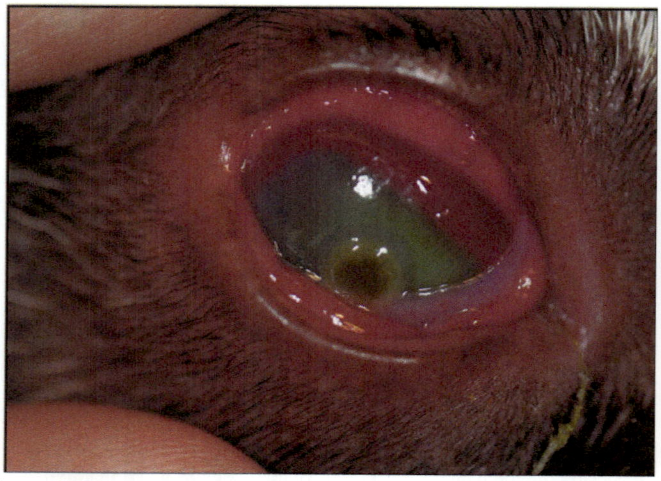

Figure 17.26 Fluorescein-stained cornea from a mixed-breed dog. Note the large pigmented ulcer.

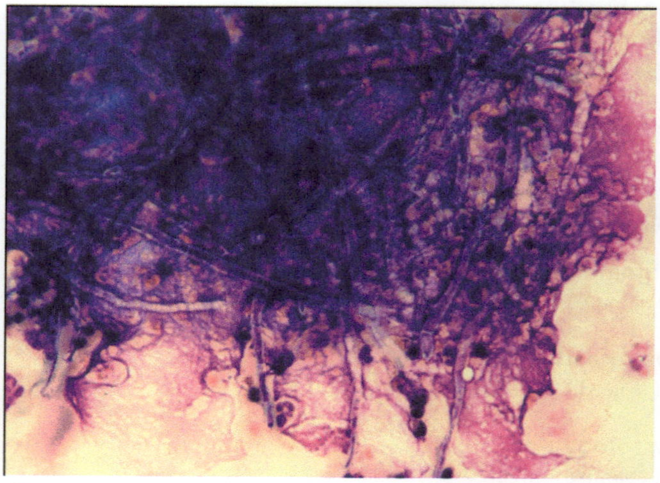

Figure 17.27 Same dog. A mat of fugal hyphae is observed, with parallel walls, septation, and branching arranged in a background of neutrophils and mucocellular debris (Wright–Giemsa, 1,000× magnification).

Inflammatory or neoplastic lesions involving adjacent tissues such as the nasal cavity or sinus can also extend into the retrobulbar space. Cytology of retrobulbar lesions can aid in the diagnosis of inflammation and bacterial or fungal infections (Walton *et al.*, 2015; Winer *et al.*, 2018). Common neoplastic retrobulbar lesions in dogs include meningioma, lymphoma, adenocarcinoma, and sarcoma (Coall *et al.*, 2022). Retrobulbar tumors in cats are overwhelmingly malignant, with the most common cytologic diagnosis of lymphoma (often secondary to extension from the nasal cavity) or carcinoma (Jones *et al.*, 2022).

SUMMARY

In conclusion, ocular cytology is a complex subject. A complete understanding of the cytology of the different structures of the healthy eye is essential so that appropriate recognition of ocular pathology, including general changes associated with inflammation, can be correctly identified.

CASES

CASE 1

Signalment/history

A mixed-breed dog presented with ocular discharge and marked reddening of the conjunctiva.

Diagnostics

Fluoroscein staining of the right eye revealed marked corneal ulceration and pigmentation (Figure 17.26). A corneal swab was performed.

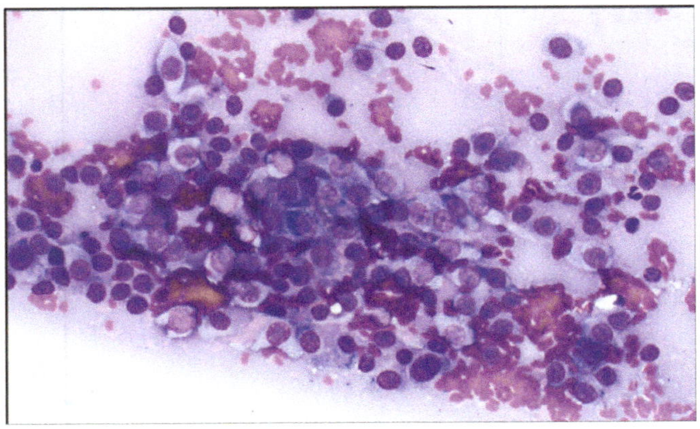

Figure 17.28 **FNA of an eyelid mass from a cat. Many pleomorphic melanocytes containing fine to coarse black melanin pigment are observed (Wright–Giemsa, 500× magnification).**

Cytology

The sample is markedly cellular and consists of a mixed inflammatory population predominated by degenerate neutrophils with few macrophages and small lymphocytes. Thick mats of fungal hyphae are observed with parallel walls, obvious septation, and perpendicular branching (Figure 17.27), consistent with fungal keratitis. Culture revealed *Aspergillus flavus.*

CASE 2

Signalment/history

A domestic shorthaired cat presented with an eyelid mass.

Diagnostics

Fine needle aspiration of the mass was performed.

Cytology

The sample is highly cellular and consists of many round to polygonal cells arranged individually and in clusters (Figure 17.28). Cells often contain fine to coarse black granular pigment, consistent with melanin. Anisocytosis and anisokaryosis are moderate and some cells contain macronucleoli. These findings are supportive of melanoma and a malignant lesion was suspected due to the degree of atypia. Excision with histopathology was recommended.

REFERENCES

Aroch I., Ofri R., Sutton G.A. (2008) Ocular manifestations of systemic diseases. In: *Slatters Fundamentals of Veterinary Ophthalmology*, 4th edn. (eds. D.J. Maggs, P.E. Miller, R. Ofri) Saunders Elsevier, St. Louis, p. 375.

Barger A.M., Skowronski M.C., MacNeill A.L. (2012) Cytologic identification of erythrophagocytic neoplasms in dogs. *Vet Clin Pathol 41*:587–589.

Bassett R.J., Burton J.J., Robson D.C. (2005) Juvenile cellulitis in an 8-month-old dog. *Aust Vet J 83*:280–282.

Bauer G.A., Spiess B.M. (1996) Lutz H. Exfoliative cytology of conjunctiva and cornea in domestic animals: A comparison of four collecting techniques. *Vet Comp Ophthalmol 6*:181–186.

Binder D.R., Sugrue J.E., Herring I.P. (2011) *Acremonium keratomycosis* in a cat. *Vet Ophthalmol 14*:111–116.

Bolzan A.A., Brunelli T.J., Castro M.B. et al. (2005) Conjunctival impression cytology in dogs. *Vet Ophthalmol 8*:401–405.

Breaux C.B., Sandmeyer L.S., Grahn B.H. (2007) Immunohistochemical investigation of canine episcleritis. *Vet Ophthalmol 10*:168–172.

Cazalot G., Regnier A., Deviers A. et al. (2011) Corneal hemangiosarcoma in a cat. *Vet Ophthalmol 14*:117–121.

Coall S.M., Premont J.E., Flatz K., Hindley K., Groth A., Billson F.M. (2022) Clinical, advanced imaging data and outcome of inflammatory and neoplastic orbital disease in 81 dogs and 16 cats in Australia (2010–2019). *Vet Ophthalmol 25*:37–50.

Cutler T.J. (2004) Corneal epithelial disease. *Vet Clin North Am Equine Pract 20*:319–343.

Dreyfus J., Schobert C.S., Dubielzig R.R. (2011) Superficial corneal squamous cell carcinoma occurring in dogs with chronic keratitis. *Vet Ophthalmol 14*:161–168.

Ewald M.M., Rankin A.J., Meekins J.M. et al. (2020) Disseminated histoplasmosis with ocular adnexal involvement in seven cats. *Vet Ophthalmol 23*:905–912.

Felten S., Matiasek K., Gruendl S., Sangl L., Hartmann K. (2018) Utility of an immunocytochemical assay using aqueous humor in the diagnosis of feline infectious peritonitis. *Vet Ophthalmol 21*:27–34.

Ferreira H., Scurrell E., Bass J., Salmon K. (2019) What is your diagnosis? Aqueous humor from a dog. *Vet Clin Pathol 48(3)*:484–486.

Fife M., Blocker T., Fife T. et al. (2011) Canine conjunctival mast cell tumors: A retrospective study. *Vet Ophthalmol 14*:153–160.

Goldreich J.E., Franklin-Guild R.J., Ledbetter E.C. (2020) Feline bacterial keratitis: Clinical features, bacterial isolates, and in vitro antimicrobial susceptibility patterns. *Vet Ophthalmol 23(1)*:90–96.

Grahn B.H., Peiffer R.L., Cullen C.L. et al. (2006) Classification of feline intraocular neoplasms based on morphology, histochemical staining and immunohistochemical labeling. *Vet Ophthalmol 9*:395–403.

Hazel S.J., Thrall M.A., Severin G.A. et al. (1985) Laboratory evaluation of aqueous humor in the healthy dog, cat, horse and cow. *Am J Vet Res 46*:657–659.

Hendrix D.V.H., Donnell R.L. (2007) Lenticular invasion by a ciliary body adenocarcinoma in a dog. *Vet Pathol 44*:540–542.

Hillström A., Tvedten H., Källberg M. et al. (2012) Evaluation of cytologic findings in feline conjunctivitis. *Vet Clin Pathol 41*:283–290.

Hindley K.E., Groth A.D., King M., Graham K., Billson F.M. (2016) Bacterial isolates, antimicrobial susceptibility, and clinical characteristics of bacterial keratitis in dogs presenting to referral practice in Australia. *Vet Ophthalmol 19*:418–426.

Jones B.A., Cotterill N., Drees R., Dietrich U.M., Purzycka K. (2022) Tumours involving the retrobulbar space in cats: 37 cases. *J Feline Med Surg 24(6)*:e116–e123.

Kaps S., Richter M., Philipp M. et al. (2005) Primary invasive ocular squamous cell carcinoma in a horse. *Vet Ophthalmol 8*:193–197.

Krehbiel J.D., Langham R.F. (1975) Eyelid neoplasms of dogs. *Am J Vet Res 36(1)*:115–119.

Labelle A.L., Hamor R.E., Barger A.M. et al. (2009) *Aspergillus flavus* keratomycosis in a cat treated with topical 1% voriconazole solution. *Vet Ophthalmol 12*:48–52.

Lavach J.D., Thrall M.A., Benjamin M.M. et al. (1977) Cytology of normal and inflamed conjunctivas in dogs and cats. *J Am Vet Med Assoc 170*:722–727.

Lu J.E., Dubielzig R. (2012) Canine eyelid granular cell tumor: A report of eight cases. *Vet Ophthalmol 15*:406–410.

Lucyshyn D.R., Vernau W., Maggs D.J. et al. (2021) Correlations between clinical signs and corneal cytology in feline eosinophilic keratoconjunctivitis. *Vet Ophthalmol 24*:620–626.

Maggs D.J. (2008) Conjunctiva. In: *Slatter's Fundamentals of Veterinary Ophthalmology*, 4th edn. (eds. D.J. Maggs, P.E. Miller, R. Ofri) Saunders Elsevier, Philadelphia, pp. 135–150.

Moore P.F. (1984) Systemic histiocytosis of Bernese Mountain Dogs. *Vet Pathol 21*:554–563.

Naisse M.P., Glover T.L., Moore C.P. et al. (1998) Detection of feline herpesvirus 1 DNA in corneas of cats with eosinophilic keratitis or corneal sequestration. *Am J Vet Res 59*:856–858.

Nevile J.C., Hurn S.D., Turner A.G. (2016) Keratomycosis in five dogs. *Vet Ophthalmol 19*:432–438.

Olbertz L., Lima L., Werner J. et al. (2012) Supposed primary conjunctival lymphoma in a dog. *Vet Ophthalmol*. doi:10.1111/j.1463–5224.2012.01027.

Pena M.T., Roura X., Davidson M.G. (2000) Ocular and periocular manifestations of leishmaniasis in dogs: 105 cases (1993–1998). *Vet Ophthalmol 3*:35–41.

Perazzi A., Bonsembiante F., Gelain M.E. et al. (2017) Cytology of the healthy canine and feline ocular surface: Comparison between cytobrush and impression technique. *Veterinary Clinical Pathology 46*:164–171.

Pirie C.G., Knollinger A.M., Thomas C.B. et al. (2006) Canine conjunctival hemangioma and hemangiosarcoma: A retrospective evaluation of 108 cases (1989–2004). *Vet Ophthalmol 9*:215–226.

Prasse K.W., Winston S.M. (1996) Cytology and histopathology of feline eosinophilic keratitis. *Vet Comp Ophthalmol 6*:74–81.

Pucket J.D., Allbaugh R.A., Rankin A.J. (2012) Treatment of dematiaceous fungal keratitis in a dog. *J Am Vet Med Assoc 240*:1104–1108.

Raskin R.E. (2010) Eye and adnexa. In: *Canine and Feline Cytology* (eds. R.E. Raskin, D.J. Meyer) Saunders Elsevier, Philadelphia, pp. 366–382.

Samuelson D.A. (2007) Eye and ear. *Textbook of Veterinary Histology*. Saunders Elsevier, Philadelphia, pp. 487–511.

Schobert C.S., Labelle P., Dubielzig R.R. (2010) Feline conjunctival melanoma: Histopathological characteristics and clinical outcomes. *Vet Ophthalmol 13*:43–46.

Schultze A.E., Ring R.D., Morgan R.V. et al. (1998) Clinical, cytologic and histopathologic manifestations of protothecosis in two dogs. *Vet Ophthalmol 1*:239–243.

Simonazzi B., Castania M., Bosco V. et al. (2009) A case of multiple unilateral corneal epithelial inclusion cysts in a dog. *J Small Anim Pract 50*:373–376.

Spinelli T.P., Bezerra L.M., de Souza B.O.F. et al. (2021) Primary conjunctival sporotrichosis in three cats from Northeastern Brazil. *Vet Ophthalmol 24(2)*:209–217.

Stades F.C., van der Woerdt A. (2013) Diseases and surgery of the canine eyelid. In: *Veterinary Ophthalmology*, 5th edn. (eds. K.N. Gelatt, B.C. Gilger, T.J. Kern) Wiley-Blackwell, Ames, p. 879.

Stiles J. (2012) Ocular infections. In: *Infectious Diseases of the Dog and Cat*, 4th edn. (ed. C.E. Greene) Saunders Elsevier, St. Louis, p. 1059.

Takiyama N., Tersaki E., Uechi M. (2010) Corneal squamous cell carcinoma in two dogs. *Vet Ophthalmol 13*:266–269.

Walton S., Martin P., Tolson C., Plumridge S., Barrs V.R. (2015) Orbital actinomycotic mycetoma caused by *Streptomyces cinnamoneus*. *JFMS Open Rep 1(1)*:2055116915589836.

Warren A.L., Summers B.A. (2007) Epithelioid variant of hemangioma and hemangiosarcoma in the dog, horse and cow. *Vet Pathol 44*:15–24.

Wegg M.L., Jeanes E.C., Pollard D., Fleming L., Dawson C. (2021) A multicenter retrospective study into endogenous causes of uveitis in cats in the United Kingdom: Ninety two cases. *Vet Ophthalmol 24*:591–598.

Wiggans K.T., Vernau W., Lappin M.R., Thomasy S.M., Maggs D.J. (2014) Diagnostic utility of aqueocentesis and aqueous humor analysis in dogs and cats with anterior uveitis. *Vet Ophthalmol 17*:212–220.

Wilcock B.P. (2007) Eye and ear. In: *Pathology of Domestic Animals, Volume 1*, 5th edn. (ed. M.G. Maxie) Saunders Elsevier, Philadelphia, pp. 459–552.

Winer J.N., Verstraete F.J.M., Cissell D.D., Le C., Vapniarsky N., Good K.L., Gutierrez C.J., Arzi B. (2018) Clinical features and computed tomography findings are utilized to characterize retrobulbar disease in dogs. *Front Vet Sci 5*:186.

Young K.M., Prasse K.W. (2007) The eyes and associated structures. In: *Diagnostic Cytology and Hematology of the Dog and Cat*, 3rd edn. (eds. R.L. Cowell, R.D. Tyler, J.H. Meinkoth, D.B. DeNicola) Mosby Elsevier, St. Louis, pp. 149–171.

Young K.M., Taylor J. (2006) Laboratory medicine: Yesterday today tomorrow: Eye on cytoplasm. *Vet Clin Pathol 35*:141.

CHAPTER 18

CYTOLOGY OF THE EAR

Cheryl Moller, Jennifer A. Neel, and K. Marcia Murphy

INTRODUCTION

The external ear functions as a conduit for sound to the middle ear and is also important for expression of behavior. The external ear is composed of the pinna (or auricle), the external auditory meatus (the entrance to the ear canal), and the cartilaginous ear canal. There is a small osseous component to the ear canal of the dog and cat, which is more developed in large animals such as horses and cattle. The external ear canal ends at the tympanic membrane (ear drum).

The convex (outer) aspect of the pinna consists of a covering of haired skin comprising epidermis, dermis, subcutis (fat, lymphatics, vessels, and nerves), and skeletal muscles, which overlie the auricular cartilage. The cartilage is elastic and contains many foramina through which blood vessels and nerves traverse (Calhoun & Stinson, 1987; Evans, 1993; Cole, 2009). The concave (inner) aspect of the pinna is more sparsely haired but also comprises epidermis, dermis, and a subcutis that is attached to the concave aspect of the auricular cartilage.

The ear canal is lined by stratified squamous epithelium, which is typically 3–5 cells thick. Variable numbers of hair follicles are present in the ear canal, the quantities of which are highly breed dependent, especially in dogs. The superficial dermis contains sebaceous glands, which open directly into hair follicles. There are also specialized, modified apocrine sweat glands (ceruminous glands) that open either into hair follicles or directly onto the surface of the epidermis. The density of ceruminous and sebaceous glands within the dermis also varies between breeds (Cole, 2009). Deeper in the dermis, there are scattered lymphoid follicles, which are important for local immunity. There are also nerves and vessels throughout the dermis and subcutis. The deepest tissues are the structural components of cartilage and trabecular bone (Figure 18.1).

As well as the dermal lymphoid tissue, the ceruminous material that resides within the ear canal is an important component of aural immunity and defense. Cerumen is acidic and composed of sloughed anucleate keratinocytes, watery ceruminous and mixed lipid sebaceous gland secretions, as well as immunoglobulins, lysozyme, and interleukins (Huang *et al.*, 1994; Cole, 2009; Crain *et al.*, 2009). The self-cleaning function of the external ear canal is an effective means of regulating the ceruminous material and is highly important for aural health. Sloughed anucleate keratinocytes migrate to the periphery of the tympanic membrane and then, along with glandular secretions and resident yeasts and bacteria, move outwards to the external auditory meatus to be shaken, scratched, or groomed out of the ear canal (Cole, 2009). Overzealous use of ceruminolytics and ear cleaners impairs this normal process (Rosychuk, 1994).

Cytologic examination of the ear canal is an important part of the diagnostic work up of otic disease in cats and dogs. Specifics of sampling this region will be discussed further below. All descriptions forthwith refer to staining characteristics with Romanowsky-type stains such as Diff-Quik® (modified rapid Romanowsky stain) or Wright–Giemsa.

In healthy dogs and cats, the normal external canal may contain yeasts, cocci, and keratinocytes. The most common yeast in the external ear canal of cats and dogs is *Malassezia pachydermatis*. The yeasts are peanut-shaped, dark basophilic, and approximately 3 µm wide and 7 µm long (Figure 18.2). There may also be 1 µm diameter dark basophilic cocci present singly, in pairs, or in small clusters. The vast

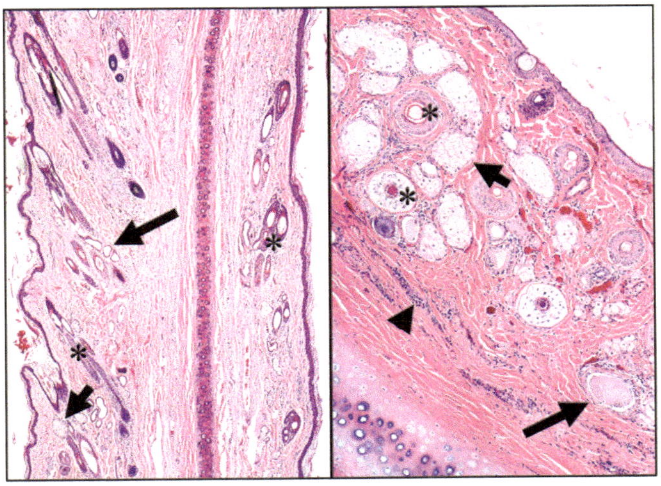

Figure 18.1 Sections of pinna and ear canal; normal structures. Left: section of normal pinna from a dog. The auricular cartilage is in the center and is covered by haired skin consisting of a thin epidermis of stratified squamous epithelium, a dermis with hair follicles (asterisks), sebaceous glands (short arrow) and ceruminous glands (long arrow), and a subcutis. Note that the hair follicles are more numerous on the convex surface (left side). Right: ear canal from a dog. This tissue shows mild hyperplastic changes (mild epidermal hyperplasia, mild dermal fibrosis) and has mild multifocal lymphoplasmacytic infiltrates (arrowhead). Note the hair follicles (asterisks), sebaceous glands (short arrow), ceruminous glands filled with inspissated secretory material (long arrow), and the structural cartilage to the lower right (H&E: left, 40× magnification; right, 100× magnification).

DOI: 10.1201/9781003258551-18

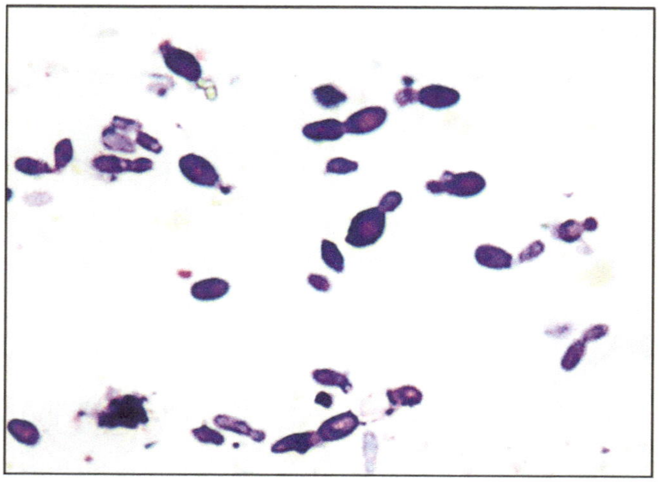

Figure 18.2 Ear swab from a cat; *Malassezia pachydermatis* yeast. Note the classic peanut or shoe print appearance of the dividing cells. The yeasts are approximately 3 × 7 μm in size and exhibit unipolar budding on a broad base forming a prominent collarette (modified Wright–Giemsa, 2,000× magnification). (Courtesy Dr. Kelli Ferris.)

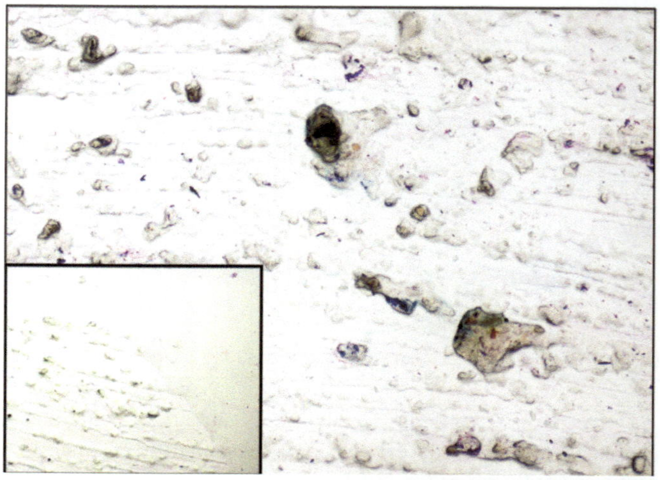

Figure 18.3 Normal ear swab from a cat; cerumen and keratin. Refractile, non- to poorly staining cerumen is admixed with angular squamous cells. Inset: immersion oil has been added to the slide and is dissolving the lipid-rich cerumen (modified Wright–Giemsa, 40× magnification; inset: 100× magnification). (Courtesy Dr. Kelli Ferris.)

majority of keratinocytes are anucleate (squames), but rare nucleated keratinocytes, also known as squamous epithelial cells, may be seen. Squames are large, angular, and flat or rolled up ('keratin bars'), and variably stain clear to pale basophilic to eosinophilic. They may contain variable numbers of very fine, bright pink to purple keratohyalin granules. Keratohyalin granules may also be free in the background. Care must be taken not to confuse these granules with cocci – bacteria are larger and typically stain a darker purple/blue (Angus, 2004). Depending on the pigmentation of the dog or cat, scattered coarse granules of brown to gold to black melanin pigment may be seen within squames or free in the background. Cerumen is lipid-rich, and therefore resists staining. It may be seen as amorphous clear material in the background, and may appear to dissolve or disappear with the addition of immersion oil (Figure 18.3).

Tater *et al.* (2003) have evaluated the cytology of the vertical ear canal of normal dogs and cats (Table 18.1). Roll preparation cytologic smears were found to be the most cellular. Dogs (n = 50) were found to have a median of 0.2 *Malassezia* spp. yeast and 3.9 keratinocytes/high-power field (hpf) (400× magnification). In addition, 42% of the dogs also had rare cocci, but the median number was 0/hpf. In cats (n = 52), approximately 8 keratinocytes/hpf were observed and there were 0.2/hpf of *Malassezia* yeast and 0.3/hpf of cocci. Rod-shaped bacteria were not seen, and are not considered a normal finding in the ears of healthy cats or dogs (Tater *et al.*, 2003). The presence of neutrophils within the ear canal is always abnormal and indicates inflammation (Ginel *et al.*, 2002).

SAMPLING

Cytologic examination is warranted for any lesion of the pinna or external ear canal. Some lesions may exfoliate poorly, such as

Table 18.1 **Cytologic findings of the external ear canal in the normal dog and cat**

	Median number per high-power field (400× magnification)	
Feature	Dog	Cat
Malassezia yeast	0.2	0.2
Cocci	0 (rare)	0.3
Keratinocytes	3.9	8

mesenchymal tumors (e.g., fibrosarcoma, hemangioma, hemangiosarcoma). Nodules can be aspirated either with or without negative pressure from an attached syringe. Swabbing ear canal nodules is unlikely to reveal the cause. Masses within the ear canal are best aspirated in a heavily sedated or anesthetized animal, facilitated via an otoscope or an otoendoscope. The aspirated material should be rapidly discharged and gently smeared across one or multiple slides. Fine needle aspiration (FNA) of the regional submandibular or retropharyngeal lymph nodes may also be indicated.

On the pinna, flat lesions may be best assessed by impression smears of any exudative or eroded/ulcerated surface, followed by careful scraping of the underlying lesion with a spatula or a dulled scalpel blade. The material may then be wiped across multiple slides. This is the most useful way of cytologically diagnosing squamous cell carcinoma (SCC).

Alopecic or crusted lesions can be assessed with hair plucks for dermatophytes or *Demodex* mites (Figure 18.4), and/or multiple superficial and deep skin scrapings in mineral oil for *Sarcoptes* or *Demodex* mites, respectively (Figure 18.5). For ceruminous debris on the pinna, a dulled blade may be used to gently collect some of the material, which is then wiped across slides without oil for staining. Organisms such as *M. pachydermitis* or *Leishmania* spp., as well as

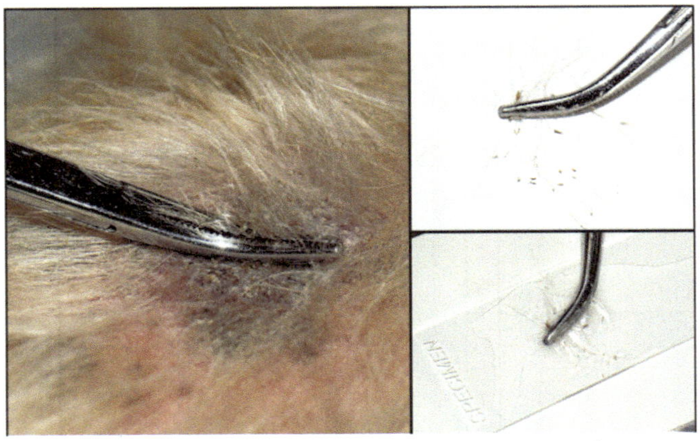

Figure 18.4 Hair pluck preparation from a dog with suspected demodicosis. Left: an area with evidence of follicular pathology (broken hairs, comedones, etc.) is selected. A sample of hair is firmly grasped with forceps, close to the skin, and is quickly plucked. Right top: a good quality sample will have a sufficient number of hairs, including the roots, to allow thorough examination. Bottom right: mineral oil is placed on a glass slide and the hairs are added. A coverslip will be placed on top to allow easy viewing with a microscope. The slide should be examined on both low-power (40×/100×) and high-power (400×) magnification.

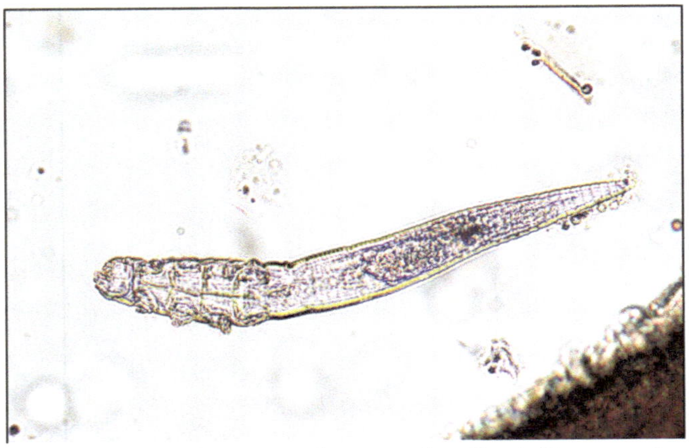

Figure 18.5 Deep skin scraping from a cat; demodicosis. The preparation shows the typical, elongated, 'cigar-shaped' appearance of *Demodex cati*. Adult mites range in length from approximately 180 to 220 μm, have a long and prominently striped abdomen, and four sets of clawed appendages. Because this mite inhabits hair follicles, hair plucks or deep scrapings are the best methods to use for screening (unstained oil mount preparation, 200× magnification).

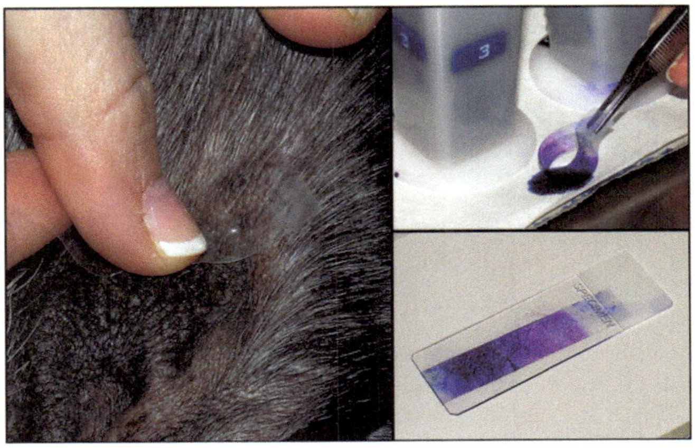

Figure 18.6 Tape strip sample preparation from the pinna of a dog. Left: tape is firmly pressed onto the lesion. Tape strip preparations are best used with drier, less exudative skin lesions. Top right: the tape strip is stained using only the third, dark blue solution of the quick stain and then briefly rinsed in water. Bottom right: the stained preparation is placed on a slide, specimen side down, and then blotted with blotting paper to removed excess liquid.

bacteria, may be identified in this way. For drier, less exudative lesions of the pinnae, tape strip sample collection is useful and less traumatic to the inflamed skin (Figure 18.6).

Cytologic examination of ceruminous and/or purulent debris is indicated for every case of otitis externa. It is also useful as a tool for monitoring response to treatment. Cytology is considered more sensitive for detecting *Malassezia* yeast and bacteria than culture (Huang *et al.*, 1994; Griffin *et al.*, 2007). Although sampling the horizontal ear canal is likely more representative of the infection, it can be difficult in an awake animal and sedation or anesthesia is not necessarily indicated for every case of otitis externa. In most cases, sampling the junction of the vertical and horizontal canals is sufficient (Angus, 2004). To optimize the sampling of the external ear canal, gently pull up on the pinna to help straighten the ear canal and then place the swab into the ear canal, angling toward the nose, and slowly advance. The swab should be rolled into the debris and then removed from the ear and rolled across glass slides. For collection of samples to search for ear mites such as *Otodectes cynotis* or *Demodex* spp., particularly in cats, a drop or two of mineral oil is placed on a separate glass microscope slide and the same swab used to collect the cytology sample is dipped into the mineral oil. The swab is then gently placed back into the ear canal and debris collected. The debris is then transferred to the same glass microscope slide containing the mineral oil by gently rolling the swab in the drop of mineral oil. Both ears should be sampled with separate swabs on separate slides, and the slides carefully labeled. Slides should be examined promptly since mites may possibly walk off the slide if left for too long.

For optimal cytologic examination, preparation of multiple slides is recommended when collecting samples from nodules or masses of the pinna or ear canal. In addition, it is always useful to keep at least one slide unstained from any type of otic cytology in case special stains are required.

Skin scrapings prepared with mineral oil are cover slipped and examined under the microscope directly. Hair plucks may be cleared with potassium hydroxide to search for dermatophytes. Other preparations should be stained. Heat fixation of the slide does not improve staining; thus rapid air-drying of smears is adequate for cytology (Toma *et al.*, 2006; Griffin *et al.*, 2007). Romanowsky-type stains such as Diff-Quik®, or similar modified rapid stains, or Wright–Giemsa are the most useful. The lipid component of cerumen may be dissolved by the alcohol in the staining process (Ginel *et al.*, 2002).

It is desirable to possess a separate set of jars of rapid stain dedicated for suspected infectious or so called 'dirty' ear cytology specimens to prevent contamination of other samples. Cytology of otic debris can be stained in the usual fashion, or, for more rapid results, a single 5–10 second dip in the counterstain (purple stain) is considered sufficient for identifying bacteria, yeast, keratinocytes, and neutrophils (Toma *et al.*, 2006). For tape preparations, jar 1 should not be used as the alcohol will remove the glue component from the tape and thus your sample.

CYTOLOGY

Cytologic examination of lesions of the external ear can be very useful to determine whether the process is inflammatory or neoplastic and, in many cases, can elucidate the etiology.

Pinna and periauricular area

Inflammatory lesions

Inflammatory lesions of the external ear may be infectious or sterile. As with any other location, the absence of detectable etiological agents on cytology does not rule out infection.

Infectious inflammation

A wide range of infectious agents may potentially be seen on smears from lesions of the pinna and periauricular area. *Malassezia* dermatitis is a common contributing factor to the clinical signs of pinnal pruritus in dogs, less commonly in cats, suffering from atopic otitis or other concurrent dermatoses. Canine leproid granuloma and leishmaniasis are two other infectious diseases with a predilection for the pinna. Other organisms that may be seen rarely on cytology of pinnal lesions from cats or dogs include yeasts such as *Blastomyces dermatitidis*, *Cryptococcus* spp., *Histoplasma capsulatum*, *Sporothrix schenckii*, other opportunistic fungi (Figure 18.7), protozoa including *Neospora caninum*, *Toxoplasma gondii*, *Trypanosoma cruzi*, the mites *Demodex*, *Sarcoptes*, and *Notoedres cati (N. cati* is seen exclusively in cats), and dermatophyte infections, which are often present elsewhere in the skin as well. The cytologic appearance of selected lesions is described below. *Otodectes cynotis* ear mites are discussed in the 'Ear Canal' section.

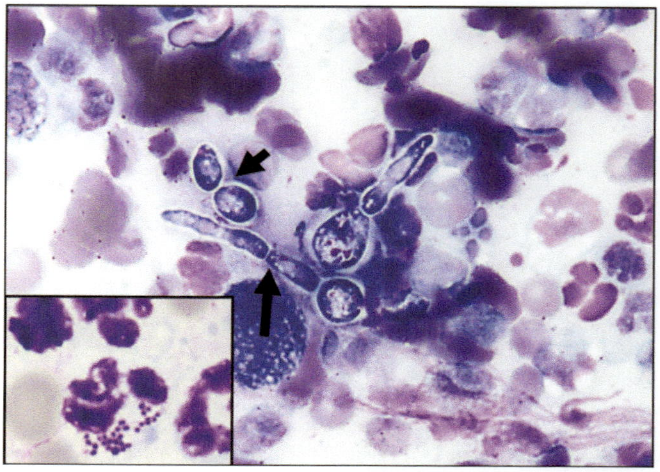

Figure 18.7 **Intact papule on the pinna of a dog on immunosuppressive therapy; opportunistic fungal infection. Fungal elements including round yeasts chained together in pseudohyphae (short arrow) and true septated hyphae (long arrow) are present on a background of macrophages and degenerate neutrophils. Inset: cytology of a ruptured and draining papule revealed only degenerate neutrophils and a secondary bacterial infection. If possible, always sample intact (nonruptured/ulcerated) lesions (Wright–Giemsa, 1,000× magnification; inset: modified Wright–Giemsa, 1,000× magnification).**

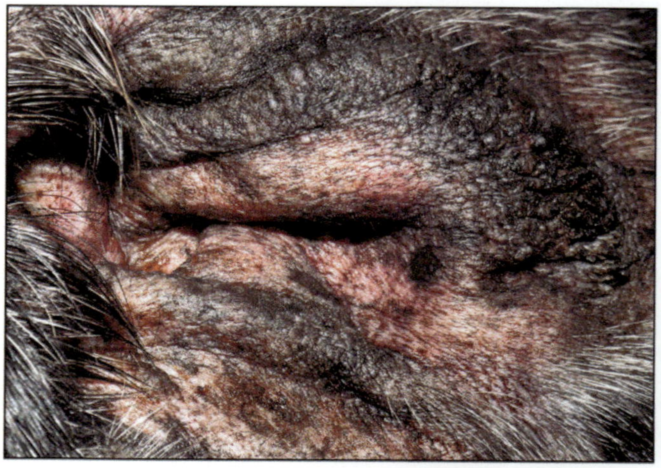

Figure 18.8 **Canine inner surface of the ear pinna; gross appearance of *Malassezia* dermatitis. The pinna is erythematous with prominent scaling, thickening, and lichenification.**

Malassezia *dermatitis*

Malassezia spp., most commonly *Malassezia pachydermatis*, are yeast organisms that can cause significant pinnal pruritus with or without ear canal involvement. The concave surface of the affected pinna is commonly erythematous, greasy or waxy (ceruminous), scaly (yellow or slate gray), crusty, and malodorous. Mild to moderate lichenification and thickening of the affected pinna may be noted, depending on chronicity (Figure 18.8). The lesions may be localized to one or both pinna, or may be generalized, affecting other parts of the animal, including the ear canals, lips, ventral neck, axillae, groin, interdigital skin, perianal area, and intertriginous areas that are warm and moist. The development of clinical signs is more common in the highly humid months, corresponding with the peak of the allergy season, but may persist into the winter. *Malassezia* dermatitis is a hypersensitivity reaction; therefore the clinical response is not related to the number of yeast organisms present but, rather, to the patient's reaction to them (Chen & Hill, 2005).

Tape strip sample collection is usually the most useful technique, causing the least irritation to the inflamed pinna. However, if the affected skin on the pinna is markedly exudative with thick ceruminous debris present, a dulled scalpel blade or spatula may be used to collect the debris and smear it onto a glass slide. In the authors' experience, the latter may cause significant irritation to the pinna, resulting in considerable self-trauma to the sampled pinna. The tape strip sample (stained in jar 3 of Romanowsky rapid stain only) or the smeared stained glass slide will reveal basophilic stained yeast ranging in size from 2.0 × 4.0 µm up to 6.0 × 7.0 µm. *Malassezia* yeast exhibit unipolar budding resulting in 'snowman', 'peanut', or 'footprint' type shapes. Inflammatory cells, most commonly neutrophils, may or may not be present, but are not a common feature of *Malassezia* dermatitis.

Leishmaniasis

Leishmania (Leishmania) infantum and *Leishmania (Leishmania) donovani* are protozoal parasites that can cause severe disease in dogs. *L. infantum* is also an important zoonotic disease. Canine leishmaniasis is endemic in Europe, Africa, South America, and Asia, and cases have been specifically reported in foxhounds in North America, as well as in imported dogs in nonendemic areas (Duprey *et al.*, 2006; Cleare *et al.*, 2014). Infection with *Leishmania* spp. can result in a spectrum of diseases, the manifestations of which depend on the interplay of parasite and host factors. The intermediate hosts of *Leishmania* are several genera of sandflies. Dogs with clinical leishmaniasis commonly have cutaneous lesions, with a predilection for more sparsely haired areas such as the muzzle and the pinna (Figure 18.9). This predilection is thought to be attributable to the biting preferences of the sandfly. Pinnal lesions range from a silvery scale with alopecia, to ulcers and, much less commonly, nodules. Lesions may be on one or both ears (Cleare *et al.*, 2014). *Leishmania (Leishmania) mexicana* can cause cutaneous disease in dogs and cats, including reported cases of pinnal lesions in cats in Texas where it is endemic (Trainor *et al.*, 2010). *Leishmania (Viannia) braziliensis* is another species which causes cutaneous lesions in dogs and cats (Brilhante *et al.*, 2019; Rivas *et al.*, 2018). Other *Leishmania* species may also sporadically cause cutaneous lesions including of the pinna in dogs and cats.

Impression smears of the exudate overlying ulcerated lesions or aspirates of the nodules typically reveal a mixed inflammatory cell population with a variable amount of hemodilution. There are macrophages with variable numbers of lymphocytes, plasma cells, and nondegenerate neutrophils. A superficial and opportunistic bacterial infection may also be seen, with predominantly cocci; some degenerate neutrophils may accompany the infection and may be seen containing phagocytized bacteria. Variable, but typically low, numbers of protozoal amastigotes are seen phagocytized by macrophages and free in the background. They are ovoid to tapered organisms, approximately 3–6 × 1.5–3.0 µm in size, with a central dark nucleus, rod-shaped kinetoplast, and pale basophilic cytoplasm (Figure 18.10).

Histologically, the pattern of the inflammation within the dermis varies, but a perivascular pattern is seen most frequently. The inflammation is pyogranulomatous to granulomatous, with macrophages and variable numbers of nondegenerate neutrophils, lymphocytes, and plasma cells. Amastigotes may be difficult to see on routine hematoxylin and eosin (H&E) staining: Giemsa stains will highlight the organisms. *Leishmania* amastigotes are approximately 3 µm in diameter, with a dark central nucleus, rod-shaped kinetoplast, and pale eosinophilic cytoplasm. They may be seen free in the dermis admixed within the inflammatory infiltrates, or phagocytized within macrophages. Although the detection of amastigotes is specific for leishmaniasis, the sensitivity of detection on histopathology is quite low. Polymerase chain reaction (PCR) assay of tissues or aspirates of lymph node, spleen, or bone marrow, or immunohistochemistry of biopsies of skin lesions are the recommended diagnostics where cytology and histopathology are negative (Cornegliani *et al.*, 2005; Giunchetti *et al.*, 2006; Cleare *et al.*, 2014; Koutinas Koutinas, 2014).

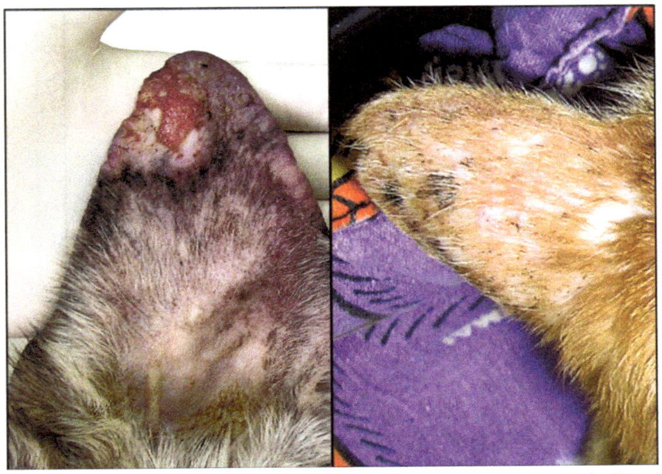

Figure 18.9 Gross appearance of leishmaniasis. Left: ear pinna of a dog; concave surface, with alopecia, erosion, ulceration, depigmentation, and hyperpigmentation. Right: ear pinna from a cat; convex surface, showing alopecia and crusting. (Courtesy Dr. Guadalupe Miro.)

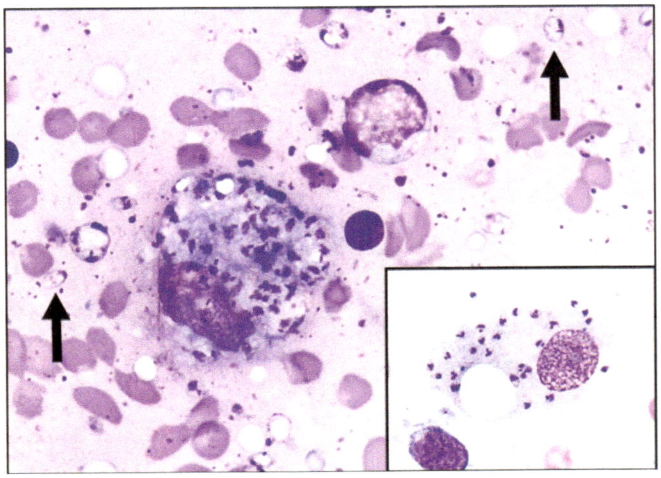

Figure 18.10 Touch imprint of an ulcerated mass on the right pinna of a cat; leishmaniasis. A large macrophage filled with amastigote forms of *Leishmania* is present on a background of protein, RBCs, and cellular debris. The organisms have a larger oval nucleus and a perpendicular, smaller, rod-shaped kinetoplast giving the image of a person hanging from a parachute. Free organisms are also noted in the background (arrows). In this case, the infection was confirmed as *L. mexicana* via RNA gene sequencing (modified Wright–Giemsa, 1,000× magnification). Inset: tissue from a foxhound, infected with *L. infantum*. A large macrophage containing amastigotes is present (Wright–Giemsa, 1,000× magnification). (American Society of Veterinary Clinical Pathology: Mystery Slide Conference, 2014, Case 8, submitted by Dr. Holly Minard.)

Mycobacteriosis

A dog-specific infection of the pinna is canine leproid granuloma. Canine leproid granuloma is a typically asymptomatic disease caused by multiple mycobacteria of the *Mycobacterium* simiae-related group (Hughes *et al.*, 2000). They are not considered zoonotic. These mycobacteria are slow-growing organisms that cause the formation of one or more firm alopecic nodules on or around the pinnae, especially on the dorsal fold of the ear (Malik *et al.*, 1998). The lesions may be ulcerated (Figure 18.11). Leproid granulomas are most frequently seen in Boxers and other short-coated breeds (Malik *et al.*, 1998). Biting flies are thought to transmit the bacteria, hence the predilection for the pinna and the more frequent occurrence in short-coated dog breeds (Smith, 1973).

Aspiration of the nodules reveals a variably cellular, mixed inflammatory cell infiltrate of epithelioid macrophages, plasma cells, lymphocytes, neutrophils, and binucleate macrophages and multinucleate giant cells (Figure 18.12). Epithelioid macrophages are macrophages with abundant pale basophilic cytoplasm and a small eccentric nucleus with a small prominent nucleolus; as the name indicates, they possess similarities to epithelial cells. The cytoplasm of epithelioid macrophages and giant cells contains clear and refractile (negative staining) rod-shaped bacteria; free bacilli may also be seen within the background (Twomey *et al.*, 2005). Mycobacteria are negative staining because their lipid cell wall resists Romanowsky-type stains (Malik *et al.*, 1998). Organism numbers vary from few to many. Acid-fast stains may be applied to air-dried and unstained smears to highlight the mycobacteria. Alternatively, stained slides that are suspect but negative may be destained and then stained with acid-fast stain (Marcos *et al.*, 2009).

Histologically, the lesions are located in the dermis and/or subcutis and are composed of sheets of epithelioid macrophages, neutrophils, fewer lymphocytes and plasma cells, and variable numbers of multinucleate giant cells. The inflammatory cell population often forms poorly circumscribed granulomas or pyogranulomas (Figure 18.13).

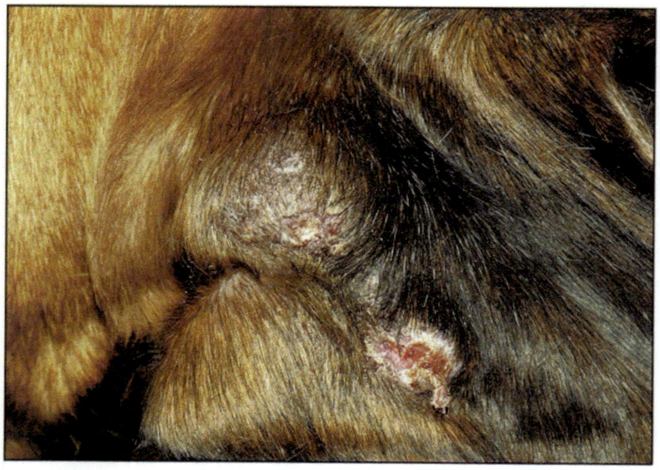

Figure 18.11 **Dorsal fold of the ear of a dog; gross appearance of leproid granulomas. A larger, partially alopecic nodule and a smaller ulcerated nodule are present. (Courtesy Dr. Frane Banovic.)**

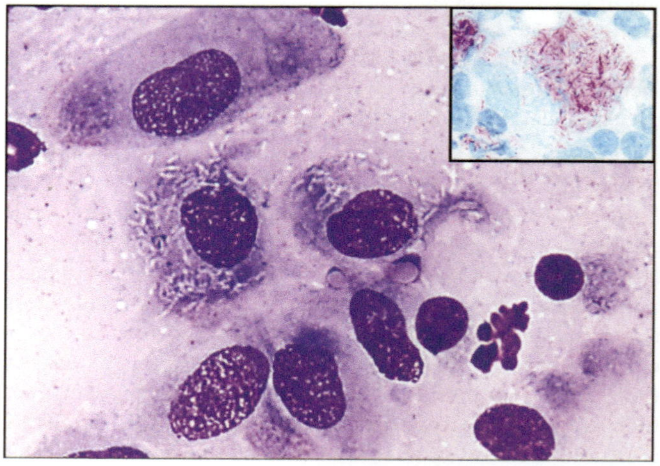

Figure 18.12 **Aspirate of a lesion on the pinna of a dog; mycobacteriosis. Epithelioid macrophages contain nonstaining bacilli. A few free bacteria are also noted in the background (modified Wright–Giemsa, 1,000× magnification). Inset: note the characteristic acid-fast staining of the organisms. Acid-fast staining may be performed on unstained or destained cytology preparations (acid-fast stain, 1,000× magnification). (Courtesy Dr. Valarie Pallatto.)**

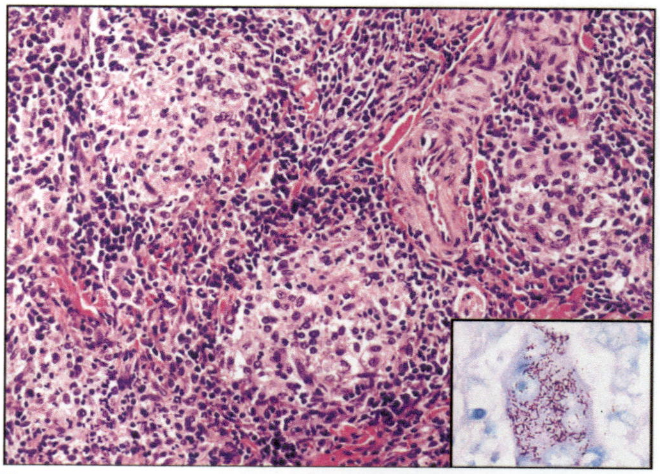

Figure 18.13 **Haired skin from the pinna of a dog; leproid granuloma. Multiple small nodules composed of epithelioid macrophages are present and are surrounded by fewer neutrophils, lymphocytes, and plasma cells (H&E, 200× magnification). Inset: a multinucleate giant cell filled with phagocytized acid-fast bacilli (acid-fast stain, 1,000× magnification).**

The cytoplasm of macrophages and giant cells contains bacilli that are negative staining and often difficult to identify on H&E stains, but are readily stained by modified acid-fast stains such as Fite stain or Ziehl–Neelsen stain (Malik *et al.*, 1998; Foley *et al.*, 2002).

The lesions usually spontaneously regress within weeks to months, although some may require treatment with surgical excision and/or anti-mycobacterial antibiotics (Malik *et al.*, 1998; Foley *et al.*, 2002). Where leproid granuloma is suspected but organisms cannot be identified on cytology or histopathology, mycobacterial PCR can be performed on Romanowsky-stained aspirate smears (not acid-fast stains) or on formalin-fixed, paraffin-embedded tissues (Reppas *et al.*, 2013).

Sterile inflammation

A variety of noninfectious conditions can cause inflammatory lesions on the pinna or periauricular region of cats and dogs. Due to the sparseness of hair, the pinnae are frequent targets of insect bites from flies (e.g. *Stomoxys calcitrans*) in dogs and mosquitoes in cats (Figure 18.14).

Nodular lesions may result. Cytologically, insect bites are characterized by a mixed inflammatory population, which is dominated by small and mature lymphocytes, with variable numbers of plasma cells in chronic lesions, and also eosinophils, which are usually predominant in mosquito bites (Nagata & Ishida, 1997). In mosquito bite hypersensitivity, free eosinophil granules may be present in the background (Power & Ihrke, 1995). Variable numbers of mast cells (especially with mosquito bites), neutrophils, and macrophages may be seen. Increased numbers of neutrophils are expected, particularly where there is ulceration and secondary infection.

Aural hematomas are frequently seen in dogs and, less commonly, in cats. They often form subsequent to head shaking due to otitis externa or the presence of a foreign body within the ear canal. Damage to auricular blood vessels results in hemorrhage between the cartilage layers or between the skin and cartilage, forming a pocket (Dye *et al.*, 2002). Aspirates contain a dense pale eosinophilic proteinaceous background with large numbers of free erythrocytes, with macrophages containing phagocytized erythrocytes and, in subacute to chronic lesions, macrophages containing gold/brown granular pigment consistent with hemosiderin (Figure 18.15). Variable neutrophilic inflammation may accompany the erythrocytes, and an occasional plump spindle cell may be seen. Removal of the inciting cause and drainage and correction of the hematoma are indicated (Joyce Day, 1997).

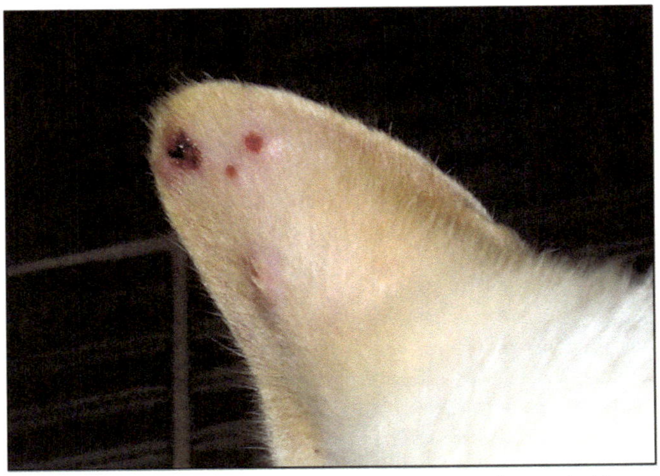

Figure 18.14 Ear pinna from a cat; gross appearance of mosquito bite hypersensitivity. One large and two smaller regions of ulceration are present. Due to the thinness of the hair in this region, the ear pinnae are often affected by insect bites.

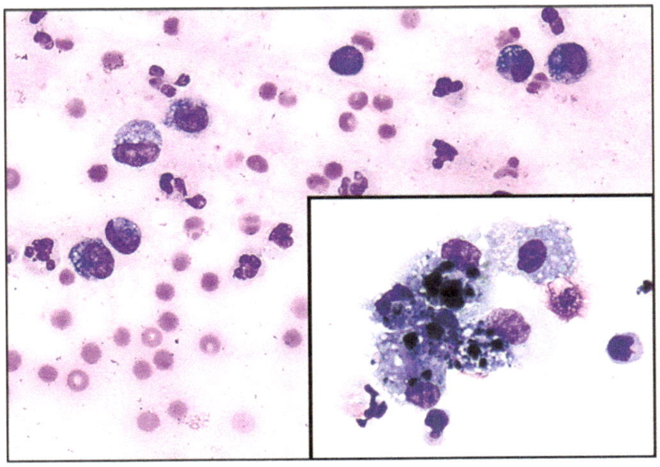

Figure 18.15 Fluid drained from the ear pinna of a dog; acute hemorrhage, aural hematoma. Many RBCs are present on a pale pink, hemolyzed background. Inflammatory cells consisting of a mix of nondegenerate neutrophils and vacuolated macrophages are also noted. In this particular case, erythrophagia is not appreciated. Grossly, the sample was hemorrhagic and failed to clot when drained. The fluctuant mass appeared 2 days previously and developed due to head shaking in response to otitis externa (Wright–Giemsa, concentrated direct preparation, 700× magnification). Inset: in this sample, coarsely clumped blue–black material within macrophages is consistent with hemosiderin and indicates an older lesion (Wright–Giemsa, 1,500× magnification). (Courtesy Dr. Ann Barger.)

Other less common sterile lesions of the pinna and periauricular region include:

- Eosinophilic plaques or granulomas, especially in cats. Lesions are composed of mainly eosinophils with accompanying nondegenerate neutrophils, macrophages, lymphocytes, plasma cells, and occasional mast cells (Bloom, 2006).
- Para-auricular abscesses can form secondary to any cause of ear canal stenosis (Rogers, 1988). Cytologically, they are composed of variably degenerate neutrophils, occasional macrophages, and anucleate squamous epithelial cells. Bacteria may be present if there is a secondary infection.
- Sterile granulomas and pyogranulomas in dogs or cats, which contain macrophages and accompanying rare to frequent neutrophils with fewer small lymphocytes and plasma cells (Santoro *et al.*, 2008). A thorough search for mycobacteria, *Leishmania*, and fungal organisms, including dermatophytes, is always indicated in such lesions, and special stains, cultures, and PCR may also be indicated.
- Feline relapsing polychondritis is a rare disease of cats that results in swollen, curled, and painful pinnae. It is thought to be an autoimmune reaction to the auricular cartilage resulting in necrosis and inflammation. Cartilage in other locations may also be affected (Delmage & Kelly, 2001; Gerber *et al.*, 2002; Baba *et al.*, 2009). Cytologic findings have not been reported but a mixed inflammatory cell infiltrate is expected.

- Frostbite, cold agglutinin disease, and vasculitis may also manifest on the tips of the pinnae.
- Systemic dermatitides such as immune-mediated, hormonal, or allergic skin diseases may also have pinnal or periauricular foliaceus. Immune-mediated diseases such as pemphigus foliaceous, pemphigus vulgaris, erythema multiforme, lupus erythematosus, dermatomyositis, bullous pemphigoid, sebaceous adenitis, and vasculitis can be seen in this region as well as elsewhere in the skin. They may present as alopecic, papular, vesicular, or ulcerated lesions. Multiple biopsies and histopathology are required for diagnosis. Hypothyroidism and hyperadrenocorticism may cause pinnal alopecia. Allergic skin disease such as atopic dermatitis, food allergy, or, rarely, contact allergy can cause alopecia, erythema, scale, or crusting lesions. In the absence of a secondary infection, cytology of suspected allergic skin disease is generally not very rewarding, typically yielding only keratinocytes and, occasionally, melanin laden cells (due to the associated hyperpigmentation). Eosinophils are only very rarely seen (KMM, personal experience).

Neoplasia and non-neoplastic mass lesions

Neoplasms of the pinnae and periauricular regions appear similar to those seen elsewhere in the skin. Metastasis to the ear appears to be very uncommon (Sula, 2012). The most common tumors seen in this region are (Bostock & Dye, 1979; Roth, 1990; Sula, 2012):

- Round cell: histiocytoma, mast cell tumor, plasmacytoma, lymphoma, melanoma, melanocytoma.
- Epithelial: SCC, cutaneous basilar neoplasm, sebaceous adenoma, sebaceous epithelioma, sebaceous carcinoma, papilloma.
- Mesenchymal: hemangioma, hemangiosarcoma, fibrosarcoma, feline sarcoids.
- Non-neoplastic mass-like lesions of the pinnae include ceruminous and sebaceous hyperplasia (see 'Ear Canal') and feline ceruminous cystomatosis. Feline ceruminous cystomatosis is a benign cystic proliferation of the ceruminous glands of the inner pinna and external ear canal. The cystic component contains brown inspissated material, which may fill the ear canal. They are grossly seen as proliferative blue/brown masses. Cytologically, the fluid is proteinaceous and basophilic (Figure 18.16), and cholesterol crystals, anucleate squamous epithelial cells, and vacuolated macrophages may be seen (Corriveau, 2012). For a description of ceruminous gland neoplasms, see 'Ear Canal' and 'Neoplasia and Non-Neoplastic Mass Lesions'.

Dentigerous cysts and dermoid cysts are lesions that may rarely be seen in the periauricular region (Sula, 2012). Dentigerous cysts contain fluid, which may be variably basophilic on smears, and there may be low numbers of vacuolated macrophages and anucleate or nucleated squamous epithelial cells (Poulet *et al.*, 1992). Dermoid cysts are congenital epidermal inclusion cysts, so cytology comprises large numbers of anucleate squamous epithelial cells and associated squamous debris (Tolbert *et al.*, 2009).

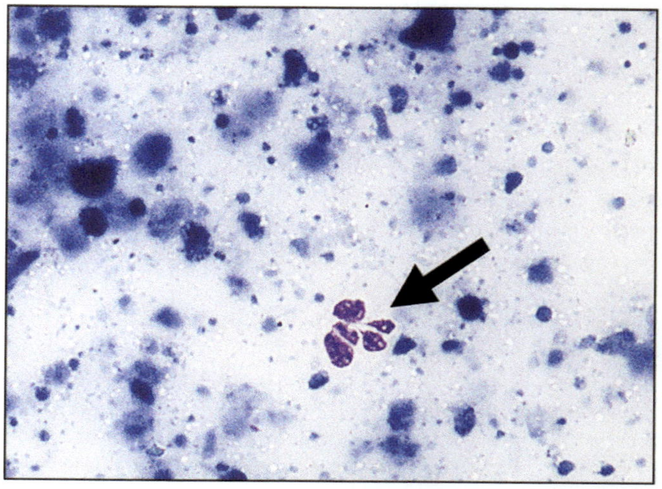

Figure 18.16 Cytologic appearance of feline ceruminous cystomatosis. The lesion is characterized by basophilic, proteinaceous fluid, which may form dense aggregates. Note the single ruptured neutrophil (arrow) (modified Wright–Giemsa, 800× magnification). (Courtesy Dr. Rebekah Gunn-Christie.)

Round cell neoplasms

Histiocytoma

Histiocytomas are benign tumors of Langerhans cells, a subtype of histiocytes located in the skin. Histiocytomas typically present as a single circular, dome-shaped, and variably alopecic mass. They have a predilection for the pinna, with most arising on the head or extremities. Young dogs less than 3 years of age are typically affected, although they may be seen in dogs of any age. This neoplasm has not been reported in cats. Cytologically, aspirates are usually moderately to highly cellular and contain large numbers of monotypic medium-sized round cells with an eccentric round to ovoid nucleus, fine chromatin, usually no distinct nucleoli, and a pale gray/blue cytoplasm with often a clearing at the periphery of the cell (Figure 18.17). Binucleate and multinucleate cells and mitotic figures are typically rare. Variable numbers of small and mature lymphocytes may also be seen admixed. Lymphocytic infiltration (T cells) is often a harbinger of imminent regression of the neoplasm. Histologically, the lesion is a nodule composed of sheets of medium-sized round cells, which are most dense superficially ('top heavy'), and often extend to the dermoepidermal junction. Mitotic figures are relatively frequent and variable numbers of small lymphocytes, occasional plasma cells, and neutrophils are interspersed (Taylor *et al.*, 1969).

Cutaneous plasmacytoma (plasma cell tumor)

Cutaneous plasmacytoma or plasma cell tumor is another round cell neoplasm that has a predilection for the pinnae in dogs. They are rare in cats. Plasmacytomas have a similar gross appearance to histiocytoma. Smears from FNAs are usually highly cellular with large numbers of round cells. The round cells typically possess a moderate nuclear to cytoplasmic (N:C) ratio and cells may exhibit moderate anisocytosis and anisokaryosis (Figure 18.18). The nucleus is round and eccentric with a variable chromatin pattern depending on the maturity of the

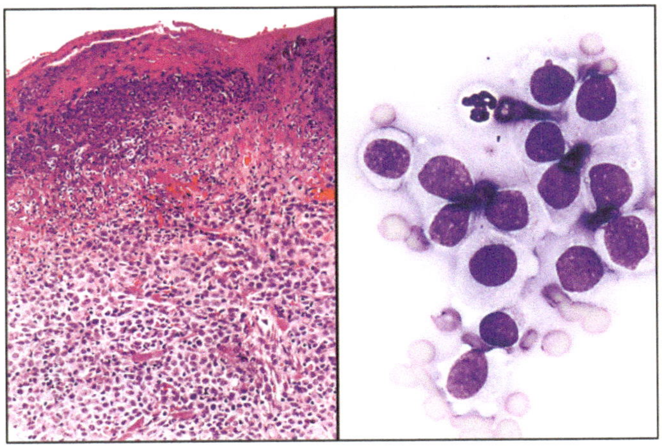

Figure 18.17 Tissue from the pinna of a dog; histiocytoma. Left: the dermis contains an expansile mass composed of sheets of medium-sized round cells. The round cells are uniform in size and have round to ovoid to reniform nuclei with pale eosinophilic cytoplasm (histiocytes). There are also very occasional small lymphocytes and neutrophils admixed. The overlying epidermis is ulcerated with an accompanying neutrophilic inflammatory response and an adherent serocellular crust (H&E, 200× magnification). Right: the classic cytologic appearance of a histiocytoma; note the pale cytoplasm, which tends to stain paler toward the outer edge of the cell, and the ruffled cytoplasmic border (modified Wright–Giemsa, 1,000× magnification).

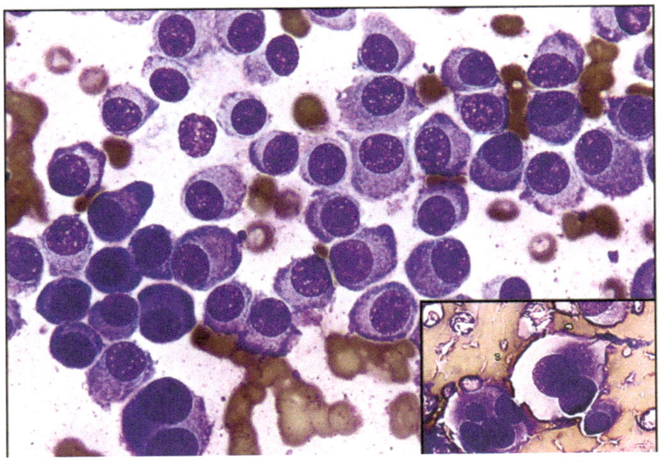

Figure 18.18 Aspirate of an ear mass in a dog; plasmacytoma. This example shows a well-differentiated plasmacytoma; cells have eccentric nuclei, coarse chromatin, basophilic cytoplasm, and variably well-developed Golgi zones. Occasional binucleated cells are present, a typical feature of this tumor type (Wright–Giemsa, 1,000× magnification). Inset: aspirate of a cutaneous mass on the pinna of a dog. As shown here, plasmacytomas can exhibit moderate to marked pleomorphism including marked anisocytosis and anisokaryosis, and multinucleation with varying sizes of nuclei. Despite the greater pleomorphism in this tumor, the expected behavior is benign (modified Wright–Giemsa, 500× magnification).

cells: stippled, slightly open, or finely clumped. Nucleoli are usually not apparent. The cytoplasm is moderately to densely basophilic and cells may have a clear region next to the nucleus (perinuclear clearing or Golgi zone). In some tumors, the periphery of the cytoplasm

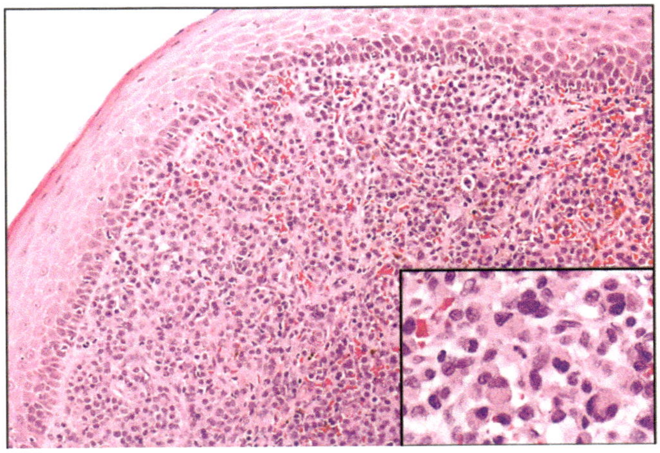

Figure 18.19 Ear mass from a dog; plasmacytoma. An expansile nodule present in the dermis is composed of sheets of plasma cells, separated from the epidermis by a thin strip of normal dermal collagen, known as a Grenz zone. Inset: the plasma cells exhibit mild anisocytosis and anisokaryosis with frequent binucleate and multinucleate cells. Despite these features, cutaneous plasmacytomas are typically behaviorally benign (H&E: main, 200× magnification; inset, 400× magnification).

may contain bright eosinophilic material, which may also be present in the background, and is thought to represent immunoglobulin. Binucleate and multinucleate cells and mitotic figures are usually frequent. Despite the pleomorphism and high mitotic rate, plasmacytomas are considered behaviorally benign and cured by complete excision. On histopathology sections, plasmacytoma is an expansile dermal tumor separated from the epidermis by a small area of normal dermal collagen (Grenz zone) composed of sheets of variably pleomorphic round cells, similar to the cytologic appearance described above (Figure 18.19).

Mast cell tumor

Mast cell tumors may be found on the pinnae of dogs and cats. Grossly, they can be nodular or plaque-like and variably alopecic. In the cat, solitary lesions are usually behaviorally benign and cured by complete excision (Molander-McCrary *et al.*, 1998). Multiple lesions may suggest disseminated mastocytosis in the cat, an aggressive and malignant syndrome (Sabattini & Bettini, 2010). In dogs, pinnal mast cell tumors are considered more aggressive than cutaneous mast cell tumors elsewhere, with a relatively high metastatic rate (Higginbotham *et al.*, 2000). Cytology of mast cell tumors is usually very cellular with large numbers of medium-sized round cells. The round cells have large numbers of dark purple round granules within the cytoplasm, which often obscure the cytoplasmic and nuclear detail. Where the nucleus can be seen, it is round with fine chromatin and typically no obvious nucleoli. Particularly in dogs, there are often variably low to high numbers of accompanying eosinophils. Free mast cell and eosinophil granules may be abundant in the background. There may also be collagen in the background, which stains palely to brightly eosinophilic (Figure 18.20). A proposed two-tier cytologic grading scheme for canine dermal mast cell tumors outlines criteria for a designation of cytologic high-grade with cytologic

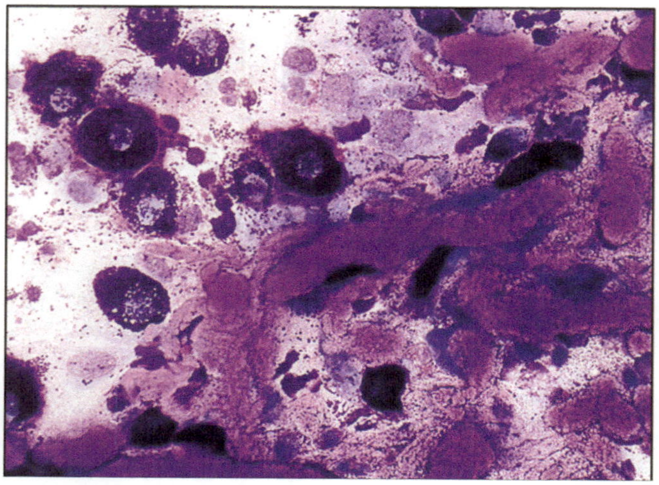

Figure 18.20 Canine skin mass; mast cell tumor with abundant collagen. Many thick, linear stands of palely to brightly eosinophilic and slightly fibrillar/granular collagen strands are admixed with well-differentiated mast cells and eosinophils. Collagen strands are occasionally seen in variable numbers in aspirates of mast cell tumor. This mast cell tumor would be consistent with a designation of cytologic low-grade (Camus *et al.*, 2016) (Wright–Giemsa, 600× magnification).

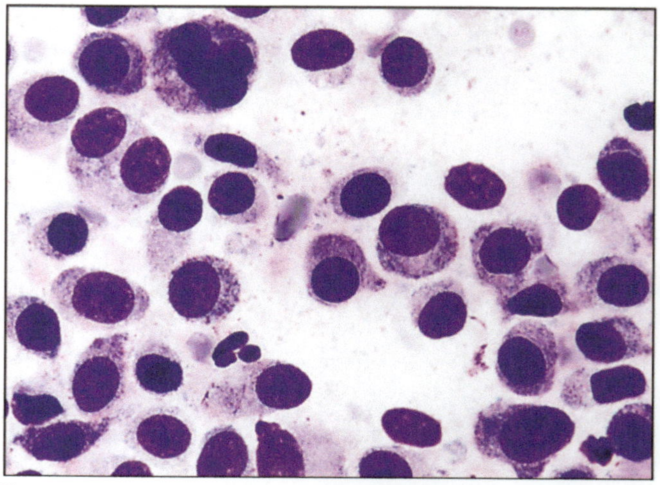

Figure 18.22 Mass on the lateral margin of the ear pinna of a 3-year-old Siamese cat; atypical mast cell tumor. These round cells are poorly granulated with only occasional cells showing a few well-delineated fine purple granules. Note the large multinucleated cell at the top of the image (Wright–Giemsa, 1,000× magnification). (Courtesy Dr. Robin Allison and Dr. Pi Jie Yang.)

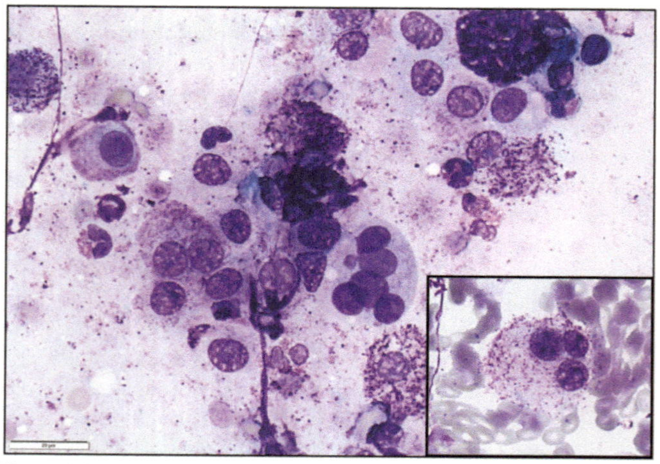

Figure 18.21 Dermal mass on the pinna of a dog; mast cell tumor with multiple criteria of malignancy (consistent with a designation of cytologic high-grade per Camus *et al.*, 2016). Mast cells are variably granulated, exhibit marked anisocytosis and anisokaryosis, with binucleate and multinucleate cells. Grading of this mass on histopathology was grade 2 (Patnaik) high grade (Kiupel) (Patnaik *et al.*, 1984; Kiupel *et al.*, 2011) (modified Wright–Giemsa, 600× magnification).

features of poor granulation (using Wright–Giemsa stain), or at least two of: mitotic figures, nuclear pleomorphism, bi- and multinucleation, and 50% variation in nuclear size (Camus *et al.*, 2016) (Figure 18.21). Although not yet widely validated, use of this grading scheme is becoming more common as veterinarians may use it for treatment planning. The Oncology-Pathology Working Group suggests caution in classifying tumors as cytologic high grade if only two criteria are used and one of them is nuclear pleomorphism or anisokaryosis, since this may overclassify mast cell tumors as high grade compared to histopathologic grading (Berlato *et al.*, 2021).

In cats, cutaneous mast cell tumors may be classified as mastocytic (appearance typical as for mast cells) or atypical/histiocytic. The atypical/histiocytic subtypes are often reported in young Siamese cats and are poorly granular, appearing more similar to histiocytes than typical mast cells (Figure 18.22).

Eosinophils and small mature lymphocytes often are admixed. This subtype may spontaneously regress (Sabattini & Bettini, 2010). The histopathologic appearance of mast cell tumors is somewhat variable, but generally consists of sheets of cells within the dermis (Figure 18.23). Unlike cytology specimens, the granules are fine and gray. Mast cell tumors can usually be confirmed (as long as they have granules) using toluidine blue or Giemsa staining, which stains the mast cell granules bright purple (metachromatic).

Melanocytomas and melanomas

Melanocytomas and melanomas may also be seen on the pinnae, particularly in cats. The majority of feline melanocytic neoplasms are behaviorally benign, but recurrence and metastasis have been reported (Miller *et al.*, 1991; Luna *et al.*, 2000). Lesions may be flattened or nodular, and are often dark brown to black (amelanotic melanomas may be pale pink). The cytology of melanocytic neoplasms is characterized by a moderate to high cellularity specimen composed of round to polygonal to spindled cells. The nucleus is typically round and most often central, with a fine sieve-like chromatin pattern, and small nucleoli may be seen. The cytoplasm is pale basophilic and contains moderate to large numbers of fine, gold to brown to black to blue/green–black granules, consistent with melanin. A differential diagnosis for melanocytic neoplasms is pigmented basal cell tumor or basilar neoplasia. Basal cell/basilar neoplasms are composed of

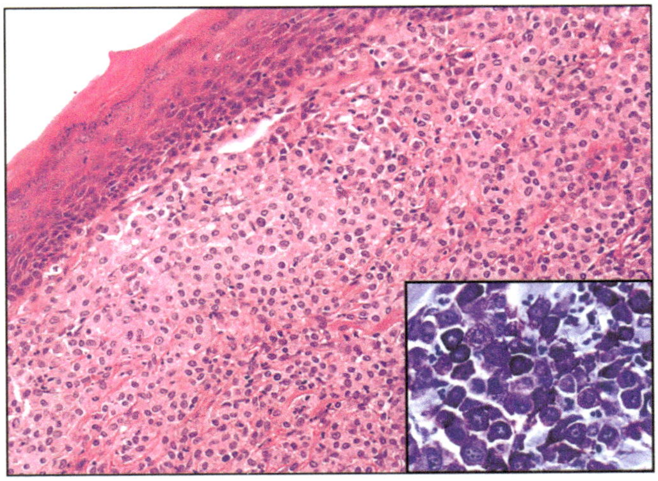

Figure 18.23 **Cutaneous mass on the pinna of a dog; mast cell tumor. Extending from below the hyperplastic epidermis throughout the superficial and mid-dermis is a mass composed of sheets of monotypic round cells. The cells exhibit mild anisocytosis and anisokaryosis and possess a round nucleus and pale eosinophilic to finely gray granular cytoplasm (mast cells). There are also occasional scattered eosinophils admixed (H&E, 200× magnification). Inset: toluidine blue staining results in the characteristic bright purple (metachromatic) color of cytoplasmic granules of the round cells, confirming the diagnosis of mast cell tumor (toluidine blue stain, 400× magnification).**

small epithelial cells, which possess a high N:C ratio and form tightly cohesive clusters, compared with melanocytic neoplastic cells, which are discrete cells with a moderate N:C ratio. In more aggressive melanocytic neoplasms, there is pleomorphism, nuclear criteria of malignancy, and reduced granularity of the cells (granules may be entirely absent in aggressive amelanotic melanomas). On histopathology, cutaneous melanocytic neoplasms typically arise in the dermis and form sheets of polygonal to spindled cells. Well-granulated tumors are often so densely pigmented that nuclear and cytoplasmic detail cannot be examined. Pleomorphism, high mitotic rate, reduced granularity, presence of neoplastic melanocytes within the epidermis (junctional activity), and vascular and lymphatic invasion are consistent with more malignant behavior (Smedley *et al.*, 2011).

Cutaneous lymphoma

Cutaneous lymphoma may be seen on the pinnae or periauricular regions of dogs and cats, but this is usually part of systemic disease. The lesions may present as nodules, or as plaques, ulcers, areas of alopecia, or scale (Sula, 2012). Cytologic preparations contain a monomorphic population of lymphocytes. The cytologic appearance varies depending on the subtype: from small to large-sized lymphocytes with a round to irregular nucleus, smooth to clumped chromatin, with or without nucleoli, and pale to deeply basophilic cytoplasm, which may be scant, have indistinct borders (veil appearance), or may be eccentric (hand-mirror or pseudopod). Moderate numbers of variably sized cytoplasmic fragments are often seen in the background. Concurrent ulceration with resultant inflammation or infection may complicate the cytologic picture and necessitate histopathology for diagnosis. As with the cytology, histopathology of cutaneous lymphoma will also vary depending on the subtype, but comprises a monomorphic population of round cells forming sheets. The neoplastic lymphocytes may be positive for CD3 (T cell) or CD79a and CD20 (B cell). The vast majority of feline and canine cutaneous lymphomas are T-cell phenotype; cutaneous B-cell lymphomas are extremely rare (Day, 1995; Ponce *et al.*, 2010).

Epithelial neoplasms

Squamous cell carcinoma

SCC is the most common neoplasm found on the pinnae of cats (Fan & de Lorimier, 2004). The majority are ultraviolet (UV) light-induced, with white cats 13 times more likely to develop pinnal SCC than pigmented cats (Dorn *et al.*, 1971). They may also be seen in the sparsely haired preauricular region, and can also be seen occasionally in dogs (Miller Shanley, 1991). The lesions are usually red, crusted, flattened lesions with ulceration. Scraping of the lesions reveals an often pleomorphic population of medium-sized to large polygonal to elongated cells present singly and in cohesive clusters (Figure 18.24). They have a moderate N:C ratio with variable and often moderate to high anisocytosis and anisokaryosis. The nucleus is round with coarse to open chromatin, often with distinct nucleoli, and the cytoplasm is pale to moderately basophilic (described as sky or robin's egg blue) and hyaline. Fine pink granules (keratohyalin granules) may be seen in the cytoplasm. Very large cells with large prominent nucleoli, binucleate and multinucleate cells, and atypical mitotic figures may be seen. Frequently, there are low to high numbers of neutrophils present, and neutrophils may be seen within the cytoplasm of the neoplastic epithelial cells (emperipolesis). Secondary bacterial infection may be seen in

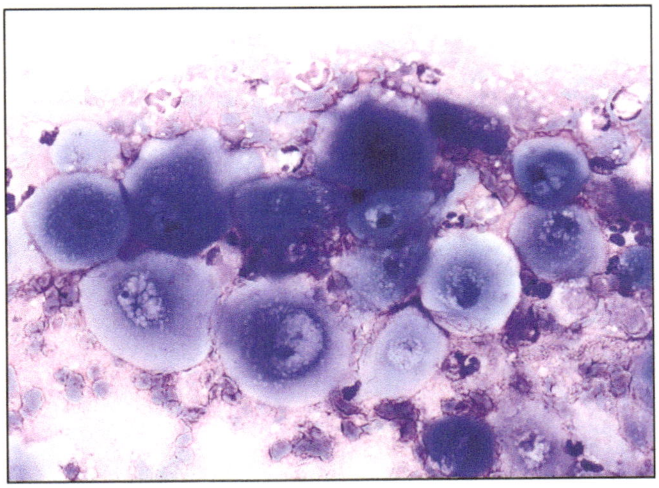

Figure 18.24 **Tissue from a dog; squamous cell carcinoma. Many large, pleomorphic, well-keratinized squamous cells are present on a background of blood and mild suppurative inflammation. Cells exhibit moderate anisocytosis and anisokaryosis, have large, pleomorphic nuclei with prominent nucleoli, and exhibit perinuclear vacuolization. Features indicating keratinization include the angular appearance of some of the cells, the pale to deep 'sky' or 'robin's egg' blue cytoplasmic color, and the waxy or ground glass appearance of the cytoplasm (Wright–Giemsa, 500× magnification).**

ulcerated lesions. Histopathology of SCC is typified by cords, islands, and trabeculae of squamous epithelial cells (Figure 18.25). There is dysmaturation characterized by abrupt cornification within islands forming concentric laminar whorls of eosinophilic keratin (keratin pearls). Pinnal SCCs are typically locally aggressive but infrequently metastasize; thus prognosis with complete surgical excision is fairly good (Lana et al., 1997).

Cutaneous basilar neoplasm ('basal cell tumor')

Cutaneous basilar neoplasms or basal cell tumors are morphological umbrella terms encompassing neoplasms of the germinal cells of the hair follicle and adnexal structures. These neoplasms may be classified as to the tissue of origin on histology, e.g. trichoblastoma for hair follicle origin and ductular adenoma as apocrine (sweat) gland origin. However, it is usually not possible to determine the tissue of origin on cytology, hence the common use of the umbrella terms. Basal cell tumors are the most common cutaneous neoplasm in the cat and are often seen on the head and neck, including the pinnae and periauricular region (Miller *et al.*, 1991). Basilar neoplasms may also be seen in dogs. They are typically seen as solitary nodules. FNAs yield moderately to highly cellular smears composed of tightly cohesive clusters of uniform small epithelial cells. Some cells may be present in linear arrays. The epithelial cells are round to slightly elongate with a high N:C ratio, a round central or eccentric nucleus, finely clumped chromatin, and basophilic cytoplasm. Nucleoli are usually not apparent (Bohn *et al.*, 2006). The cytoplasm may contain fine, gold to brown to black granules consistent with melanin; therefore a melanocytic neoplasm is a differential for pigmented tumors (Figure 18.26; Stockhaus *et al.*, 2001). Histopathology sections of basilar neoplasia reveal an expansile, dermal mass composed of lobules of small, uniform epithelial cells (Figure 18.27). Cystic areas may be present within the mass (Bohn *et al.*, 2006). Basal cell tumors are usually behaviorally benign but may be locally aggressive (Day *et al.*, 1994). Some basal cell tumors in dogs can grow quite large.

Sebaceous adenoma/epithelioma/carcinoma

Sebaceous neoplasms may also be seen on the pinnae of dogs and, less frequently, cats. They are most often small, cauliflower-like masses. Aspiration of sebaceous proliferations reveals multiple cohesive clusters of uniform, small to medium-sized epithelial cells, which have uniformly and finely vacuolated cytoplasm. Acinar or tubular structures may be seen, which can contain a central aggregate of amorphous eosinophilic secretory material. The N:C ratio is typically low to moderate, with a central nucleus possessing dense chromatin and no obvious nucleoli. The background is often pale eosinophilic to basophilic, and proteinaceous with scattered clear lipid vacuoles. Sebaceous hyperplasia cannot be differentiated from adenoma on cytology.

Sebaceous epitheliomas also appear similar, although representative smears typically contain a predominance of basal-type epithelial cells (similar to those described above for basal cell and basilar tumors; Figure 18.28). Sebaceous adenocarcinomas are rare, and they often have multiple criteria of malignancy with increased anisocytosis and anisokaryosis, high N:C ratios, multinucleated cells, and prominent nucleoli. There may be few lipid vacuoles in the cytoplasm to indicate their identity (Dickinson & Young, 2005). With sebaceous

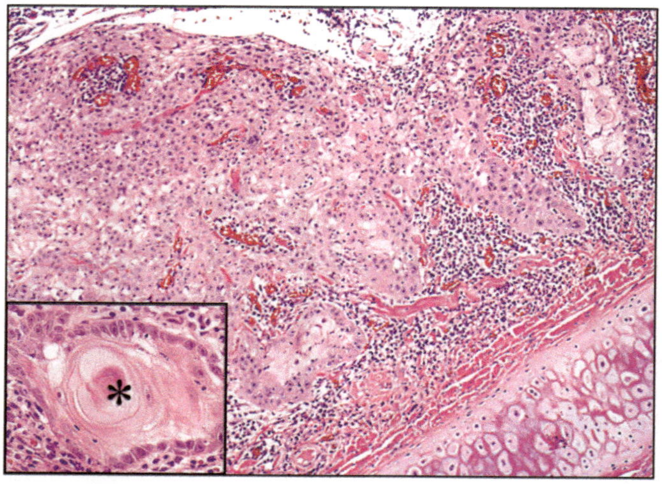

Figure 18.25 Ulcerated mass on the pinna of a cat; squamous cell carcinoma. The dermis is expanded and infiltrated by clusters of epithelial cells forming trabeculae and nests. There are frequent clusters with abrupt keratinization and keratin pearls. There are also moderate numbers of neutrophils and lymphocytes with fewer plasma cells in the surrounding dermis. Note that there is also complete loss of normal epidermis (ulceration) with a partially adherent exudate on the surface. Neoplastic cells do not infiltrate the cartilage. Inset: note the moderate anisocytosis and anisokaryosis in the neoplastic epithelial cell population and the large central area of abrupt cornification with keratin pearl formation (asterisk). There are mixed inflammatory cells in the surrounding dermis (H&E: main, 100× magnification; inset, 400× magnification).

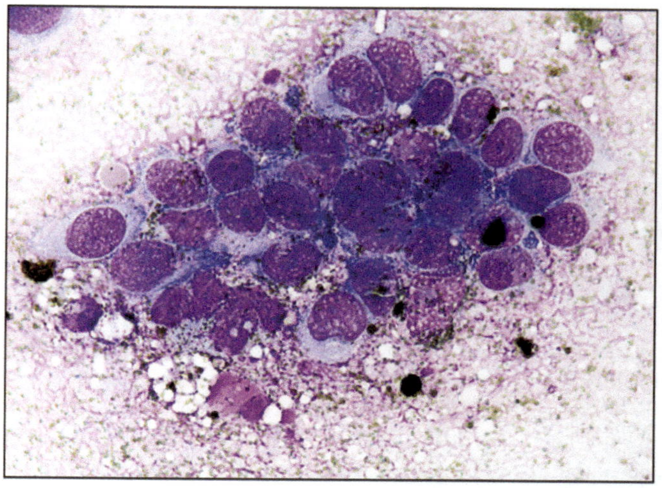

Figure 18.26 Aspirate of a mass on the pinna of a cat; pigmented basal cell tumor/basilar neoplasm. A cluster of mildly pleomorphic epithelial cells is present on a background of protein and free melanin granules. The epithelial cells are medium in size with mild anisocytosis and anisokaryosis. They have round to oval nuclei, visible nucleoli, and a thin rim of moderate basophilic cytoplasm containing variable numbers of melanin granules. Pigmented basilar neoplasms can easily be mistaken for melanoma (Wright–Giemsa, 1,000× magnification).

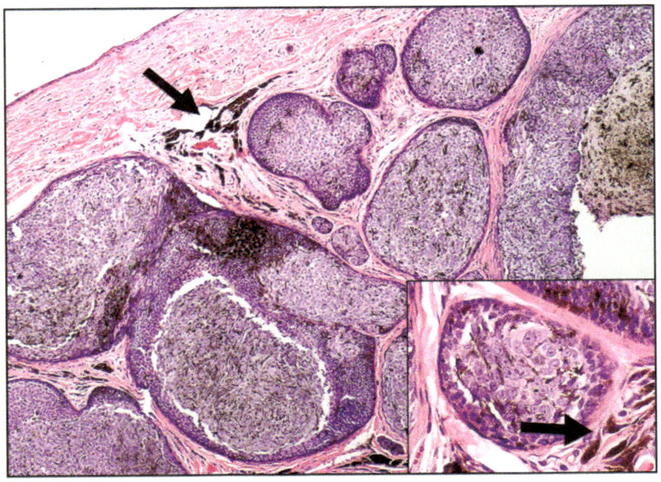

Figure 18.27 Mass on the pinna of the ear of a cat; basilar neoplasm, trichoblastoma. The dermis is expanded by multifocal well-demarcated lobules of uniform epithelial cells. At the periphery of the lobules, the epithelial cells are smaller, more hyperchromatic, and have a high N:C ratio (basilar). Toward the center of the lobule, they are slightly larger, paler, with a moderate to high N:C ratio (parabasal). Many of the epithelial cells contain a small to moderate amount of brown/black granular pigment in the cytoplasm (melanin). Macrophages containing phagocytized melanin (melanomacrophages) are present in the surrounding dermis (arrow). Inset: islands of follicular epithelial cells containing melanin pigment. Note the melanomacrophages (arrow) in the surrounding dermis. These neoplasms are typically cured by complete excision (H&E: main, 100× magnification; inset, 400× magnification).

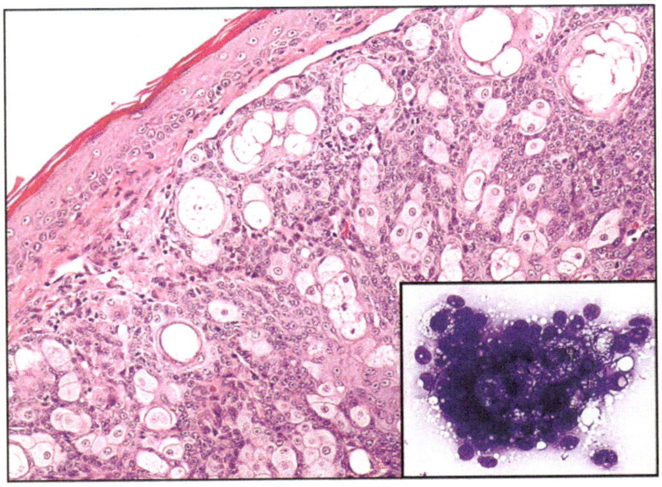

Figure 18.28 Mass on the ear of a dog; sebaceous epithelioma. Expanding the dermis is a densely cellular mass composed of sheets and lobules of polygonal epithelial cells. Epithelial cells are predominantly small and hyperchromatic with a high N:C ratio (basilar cells), that occasionally abruptly differentiate into larger cells with pale foamy cytoplasm, consistent with sebaceous epithelial cells. Frequent ductal differentiation is seen. Occasional mitotic figures are present. The overlying epidermis is unaffected. The predominance of basilar cells is the reason this is diagnosed as a sebaceous epithelioma rather than an adenoma (H&E, 200× magnification). Inset: aspirate from the same tumor showing a cluster of small basophilic basilar epithelial cells with a focus of larger, foamy sebaceous cells at the center (Wright–Giemsa, 500× magnification).

hyperplasia and adenomas, surgical excision is usually curative and regrowth rare. Adenocarcinoma is more aggressive, invasive, and may metastasize (Scott & Anderson, 1990). On histopathology sections, sebaceous hyperplasia forms lobules of mature, finely vacuolated, sebaceous epithelial cells around a central duct, with a single layer of basal reserve cells. Adenomas are similar, forming solid lobules of sebaceous epithelial cells, while sebaceous epitheliomas have a predominance of basal reserve cells, with multiple areas of sebaceous differentiation. Adenocarcinomas are poorly circumscribed multilobular masses of pleomorphic and atypical epithelial cells, which may have few lipid vacuoles within the cytoplasm (Goldschmidt *et al.*, 1998).

Papillomas

Papillomas are benign neoplasms of the epidermis. They are fairly common in dogs but very rare in cats (Munday *et al.*, 2007). In younger dogs they are often induced by canine papillomavirus and in older dogs they are more often spontaneous (Sula, 2012). They may be nodular or exophytic. Cytology may be variably cellular and contain uniform, small to medium-sized, polygonal to slightly elongated epithelial cells present singly or in clusters. They typically possess a moderate N:C ratio with a central nucleus, finely clumped chromatin, and no obvious nucleoli. The cytoplasm may vary from moderately to palely basophilic, and may be somewhat hyaline or contain pink granules, depending on the stage of keratinization of the proliferating cells. Papillomas caused by papillomavirus typically contain a dusty magenta cytoplasm and may have visible nucleoli. Viral inclusions are usually absent (Sprague & Thrall, 2001). On histopathology, some epithelial cells may contain shrunken dark nuclei surrounded by a clear halo (koilocytes) and, in papillomavirus-induced papillomas, rare cells may have basophilic intranuclear viral inclusions (Figure 18.29; Goldschmidt *et al.*, 1998). Complete excision is typically curative, but additional lesions may appear elsewhere, especially when they are induced by papillomavirus.

Mesenchymal lesions

Hemangioma/hemangiosarcoma

The vascular neoplasms hemangioma and hemangiosarcoma can be seen on the pinnae and the sparsely haired preauricular region of cats and, less frequently, dogs. These tumors are most often UV light-induced (Nikula *et al.*, 1992). They appear as red, flattened to raised lesions. Hemangiosarcomas are more often seen in cats, while hemangiomas are more common in dogs (Sula, 2012). FNA or scrapings of vascular tumors are largely unrewarding due to their very nature. A background of hemodilution with macrophages exhibiting erythrophagia or containing hemosiderin may be seen. Plump polygonal to spindled cells may also be seen, but often diagnosis is not definitive and histopathology is required.

Hemangiomas are typified histologically by a fairly well-demarcated dermal mass of uniform plump cuboidal to spindled cells forming vascular channels that contain variable numbers of erythrocytes (Figure 18.30). Hemangiosarcomas are invasive and exhibit cellular and nuclear atypia, and cells may form solid sheets, requiring a careful search to find vascular channels. Hemangiomas are cured by complete excision. Hemangiosarcomas frequently recur, but metastasis of

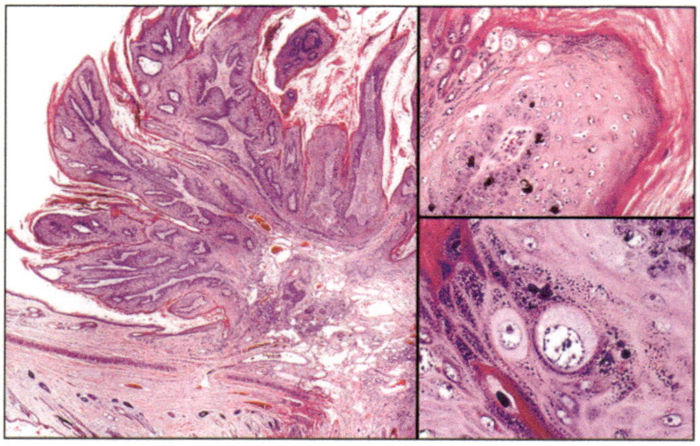

Figure 18.29 Exophytic mass on the ear pinna of a dog; papilloma. Left: the subgross appearance of the mass. Note the growth of the pattern is in an upward and inward manner typical of a viral-induced papilloma. The epidermis is markedly hyperplastic and thrown into exaggerated folds with deep rete pegs (exophytic). Upper right: there is moderate to marked anisocytosis and anisokaryosis of keratinocytes, particularly in the stratum spinosum. Lower right: scattered hypertrophic individual keratinocytes are rounded up and have an expanded pale watery to granular cytoplasm (koilocytes) (H&E: left, subgross image; upper right, 200× magnification; lower right, 400× magnification).

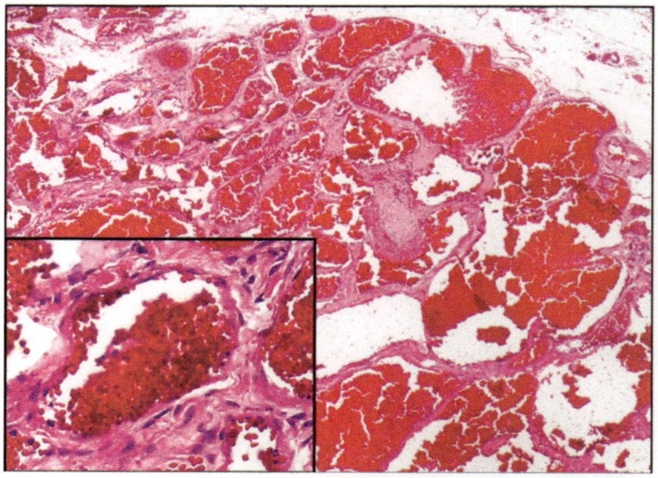

Figure 18.30 Mass at the base of the ear from a dog; hemangioma. The dermis is markedly expanded by a well-demarcated mass composed of uniform spindle cells forming blood-filled vascular channels, which are quite uniform in size. Inset: a higher-power view of a vascular channel. The spindle cells forming the stroma can be clearly seen, as can the flattened endothelial cells lining the channel. FNA would yield chiefly fresh blood and, possibly, a few uniform spindle cells (H&E: main, 40× magnification; inset, 200× magnification).

cutaneous lesions is not considered to occur commonly (Miller *et al.*, 1992).

Fibrosarcoma/soft tissue sarcoma

Fibrosarcomas and soft tissue sarcomas are malignant neoplasms derived from soft connective tissues (Dennis *et al.*, 2011). Fibrosarcomas can occur on the pinnae, particularly in cats (nonvaccine-associated; Gross *et al.*, 2005). The lesions are firm and raised and may have indistinct margins. FNAs of fibrosarcomas are often poorly cellular. High yielding specimens, such as impression smears or scrapings of biopsies, contain a population of medium-sized to large spindled cells, which may be pleomorphic. Neoplastic fibroblasts have an ovoid to elongate nucleus, often with an open chromatin pattern, one to multiple nucleoli, and pale basophilic cytoplasm that is wispy and may be bipolar.

Although nomenclature is often in flux, currently for dogs, fibrosarcomas come under the collective term of cutaneous/subcutaneous soft tissue sarcoma (may also be called spindle cell tumor of soft tissue), along with perivascular wall tumor/hemangiopericytoma and (peripheral) nerve sheath tumor. They are termed collectively since although they may exhibit different morphological patterns chiefly appreciable on histopathology, the patterns do not always correlate with cell type of origin on a panel of immunohistochemical stains or electron microscopy. In any case, their behavior is not influenced by morphological patterns/subtypes but they are all generally predictable by the same histopathologic grading scheme, which is applicable only to dogs (Dennis *et al.*, 2011). Aspirates of canine soft tissue sarcomas are typically high-yield. They yield clumps and individualized medium- to large-sized spindle cells which possess moderate N:C ratio with an ovoid nucleus, dense chromatin, small nucleoli, and pale to moderately basophilic wispy cytoplasm, sometimes with low numbers of fine clear vacuoles or a light dusting of pink material. Scattered binucleate and multinucleate cells may be seen, and multinucleate cells may have peripheral nuclei ('crown cells'). Clumps are associated with a small amount of pink fibrillar matrix. On histopathology, soft tissue sarcoma is seen within the dermis as an infiltrative and poorly demarcated mass composed of interlacing bundles of often pleomorphic spindle cells forming streams and whorls (Figure 18.31). Fibrosarcomas/soft tissue sarcomas in both cats and dogs are locally aggressive so recurrence is common, especially for feline fibrosarcomas and grade II and III canine soft tissue sarcomas with close surgical margins, but they all infrequently metastasize (Hendrick *et al.*, 1995; Dennis *et al.*, 2011).

Feline sarcoids

Feline sarcoids are masses formed by proliferating fibroblasts induced by infection with bovine papillomaviruses (Sula, 2012). They are most frequently seen in young male cats in rural areas. The pinna is a common site for these masses (Gross *et al.*, 2005). The lesions are likely poorly exfoliative on aspiration, but scrapings may be adequately cellular. The cytology would be consistent with a mesenchymal cell proliferation, with plump spindled to polygonal cells with wispy pale basophilic cytoplasm, which may show some atypia. Histopathology of feline sarcoids typically shows an expansile and poorly demarcated mass of mesenchymal cells sometimes forming whorls. The characteristics that assist differentiation of feline sarcoid from soft tissue sarcomas are lining up of cells at the dermoepidermal junction perpendicular to the basement membrane ('picket fence' appearance) and involvement of the epidermis with hyperplasia and prominent rete ridges. Papillomavirus DNA may be isolated from fresh/frozen tissues with PCR (Gross *et al.*, 2005).

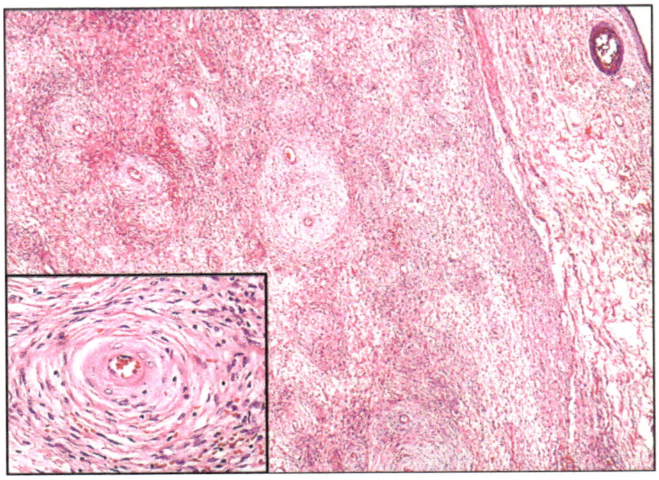

Figure 18.31 Mass on the ear pinna of a dog; soft tissue sarcoma, grade 2. The middle to deep dermis is markedly expanded by a fairly well-demarcated and nonencapsulated mass composed of streams and whorls of neoplastic mesenchymal cells. The mesenchymal cells are spindled to stellate and frequently are arranged in concentric perivascular whorls around blood vessels. Such a pattern is characteristic of perivascular wall tumors; however, immunohistochemistry is required to further distinguish the soft tissue sarcoma subtypes. In practice, the subtype does not typically influence the prognosis, as soft tissue sarcomas behave in similar ways. Inset: A high-power view of a blood vessel surrounded by concentric whirls of neoplastic spindle cells (H&E: main, 40× magnification; inset, 200× magnification).

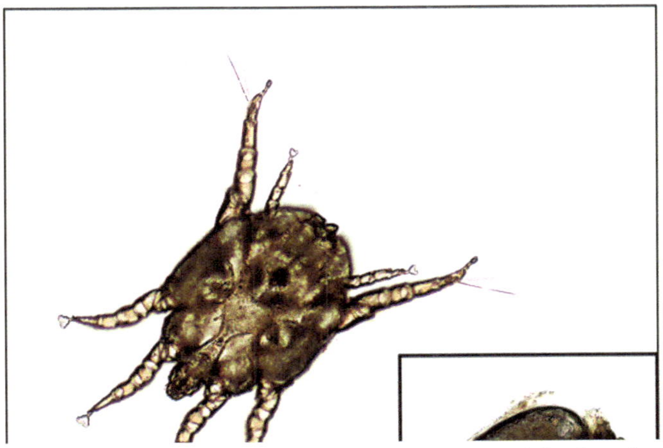

Figure 18.32 Ear swab from a cat; otodectic mange. An adult mite and egg (inset). Mites are not considered part of the normal flora of the external ear canal: even a single mite or egg warrants treatment (oil preparation: main, 100× magnification; inset, 200× magnification). (Courtesy Dr. Kelli Ferris.)

Ear canal

Inflammatory lesions

Inflammatory diseases of the ear canal can develop from the external environment, via the hematogenous route, or, uncommonly, via extension from the middle ear through a ruptured tympanic membrane.

Infectious

Ear mites

The ear mite *Otodectes cynotis* is the cause of approximately 50% of cases of otitis externa in cats. As few as two or three mites can trigger otitis via a type I (immediate) hypersensitivity response (Weisbroth *et al.*, 1974; Powell *et al.*, 1980). *O. cynotis* can also infect dogs. Otodectic mange is variably pruritic and the consistency of the cerumen is variable. Mites may be seen grossly in the ear canal as tiny white specks that move. Swabs from infected animals yield variable numbers of mites. On cytology, *O. cynotis* adult mites are up to 450 μm long and 280 μm wide with a round body, a thick chitinous exoskeleton, jointed appendages with two pairs rostrally and two pairs caudally, and tapered biting mouthparts (Loshe *et al.*, 2002). Adults, nymphs, or eggs (100 × 210 μm) may be seen (Figure 18.32). The presence of even one mite or egg indicates infection. Examination of stained ear swab cytology is also useful to assess any secondary infections. Treatment of ear mites is by application of topical acaricides (Angus, 2004).

Bacterial and fungal infections

Bacterial and fungal infections of the external ear canal are almost always secondary to an underlying allergic inflammatory disease or, less commonly, a foreign body, which alters the permeability of the epidermis in the ear canal and results in a change in the otic microenvironment (Murphy, 2001). Pinnal conformation, the presence of hair within the ear canal, external temperature, and humidity have not been found to correlate with the risk for otitis externa (Grono, 1970a, 1970b; Huang & Huang, 1999; Yoshida *et al.*, 2002; Cole, 2009).

The most common microorganisms involved in ear diseases are the cocci *Staphylococcus pseudintermedius* in dogs and *Staphylococcus aureus* and *S. pseudintermedius* in cats, *M. pachydermatis* yeasts, and *Pseudomonas aeruginosa* rods (Guillot & Bond, 1999; McEwan, 2000; Petersen *et al.*, 2002; Nardoni *et al.*, 2005). Although a variety of saprophytic fungi can be cultured from the ears of dogs and cats, pathogenic infections caused by fungi other than *Malassezia* are rare (Figure 18.33). Pathogenic fungal infections (otomycosis) have been reported with *Candida albicans*, *Aspergillus* spp., *Sporothrix schenkii*, and the dermatophyte *Microsporum canis* in Persian cats (Dion Speckmann, 1978; McKellar et al., 1990; Godfrey, 2000; Coyner, 2010; Ghibaudo Peano, 2010; Goodale et al., 2016). Other fungal infections including *Cryptococcus* spp. causing otitis interna in a cat have been rarely reported (Paulin *et al.*, 2012).

Cytology of otitis externa typically contains a background of anucleate squamous epithelial cells with associated debris. The microorganisms seen will vary but are most often cocci (Figure 18.34) and/or peanut-shaped *Malassezia* yeasts (in numbers above that considered 'normal' in the ear canal: see Table 18.1; Figure 18.35). There may also be variably degenerate neutrophils present, indicating inflammation. Bacterial rods may be seen in some cases (Figure 18.36), typically associated with more severe inflammatory responses (Figure 18.37). Rarely, *Candida* spp. yeasts, pseudohyphae, or hyphae may be seen or, with *Aspergillus*, septate, branching hyphae. Cytology will allow selection of appropriate antibiotic or antifungal medications, as well as guide the requirement for anti-inflammatory therapy (presence and numbers of neutrophils). A reproducible, semiquantitative method of

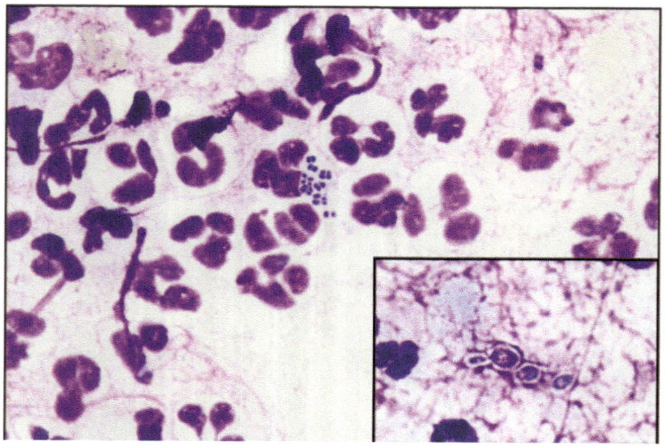

Figure 18.33 Swab from the ear of a dog; concurrent bacterial and fungal infections. The majority of the slide shows numerous degenerate neutrophils with many intra- and extracellular paired cocci bacteria. Inset: also present are rare, small, round to oval yeasts, occasionally forming chains (pseudohyphae). Although not cultured in this case, the most likely agent is *Candida* (modified Wright–Giemsa, 1,000× magnification). (Courtesy Dr. Frane Banovic.)

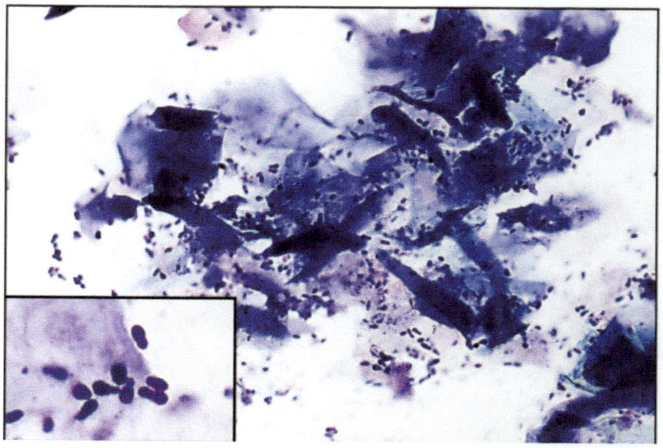

Figure 18.35 Discharge from the ear canal of a dog; yeast otitis. Clumps of angular keratinized squamous cells are present together with numerous peanut/shoeprint-shaped *Malassezia* spp. yeasts. Yeasts are adhered to the squamous cells and are present in the background. Inset: high-power appearance of the yeast (modified Wright–Giemsa: main, 500× magnification; inset, 1,000× magnification). (Courtesy Dr. Valarie Pallatto.)

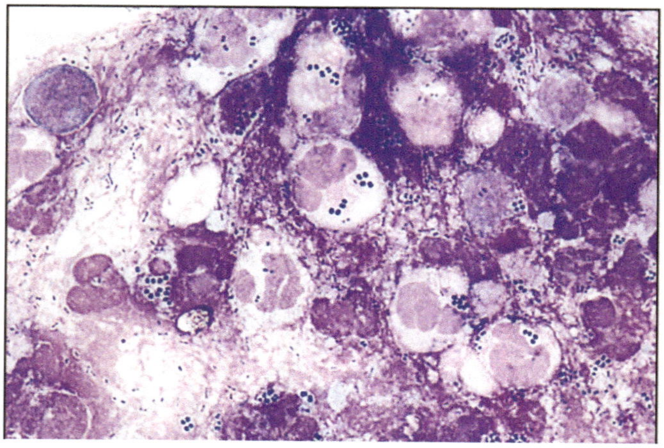

Figure 18.34 Discharge from the ear canal of a dog; suppurative inflammation with intralesional cocci bacteria. Sheets of degenerate neutrophils with myriad intra- and extracellular cocci, often in pairs, are present. This dog presented for vestibular disease. Culture of fluid from the middle ear grew *Providencia stuartii* (a Gram-negative bacillus) and *Staphylococcus pseudintermedius* (Wright–Giemsa, 1,000× magnification).

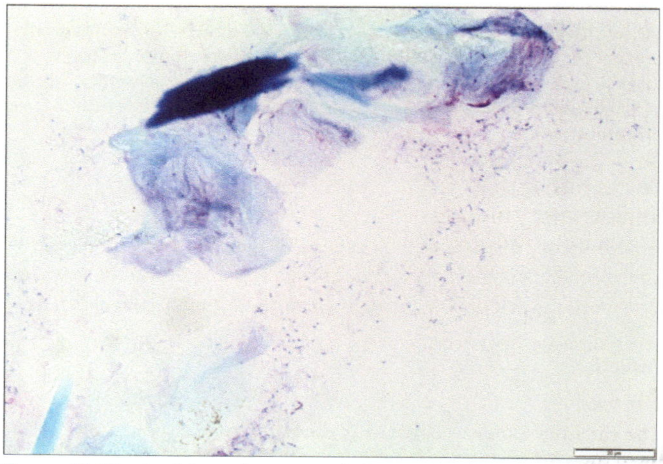

Figure 18.36 Swabfrom the ear canal of a dog; mixed bacteria. Scattered and clumps of anucleate keratinocytes with occasional melanization (bottom; black/golden granules) and mixed bacteria: cocci and bacilli (rods) (modified Wright–Giemsa: 600× magnification).

evaluating ear cytology may be utilized for assessing severity of otitis externa, as well as to monitor response to treatment (Table 18.2).

Histological assessment of otitis externa is usually only performed following total ear canal ablation. Variable numbers of anucleate squamous epithelial cells, cocci, yeasts, or rods are present in the canal. The epidermis is often moderate to markedly thickened (hyperplastic) and may have variable thickening of the stratum corneum (orthokeratotic or parakeratotic hyperkeratosis). Intercellular edema (spongiosis) or intracellular edema (ballooning degeneration) may be seen, and there are frequently moderate numbers of neutrophils traversing (exocytosing) the epidermis into the canal. There may be erosion or ulceration of the epidermis. Hair follicles may also be affected. The subjacent dermis frequently has moderate to high numbers of lymphocytes and plasma cells in a perivascular, periadnexal, or diffuse pattern (Figure 18.38). The inflammation may form discrete aggregates of lymphocytes (lymphoid follicles). There may also be hyperplasia of ceruminous glands and/or sebaceous glands (Figure 18.39).

Noninfectious lesions

Excessive cerumen may, occasionally, be the result of noninfectious causes. Overexuberant use of ear cleaners can macerate the ear canal and impair the migration of anucleate squamous epithelial cells. Ear swab cytology is composed only of squamous epithelial cells, which

Table 18.2 **Scale for use in the cytologic evaluation of otitis externa**

Scale	Description
0	No bacteria, yeast, or inflammatory cells (normal)
1+	Occasional bacteria or yeast (may be normal), or inflammatory cells seen on careful detection
2+	Bacteria, yeast, or inflammatory cells present in low numbers but detectable rapidly without difficulties
3+	Bacteria, yeast, or inflammatory cells present in larger numbers but detectable rapidly without difficulties
4+	Massive amount of bacteria, yeast, or inflammatory cells present and detectable rapidly without difficulties

From: Budach SC, Mueller RS (2012) Reproducibility of a semiquantitative method to assess cutaneous cytology. *Vet Dermatol* 23:426–480.

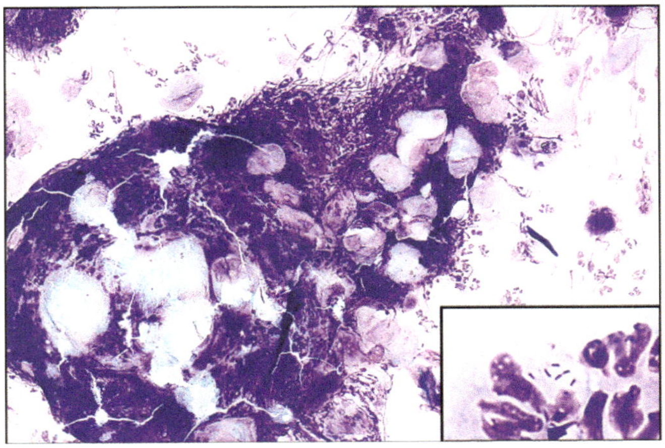

Figure 18.37 **Discharge from the ear canal of a dog; suppurative inflammation with intralesional bacilli. A large clump of material composed of anucleate keratinocytes (pale to bright blue angular structures) admixed with many neutrophils is present. Inset: neutrophils are degenerate and occasionally contain bacilli (Wright–Giemsa: main, 200× magnification; inset: 1,000× magnification).**

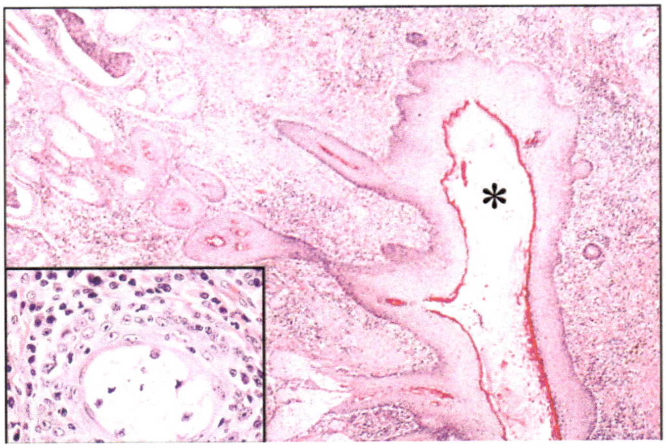

Figure 18.38 **Ear canal from an American Cocker Spaniel dog; lymphoplasmacytic otitis externa. The ear canal (asterisk) is markedly stenotic and filled with cerumen and keratinous debris. The epidermis is markedly thickened. The dermal changes are characterized by a moderate to marked lymphoplasmacytic inflammatory response with ceruminous hyperplasia. The dermal collagen is abundant and dense, indicating fibrosis. Inset: an island of sebaceous cells is surrounded by lymphoplasmacytic inflammation. This dog presented for a total ear canal ablation for treatment of chronic otitis.** ***Staphylococcus pseudintermedius*** **and** ***Pseudomonas aeruginosa*** **were cultured from the ear canal (H&E: main, 40× magnification; inset: 400× magnification).**

are predominantly anucleate. The treatment is to simply decrease the frequency of ear cleaner use (Rosychuk, 1994).

Primary secretory otitis media in the Cavalier King Charles Spaniel (Figure 18.40) can extend out into the external ear canal if the tympanic membrane is ruptured. The ear canal contains a variably colored viscous plug, which cytologically is composed of mucus (Figure 18.41), which stains Alcian blue and periodic acid-Schiff positive, and sometimes, variable numbers of neutrophils and macrophages (Weinstein *et al.*, 2016). Rarely, yeasts, cocci, or epithelial cells are also seen in the plug material (Stern-Bertholtz *et al.*, 2003).

Cholesterol granulomas have been rarely reported in the middle ears of dogs and cats. In these lesions, granuloma formation is secondary to the presence of cholesterol (acicular clefts) which accumulates due to cellular breakdown and lack of clearance, and acts like a foreign body. They cause disease from space-occupying lesion effects (Fliegner *et al.*, 2007). Note that acicular clefts can form secondary to any cause of otitis media and are not diagnostic for cholesterol granuloma (Sula *et al.*, 2014).

Proliferative, necrotizing otitis externa is an uncommon disease of young cats <5 years of age. Grossly, the lesions appear as dark brown to black, friable, and somewhat exophytic to plaque-like masses, which cover the concave surface of the pinna and often extend into the ear canal. The ear canal may be filled with exfoliated material. The cytology has not been described, but histologically the lesions possess a thickened (acanthotic) epidermis with a thickened cornified layer with retained nuclei (parakeratotic hyperkeratosis). The outer root sheath of hair follicles is thickened with many shrunken, dark pink keratinocytes with shrunken dark nuclei (apoptosis). Apoptosis or necrosis of the epidermis between hair follicles is not seen. The openings of hair follicles are filled with nucleated squamous epithelial cells, neutrophils, and cellular debris. There is also variable mixed inflammation in the dermis (Mauldin *et al.*, 2007). The cause of this lesion is unknown but it is thought to involve a T-lymphocyte-mediated autoimmune response with induction of keratinocyte apoptosis (Videmont & Pin, 2010). The masses usually resolve spontaneously after a variable period of time (Mauldin *et al.*, 2007).

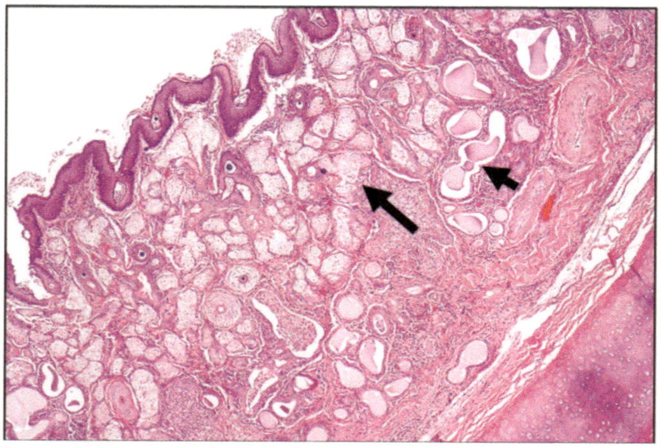

Figure 18.39 External ear canal from a dog; proliferative otitis externa. The epidermis is moderately thickened and folded with pronounced rete ridges. There is marked ceruminous (short arrow) and sebaceous (long arrow) gland hyperplasia. An accompanying mild lymphoplasmacytic inflammatory response is also present (H&E, 40× magnification).

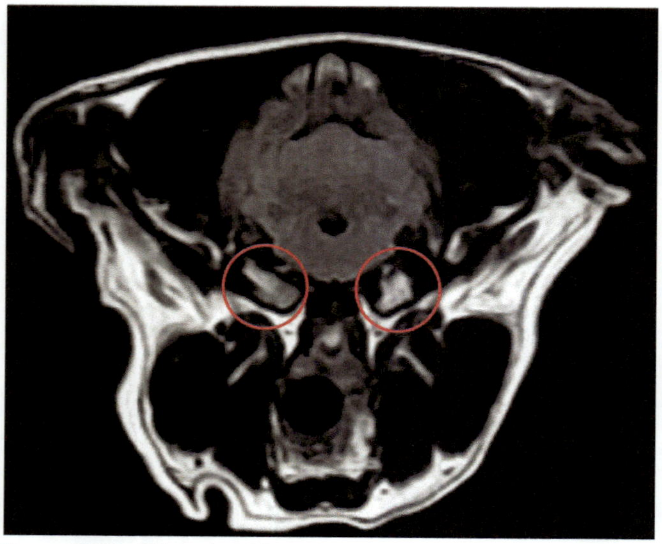

Figure 18.40 Bilateral middle ear lesions of a Cavalier King Charles Spaniel; primary secretory otitis media. MRI T2w FLAIR image showing material in both tympanic bullae (red circles). Radiologist description: the tympanic bullae are filled with T1-weighted hypointense, T2-weighted hyperintense, T2 FLAIR hyperintense, non-contrast enhancing material bilaterally with no overt increased mucosal contrast enhancement. (Courtesy Dr. Caitlin Doran and Dr. Yu Hung (Alex) Hsieh.)

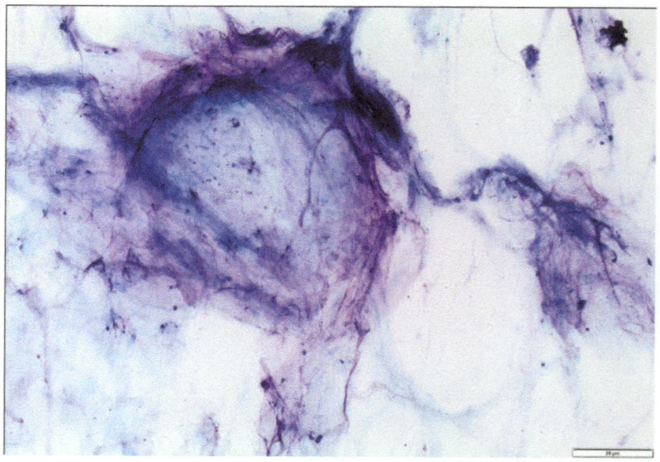

Figure 18.41 Bilateral middle ear lesions of a Cavalier King Charles Spaniel; primary secretory otitis media. Fine needle aspiration was performed of the material in the middle ear which yielded abundant mucus (modified Wright–Giemsa, 100× magnification).

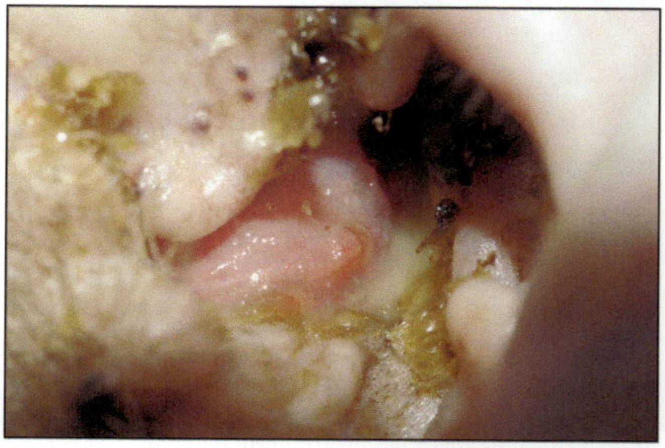

Figure 18.42 Otoscopic view of the external ear canal of a cat; inflammatory polyp. The smooth, pink, proliferative tissue of an inflammatory polyp is visualized through the otoscope.

Neoplastic and non-neoplastic mass lesions

Neoplasms and non-neoplastic mass lesions of the ear canal are reportedly uncommon tumors in dogs and cats. Unique to this location are ceruminous gland neoplasms and proliferations, endolymphatic sac tumor, as well as inflammatory polyps and aural cholesteatomas. Other neoplasms reported in the external ear canal appear similar to those of the pinnae (see above) and elsewhere in the skin. Round cell tumors include histiocytoma, plasmacytoma, and melanoma. Epithelial tumors include sebaceous adenoma, sebaceous adenocarcinoma, SCC, and papilloma. Mesenchymal tumors of the ear canal include sarcoma and hemangiosarcoma. It is worth noting that SCC of the ear canal is an aggressive neoplasm and is more aggressive than ceruminous adenocarcinoma in both dogs and cats (London *et al.*, 1996).

Polyps

Inflammatory or nasopharyngeal polyps may be found in the ear canal of cats and, rarely, dogs (Figure 18.42, Anderson *et al.*, 2000; Fan & Lorimier, 2004). Polyps are hyperplastic masses, not neoplasms. In cats they may be found in the ear canals (usually originating from the middle ear but can be found in the external canal if the tympanic membrane ruptured), nasopharynx, or tympanic bulla (Hoppers *et al.*, 2020). In dogs, external ear canal origin appears to be

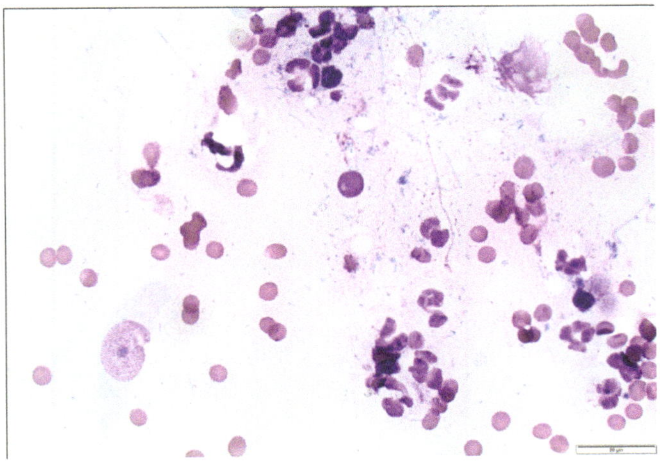

Figure 18.43 **Fine needle aspirate from a mass in the ear canal of a cat; inflammatory (nasopharyngeal) polyp. A columnar epithelial cell with indistinct cilia (bottom left) with mildly degenerate neutrophils and bacilli (modified Wright–Giemsa; 600× magnification).**

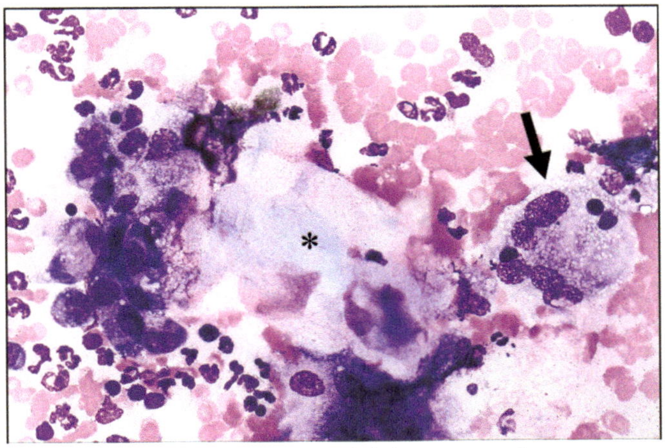

Figure 18.44 **Tissue from a dog; aural cholesteatoma with pyogranulomatous inflammation. A central clump of anucleate keratinocytes (asterisk) is present on a background of mixed inflammation and blood. Nondegenerate neutrophils and macrophages predominate, but occasional multinucleated giant cells (arrow) are also present. When tissue is exposed to keratin, it elicits a significant suppurative to pyogranulomatous inflammatory response (foreign body-type reaction) (Wright–Giemsa, 500× magnification).**

most common (Schuldenfrei *et al.*, 2023). The inciting cause of polyps is unknown. They are most frequently seen in cats <3 years of age but may occur at any age (Veir *et al.*, 2002). Polyps may arise in one ear, or bilaterally (Hoppers *et al.*, 2020). The polypoid portion can be visualized with an otoscope or otoendoscope and is attached by a thin stalk. FNA of inflammatory polyps yields a mixed inflammatory cell population comprising macrophages, small mature lymphocytes, neutrophils, occasional plasma cells, and sometimes multinucleate giant cells. There are also large polygonal squamous epithelial cells or smaller epithelial cells singly or in small clusters. In some polyps there may be a population of uniform columnar and, possibly, ciliated epithelial cells, which may be present in linear array, indicating respiratory differentiation (Figure 18.43; De Lorenzi *et al.*, 2005).

Histologically, polyps comprise a mass of loose fibrovascular tissue with admixed lymphocytes and plasma cells and, possibly, neutrophils and macrophages, covered by a stratified squamous to ciliated columnar epithelium (Lane *et al.*, 1981). Surgical removal via traction or avulsion is usually recommended, but if there is involvement of the tympanic bulla, recurrence is more frequent and a bulla osteotomy may be required (Veir *et al.*, 2002).

Aural cholesteatoma

Aural cholesteatomas, also known as keratinizing cysts, are non-neoplastic masses that form in the middle ear of dogs, but they may extend into the external ear if the tympanic membrane is ruptured. They can also extend into the inner ear and cause otitis interna and meningoencephalitis (Newman *et al.*, 2015). Aural cholesteatomas may be congenital or acquired. Acquired aural cholesteatomas are commonly associated with chronic otitis media and appear as pearl-like nodules. The cytology is consistent with a keratinizing cyst, with large numbers of anucleate squamous epithelial cells and squamous debris (Figure 18.44). Inflammation may also be present, with variable numbers of neutrophils and macrophages. Secondary yeast and/or cocci may also be seen.

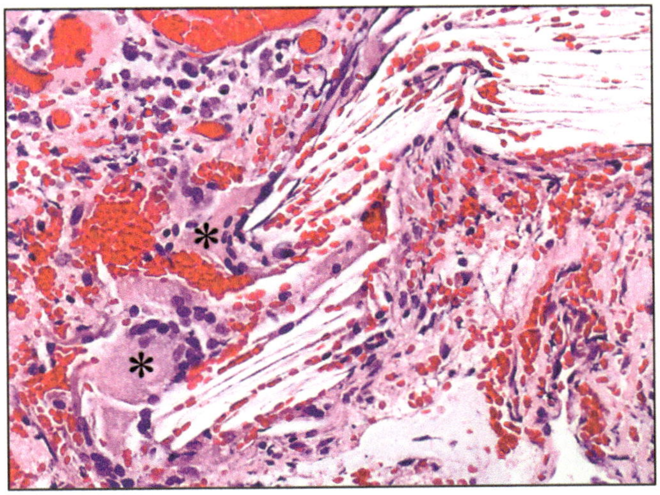

Figure 18.45 **Mass from the middle ear canal of a cat; cholesteatoma. This mass was friable and broke into pieces when it was surgically removed from the middle ear. The mass contains acicular cholesterol crystals surrounded by multinucleate giant cells (asterisks), indicating cell membrane breakdown. Anucleate squames, characteristic of this lesion, are not captured in this image. Extension into the external ear canal can be seen when there is rupture of the tympanic membrane (H&E, 400× magnification).**

The histopathology of aural cholesteatoma is described as a cystic lesion lined by a stratified squamous epithelium with a thick stratum corneum. The epithelium often shows differentiation to ciliated columnar epithelium. The subjacent dermis may have fibrosis, with some lymphocytes and plasma cells and usually low numbers of macrophages and neutrophils (Figure 18.45). The cystic space contains free anucleate squames (Hardie *et al.*, 2008).

Ceruminous gland neoplasms

Ceruminous glands are modified sweat glands found in the external ear canal. Ceruminous gland neoplasms are more often malignant in cats and benign in dogs (Fan & Lorimier, 2004). Cocker Spaniels appear predisposed to these neoplasms (Moisan & Watson, 1996). Adenomas are small, pedunculated, brown, irregular, firm, well-circumscribed nodules within the ear canal (Figure 18.46). Multiple adenomas are often seen. Adenocarcinomas may be nodular to flattened and plaque-like, with indistinct margins, and ulceration may be present. These neoplasms are associated with chronic otitis externa (Moisan & Watson, 1996).

The cytology of ceruminous gland adenomas is dominated by cohesive clusters of small to medium-sized round to polygonal epithelial cells. Clusters are regular and may appear mosaic-like. The cells possess a low to moderate N:C ratio with a round to oval nucleus, finely clumped chromatin, and a single prominent nucleolus. The cytoplasm ranges from pale to moderately basophilic. The degree of anisocytosis and anisokaryosis is usually mild, but may be moderate when there is a secondary bacterial infection present, and may result in misdiagnosis of adenocarcinoma. In the background there may be blue to black, variably smooth to coarse granular material, which can resemble melanin but represents secretions from ceruminous ducts (Figure 18.47; De Lorenzi *et al.*, 2005). Adenomas cannot be reliably differentiated from hyperplasia on cytology.

Histopathology of ceruminous gland adenoma reveals a polypoid to papillary dermal mass that is expansile and well-demarcated. The mass is composed of uniform cuboidal to columnar epithelial cells present in tubules, papillary clusters, and acini, contained by an intact basement membrane. The individual cells have a moderate to high N:C ratio with a round to ovoid nucleus, stippled chromatin, and a single, small prominent nucleolus. The cytoplasm is pale eosinophilic. The lumens of acini contain pale basophilic to brown, finely granular material admixed with few neutrophils and nuclear and cellular debris (Figure 18.48). Mitotic figures are infrequent to rare. Variable numbers of lymphocytes, plasma cells, neutrophils, and macrophages are present in the surrounding dermis (Moisan & Watson, 1996).

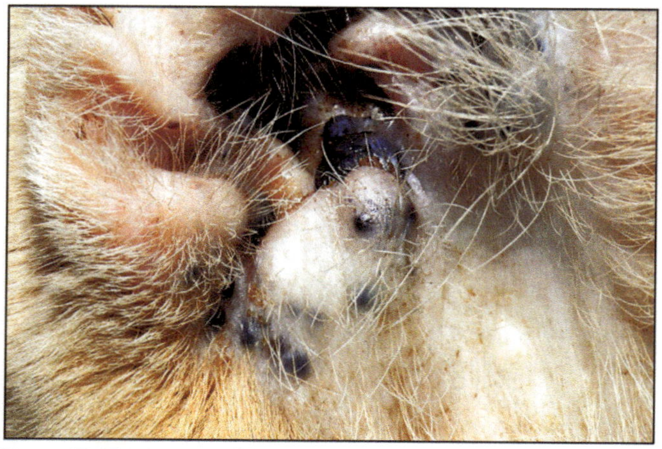

Figure 18.46 Opening of the ear canal of a cat; ceruminous gland adenomas. One large and several small darkly pigmented masses are present. (Courtesy Dr. Frane Banovic.)

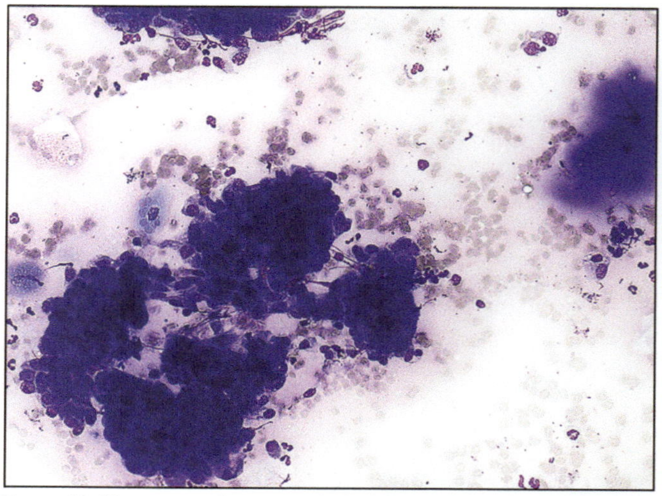

Figure 18.47 Mass in the ear canal of a dog; ceruminous gland adenoma. Clusters of deeply basophilic epithelial cells are present. Cells are uniform in appearance with round to oval nuclei and moderate amounts of deeply basophilic cytoplasm. To the right, there is a small lake of amorphous extracellular blue material consistent with ceruminous secretions. Mild suppurative inflammation is also present (Wright–Giemsa, 250× magnification).

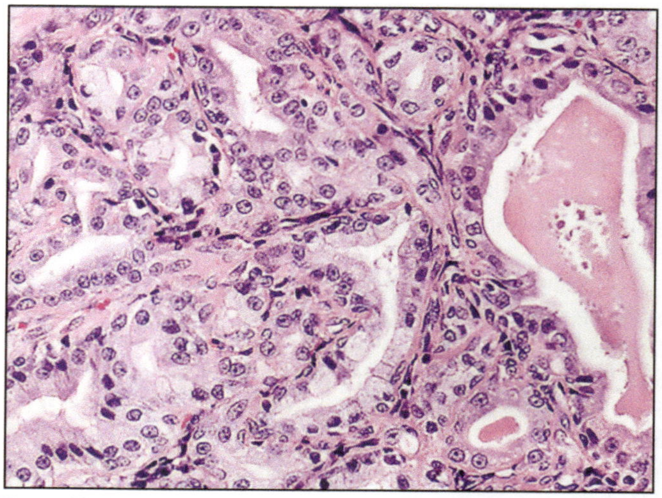

Figure 18.48 Polypoid mass in the ear canal of a cat; ceruminous adenoma. Expanding the dermis is a neoplasm composed of uniform cuboidal epithelial cells forming tubules and acini. The cells exhibit mild anisocytosis and anisokaryosis. Occasional acini contain pale eosinophilic amorphous material within the lumen (cerumen) (H&E, 300× magnification).

Ceruminous gland adenocarcinomas have multiple cellular criteria of malignancy in cytology samples including marked anisocytosis and anisokaryosis, coarse chromatin, large nuclei, macronucleoli, and binucleate and multinucleate cells (Figure 18.49). Variable numbers of neutrophils with cocci bacteria and amorphous basophilic debris

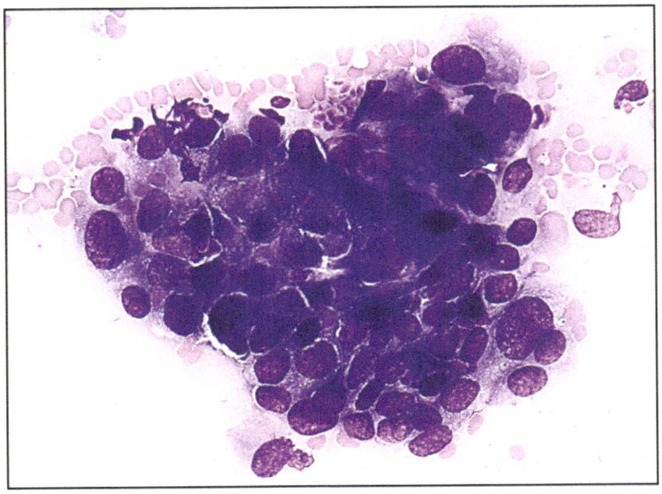

Figure 18.49 Mass in the ear canal of a dog; ceruminous gland adenocarcinoma. This tumor shows significant pleomorphism with moderate anisocytosis and anisokaryosis, cellular crowding, nuclear molding, and visible nucleoli. Biopsy confirmed a ceruminous gland adenocarcinoma (modified Wright–Giemsa, 500× magnification). (Courtesy Dr. Rebekah Gunn-Christie.)

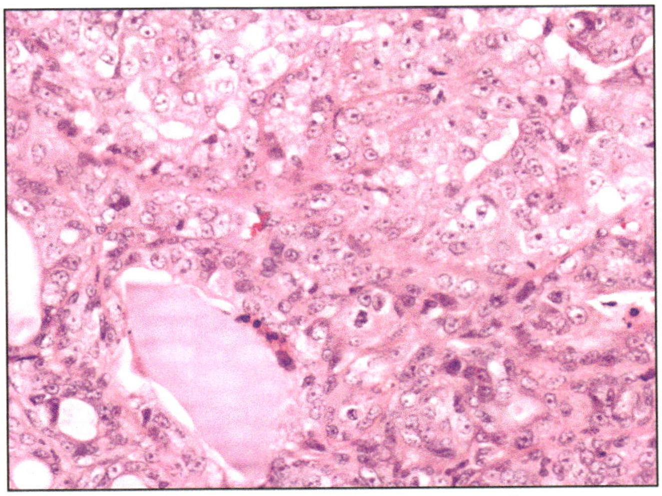

Figure 18.50 Ear canal mass from a dog; ceruminous adenocarcinoma. The dermis is infiltrated by a poorly demarcated neoplasm composed of epithelial cells forming jumbled clusters, nests, and acini. Occasional acini contain pale amphophilic material within the lumen (cerumen) (H&E, 400× magnification).

(necrosis) are often observed. Blue to black extracellular material/granules may be present in the background (ductal secretions). Cell clusters may be regular and mosaic-like, as in adenomas, or nuclear molding may be present. A useful feature to assist differentiation from adenomas is the presence of acinar clusters in adenocarcinomas (De Lorenzi *et al.*, 2005). Take care with interpretation of cellular atypia in the presence of inflammation and bacterial infection. Ceruminous gland neoplasms are frequently accompanied by otitis externa, which can complicate differentiation of adenoma from adenocarcinoma.

Histologically, adenocarcinomas are exophytic to polypoid dermal masses, which are locally invasive through the dermis and subjacent stroma but do not usually invade through the auricular cartilage. Epidermal invasion may be seen. Adenocarcinomas form tubules, nests, acini, and sheets. Individual cells often exhibit loss of polarity, where the nucleus is no longer at the basolateral aspect of the acinus. Multiple cellular criteria of malignancy are typical with marked anisocytosis and anisokaryosis and frequent mitotic figures (up to 10/hpf). Areas of necrosis and mixed inflammation are usually present (Figure 18.50). Transition to squamous epithelial cells with abrupt keratinization may be seen (squamous differentiation). Tumors may occasionally be mixed, with chondroid metaplasia reported (Moisan & Watson, 1996). Surgical removal usually requires total ear canal ablation, but invasion through the tympanic membrane into the middle ear appears to be rare. The reported frequency of metastasis varies between references, with older references citing up to 50% metastasis rates and more recent references suggesting that metastasis is less common (Legendre & Krahwinkel, 1981; London *et al.*, 1996; Moisan & Watson, 1996). Reported sites of metastasis are regional lymph nodes, lungs, and abdominal organs (Legendre & Krahwinkel, 1981). FNA of submandibular and retropharyngeal lymph nodes may be warranted as part of the clinical staging.

Endolymphatic sac tumor

Endolymphatic sac tumors have been rarely described in dogs. They arise from the posterior wall of the temporal bone in the inner ear, and may be found in the inner or middle ear. These tumors are locally invasive and can cause lysis of the temporal bone, but metastasis has not been reported. Histologically, they are comprised of one to two layers of well-differentiated cuboidal epithelial cells forming papillary projections on a thin fibrovascular stalk (Barnes *et al.*, 2017). To the authors' knowledge, cytology of these tumors has not yet been described.

CASES

CASE 1

Signalment/history

A 3.5-year-old, spayed female Jack Russell Terrier with a history of recurrent ear infections. She was adopted by her owners when she was 12 weeks of age and has suffered with ear problems her entire life. She was noted to have an ear infection the day she was adopted. There is no seasonal improvement or worsening of the clinical signs. The owners also report that the dog's stools are soft, making it difficult to pick them up, and she will vomit intermittently (approximately once weekly) with no other signs of illness.

Physical examination

All abnormal findings are limited to the ears. The concave surface of each pinna is erythematous and swollen, with mild to moderate lichenification and hyperpigmentation, and a malodorous ceruminous scaling and crusting are present (Figure 18.51). The pinnae are sensitive to touch. Otoscopic examination reveals mild hyperplasia of

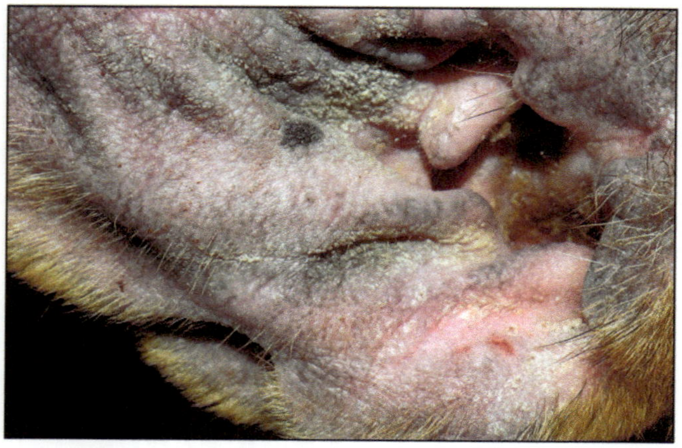

Figure 18.51 Ear pinna from a dog with a history of ear infections and allergies. The pinna is erythematous and swollen with mild to moderate lichenification, hyperpigmentation, ceruminous scaling, and crusting.

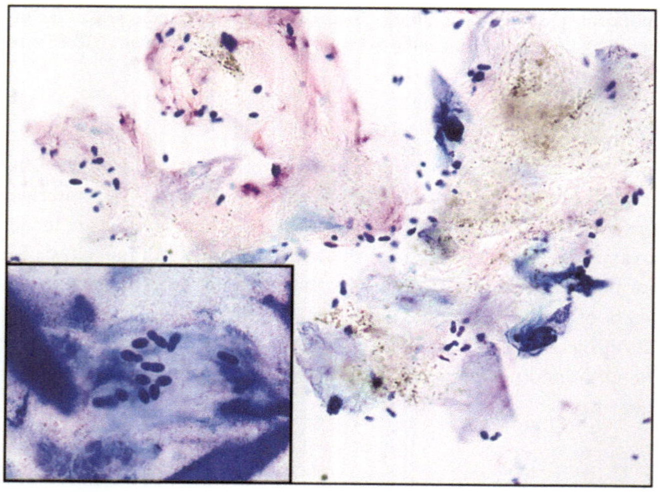

Figure 18.52 Canine ear pinna and canal cytology preparations; *Malassezia* spp. dermatitis. Clumps of keratinized epithelial cells with adhered *Malassezia* spp. yeast are present. Note the small, brown round to rice-shaped melanin granules in the keratinocytes; these should not be mistaken for bacteria. Inset: tape preparation from the same patient showing basophilic keratinocytes with adhered yeast and keratin bars (modified Wright–Giemsa: main, 500× magnification; inset: 1,000× magnification).

the lining of each ear canal with a moderate amount of light brown ceruminous, malodorous debris clinging to the lining of each ear canal. Each tympanic membrane is intact and normal.

Cytology

Cytology samples were collected from the pinna using the tape strip technique and from the ear canals using a cotton tipped applicator (Figure 18.52). Cytology results showed 4+ *Malassezia* spp. yeast from the left pinna, 1+ *Malassezia* spp. yeast from the right pinna, 2+ *Malassezia* spp. yeast from the left ear canal, and 3+ *Malassezia* spp. yeast from the right ear canal.

Management/outcome

The dog was placed on a strict diet trial using a limited antigen kangaroo and oatmeal diet (Iams Veterinary Formula Skin & Coat Plus Response KO diet) to rule in/out food allergies as a primary or contributing factor in her allergic ear disease. The ear canal infections were treated with topical Posatex Otic Suspension (Merck Animal Health; 1.0% orbifloxacin, 0.1% mometasone furoate monohydrate, and 0.1% posaconazole, otic suspension) in each ear canal (0.2 ml q24h for 21 days). The *Malassezia* spp. dermatitis of the pinnae was treated by cleaning the pinnae daily with Epi-Otic (Virbac Animal Health; 2.7% lactic acid and 0.1% salicylic acid) ear cleanser on a cotton ball, allowing 2 minutes contact time. The pinnae were then wiped clean and dry using dry cotton balls and then 1–2 drops of Posatex were applied daily for 7 days and then twice weekly for 7 days. Once the infections were cleared, the food trial was continued for another 21 days with weekly ear cleaning of the ear canals as the only treatment.

The ear infections completely resolved with the treatment plan above and did not recur 3 weeks after medications were ceased. On food rechallenge with her previous diet, her pinnae and ear canals became erythematous within 2–3 days, which resolved when the rechallenge was discontinued. The dog has been maintained on the KO diet without further flaring of the clinical signs. Interestingly, the gastrointestinal issues also completely resolved while on the food trial, and flared on food rechallenge.

Discussion

This case illustrates how factors influencing the microenvironment of the ear can predispose individuals to developing *Malassezia* spp. yeast overgrowth/infection. In this case, food allergies resulting in inflammation and altered sebum production of the pinnae and ear canal allowed overgrowth of yeasts, which, themselves, are capable of eliciting a hypersensitivity reaction. Eliminating both the yeast infection and the predisposing factor (food allergy in this case) is necessary for clinical resolution (Murphy, 2001).

CASE 2

Signalment/history

A 15-month-old, female spayed Maine Coon cat with a 3-month history of a unilateral left ear problem. The cat was adopted from a Maine Coon breeder as a young kitten. She appeared to be healthy at that time. Three months ago the owner noted that the cat appeared to be sensitive when her left ear was touched, and purulent debris was found on otoscopic examination.

Cytology/initial treatment

Ear cytology using a cotton tipped applicator revealed numerous inflammatory cells (4+) and cocci (2+) (Figure 18.53). Tresaderm (Merial; 40 mg thiabendazole, 1 mg dexamethasone, 3.2 mg neomycin/ml of solution) ear medication was prescribed (0.15 ml in the ear daily for 14 days) and the cat appeared to be more comfortable. Neither repeat cytology nor repeat otoscopic examination was

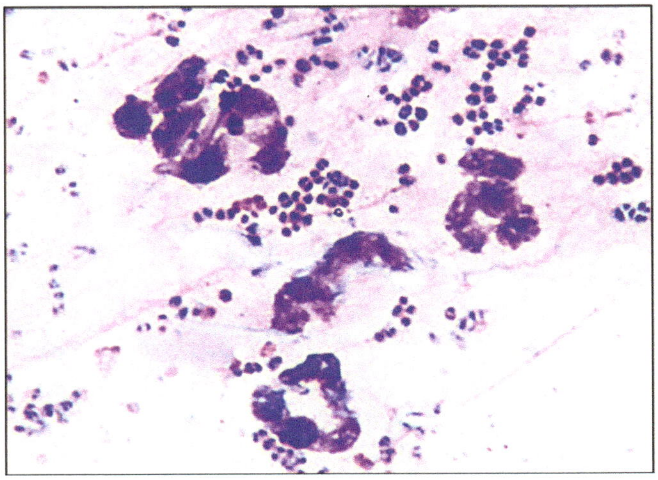

Figure 18.53 Ear cytology from a young adult cat with a history of unilateral ear sensitivity. Many degenerate neutrophils and myriad cocci are present on a proteinaceous background (modified Wright–Giemsa, 1,500× magnification).

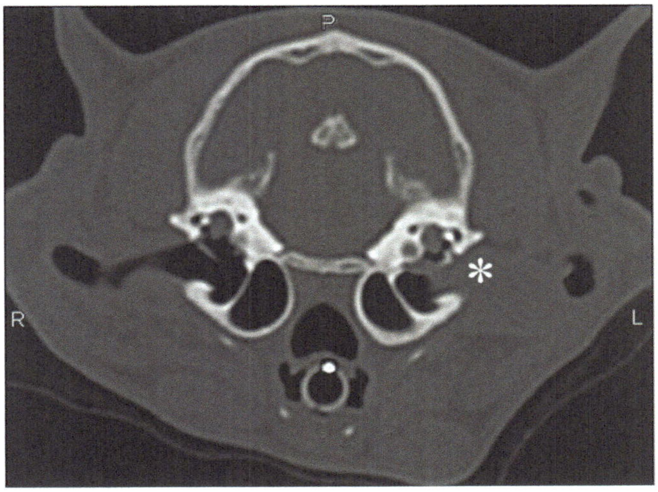

Figure 18.54 Image from a CT scan of a young adult cat with a history of unilateral ear sensitivity. The left ear canal is filled with a soft tissue attenuating structure (asterisk) that extends from the vertical canal into the middle ear. An inflammatory polyp is most likely.

performed. Within 2–3 weeks of discontinuing the Tresaderm, the ear infection was documented to have recurred. At the last recheck visit, the cat had been treated with the Tresaderm once again for 14 days, with clinical improvement noted; however, on otoscopic examination, the ear canal remained full of purulent debris. Otic cytology was repeated and numerous inflammatory cells were found with no evidence of infection (no cocci, rods, or yeast found). An inflammatory polyp was suspected and the cat was scheduled for a bulla CT scan, gentle cleaning of the ear canal, and possible traction extraction of the polyp.

Imaging

On the CT scan, the left ear canal was reported to be full of a soft tissue attenuating structure (Figure 18.54). The structure extended through the tympanic membrane into the middle ear and came in contact with the outer osseous wall of the cochlea. The remainder of the tympanic bulla and the inner ear were normal.

Management/outcome

On otoscopic examination, following gentle removal of the purulent debris from the ear canal, a pink fleshy mass was noted and was removed from the canal using hemostats and traction avulsion. Subsequent histopathologic evaluation of the mass confirmed a nasopharyngeal polyp with lymphoplasmacytic inflammation (Figure 18.55).

Immediately following the procedure, the cat was placed on oral prednisolone at a tapering dose for 8 weeks: 2 mg/kg daily for 14 days, 1 mg/kg daily for 14 days, 0.5 mg/kg daily for 14 days, and 0.5 mg/kg on alternate days for 14 days. She was rechecked at 1 week, 6 weeks, 3 months, and 1 year post-removal of the mass and has recovered without incident. She is playful, interacts with the family, and shows no evidence of recurrence of the polyp.

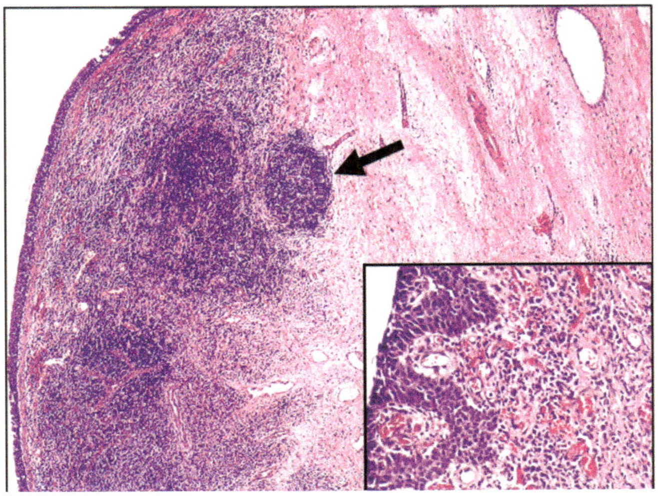

Figure 18.55 Section of a mass retracted from the ear canal of a cat; nasopharyngeal polyp. The mass is composed of fibrous connective tissue lined by pseudostratified to cuboidal epithelium. Multifocal aggregates of lymphocytes are present and occasionally form follicles (arrow). Inset: below the pseudostratified epithelium, a mixed inflammatory infiltrate is present. Lymphocytes predominate, but lesser numbers of plasma cells, macrophages, and neutrophils are also present as are many vascular structures (H&E: main, 40× magnification; inset: 200× magnification).

Discussion

In this case, the species, age (young), and recurrent, unilateral nature of the clinical signs should all lead to suspicion of an underlying lesion, most likely an inflammatory polyp. While inflammatory polyps can often be visualized by otoscopic or oropharyngeal examination, advanced imaging can also be helpful for evaluation of middle ear involvement and therapeutic planning (traction avulsion versus ventral bulla osteotomy). Although recurrence may be more likely with traction avulsion, many clinicians prefer this simpler approach and reserve ventral bulla osteotomy for cases in which there is middle ear involvement or with recurrence following traction avulsion. Use of corticosteroids may decrease the risk of recurrence (Fan & de Lorimier, 2004).

CASE 3

Signalment/history

An 11.5-year-old, neutered male American Cocker Spaniel with a long history of ear and skin problems related to atopic otitis/dermatitis. His skin allergy signs are well controlled with oral cyclosporine (5 mg/kg) daily and a limited antigen venison and potato diet (Hill's Prescription Diet d/d Canine Skin Support Potato & Venison Formula); however, his ears still flare from time to time, usually after he is boarded. Approximately 6 weeks ago, the owner noted a small mass on the left pinna. At first the dog was not bothered by the mass, but the owner is concerned because the mass is increasing in size and is more red and irritated than previously noted. Now it does seem to bother the dog, and he will scratch at the left pinna and occasionally bleeding from the growth is noted.

Physical examination

On physical examination, other than the mass on the pinna, there is no evidence of inflammation or infection involving the ears. A 3.5 × 2 cm mass is located on the concave surface of the left pinna, just before the entrance to the external ear canal (Figure 18.56). The mass is multilobulated, malodorous, eroded, and exudative with necrotic tissue and a cream colored substance/exudate.

Cytology

Cytologic findings based on FNA of the mass reported carcinoma with ceruminous adenocarcinoma being a strong consideration given the location, although no secretory material was observed (Figure 18.57).

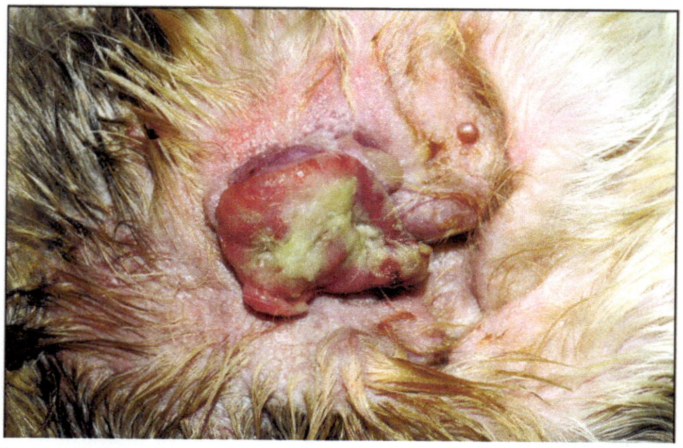

Figure 18.56 Concave surface from the ear pinna of a dog; carcinoma. A large, fleshy, erythematous and multilobulated mass is present near the entrance to the external ear canal. Erosions and surface exudation are present on the mass and erythema in the surrounding tissues is also noted.

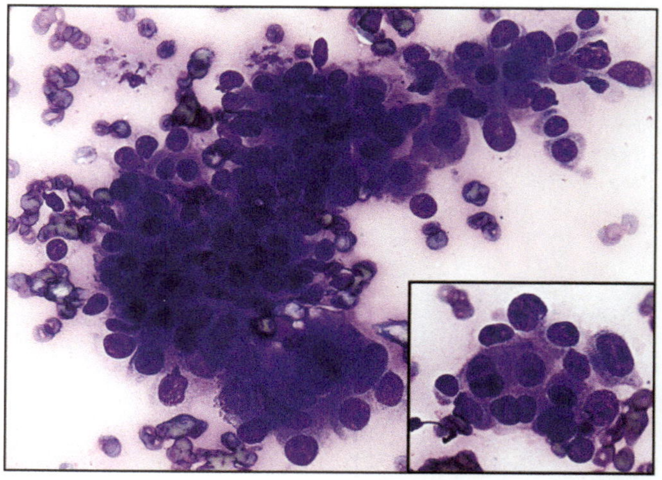

Figure 18.57 Cytology of a mass from the ear pinna of a dog; carcinoma. Clusters of deeply basophilic and jumbled epithelial cells are present. Cells exhibit mild to moderate anisocytosis and anisokaryosis, have a high and variable N:C ratio, and moderately basophilic cytoplasm. Nuclear molding is noted. Inset: cells have large, oval, deeply basophilic nucleoli. Although no material suggestive of glandular secretions is present, given the location, a ceruminous adenocarcinoma would be the top consideration (Wright-Giemsa, 500× magnification).

Management/outcome

The mass was surgically removed. Histopathologic evaluation reported a poorly differentiated carcinoma with nine mitotic figures/10 hpf and 6 mm lateral by 1.5 mm deep margins. The owners declined further staging or treatment concerning the neoplasm. At 6-month follow-up, the dog continued to do well, with no recurrence of the mass noted, and his allergies remained well controlled.

Discussion

This case illustrates the critical role cytology plays in the clinical evaluation of mass lesions. Although evaluation of the cytology preparation did not allow for specific identification of the neoplasm type, the mass could be identified as a carcinoma, which is helpful in planning for the removal of the mass and additional diagnostics (staging, declined in this case). In this particular case, histopathology was also unable to specifically identify the type of carcinoma, but still provided valuable information regarding surgical margins and mitotic index, a measure of tumor proliferation.

REFERENCES

Anderson D.M., Robinson R.K., White R.A. (2000) Management of inflammatory polyps in 37 cats. *Vet Rec 147*:684–687.

Angus J.C. (2004) Otic cytology in health and disease. *Vet Clin North Am Small Anim Pract 34*:411–424.

Baba T., Shimizu A., Ohmuro T. et al. (2009) Auricular chondritis associated with systemic joint and cartilage inflammation in a cat. *J Vet Med Sci 1*:79–82.

Barnes K.J., Clear V., Youmans K. et al. (2017) Endolymphatic sac tumor in two dogs. *Vet Pathol 54*:683–685.

Berlato D., Bulman-Fleming J., Clifford C.A. et al. (2021) Value, limitations, and recommendations for grading of canine cutaneous mast cell tumors: A consensus of the Oncology-Pathology Working Group. *Vet Pathol 58*:858–863.

Bloom P.B. (2006) Canine and feline eosinophilic skin diseases. *Vet Clin North Am Small Anim Pract 36*:141–160.

Bohn A.A., Wills T., Caplazi P. (2006) Basal cell tumor or cutaneous basilar epithelial neoplasm? Rethinking the cytologic diagnosis of basal cell tumors. *Vet Clin Pathol 35*:449–453.

Bostock D.E., Dye M.T. (1979) Prognosis after surgical excision of fibrosarcomas in cats. *J Am Vet Med Assoc 175*:727–728.

Brilhante A.F., Lima L., Zampieri R.A. et al. (2019) *Leishmania (Viannia) braziliensis* type 2 as probable etiological agent of canine cutaneous leishmaniasis in Brazilian Amazon. *Plos One 14*:e0216291.

Calhoun M.L., Stinson A.W. (1987) Integument. In: *Textbook of Veterinary Histology* (eds. H.D. Dellmann, E.M. Brown) Lea & Febiger, Philadelphia, pp. 382–415.

Camus M.S., Priest H.L., Koehler J.W. et al. (2016) Cytologic criteria for mast cell tumor grading in dogs with evaluation of clinical outcome. *Vet Pathol 53*:1117–1123.

Chen T.A., Hill P.B. (2005) The biology of *Malassezia* organisms and their ability to induce immune responses and skin disease. *Vet Dermatol 16*:4–26.

Cleare E., Mason K.V., Mills J. et al. (2014) Remaining vigilant for the exotic: Cases of imported canine leishmaniosis in Australia 2000–2011. *Aust Vet J 92*:119–127.

Cole L.K. (2009) Anatomy and physiology of the canine ear. *Vet Dermatol 20*:412–421.

Cornegliani L., Fondevila D., Vercelli A. et al. (2005) PCR technique detection of *Leishmania* spp. but not *Mycobacterium* spp. in canine cutaneous 'sterile' pyogranuloma/granuloma syndrome. *Vet Dermatol 16*:233–238.

Corriveau L.A. (2012) Use of a carbon dioxide laser to treat ceruminous gland hyperplasia in a cat. *J Feline Med Surg 14*:413–416.

Coyner K. (2010) Otomycosis due to *Aspergillus* spp. in a dog: Case report and literature review. *Vet Dermatol 21*:613–618.

Crain N., Nelson B.L., Barnes E.L. et al. (2009) Ceruminous gland carcinomas: A clinicopathologic and immunophenotypic study of 17 cases. *Head Neck Pathol 3*:1–17.

Day D.G., Couto C.G., Weisbrode S.E. et al. (1994) Basal cell carcinoma in two cats. *J Am Anim Hosp Assoc 30*:265–269.

Day M.J. (1995) Immunophenotypic characterization of cutaneous lymphoid neoplasia in the dog and cat. *J Comp Pathol 112*:79–96.

De Lorenzi D., Bonfanti U., Masserdotti S. et al. (2005) Fine-needle biopsy of external ear canal masses in the cat: Cytologic results and histologic correlations in 27 cases. *Vet Clin Pathol 34*:100–105.

Delmage D.A., Kelly D.F. (2001) Auricular chondritis in a cat. *J Small Anim Pract 42*:499–501.

Dennis M.M., McSporran K.D., Bacon N.J. et al. (2011) Prognostic factors for cutaneous and subcutaneous soft tissue sarcomas in dogs. *Vet Pathol 48*:73–84.

Dickinson R.M., Young K.M. (2005) Cutaneous mass aspirate from a golden retriever: "glandular guile". *Vet Clin Pathol 34*:421–424.

Dion W.M., Speckmann G. (1978) Canine otitis externa caused by the fungus *Sporothrix schenkii*. *Can Vet J 19*:44–45.

Dorn C.R., Taylor D.O., Schneider R. (1971) Sunlight exposure and risk of developing cutaneous and oral squamous cell carcinoma in white cats. *J Natl Cancer Inst 46*:1073–1078.

Duprey Z.H., Steurer F.J., Rooney J.A. et al. (2006) Canine visceral leishmaniasis, United States and Canada, 2000–2003. *Emerg Infect Dis 12*:440–446.

Dye T.L., Teague H.D., Ostwald Jr D.A. et al. (2002) Evaluation of a technique using the carbon dioxide laser for the treatment of aural hematomas. *J Am Anim Hosp Assoc 38*:385–390.

Evans H.E. (1993) The ear. In: *Miller's Anatomy of the Dog* (ed. H.E. Evans) Saunders, Philadephia, pp. 988–1008.

Fan T.M., de Lorimier L.P. (2004) Inflammatory polyps and aural neoplasia. *Vet Clin North Am Small Anim Pract 34*:489–509.

Fliegner R.A., Jubb K.V.F., Lording P.M. (2007) Cholesterol granuloma associated with otitis media and destruction of the tympanic bulla in a dog. *Vet Pathol 44*:547–549.

Foley J.E., Borjesson D., Gross T.L. et al. (2002) Clinical, microscopic, and molecular aspects of canine leproid granuloma in the United States. *Vet Pathol 39*:234–239.

Gerber B., Crottaz M., von Tscharner C. et al. (2002) Feline relapsing polychondritis: Two cases and a review of literature. *J Feline Med Surg 4*:189–194.

Ghibaudo G., Peano A. (2010) Chronic monolateral otomycosis in a dog caused by *Aspergillus ochraceus*. *Vet Dermatol 21*:522–526.

Ginel P.J., Lucena R., Rodriguez J.C. et al. (2002) A semiquantitative cytological evaluation of normal and pathological samples from the external ear canal of dogs and cats. *Vet Dermatol 13*:151–156.

Giunchetti R.C., Mayrink W., Genaro O. et al. (2006) Relationship between canine visceral leishmaniosis and the *Leishmania (Leishmania) chagasi* burden in dermal inflammatory foci. *J Comp Pathol 135*:100–107.

Godfrey D. (2000) *Microsporum canis* associated with otitis externa in a Persian cat. *Vet Rec 147*:50–51.

Goldschmidt M.H., Dunstan R.W., Stannard A.A. et al. (1998) *Histological Classification of Epithelial and Melanocytic Tumors of the Skin of Domestic Animals*, Vol. III, 2nd edn. Armed Forces Institute of Pathology, Washington DC.

Goodale E.C., Outerbridge C.A., White S.D. (2016) Aspergillus otitis in small animals – A retrospective study of 17 cases. *Vet Dermatol 27*:3–e2.

Griffin J.S., Scott D.W., Erb H.N. (2007) *Malassezia* otitis externa in the dog: The effect of heat-fixing otic exudate for cytological analysis. *J Vet Med 54*:424–427.

Grono L.R. (1970a) Studies of the microclimate of the external auditory canal in the dog. I. Aural temperature. *Res Vet Sci 11*:307–311.

Grono L.R. (1970b) Studies of the microclimate of the external auditory canal in the dog. III. Relative humidity within the external auditory meatus. *Res Vet Sci 11*:316–319.

Gross T.L., Ihrke P.J., Walder E.J. et al. (2005) Fibrous tumors. *Skin Diseases of the Dog and Cat: Clinical and Histopathologic Diagnosis*, 2nd edn. Blackwell Science, Oxford, pp. 730–731.

Guillot J., Bond R. (1999) *Malassezia pachydermatis*: A review. *Med Mycol 37*:295–306.

Hardie E.M., Linder K.E., Pease A.P. (2008) Aural cholesteatoma in twenty dogs. *Vet Surg 37*:763–770.

Hendrick M.J., Schofer F.S., Goldschmidt M.H. (1995) Comparison of fibrosarcomas that developed at vaccination sites and at nonvaccination sites in cats: 239 cases (1991–1992). *J Am Vet Med Assoc 205*:1425–1429.

Higginbotham M.L., Henry C.J., Watson Z. et al. (2000) Biological behavior of canine aural mast cell tumors. In: *Proceedings of the 20th Annual Meeting of the Veterinary Cancer Society*. Pacific Grove, p. 52.

Hoppers S.E., May E.R., Frank L.A. (2020) Feline bilateral inflammatory aural polyps: A descriptive retrospective study. *Vet Dermatol 31*:385–e102.

Huang H.P., Fixter L.M., Little C.J.L. (1994) Lipid content of cerumen from normal dogs and otitic canine ears. *Vet Rec 134*:380–381.

Huang H.P., Huang H.M. (1999) Effects of ear type, sex, age, body weight, and climate on temperatures in the external acoustic meatus of dogs. *Am J Vet Res 60*:1173–1176.

Hughes M.S., James G., Ball N. et al. (2000) Identification by 16S rRNA gene analyses of a potential novel mycobacterial species as an etiological agent of canine leproid granuloma syndrome. *J Clin Microbiol 38*:953–959.

Joyce J.A., Day M.J. (1997) Immunopathogenesis of canine aural haematoma. *J Small Anim Pract 38*:152–158.

Kiupel M., Webster J.D., Bailey K.L. et al. (2011) Proposal of a 2-tier histologic grading system for canine cutaneous mast cell tumors to more accurately predict biological behavior. *Vet Pathol 48*:147–155.

Koutinas A.F., Koutinas C.K. (2014) Pathologic mechanisms underlying the clinical findings in canine leishmaniosis due to *Leishmania infantum/chagasi*. *Vet Pathol 51*:527–538.

Lana S.E., Ogilvie G.K., Withrow S.J. et al. (1997) Feline cutaneous squamous cell carcinoma of the nasal planum and the pinnae: 61 cases. *J Am Anim Hosp Assoc 33*:329–332.

Lane J.G., Orr C.M., Lucke V.M. et al. (1981) Nasopharyngeal polyps arising in the middle ear of the cat. *J Small Anim Pract 22*:511–522.

Legendre A.M., Krahwinkel D.J. Jr (1981) Feline ear tumors. *J Am Anim Hosp Assoc 17*:1035–1037.

London C.A., Dubilzeig R.R., Vail D.M. et al. (1996) Evaluation of dogs and cats with tumors of the ear canal: 145 cases (1978–1992). *J Am Vet Med Assoc 208*:1413–1418.

Loshe J., Rinder H., Gothe R. et al. (2002) Validity of species status of the parasitic mite *Otodectes cynotis*. *Med Vet Entomol 16*:133–138.

Luna L.D., Higginbotham M.L., Henry C.L. et al. (2000) Feline non-ocular melanoma: A retrospective study of 23 cases (1991–1999). *J Feline Med Surg 2*:173–181.

Malik R., Love D.N., Wigney D.I. et al. (1998) Mycobacterial nodular granulomas affecting the subcutis and skin of dogs (canine leproid granuloma syndrome). *Aust Vet J 76*:403–407.

Marcos R., Santos M., Santos N. et al. (2009) Use of destained cytology slides for the application of routine special stains. *Vet Clin Pathol 38*:94–102.

Mauldin E.A., Ness T.A., Goldschmidt M.H. (2007) Proliferative and necrotizing otitis externa in four cats. *Vet Dermatol 18*:370–377.

McEwan N.A. (2000) Adherence by *Staphylococcus intermedius* to canine keratinocytes in atopic dermatitis. *Res Vet Sci 68*:279–283.

McKellar Q.A., Rycroft A., Anderson L. et al. (1990) Otitis externa in a foxhound pack associated with *Candida albicans*. *Vet Rec 127*:15–16.

Miller M.A., Nelson S.L., Turk J.R. et al. (1991) Cutaneous neoplasia in 340 cats. *Vet Pathol 28*:389–395.

Miller M.A., Ramos J.A., Kreeger J.M. (1992) Cutaneous vascular neoplasia in 15 cats: Clinical, morphologic, and immunohistochemical studies. *Vet Pathol 29*:329–336.

Miller W.H. Jr, Shanley K.J. (1991) Bilateral pinnal squamous cell carcinoma in a dog with chronic otitis externa. *Vet Dermatol 2*:37–39.

Moisan P.G., Watson G.L. (1996) Ceruminous gland tumors in dogs and cats: A review of 124 cases. *J Am Anim Hosp Assoc 32*:448–452.

Molander-McCrary H., Henry C.J., Potter K. et al. (1998) Cutaneous mast cell tumors in cats: 32 cases (1991–1994). *J Am Anim Hosp Assoc 34*:281–284.

Munday J.S., Hanlon E.M., Howe L. et al. (2007) Feline cutaneous viral papilloma associated with human papillomavirus type 9. *Vet Pathol 44*:924–927.

Murphy K.M. (2001) A review of techniques for the investigation of otitis externa and otitis media. *Clin Tech Small Anim Pract 16*:236–241.

Nagata M., Ishida T. (1997) Cutaneous reactivity to mosquito bites and its antigens in cats. *Vet Dermatol 8*:19–26.

Nardoni S., Macianti F., Rum A. et al. (2005) Isolation of *Malassezia* species from healthy cats and cats with otitis. *J Feline Med Surg 7*:141–145.

Newman A.W., Estey C.M., McDonough S. et al. (2015) Cholesteatoma and meningoencephalitis in a dog with chronic otitis externa. *Vet Clin Pathol 44*:157–163.

Nikula K.J., Benjamin S.A., Angleton G.M. (1992) Ultraviolet radiation, solar dermatosis, and cutaneous neoplasia in beagle dogs. *Radiat Res 129*:11–18.

Patnaik A.K., Ehler W.J., MacEwen E.G. (1984) Canine cutaneous mast cell tumor: Morphologic grading and survival time in 83 dogs. *Vet Pathol 21*:469–474.

Paulin J., Morshed M., Armién A.G. (2012) Otitis interna induced by *Cryptococcus neoformans* var. *grubii* in a cat. *Vet Pathol 50*:260–263.

Petersen A.D., Walker R.D., Bowman M.M. et al. (2002) Frequency of isolation and antimicrobial susceptibility patterns of *Staphylococcus intermedius* and *Pseudomonas aeruginosa* isolates from canine skin and ear samples over a 6-year period (1992–1997). *J Am Anim Hosp Assoc 38*:407–413.

Ponce F., Marchal T., Magnol J.P. et al. (2010) A morphological study of 608 cases of canine malignant lymphoma in France with a focus on comparative similarities between canine and human lymphoma morphology. *Vet Pathol 47*:414–433.

Poulet F.M., Valentine B.A., Summers B.A. (1992) A survey of epithelial odontogenic tumors and cysts in dogs and cats. *Vet Pathol 29*:369–380.

Powell M.B., Weisbroth S.H., Roth L. et al. (1980) Reaginic hypersensitivity in *Otodectes cynotis* infestation of cats and mode of feeding. *Am J Vet Res 41*:877–882.

Power H.T., Ihrke P.J. (1995) Selected feline eosinophilic skin diseases. *Vet Clin North Am Small Anim Pract 25*:833–850.

Reppas G., Fyfe J., Foster S. et al. (2013) Detection and identification of mycobacteria in fixed stained smears and formalin-fixed paraffin-embedded tissues using PCR. *J Small Anim Pract 54*:638–646.

Rivas A.K., Alcover M., Martínez-Orellana P. et al. (2018) Clinical and diagnostic aspects of feline cutaneous leishmaniosis in Venezuela. *Parasit Vectors 11*:141–155.

Rogers K.S. (1988) Tumors of the ear canal. *Vet Clin North Am Small Anim Pract 18*:859–868.

Rosychuk R.A.W. (1994) Management of otitis externa. *Vet Clin North Am Small Anim Pract 24*:921–952.

Roth L. (1990) Rhabdomyoma of the ear pinna in four cats. *J Comp Pathol 103*:237–240.

Sabattini S., Bettini G. (2010) Prognostic value of histologic and immunohistochemical features in feline cutaneous mast cell tumors. *Vet Pathol 47*:643–653.

Santoro D., Prisco M., Ciaramella P. (2008) Cutaneous sterile granulomas/pyogranulomas, leishmaniasis and mycobacterial infections. *J Small Anim Pract 49*:552–561.

Schuldenfrei M.D., Lam A.T.H., Outerbridge C.A. et al. (2023) Evaluation of aural masses submitted as inflammatory polyps in 20 dogs (2000–2020). *Vet Dermatol 34*:77–86.

Scott D.W., Anderson W.I. (1990) Canine sebaceous gland tumors: A retrospective analysis of 172 cases. *Canine Pract 15*:19–27.

Smedley R.C., Spangler W.L., Esplin D.G. et al. (2011) Prognostic markers for canine melanocytic neoplasms: A comparative review of the literature and goals for future investigation. *Vet Pathol 48*:54–72.

Smith R.I.E. (1973) Canine skin tuberculosis. *Rhodesian Vet J 3*:63–64.

Sprague W., Thrall M.A. (2001) Recurrent skin mass from the digit of a dog. *Vet Clin Pathol 30*:189–192.

Stern-Bertholtz W., Sjostrom L., Hakanson N.W. (2003) Primary secretory otitis media in the cavalier King Charles spaniel: A review of 61 cases. *J Small Anim Pract 44*:253–256.

Stockhaus C., Teske E., Rudolph R. et al. (2001) Assessment of cytological criteria for diagnosing basal cell tumours in the dog and cat. *J Small Anim Pract 42*:582–586.

Sula M.J.M. (2012) Tumors and tumorlike lesions of dog and cat ears. *Vet Clin North Am Small Anim Pract 42*:1161–1178.

Sula M.M., Njaa B.L., Payton M.E. (2014) Histologic characterization of the cat middle ear: In sickness and in health. *Vet Pathol 51*:951–967.

Tater K.C., Scott D.W., Miller W.H. Jr et al. (2003) The cytology of the external ear canal in the normal dog and cat. *J Vet Med 50*:370–374.

Taylor D.O.N., Dorn C.R., Luis O.H. (1969) Morphologic and biologic characteristics of the canine cutaneous histiocytoma. *Cancer Res 29*:83–92.

Tolbert K., Brown H.M., Rakich P.M. et al. (2009) Dermoid cysts presenting as enlarged thyroid glands in a cat. *J Feline Med Surg 11*:717–719.

Toma S., Cornegliani L., Persico P. et al. (2006) Comparison of 4 fixation and staining methods for the cytologic evaluation of ear canals with clinical evidence of ceruminous otitis externa. *Vet Clin Pathol 35*:194–198.

Trainor K.E., Porter B.F., Logan K.S. et al. (2010) Eight cases of feline cutaneous leishmaniasis in Texas. *Vet Pathol 47*:1076–1081.

Twomey L.N., Wuerz J.A., Alleman A.R. (2005) A 'down under' lesion on the muzzle of a dog. *Vet Clin Pathol 34*:161–163.

Veir J.K., Lappin M.R., Foley J.E. et al. (2002) Feline inflammatory polyps: Historical, clinical, and PCR findings for feline calici virus and feline herpes virus-1 in 28 cases. *J Feline Med Surg 4*:195–199.

Videmont E., Pin D. (2010) Proliferative and necrotising otitis in a kitten: First demonstration of T-cell-mediated apoptosis. *J Small Anim Pract 51*:599–603.

Weinstein N.M., Boes K.M., Mauldin E. et al. (2016) What is your diagnosis? Middle ear material from a dog. *Vet Clin Pathol 45*:195–196.

Weisbroth S.H., Powell M.B., Roth L. et al. (1974) Immunopathology of naturally occuring otodectic otoacariasis in the domestic cat. *J Am Vet Med Assoc 165*:1088–1093.

Yoshida N., Naito F., Fukata T. (2002) Studies of certain factors affecting the microenvironment and microflora of the external ear of the dog in health and disease. *J Vet Med Sci 64*:1145–1147.

CHAPTER 19

BONE MARROW ASPIRATION AND BIOPSY

Emmeline Tan and Dorothee Bienzle

INDICATIONS

Bone marrow examination has a central role in the diagnosis of hematologic and infectious conditions, and for detecting and staging potentially metastatic neoplasms. Ideally, both marrow aspiration cytology and core (trephine) biopsy should be performed; the former facilitates detailed cell morphology assessment, differential cell counting, and identification of infectious agents, while the latter enables determination of overall cellularity, hemosiderin stores, and tissue architecture. Any abnormal complete blood cell count (CBC) finding that cannot be explained by extramedullary causes is a primary indication for marrow evaluation. Specific examples of CBC abnormalities that should prompt marrow examination include persistent and unexplained cytopenia (non-regenerative anemia, neutropenia, or thrombocytopenia); dysplasia in one or several cell lines (Figure 19.1); inappropriate or persistent rubricytosis (Figure 19.2); ovalocytosis (Figure 19.3); and the presence of blasts or other atypical cells in circulation (Figures 19.4, 19.5). Assessment of marrow to investigate possible lytic lesions or metastatic neoplasms constitutes a secondary indication. Marrow aspiration and biopsy are relatively invasive procedures and, therefore, indications should be clearly established. Marrow samples should be interpreted in light of the history, physical examination, concurrent CBC findings, and results of ancillary diagnostic assays such as serum biochemistry, infectious disease serology, and imaging.

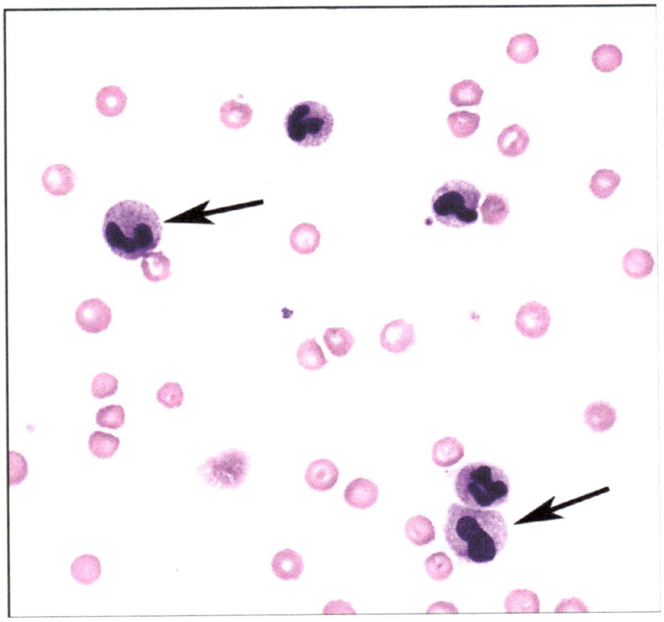

Figure 19.1 Blood smear from a dog with neutropenia, non-regenerative anemia, and neutrophil dysplasia. Note large hyposegmented neutrophils with condensed chromatin (arrows), 600× magnification.

CONTRAINDICATIONS

There are no absolute contraindications for marrow aspiration and biopsy; however, relative contraindications, such as those pertaining to patient tolerance of general anesthesia or sedation, may exist. Thrombocytopenia is of limited concern as a contraindication for the procedure since hemorrhage into the confined marrow space is usually self-limiting; however, soft tissue trauma during access to bone should be carefully minimized in animals with thrombocytopenia or coagulopathy. In humans, non-major bleeding occurred in 0.19% of marrow biopsies, and was linked to thrombocytopenia rather than

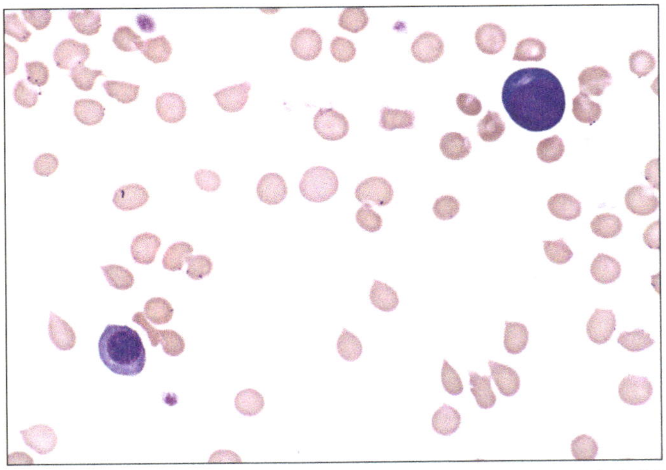

Figure 19.2 Blood smear from a dog with persistent neutropenia (0.5–0.9 × 10^9/L), anemia (hematocrit 0.20–0.29 L/L), thrombocytopenia (45–62 × 10^9/L), low-grade rubricytosis, and atypical cells, 600× magnification. Clinical assessment failed to reveal infection or inflammation, and a diagnosis of chronic neutrophilic leukemia was established.

DOI: 10.1201/9781003258551-19

anticoagulant therapy (Moore & Kotchekov, 2021). Reduced immune competency due to neutropenia warrants additional precaution to reduce potential bacterial exposure, but in most animals with persistent neutropenia, assessment of marrow is an essential component of establishing a diagnosis. The risk of bone fracture is considered low and should be minimized by the use of biopsy needles that are proportional to the size of the patient, and consideration of potential preexisting bone structural abnormalities such as osteoporosis.

SAMPLE COLLECTION

The flat bones (skull, vertebrae, sternebrae, pelvis, ribs) and the proximal part (metaphysis) of the long bones retain active hematopoiesis throughout life and are therefore suited for obtaining representative samples. The most aspirated sites in dogs and cats are the proximal humerus, the sternum, the iliac crest, and the trochanteric fossa of the femur (Figure 19.6). Due to the challenge of correct needle placement in awake and mobile animals, especially smaller dogs and cats, patients are typically sedated or anesthetized unless they have a very placid nature or are critically ill, in which case light or no sedation with local anesthesia may suffice. Historically, aspirates of the manubrium of the sternum were avoided in dogs and cats due to the perceived risk of penetrating the thoracic cavity. However, the sternum is commonly aspirated in humans because of limited overlying soft tissue compared to other sites, the thinner nature of the sternal cortical bone, and because hematopoiesis remains active at this site throughout adulthood (Tomasian & Jennings, 2022). For similar reasons, the sternum is also favored by some clinicians in dogs and cats as a site for aspiration and has yielded samples that are of comparable cellularity

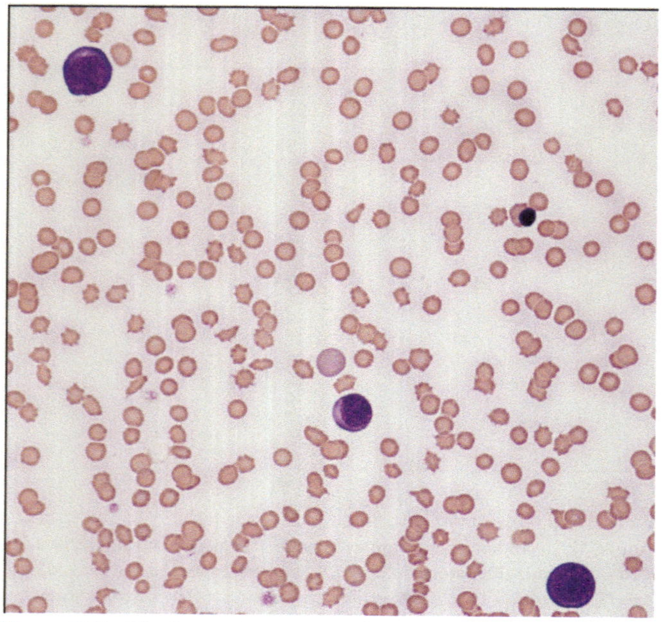

Figure 19.3 **Blood smear from a cat with rubricytosis, 400× magnification.**

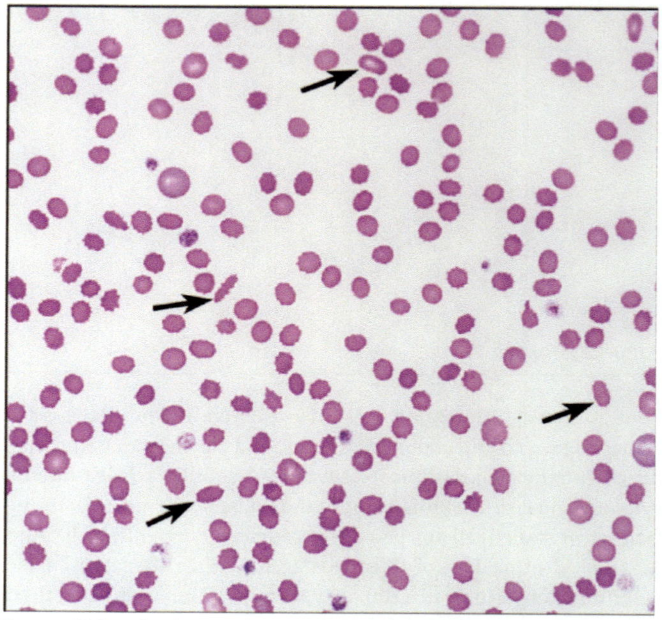

Figure 19.4 **Blood smear from a dog with non-regenerative anemia characterized by ovalocytosis and acanthocytosis (arrows), 400× magnification.**

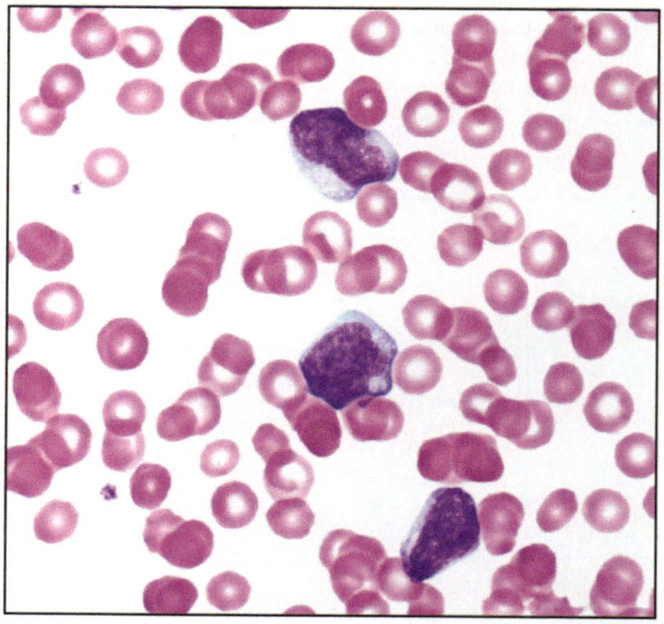

Figure 19.5 **Blood smear from a dog with anemia, thrombocytopenia, and blasts, 1,000× magnification.**

to those from the iliac crest and humerus (Defarges *et al.*, 2013). The sternum is not suitable for core biopsy.

Obtaining good quality marrow samples requires sterile procedure and appropriate equipment. The skin is aseptically prepared, local anesthetic is infiltrated into the skin, subcutaneous tissue, and periosteum, and a small skin incision is made. Sternal aspirates can be collected with a regular 20-gauge hypodermic needle due to the thin

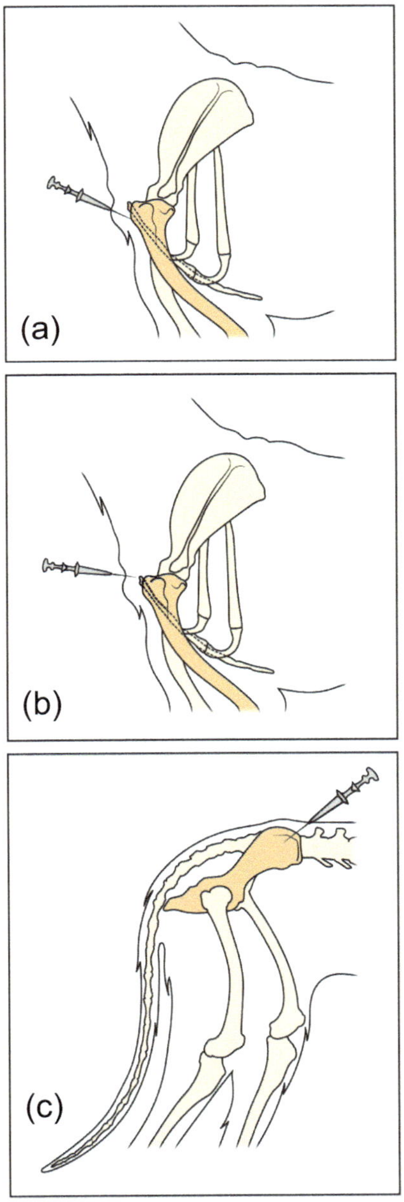

Figure 19.6 **Sites for marrow aspiration include proximal humerus (a); manubrium of sternum (b); and iliac crest (c).**

cortex of this bone. This can be very helpful in critically ill patients not suited for general anesthesia, or in obese patients where other sites are difficult to precisely locate. Penetrating the sternal marrow cavity with a hypodermic needle requires much less force than penetration of the cortex of pelvic, humeral, or femoral bone. Typically, only 0.1 to 0.3 mL of sternal marrow can be aspirated but that is sufficient for preparing multiple slides. To aspirate marrow from other sites, special needles of hardened steel (e.g. Rosenthal needles) with a stylet that occludes the lumen during bone penetration are required. Such needles must be sharp, the stylet must be precisely aligned with the shaft of the needle, and considerable force is needed to gradually advance the needle with forth-and-back rotation through the bone cortex. Single-use needles are popular because they are consistently sharp and do not require re-sterilization, but their use is more costly. Multi-use needles can be sharpened and autoclaved for multiple aspirations. Once the needle is seated firmly in bone, the stylet is removed, and a 6 or 12 mL syringe containing a few drops of 1% ethylenediaminetetraacetic acid (EDTA) is tightly attached. Vigorous aspiration with the syringe creates negative pressure that disrupts sinusoids and dislodges cells in the marrow cavity to yield gradually appearing, thick bloody fluid in the syringe. Generally, 0.2 to 0.5 mL of marrow in the syringe is sufficient for at least 5 smears, and the remaining fluid may be placed in EDTA-containing tubes for automated hematology analysis, flow cytometry, and/or PCR. Aspirating greater volumes of marrow induces progressively more hemorrhage from disrupted sinusoids, and is not recommended due to dilution of marrow cells. Marrow can be aspirated without EDTA in syringes if the operator is experienced, the samples are obtained quickly, and slides are prepared rapidly before the sample clots.

For core biopsy, a longer and wider needle suitable for cutting a core of marrow containing trabecular bone with interspersed hematopoietic and adipose tissue is required (e.g. 11-, 13-, or 15-gauge Jamshidi needle). Marrow core biopsy should be performed prior to or at a different site than marrow aspiration to avoid areas with hematopoietic architecture disrupted from aspiration. The skin at the chosen site is aseptically prepared and infiltrated with local anesthetic as for aspiration, a stab incision is made, and the core biopsy needle with stylet in place is 'drilled' into the cortex using steady pressure with forth-and-back rotation at approximately a right angle to the site of bone penetration. Once the needle is seated firmly in the cortical bone, the stylet is removed, and the 'empty' needle is advanced for 2 to 3 cm to cut out a cylindrical core of marrow tissue. Penetration of the distant cortical bone by the needle without the stylet in place is very difficult; therefore, there is little danger from advancing the empty needle for 3 to 4 cm in the marrow cavity of a medium-size dog. Next, it is attempted to break off the distal part of the cylindrical core by rotation and slight lateral movements of the needle. Once it is thought that a core has been captured in the lumen, the needle is gradually retracted from the bone. The core itself is recovered from the lumen of the needle by gentle retrograde propulsion with a blunt wire, which is supplied with the core biopsy needle. The needle itself is tapered toward the tip to facilitate retention of the core; therefore, pushing the core out forward would crush the tissue. Further details on marrow collection techniques are available elsewhere (Bienzle, 2012, Abrams-Ogg *et al.*, 2012, Defarges *et al.*, 2013).

SLIDE PREPARATION

Slides should be prepared immediately after sample collection. A drop of marrow is expelled onto one end of a slide, the slide is tilted to let blood run off onto absorbent paper (marrow particles will adhere to the glass slide), and then a second slide is backed into the remaining marrow drop and pulled forward at approximately a 45° angle, analogous to preparing a feather-edge blood film. In addition to preparing feather-edge type blood films where marrow particles are maintained aggregated, several 'squash' type of films should also be prepared by gently dropping a second slide perpendicular to the first slide on the drop of marrow remaining after blood has run off, and pulling that slide forward. In this type of smear, particles are spread apart to facilitate individual cell recognition (Figure 19.7). Two to three of each type of smear should be prepared and rapidly air-dried, either with the aid of a small fan or by vigorously waving slides in the air. Removing blood prior to preparing smears concentrates hematopoietic elements and hastens slide drying, thereby improving cell preservation. It is difficult to impossible to prepare good films from clotted samples though clots may be fixed in formalin for subsequent paraffin embedding and sectioning.

Alternatively to immediate film preparation, aspirated marrow can be placed in a glass or Petri dish that is then tilted to separate the pale yellowish marrow particles from blood. Particles are then retrieved using a pipette, microhematocrit tube, or hypodermic needle, placed on a slide, and films are prepared as above. Aspirated marrow remaining in the syringe should be placed in a 3 mL EDTA tube and submitted along with the slides in case additional slides need to be prepared or special tests are anticipated. Normal marrow aspirates have cell concentrations >50,000/μL; therefore, even a small volume of marrow can yield abundant cells for flow cytometry, immunochemistry, or assessment by PCR (Tan *et al.*, 2014a).

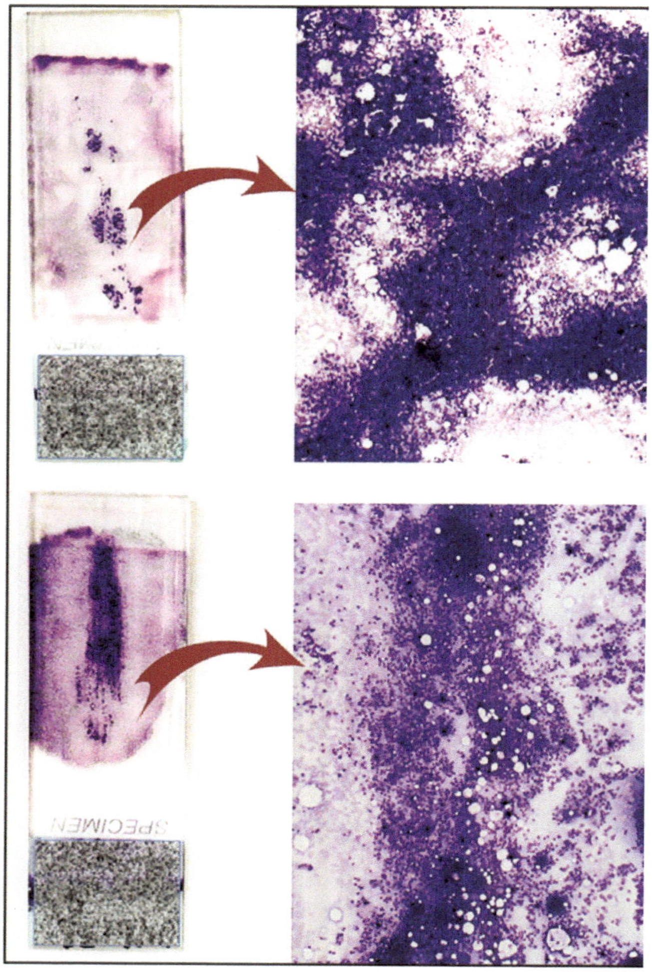

Figure 19.7 **Marrow aspirate films with poorly spread dense particles (top) and well-spread particles (bottom). Images on right at 50× magnification.**

If there is doubt about the quality of the marrow aspirate, or particles are not grossly visible, it is advisable to stain one slide with a quick-type Romanowsky stain (e.g. Dip Quick®, Jorvet) before recovering the patient from general anesthesia. A good quality marrow film should have grossly apparent granular material and cell-dense areas admixed with blood (Figure 19.8). Microscopically, there should be abundant particles and hematopoietic cells. If slides are not cellular, aspiration should be repeated. Unsuccessful aspiration or poorly cellular samples are not necessarily a result of poor technique but are more likely to reflect marrow diseases such as myelofibrosis, myelophthisis, or aplastic anemia (Donald & Kakkar, 2021). In these cases, marrow core biopsy is required for diagnosis.

Whole anti-coagulated marrow can be assessed in automated hematology analyzers if grossly visible clots are first manually removed (for example with wooden applicator sticks). Analysis of nucleated cells by size and peroxidase content in instruments such as the Advia 2120 (Siemens) or by light scatter and fluorescence in the Sysmex XT2000iV yields rapid information about sample cellularity, cell types, reticulocyte concentration, and cell distribution (Figure 19.9, Tan *et al.*, 2014a; Criswell *et al.*, 2018; Pernecker *et al.*, 2017).

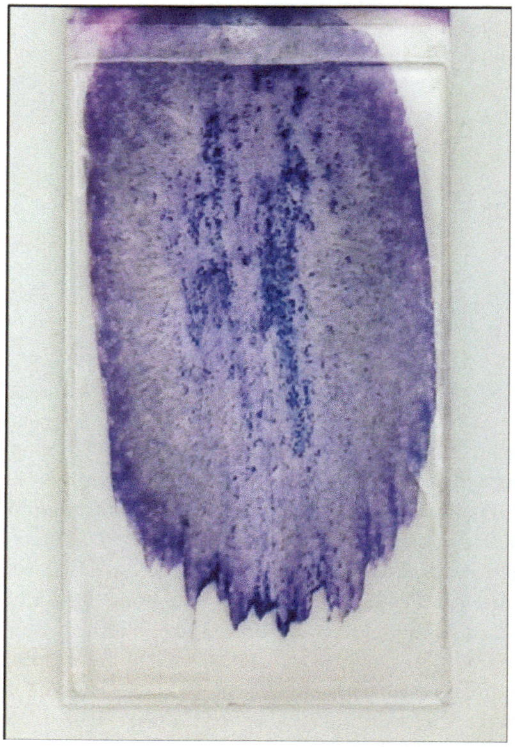

Figure 19.8 **Example of well-prepared BM aspirate smear, showing darker purple BM particles surrounded by blood.**

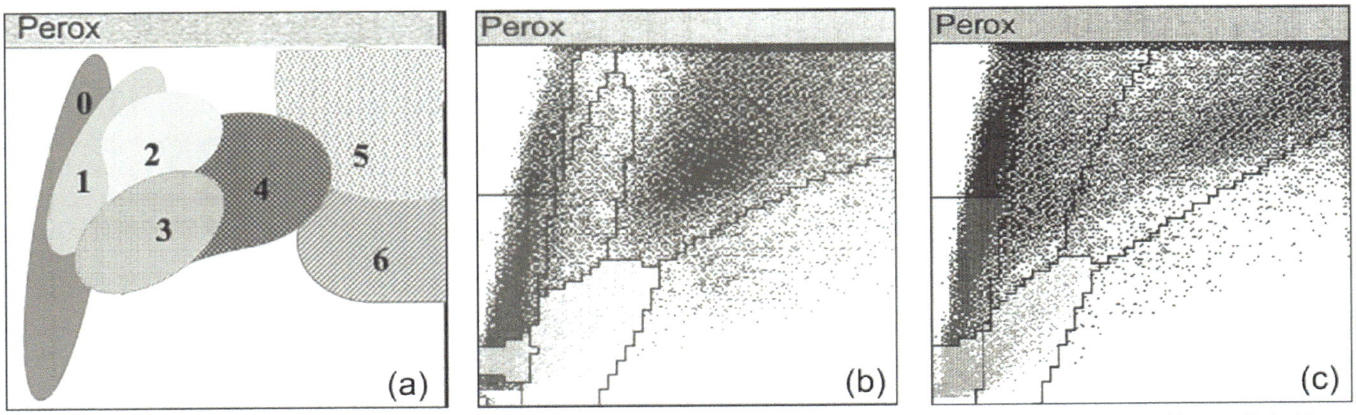

Figures 19.9a–c Analysis of marrow aspirates in the automated hematology analyzer Advia 2120 yields differential cell estimates. (a) 0 = Cells lacking peroxidase activity are lymphocytes and large unstained cells (LUC); 1 and 2 = large cells with low peroxidase activity are immature granulocytic cells; 3 = medium-size cells with low to moderate peroxidase activity are monocytic cells; 4 = medium-size cells with moderate to high peroxidase activity are likely metamyelocytes; 5 = large cells with high peroxidase activity are likely band neutrophils; 6 = medium-size cells with high peroxidase activity are likely segmented neutrophils. (b) Granulocytic hyperplasia with numerous mature granulocytes. (c) Acute myeloid leukemia with partial neutrophil differentiation.

CORE BIOPSY PROCESSING

Core biopsies may be collected first from the same site used subsequently for aspiration, or from a different site. Once the core has been extruded retrogradely from the needle lumen, it should be handled gently to avoid introducing artifact. The length of a fresh core should be at least 1.5 cm in cats and small dogs, and 2–3 cm in medium to large dogs, to yield an adequate sample prior to formalin fixation, which induces ~10% tissue shrinkage. Cores from normal marrow are reddish (Figure 19.10 [top]), and those from fibrotic or leukemic marrow are typically whitish. Histologically, good quality biopsy sections should contain at least 3 inter-trabecular spaces free of artifact; therefore, larger cores are likely of better diagnostic quality since they contain a greater number of inter-trabecular spaces (Abrams-Ogg *et al.*, 2012).

Biopsy sections of marrow allow determination of cellularity, cell density and adequacy of iron stores, and identification of fibrosis, lymphoid aggregates, megakaryocyte clustering, metastatic tumors, and other focal lesions. Myelofibrosis is rarely identified in marrow aspirates since samples from fibrotic marrow are typically poorly cellular, and the extent of fibrosis cannot be determined without core biopsy. Individual hematopoietic cell identification is more challenging on hematoxylin and eosin (H&E) stained sections than on cytology preparations. Marrow cellularity is a measure of the ratio of hematopoietic to adipose tissue, and correlates with hematopoietic activity. While marrow adipose tissue morphologically appears relatively homogeneous, differential responsiveness to metabolic hormones, reciprocal effects on bone density, interaction with marrow stromal cells, and regulation of hematopoiesis have recently been recognized (Li & MacDougald, 2021b). Neonates normally have marrow cellularity exceeding 90%, and with progressive age this percentage decreases to approximately 10% in healthy geriatric animals (Travlos, 2006). Increased cellularity or hyperplasia is usually a response to increased peripheral cell demand because of the shortened lifespan of blood cells (e.g. immune-mediated anemia) or chronic inflammation (e.g. pyoderma). Decreased cellularity or atrophy (often inaccurately called 'hypoplasia') results from toxic, autoimmune, infectious, drug-mediated, or other injury to hematopoietic precursor cells.

When submitting both aspirate cytology and core biopsy samples, it is essential to keep cytology slides separated from formalin jars. Exposure of cytology slides to formalin fumes alters or obliterates subsequent staining and severely reduces their diagnostic utility (Figure 19.11).

CYTOLOGICAL FEATURES OF HEALTHY MARROW

Diagnostic examination of marrow films is performed in a systematic fashion noting the cellularity and quality of the preparation, number of particles, relative proportion and morphology of each cell type, presence of iron stores (dogs), metastatic or other non-hematopoietic cells, and infectious agents. Particle cellularity is determined on 'feather-edge' type smears, and corresponds well to overall cellularity in biopsy sections (Riley *et al.*, 2009). Differential nucleated cell counts (minimally 500 cells) should be performed as a quantitative and objective means of evaluation, and should reflect multiple slides and areas since cell composition can vary focally. Summary statistics for hematopoietic cells in healthy dogs and cats have been published (Mischke & Busse, 2002, Tan *et al.*, 2014a) and reflect the normally pyramidal cell maturation of homeostatic hematopoiesis. Maturing post-mitotic granulocytes and late stage rubricytes predominate, with fewer immature cells and relatively few blasts (Table 19.1). The granulocytic-to-erythrocytic cell ratio (G:E) is more accurately determined from differential cell counts rather than estimates. The G:E is sometimes referred to as the myeloid-to-erythroid (M:E) cell ratio; however, since 'myeloid' refers to all marrow cells that are descended from common precursors and have plasticity in morphological features, the term 'G:E' is more precise and preferred by the authors. The

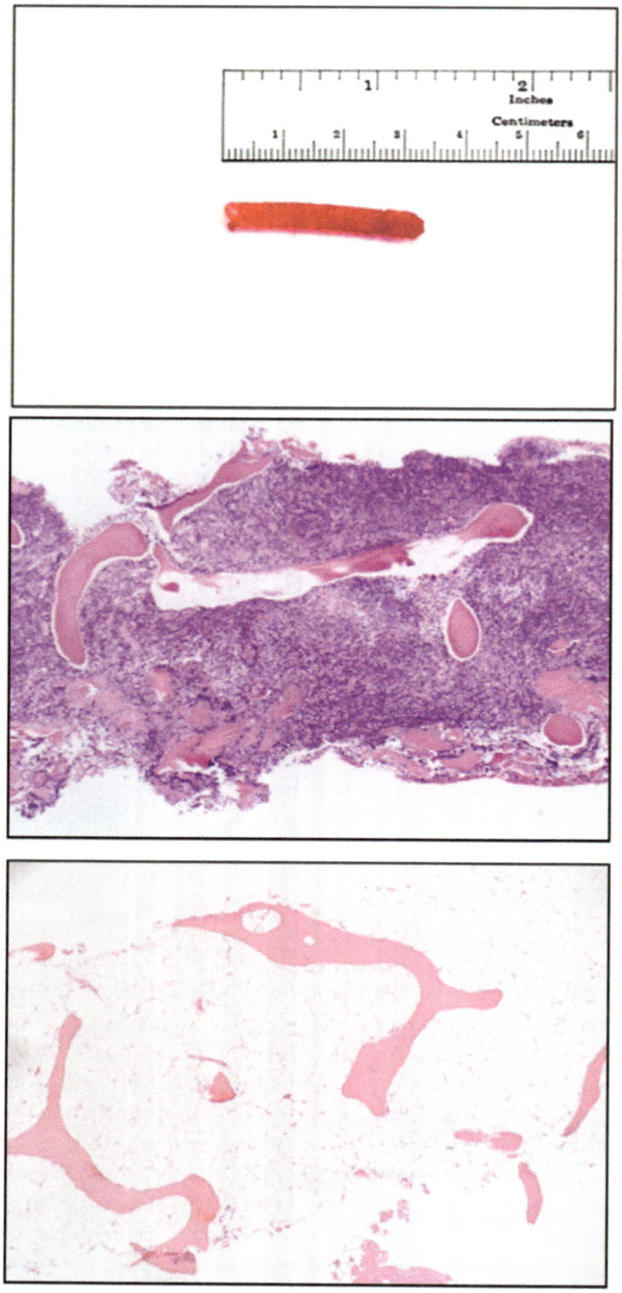

Figure 19.10 **(top) A good quality marrow core should be reddish and at least 2 cm in length. (middle) Hypercellular marrow from adult dog with non-regenerative immune-mediated anemia. The sample is >95% cellular, with little to no visible fat. (bottom) Hypocellular marrow from a dog with severe hematopoietic atrophy. Cellularity is <5%. Magnification 50×.**

G:E for healthy dogs and cats ranges from ~0.8 to 2.0. An increased G:E cell suggests granulocytic hyperplasia and/or erythrocytic atrophy, while a decreased G:E suggests granulocytic atrophy or erythrocytic hyperplasia.

GRANULOCYTIC CELLS

In health, a segmented neutrophil derives from a myeloblast in 6 to 7 days. This time may be reduced during intense demand for neutrophils such as acute inflammation. The earliest recognizable granulocytic precursor is the *myeloblast*, which is a large round cell with a round central nucleus and high nuclear to cytoplasmic (N:C) ratio (Figure 19.12). Nuclear chromatin is finely stippled with a single nucleolus or several nucleoli. As the myeloblast differentiates, magenta-stained primary granules become apparent in the cytoplasm. *Promyelocytes* (progranulocytes) have primary granules, lower N:C, and nucleoli are no longer visible. In *myelocytes*, primary granules are no longer noticeable, secondary granules appear that characterize the type of granulocyte differentiation (neutrophil, eosinophil, or basophil), and nuclei are smaller with more condensed chromatin. Cells are mitotically active during these three stages, which together comprise the granulocyte mitotic pool.

Nuclear indentation is first detectable in *metamyelocytes* that initially have a slightly reniform nuclear shape, and then progressively more indentation leading to band-shaped nuclei. Metamyelocytes no longer divide. *Band* granulocytes have horseshoe- or S-shaped nuclei; if indentation in any area of the nucleus exceeds 2/3 diameter of any other area of the nucleus, the cell is classified as a *segmented* granulocyte. Metamyelocytes, band, and segmented granulocytes comprise the maturing post-mitotic component of granulocytic cells. With progressive maturation, chromatin becomes increasingly condensed and clumped. Segmented neutrophils have pale pink (dogs) or faint blue to blue–gray cytoplasm (cats), while mature segmented eosinophils and basophils are recognizable by their respective prominent secondary granules. Post-mitotic cells represent the majority of granulocytic cells in normal marrow, and typically the mitotic-to-post-mitotic cell ratio is ~1:4 to 1:8 in dogs and cats. The more mature granulocytes (bands and segmented neutrophils) can be released from the marrow at times of need, and are known as the 'marrow granulocyte reserve' (MGR). The release of metamyelocytes and more immature forms reflects increased severity of demand for peripheral granulocytes or disturbed homeostatic granulopoiesis. The MGR represents approximately 3 to 5 days of neutrophil supply.

ERYTHROCYTIC CELLS

The earliest recognizable erythrocyte precursor is the *rubriblast*. This is a large, round cell with a high N:C and a round nucleus surrounded by a rim of deeply basophilic cytoplasm (Figure 19.13). Nuclear chromatin is stippled and nucleoli, usually single but sometimes multiple, are prominent. Rubriblasts are distinct from myeloblasts by their darker blue cytoplasm and slightly smaller size, but in dense cell preparations with less-than-optimal cell spreading and drying, it can be challenging to differentiate rubriblasts from myeloblasts. *Prorubricytes* are slightly smaller, with inconspicuous nucleoli and more clumped chromatin. As rubricytes mature, there is a gradual reduction in cell size, decrease in N:C, and progressive nuclear

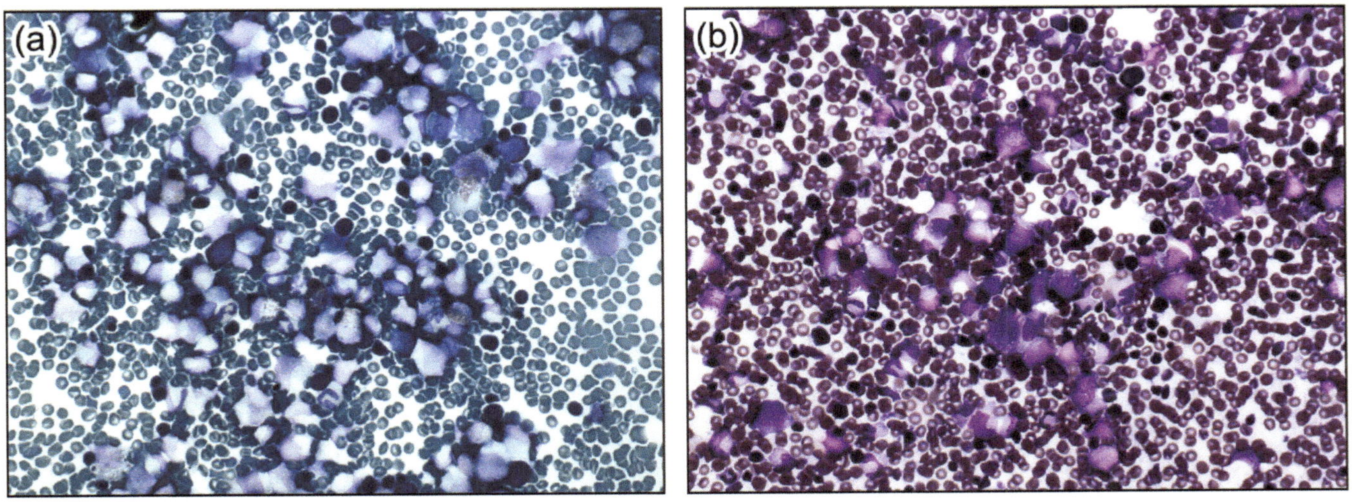

Figure 19.11 Formalin fume exposure alters Romanowsky-type staining properties of cells. (a) Marrow smear stained after shipment in a sealed plastic bag with a jar of formalin. (b) Smear from the same sample shipped separate from formalin jar. Both images 600× magnification.

Table 19.1 **Differential cell counts in bone marrow aspirate smears of healthy dogs and cats**

Cell type	Dogs; n = 92, mean % ± SD[A]	Dogs; n = 43, mean % ± SD[B]	Cats; n = 7, mean % ± SD[C]
Neutrophil segmenter	3.32 ± 1.85	13.59 ± 4.3	12.86 ± 4.85
Neutrophil band	26.1 ± 5.82	11.31 ± 2.87	14.1 ± 1.30
Neutrophil metamyelocyte	5.80 ± 1.71	7.65 ± 2.46	10.06 ± 3.20
Neutrophil myelocyte	2.76 ± 0.98	5.64 ± 2.15	4.31 ± 2.49
Promyelocyte	2.27 ± 0.99	3.23 ± 1.40[d]	1.74 ± 1.04
Myeloblast	0.11 ± 0.14		0.08 ± 0.16
Eosinophil segmenter	0.20 ± 0.22	1.95 ± 0.88[e]	0.6 ± 0.20
Eosinophil band	1.30 ± 0.97		0.49 ± 0.40
Eosinophil metamyelocyte	0.85 ± 0.62		0.54 ± 0.39
Eosinophil myelocyte	0.57 ± 0.47		0.60 ± 0.42
Rubriblasts and prorubricytes	4.43 ± 1.23	2.48 ± 1.06	1.17
Early rubricytes	5.06 ± 2.66	23.05 ± 5.48[f]	4.02[g]
Late rubricytes	26.0 ± 6.20		
Metarubricytes	9.53 ± 3.63	21.90 ± 5.67	17.57
Monoblasts/promonocytes	0.37 ± 0.34	1.02 ± 0.55	NR
Macrophages	0.22 ± 0.24	NR	NR
Plasma cells	2.98 ± 1.65	1.46 ± 1.01	0.8
Lymphocytes	6.39 ± 3.75	4.38 ± 1.76	16.13
Basophils	0 ± 0.01	NR	0.4
Megakaryocytes	0.13 ± 0.13	20.07 ± 11.39[g]	NR
G:E ratio	1.08 ± 0.61	0.89 ± 0.28	1.63 ± 0.35

[a] Mischke & Busse, 2002.
[b] Tan et al., 2014.
[c] Jain, 1993.
[d] Promyelocytes and myeloblasts enumerated together.
[e] Enumerated together as 'eosinophils and precursors'.
[f] Enumerated together as 'rubricytes'.
[g] Per non-contiguous 100× magnification field.
NR = not reported.

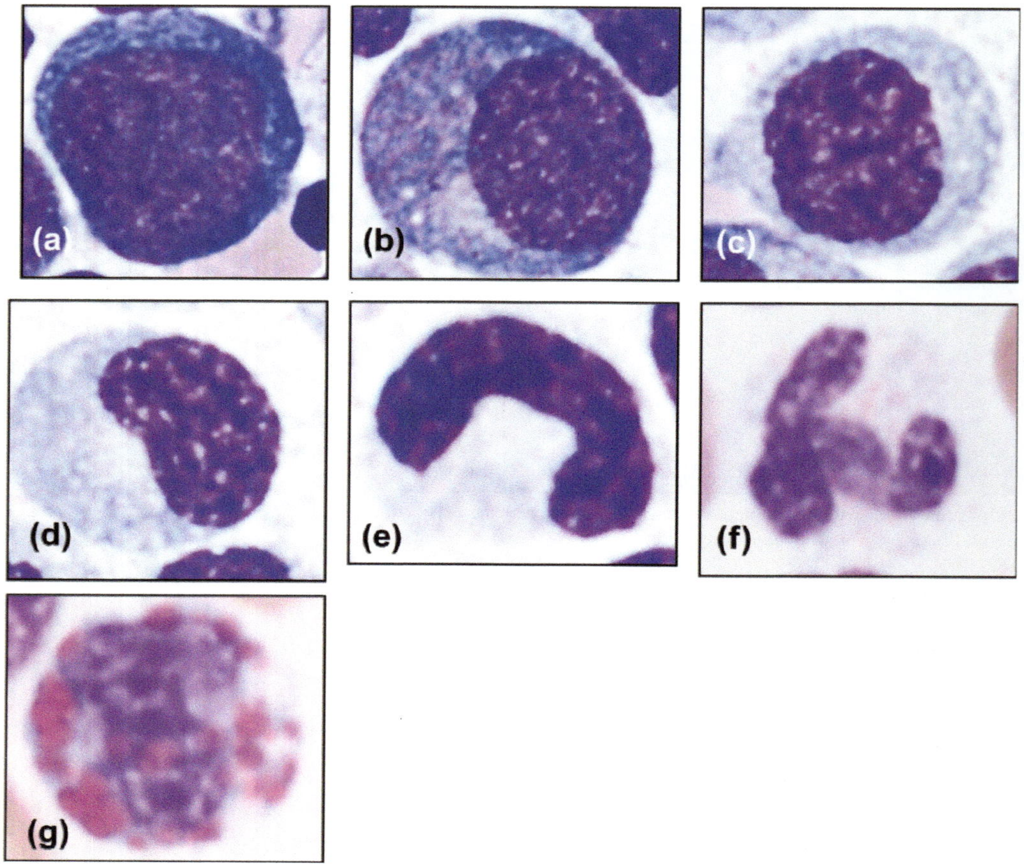

Figure 19.12 The granulocytic cell mitotic pool is comprised of (a) myeloblast, (b) promyelocyte, and (c) myelocyte. The post-mitotic pool is comprised of (d) metamyelocyte, (e) band neutrophil, and (f) segmented neutrophil. Eosinophilic (g) precursors are recognized by the appearance of characteristic secondary granules. Approximately 2,000× magnification.

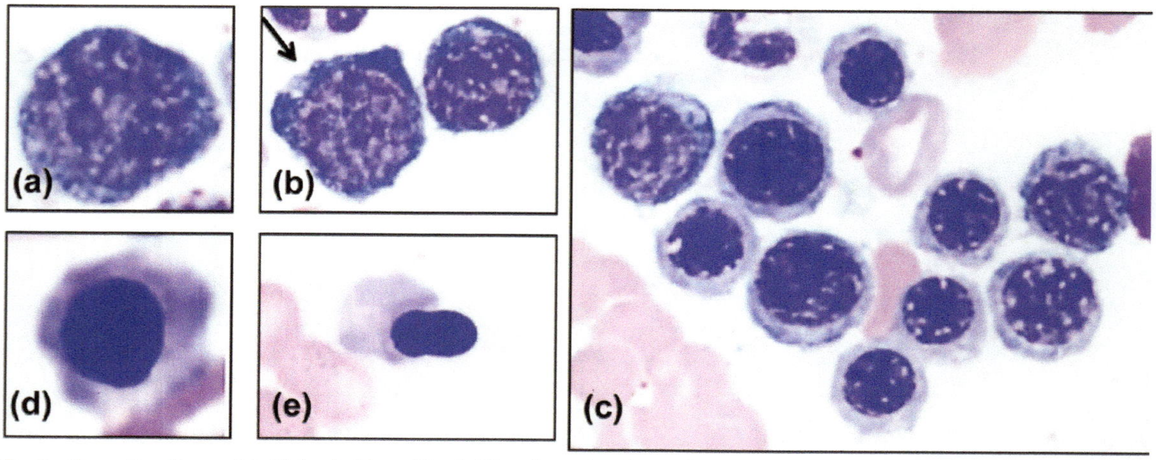

Figure 19.13 Erythrocytic cells consist of (a) rubriblast, (b) rubriblast (arrow) and prorubricyte, (c) rubricytes of various stages, (d) metarubricyte, and (e) metarubricyte in the process of nuclear extrusion. Magnification 1,000–1,500×.

condensation with a concurrent increase in cytoplasmic hemoglobin content. *Rubricytes* are divided into basophilic and polychromatophilic depending on the degree of hemoglobinization. The last nucleated stage is the *metarubricyte*, which contains a pyknotic nucleus and light orange-pink (polychromatophilic) cytoplasm. Mitosis no longer occurs at this stage. The nucleus of metarubricytes is extruded immediately prior to traverse of the marrow sinusoids and release into circulation as *polychromatophilic erythrocytes* (reticulocytes). At this stage, most organelles have disappeared, but hemoglobin synthesis continues until transition into mature erythrocytes. Consistent identification of individual rubricyte maturational stages can be challenging since cells evolve gradually; hence the authors favor classification of rubricytes during differential cell counting into four stages: rubriblast/prorubricyte, early rubricyte, late rubricyte, and metarubricyte (Table 19.1).

In vivo, erythropoiesis occurs extra-sinusoidally within specific erythropoietic niches that provide both negative and positive regulatory signals for cell proliferation and differentiation. Microscopically, these so-called erythroblastic islands comprise a central macrophage ('nurse cell') surrounded by 4 to 30 erythroid precursors of various stages (Li *et al.*, 2021a). Erythroblastic islands are occasionally observed in normal marrow films (Figure 19.14).

MEGAKARYOCYTES

The maturing megakaryocyte undergoes several rounds of nuclear endomitosis and endoduplication, resulting in progressively larger cells with greater cytoplasmic volume and increasingly lobulated nuclei. Mature megakaryocyte nuclei are composed of individual round lobules that remain connected to each other. With progressive age, megakaryocyte nuclear lobules condense and become folded. In general, megakaryocytes with large nuclei and a small amount of cytoplasm have replicative ability, while those with abundant cytoplasm give rise to platelets and no longer divide. Cytoplasmic maturation involves the production of granules that are imparted to platelets when they are released as cytoplasmic fragments. Granules impart a progressively pinker and stippled appearance to the cytoplasm of mature megakaryocytes. Mature megakaryocytes are very large (50–200 μm) and polyploid (up to 128N ploidy) and are best enumerated at low magnification (Figure 19.15). In animals without hematological disease, 3 to 8 megakaryocytes per particle are typical.

OTHER CELLS

Monocytic cells comprise a very low percentage of nucleated cells in marrow. The earliest recognizable form is the *monoblast*, which has an oval to slightly indented nucleus surrounded by a scant amount of dark blue cytoplasm. The N:C of monoblasts is generally lower than that of myeloblasts. *Promonocytes* have indented to irregular-shaped nuclei, gray-blue cytoplasm devoid of granules, and possibly a few cytoplasmic small vacuoles. *Monocytes* in marrow aspirates have horseshoe- or butterfly-shaped nuclei and light gray-blue cytoplasm that may contain a few small vacuoles, similar to monocytes in blood.

Plasma cells and small lymphocytes are morphologically similar as in other tissues and comprise a small percentage of cells in the marrow of dogs (Table 19.1). In healthy young cats, lymphocytes can make up ~15–20% of marrow nucleated cells, but this proportion decreases with progressive age. Macrophages containing metarubricyte nuclei and hemosiderin are regularly observed in marrow films, and rare individual mast cells may also be present.

IRON

With Romanowsky-type stains, hemosiderin appears as brown-black to gray-black aggregates in macrophages or extracellularly in the thick areas of marrow granules (Figure 19.16). Hemosiderin may also be noted as more dispersed finely granular green-brown pigment in individual macrophages. Prussian blue stain is useful to highlight iron in cytology or histology preparations. In humans, absence of stainable iron is only confidently reported when at least seven marrow particles in a sample lack stainable iron, which often requires evaluation of more than one slide (Chauffaille *et al.*, 2019). Iron stores may be better assessed in marrow biopsy sections since they contain more hematopoietic cells than aspirates but decalcification can also reduce stainable iron (Riley *et al.*, 2009). Lack of coarse iron in marrow may be associated with but is not necessarily indicative of iron

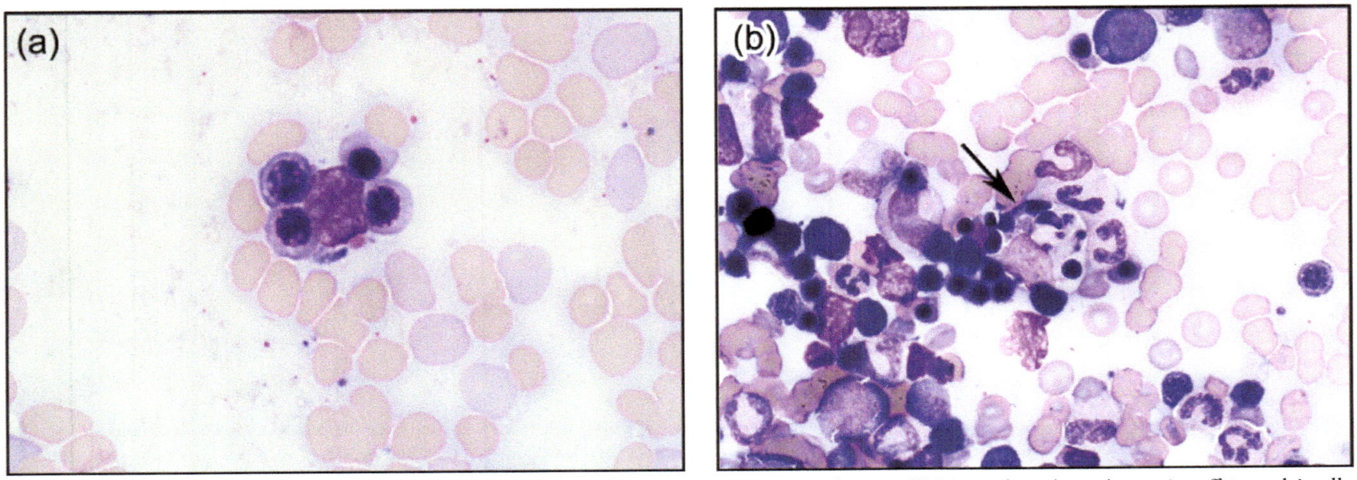

Figures 19.14 **(a) Erythroblastic island with central macrophage ('nurse cell'), 1,000× magnification. (b) Macrophage (arrow) contains effete nuclei, cell debris, and heme pigments, and is surrounded by rubricytes, 600× magnification.**

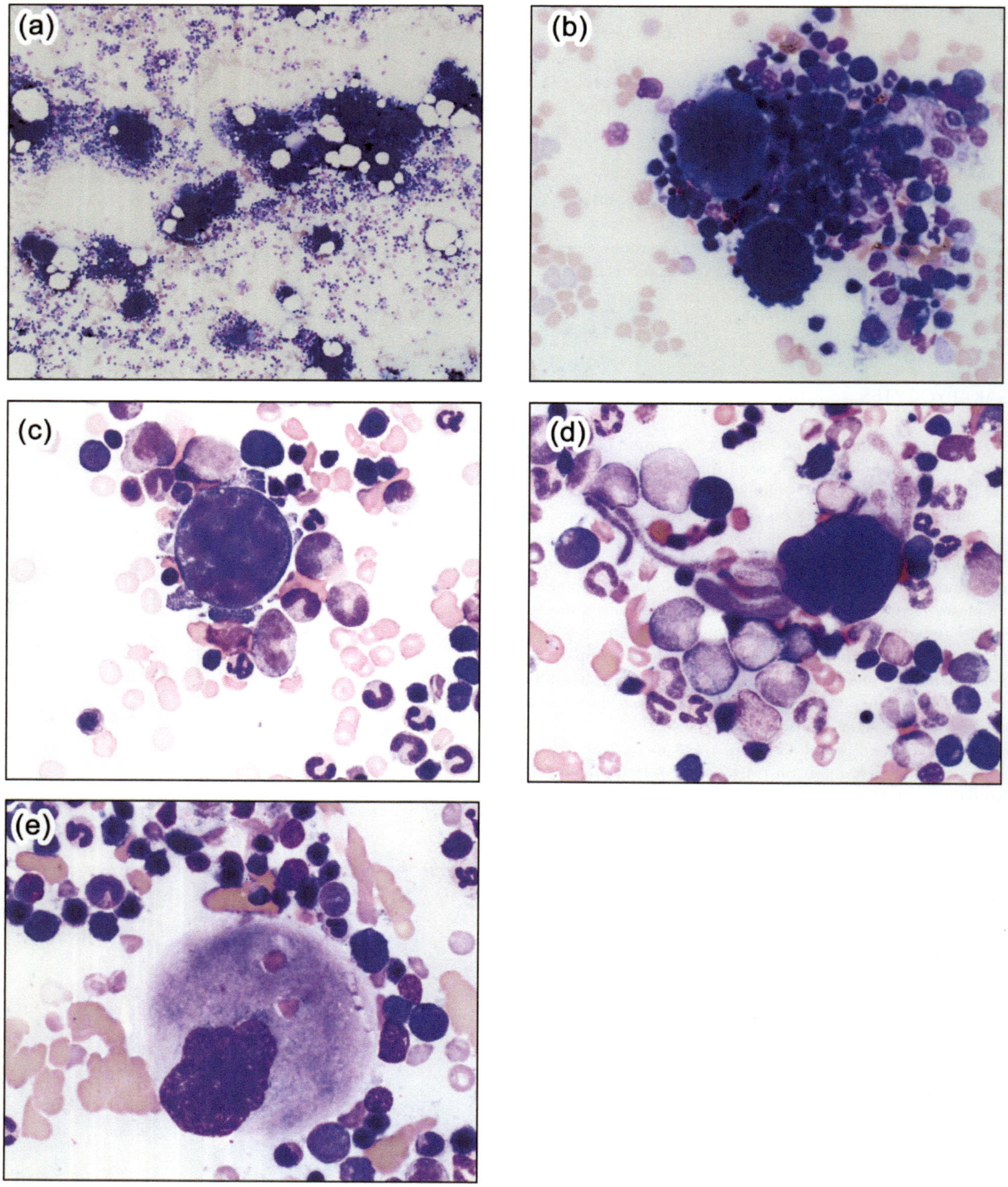

Figures 19.15 (a) Megakaryocytes are best enumerated at low magnification. This sample is from a dog with megakaryocytic hyperplasia and immune-mediated thrombocytopenia, 100× magnification. (b) Immature megakaryocytes have large nuclei and a moderate amount of cytoplasm, 200× magnification. (c) Megakaryocyte in endomitosis, 400× magnification. (d) Release of elongated proplatelets from the megakaryocyte, 400× magnification. (e) Mature megakaryocyte with condensed and fused nuclear lobes and abundant pink granular cytoplasm, 400× magnification.

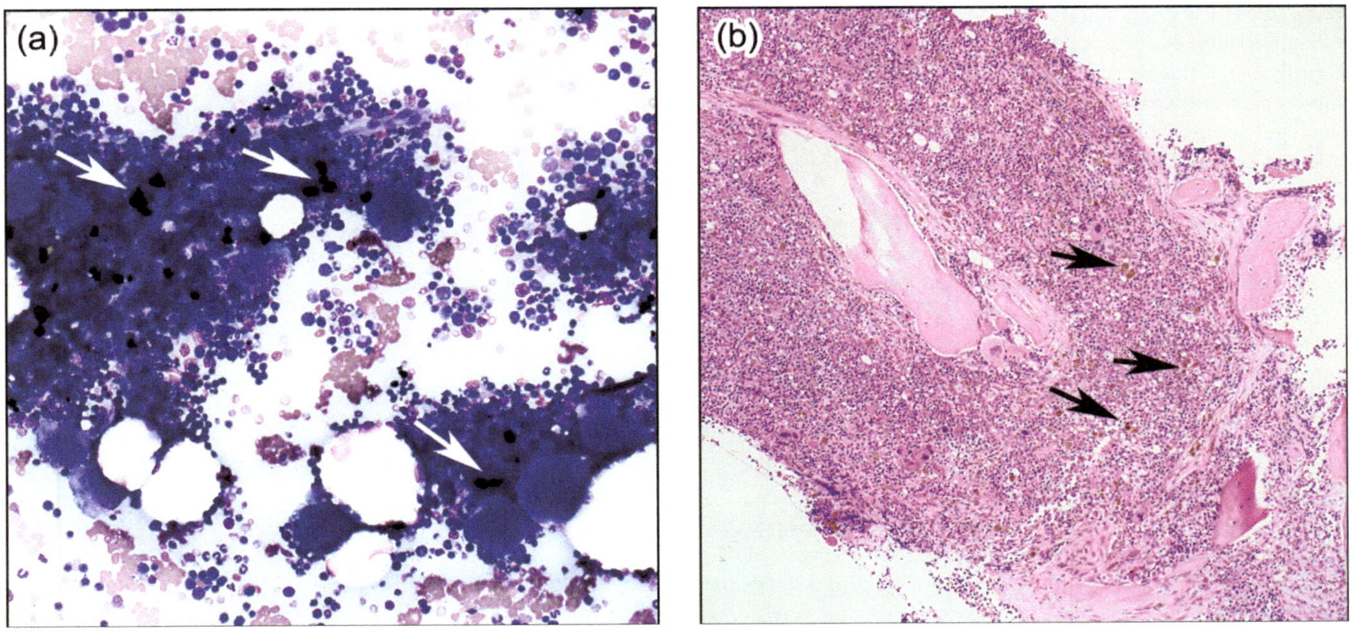

Figures 19.16a, b Iron (arrows) appears dark black on Wright stain (a) and brown-gold on H&E stained sections (b), both at 100 magnification.

deficiency anemia in humans and dogs (Barron *et al.*, 2001; Thomason & Almiski, 2009; Pawsat *et al.*, 2023). A scoring system for iron in canine marrow aspirates has been reported with scores for stainable iron correlating well with other parameters of iron availability such as reticulocyte hemoglobin content (Pawsat *et al.*, 2023). Iron is normally absent in feline marrow.

Iron deficiency should be suspected from CBC indicators such as hypochromic reticulocytes, hypochromic microcytic or normocytic erythrocytes, increased erythrocyte fragmentation, and anemia, and should be confirmed by measurement of serum iron and ferritin concentration, iron binding capacity, and low iron scores on marrow slides. Decreases in erythrocyte volume and development of anemia occur relatively late in iron deficiency.

HEMATOPOIETIC ABNORMALITIES

Erythroid hyperplasia

Erythroid hyperplasia (Figure 19.17) results from up-regulated erythropoiesis and is characterized by normal or increased marrow cellularity with a relative or absolute increase in erythroid cells, reduced G:E, and increased reticulocyte concentration in peripheral blood. It is most commonly a response to increased demand for erythrocytes, such as in immune- or toxin-mediated hemolytic anemia, blood loss, or chronic hypoxia. An increase in blood reticulocytes occurred within 48 hours and lasted 12–14 days in humans given a single injection of erythropoietin (Pérez-Ruixo *et al.*, 2008). Similarly, in rats one erythropoietin injection caused an increase in early rubricytes by 24 hours, late rubricytes at 72 hours, and peripheral blood reticulocytosis at 72–96 hours (Xu *et al.*, 2022). These time frames correspond to those observed in dogs and cats where marrow erythroid hyperplasia is not evident until at least 48 hours after onset of anemia due to hemorrhage. The magnitude and timing of the erythropoietic response to anemia depend on the body condition of the animal, the abundance of iron and other nutrients, the severity and rapidity of onset of anemia, whether blood loss is external or internal, and the presence of concurrent illness. Regenerative anemias, such those typically associated with immune-mediated hemolytic anemia (IMHA) or blood loss in

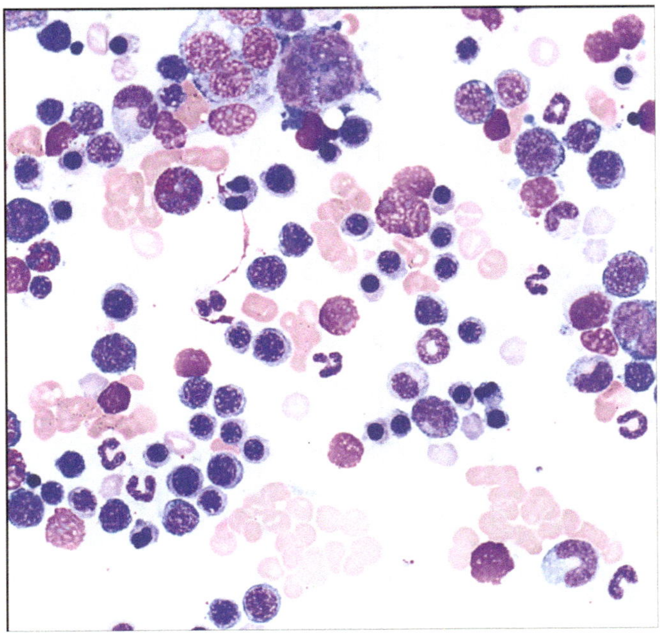

Figure 19.17 Erythrocytic hyperplasia in a dog with blood loss anemia, 400× magnification.

young animals, are not indications for marrow evaluation since there is usually evidence of an appropriate response on the CBC. The cause of anemia in such cases can be diagnosed from a thorough history, blood smear evaluation (e.g. spherocytes), or imaging (e.g. splenic hemangiosarcoma).

Erythropoiesis may be hyperplastic but nevertheless ineffective, as indicated by lack of blood reticulocytosis and persistence of anemia. Hyperplastic but ineffective erythropoiesis may occur with severe iron deficiency, immune destruction of rubricytes, myelodysplasia, cobalamin deficiency, and other conditions (Lutz *et al.*, 2013). Erythroid hyperplasia may also be accompanied by '*incomplete maturation*' where there is an abundance of early and late rubricytes, and there may be metarubricytes, but a paucity of reticulocytes (Figure 19.18).

Erythroid atrophy

Erythroid atrophy is characterized by normal to decreased marrow cellularity with a relative or absolute reduction in erythroid cells. As a result, in most cases the G:E is increased, and if animals have erythroid atrophy concurrent with inflammation and granulocytic hyperplasia, the G:E cell ratio may be extremely high (Figure 19.19). Causes of erythroid atrophy include chronic kidney disease, other chronic illness, systemic viral infection, erythroid precursor cell injury, myelodysplasia, myeloid neoplasia (Figure 19.20), and in rare cases antibodies to erythropoietin, usually subsequent to treatment with recombinant erythropoietin. Erythroid atrophy results in non-regenerative or poorly regenerative anemia.

Non-regenerative immune-mediated anemia (NRIMA) and precursor-targeted immune-mediated anemia (PIMA) are conditions with overlapping diagnostic features (Lucidi *et al.*, 2021; Woolhead *et al.*, 2021). An immune-mediated etiology is suggested by increased immunoglobulin or phosphatidylserine detection on marrow rubricytes, though validated diagnostic tests with high specificity to confirm this pathogenesis remain elusive. In dogs with severe non- or poorly regenerative anemia, a lack of peripheral blood spherocytosis and hemolysis, and increased frequency of rubricyte phagocytosis by marrow macrophages, NRIMA/PIMA should be suspected. Immune dysregulation secondary to thymoma has also been associated with erythroid atrophy and marrow pan-atrophy. These findings support immune mechanisms contributing

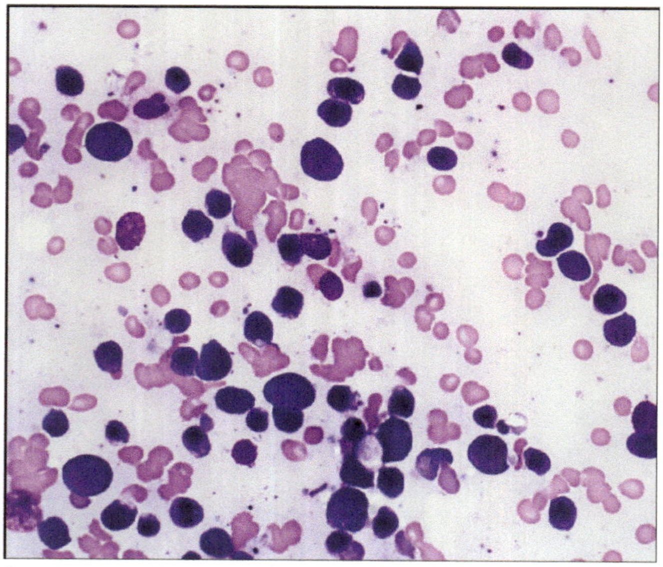

Figure 19.18 Erythrocytic hyperplasia with incomplete maturation in a dog, 400× magnification. There is a relative paucity of polychromatic cells despite a large number of rubricytes.

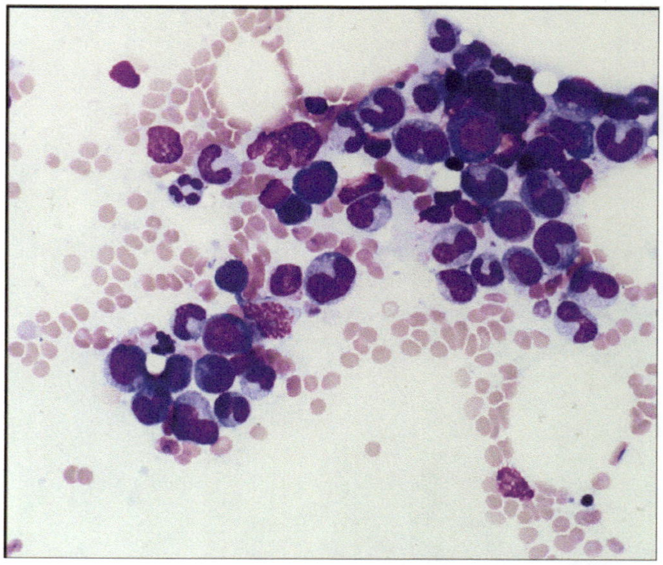

Figure 19.19 Granulocytic hyperplasia and erythrocytic atrophy in a dog with chronic inflammation, 400× magnification.

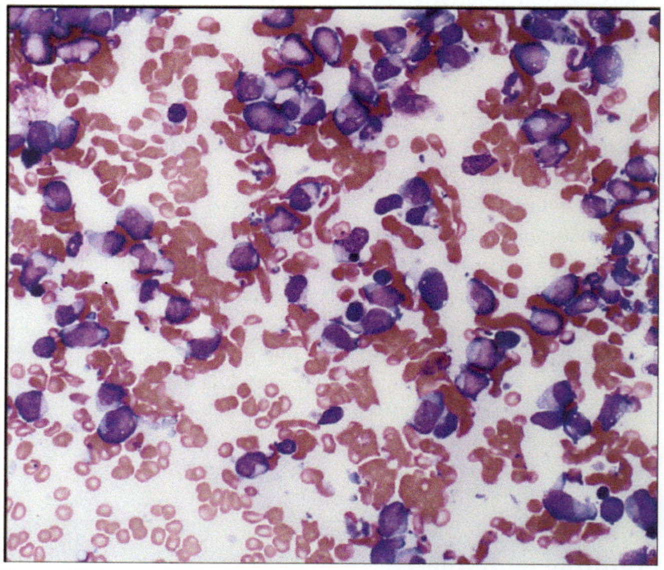

Figure 19.20 Marrow smear from a dog with acute myeloid leukemia (WBC 185 × 10^9/L, 400× magnification. There is lack of maturation to band and segmented neutrophils, and a paucity of rubricytes.

to some cases of erythroid atrophy. Animals that recover from erythroid atrophy have a transient shift toward early rubricytes prior to re-establishment of orderly and complete maturation. Persistent erythroid atrophy and anemia in conjunction with dysplastic features in hematopoietic cells should prompt consideration of myelodysplastic syndrome (MDS).

Immune-mediated cytopenia (IMC) in cats manifests with anemia and frequently also with neutropenia or thrombocytopenia. There may be erythrocyte and/or leukocyte and/or platelet agglutination on blood smears (Figure 19.21). Marrow findings are similarly diverse, and hyperplasia, atrophy, and dysplasia with or without myelofibrosis may all occur. Blood lymphocytes are often in the high normal range or increased, and frequently also increased in marrow from cats with IMC. While T-lymphocytes typically predominate, plasma cells and B-lymphocytes are also present (Figure 19.22).

Some cats infected with feline leukemia virus (FeLV) subgroup C develop pure red cell aplasia (PRCA) characterized by profound, nonregenerative anemia with normal granulocyte and platelet concentrations. Marrow aspirates show a near complete absence of erythrocytic cells with normal granulopoiesis and megakaryopoiesis. FeLV-C binds to and impairs the function of the cell surface receptor FLVCR1, which is a heme exporter important in protecting erythroid progenitors against the toxic effects of heme (Khan & Quigley, 2013).

Dyserythropoiesis

Dyserythropoiesis is abnormal erythrocyte maturation and/or morphology. Examples include megaloblastic cells, rubricytes with abnormal nuclear shapes or multiple nuclei, premature pyknosis, and siderotic inclusions in rubricytes (Figure 19.23). Megaloblastic cells result from asynchronous DNA synthesis and cell growth yielding abnormally large cells with relatively small nuclei. Megaloblastic erythropoiesis gives rise to peripheral blood macrocytosis. In humans, megaloblastosis is most commonly due to cobalamin and/or folate deficiency from impaired absorption (chronic pancreatitis or malabsorptive disorders), dietary scarcity, lack of intrinsic factor, or a defective cubam transporter. Affected individuals typically have mild anemia and also neutrophil hypersegmentation. Anemia and neutrophil hypersegmentation but not macrocytosis were reported in dogs with intestinal cobalamin malabsorption due mutations in the *CUBN* gene (Imerslund-Gräsbeck-like syndrome) (Lutz *et al.*, 2013; Sancho *et al.*, 2021). Similar changes do not appear to occur in dogs with hypocobalaminemia or hypofolatemia secondary to intestinal disease (Stanley *et al.*, 2019).

Megaloblastic erythropoiesis is a feature of some FeLV infections, and typically manifests with macrocytosis, anemia, and other cytopenias. Macrocytosis precedes anemia, and is considered a harbinger of FeLV-associated myelodysplastic syndrome (MDS) (Hisasue *et al.*, 2009).

Peripheral blood macrocytosis and megaloblastic change in marrow occurs in some toy and miniature poodles (Canfield & Watson, 1989). Marrow abnormalities are confined to erythroid cells and include megaloblastosis, multinucleation, abnormal mitoses, occasional sideroblasts, and multiple and abnormally shaped Howell-Jolly bodies. Dogs are usually not anemic, and the condition is not associated with cobalamin or folate deficiency (Boyd & Best, 2018).

Granulocytic hyperplasia

Granulocytic hyperplasia results from increased granulopoiesis and is characterized by normal or increased marrow cellularity and an increased G:E. Granulocytic hyperplasia may be effective resulting in granulocytosis, or ineffective with granulocytopenia despite marrow hyperplasia.

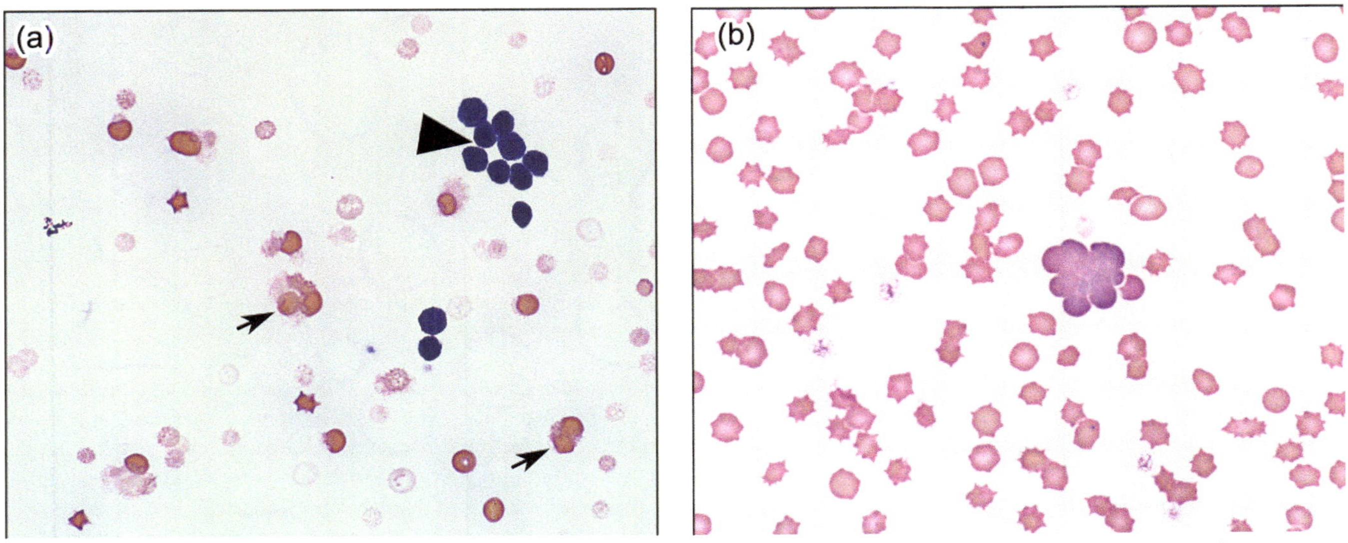

Figures 19.21a, b (a) Blood smear from a cat with anemia, neutropenia, and thrombocytopenia, 400× magnification. There was leukoagglutination (arrowhead), erythrocyte agglutination (arrow), and marked hemolysis. (b) Blood smear from a cat with anemia and neutropenia showing agglutination of polychromatophilic cells, 600× magnification.

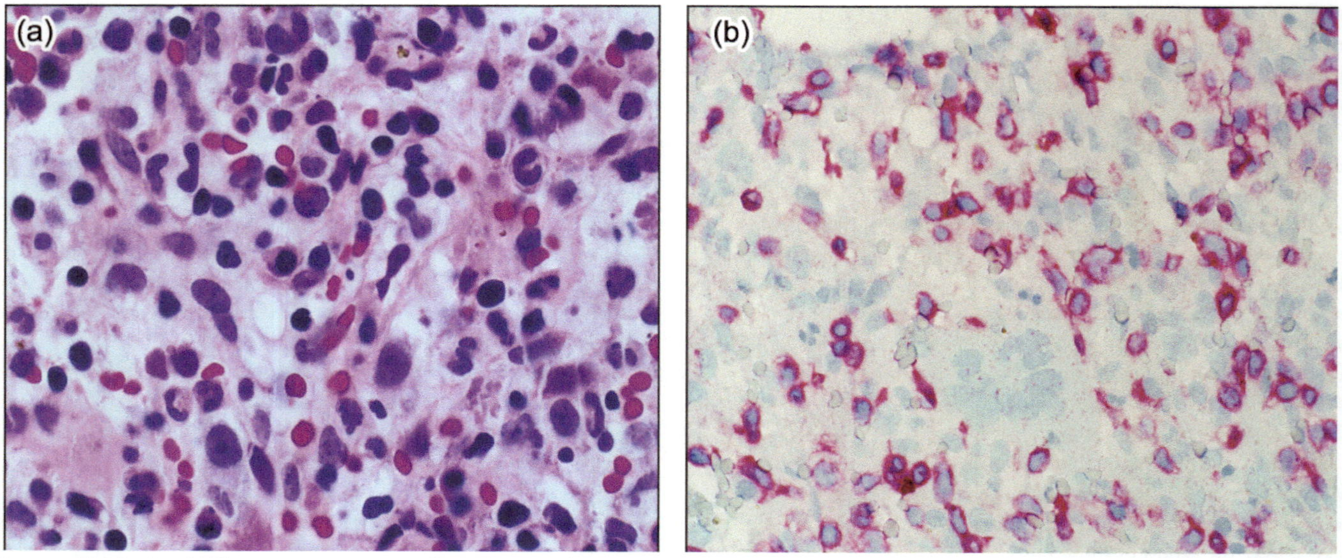

Figures 19.22a, b (a) The marrow core section from the cat with immune-mediated cytopenia in Figure 19.21a contains numerous small lymphocytes, plasma cells, and few metarubricytes, 600× magnification. (b) Immunohistochemical staining identifies lymphocytes as CD3 positive. Only rare CD79a positive lymphocytes were present (not shown), 600× magnification.

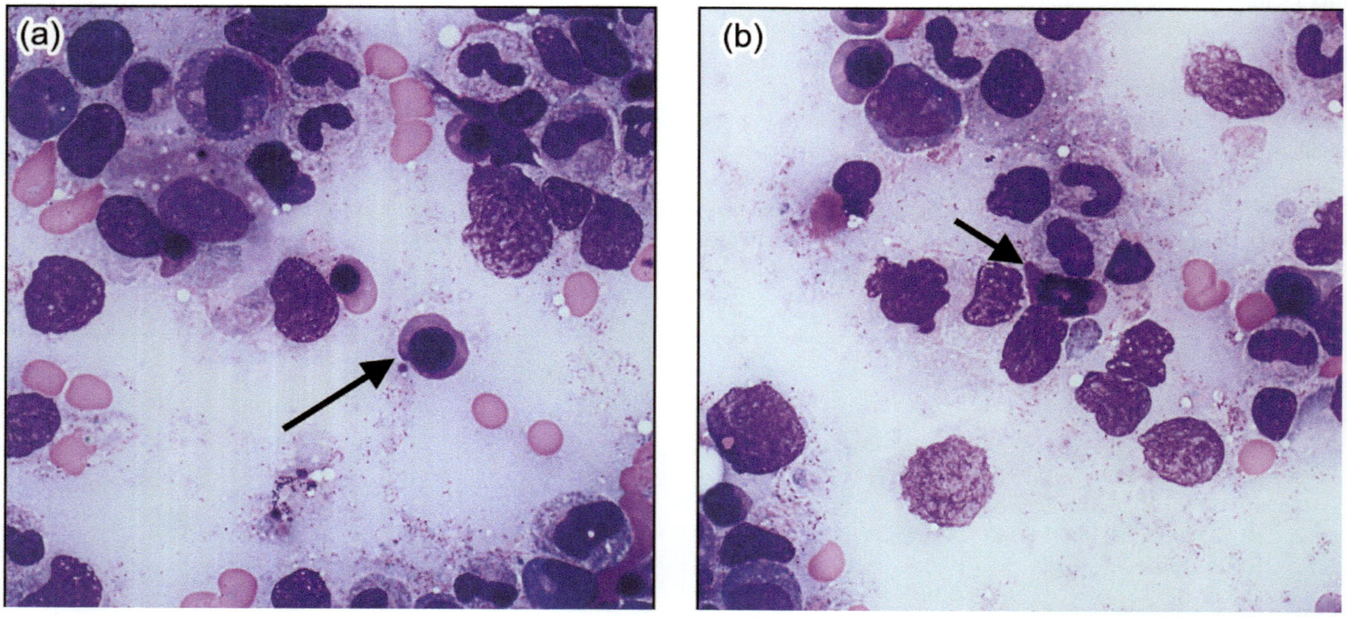

Figures 19.23a, b Marrow smear from a dog with anemia, 1,000× magnification. Rubricytes have dysplastic changes indicated by cells with fully hemoglobinized cytoplasm but large immature nuclei (a, arrow) and mitotic metarubricytes (b, arrow).

Neutrophil hyperplasia

Effective marrow neutrophil hyperplasia results from a persistently increased peripheral demand for neutrophils due to inflammation in conditions such as infection, sepsis, tissue necrosis, immune-mediated disease, and malignancy. Cytokines produced during inflammation increase neutropoiesis. Marrow neutrophils may have toxic changes in severe inflammatory disease or during recovery from marrow injury. Such changes reflect accelerated maturation with disturbed organelle formation. When tissue demand exceeds marrow storage of segmented neutrophils, band neutrophils and progressively more immature granulocytes are released, which results in a left shift in marrow granulopoiesis. If an inflammatory cause for neutrophilia is apparent, marrow evaluation is not indicated.

Ectopic production of granulocyte colony-stimulating factor (G-CSF) and/or granulocyte-macrophage colony-stimulating factor (GM-CSF) is a rare cause of neutrophilia (Petterino *et al.*, 2011). In such cases neutrophilia may be extreme (>100 × 10^9/L) and differentiation from chronic neutrophilic leukemia (CNL) is warranted. Paraneoplastic leukocytosis differs from CNL by the absence of immature circulating cells, anemia, and thrombocytopenia in the former.

Inherited neutrophil disorders that cause neutrophil hyperplasia include canine and feline leukocyte adhesion deficiency (LAD) and cyclic hematopoiesis (CH). The most common form of LAD is due to an autosomal recessive mutation in the gene that encodes CD18, part of the beta-2 integrins. Neutrophils lacking integrin expression are unable to leave the vasculature, and ensuing bacterial infection and inflammation cause massive neutrophilia and premature death (Bauer *et al.*, 2004). Most reported cases are in Irish setters though mixed breed dogs and cats can also be affected (Zimmerman *et al.*, 2013; Bauer *et al.*, 2017). Cyclic hematopoiesis occurs in collies and collie-like dogs and is due to a mutation in the gene coding for an adapter protein subunit important in the trafficking of proteins such as neutrophil elastase (Lee *et al.*, 2022). Affected dogs have 10–14-day cycles of neutropenia followed by recovery that correspond to periods of marrow neutrophilic atrophy followed by hyperplasia.

Ineffective neutrophil hyperplasia may be seen in steroid-responsive or immune-mediated neutropenia (IMN), where the marrow may be hypercellular with abundant early to band stage neutrophils but a paucity of segmented neutrophils (Perkins *et al.*, 2004). As with NRIMA/PIMA, diagnosis is based on exclusion of other causes of neutropenia and response to immunosuppressive therapy. Ineffective neutrophilic hyperplasia with dysplasia may also be a feature of MDS in dogs.

Eosinophil hyperplasia

Eosinophil hyperplasia results from a persistent demand for eosinophils in hypersensitivity or allergy, inflammation, dermatopathy (feline eosinophilic granuloma complex), parasitism, or due to paraneoplastic cytokine production. Eosinophils transit through the vasculature rapidly but have prolonged tissue survival in the presence of interleukin (IL) 5; hence blood eosinophil concentration may not reflect increased marrow eosinopoiesis. Tumor production of cytokines, in particular T-cell lymphoma, may result in eosinophil hyperplasia.

When a cause of persistent eosinophilia is not identified, primary 'hypereosinophilic syndrome' (HES) should be considered. Humans with primary HES may have mutations in growth factors like Fip1-like 1 (FI1L1) or platelet-derived growth factor receptor-α (PDGFRA), clonal T lymphocytes (without lymphoproliferative disease), and increased risk of developing acute myeloid leukemia (AML) (Klion, 2022). Genetic changes are not found in approximately 40% of humans with primary HES, and the condition is then designated 'idiopathic' HES. A higher proportion of such patients than those without HES nevertheless progress to AML. Idiopathic HES in cats (Beaumier *et al.*, 2022) and dogs (Casamian-Sorrosal *et al.*, 2020) is characterized by marrow eosinophil hyperplasia, and infiltration and injury of organs such as the heart and lung. Whether there is an underlying genetic abnormality or an increased risk of progression to myeloid neoplasia is unknown.

Granulocytic atrophy

In granulocytic atrophy the marrow is normo- or hypocellular, and erythroid cells are normal or increased, resulting in a low G:E. In all instances, granulocytic atrophy implies neutrophilic atrophy. Genetic causes of neutropenia are uncommon, and generally identified in young animals. Acquired granulocytic atrophy may be due to direct cytotoxic precursor cell injury from drugs such as doxorubicin, hydroxyurea, and vinblastine; idiosyncratic drug reactions to benzimidazole anthelmintics (fenbendazole, albendazole, and levamisole); anti-epileptic medication (phenobarbital, primidone, and phenytoin); griseofulvin, cephalosporin, sulphonamide, methimazole, carprofen, estrogenic compounds such as diethylstilbestrol; valacyclovir and chloramphenicol; and infection with parvo- and other viruses. Marrow cytologic findings are variable depending on the stage and severity of atrophy. There may be a near complete absence of granulocytic cells or there may be a predominance of early precursor cells. If myeloblasts and promyelocytes prevail over differentiated neutrophils in marrow, distinction from AML is important, and repeated CBC, and possibly repeated marrow assessment, is required. In particular, cats recovering from parvovirus infection or cytotoxic injury can have markedly left-shifted granulocytic atrophy that can be difficult to distinguish from AML.

Immune-mediated neutropenia is uncommon in dogs and may be part of IMC in cats. Complete absence of granulocytic cells is termed pure white cell aplasia (PWCA) and is thought to result from immune destruction of myelomonocytic precursor cells comparable to PRCA (Weiss & Henson, 2007). Pure white cell aplasia appears to be rare in animals and humans, and has been associated with thymoma in humans (Céspedes López *et al.*, 2022).

There are many potential causes of granulocytic atrophy. Since lack of production of neutrophils is incompatible with life, the cause of any persistent neutropenia needs to be identified. History and physical examination can rule out most infectious and drug-related causes. If marrow is found to have markedly left-shifted granulopoiesis but normal erythropoiesis and megakaryopoiesis, an early stage of recovery from injury is most likely. Serial hematological assessments are necessary to monitor recovery.

Dysgranulopoiesis

Dysgranulopoiesis refers to abnormalities in granulocyte maturation and morphology, while *dysmyelopoiesis* refers to abnormalities in any hematopoietic cell lineage. Examples of dysgranulopoiesis are giant neutrophils, abnormal nuclear shapes, abnormal segmentation, hyposegmentation, and hypersegmentation (Figure 19.24). Non-neoplastic causes of dysgranulopoiesis are drug-induced toxicity, sepsis, and cobalamin deficiency. Rapidly regenerating granulocytes may also transiently have dysplastic features. Granulocyte dysplasia is a common feature of MDS and AML, and it can be challenging to distinguish a rapidly regenerating marrow with some dysplastic features from myeloid neoplasia.

Megakaryocyte hyperplasia

Thrombopoietin (TPO) and its receptor MPL regulate megakaryopoiesis and all stages of platelet production except platelet release

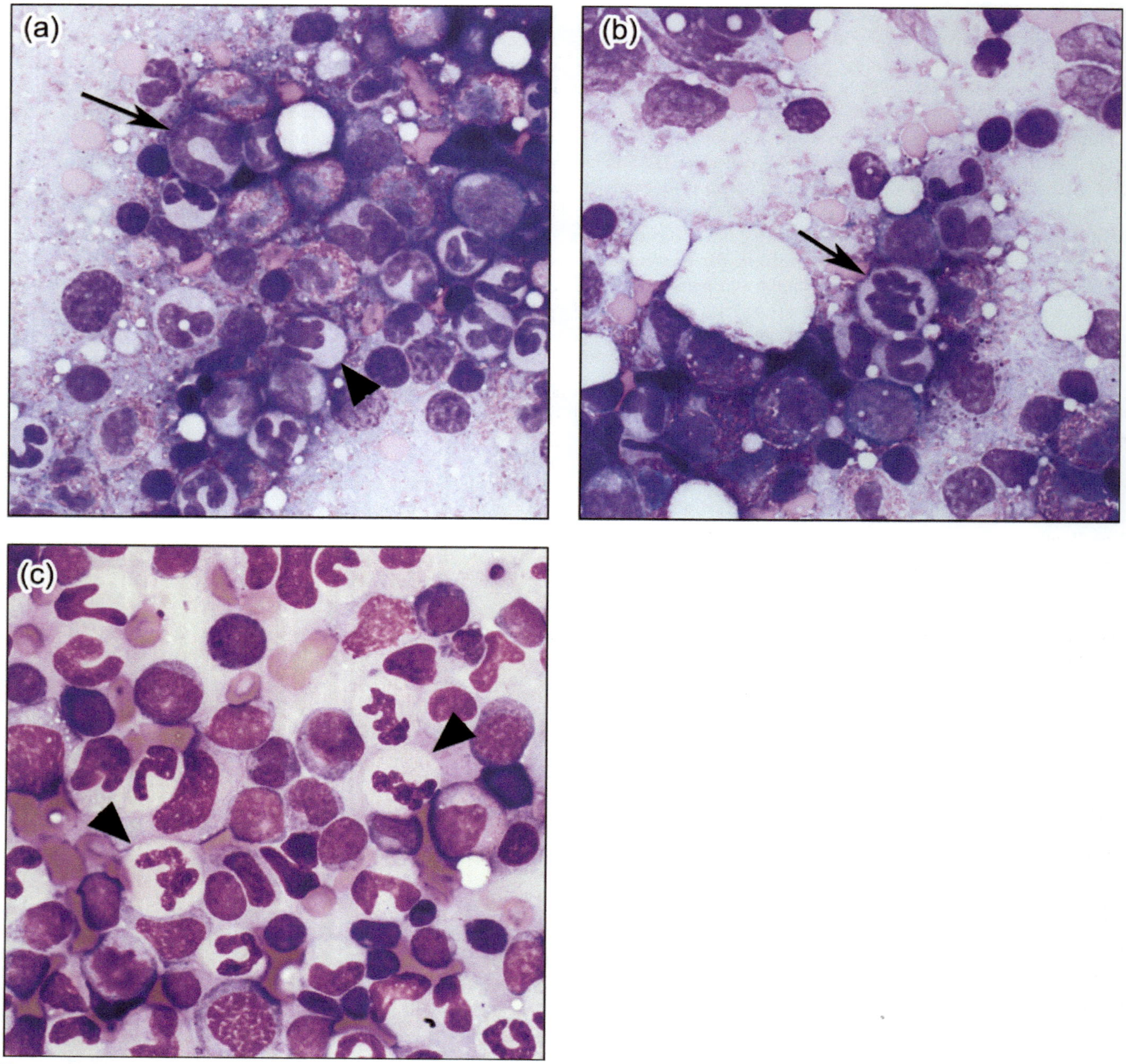

Figures 19.24a–c Marrow smears from a dog with neutropenia, 1,000× magnification. There is dysgranulopoiesis as indicated by (a) giant metamyelocytes (arrow) and hypersegmented neutrophils (arrowhead); (b) mitotic neutrophils with fully granular cytoplasm (arrow), and (c) abnormally segmented neutrophils.

(Hitchcock *et al.*, 2021). Serum concentration of TPO is inversely proportional to platelet mass; thus conditions with increased destruction or consumption of platelets cause megakaryocytic hyperplasia. In many instances, megakaryocyte hyperplasia is left shifted, and immature megakaryocytes with a high nuclear to cytoplasmic ratio predominate (Figure 19.25). In immune-mediated thrombocytopenia (ITP) platelet lifespan is severely shortened, and a competent marrow responds with massive megakaryocyte hyperplasia. Chronic intravascular coagulation, vasculitis, and early stages of rickettsial infection (e.g. *Ehrlichia canis*) can also induce megakaryocyte hyperplasia. However, as noted above, marrow aspiration is not indicated when a cause of cytopenia has been identified or is strongly suspected (Gunduz *et al.*, 2014).

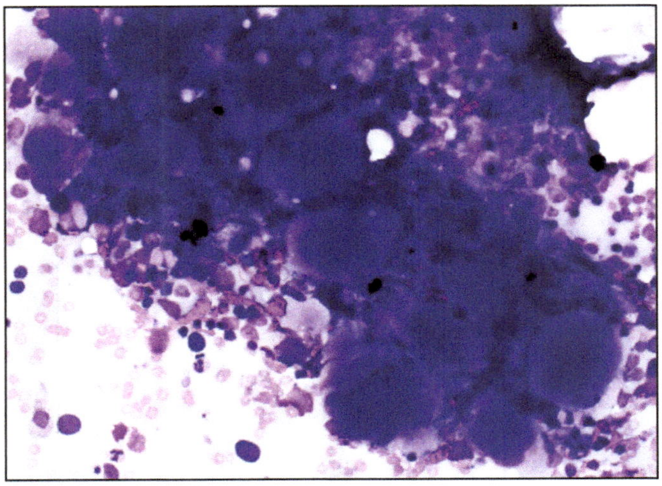

Figure 19.25 Marked megakaryocytic hyperplasia in a dog with immune-mediated thrombocytopenia, 200× magnification.

Megakaryocyte hyperplasia can result in thrombocytosis in chronic inflammatory disorders and iron deficiency. The effect of iron deficiency on megakaryocyte development appears to be independent of TPO but the exact mechanism is not clearly defined (Evstatiev *et al.*, 2014). Tumors can also induce thrombocytosis, and carcinomas were most commonly associated with thrombocytosis in dogs (Cheney *et al.*, 2022; Neel *et al.*, 2012). Megakaryocyte hyperplasia is a common feature of MDS, and is the predominant abnormality in essential thrombocythemia (ET), a myeloproliferative neoplasm.

Megakaryocyte atrophy

Relative to other hematopoietic cells, megakaryocytes occur at low frequency in marrow. Therefore, it may be difficult to appreciate megakaryocyte atrophy in poorly cellular marrow aspirates or those lacking particles. Accurate enumeration of megakaryocytes is therefore better performed on histological sections than cytology films (Travlos, 2006). Presumed immune-mediated megakaryocyte atrophy has been reported in a few dogs (Lachowicz *et al.*, 2004).

Dysmegakaryopoiesis

Micro-megakaryocytes, megakaryocyte hypo- or hyper-lobulation, anisokaryosis, and nuclear separation signify dysmegakaryopoiesis (Figure 19.26). Dysmegakaryopoiesis may accompany accelerated platelet production such as in immune-mediated thrombocytopenia and is often the most prominent feature of MDS. Due to their large size, megakaryocytes may not flatten well on cytology preparations on glass slides, and cellular detail may therefore be difficult to appreciate. Hence, megakaryocyte number and morphology are better assessed on histopathology sections.

Bone marrow infections

There are certain infectious agents that preferentially locate to marrow. *Leishmania* is a protozoan that may be observed in marrow and no other locations (Figure 19.27). *Cytauxzoon* involves marrow as one of many sites of infection (Figure 19.28), and fungal infections such as histoplasmosis may be diagnosed from marrow aspirates. Some strains of FeLV induce severe myelofibrosis with lymphoid aggregates,

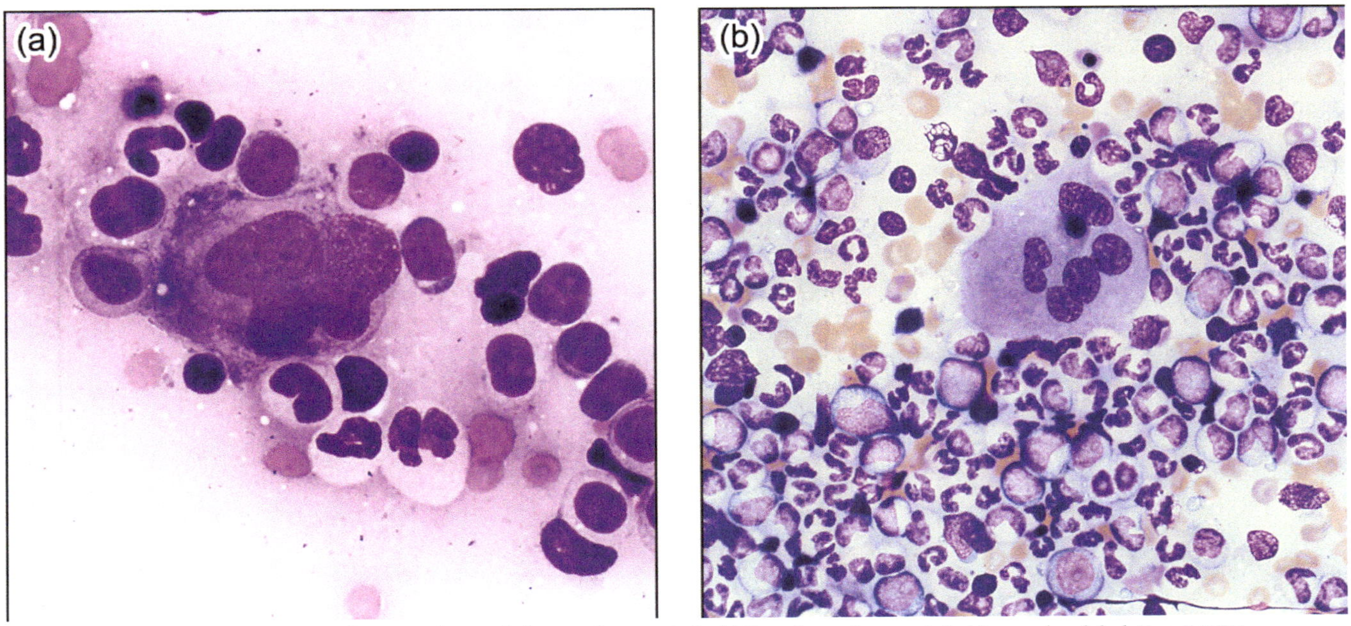

Figures 19.26a, b Marrow aspirates from two dogs with dysmegakaryopoiesis. (a) Dwarf megakaryocyte lacking nuclear lobulation, 1,000× magnification. (b) Disconnected nuclear lobes of various sizes, 400× magnification.

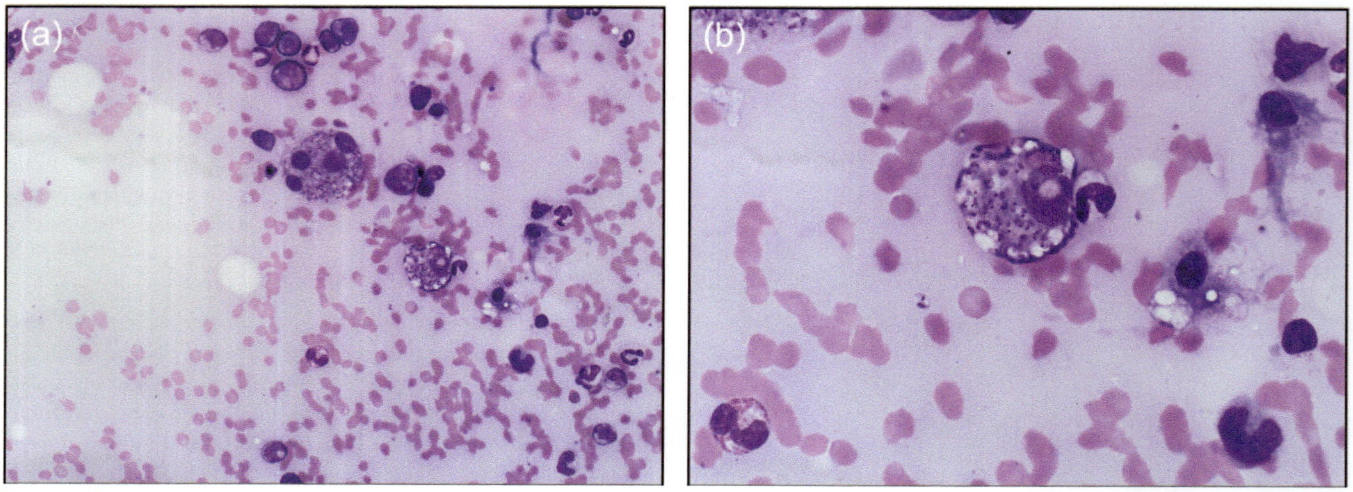

Figures 19.27a, b **Marrow aspirate from a dog with epistaxis, ulcerative dermatitis, and emaciation shows *Leishmania amastigotes* in macrophages (a, 200× magnification; b, 600× magnification).**

iron accumulation, erythroid atrophy, and anemia (Figure 19.29). Chronic bartonellosis may result in granulomatous inflammation of the marrow, similar to other organs.

Myeloid neoplasia

Myeloid neoplasms are broadly categorized into acute myeloid leukemia (AML), myeloproliferative neoplasm (MPN), and myelodysplastic syndrome (MDS), in accordance with criteria proposed by the World Health Organization (WHO) for humans (Khoury *et al.*, 2022). Categorization is based on morphologic, genetic, and/or immunophenotypic features, but it is increasingly recognized that there is extensive overlap between categories in the underlying genetic lesions and the phenotype. The blast cell count remains a key indicator. The general approach put forth in the 2022 WHO classification of myeloid neoplasms in humans consists of the triad of lineage attribution (morphology and immunophenotype), dominant clinical attributes (acute vs chronic, cytopenia vs cytosis, blast proportion, dysplasia), and biological attributes (gene fusions, rearrangements, mutations). In animals, lineage attributes can be determined with standard hematology analysis incorporating light scatter and impedance, microscopic assessment, cytochemistry, and flow cytometry (Meichner *et al.*, 2020). Clinical attributes are readily derived from history, laboratory results analyzed over time, and marrow interpretation. The biological attributes are more challenging to determine in animals. Precursor conditions for myeloid neoplasia in humans are clonal hematopoiesis of indeterminate potential (CHIP) and clonal cytopenia of undetermined significance (CCUS). These conditions increase in frequency with progressive age and pose a risk for progression to myeloid neoplasia. They likely also occur in animals. Though clonal rearrangements in lymphocyte antigen receptor genes have been noted in dogs with AML, the frequency and nature of clonal hematopoiesis in dogs or cats remain undetermined (Stokol *et al.*, 2017). Albeit, sequencing technologies, analytic pathways, and reference databases are gradually building, which will enable the addition of biological features to the categorization of myeloid neoplasms in dogs in the near future (Harris *et al.*, 2022).

The diagnosis of myeloid neoplasia in animals is often challenging with only routine diagnostic test results and history. Careful integration of history, imaging, hematologic, and marrow findings is needed, and the use of immunophenotyping by flow cytometry (FC), immunohistochemistry (IHC), and/or immunocytochemistry (ICC) is very helpful in characterizing morphologically ambiguous cells. The lineage of blasts can usually not be determined by morphology alone since there is overlap in the appearance of lymphoid blasts, myeloblasts, monoblasts, rubriblasts, and megakaryoblasts. It is essential that the persistent nature of cytopenia is verified, and that other causes of increased blasts, such as drug-toxicity and

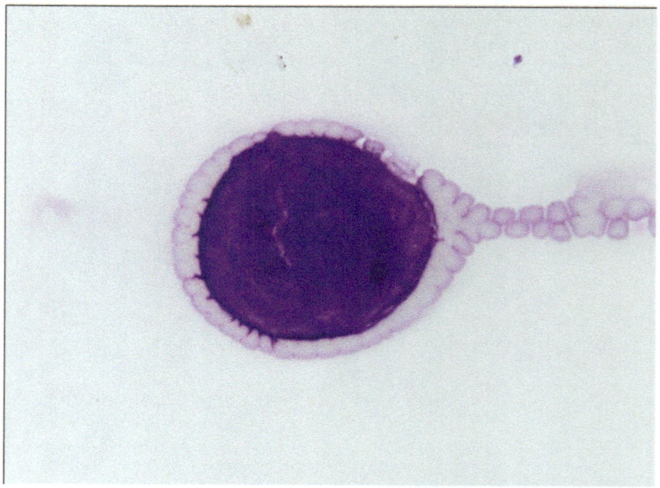

Figure 19.28 **Marrow aspirate from a severely ill and anemic cat contains a *Cytauxzoon* schizont, 200× magnification. Image provided by J. Tarigo, University of Georgia.**

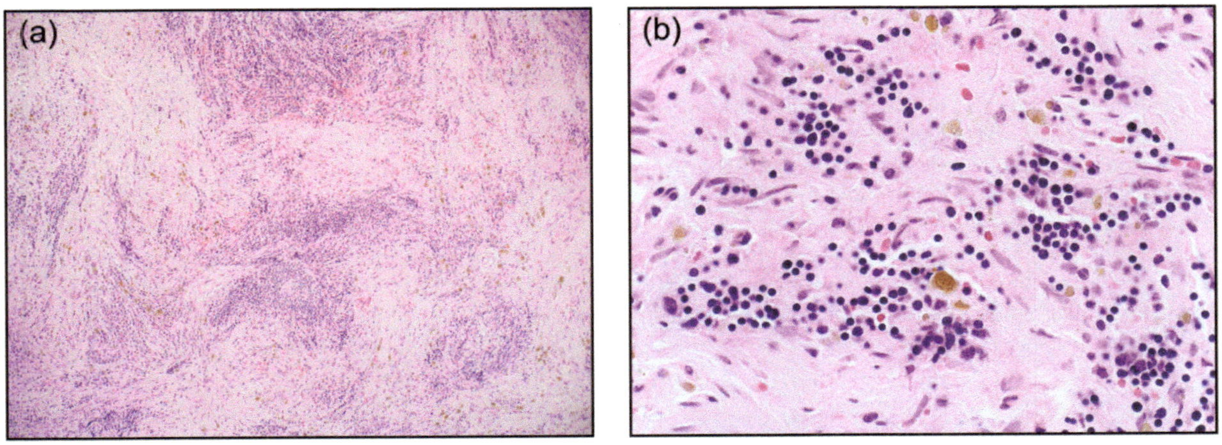

Figures 19.29a, b Marrow core section from a feline leukemia virus-seropositive cat with severe anemia and lymphocytosis; H&E: a, 200× magnification; b, 600× magnification. There is marked myelofibrosis (precluding marrow aspiration) with numerous aggregates of lymphocytes and coarse iron.

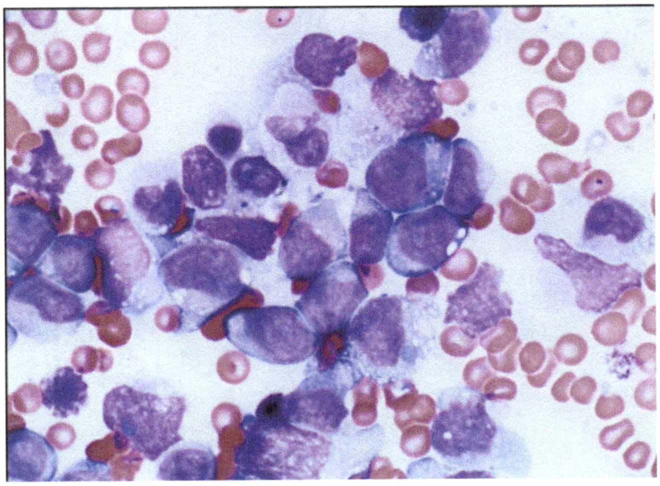

Figure 19.30 Marrow smear from a dog with non-regenerative anemia and acute myeloid leukemia consists predominantly of undifferentiated blasts, 1,000× magnification.

infection, are ruled out before a diagnosis of myeloid neoplasia is made.

Broadly, AML is defined by persistent cytopenia and ≥20% blasts in blood or marrow. Patients with AML often present with acute illness, but may have had cytopenia or cytosis for weeks or months prior. The proportion of blasts in blood or marrow can range from 20 to 100%, the leukocyte count may be low or extremely high, the marrow may be hypo- or hypercellular, and cells may be dysplastic (Figure 19.30). These variable features reflect the biologic heterogeneity of AML, and pose a diagnostic challenge, in particular in cases with 20–40% blasts. There may be partial differentiation into recognizable progeny cells that allow morphologic subcategorization as 'AML with neutrophilic, eosinophilic, monocytic, erythrocytic etc. differentiation' (Figures 19.31, 19.32). It is unclear at this time whether subcategories of AML have different prognoses. While the diagnosis of AML is usually assigned a guarded prognosis, some dogs with AML have responded to combination chemotherapy and survived months to a year (Matsuyama *et al.*, 2023; Tan *et al.*, 2014b). Detection

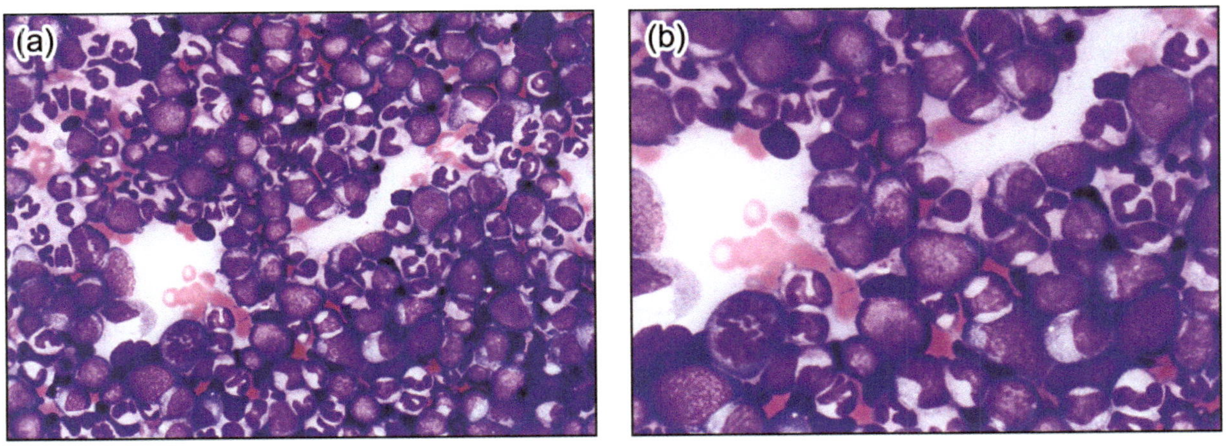

Figures 19.31a, b Marrow smear from a dog with acute myeloid leukemia, partial neutrophilic differentiation, 600× (a) and 1,000× (b) magnification. A 500-cell differential count yielded 46% blast cells.

of alkaline phosphatase or peroxidase activity (Figure 19.9) may be helpful to identify myelomonocytic or monocytic and myeloblast cells, respectively (Stokol *et al.*, 2015).

Myeloproliferative neoplasms are the former chronic leukemias, and are defined by marked cytosis of one cell type, mild cytopenia of other cell types, and ≤5% blast cells in marrow (Figure 19.33). The MPNs are rare in dogs and cats, and it is more likely that a patient with an extremely high neutrophil or eosinophil count has paraneoplastic leukocytosis than an MPN. The pathogenesis of MPN in humans consists of either the constitutive activation of mutated cytokine receptors or independence from normal cytokine regulation (Li *et al.*, 2023). It is likely that MPN in animals have similar pathogenic mechanisms. Subcategorization of MPN is according to the prevailing proliferating cell type into polycythemia vera, chronic neutrophilic or eosinophilic leukemia, essential thrombocythemia, etc. The MPN may manifest with hemoglobin concentration >200g/L and leukocyte counts $>200 \times 10^9$/L, and secondary tumor burden effects such as splenomegaly and vascular accidents in the brain, retina, or spleen may precipitate initial clinical assessment.

Myelodysplastic syndrome is a broad category of hematopoietic conditions characterized by persistent cytopenia, hypercellular marrow, and dysplasia. The proportion of blast cells in the marrow is between 5 and 20% (Figure 19.34). Hence, the marrow is responding inappropriately and ineffectively to peripheral

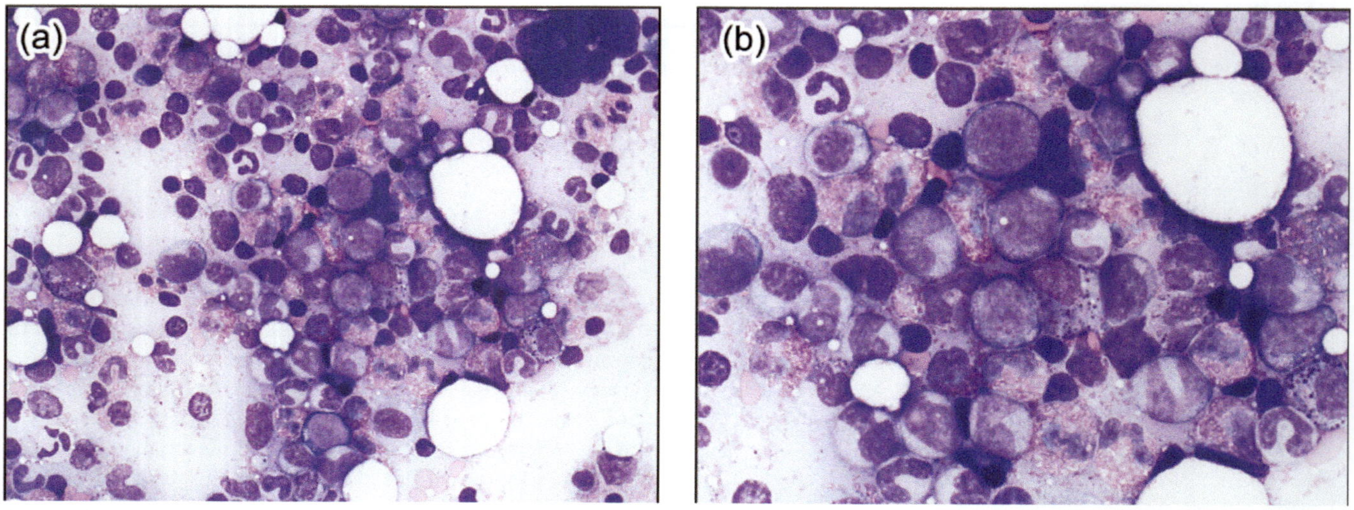

Figure 19.32 Dog with acute myeloid leukemia, partial eosinophilic and basophilic differentiation, 600× (a) and 1,000× (b) magnification. A 500-cell differential count yielded 24% blast cells.

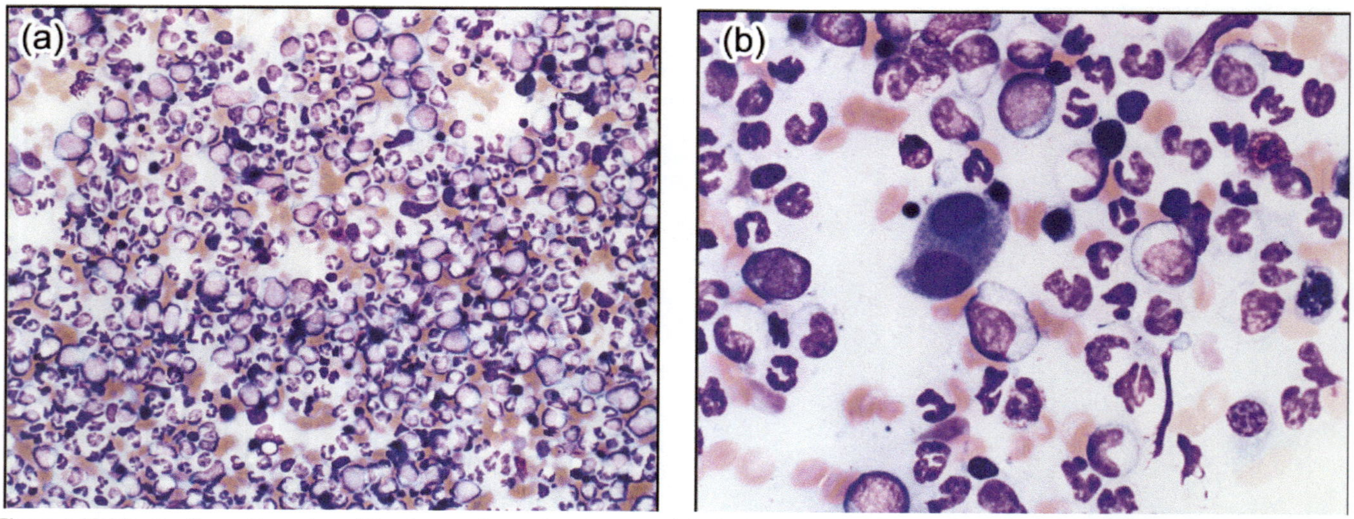

Figures 19.33a, b Dog with myeloproliferative neoplasm, chronic neutrophilic leukemia; 200× (a) and 600× (b) magnification. The dog had mild anemia and a WBC count of 89×10^9/L with no blast cells in circulation. A 500-cell marrow differential count yielded 5% blast cells.

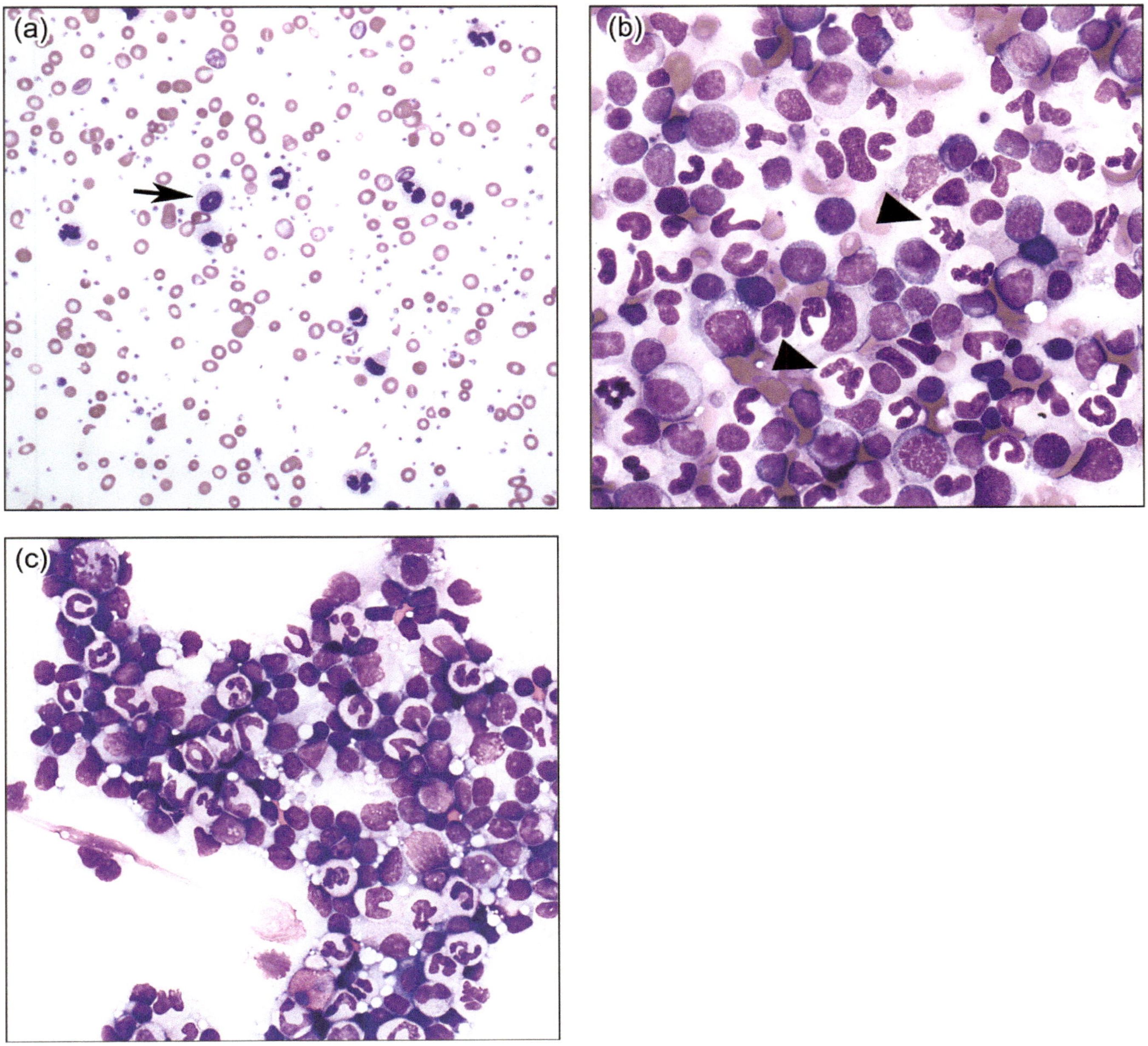

Figures 19.34a–c Dog with myelodysplastic syndrome. (a) The blood smear shows marked anisocytosis, anemia, and acanthocytosis; 200× magnification. There are occasional dysplastic granulocytes (arrow). (b) In the marrow there are abnormally segmented neutrophils (arrowhead); 600× magnification. (c) A lymph node aspirate also contains numerous dysplastic granulocytes; 600× magnification.

demand. In humans, specific cytogenetic changes and mutations allow stratification of patients with MDS into prognostically meaningful categories (Li *et al.*, 2023). Similar tests are not yet available for animals; therefore, providing a prognosis for MDS is challenging. Some cases of MDS in dogs progress to AML, others remain static and may become transfusion dependent, and in some cases the cytopenia improves with prolonged immunosuppression. Recently recognized in humans, VEXAS (vacuoles, mutated E1 ubiquitin activating enzyme, x chromosomal location, autoinflammation, somatic mutation) is a syndrome characterized by adult onset of anemia and/or other cytopenia, MDS, variably severe autoinflammation, and clonal hematopoiesis (Gutierrez-Rodrigues *et al.*, 2023). Patients generally improve with immunosuppression, and it could be speculated that some dogs with MDS responsive to immunosuppression may have a condition with similar pathogenesis.

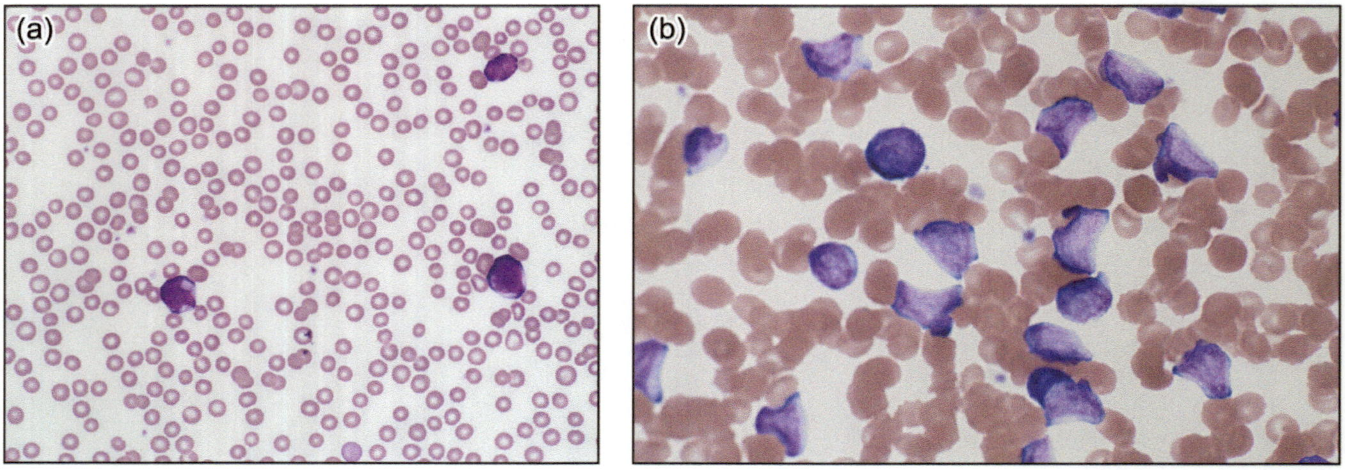

Figure 19.35 Dog with acute lymphoblastic leukemia has pancytopenia with a moderate number of blasts on the blood film (a); 400x magnification. (b) The marrow consists of nearly 100% blasts that expressed CD21 on flow cytometry indicating B-cell type; 600x magnification.

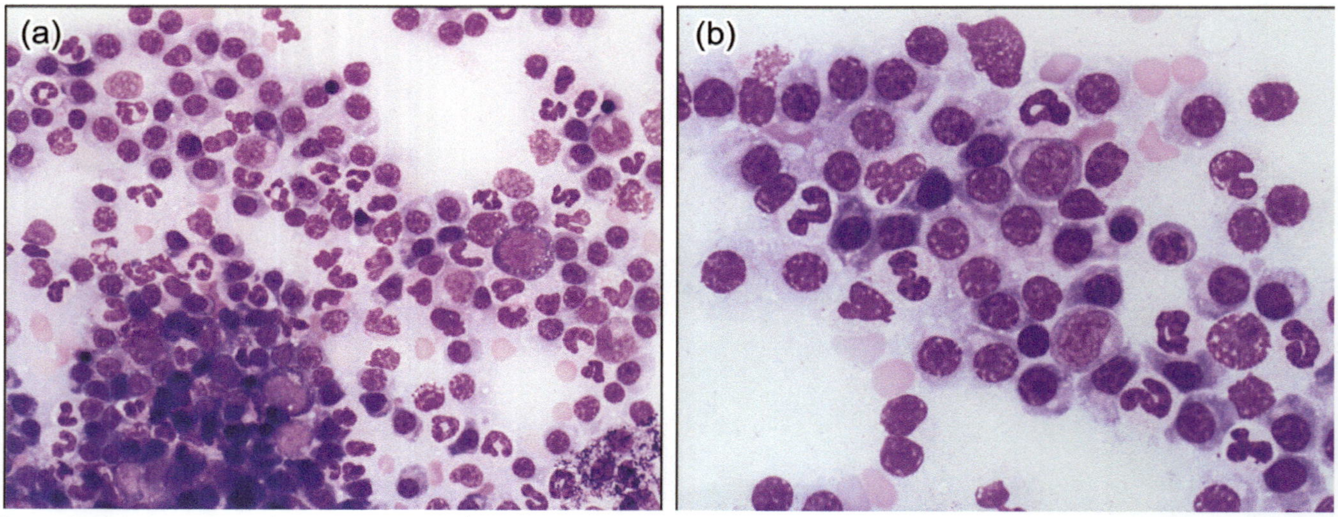

Figure 19.36 Marrow smear from a dog with monoclonal gammopathy and hypercalcemia; 400× (a) and 600× (b) magnification. There are numerous morphologically unremarkable plasma cells among hematopoietic cells.

Morphologically, MDS should be subcategorized according to the proportion of blast cells and the prevailing cytopenia into refractory anemia with excess blasts (RAEB), refractory neutropenia with excess blasts (RNEB), etc. (Khoury *et al.*, 2022). Myelofibrosis is frequently a component of MDS, but the prognostic implication thereof is undefined.

Non-myeloid neoplasms in bone marrow

Non-myeloid neoplasms that may arise in or involve marrow include acute lymphocytic leukemia (ALL, Figure 19.35), some types of lymphoma, mast cell tumors, multiple myeloma (Figure 19.36), histiocytic sarcoma (Figure 19.37), carcinoma (Figure 19.38), and others (Pinard *et al.*, 2021). Acute lymphocytic leukemia may be difficult to distinguish morphologically from poorly differentiated myeloid leukemia since both are composed of nearly 100% blast cells. However, immunophenotyping usually allows detection of B- (CD20, CD21, CD79a, Pax-5) or T-cell markers (CD3, CD5) on ALL cells.

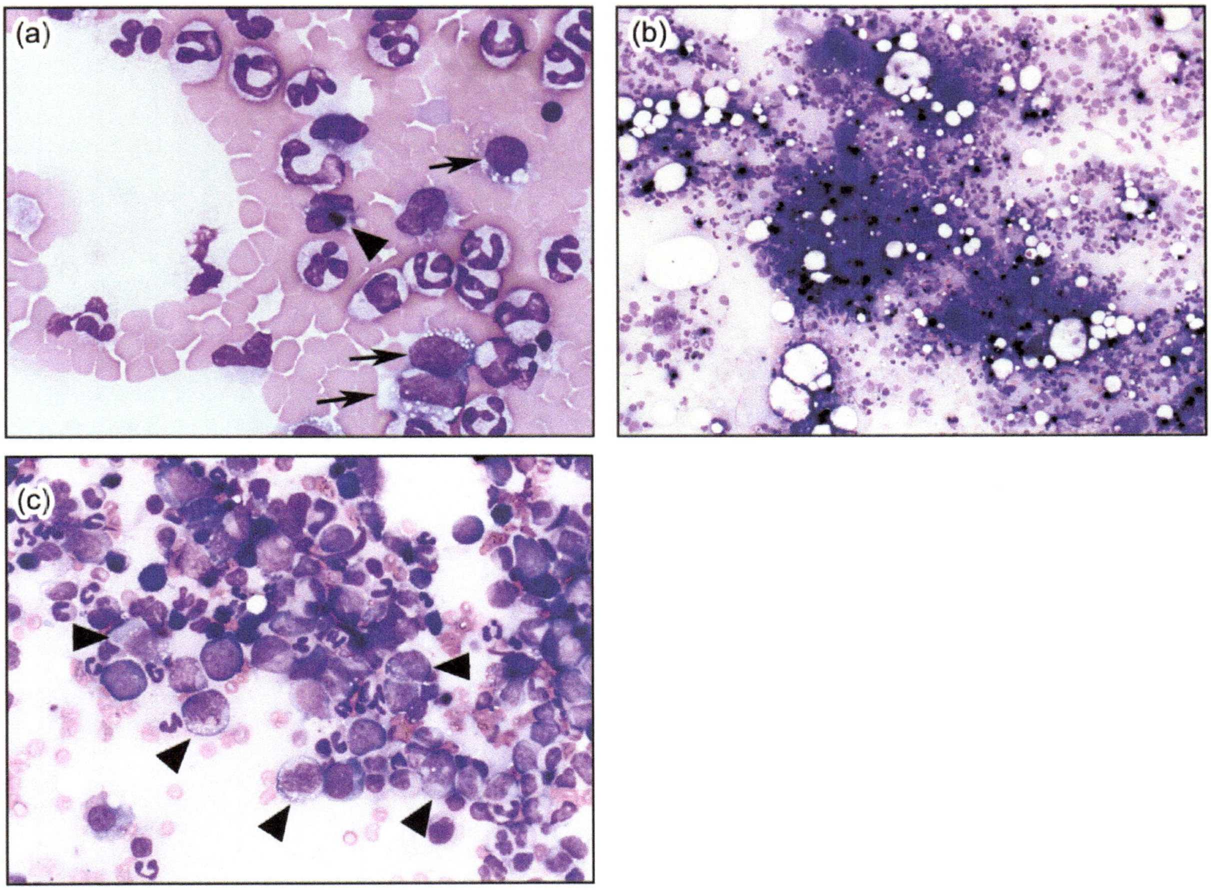

Figure 19.37 Blood film from a dog with mild anemia and histiocytic sarcoma. (a) At the feather tip of the blood film are large round histiocytes with cytoplasmic vacuoles (arrow), and one cell contains heme pigment (arrowhead); 600× magnification. (b) A marrow aspirate shows abundant coarse iron and high cellularity; 100× magnification. (c) There are scattered histiocytes (arrowhead) among hematopoietic cells; 400× magnification. Histiocytes are neither frequent nor easily identified.

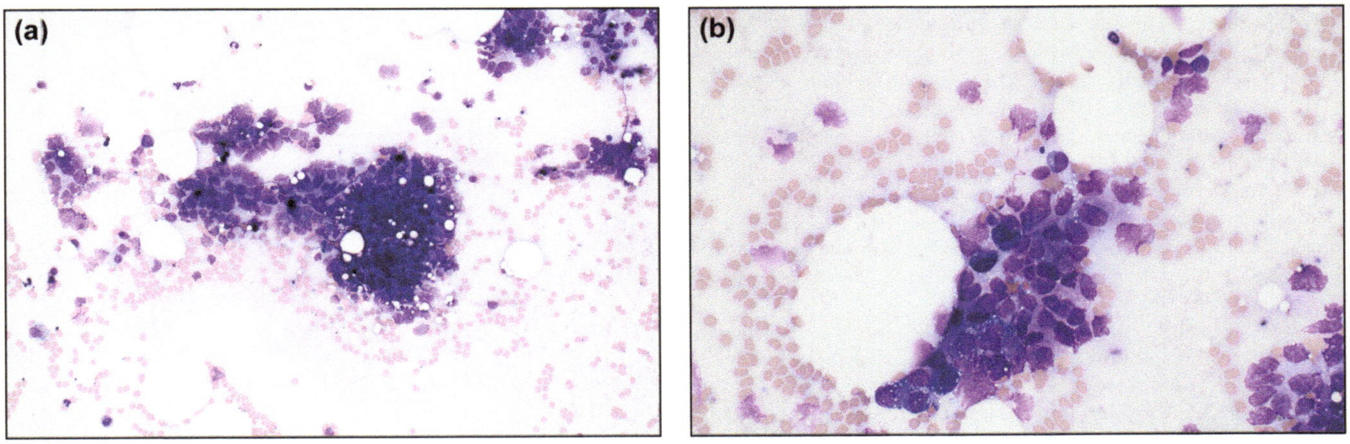

Figure 19.38 Sternal marrow aspirate from a dog with mild anemia and disseminated intravascular coagulation of unknown cause. (a) There are cohesive clusters of non-hematopoietic (epithelial) cells amidst extracellular hemosiderin and a few hematopoietic cells; 200× magnification. Viability among the cohesive cells is variable. (b) The cohesive cells, when intact, have a nuclear to cytoplasmic ratio >1 and dark basophilic cytoplasm with fine vacuoles; 400× magnification. The epithelial cell clusters were noted in two of ten slides evaluated, and were often of limited viability. The interpretation was 'carcinoma of unknown origin metastatic to marrow'.

REFERENCES

Abrams-Ogg A., Defarges A., Foster R.A. et al. (2012) Comparison of canine core bone marrow biopsies from multiple sites during different techniques and needles. *Vet Clin Pathol 41(2)*:235–242.

Barron B.A., Hoyer J.C., Tefferi A. (2001) A bone marrow report of absent stainable iron is not diagnostic of iron deficiency. *Ann Hematol 80(3)*:166–169.

Bauer T.R., Yu-Chen G., Creevy K.E. et al. (2004) Leukocyte adhesion deficiency in children and Irish Setter dogs. *Ped Res 55*:363–367.

Bauer T.R. Jr, Pratt S.M., Palena C.M., Raj K., Giger U. (2017) Feline leukocyte adhesion (CD18) deficiency caused by a deletion in the integrin β^2 (ITGB2) gene. *Vet Clin Pathol 46(3)*:391–400.

Beaumier A., Batista Linhares M., Rush J.E., Piedra-Mora C. (2022) Hypereosinophilic syndrome with cardiac infiltration and congestive heart failure in a cat. *J Vet Cardiol 41*:11–17.

Bienzle D. (2012) Collection and interpretation of bone marrow samples. In: *Manual of Small Animal Haematology and Haemostasis*, 2nd edn. (eds. M. Day, A. Mackin, J. Littlewood) British Small Animal Veterinary Association, Gloucester, pp. 21–30.

Boyd S.P., Best M.P. (2018) Persistent reticulocytosis in a case of poodle macrocytosis. *Vet Clin Pathol 47(3)*:400–406.

Canfield P.J., Watson A.D. (1989) Investigations of bone marrow dyscrasia in a poodle with macrocytosis. *J Comp Pathol 101(3)*:269–278.

Casamian-Sorrosal D., Silvestrini P., Blake R. et al. (2020) Clinical features and long-term follow-up of 70 cases of canine idiopathic eosinophilic lung disease. *Vet Rec 187(8)*:e65.

Céspedes López R., Amutio Díez E., Martín Martitegui X. et al. (2022) Pure white cell aplasia an exceptional condition in the immunological conundrum of thymomas: Responses to immunosuppression and literature review. *Clin Case Rep 10(5)*:e05742.

Chauffaille M.L.L.F., Perazzio A.B., Gouvea C.P. (2019) Marrow iron staining should always be performed to diagnose Myelodysplastic/myeloproliferative neoplasia with ring sideroblasts and thrombocythemia. *Hematol Transfus Cell Ther 41(3)*:279–280.

Cheney A., Woolcock A.D., Mukhopadhyay A., Knapp D., Moore G.E. (2022) Interleukin-6 and thrombopoietin concentrations in dogs with carcinoma with and without thrombocytosis *J Vet Intern Med 36(1)*:227–233.

Criswell K.A., Bock J.H., Johnson K. et al. (2018) Validation of Sysmex XT-2000iV analyzer-generated quantitative bone marrow differential counts in cynomolgus monkeys, Beagle dogs, and CD-1 mice. *Vet Clin Pathol 47*:539–555.

Defarges A., Abrams-Ogg A., Foster R.A., Bienzle D. (2013) Comparison of sternal, iliac, and humeral bone marrow aspiration in Beagle dogs. *Vet Clin Pathol 42(2)*:170–176.

Donald S., Kakkar N. (2021) Dry tap on bone marrow aspiration: A red flag. *J Hematopathol 14*:125–130.

Evstatiev R., Bukaty A., Jimenez K. et al. (2014) Iron deficiency alters megakaryopoiesis and platelet phenotype independent of thrombopoietin. *Am J Hematol 89(5)*:527–529.

Gunduz E., Kivanc B.K., Arik D. et al. (2014) Bone marrow examination in patients with immune thromobocytopenia: Is there anything different in older patients? *Europ J Haematol 92(2)*:157–160.

Gutierrez-Rodrigues F., Kusne Y., Fernandez J. et al. (2023) Spectrum of clonal hematopoiesis in VEXAS syndrome. *Blood*. doi: 10.1182/blood.2022018774.

Harris R.A., Rout E.D., Yoshimoto J.A., Avery P.R., Avery A.C. (2022) Using digital RNA counting to establish flow cytometry diagnostic criteria for subtypes of CD34+ canine acute leukaemia. *Vet Comp Oncol 20(3)*:710–719.

Hisasue M., Nagashima N., Nishigaki K. et al. (2009) Myelodysplastic syndromes and acute myeloid leukemia in cats infected with feline leukemia virus clone33 containing a unique long terminal repeat. *Internat J Cancer 124*:1133–1141.

Hitchcock I.S., Hafer M., Sangkhae V., Tucker J.A. (2021) The thrombopoietin receptor: Revisiting the master regulator of platelet production *Platelets 32(6)*:770–778.

Khan A.A., Quigley J.G. (2013) Heme and FLVCR-related transporter families SLC48 and SLC49. *Molecular Aspects of Medicine 34(2–3)*:669–682.

Khoury J.D., Solary E., Abla O. et al. (2022) The 5th edition of the World Health Organization classification of haematolymphoid tumours: Myeloid and histiocytic/dendritic neoplasms. *Leukemia 36(7)*:1703–1719.

Klion A.D. (2022) Approach to the patient with suspected hypereosinophilic syndrome *Hematology Am Soc Hematol Educ Program 2022(1)*:47–54.

Lachowicz J.L., Post G.S., Moroff S.D., Mooney S.C. (2004) Acquired amegakaryocytic thrombocytopenia--Four cases and a literature review *J Small Anim Pract 45(10)*:507–514.

Lee G.K.C., Barbosa C., Andersen G. et al. (2022) Cyclic hematopoiesis in a mixed-breed dog: Case report and brief review *J Vet Diagn Invest 34(6)*:1006–1009.

Li N., Chen M., Yin C.C. (2023) Advances in molecular evaluation of myeloproliferative neoplasms *Semin Diagn Pathol 40(3)*:187–194.

Li W., Guo R., Song Y. et al. (2021a) Erythroblastic island macrophages shape normal erythropoiesis and drive associated disorders in erythroid hematopoietic diseases. *Front Cell Dev Biol 8*:613885.

Li Z., MacDougald O.A. (2021b) Preclinical models for investigating how bone marrow adipocytes influence bone and hematopoietic activity. *Best Pract Res Clin Endocrinol Metab 35*:101547.

Lucidi C.A., Gerlach J.A., Jutkowitz A., Scott M.A. (2021) Immunoglobulin G and phosphatidylserine in regenerative and nonregenerative immune-mediated anemias of dogs. *J Vet Intern Med 35(6)*:2713–2721.

Lutz S., Sewell A.C., Reusch C.E., Kook P.H. (2013) Clinical and laboratory findings in border collies with presumed hereditary juvenile cobalamin deficiency. *J Am Anim Hosp Assoc 49(3)*:197–203.

Matsuyama A., Beeler-Marfisi J., Wood R.D. et al. (2023) Treatment of myeloid neoplasia with doxorubicin and cytarabine in 11 dogs. *Vet Comp Oncol 21(1)*:54–61.

Meichner K., Stokol T., Tarigo J. et al. (2020) Multicenter flow cytometry proficiency testing of canine blood and lymph node samples *Vet Clin Pathol 49(2)*:249–257.

Mischke R., Busse L. (2002) Reference values for the bone marrow aspirates in adult dogs. *J Vet Med A Physiol Pathol Clin Med 49(10)*:499–502.

Moore M., Kotchetkov R. (2021) Anticoagulation and bone marrow biopsy: Is it safe to proceed? *Hematoly 26*:206–209.

Neel J.A., Snyder L., Grindem C.B. (2012) Thrombocytosis: A retrospective study of 165 dogs. *Veterinary Clinical Pathology 41(2)*:216–222.

Pawsat G.A., Fry M.M., Behling-Kelly E. et al. (2023) Bone marrow iron scoring in healthy and clinically ill dogs with and without evidence of iron-restricted erythropoiesis. *Vet Clin Pathol*. doi: 10.1111/vcp.13209.

Pérez-Ruixo J.J., Krzyzanski W., Hing J. (2008) Pharmacodynamic analysis of recombinant human erythropoietin effect on reticulocyte production rate and age distribution in healthy subjects. *Clin Pharmacokinet 47(6)*:399–415.

Perkins M.C., Canfield P., Churcher R.K., Malik R. (2004) Immune-mediated neutropenia suspected in five dogs. *Aust Vet J 82(1–2)*:52–7.

Pernecker I., Bauer N.B., Johannes S. et al. (2017) Comparison of the Sysmex XT-2000iV with microscopic differential counts of canine bone marrow. *J Vet Diagn Invest 29*:148–153.

Petterino C., Luzio E., Baracchini L. et al. (2011) Paraneoplastic leukocytosis in a dog with a renal carcinoma. *Vet Clin Pathol 40(1)*:89–94.

Pinard C.J., Ludwig L., Egan R. et al. (2021) Primary bone marrow T-cell lymphoma in a Golden Retriever *Vet Clin Pathol 50(1)*:142–150.

Riley R., Williams D., Ross M. et al. (2009) Bone marrow aspirate and biopsy: A pathologist's perspective. II: Interpretation of bone marrow aspirate and biopsy. *J Clin Lab Anal 23(5)*:259–307.

Sancho I.M., Holmes A., Adamantos S. (2021) Imerslund-Grasbeck syndrome in a cross-breed dog. *J Small Anim Pract 62(8)*:709–711.

Stanley E., Appleman E., Schlag A., Siegel A. (2019) Relationship between cobalamin and folate deficiencies and anemia in dogs. *J Vet Intern Med 33(1)*:106–113.

Stokol T., Schaefer D.M., Shuman M., Belcher N., Dong L. (2015) Alkaline phosphatase is a useful cytochemical marker for the diagnosis of acute myelomonocytic and monocytic leukemia in the dog *Vet Clin Pathol 44(1)*:79–93.

Stokol T., Nickerson G.A., Shuman M., Belcher N. (2017) Dogs with acute myeloid leukemia have clonal rearrangements in T and B cell receptors. *Front Vet Sci 4*:76.

Tan E., Abrams-Ogg A., Defarges A., Bienzle D. (2014a) Automated hematologic analysis of bone marrow aspirate samples from healthy Beagle dogs. *Vet Clin Pathol 43(3)*:342–351.

Tan E., Abrams-Ogg A.C., Defarges A., Bienzle D. (2014b) Automated analysis of bone marrow aspirates from dogs with haematological disorders. *J Compar Pathol 151(1)*:67–79.

Thomason R.W., Almiski M.S. (2009) Evidence that stainable bone marrow iron following parenteral iron therapy does not correlate with serum iron studies and may not represent readily available storage iron. *Am J Clin Pathol 131(4)*:580–585.

Tomasian A., Jennings J.W. (2022) Bone marrow aspiration and biopsy: Techniques and practice implications. *Skeletal Radiol 51(1)*:81–88.

Travlos G.S. (2006) Normal structure, function and histology of the bone marrow. *Toxicol Pathol 34*:248–262.

Weiss D.J., Henson M. (2007) Pure white cell aplasia in a dog. *Vet Clin Pathol 36(4)*:373–5.

Woolhead V.L., Szladovits B., Chan A., Swann J.W., Glanemann B. (2021) Breed predispositions, clinical findings, and prognostic factors for death in dogs with nonregenerative immune-mediated anemia. *J Vet Intern Med 35(1)*:252–260.

Xu P., Wong R.S.M., Krzyzanski W., Yan X. (2022) Dynamics of erythroferrone response to erythropoietin in rats. *Front Pharmacol 13*:876573.

Zimmerman K.L., McMillan K., Monroe W.E., et al. (2013) Leukocyte adhesion deficiency type I in a mixed-breed dog. *J Vet Diagn Invest 25(2)*:291–6.

INDEX

Page numbers in *italic* indicate figure and **bold** indicate table respectively